The Oxford Handbook of
Rehabilitation Psychology

OXFORD LIBRARY OF PSYCHOLOGY

EDITOR-IN-CHIEF

Peter E. Nathan

AREA EDITORS:

Clinical Psychology
David H. Barlow

Cognitive Neuroscience
Kevin N. Ochsner and Stephen M. Kosslyn

Cognitive Psychology
Daniel Reisberg

Counseling Psychology
Elizabeth M. Altmaier and Jo-Ida C. Hansen

Developmental Psychology
Philip David Zelazo

Health Psychology
Howard S. Friedman

History of Psychology
David B. Baker

Industrial/Organizational Psychology
Steve W. J. Kozlowski

Methods and Measurement
Todd D. Little

Neuropsychology
Kenneth M. Adams

Personality and Social Psychology
Kay Deaux and Mark Snyder

OXFORD LIBRARY OF PSYCHOLOGY

Editor in Chief PETER E. NATHAN

The Oxford Handbook of Rehabilitation Psychology

Edited by

Paul Kennedy

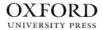
UNIVERSITY PRESS

OXFORD
UNIVERSITY PRESS

Oxford University Press, Inc., publishes works that further
Oxford University's objective of excellence
in research, scholarship, and education.

Oxford   New York
Auckland   Cape Town   Dar es Salaam   Hong Kong   Karachi
Kuala Lumpur   Madrid   Melbourne   Mexico City   Nairobi
New Delhi   Shanghai   Taipei   Toronto

With offices in
Argentina   Austria   Brazil   Chile   Czech Republic   France   Greece
Guatemala   Hungary   Italy   Japan   Poland   Portugal   Singapore
South Korea   Switzerland   Thailand   Turkey   Ukraine   Vietnam

Published by Oxford University Press, Inc.
198 Madison Avenue, New York, New York 10016
www.oup.com

Library of Congress Cataloging-in-Publication Data

The Oxford handbook of rehabilitation psychology / edited by Paul Kennedy.
  p. cm.
  ISBN 978–0–19–973398–9
1. Rehabilitation—Psychological aspects—Handbooks, manuals, etc.   2. People with disabilities—
Rehabilitation—Psychological aspects—Handbooks, manuals, etc. I. Kennedy, Paul, 1959-
RM930.O936 2012
616.89'1523—dc23
2012013261

9 8 7 6 5 4 3 2 1
Printed in the United States of America
on acid-free paper

SHORT CONTENTS

OXFORD LIBRARY OF PSYCHOLOGY

The *Oxford Library of Psychology*, a landmark series of handbooks, is published by Oxford University Press, one of the world's oldest and most highly respected publishers, with a tradition of publishing significant books in psychology. The ambitious goal of the *Oxford Library of Psychology* is nothing less than to span a vibrant, wide-ranging field and, in so doing, to fill a clear market need.

Encompassing a comprehensive set of handbooks, organized hierarchically, the *Library* incorporates volumes at different levels, each designed to meet a distinct need. At one level are a set of handbooks designed broadly to survey the major subfields of psychology; at another are numerous handbooks that cover important current focal research and scholarly areas of psychology in depth and detail. Planned as a reflection of the dynamism of psychology, the *Library* will grow and expand as psychology itself develops, thereby highlighting significant new research that will impact on the field. Adding to its accessibility and ease of use, the *Library* will be published in print and, later on, electronically.

The *Library* surveys psychology's principal subfields with a set of handbooks that capture the current status and future prospects of those major subdisciplines. This initial set includes handbooks of social and personality psychology, clinical psychology, counseling psychology, school psychology, educational psychology, industrial and organizational psychology, cognitive psychology, cognitive neuroscience, methods and measurements, history, neuropsychology, personality assessment, developmental psychology, and more. Each handbook undertakes to review one of psychology's major subdisciplines with breadth, comprehensiveness, and exemplary scholarship. In addition to these broadly-conceived volumes, the *Library* also includes a large number of handbooks designed to explore in depth more specialized areas of scholarship and research, such as stress, health and coping, anxiety and related disorders, cognitive development, or child and adolescent assessment. In contrast to the broad coverage of the subfield handbooks, each of these latter volumes focuses on an especially productive, more highly focused line of scholarship and research. Whether at the broadest or most specific level, however, all of the *Library* handbooks offer synthetic coverage that reviews and evaluates the relevant past and present research and anticipates research in the future. Each handbook in the *Library* includes introductory and concluding chapters written by its editor to provide a roadmap to the handbook's table of contents and to offer informed anticipations of significant future developments in that field.

An undertaking of this scope calls for handbook editors and chapter authors who are established scholars in the areas about which they write. Many of the nation's and world's most productive and best-respected psychologists have agreed to edit *Library* handbooks or write authoritative chapters in their areas of expertise.

For whom has the *Oxford Library of Psychology* been written? Because of its breadth, depth, and accessibility, the *Library* serves a diverse audience, including graduate students in psychology and their faculty mentors, scholars, researchers, and practitioners in psychology and related fields. Each will find in the *Library* the information they seek on the subfield or focal area of psychology in which they work or are interested.

Befitting its commitment to accessibility, each handbook includes a comprehensive index, as well as extensive references to help guide research. And because the *Library* was designed from its inception as an online as well as a print resource, its structure and contents will be readily and rationally searchable online. Further, once the *Library* is released online, the handbooks will be regularly and thoroughly updated.

In summary, the *Oxford Library of Psychology* will grow organically to provide a thoroughly informed perspective on the field of psychology, one that reflects both psychology's dynamism and its increasing interdisciplinarity. Once published electronically, the *Library* is also destined to become a uniquely valuable interactive tool, with extended search and browsing capabilities. As you begin to consult this handbook, we sincerely hope you will share our enthusiasm for the more than 500-year tradition of Oxford University Press for excellence, innovation, and quality, as exemplified by the *Oxford Library of Psychology*.

Peter E. Nathan
Editor-in-Chief
Oxford Library of Psychology

ABOUT THE EDITOR

Paul Kennedy

Paul Kennedy is Professor of Clinical Psychology at the University of Oxford and Trust Head of Clinical Psychology based at the National Spinal Injuries Centre, Stoke Mandeville Hospital, in the United Kingdom. He has published over 100 scientific papers for peer-reviewed journals and written and edited a number of books on clinical health psychology and physical disability. He is the founding chair of both the Multi-Disciplinary Association of Spinal Cord Injury Professionals (MASCIP) and the European Spinal Psychologists Associations (ESPA). In 2002, he was awarded a distinguished service award by the American Association of Spinal Cord Injury Psychologists and Social Workers, and, in 2005, made a visiting fellow of the Ministry of Science and Medical Research in Australia. In 2009, he was given the Chairman's Award (Buckinghamshire Hospitals NHS Trust) as part of the National Spinal Injuries Centre's CARF Team. In 2011, he was presented with the Guttmann prize by the Deutschprachige Medizinische Gesellschaft fur Paraplegie (DMPG—German-speaking society of Paraplegia).

ACKNOWLEDGMENTS

It has been a pleasure working on this project, which was greatly helped by the enthusiasm of the many others involved. I would like to thank all the chapter authors for their excellence, responsiveness and good humor.

Appreciation is also due to the New York Office of Oxford University Press, especially Sarah Harrington and Chad Zimmerman for their help and unstinting support. In the production stages Nisha Selvaraj from Newgen Knowledge Works has been great as has Angela Fox in the early planning stages. Finally, I would like to thank the people who make my life special, a great big thank you to Oonagh, Julia, and Dermot, to whom this book is dedicated with love and gratitude.

CONTRIBUTORS

Stephen D. Anton
Department of Clinical and Health
Psychology and Department of Aging
and Geriatric Research
University of Florida
Gainesville, Florida

Donita E. Baird
Psychological and Behavioural Medicine
Unit, Monash Medical Centre School of
Psychology, and Psychiatry,
Monash University
Melbourne, Australia

Jane Barton
Community Stroke Team
Sheffield Health and Social Care
NHS Foundation Trust
Sheffield, United Kingdom

Paul Bennett
Department of Psychology
University of Swansea
Swansea, United Kingdom

Carol Blessing
Employment and Disability Institute
Cornell University
Ithaca, New York

Susanne M. Bruyère
Employment and Disability Institute
Cornell University
Ithaca, New York

Yue Cao
Department of Health Sciences and
Research
Medical University of South Carolina
Charleston, South Carolina

Nancy C. Cheak-Zamora
Department of Health Psychology
University of Missouri
Columbia, Missouri

Yuying Chen
Department of Physical Medicine and
Rehabilitation
University of Alabama at Birmingham
Birmingham, Alabama

Julie Chronister
Department of Counseling
San Francisco State University
San Francisco, California

David M. Clarke
Psychological and Behavioural Medicine
Unit, Monash Medical Centre School of
Psychology, and Psychiatry,
Monash University
Melbourne, Australia

Laura Coffey
School of Nursing
Dublin City University
Dublin, Ireland

Ashley Craig
Rehabilitation Studies Unit
University of Sydney Medical School
Sydney, Australia

Linda A. Cronin
Freelance writer
Cedar Grove, New Jersey

Kathleen K. M. Deidrick
Department of Health Psychology
Thompson Center for Autism and
Neurodevelopmental Disorders
University of Missouri
Columbia, Missouri

Geoff Denham
Department of Counselling and
Psychological Health
La Trobe University
Melbourne, Australia

Deirdre M. Desmond
Department of Psychology
National University of Ireland Maynooth
Maynooth, Ireland

Elena Harlan Drewel
Department of Health Psychology
Thompson Center for Autism and
Neurodevelopmental Disorders
University of Missouri
Columbia, Missouri

Timothy R. Elliott
Department of Educational Psychology
Texas A&M University
College Station, Texas

Maarten J. Fischer
Department of Clinical Oncology
Department of Medical Psychology
Leiden University Medical Center
Leiden, the Netherlands

Robert G. Frank
College of Public Health and
Department of Psychology
Kent State University
Kent, Ohio

Pamela Gallagher
School of Nursing
Dublin City University
Dublin, Ireland

Adam T. Gerstenecker
Department of Psychology
University of Louisville
Louisville, Kentucky

Douglas Gibson
Department of Psychiatry
Virginia Commonwealth University
Richmond, Virginia

Thomas P. Golden
Employment and Disability Institute
Cornell University
Ithaca, New York

Kristofer J. Hagglund
Department of Health Psychology
University of Missouri
Columbia, Missouri

Stephanie L. Hanson
College of Public Health & Health
Professions
University of Florida
Gainesville, Florida

Solam T. Huey
James J. Peters VA Medical Center
Bronx, New York

Ebonee T. Johnson
Department of Rehabilitation Psychology
University of Wisconsin
Madison, Wisconsin

Adrian A. Kaptein
Department of Medical Psychology
Leiden University Medical Center
Leiden, the Netherlands

Paul Kennedy
Oxford Institute of Clinical Psychology
Training
University of Oxford
Oxford, United Kingdom

Thomas R. Kerkhoff
Department of Clinical and Health
Psychology
University of Florida
Gainesville, Florida

Hanoch Livneh
Rehabilitation Counseling Program
Portland State University
Portland, Oregon

Malcolm MacLachlan
School of Psychology and Centre
for Global Health
Trinity College Dublin
Dublin, Ireland

Benjamin T. Mast
Department of Psychology
University of Louisville
Louisville, Kentucky

Erin Martz
Oregon State Hospital and Rehability
Portland State University
Portland, Oregon

Michelle A. Meade
Department of Physical Medicine and
Rehabilitation
Center for Managing Chronic Disease
University of Michigan
Ann Arbor, Michigan

Charles T. Merbitz
Department of Applied Behavior Analysis
The Chicago School of Professional
Psychology
Chicago, Illinois

Nancy Hansen Merbitz
Merbitz Health and Wellness Services
Pontiac, Illinois

Jeri Morris
Department of Psychology
Roosevelt University
Chicago, Illinois

Elias Mpofu
Department of Rehabilitation
Counselling
University of Sydney
Sydney, Australia

Fiadhnait O'Keeffe
Department of Psychology
National Rehabilitation Hospital, Dun
Laoghaire
Co, Dublin, Ireland

Kenneth I. Pakenham
School of Psychology
University of Queensland
Brisbane, Australia

Michael G. Perri
Department of Clinical and Health
Psychology
University of Florida
Gainesville, Florida

Kathryn Nicholson Perry
School of Psychology
University of Western Sydney
Sydney, Australia

Sukyeong Pi
Employment and Disability
Institute
Cornell University
Ithaca, New York

Joseph F. Rath
Rusk Institute of Rehabilitation
Medicine
New York University School
of Medicine
New York, New York

Craig Ravesloot
Rural Institute on Disabilities
University of Montana
Missoula, Montana

Stephanie A. Reid-Arndt
Department of Health Psychology
University of Missouri
Columbia, Missouri

J. Scott Richards
Department of Physical Medicine and
Rehabilitation
University of Alabama at
Birmingham
Birmingham, Alabama

Elizabeth J. Richardson
Department of Physical Medicine and
Rehabilitation
University of Alabama, Birmingham
Birmingham, Alabama

Judy P. Ripsch
Department of Counseling Psychology
The Chicago School of Professional
Psychology
Chicago, Illinois

Patricia A. Rivera
Department of Veterans Affairs Medical
Center
Birmingham, Alabama

Bruce Rybarczyk
Department of Psychology
Virginia Commonwealth University
Richmond, Virginia

Margreet Scharloo
Department of Medical Psychology
Leiden University Medical Center
Leiden, the Netherlands

Tom Seekins
Rural Institute on Disabilities
University of Montana
Missoula, Montana

Andrea Shamaskin
Department of Psychology
Virginia Commonwealth University
Richmond, Virginia

Elisabeth Sherwin
Department of Psychology
University of Arkansas at Little Rock
Little Rock, Arkansas

Emilie F. Smithson
The National Spinal Injuries Centre
Stoke Mandeville Hospital
Buckinghamshire, United Kingdom

William Stiers
Department of Physical Medicine and
Rehabilitation
The Johns Hopkins University
Baltimore, Maryland

Robyn L. Tate
Rehabilitation Studies Unit
Northern Clinical School
University of Sydney Medical School
Sydney, Australia

Esther van den Ende
Rijnlands Rehabilitation Center
Leiden, the Netherlands

Sara Van Looy
Employment and Disability Institute
Cornell University
Ithaca, New York

Stephen T. Wegener
School of Medicine
Department of Physical Medicine and
    Rehabilitation
Johns Hopkins University
Baltimore, Maryland

CONTENTS

PART 1

Perspectives in Rehabilitation Psychology

Rehabilitation Psychology: Introduction, Review, and Background

Paul Kennedy

Abstract

This chapter provides an overview of the different areas of rehabilitation psychology addressed in this book. Rehabilitation psychology is a growing field in professional practice; it involves the application of psychological knowledge and skills to the understanding and treatment of individuals with physical disabilities, with the aim of optimizing outcomes in terms of health, independence, and daily functioning, and of minimizing secondary health complications. Several conceptual frameworks of disability and their relation to clinical practice are discussed. These include the biopsychosocial model (Engel, 1980), in which a combination of biological, social, and psychological factors contribute to physical health and illness; the World Health Organization's International Classification of Functioning, Disability, and Health; the integrated framework of Wright (1960, 1983); Trieschmann's (1988) model, based on her work on spinal cord injuries; and the ABC model of rehabilitation psychology (Cox et al., 2010). The chapter ends with an overview of this book's remaining chapters.

Key Words: Rehabilitation psychology, biopsychosocial model, health trends, roles, conceptual frameworks, and interventions.

This book deals with the emotional, psychosocial, and psychological factors associated with the rehabilitation and treatment of people with physical disabilities. An understanding of the relevant psychological processes and associated interventions is critical in enabling individuals and society to manage the consequences of disability and chronic disease. This chapter begins by presenting some of the established definitions of rehabilitation psychology before offering the health and population context that has contributed to the development of rehabilitation psychology over the past 60 years. It will then review the conceptual framework of disability and present the models that underpin practice. The chapter finishes with an overview of the contents of this book, provided by contributors who have assembled an excellent guide to the best evidence-based practices and approaches that

support physical rehabilitation, improve individual well-being, and encourage organizational and professional development in the growing field of applied psychology.

Scherer et al. (2004) define rehabilitation psychology as a specialty area of practice within the broad field of psychology. Rehabilitation psychology is the application of psychological knowledge and understanding on behalf of individuals with disabilities and societies and includes activities such as research, clinical practice, teaching, public education, development of social policy and advocacy. More recently, Stiers, Perry, Kennedy, and Scherer (2011) defined rehabilitation psychology practice as a specialty within a domain of professional health service psychology that applies psychological knowledge and skills on behalf of individuals with physical and cognitive impairment and chronic health conditions with the goal of maximizing their health and welfare, independence and choice, functional abilities, and social role participation while minimizing secondary health complications. Rehabilitation psychologists provide a broad range of services across diverse settings to a variety of health consumers, and they have worked over the past decades to expand clinical services across the full range of health care provision. In Europe and Australia, rehabilitation psychology is not generally recognized as a specialty by that name, and many psychologists working with persons with disabilities are called clinical psychologists, clinical health psychologists, health psychologists, or neuropsychologists, despite the specialized work they do that would be called rehabilitation psychology in the United States.

Rehabilitation psychology, one of the first applied clinical specialties in professional psychology in the United States, has embodied the broader pursuit of psychology as a health care profession for the past 50 years (Brown, DeLeon, Loftis, & Scherer, 2008). The growth of rehabilitation psychology has resulted, in large part, from advancing technologies that have led to an increased incidence in people surviving catastrophic injuries and illnesses who would not have survived them in previous generations. As the number of survivors increased, so did the incidence of life-long and complex physical, mental, and emotional disabilities previously not encountered in the profession of psychology. Largely because of continued advancements in acute care more generally, relatively new types of injuries from recent war fronts, and a general increase in life-expectancy, the role of and need for rehabilitation psychologists specifically trained to assist these individuals has grown tremendously (Cox, Hess, Hibbard, Layman, & Stewart, 2010).

Although advances have often been heralded by war—ancient, modern, and recent—new challenges have been presented by the changing spectrum of common diseases and overall increased longevity. The number of individuals over 65 is expected to double in the United States from 40 to 80 million by 2050, a projected growth of 135%. The number of seniors over 85 years of age is similarly expected to increase by 350% during this same period. With this growth, an increased incidence of age-related physical and mental impairments, limitations, and disabilities is foreseen (U.S. Census Bureau, 2004). According to the Health Survey of England (Joint Health Service Unit, 2002), 18% of men and women aged 16 and over reported having one or more of five types of disability (locomotor, personal care, sight, hearing, and communication), and 5% of adults were found to have a serious disability. In 2001, care providers to individuals with chronic conditions accounted for 83% of health care spending in the United States (Anderson & Horvath, 2002).

In surveying future trends in global health, the World Health Organization (WHO) predicted that the four leading causes of death in 2030 are projected to include HIV/AIDS, unipolar depressive disorders, ischemic heart disease, and road traffic accidents (Mathers & Loncar, 2006). As Brown, DeLeon, Loftis, and Scherer (2008) highlight, each of these conditions and their associated impairments are significantly impacted by behavioral lifestyle habits and psychological principles and interventions. Rehabilitation psychologists are involved in a range of interventions that include the provision and support of psychotherapy, the reduction of distress and improvement of quality of life, the engagement of patients with treatment protocols and recommendations, the reduction of catastrophic thinking and despair, the fostering of the principles of normalization, and the provision of education and training.

The biopsychosocial model (Engel, 1980) has provided a broad conceptual framework for the wider development of rehabilitation psychology, as well as promoting a more collaborative framework within the delivery of health care for people with chronic physical disabilities. Although Suls and Rothman (2004) suggest that the biopsychosocial model holds to the idea that biological, psychological, and social processes are integrally and interactively involved in physical health and illness, the full potential for the model remains untapped. They have also suggested that, in the past three decades, basic and applied research across a range of substantive areas has affirmed the value of biopsychosocial perspective and demonstrated how biological, psychological, and social processes operate together to affect physical health outcomes. However, there remains the sense that the optimism expressed by Frank, Gluck, and Buckelew (1990) in describing rehabilitation psychology as psychology's greatest opportunity has also yet to be fulfilled. Nevertheless, the success of the biopsychosocial approach can be seen in both the substantial growth in government support for health-related behavioral and psychological research, and the considerable increase in the extent to which citations of behavior have appeared in medical journals (Suls & Rothman, 2004).

The WHO's International Classification of Functioning, Disability, and Health (the ICF) describes a model of disability that has attempted to be more respectful of the needs of individuals with disability than the one it replaced (WHO, 2001). The present ICF replaces the older WHO framework, which included the terms *impairment, disability,* and *handicap*. The newer model recognizes the importance of context and frames disability as a person–task–environmental interaction, rather than something located within an individual. It strives to encompass what a person can or cannot do, covering not only bodily functions and structures but also activities and participation, together with environmental and other contextual factors. Functioning and disability are conceived of as multidimensional concepts relating to the body functions and structures of people, the activities they do, the areas of life in which they participate, and the factors in the environment that affect these experiences (see Figure 1.1).

Masala and Petretto (2008) reviewed conceptual elaborations on disablement in the 20th century and found that the current WHO ICF model has been translated and recognized in 191 countries. The ICF model also incorporates contributions from self-advocacy associations and is now recognized by most clinicians, thus enjoying a higher visibility than most other conceptual models. Rauch, Ceiza, and Stucki (2008) have developed ICF tools for rehabilitation management in clinical practice. These tools allow for the description of a functioning state, the illustration of the patient's experience of functioning, and the relationship between rehabilitation goals and appropriate intervention targets. These ICF tools support a common understanding of functioning and the communication between team members in multidisciplinary rehabilitation.

Beatrice A. Wright is perhaps the most important thinker in this field, and she has integrated a broad biopsychosocial framework with social participation and the inclusion of perspectives from people with disabilities. When her *Physical Disability: A Psychological Approach* was published in 1960, it was among the first theory-driven psychological statements on the subject, steeped in the best scholarly traditions of the day, in full command of the extant literature, and enriched with observations relevant to both academicians and practitioners (Dunn & Elliott, 2005). Wright's text, with its deep, well-written integration of conceptual models, clinical practice issues, and personal observations, has given rehabilitation psychologists much to anchor on in the 50 years since it was written. With an insight that was ahead of her time, Wright (1960, 1983) highlighted the negative consequences of not treating people with disabilities as individuals. She commented upon the contribution of coping to broader psychosocial outcomes and noted the importance of accepting one's disability as non-devaluating. Her 20 value-laden beliefs (Wright, 1983) and principles that underlie the rehabilitation process include individual characteristics, disability–environment interaction, multiprofessional involvement, and the importance of client autonomy. Dunn and Elliott (2005) concluded that her work has clearly contributed to knowledge in rehabilitation psychology and helped to construct the views of how people live with disabilities. The work's impact and importance go beyond the intellectual and the academic because it helped to shape the clinical orientation of a generation of practitioners.

In the early 1980s, when I started working as a clinical psychologist with people with disabilities, I found that Wright's writing helped frame an understanding of the experience of disability that has helped me across many different settings. Other contributions in my own development as an applied practitioner were the writings of Muriel Lezak and Roberta Trieschmann. *Neuropsychological Assessment*, first published by Lezak in 1976 and with the latest edition being published in 2004, is one of those few academic texts to be used regularly by both experienced practitioners and those new to the field. Like many aspiring clinical neuropsychologists, I was never far from a copy of this book, which provided a clinically sensible review of assessment tools, theoretical frameworks for understanding complex neuropsychological phenomena, and clinical insights.

Finally, from my own perspective, I found that Trieschmann's (1988) work on spinal cord

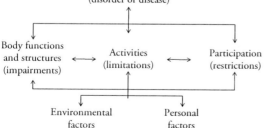

International classification of functioning, disability and health (ICF)

Health condition (disorder or disease)

Body functions and structures (impairments) ←→ Activities (limitations) ←→ Participation (restrictions)

Environmental factors   Personal factors

Figure 1.1 Concepts of disability.

injuries effectively integrated the individual context in society. This aided my early work with spinal cord injured patients in the early 1980s. She suggested that if rehabilitation is the process of teaching the person to live with his or her disability, then the environment and the multiple factors that influence behavior become the concern of everyone in the rehabilitation team. Behavior (B), health, and rehabilitation adjustment are a function of the integration of the psychosocial (P), biological-organic (O), and environmental (E) factors. She proposed the following behavioral equation for rehabilitation success: $B = f (P \times O \times E)$.

Thus, the rehabilitation process should provide the individual with the skills needed to function as a self-sufficient adult in the family, work setting, community, and society in general. Taken together, these conceptual frameworks provide paradigms that have enabled the growth, knowledge, and understanding of psychological applications in physical rehabilitation.

When I was involved in setting up the first clinical psychology service for people with spinal cord injuries in the London Spinal Unit in the early '80s, I received a very helpful letter from a clinical psychologist by the name of Dr. Robert McGovern, who worked in the Veterans Administration medical center in Cleveland, Ohio. He described the key aspects of the role as including:

- The provision of support for psychotherapy
- The organization of educational and therapeutic groups
- The provision of support to family members
- The facilitation of peer support systems
- The provision of marital and sexual counselling
- The provision of training to rehabilitation staff

At the time, I found this helpful in establishing a new clinical service, and now much of this advice remains remarkably relevant.

Recently Cox, Hess, Hibbard, Layman, and Stewart (2010) proposed a similar but more comprehensive conceptual model of interventions. The ABCs of rehabilitation psychology interventions are (A) adjustment, (B) behavioral interventions, and (C) cognitive remediation, compensatory skills building, and consultation and advocacy. Adjustment-based psychotherapy is at the heart of the therapeutic process, as it typically serves as both the umbrella and the net for the Bs and Cs of subsequent interventions. Acute stress disorder, anxiety and depression, work and family adjustment, and behavioral interpersonal changes are commonly addressed by adjustment psychotherapy.

Rehabilitation psychologists use a variety of psychotherapeutic processes on an individual, group, and family level. Interventions have been drawn from formulations based on cognitive-behavioral therapy frameworks, supportive psychotherapy, and coping (e.g., coping effectiveness training). Cox et al. referred to behavioral interventions (B) that are aimed at addressing the individual's altered behaviors secondary to disability onset while enhancing interpersonal skills. These behavioral interventions would include strategies to manage challenging behavior, interventions to enhance adherence to rehabilitative regimes, and the management of emotional distress, apathy, and substance abuse. The several Cs in Cox et al.'s 2010 models refer to cognitive remediation, that includes cognitive retraining, attention training, and error-correcting feedback. Compensatory skills are about acquiring new strategies for minimizing disability. Consultation in advocacy includes work with teams and community staff who advocate for ethically sound and culturally sensitive interventions to maximize the individual's quality of life and independent living in the community.

These ideas and many others are developed and elaborated on in the rest of this book. The remainder of part one provides further perspectives on rehabilitation psychology.

In chapter 2, Elizabeth Sherwin provides a comprehensive account of the large and disparate literature on the history of rehabilitation psychology. In response to the One-World theme of the 21st century, she calls for the internationalization of rehabilitation psychology as a necessity, and comments on the need to collaborate with health psychologists and develop a greater focus on community-based rehabilitation. In chapter 3, Joseph Rath and Timothy Elliot consider the illustrative psychological models that have been influential in rehabilitation psychology. They review the current status of these models, describe their impact on clinical practice, and propose a more dynamic model for understanding positive growth following disability.

In chapter 4, Hanoch Livneh and Erin Martz explore the conceptual and empirical approaches to the study of psychosocial adaptation and chronic illness and disability. They make a number of suggestions that increase the conceptual coherence associated with adaptation and provide a number of insightful empirical recommendations.

Yuying Chen and Yue Cao, in chapter 5, explain how rehabilitation psychology is enriched by epidemiological approaches. The knowledge of health and disease at the population level helps set viable goals, the appropriate tools and methodology help identify long-term rehabilitation outcomes, and measurement scales help assess psychosocial functioning and quality of life.

In chapter 6, Nancy Merbitz, Charles Merbitz, and Judy Ripsch further develop the theme of rehabilitation outcomes by reviewing the dominant trends in outcomes and assessment. They describe how research methods from the quality improvement tradition transform processes and outcomes in rehabilitation. They also provide a discourse on how some of society's contextual factors need to be taken into account when considering rehabilitation outcomes.

In the next chapter, Emilie Smithson and I demonstrate how psychological theory has provided an ideal framework on which to structure the provision of person-centered rehabilitation and engage the patient in taking responsibility and ownership of treatment plans in the rehabilitation context. We also review the application of goal planning in hospital-based rehabilitation settings.

In chapter 8, Craig Ravesloot and Tom Seekins review the emerging role for rehabilitation psychologists in the delivery of community-based rehabilitation services. They highlight the goal of the rehabilitation psychologist in developing participation across vocational, health care, and educational domains. Patricia Rivera extends our awareness of community issues from the perspective of family care givers. In chapter 9, she highlights the increased recognition of family caregivers in rehabilitation research and provides an overview of interventions that positively impact caregiver well-being.

In chapter 10, Kathleen Deidrick and Elena Drewel broaden our understanding of family issues by focusing on the role of the rehabilitation psychologist in supporting children with chronic health conditions, and they draw attention to the limitations in existing research in this field. In the last chapter of this section, Adam Gerstenecker and Benjamin Mast examine the role of rehabilitation psychologists working with older adults. They explore the core concepts in geriatric rehabilitation and highlight the predictors of successful outcomes. They also review approaches to assessing cognitive impairment and depression and provide information on specific interventions for treating depression in geriatric rehabilitation patients.

In part two, we explore clinical contexts and their applications. In chapter 12, Kenneth Packenham presents information on multiple sclerosis that includes etiology, symptoms, and treatment, followed by a discussion of coping with multiple sclerosis and a review of psychosocial interventions. In chapter 13, Jane Barton then reviews the psychological experience of strokes and the psychological factors that are important in rehabilitation and recovery. In chapter 14, Robyn Tate provides an overview of the current clinical and research literature on traumatic brain injury as it pertains to rehabilitation psychology. This chapter also reports the results of systematic reviews on the types and effectiveness of interventions for cognitive, behavioral, and emotional disorders encountered after traumatic brain injuries. Jeri Morris (chapter 15) looks at the practice of neurorehabilitation in post acute rehabilitation. She provides a historical perspective and reviews the evidence-based findings in studies of cognitive rehabilitation, as well as providing a commentary on the complexities involved in the rehabilitation of brain injured individuals. In chapter 16, Emilie Smithson and I discuss the psychological, social, and physical issues related to spinal cord injury and explore psychological interventions utilized by rehabilitation psychologists in this setting.

Persistent and chronic pain is a major clinical theme in rehabilitation psychology. In chapter 17, Elizabeth Richardson and Scott Richards explore the complex interface of cognition, behavior, and pathophysiology in persistent pain and its psychological and behavioral comorbidities. Margreet Scharloo and her colleagues explore chronic and obstructive pulmonary disease in chapter 18, describing comprehensive pulmonary rehabilitation programs and the efficacy of cognitive-behavioral interventions. In chapter 19, Paul Bennett identifies the key goals for cardiac rehabilitation programs and considers the comparative impact of education and behaviorally based interventions. In chapter 20, Deirdre Desmond and her colleagues explore individual impact to limb loss and highlight the critical psychological and social issues in amputation. In chapter 21, Bruce Rybarczyk and colleagues present the myriad of psychological challenges faced by individuals undergoing solid organ transplantation. This chapter describes the most common transplantations and uses case studies to illustrate the role of rehabilitation psychologists in preoperative evaluation and treatments used to facilitate adjustment to transplantation.

In the final chapter in part two, Baird and Clarke describe diabetes and its optimal management within a biopsychosocial framework. This includes health delivery factors, treatment adherence and psychological therapies that integrate disease self-management and emotions.

In part three, the book addresses broader professional issues associated with rehabilitation psychology and future challenges. It begins with William Stiers and Kathryn Nicholson Perry presenting the issues of education and training in the specialty of applied rehabilitation psychology. They explore selection, the structures and processes of training programmes, and the competencies expected of successful trainees. In chapter 24, Thomas Kerkhoff and Stephanie Hanson consider ongoing challenges in applied health care ethics from an international perspective. They describe the emerging professional competence movement within psychology and the role of ethics in developing and maintaining functional professional competencies. Vocational, training, and social integration are reviewed in chapter 25 by Carol Blessing and her colleagues. They explore the importance of community citizenship and valued roles for people with disabilities, as well as the positive impact of social integration and inclusion on quality of life. They provide an overview of historical and philosophical issues and discuss the importance of vocational training in leading to successful employment outcomes. Ashley Craig looks at resilience in people with physical disabilities in chapter 26. He defines resilience as a process of involving a person in maintaining stable psychological, social, and physical functioning while adjusting to the affects of physical disability and subsequent impairment. He reviews the protective factors in physical disability and the challenges for resilience research in people with disabilities. The expert patient and the self-management of chronic conditions and disabilities is the theme of chapter 27, by Michelle Meade and Linda Cronin. They review the theories, programs, components, and issues that inform the development of self-managing skills, as well as the roles for rehabilitation psychologists in supporting this development.

The demographic shifts that include more elderly population and those living with chronic medical conditions have been referred to; in chapter 28, Cheak-Zamora and her colleagues address health legislation and public policies as they pertain to these issues. Significant policy, procedure, and practice changes are essential to solving growing demographic changes and increasing costs.

They propose that rehabilitation psychologists have a clear vantage point to help guide movement toward more integrated health care models that value health promotion, prevention, and collaborative care. The theme of prevention is developed further by Stephen Anton and Michael Perri in chapter 29. They focus on the critical role that eating and exercise behaviors have in the prevention of cardiovascular disease and diabetes. Disability and cultural issues are addressed in chapter 30 by Elias Mpofu and his colleagues. They explain how communities differ in the extent to which they enable the full inclusion of others. They also explore the cultural foundations of rehabilitation and discuss sociocultural differences. In chapter 31, Malcolm MacLachlan considers the role of rehabilitation psychology in the context of global health. He reviews the relationship among rehabilitation psychology and disability, public health, and global health. This chapter addresses how human resources for health crises effect rehabilitation in low-income countries and how advocacy and networking are being used to provide a stronger and more effective evidence-base for addressing the challenges facing people with disabilities in low-income countries in general and in Africa in particular.

References

Anderson, G. F., & Horvath, J. (2002). *Chronic conditions: Making the case for ongoing care.* Prepared by Partnership for Solutions, JohnHopkinsUniversity, for the Robert Wood Johnson Foundation. Retrieved September 15, 2011, from http://www.partnershipforsolutions.org/DMS/files/chronicbook2002.pdf.

Brown, K. S., DeLeon, P. H., Loftis, C. W., & Scherer, M. J. (2008). Rehabilitation psychology: Realising the true potential. *Rehabilitation Psychology, 53,* 111–121.

Cox, D. R., Hess, D. W., Hibbard, M. R., Layman, D. E., & Stewart, R. K. (2010). Specialty practice in rehabilitation psychology. *Professional Psychology: Research and Practice, 41,* 82–88.

Dunn, D. S., & Elliott, T. R. (2005). Revisiting a constructive classic: Wright's Physical Disability: A Psychosocial Approach. *Rehabilitation Psychology, 50,* 183–189.

Engel, G. L. (1980). The clinical application of the biopsychosocial model. *American Journal of Psychiatry, 137,* 535–544.

Frank, R. G., Gluck, J. P., & Buckelew, S. (1990). Rehabilitation: Psychology's opportunity. *American Psychologist, 45,* 757–761.

Joint Health Service Unit (2002). Health Survey for England 2002. Joint health surveys unit national centre for social research department of Epidemiology and public health at the royal free and university college medical school, 2003. Retrieved September 15, 2011, from http://www.dh.gov.uk/en/Publicationsandstatistics/Publications/ Publicati ons Statistics/DH_4078027.

Lezak, M. D. (1976). *Neuropsychological Assessment.* New York: Oxford University Press.

Masala, C., & Petretto, D. R. (2008). From disablement to enablement: conceptual models of disability in the 20th century. *Disability Rehabilitation, 30,* 1233–1244.

Mathers, C. D., & Loncar, D. (2006). Projections of global mortality and burden of disease from 2002 to 2030. *Public Library of Science Medicine, 3,* e442. Retrieved September 15, 2011, from http://www.medicine.plosjournals.org/perlserv?request=getdocument&doi=10.1371%2Fjournal.pmed.0030442.

Rauch, A., Ceiza, A., & Stucki, G. (2008). How to apply the International Classification of Functioning, Disability and Health (ICF) for rehabilitation management in clinical practice. *European Journal of Physical and Rehabilitation Medicine, 44,* 329–342.

Scherer, M. J., Blair, K. L., Banks, M. E., Brucker, B., Corrigan, J., & Wegener, S. (2004). Rehabilitation Psychology. In W. E. Craighead & C. B. Nemeroff (Eds.), *The Concise Corsini Encyclopedia of Psychology and Behavioural Science* (3rd ed., pp. 801–802).Hoboken, NJ: Wiley. Retrieved September 15, 2011, from http://www.apa.org/divisions/div22/RPdef.html.

Stiers, W., Perry, K. N., Kennedy, P., & Scherer, M. J. (2011). Rehabilitation psychology. In P. R. Martin, F. M. Cheung, M. C. Knowles, M. Kyrios, J. B. Overmier, and J. M. Prieto (Eds.), *IAAP Handbook of Applied Psychology* (pp. 573–587). Oxford, UK: Wiley-Blackwell.

Suls, J., & Rothman, A. (2004). Evolution of the biopsychosocial model: Prospects and challenges for health psychology. *Health Psychology, 23,* 119–125.

Trieschmann, R. (1988). *Spinal cord injuries: Psychological, social and vocational rehabilitation* (2nd ed.). New York: Demos Publications.

US Census Bureau (2004). American community survey: Selected social characteristics 2004. Retrieved September 15, 2011, from http://factfinder.census.gov/servlet/ADPTable?_bm=y&-qr_name=ACS_2004_EST_G00_DP2&geo_id=01000US&ds_name=ACS_2004_EST_G00_&_lang=en.

World Health Organisation. (2001). *International classification of functioning, disability and health.* Genvea, Switzerland: World Health Organisation.

Wright, B, A. (1960). *Physical disability: A psychosocial approach.* New York: Harper and Row.

Wright, B. A. (1983). *Physical disability: A psychosocial approach* (2nd ed.). New York: Harper and Row.

A Field in Flux: The History of Rehabilitation Psychology

Elisabeth Sherwin

Abstract

Rehabilitation psychology is a field in flux. With roots in the early legislation to protect those injured in the course of their job or duty (or both), the field now faces those very same issues again: (welfare) legislation of health care and provision of services to those injured in the course of their job and/or duty. This chapter outlines the path from then to now, and addresses the struggles and milestones the field has faced and crossed. Finally, in an attempt to place the field in a bigger context, a modest review of rehabilitation psychology efforts around the world is presented.

Key Words: Rehabilitation psychology, history, international, future.

Summarizing the history of rehabilitation psychology requires reviewing a large and disparate literature. Some sources address the developmental aspects of the field: first meetings, the establishment of a professional organization, debates over training, discussions of future direction. Others identify influences on the field: theoretical sources and new directions, innovative technologies and therapies. The purpose of this chapter is to attempt to summarize all these topics, as well as to internationalize the history: too often, the story reads as if rehabilitation psychology exists solely in the United States. A modest review of these other worlds adds to our understanding of the universal and the unique in the psychology of rehabilitation.

However, before delving into the history of it all, a note must be made: psychology has left its imprint on both the rehabilitation process (e.g., Angelo, Leonard, Majovsky, & Muir, 1991; Petronio, 1992; Kreutzer & Kolakowsky-Hayner, 1999; Dunn & Dougherty, 2005; Gzil, Lefeve, Cammelli, Pachoud, Ravaud, & Leplege 2007) and on our understanding of the experience of living with a disability (e.g., Dunn, 2000; Dunn, Uswatte, & Elliott, 2009;

Katz, Shurka, & Florian, 1978; Florian & Shurka, 1983; Itzhaky & Schwartz, 1998; Roer-Strier, 2002; Heiman & Precel, 2003; Peterson & Elliott, 2008; van Kampen, van Zijverden, & Emmett, 2008). In 2003, the April issue of the *American Psychologist* was largely devoted to the relationship between these two concepts. Titled "A New Model of Disability," its opening article was "Discourse on Disability and Rehabilitation Issues" (Pledger, 2003, pp. 279–284). Whether clearly attempting to address the divide (Melia, Pledger, & Wilson, 2003, pp. 285–288; Olkin & Pledger, 2003, pp. 296–304) or broaden the definitions (Tate & Pledger, 2003, pp. 289–295; Gill, Kewman, & Brannon, 2003, pp. 305–312), all highlight the fact that the disability and rehabilitation processes are not mutually exclusive. This fact is a theme that runs throughout the history of rehabilitation psychology (Elliott & Gramling, 1990; Scherer, 2010; Stubbins, 1989; Thomas & Chan, 2000): where does rehabilitation psychology stop and rehabilitation counseling start (e.g., Emener, 1986; Jansen & Fulcher, 1982; Mugford, 1975)? Is rehabilitation psychology a specialty in clinical psychology, counseling psychology, or neither (Elliott & Shewchuk, 1996; Mullins, Ozolins, & Morris, 1988; Wegener, Elliott, & Hugglund, 2000)? Where do other clinicians in the rehabilitation setting fit in (Holland & Whalley, 1981; Jackson, 1980; Matarazzo, 1994; Thomas, Gottlieb, & Kravetz, 1974)? Some of these questions are more easily answered today. For example, over time, rehabilitation psychologists have ceded vocational issues to counselors and psychologists specializing in vocational rehabilitation (Elliott & Leung, 2005; Fraser & Johnson, 2010; Savickas & Baker, 2005) and neuropsychologists have emerged as constituting their own specialty (Boake, 2008). The struggle (and its at times arbitrary delineation of identity and turf) is the result of the multidisciplinary origins of the field (Stubbins, 1989).

The Facts

In the Beginning

Peterson and Aguilar (2004), in an ambitious undertaking, chart the emergence of rehabilitation counseling from the early days of ancient Greece and Rome to the modern age. The perception of disability alternated between something to be borne stoically to a punishment from God, and active interventions were few until the days of Dorothea Dix and the movement to reform treatment for individuals with mental illness. Her efforts and the visibility of veterans with physical disability after the Civil War led to the first federal funding of rehabilitation. But these efforts were few and paltry, and the bulk of caring for those with physical disabilities (and mental illness) fell to philanthropic (often religion-based) organizations (pp. 50–54).

In the 19th and early 20th century, several landmark events were associated with the eventual emergence of rehabilitation psychology. Among the earliest was the establishment, in 1908, of the Cleveland Rehabilitation Center, "the first modern rehabilitation facility" and the enactment of the first workers' compensation law, the *Federal Employee's Compensation Act* (FECA). Although spotty in its coverage and often challenged in application, it initiated funding by the federal government to facilitate the well-being of its employees. After World War I, the *Smith-Hughes Act* (1917) directed funds for the vocational education of veterans. The *Soldiers Rehabilitation Act* (1918) established federal funding for rehabilitation of veterans, albeit primarily vocational. This benefit was expanded in the *Civilian Vocational Rehabilitation Act* (1920), with the federal government requiring state involvement by offering matching funds. In 1921, the

Veterans Bureau (a precursor of the Department of Veteran Affairs) was established by consolidating several agencies (Larson & Sachs, 2000). Despite an early (failed) effort to abolish federal funding for vocational rehabilitation services, Franklin Delano Roosevelt went on to establish the *Social Security Act* in 1935, which was "the first permanent source of federal funding relate to vocational issues" (Peterson & Aguilar, 2004, p. 57).

Although the years between the world wars were rich in federal legislation regarding rehabilitation, their focus was largely vocational. It was World War II that served as the major catalyst for many fields in psychology, including rehabilitation, and the parameters of what rehabilitation included were enlarged. The needs of returning veterans overwhelmed society, and many professions were drawn into the fray to address them (Elliott & Rath, 2011). In 1947, the American Medical Association's Advisory Board of Medical Specialties approved physical medicine as a specialty board ("History of Physical Medicine and Rehabilitation," 2011). In 1948, the "first center to utilize the emerging science of rehabilitative medicine in the treatment of individuals with disabilities" was established by Howard Rusk (Rusk, 1977a,b, as cited in Peterson & Aguilar, 2004, p. 55). In 1954, the Vocational Rehabilitation Act was instituted and, in addition to establishing benefits for a host of vulnerable populations, it also "provided major funding for research and demonstration grants. It also led to the creation of graduate programs in rehabilitation counseling...." (Peterson & Aguilar, 2004, p. 58).

Self-determination

With the passing of the Vocation Rehabilitation Act in 1954, a slew of universities opened graduate training programs in rehabilitation counseling. Funded by the Vocational Rehabilitation Administration, their focus was to be on vocational rehabilitation counseling (Olshansky & Hart, 1967). However, in 1957, Olshansky reviewed some of the programs, only to find that "training in psychology dominated all the programs and that only token attention was given to the area of occupations and the realities of the labor market" (Olshansky & Hart, 1967, p. 28). The role of psychology in the emerging field of rehabilitation counseling is not surprising. In part, it stemmed from the informal "retreading" that psychologists undertook, many of whom were not necessarily trained in clinical or counseling psychology.

One such figure was Beatrice Wright, who trained as a social psychologist with Kurt Lewin, but was employed as a counselor by the United States Employment Service to provide veterans with vocational guidance. Another Lewin protégée was Roger Barker, who along with Beatrice Wright and others authored *Adjustment to Physical Handicap and Illness: A Survey of the Social Psychology of Physique and Disability* in 1946.[1] See Table 2.1 for the Table of Contents of this early compilation on psychology and disability. Other psychologists have included George N. Wright, past president of the division (1983–1984), who was instrumental in facilitating the establishment of several international graduate rehabilitation psychology programs and who focused on vocational rehabilitation counseling (G. N. Wright, 1989); John McGowan, a counseling psychologist who would co-author with Thomas Porter (McGowan & Porter, 1967) *An Introduction to the Vocational Rehabilitation Process: A Training Manual*; and Lloyd Lofquist, trained as a counseling psychologist, on faculty at the department of psychology at the University of Minnesota, who wrote extensively about rehabilitation counseling, including an early (Lofquist, 1959) operational definition of rehabilitation counseling.

As those serving individuals with disabilities grew in numbers, a special interest group within the American Psychological Association (APA) was formed; this group was officially recognized in 1949. The group's name, The National Council on Psychological Aspects of Physical Disability was changed in 1956, and "physical" was dropped from it title in order to broaden its membership. In 1958, the special interest group became the Division of

Table 2.1 Partial table of contents for adjustment to physical handicap and illness: A survey of the social psychology of physique and disability

Somatopsychological aspects of normal variations in physique

Somatopsychological significance of crippling

Psychology of the tubercular

Somatopsychological significance of impaired hearing

Social psychology of acute illness

Employment of the disabled

Bibliographies of literature on the somatopsychological significance of physique

From Barker, Wright, & Gonick, 1946.

Psychological Aspects of Disability (Thomas, 2004), changing to Division 22, Rehabilitation Psychology in 1971 (B. A. Wright, 1993). Earlier that same year, with financial support from James Garrett, the associate director of the Office of Vocational Rehabilitation (OVR) in the Department of Health, Education, and Welfare, the first conference on what was to become rehabilitation psychology was held in Princeton, New Jersey (Larson & Sachs, 2000). The conference focused on "The Roles of Psychology and Psychologists in Rehabilitation," and its planning committee was chaired by Victor Raimy (who edited the proceedings for the famous Boulder conference that conceived the research-practitioner model that still guides training in clinical psychology) (Raimy, 1950). The attendee list included all members of the special interest group, as well as a host of others affiliated with other divisions of APA, federal agency administrators, and individuals affiliated with the caring professions (e.g., social work, nursing, physical therapy, occupational therapy, etc.) (Elliott & Rath, 2011).

Unexpectedly, the conference could not agree on a definition of rehabilitation (B. A. Wright, 1993). However, Wright (B. Wright, 1959), who edited the proceedings (see Table 2.2), identified 12 guiding principles that would "capture the distinctive character of rehabilitation as a movement and philosophy" (p. 64). These 12 principles were identified as universal, in that they were not unique to physical rehabilitation: (1) A human being merits respect, irrespective of disabilities; (2) membership in society should be available to all human beings, irrespective of disabilities; (3) emphasis should be placed on an individual's assets, with effort applied to ameliorating pathological processes in the physical and mental make-up; (4) behavior is a function of the person and environment; (5) treatment should be comprehensive, including the physical and the psychosocial; (6) treatment should be tailored to the individual's needs; (7) the patient, to the degree possible, should have an active role in his or her own rehabilitation process; (8) society has an obligation to provide for the needs of all its members, including those with disability; (9) solutions for disability require interdisciplinary and interagency integration; (10) rehabilitation is a continuous process; (11) psychological factors are inherently part of the rehabilitation process; and (12) rehabilitation, because of its complex nature, requires constant reevaluation (pp. 27–28). Despite the non–gender neutral language (a product of its time), these principles have withstood the test of time. As Wright (1993) accurately assessed nearly

Table 2.2 Partial table of contents of the proceedings of the Conference on Psychology and Rehabilitation

Background and organization of the institute The scope and nature of rehabilitation	Beatrice Wright for the American Psychological Association
The roles and functions of psychologists in rehabilitation	
Preparing psychologists for work in rehabilitation	
Interprofessional relations	
Psychological research in rehabilitation	
A word in conclusion	
Rehabilitation today and tomorrow	Mary E. Switzer
Next steps in rehabilitation	Howard A. Rusk
Appendix I. Participants in the institute	
Appendix II. Committee members	
Appendix III. Bibliographies	
A. Psychological aspects of disability	
B. Interprofessional relations	
C. Training of psychologists	
Appendix IV. Research topics	

From Wright, 1959.

40 years later, these principles will "accord well with the spirit of the Independent Living Movement launched in the 1970s" (p. 64).

Larson and Sachs (2000) (whose review of the history of Division 22 is the touchstone for many histories of the Division or of rehabilitation psychology) suggest that the difficulties in agreeing on a definition of rehabilitation stemmed from the debate on whether to include mental disorders in the purview of rehabilitation psychology or remain focused on physical ones. The presence—and subsequent removal—of the word "physical" from the title of the Council that was the precursor to Division 22 is a reflection of this struggle (p. 40). As they note, the reality of the multidisciplinary nature of rehabilitation made such tension inevitable. The more philosophical and training orientations, the more divergent the perspectives on the nature and scope of rehabilitation. More easily reached was consensus regarding the import of *vocation*, gainful employment of any type in the lives of individuals undergoing rehabilitation. Psychology in the rehabilitation setting was also addressed, with an understanding that it may take on a more informal and flexible nature in response to the needs of the individual and the setting in which delivered. Finally, the issue of training of rehabilitation psychologists was addressed: training at the doctoral level was identified, and an outline of curricular requirements developed (p. 40–41).

A second conference, held a year later at Clark University, was also sponsored by the Office of Vocational Rehabilitation. Larson and Sachs (2000) describe it, relying on the proceedings edited by Leviton (1959).[2] This conference was more structured than the seminal one a year earlier. Of note was Myerson's call for the development of a comprehensive theory of rehabilitation that would integrate the person, the disability, the social setting, and the rehabilitation process itself, all of which should be perceived as open and amenable to change. Moreover, Myerson urged the pursuit of sustained programs of research, rather than single studies or case studies (Larson & Sachs, p. 41).

Indeed, the following year, in 1960, a third conference was convened in Miami, with research as its focus. Elliott and Rath (2011) note that the attendee list reflected this focus, namely, identifying and delineating a research agenda that represented the unique interests of psychology in rehabilitation, as well as that of rehabilitation as a whole. Although clinicians were heavily represented, luminaries (or soon to be) such as Leona Tyler, Cecil Patterson, George England, and Donald Patterson, as well as John Darley and Lloyd Lofquist, worked with others renowned for their achievements in social psychology, such as Tamara Dembo, Richard Lazarus, Harold Kelley, Albert Hastorf, Edward Jones, and John Thibaut. Other experts present were Orval Mowrer, with his work in learning theory, and Lee Cronbach in psychometrics. The proceedings were edited by Lofquist (1960; see Table 2.3).

A fourth conference, in 1970, was convened in Monterey, California and focused on the psychological aspects of disability. In contrast to the first two, this one was not initiated by the Office of Vocational Rehabilitation, but was funded by the APA. Of further note, this was the first conference in which students participated. Among novel issues raised were the impact of race, ethnicity, and poverty on rehabilitation. Another development was Leviton's paper on the patient–professional relationship. The insider–outsider paradigm was applied to the relationship to highlight the differing perspective on the nature and experience of disability (Larson & Sachs, 2000). The proceedings were summarized by Neff (1971; see Table 2.4).

The issues addressed in these conferences, particularly the identity of rehabilitation psychology, training, and the nature and focus of research continue to be a subjects of debate till this very day.

The Many Identities of Rehabilitation Psychology

"One of the more remarkable and intriguing stories in the evolution of rehabilitation psychology is.... [i]ts ambivalent relationship with the highly-influential rehabilitation counseling profession (indeed, to this day, many psychologists in some specialty areas mistakenly equate rehabilitation psychology with rehabilitation counseling)" (Elliott & Rath, 2011. This struggle expresses itself in writings on both sides of the aisle.

Vocational Counseling

Lofquist, who edited the proceedings for the Miami conference in 1960, a counseling psychologist by training, is firmly identified by his writing in the field of rehabilitation counseling. Already in 1959, he argued that "rehabilitation counseling is not a specialty separate from, or different from, counseling psychology, but rather *is* counseling psychology plus an overlay of medical and paramedical knowledge necessary in the particular setting in which the counselor practices" (p. 7). However, when "talk[ing] about counseling psychology, he is referring to *vocational* counseling—i.e., counseling oriented toward vocational planning—not therapeutic counseling—not to clinical counseling" (p. 7). Within a decade, Jaques (1970) expanded the definition of a rehabilitation counselor to include assisting the client to understand existing problems and potentials and helping the client make effective use of personal and environmental resources for his or her best possible vocational, personal, and social adjustment. Fraser and Johnson (2010) describe the "VR [vocational rehabilitation] counselor...[as] usually an individual with a master's degree in rehabilitation counseling" (p. 357). (Of note is the emergence of the "employment counselor," a field of expertise under the auspice of the counseling profession; see http://www.employmentcounseling.org/). The questions

Table 2.3 Partial table of contents of the proceedings for Conference on Psychological Research and Rehabilitation

Introduction	Lloyd H. Lofquist
Cognitive processes, cognitive theories, and rehabilitation	Franklin C. Shontz
Differential psychology and rehabilitation	George W. England
Learning, behavior, and rehabilitation	Lee Meyerson, John L. Michael, O. Hobart Mowrer, Charles E. Osgood and Arthur W. Staats
Personality, motivation, and clinical phenomena: Some implications of social psychological theory for research on the handicapped	Emory L. Cowen Harold H. Kelley, Albert H. Hastorf, Edward E. Jones, John W. Thibaut and William M. Usdane
Editorial comment	Lloyd H. Lofquist

From Lofquist, 1960.

Table 2.4 Partial table of contents of the Conference Proceedings on the Psychological Aspects of Disability

Cognitive and motor aspects of handicapping conditions in the neurologically impaired	Leonard Diller
Physical disability and personality	Franklin C. Shontz
Behavioral methods in rehabilitation	Wibert E. Fordyce
Rehabilitation and work	Walter S. Neff
The social psychology of disability	Bernard Kutner
Rehabilitation and poverty	George J. Goldin
Race, ethnicity, social disadvantagement, and rehabilitation	Edmund W. Gordon
Professional–client relations in a rehabilitation hospital setting	Gloria L. Leviton
Research utilization in rehabilitation	Everett M. Rogers
Rehabilitation psychologists: Roles and functions	Donald Brieland
Psychologists in rehabilitation: Manpower and training	Shalom E. Vineberg
State of the art: An overview	Joan H. Criswell
The state of the art: Rehabilitation Research Utilization Conference planning committee	William M. Usdane

From Neff, 1971.

that arise then are: What is a rehabilitation psychologist? What is a rehabilitation counselor? What is a vocational counselor?

In the early days, the training was less important than the job undertaken; recall Beatrice Wright, who trained in social psychology yet served as a vocational counselor. However, by 1967, Olshansky and Hart were querying whether it was "psychologists in vocational rehabilitation or vocational rehabilitation counselors" (p. 28). They clearly advocated that it was the latter as they believed that "the state vocational rehabilitation agency is not a clinic for the treatment of psychological disorders" (p. 28). And, although "psychological sophistication is basic to the counselor's role...the focus [is] on vocational guidance, and helping 'the client move toward the world of work'" (p. 28). Today, the ideal vocational counselor has graduate training in rehabilitation psychology and acquired expertise (as reflected by certification) in vocational counseling (Fraser & Johnson, 2010, p. 358). Thus, theoretically, individuals with graduate training in clinical and counseling rehabilitation psychology may all serve as vocational counselors if they have the appropriate certification, which ensures the competencies Olshansky and Hart (1967) were concerned about.

What remains is to delineate (or untangle), if possible, the identity of the rehabilitation psychologist and the rehabilitation counselor. This effort is reflected in writings about the field by its proponents, as well as by their respective debates over professional training.

Rehabilitation Psychology and Rehabilitation Counseling

The primary (and primal) struggle appears to be between rehabilitation counselors and rehabilitation psychologists. A recent definition of rehabilitation psychology states that it "is a specialty area within psychology that focuses on the study and application of psychological knowledge and skills on behalf of individuals with disabilities and chronic health conditions in order to maximize health and welfare, independence and choice, functional abilities and social role participation across the lifespan" (Scherer, 2010, p. 1444). In contrast, rehabilitation counseling "emerged as a full time occupation (Leahy & Szymanski, 1995, p. 164) from federal mandate responding to a need among individuals with disabilities. Rehabilitation counseling is defined "as a profession that assists persons with disabilities in adapting to the environment, assists environments in accommodating the needs of the individual, and works toward full participation of persons with disabilities in all aspects of society, especially work" (Szymanski, 1985, p. 3).

A careful reading of these respective definitions (and there are numerous others), suggests that both provide services to the same population—individuals with disabilities. However, rehabilitation counselors could be found working with individuals with developmental or learning disabilities and individuals struggling with substance abuse, whereas rehabilitation psychologists initially largely confined their services to physical disabilities, chronic health conditions, and cognitive disabilities that are not congenital (Brieland, 1971). However, this distinction no longer holds, according to Elliott and Rath (2011). Moreover, rehabilitation psychologists, according to some, are first and foremost (clinical or counseling) psychologists (Elliott & Gramling, 1990; Wegener, Hagglund, & Elliott, 1998; Wegener et al., 2000). Rehabilitation counselors, on the other hand, do not rest on a broad, universal theoretical base, such as psychology. Rather, their base is cobbled from the respective duties and roles they fulfill: guidance counselor (school psychology, education), therapist (psychology), case manager, case coordinator (social work), clinical life reviewer, psychometrician, educator, team member, social and family relator, placement counselor, community and client advocate (law), life engagement counselor (recreational therapy), long-term conservator, and clinician (Whitehouse, 1975).

TRAINING

Rehabilitation Counseling

Differences in philosophy and orientation are also reflected in the training process of rehabilitation psychologists compared to rehabilitation counselors. While clinical and counseling psychologists held their first conference on graduate training models in 1950, and rehabilitation psychology in 1959 and 1960, rehabilitation counseling held its first conference in 1941 (McAlees,1975). Like graduate programs in clinical and counseling psychology that are accredited by the APA, rehabilitation counseling programs are accredited by the Council on Rehabilitation Education, established in 1971 and incorporated in 1972 (http://www.core-rehab.org/WhatisCORE.html). Historically, rehabilitation counselors were master's degree level professionals (Maki, Berven, & Allen, 1985, p. 146), however this has changed in recent years (Maki, Berven, &

Peterson, 2003) with the emergence of doctoral programs that train individuals to serve as educators in graduate programs in rehabilitation counseling. And, although the primary focus of rehabilitation counseling used to be vocational counseling, the role of therapy had evolved sufficiently for Maki and Delworth (1995) to write about the growing need for clinical supervision. Others have focused on the growing need to assess the impact of multicultural training programs on the functioning of rehabilitation counselors, in order to ensure cross-cultural competencies (Rubin, Davis, Noe, & Turner, 1996). As a graduate student noted, "[h]istory shows that the profession has come to the point of realizing that the client is the focus of the process" (Hennessey, 2001, p. 156).

Moreover, training in research, once the purview of psychology, has been integrated into the training and identity of rehabilitation counseling. The scientist-practitioner model, developed in Boulder (Raimy, 1950) and the hallmark of training in clinical and counseling psychology, has been implemented in the graduate curriculum of rehabilitation counseling (Bellini & Rumrill, 1999). It has also remained on the cutting edge of training delivery, as Leech and Holcomb (2004) described the development of an online master's degree program in rehabilitation counseling. The program was established to address both the needs of a largely rural state and as a "mechanism for leveling the playing field for students with disabilities as well as for nontraditional students seeking to advance their education" (p. 136). And despite the encroaching overlap in training and domain with rehabilitation psychology, Leierer, Strohmer, Blackwell, Thompson, and Donnay's (2008) testing of the Rehabilitation Counselor Scale in the Revised Strong Interest Inventory indicated that there is "support for the concept that the profession of rehabilitation counseling is a well-defined occupation whose members possess interest patterns that are distinctly different from people in general" (p. 73).

Rehabilitation Psychology

The clearer, more defined, the identity, the easier it is to recruit and initiate. In 1959, Wright summarized the Princeton Conference recommendations on "[p]reparing psychologists to work in rehabilitation" (p. 45). Four guiding propositions were outlined: "(1) The scope of rehabilitation requires psychologists trained at the doctoral level ... (2) The roles and functions of psychologists in rehabilitation do not require the creation of a separate specialty... (3) All branches of psychology have contributions to make to rehabilitation.... (4) Rehabilitation has basic contributions to make to psychology in general" (pp. 45–48). Three training formats thus arose: (1) building on the existing structure of clinical and counseling doctoral programs, content on disability rehabilitation is added to the curriculum. However, this was immediately identified as a problematic solution considering the heavy load of core classes already required; thus, the next two formats: (2) maintaining the current format of clinical and counseling curriculum and introducing content relevant to rehabilitation during the course of a specialized internship, and (3) designing a specialized doctoral program solely for rehabilitation (p. 47–48). The conference did not commit to a solution. Inevitably, the second format has been the road most traveled.

Some 30 years later, Elliott and Gramling (1990) bemoaned the fact that the "lack of clarity regarding roles, functions, and research of psychologists in inpatient and outpatient rehabilitation settings has hampered efforts to establish guidelines for training graduate students to work in rehabilitative settings" (p. 762). In the years since the Princeton conference, others have expressed similar concerns. Shontz and Wright (1980) declared that rehabilitation psychology is a field distinct from behavioral medicine and that "it is no longer possible to learn rehabilitation psychology through an internship or an on-the-job training program" (p. 992). They advocated specialized training during graduate school, but stated that this training may be part of a separate program of graduate study or as a specialty within other programs—in essence, no more authoritative than the recommendations extended in 1959. Eisenberg and Jensen (1987) wondered if rehabilitation psychologists in medical settings were redundant, and although they were reassured that they were not, the authors concluded that "[u]ntil the ambiguous identity of rehabilitation psychology is clarified, attempts to delimit the roles and functions of this subspecialty will continue to be frustrated" (p. 477).

The supremacy of core training in clinical or counseling psychology in rehabilitation psychology (which in 1959 was only one of three possible scenarios) was put forth by Grzesiak by 1981, and was to be reiterated by Wegener, Hagglund, and Elliott (1998). Two years later, Thomas and Chan (2000) challenged Wegener, Hagglund, and Elliott's contention. This exchange (which continued in a rebuttal by Wegener, Elliott, and Hagglund [2000])

reflects the primal struggle between rehabilitation psychology and rehabilitation counseling. Thomas and Chan (2000) focused on the breadth and scope of rehabilitation psychology acknowledged by Shontz and Wright (1980), and contended that this breadth supports graduate training in counseling as a legitimate portal to rehabilitation psychology. Specifically, citing research (Leung, Sakata, & Ostby, 1990) that indicates that few graduate programs in *clinical and counseling psychology* offer courses in rehabilitation (such as those recommended by the conference in 1959 (Wright, 1959, p. 49–50) or subsequently (e.g., Shontz & Wright, 1980, p. 922–923)), Thomas and Chan (2000) conclude that graduate programs in *rehabilitation counseling* are closer to the 1959 recommendations, and therefore they are equally viable portals to the profession of rehabilitation psychology.

The heart of the matter is whether a rehabilitation psychologist is a psychologist first (with a doctorate in clinical or counseling psychology) or whether rehabilitation training and experience take precedence. Elliott (2002), in his 2001 presidential address to the members of the Division of Rehabilitation Psychology, stated unequivocally that "by definition, rehabilitation psychology is an applied extension of the larger domain of psychology" (p. 132). Moreover, he noted that "it is imperative that... [rehabilitation psychologists] stay grounded in our scientific heritage and current in our use of available theories, techniques, and technologies" (p. 138). Nearly a decade later—and close to half a century after the seminal conference at Princeton—the issue of training has not been resolved. Hibbard and Cox (2010) note that "doctoral preparation remains the minimal competency expectation of today's rehabilitation psychologist" (p. 469). Furthermore, "rehabilitation psychologists emerge from clinical, counseling, school, neuropsychology, and health psychology backgrounds" (p. 469).

Despite this confusion, efforts have been made to enhance the clinical experience of psychologists entering the field of rehabilitation psychology and increase their expertise in rehabilitation. In 1992, the Conference on Postdoctoral Training in Professional Psychology in Ann Arbor, Michigan, was attended by members of the APA's Division 22 (Rehabilitation Psychology) and of the American Congress of Rehabilitation Medicine (ACRM) to delineate a joint model for postdoctoral training in rehabilitation psychology (Patterson & Hanson, 1995). The prerequisites were clearly within the purview of psychology: completion of all requirements for a doctoral degree from a program accredited by the APA or the Canadian Psychological Association (CPA), and completion of a similarly accredited internship. In 2007, Stiers and Stucky (2008) surveyed internship sites that met criteria for training in rehabilitation psychology: an Association of Psychology Postdoctoral and Internship Center (APPIC) listing "rehabilitation psychology" or "physical disability" as a specialty (p. 537). Their findings were not encouraging: "at sites where psychology training involved rehabilitation populations, the majority did not teach rehabilitation psychology, and of those sites that did there was not usually a *focus* on rehabilitation psychology, and faculty were either not board certified or were board certified in something other than rehabilitation psychology" (p. 542). Comparing the results to the guidelines established by Division 22 and ACRM over 10 years earlier (Patterson & Hanson, 1995), Stiers and Stucky noted that only 63% of postdoctoral sites actually met the full recommended criteria for postdoctoral training, and only 21% of the resident sites formally taught the full complement of competencies for certification by the American Board of Rehabilitation Psychology (established in 1995). Perhaps most distressing for those advocating the necessity of a basis in graduate training in psychology (see Elliott & Warren, 2007) was that only 74% sites required that residents be graduates of APA-accredited intern programs.

Summary

In short, many roads lead to rehabilitation psychology (to paraphrase Thomas & Chan, 2000). The distinctions rest on level of graduate training (master's degree vs. a Ph.D. or Psy.D.), historical and philosophical roots (vocation vs. psychology), and focus on training (psychology with additional training and experience in rehabilitation, as opposed to a clear disability and rehabilitation). Although the divide seems both insurmountable and miniscule, it may come down to membership— rehabilitation counselors may belong to the American Rehabilitation Counseling Association (in 1971, members were primarily from private rehabilitation agencies [Brieland, p. 276]), the National Rehabilitation Counseling Association (the preferred professional organization; its members were primarily employed by state divisions of rehabilitation [Brieland, 1971, p. 2760]), or Division 22 of the APA (primarily counselors employed by the Veterans Administration [Brieland, 1971, p. 277]).

Psychologists are more likely to join Division 22 and the ACRM.

Themes and Variations—North America
Forces at Play
THEORETICAL UNDERPINNINGS

As noted, from the start, the actors central to the emerging field were a diverse lot: counseling psychologists, clinical psychologists, social psychologists, civil servants, and a host of professionals affiliated with the medical world. Of those, the voices heard most frequently were those with a background in social psychology. This may be in part a by-product of the academic roots and affiliations of the authors, who often had theory to guide them and the compulsion to publish. Kurt Lewin's (1935) conceptualization of behavior as a function of both the person and the environment ($B = f(PE)$) (Lewin, Heider, & Heider, 1936) still guides rehabilitation psychology. This can be directly related to the early influence of Lewin's graduates, who permeated the field in its early years. Thus, Kurt Lewin's experimental social psychology laboratory produced Beatrice Wright, whose name is synonymous with rehabilitation psychology (Brodwin, 2010; Davis, 2011) and who is the author of the seminal *Psychology and Rehabilitation* (1959) and *Physical Disability: A Psychological Approach* (1960), which in its second edition, was re-titled *Physical Disability: A Psychosocial Approach* (1983). Her background in social psychology is reflected in the theoretical orientation in which she grounds her writings (Wright, 1972, 1989).

Moreover, Lewin's (1935) writings on minority group experiences (arising from his own minority status as a Jew in Germany during the early years of the Nazi regime) also outlined the concept of the insider–outsider (Dembo, 1964) that also heavily influenced the understanding of disability. Dembo, who identified herself as a Lewinian, explicitly acknowledged her application of Lewin's perspective to rehabilitation (1982), authored *Sensitivity of One Person to Another* (1964), and had earlier co-authored *Adjustment to Misfortune: A Problem of Social-Psychological Rehabilitation* (1956) with Wright (Dembo, Leviton, & Wright, 1956). Other contributions from Lewin's graduates include Gloria Ladieu's (later Leviton) *Studies in Adjustment to Visible Injuries: Evaluation of Help by the Injured* (Ladieu, Hanfmann and Dembo, 1947) and *Studies in Adjustment to Visible Injuries: Social Acceptance of the Injured* (Ladieu, Adler, & Dembo, 1948); Roger Barker, who co-authored *Adjustment to*

Physical Handicap and Illness: A Survey of the Social Psychology of Physique and Disability with Wright and Gonick in 1946, and authored *The Social Psychology of Physical Disability* in 1952.. Not only were Lewin's disciples prolific individually, they also often collaborated, for example: Ladieu and Dembo (1947, 1948), Dembo and Wright (1948), Dembo, Ladieu-Leviton, and Wright (1952, 1956); and Dembo, Diller, Gordon, Leviton, and Sherr (1973). The influence of social psychology continues and is reflected in such works such as Dunn's (2000) chapter on social psychological issues in disability, and the emerging literature marrying positive psychology with disability and rehabilitation; examples here include Dunn and Dougherty's (2005) commentary on "Prospects for a positive psychology of rehabilitation" and Dunn, Uswatte, and Elliott's (2009) chapter on happiness, resilience and positive growth following physical disability. The rich interdisciplinary nature of rehabilitation psychology (Stubbins, 1989) also includes contributions from clinical psychology, counseling psychology, and the neurosciences (see Elliott & Rath, 2011] for an excellent summary of the impact of these respective fields).

THE REAL WORLD

Since rehabilitation psychology has its roots in vocational and rehabilitation counseling, and these fields have their roots in federal legislation, it is not surprising that rehabilitation psychology has also involved itself with public health and policy. The passage of the Americans with Disabilities Act (ADA) in 1990 influenced the types of services provided by psychologists. The field responded, with Pape and Tarvydas (1993) declaring that "new or upgraded psychological knowledge and skill will be necessary to assist persons with disabilities, employers, coworkers, and the rehabilitation team" (p. 118) in the implementation of the Act. They concluded that the "law...provides an enormous opportunity for psychologists to expand their practices into the larger community beyond their offices and hospitals" (p. 128). Of note is that the target population was psychologists in general, not specifically rehabilitation psychologists. However, the model of enhanced training that Pape and Tarvydas (1993) proposed is based on a three-tier core, with rehabilitation principles, knowledge, and function as the base; then disability concepts, functions, and knowledge; and culminating with ADA knowledge and functions (pp. 123–125). Ironically, they felt that, in the short term, rehabilitation psychologists would need to turn to the rehabilitation counselors for assistance regarding aspects of the Act (p. 126).

Four years later, Elliott and Klapow (1997) responded to the radical changes in health care reimbursement and called for them to be addressed by both practicing and academic psychologists, warning that failure to respond to the crisis would result in the diminishment of psychology in health care (p. 256). Their recommendations were to implement changes in professional identity (e.g., "broaden professional options...by emphasizing behavioral science expertise versus mental health service provision" [p. 265]) and in training (e.g., integrating market trends into curriculum, introducing cross-disciplinary evaluation assessment practices, reducing the number of predoctoral clinical hours required for internship placement, and expecting greater preparation in administrative, consultive, and evaluative skills [p. 266]). Elliott and Frank (2000) urged an evaluation of the cost-effectiveness of treatment offered by high- versus low-cost (doctoral vs. nondoctoral) providers: namely, to guide the respective service provider to the role that maximizes the ratio of training and cost to outcome of treatment (p. 647). They also acknowledged that the growing movement toward prescription privileges for psychologists may add another arena in which doctoral-level rehabilitation psychologists may find a niche. They suggest that prescription privileges may be "particularly cost effective in outpatient, community-based programs and to people in rural, inner-city, and other underserved areas" (p. 648). Within these new horizons, the authors warned of the (inevitable) competition to provide clinical services that will ensue as a result of changes in payment systems. They suggested that in the search for new treatment models and roles lies the hope for the future of rehabilitation psychologists. However, to "realize these roles, rehabilitation psychologists must remember their primary identity as scientists in the pursuit of refining clinical practice" (p. 651).

Echoing Elliott and Klapow (1997), Glueckauf (2000) offered principles and strategies for unifying doctoral education in rehabilitation and heath care psychology. Responding to the changes in treatment delivery imposed by managed care on a host of subspecialties in psychology (rehabilitation, neuropsychology, health, pediatric, and clinical geopsychology), he offered four principles: (1) the client is a hub of a wheel, and the client and the family are the focus of service; (2) psychologists must have a dynamic role orientation that rejects the old model of an in-house, clinical scientist or medical school clinician; (3) training in research should be linked to evaluation of the effectiveness of psychological services; and (4) it is vital to promote increasing awareness and proficiency in provision of care to a diverse ethnic population, along with recruiting ethnic minorities into the field and increasing the number of ethnic minority faculty (pp. 621–622).

The push to move rehabilitation psychologists from their safe academic ivory towers, rehabilitation hospitals, and inpatient centers continued. Gill, Kewman, and Brannon (2003) addressed the growing need for psychologists working with individuals with disabilities to involve themselves in improving disability policies (p. 305). They called on psychologists to reframe how psychology approaches disability and disability problems, relationships with consumers, and the responsibilities of psychologists regarding disability issues and implementation of disability policy agendas. They acknowledged that these changes will require changes in training policies, and the efforts to implement the reframing may be hampered or facilitated by external forces, such as reimbursement policies. They urged psychologists to form coalitions with consumer groups "to promote disability policy enlightened by the knowledge and perspectives of the groups involved" (p. 311).

On the 50th anniversary of the organization of Division 22, Brown, DeLeon, Loftis, and Scherer (2008) urged rehabilitation psychologists to realize their potential and "develop and promote in the public's consciousness the type of rehabilitation care that every one…would desire be readily available for him- or herself and their families" (p. 119). The fulfillment of this potential will require pursuing the opportunities inherent in the changing world of health care delivery, and these authors suggest that psychologists should involve themselves with the growing use of technology. They provided two examples: electronic medical records and assistive technology (AT) devices. For the former, they exhort rehabilitation psychologists to be "vigilant and provide input into the impact of such systems not only on privacy but also on accessibility features for use by individuals with disabilities" (p. 114). As to the latter, they note that rehabilitation psychologists "must recognize that support for a person with a disability through AT, environmental accommodation, and so forth must be adapted to the individual's needs ad preferences, rather than having the individual having to adapt to the existing structure of support" (p. 115). Rehabilitation psychologists

are also in a position to use their expertise to treat the rise in chronic diseases (Frank & Elliott, 2000) by promoting "proactive leadership in multidisciplinary teams and in the large health care environment" (p. 116). By taking the lead in recognizing and addressing health care disparities and their unequal impact on individuals with disabilities and their caregivers, psychologists can levy their training to bring about change. Finally, in order to institutionalize these changed roles and responsibilities, rehabilitation psychology will have to re-evaluate the models of training currently in place and assess their suitability to this new era of health care delivery.

Responding to the realities of managed health care, the changing world of technology, and the interminable wars (Packard, 2007) has propelled rehabilitation psychology to address the health of the public at large—not just individuals with disabilities. Indeed, the paradigm shift from "disabled individuals" to "individuals with disability" (and indeed the rejection of the medical model of disability [Pledger, 2003; Thomas, 2004]) reintegrates individuals with disability into the community, into the public sphere. While public health professionals focus on communities (even countries), rehabilitation psychology focuses on the individual, at most addressing the needs of the individual's family and/or caregivers. These different foci can be bridged. Lollar (2008) identifies four such bridges: the first bridge arises from an equal emphasis being placed on science, health and well-being, and environmental factors. Both public health and psychology employ classification systems: psychology's system rests on the *Diagnostic and Statistical Manual* (DSM) and public health's on the *International Classification of Diseases*, and now the *International Classification of Functioning, Disability and Health* (ICF) as well. The latter serves as the first bridge to be used as a "conceptual framework" by rehabilitation psychologists to code functioning in different domains.

The second bridge emerges from the joint attention paid to secondary conditions and their impact. By preventing secondary conditions for individuals living with disability, both public and health and rehabilitation are promoted. The third bridge, the Healthy People Agenda, originates with public health but impacts rehabilitation psychology. The fourth bridge is education and training that will allow the building of even more bridges, thereby enhancing the health of the individual and his or her community—the ultimate goal of both disciplines (Stiers, Perry, Kennedy, & Scherer, 2011, p. 583).

Themes and Variations—International

There is no doubt that rehabilitation psychologists practice outside of the United States, as evidenced by their attendance at annual conferences held by the APA or the ACRM, and at meetings held by international organizations such as the International Brain Injury Association or the World Health Organization. However, documenting the world of international rehabilitation psychology is challenging for several reasons: many foreign rehabilitation psychologists publish in their native-language journals and these are less likely to appear in search engines such as EBSCO; when foreign practitioners publish in English-language journals, the content addressed in these publications is not necessarily specific to their native community; and finally, because a large part of the world is struggling to survive poverty and strife, publishing clinical practice experiences or conducting research for academic reasons is low on the list of priorities.

The following is a very modest effort to document the efforts of the international rehabilitation psychology community. The endeavor is constrained by the reasons listed above, and by the author's research and foreign language skills.

North America
CANADA

Canada is unique in two ways: since 1966, it has had a universal health care plan, and the responsibility for health and welfare is shared between the federal government and the provinces (the equivalent of the states in the United States). The health care program was based on five principles, including universality of eligibility. Although many services are offered and individuals with disabilities are participants in the Charter of Rights and Freedoms, the system has struggled with defining the scope of rehabilitation services and with subsidizing them: "This requires the development of a normative foundation for analyzing the goals of respect, participation, and accommodation that will result in consistent policy objectives" (Jongbloed, 2003, p. 208).

In a review of the history of rehabilitation counseling, Rudman (2004) described the professionals involved in providing rehabilitation services to individuals with disabilities. Similar to the United States, Canada also has certified rehabilitation counselors. Interestingly, however, and as opposed to the United States, where the catalysts for certification were professional organizations (McAlees, 1975), demand for certification came from Canadian consumers and was not initiated by the profession. After careful evaluation, "a certification process, based on competencies defined in the U.S. certification process" (Rudman, 2004, p. 85) was eventually adopted in 1990. Of note was that while a common core of knowledge seems to be shared with the United States, training needs and the weight associated with each domain of knowledge was different for Canadian counselors. Ethical standards, planning for rehabilitation services, vocational implications of disabilities, medical aspects of disabilities, and functional capacities of individuals with disabilities (pp. 85–86) were rated as having highest import. The Canadian standards were adapted to reflect the local educational system and include educational and work experience. The Canadian equivalent of vocational counselor is the *certified vocational evaluator*, which, as in the United States, is an area of expertise for the rehabilitation counselor. In addition, another baccalaureate-based degree is that of the *registered rehabilitation professional*, which requires education, work experiences and references, and continuing education but no certification examination.

South America
MEXICO

As part of the international section in *Rehabilitation Psychology*, in 2004, Marshall et al. summarized a series of studies conducted in Southern Mexico. The purpose of the studies was to "conduct exploratory research, descriptive in design, and thereby document the needs of indigenous people with disabilities in different geographic regions of the state of Oaxaca, Mexico" (p. 15). In their summary, the authors noted that "[r]ehabilitation psychology does not exist in Mexico" (p. 16), and that "[t]he absence of the field and its professionals arose from the lack of university programs, at the state or national level, to provide training in psychologists or educators for social or vocational rehabilitation. Access to rehabilitation services that are available is constrained by insurance and funds. The authors encouraged continued collaboration because understanding the cultural perspectives of the peoples of both countries can provide meaningful information for the development and enhancement of appropriate rehabilitation training and service activities" (Marshall et al., 2004, p. 19).

Although review of the literature indicates that there are some efforts to the provision of rehabilitation psychology (e.g., Garay-Sevilla et al., 1995; Luque-Coqui et al., 2003), they are too few. However, in 2006, the University of North Texas received a grant to partner with the Autonomous University of Guadalajara ("UNT department receives," retrieved April 21, 2011) to introduce a master's degree program in rehabilitation counseling.

Europe

The European Union has an umbrella organization for all psychologists, the European Federation of Psychologists' Associations (EFPA; http://www.efpa.eu), which has 35 member countries. It also established an overarching accreditation of psychologists, EuroPsy (http://www.europsy-efpa.eu), which has been in effect since 2010. Supplementing national standards, it "presents a benchmark or a set of European standards for Psychology that will serve as the basis for evaluating the academic education and professional training of psychologists across the different countries of the EU, and other countries within EFPA" (EFPA, 2009, p. 6). Rehabilitation psychology is not among the areas of practice and specialization. However, clinical and health psychology are identified as areas of practice.

UNITED KINGDOM
Britain

The British Psychological Society does not include a division of rehabilitation psychology; it does, however, have divisions of clinical and health psychology. The members of the Division of Health Psychology are involved in the promotion and maintenance of health, the prevention and management of illness, the identification of psychological factors contributing to physical illness, the improvement of the health care system, and the formulation of health policy (see http://dhp.bps.org.uk/). Some of these goals overlap with those of rehabilitation psychology as defined in the United States.

Despite issues of labeling, Britain produced two renown figures in the field of physical rehabilitation. Both came to the forefront as the result of the devastation of World War II: Sir Ludwig Guttman and Oliver Zangwill. Sir Ludwig Guttman, a neurologist and a refugee from Nazi Germany, was asked in 1943 to head the spinal cord injury unit for injured soldiers at Stoke Mandeville hospital. "His conviction that patients [with a spinal cord injury] could move from the situation of being desperate and dependent and become active members of society again" (Lomi, Geroulanos, & Kekatos, 2004, p. 2) was a driving force behind his innovative rehabilitation programs, which included the integration of sports into the treatment plan.

Oliver Zangwill played "a pivotal role in the emergence of neuropsychology in Britain after World War II" (Collins, 2006, p. 89). His work as a psychologist at the Brain Injuries Unit in Edinburgh Scotland precipitated his research, where attention was devoted to the "study and assessment of specific patterns of cognitive disability associated with cerebral injury or disease" (Zangwill, 1945, p. 248). The focus on assessment led to the pursuit of psychological techniques to facilitate neuropsychiatric diagnosis, with the goal to "adapt, where possible, general psychological principles and methods to concrete problems of re-education and resettlement" (p. 248), namely, rehabilitation. His subsequent work at the School of Clinical Medicine at Oxford facilitated the merging of neurology and psychological assessment.

Ireland

In 2008, Johnstone, Walsh, Carton, and Fish outlined the condition and needs of individuals with acquired disabilities in Ireland. In contrast to the attention devoted to intellectual disabilities, Ireland was lacking in services for individuals with acquired disabilities (physical and cognitive). However, since 1999, a series of events have increased public awareness of disability issues: that year the National Disability Authority was established, the European Commission declared 2003 as the Year of Individuals with Disabilities, and, in 2005, the Irish Disability Bill was legislated. The Irish government and respective professional organizations have identified the need for specialization in rehabilitation. Johnstone et al. (2008) urged psychologists in Ireland to join the movement and position themselves to provide the necessary services. The authors note some positive advances that suggest this process is commencing, but it is still in its infancy (p. 715).

SPAIN

The Spanish Psychological Association, established in 1980, like other European counterparts, does not include a division of rehabilitation psychology. Again, like others, it recognizes health psychology and clinical psychology as specializations. The purview of a health psychologist includes, among other things "officially deal[ing] with all psychological problems linked to the illness process (diagnosis, suffering, treatment, cure/chronification, rehabilitation). Thus, Health Psychology may deal with psychological impact of a serious disease diagnosis, or psychosocial impact of a hospitalization, or psychological training, in order to facilitate a post-surgery recovering [*sic*], or life quality in treatments with very aggressive side effects" (Spanish Psychological Association, 2011). This definition seems to echo the responsibilities (among others) of a rehabilitation psychologist.

However a review of research in clinical and health psychology during the last decade of the 20th century reveals that publications in areas that would be identified as rehabilitation psychology *per se* do not exist (Sanz, 2001). Reviewing literature published during that time and surveying the university professors who wrote them revealed 85 different research trends. Whereas only 16.6% of the faculty identified their area of research as health psychology, that group generated the highest percentage in research trends (31.7%) (p. 158). These trends can be grouped into etiology and explanatory models (e.g., type A), assessment and diagnosis (e.g., quality of life, translation of scales into Spanish), health intervention (health promotion and prevention of illness), and intervention in illness. The last trend has generated the most studies, and areas of interest were particularly focused on children's bronchial asthma and a more general model of the relationship between stress and psychophysiological disorders. Hypertension has also received attention, as has the development and assessment of procedures to reduce the stressful impact of hospitalization and surgery (p. 172).

Like other countries that have emerged from totalitarian regimes, academic psychology (and therefore the flow of publications in general, and clinically oriented ones in particular) is still evolving (p. 152). Moreover, and this may be applied to other non–English speaking countries, the bulk of publications are in the official languages of Spain (p. 154) and disseminated through national journals (72.6%, p. 158). Only 20.8% of all publications in clinical and health psychology were concentrated in international, English-language journals, thereby diminishing their impact in the English-speaking world. In fact, a search of *The Spanish Journal of Psychology* elicited only one citation concerning rehabilitation (Rodríguez & San Gregorio, 2005), *Psychosocial Adaptation in Relatives of Critically Injured Patients Admitted to an Intensive Care Unit.*

GERMANY

In a review of the German Psychological Society web page (http://www.dgps.de/en/dgps) shows a pattern similar to that seen in Britain and the EFPA: although sections (divisions) of health psychology and clinical psychology and psychotherapy

exist, rehabilitation psychology is not among them. However, in a 2004 section on international rehabilitation in the *Journal of Rehabilitation Psychology,* Gauggel, Heinman, Bocker, Lammler, Borschelt, and Steinhagen-Thiessen published an article on patient–staff agreement on Barthel Index scores at admission and discharge of elderly stroke patients.

SCANDINAVIA

The Norwegian Psychological Association, which has already adopted EFPA's EuroPsy, functions both as a trade union and an independent political body. Language barriers prevent any further assessment of its structure. In this socialized climate, rehabilitation is expected to abound, but, based on literature searches, details are scant (e.g., Vik, Lilja, & Nygard, 2007, *The influence of the environment on participation subsequent to rehabilitation as experienced by elderly people in Norway,* published in the *Scandinavian Journal of Occupational Therapy.*)

Middle East
ISRAEL

The largest international body of published literature on the development or emergence of rehabilitation psychology, training, and function is from Israel. With the help of rehabilitation educators from the United States, a master's degree program in rehabilitation psychology was established at Bar Ilan University in 1969 (Katz & Kravetz, 1989). Although rehabilitation was practiced in Israel even before the State was established, it was largely the purview of social workers. However, a visit by George N. Wright changed that. Wright was "involved in several international initiatives (including in Japan, Australia, and Saudi Arabia, [Wright, 1989]) in the field of rehabilitation counseling, from the late 1960s until about 1990" (K. Thomas, personal communication, July 8, 2010). A visit to Israel in 1963 convinced him that the model of graduate training in rehabilitation counseling, already in place in the United States (and at the University of Wisconsin-Madison, Wright's home department), could be adapted to meet the needs of the State of Israel (Katz & Kravetz, 1989). The decision to append the training in rehabilitation to a psychology program was anchored in the fact that rehabilitation counseling in the United States "adhere[d] to a psychological model of human service delivery" (p. 240). Bar Ilan University, the site of the first program in clinical psychology in Israel, was selected and the department of psychology was receptive.

In addition to the underpinnings of psychology in rehabilitation, there were also pragmatic reasons to affiliate with a department of psychology. Because of the existing set of specializations already in place, the new program required the addition of only a few new courses. Shlomo Katz became the first coordinator of the program, and Shlomo Kravetz joined later. Both were graduates of the master's degree program at Bar Ilan University (in 1965 and 1969, respectively). Both pursued doctoral training in rehabilitation counseling at the University of Wisconsin-Madison (graduating in 1969 and 1973), respectively.

Despite its roots in rehabilitation counseling, the program at Bar Ilan University evolved into specialized training for psychologists rather than into "an independent profession of vocational rehabilitation counselors" (p. 241.) This process was not part of the counseling–psychology struggle described elsewhere in this chapter. Rather, it was a by-product of program's hosting within a psychology department (a decision largely based on practical reasons) and the evolving reality of Israeli licensure of psychologists. Since the students were awarded master's degree in psychology they had to be prepared to meet the requirements, professional and legal, of licensure in psychology. However, these same pioneer students and faculty were then responsible for the formation of the rehabilitation psychology division within the Israel Psychology Association, and this then "served as the source for the legal mechanism and regulations governing the licensing of rehabilitation psychologists" (p. 241). In this, the program at Bar-Ilan mirrored the efforts of psychology in the United States to identify rehabilitation psychology as an area of expertise within psychology (e.g., Elliott & Warren, 2007); Wegener et al., 1998).

The political situation in Israel has influenced the focus of rehabilitation in Israel. For example, Katz and Kravetz (Katz, Galatzer, & Kravetz, 1978), two of the founding fathers of the program at Bar Ilan, described a sheltered workshop for "brain-damaged war veterans [sic]", that is still in existence in Tel Aviv, more than 50 years later. Galatzer was also on faculty at Bar Ilan, along with Victor Florian (whose contributions to rehabilitation studies are too many to list here) and Eli Vakil, who described the state of neuropsychology in Israel and tied its emergence to the clinical rehabilitation of veterans with brain injuries (1994).

In 1993, Florian described rehabilitation psychology in Israel, which was by then was firmly identified with psychology, but with a scope of practice as broad as that of rehabilitation counselors: "[t]hey

work with a variety of disabilities including mental retardation, brain injury, spinal cord injury, chronic heart disease, cancer, drug addiction, and psychiatric problems" (p. 12). These roles are reflected in publications that have emerged from the profession in Israel, often with the contributions of the faculty at Bar Ilan: Katz and Kravetz,(1980), *The relationship between post-elementary educational and vocational frameworks and the vocational and economic status of hearing impaired individuals;* Shurka (who acknowledges Victor Florian), (1984), *Attitudes towards disability and rehabilitation among political and professional leaders in Israeli development towns;* Florian and Kehat, (1987), *Changing high school students' attitudes toward disabled people*; Drory, Florian and Kravetz, (1991), *Sense of coherence: Sociodemographic variables and perceived psychological and physical health;* Kravetz and Katz, (1994), *Attitudes toward Israeli war veterans with disabilities: Combat versus noncombat military service and responsibility for the disability;* Roe, Hasson-Ohayon, Lachman and Kravetz , (2007), *Selecting and implementing evidence-based practices in psychiatric rehabilitation services in Israel: A worthy and feasible challenge*; Roe, Gross, Kravetz, Baloush-Kleinman and Rudnick, (2009), *Assessing psychiatric rehabilitation service (PRS) outcomes in Israel: Conceptual, professional and social issues;* Rihtman, Tekuzener, ParushTenenbaum, Bachrach, and Ornoy, (2010), *Are the cognitive functions of children with Down syndrome related to their participation.*

Asia
Japan

Although the Japanese Psychological Association was established in 1927, it does not appear to have any divisions or specializations. Furthermore, although G. N. Wright (1989) notes that the Japan's Women's University established a rehabilitation counselor education program, a search on the university's website found no mention of the program or of its founder, Professor Yoko Kojima-Cassels.

AUSTRALASIA
Australia

In 1944, the Australian Psychological Society began as a branch of the British Psychological Society. In 1966, it was incorporated as the Australian Psychological Society Limited (http://www.psychology.org.au/about/governance/). The organization is divided into nine colleges, and although there is no college of rehabilitation psychology, there is a college of health psychology: "Health psychologists specialise in understanding the relationships between psychological factors (e.g., behaviours, attitudes, beliefs) and health and illness. Health psychologists practice in two main areas: health promotion (prevention of illness and promotion of healthy lifestyles) and clinical health (application of psychology to illness assessment, treatment, and rehabilitation)" (see http://www. groups.psychology.org.au/chp/). There is also an interest group in rehabilitation psychology (http:// www.groups.psychology.org.au/rpig/). Although rehabilitation psychology is only an interest group at this point, its roots appeared relatively early (e.g., Kendall and Marshall's (2004) article that appeared in APA's *Rehabilitation Psychology* titled *"Factors that prevent equitable access to rehabilitation for Aboriginal Australians with disabilities: The need for culturally safe rehabilitation"*) there is no doubt that, based on publications, rehabilitation psychology is alive and well in Australia, as evidenced by a number of articles published in 2010: Dorstyn, Mathias, and Denson, (2010). *Psychological intervention during spinal rehabilitation: a preliminary study*; Galvin, Froude, and McAleer (2010). *Children's participation in home, school and community life after acquired brain injury*; Turner and Andrewes, D. (2010). *Assessing the cognitive regulation of emotion in depressed stroke patients*; Wales, Matthews, and Donelly (2010). *Medically unexplained chronic pain in Australia: difficulties for rehabilitation providers and workers in pain.*

Its accrediting arm, the Australian Psychology Accreditation Council (http://www.apac.psychology.org.au/) oversees Australasia, and includes Hong Kong, Malaysia, and Singapore.

ASIA PACIFIC DISABILITY REHABILITATION JOURNAL

The journal *Rehabilitation Psychology*, the flagship journal of the division of rehabilitation psychology of the APA, is an excellent mirror of the cutting-edge issues facing rehabilitation psychologists. However, its very pedigree may be daunting to authors outside of North America and/or unaffiliated with a leading foreign university. In contrast, the *Asia Pacific Disability Rehabilitation Journal* (APDRJ), was established in 1997 with the support of Action for Disability in the United Kingdom; CORDAID, in the Netherlands, joined Action for Disability as a sponsor some years later. With the support of these two donors, two issues of the journal were brought out each year and distributed free of cost to readers, 60% of whom were from developing countries. The journal was for private circulation, meant for researchers, planners, administrators, professionals, donor organizations, and implementing agencies involved in disability and community-based rehabilitation. The AIFO, a donor from Italy, began hosting the journal and its back issues on their website from 2001. In 2011, the journal changed its name to *Disability, CBR, and Inclusive Development* ("Journal history" 2011).

This publication appears to span the whole world, particularly the less fortunate regions such as South Asia (Thomas and Thomas, 2002, *Status of women with disabilities in South Asia*), Nepal (Boyce and Paterson, 2002, *Community based rehabilitation for children in Nepal*) , Mongolia (Sharma and Deepak, 2002, *A case study of the community based rehabilitation programme in Mongolia*) China (Tasiemski, Nielsen, and Wilski, 2010, *Quality of life in people with spinal cord injury - earthquake survivors from Sichuan province in China*), Indonesia (Schuller, et al., 2010, *The way women experience disabilities and especially disabilities related to leprosy in rural areas in south Sulawesi, Indonesia*), Bhutan (Dorji and Solomon, 2009, *Attitudes of health professionals toward persons with disabilities in Bhutan*) Thailand (Chinchai and Wittayanin, 2008, *Influence of the home visit programme on the functional abilities and quality of life of people with spinal cord injury in Thailand*), Sri Lanka (Chappell and Sirz, 2003, *Quality of life following spinal cord injury for 20–40 year old males living in Sri Lanka*), Africa (Monk and Wee, 2008, *Factors shaping attitudes towards physical disability and availability of rehabilitative support systems for disabled persons in rural Kenya*) and East Europe (Turmusani, 2002, *Disability and development in Kosovo: the case for community based rehabilitation*).

The journal also attends to culture (Nagata, 2008, *Disability and development: is the rights model of disability valid in the Arab region? An evidence-based field survey in Lebanon and Jordan*), and offers extensive coverage to leprosy, a disease the west has long forgotten (e.g., Iyor ,2010, *Beliefs and attitudes about leprosy of non-leprosy patients in a reversely integrated hospital;* Nicholls and Smith, 2002, *Developments and trends in rehabilitation in leprosy.*) In sum, in its short time in existence *Asia Pacific Disability Rehabilitation Journal* has offered an outlet and served as a resource for those professionals on the front line.

Conclusion
The Future

It is appropriate to start a discussion of the future of rehabilitation after concluding a summary of the *Asia Pacific Disability Rehabilitation Journal*. The journal instantiates two major issues that rehabilitation psychology needs to face: the first is its ethnocentric world. APDRJ is the antithesis of this phenomena: it reflects both a diverse authorship and a diverse world. The internationalization of rehabilitation psychology is a necessity, both to bring new ideas to old problems and to be truly inclusive, not according to the traditional in–out bias of those with and without a disability, but at a deeper level encompassing all those who struggle with disability and those who don't, and all those who provide services, not just those in the Western world and its satellites. Thus, recruiting manuscripts from individuals who would not consider publishing in the more traditional outlets of rehabilitation psychology is essential. Moreover, partnering across cultures and languages is more effective in discovering both the universal and unique.

A second goal that rehabilitation psychology should set for itself is that of reaching out to different health care systems to learn how psychologists practice and provide services under different scenarios. The debate over public health care in the United States can and should be influenced through learning from countries where public health care already exists (e.g., Britain, Canada, Scandinavia). The best and the worst can be identified and the growing pains minimized. Here, rehabilitation psychologists may need to collaborate with health psychologists; prevention is less expensive than a cure, and effective partnership may decrease the need for the services of rehabilitation psychologists in certain areas, thus freeing them to focus on the growing population of veterans from military operations (e.g., Iraq and Afghanistan).

The rehabilitation needs of returning veterans are complex. More soldiers are surviving their injuries, and the system and services put in place for veterans from previous wars are becoming overwhelmed (Brown, 2008; McCrae et al., 2008). The scope, complexity, and duration of services needed can be expected to challenge rehabilitation psychology. The development and refinement of tele-health interventions may compensate for the gap between needs and those available to address for them (e.g., Wade & Wolfe, 2005). Additionally, attention will need to be devoted to gender issues in rehabilitation (e.g., Thurer, 1982). Gender differences have not been properly addressed in rehabilitation psychology. Attention has been devoted to issues of adjustment to breast cancer or other "female" illnesses, and attention has been devoted to generic adjustment to disability. However the growing number of female veterans requiring rehabilitation must push the field to inspect its biases about issues that confront a woman when learning to live with a disability. Also, echoing the change of name of the *Asia Pacific Disability Rehabilitation Journal* to *Disability, CBR, and Inclusive Development*, rehabilitation psychology should focus on community-based rehabilitation, because the natural state and place for the individual with disability is in the community, as part of society (Wright, B., 1959).

Finally, rehabilitation psychology might consider picking up where George N. Wright left off; that is, to "make a global impact: . . . . Training international students (Chen, Ong, & Brodwin, 2008) in a model of rehabilitation psychology which considers the psychological understanding of the individual with a disability and handicap to be an important adjunct to the medical, social, and vocational knowledge required for the provision of effective and efficient rehabilitation services" (Wright, 1989, p. 240). This vision can then carry over to advocacy and development of policy that will promote optimal quality of life.

Acknowledgments

Tim Elliott deserves a very special mention for encouraging me to write this chapter, as well as for being a lifelong mentor and friend. I wish to offer my thanks to Professors Norm Berven, Kenneth Thomas and David Rosenthal of the Department of Rehabilitation Psychology and Special Education at the University of Wisconsin-Madison. In Israel my thanks go to Professors Shlomo Katz and Solomon Kravetz of Bar Ilan University. A heartfelt thank you goes to Chad Zimmerman, for his patience and sense of humor. And, last but not least, a million thanks to the intrepid folks at the Ottenheimer Library at the University of Arkansas at Little Rock, without whom I could never have completed this chapter.

Notes

1. In the course of researching this chapter, I found two versions of the sequence of authorship for this manuscript. All listed Barker as the first author, but there was disagreement about the second author. All were retrieved from EBSCO. The first has Barker as first author and Gonick as second, with Wright as

third: i.e., Barker, R., Gonick, M., Wright, B., & Social Science Research, C. (1946). *Adjustment to Physical Handicap and Illness: A Survey of the Social Psychology of Physique and Disability.* This reference was retrieved by EBSCO from SocINDEX. The second, retrieved from PsycINFO and PsycBooks, listed Wright as the second author and Gonick as the third: Barker, R. G., Wright, B. A., & Gonick, M. R. (1946). *Adjustment to Physical Handicap and Illness: A Survey of the Social Psychology of Physique and Disability.* New York: Social Science Research Council. doi:10.1037/11780–000. PsycINFO also references this manuscript as a journal article: Barker, R. G., Wright, B. A., & Gonick, M. R. (1946). Adjustment to physical handicap and illness: a survey of the social psychology of physique and disability. *Social Science Research Council Bulletin,* 55. Retrieved from EBSCO*host*. I chose to employ the citation that includes the doi, for ease of retrieval. Finally, I could find no record of a second edition, published in 1953, with Meyerson (at times spelled Myerson, see Larson & Sachs, 2000, p. 54) as coauthor, as noted in Dunn's (2000) references (p. 580).

2. Despite my best efforts, I was unable to obtain a copy of the proceedings edited by Leviton from the conference held at Clark University in 1959. Therefore, I had to rely on Larson and Sachs' (2000) summary of the event and could not present the Table of Contents.

References

Angelo, J. A., Leonard, C., Majovski, L., & Muir, C. A. (1991). Using psychological approaches to improve rehabilitation results. *Journal of Insurance Medicine, 23,* 233–235.

Barker, R. G., Wright, B. A., & Gonick, M. R. (1946). Adjustment to physical handicap and illness: A survey of the social psychology of physique and disability. *Social Science Research Council Bulletin, 55.* doi:10.1037/11780-000.

Barker, R. G., & Wright, B. A. (1952). The social psychology of adjustment to physical disability. In J. F. Garrett & J. F. Garrett (Eds.), *Psychological aspects of physical disability* (pp. 18–32). (Office of Vocational Rehabilitation, Rehabilitat. Serv. Ser. No. 210). Oxford England: U.S. Government Printing Office. Retrieved from EBSCO*host*.

Bellini, J. L., & Rumrill, P. D. (1999). Implementing a scientist-practitioner model of graduate-level rehabilitation counselor education: Guidelines for enhancing curricular coherence. *Rehabilitation Education, 13,* 261–275.

Boake, C. (2008). Clinical neuropsychology. *Professional Psychology: Research and Practice, 39,* 234–239. doi: 10.1037/0735–7028.39.2.234.

Boyce, W., & Paterson, J. (2002). Community based rehabilitation for children in Nepal. *Asia Pacific Disability Rehabilitation Journal,* 67–81. Retrieved from EBSCO*host*.

Brieland, D. (1971). Rehabilitation psychologists: Roles and functions. In W. S. Neff (Ed.), *Rehabilitation psychology* (pp. 276–286). Washington DC: American Psychological Association.

Brodwin, M. G. (2010). DVD review: Practical wisdom: Positive rehabilitation psychology and the legacy of Beatrice Wright by Henry McCarthy. *Rehabilitation Education, 24,* 167–169. Retrieved from EBSCO*host*.

Brown, K. S., DeLeon, P. H., Loftis, C. W., & Scherer, M. J. (2008). Rehabilitation psychology: Realizing the true potential. *Rehabilitation Psychology, 53,* 111–121. doi: 10.1037/0090–5550.53.2.111.

Brown, N. D. (2008). Transition from Afghanistan and Iraqi battlefields to home: An overview of selected war wounds and the federal agencies assisting soldiers regain their health. *American Association of Occupational Health Nurses Journal, 56,* 343–346.

Chappell, P., & Sirz, S. (2003). Quality of life following spinal cord injury for 20–40 year old males living in Sri Lanka. *Asia Pacific Disability Rehabilitation Journal, 14,* 162–178. Retrieved from EBSCO*host*.

Chen, R. K., Ong, L. Z., & Brodwin, M. G. (2008). Making a global impact: The United States' role in training international students as rehabilitation counselors and educators. *Rehabilitation Education, 22,* 193–202.

Chinchai, P., & Wittayanin, W. (2008). Influence of the home visit programme on the functional abilities and quality of life of people with spinal cord injury in Thailand. *Asia Pacific Disability Rehabilitation Journal, 19,* 50–59. Retrieved from EBSCO*host*.

Collins, A. F. (2006). An intimate connection: Oliver Zangwill and the emergence of neuropsychology in Britain. *History of Psychology, 9,* 89–112. doi: 10.1037/1093–4510.9.2.89.

Davis, A. (2011). Practical wisdom: Positive rehabilitation psychology and the legacy of Beatrice Wright. *Counseling Today, 53,* 26–27. Retrieved from EBSCO*host*.

Dembo, T. (1964). Sensitivity of one person to another. *Rehabilitation Literature, 25,* 231–235. Retrieved from EBSCO*host*.

Dembo, T. (1982). Some problems in rehabilitation as seen by a Lewinian. *Journal of Social Issues, 38,* 131–139. Retrieved from EBSCO*host*.

Dembo, T., Diller, L., Gordon, W. A., Leviton, G., & Sherr, R. (1973). A view of rehabilitation psychology. *American Psychologist, 28,* 719–722. doi:10.1037/h0035761.

Dembo, T., Ladieu-Leviton, G., & Wright, B. A. (1952). Acceptance of loss— amputations. In J. F. Garrett & J. F. Garrett (Eds.), *Psychological aspects of physical disability* (pp. 80–96). (Office of Vocational Rehabilitation, Rehabilitat. Serv. Ser. No. 210). Oxford England: U.S. Government Printing Office. Retrieved from EBSCO*host*.

Dembo, T., Leviton, G. L., & Wright, B. A. (1956). Adjustment to misfortune: A problem of social-psychological rehabilitation. *Artificial Limbs, 3,* 4–62.

Dorji, S., & Solomon, P. (2009). Attitudes of health professionals toward persons with disabilities in Bhutan. *Asia Pacific Disability Rehabilitation Journal, 20,* 32–42. Retrieved from EBSCO*host*.

Dorstyn, D., Mathias, J., & Denson, L. (2010). Psychological intervention during spinal rehabilitation: A preliminary study. *Spinal Cord, 48,* 756–761. doi:10.1038/sc.2009.161.

Drory, Y., Florian, V., & Kravetz, S. (1991). Sense of coherence: Sociodemographic variables and perceived psychological and physical health. *Psikhologyah: Ktav et madai Yisraeli le'iyun ulemehk'ar, 2,* 119–125.

Dunn, D. S. (2000). Social psychological issues in disability. In R. G. Frank & T. R. Elliott (Eds.), *Handbook of rehabilitation psychology* (pp. 565–584). Washington DC: American Psychological Association.

Dunn, D. S., & Dougherty, S. B. (2005). Prospects for a positive psychology of rehabilitation. *Rehabilitation Psychology, 50,* 305–311.

Dunn, D. S., Uswatte, G., & Elliott, T. R. (2009). Happiness, resilience, and positive growth following physical disability: Issues for understanding, research, and therapeutic intervention. In S. J. Lopez & C. R. Snyder (Eds.), *Oxford handbook of positive psychology* (2nd ed., pp. 651–664). New York: Oxford University Press.

Eisenberg, M. G., & Jensen, M. (1987). Rehabilitation psychologists in medical settings: A unique subspecialty or a redundant one? *Professional Psychology: Research and Practice, 18,* 475–478.

EFPA. (2009). *EuroPsy Regulation December 2009.* http://www.europsy-efpa.eu/regulations.

Elliott, T. R. (2002). Defining our common ground to reach new horizons. *Rehabilitation Psychology, 47,* 131–143. doi: 10.1037/0090-5550.47.2.131.

Elliott, T. R., & Frank, R. G. (2000). Afterward: Drawing new horizons. In R. G. Frank & T. R. Elliott (Ed.), *Handbook of rehabilitation psychology* (pp. 645–653). Washington DC: American Psychological Association.

Elliott, T. R., & Gramling, S. E. (1990). Psychologists and rehabilitation: New roles and old training models. *American Psychologist, 45,* 762–765.

Elliott, T. R., & Klapow, J. C. (1997). Training psychologists for a future in evolving health care delivery systems: Building a better Boulder model. *Journal of Clinical Psychology in Medical Settings, 4,* 255–267.

Elliott, T. R., & Leung, P. (2005). Vocational rehabilitation: History and practice. In W. B. Walsh & M. L. Savickas (Eds.), *Handbook of vocational psychology: Theory, research and practice* (2nd ed., pp. 319–342). Mahwah, NJ: Lawrence Erlbaum Associates.

Elliott, T., & Rath, J. (2011). Rehabilitation psychology. In E. Altmaier & J. I. Hanson (Eds.), *The Oxford handbook of counseling psychology* (pp. 679–702). New York: Oxford University Press.

Elliott, T. R., & Shewchuck, R. M. (1996). Defining health and well-being for the future of counseling psychology. *The Counseling Psychologist, 24,* 743–750.

Elliott, T. R., & Warren, A. M. (2007). Why psychology is important in rehabilitation. In P. Kennedy (Ed.), *Psychological management of physical disabilities: A practitioner's guide* (pp.16–39). New York: Routledge/Taylor & Francis Group.

Emener, W. G. (1986). Historical perspectives: Introduction commentary. In W. G. Emener (Ed.), *Rehabilitation counselor preparation and development: Selected critical issues* (pp. 5–8). Springfield, IL: Charles C. Thomas.

Florian, V. (1993). Rehabilitation psychology in Israel. *Rehabilitation Psychology News, 20,* 12.

Florian, V., & Kehat, D. (1987). Changing high school students' attitudes toward disabled people. *Health and Social Work, 12,* 57–63.

Florian, V., & Shurka, E. (1983). Non-disabled opinions on sexual activities and family roles for disabled persons, and disabled persons' views of these opinions. *International Journal of Rehabilitation Medicine, 5,* 17–20.

Frank, R. G., & Elliott, T. R. (2000). Rehabilitation psychology: Hope for a psychology of chronic conditions. In R. G. Frank and T. R. Elliott (Ed.), *Handbook of rehabilitation psychology* (pp. 3–8). Washington DC: American Psychological Association.

Fraser, R. T., & Johnson, K. (2010). Vocational rehabilitation. In R. B. Frank, M. Rosenthal & B. R. Caplan (Eds.), *Handbook of rehabilitation psychology* (2nd ed., pp. 357–363). Washington DC: American Psychological Association.

Galvin, J., Froude, E., & McAleer, J. (2010). Children's participation in home, school and community life after acquired brain injury. *Australian Occupational Therapy Journal, 57,* 118–126. Retrieved from EBSCO*host.*

Garay-Sevilla, M., Nava, L., Malacara, J., Huerta, R., Díaz de León, J., Mena, A., & Fajardo, M. (1995). Adherence to treatment and social support in patients with non-insulin dependent diabetes mellitus. *Journal of Diabetes and Its Complications, 9,* 81–86. Retrieved from EBSCO*host.*

Gauggel, S., Heinmann, A. W., Bocker, Lammer, G., Borchelt, M., & Steinhagen- Thiessen, E. (2004). Patient-staff agreement on Barthel Index scores at admission and discharge in a sample of elderly stroke patients. *Journal of Rehabilitation Psychology, 49,* 21–27. doi: 10.1037/00900-5550.49.1.21.

Gill, C. J., Kewman, D. G., & Brannon, R. W. (2003). Transforming psychological practice and society. *American Psychologist, 58,* 305–312. doi: 10.1037/0003–066X.58.4.305.

Glueckauf, R. L. (2000). Doctoral education in rehabilitation and health care psychology: Principles and strategies for unifying subspecialty training. In R. G. Frank & T. R. Elliott (Ed.), *Handbook of rehabilitation psychology* (pp. 615–627). Washington DC: American Psychological Association.

Grzesiak, R. C. (1981). Rehabilitation psychology, medical psychology, health psychology and behavioral medicine. *Professional Psychology, 12,* 411–413.

Gzil, F., Lefeve, C., Cammelli, M., Pachoud, B., Ravaud, J. F., & Leplege, A. (2007). Why is rehabilitation not yet fully person-centered and should it be more person-centered? *Disability and Rehabilitation, 29,* 1616–1624.

Heiman, T., & Precel, K. (2003). Students with learning disabilities in higher education: Academic strategies profile. *Journal of Learning Disabilities, 36,* 248–258.

Hennessey, M. (2001). Student paper. What is rehabilitation counseling?: A student's perspective on professional identity. *Work, 17,* 151–156. Retrieved from EBSCO*host.*

Hibbard, M. R., & Cox, D. R. (2010). Competencies of a rehabilitation psychologist. In R. B. Frank, M. Rosenthal, & B. R. Caplan (Eds.), *Handbook of rehabilitation psychology* (2nd ed., pp. 467–475). Washington DC: American Psychological Association.

History of Physical Medicine and Rehabilitation. (2011). Retrieved April 10, 2011, from http://www.mcw.edu/physicalmedicine/history.htm.

Holland, L. K., & Whalley, M. J. (1981). The work of a psychiatrist in a rehabilitation hospital. *British Journal of Psychiatry, 138,* 222–229.

Itzhaky, H., & Schwartz, C. (1998). Empowering the disabled: A multidimensional approach. *International Journal of Rehabilitation Research, 21,* 301–310.

Iyor, F. (2010). Beliefs and attitudes about leprosy of non-leprosy patients in a reversely integrated hospital. *Asia Pacific Disability Rehabilitation Journal, 21,* 92–100. Retrieved from EBSCO*host.*

Jackson, J. L. (1980). The emerging role of the administrative technician in the rehabilitation process. *Rehabilitation Literature, 41,* 284–288.

Jaques, M. E. (1970). *Rehabilitation counseling: Scope and services.* Oxford, England: Houghton Mifflin. Retrieved from EBSCO*host.*

Jansen, M. A., & Fulcher, R. (1982). Rehabilitation psychologists: Characteristics and scope of practice. *American Psychologist, 37,* 1282–1283.

Johnstone, B., Walsh, J., Carton, S., & Fish, R. (2008). Rehabilitation psychology: Meeting the needs of individuals with acquired disabilities in Ireland. *Disability and Rehabilitation, 30,* 709–715.

Jongbloed, L. (2003). Disability policy in Canada: An overview. *Journal of Disability Policy Studies, 13,* 203–209. Retrieved from EBSCO*host*.

"Journal history." (2011). Retrieved on April 21, 2011, from http://dcidj.org/about/history.

Katz, S., Galatzer, A., & Kravetz, S. (1978). The physical, psych-social and vocational effectiveness of a sheltered workshop for brain-damaged war veterans. *Scandinavian Journal of Rehabilitation Medicine, 10,* 51–57.

Katz, S., & Kravetz, S. (1980). The relationship between post-elementary educational and vocational frameworks and the vocational and economic status of hearing impaired individuals. *International Journal of Rehabilitation Research. [Internationale Zeitschrift Für Rehabilitationsforschung. Revue Internationale De Recherches De Réadaptation], 3,* 244–246. Retrieved from EBSCO*host*.

Katz, S., & Kravetz, S. (1989). The rehabilitation psychology program at Bar Ilan University, Israel. *Rehabilitation Education, 3,* 239–243.

Katz, S., Shurka, E., & Florian, V. (1978). The relationship between physical disability, social perception, and psychological distress. *Scandinavian Journal of Rehabilitation Medicine, 10,* 109–113.

Kendall, E., & Marshall, C. A. (2004). Factors that prevent equitable access to rehabilitation for Aboriginal Australians with disabilities: The need for culturally safe rehabilitation. *Rehabilitation Psychology, 49,* 5–13. doi: 10.1037/0090-5550.49.1.5.

Kravetz, S., & Katz, S. (1994). Attitudes toward Israeli war veterans with disabilities: Combat versus noncombat military service and responsibility for the disability. *Rehabilitation Counseling Bulletin, 37,* 371–379.

Kreutzer, J. S., & Kolakowsky-Hayner, S. A. (1999). Laws of the house of rehab: A guide to managing psychological distress and promoting benefit from rehabilitation. *NeuroRehabilitation, 19,* 91–102.

Ladieu, G., Adler, D. L., & Dembo, T. (1948). Studies in adjustment to visible injuries: Social acceptance of the injured. *Journal of Social Issues, 4,* 55–61. Retrieved from EBSCO*host*.

Ladieu, G., Hanfmann, E., & Dembo, T. (1947). Studies in adjustment to visible injuries: Evaluation of help by the injured. *The Journal of Abnormal and Social Psychology, 42,* 169–192. doi:10.1037/h0055914.

Larson, P. C., & Sachs, P. R. (2000). A history of Division 22 (Rehabilitation Psychology). In D. A. Dewsbury (Ed.), *Unification through division: Histories of the divisions of the American Psychological Association* (Vol. V, pp. 33–58). Washington DC: American Psychological Association.

Leahy, M. J., & Szymanski, E. (1995). Rehabilitation counseling: Evolution and current status. *Journal of Counseling and Development, 74,* 153–166. Retrieved from EBSCO*host*.

Leech, L. L., & Holcomb, J. M. (2004). Leveling the playing field: The development of a distance education program in rehabilitation counseling. *Assistive Technology, 16,* 135–143.

Leier, S. J., Strohmer, D. C., Blackwell, T. L., Thompson, R. C., & Donnay, D. A. C. (2008). The Rehabilitation Counselor Scale: A new scale for the revised Strong Interest Inventory. *Rehabilitation Counseling Bulletin, 51,* 68–75. doi: 10.1177/0034355207311341.

Leung, P., Sakata, R., & Ostby, S. (1990). Rehabilitation psychology professional training: A survey of APA accredited programs. *Rehabilitation Education, 4,* 177–183.

Leviton (1959). *The relationship between rehabilitation and psychology: Proceedings of a conference sponsored by the Office of Vocational Rehabilitation.* Worcester, Massachusetts: Clark University, June 11–13.

Lewin, K. (1935). Psycho-sociological problems of a minority group. *Character and Personality, 3*(3), 175–187. Retrieved from EBSCO*host*.

Lewin, K., Heider, F., & Heider, G. (1936). Formulation of law and representation of situation. In K. Lewin, F. Heider, & G. Heider (Eds.), *Principles of topological psychology* (pp. 8–13). New York: McGraw-Hill. doi:10.1037/10019-002.

Lofquist, L. H. (1959). An operational definition of rehabilitation counseling. *Journal of Rehabilitation, 25,* 7–9.

Lofquist, L. H. (Ed.). (1960). *Psychological research and rehabilitation.* Washington DC: American Psychological Association. doi:10.1037/10041-001.

Lollar, D. (2008). Rehabilitation psychology and public health: Commonalities, barriers and bridges. *Rehabilitation Psychology, 53,* 122–127. doi: 10.1037/0090-5550.53.2.122.

Lomi, C., Geroulanos, S., & Kekatos, E. (2004). Sir Ludwig Guttmann—"The de Coubertin of the paralysed." *Journal of the Hellenic Association of Orthopaedic and Traumatology, 55.* Retrieved from http://www.acta-ortho.gr/v55t1_6.html.

Luque-Coqui, M., Chartt, R., Tercero, G., Hernández Roque, A., Romero, B., & Morales, F. (2003). [Self-esteem in Mexican pediatric patients on peritoneal dialysis and kidney transplantation]. *Nefrología: Publicación Oficial De La Sociedad Española Nefrología, 23,* 145–149. Retrieved from EBSCO*host*.

Maki, D. R., Berven, N. L., & Allen, H. A. (1985). Doctoral study in rehabilitation counseling: Current status. *Rehabilitation Counseling Bulletin, 28,* 146–154.

Maki, D. R., Berven, N. L., & Peterson, D. B. (2003). Doctoral study in rehabilitation: III. Status and trends. *Rehabilitation Counseling Bulletin, 46,* 136–146.

Maki, D., & Delworth, U. (1995). Clinical supervision: A definition and model for the rehabilitation counseling profession. *Rehabilitation Counseling Bulletin, 38,* 282–293. Retrieved from PsycINFO database.

Marshall, C. A. Burros, H. L., Gotto, G., McAllan, L., Martinez P. V., Juarez, L. G., & Rey F. P. (2004). The United States and Mexico: Creating partnerships in rehabilitation. *Rehabilitation Psychology, 49,* 14–20. doi: 10.1037/0090-5550.49.1.14.

Matarazzo, J. D. (1994). Psychology in medical school: A personal account of a department's 35-year history. *Journal of Clinical Psychology, 50,* 7–36.

McAlees, D. C. (1975). Toward a new professionalism: Certification and accreditation. *Rehabilitation Counseling Bulletin, 18,* 160–165. Retrieved from EBSCO*host*.

McCrae, M., Pliskin, N., Barth, J., Cox, D., Fink, J., French, L., et al. (2008). Official position of the military TBI task force on the role of neuropsychology and rehabilitation psychology in the evaluation, management, and research of military veterans with traumatic brain injury. *The Clinical Neuropsychologist, 22,* 10–26. doi: 10.1080/13854040701760981.

McGowan, J. F., & Porter, T. L. (1967). *An introduction to the vocational rehabilitation process. A training manual.* Rehabilitation Service Series No. 68–32. Washington, DC: Superintendent of Documents, U.S. Government Printing Office, http://www.eric.ed.gov/ERICWebPortal/search/detailmini.jsp?_nfpb=true&_&ERICExtSearch_SearchValue_0=ED042011&ERICExtSearch_SearchType_0=no&accno=ED042011.

Melia, R. P., Pledger, C., & Wilson, R. (2003). Disability and rehabilitation research: Opportunities for participation, collaboration, and extramural funding for psychologists. *American Psychologist, 58,* 285–288. doi: 10.1037/0003-066X.58.4.285.

Monk, J., & Wee, J. (2008). Factors shaping attitudes towards physical disability and availability of rehabilitative support systems for disabled persons in rural Kenya. *Asia Pacific Disability Rehabilitation Journal, 19,* 93–113. Retrieved from EBSCO*host.*

Mugford, T. (1975). Vocational rehabilitation counseling: An interpersonal approach. *Dissertation Abstracts International, 35,* 5824.

Mullins, L.L., Ozolins, M., & Morris, C. R. (1988). Clinical psychology and cost effective rehabilitation: A behavioral medicine approach. *Oklahoma State Medical Association, 81,* 341–345.

Nagata, K. (2008). Disability and development: Is the rights model of disability valid in the Arab region? An evidence-based field survey in Lebanon and Jordan. *Asia Pacific Disability Rehabilitation Journal, 19,* 60–78. Retrieved from EBSCO*host.*

Neff, W. S. (Ed.). (1971). *Rehabilitation psychology.* Washington DC: American Psychological Association. doi: 10.1037/10043-000.

Nicholls, P., & Smith, W. (2002). Developments and trends in rehabilitation in leprosy. *Asia Pacific Disability Rehabilitation Journal,* 92–99. Retrieved from EBSCO*host.*

Olkin, R., & Pledger, C. (2003). Can disability studies and psychology join hands? *American Psychologist, 58,* 296–304. doi: 10.1037/0003-066X.58.4.296.

Olshansky, S., & Hart, W. R. (1967). Psychologists in vocational rehabilitation or vocational rehabilitation counselors? *Journal of Rehabilitation, 33,* 28–29.

Packard, E. (2007). Serving those who serve. A closer look at division 22: A growing field meets the challenges of war. *Monitor on Psychology, 38,* 54.

Pape, D. S. A., & Tarvydas, V. M. (1993). Responsible and responsive rehabilitation consultation on the ADA: The importance of training for psychologists. *Rehabilitation Psychology, 38,* 117–131.

Patterson, D. R., & Hanson, S. L. (1995). Joint Division 22 and ACRM guidelines for postdoctoral training in rehabilitation psychology. *Rehabilitation Psychology, 40,* 299–310.

Peterson, D. B., & Aguilar, L. J. (2004). History and systems: United States. In T. F. Riggar & D. R. Maki (Eds.), *Handbook of rehabilitation counseling* (pp. 50–75). New York: Springer.

Peterson, D. B., & Elliott, T. R. (2008). Advances in conceptualizing and studying disability. In T.F. Riggar & D. R. Maki (Eds.), *The handbook of rehabilitation counseling* (pp. 50–75). New York: Springer.

Petronio, L. (1992). Theoretical considerations of the rehabilitation process. *Annali dell'Istituto Superiore di Sanità, 28,* 309–310.

Pledger, C. (2003). Discourse on disability and rehabilitation issues: Opportunities for psychology. *American Psychologist, 58,* 279–284. doi: 10.1037/0003-066X.58.4.279.

Raimy, V. C. (Ed.). (1950). *Training in clinical psychology.* New York: Prentice- Hall, Inc.

Rihtman, T., Tekuzener, E., Parush, S., Tenenbaum, A., Bachrach, S., & Ornoy, A. (2010). Are the cognitive functions of children with Down syndrome related to their participation? *Developmental Medicine and Child Neurology, 52,* 72–78. Retrieved from EBSCO*host.*

Roe, D., Gross, Y., Kravetz, S., Baloush-Kleinman, V., & Rudnick, A. (2009). Assessing psychiatric rehabilitation service (PRS) outcomes in Israel: Conceptual, professional and social issues. *The Israel Journal of Psychiatry Related Sciences, 46,* 103–110.

Roe, D., Hasson-Ohayon, I., Lachman, M., & Kravetz, S. (2007). Selecting and implementing evidence-based practices in psychiatric rehabilitation services in Israel. *The Israel Journal of Psychiatry Related Sciences, 44,* 47–53.

Rodríguez, A., & San Gregorio, M. (2005). Psychosocial adaptation in relatives of critically injured patients admitted to an intensive care unit. *The Spanish Journal of Psychology, 8,* 36–44. Retrieved from EBSCO*host.*

Roer-Strier, D. (2002). University students with learning disabilities advocating for change. *Disability and Rehabilitation, 24,* 914–924.

Rubin, S. E., Davis, E. L., Noe, S. R., & Turner, T. N. (1996). Assessing the effects of continuing multicultural rehabilitation counseling education. *Rehabilitation Education, 10,* 115–126.

Rudman, R. (2004). History and systems: Canada. In T. F. Riggar & D. R. Maki (Eds.), *Handbook of rehabilitation counseling* (pp. 76–87). New York: Springer.

Sanz, J. (2001). The decade 1989–1998 in Spanish psychology: An analysis of research in personality, assessment, and psychological treatment (Clinical and Health Psychology). *The Spanish Journal of Psychology, 4,* 151–181.

Savickas, M. L., & Baker, D. B. (2005). The history of vocational psychology: Antecedents, origin, and early development. In W. B. Walsh & M. L. Savickas (Eds.), *Handbook of vocational psychology: Theory, research and practice* (2nd ed., pp. 15–50). Mahwah, NJ: Lawrence Erlbaum Associates.

Scherer, M. J. (2010). Rehabilitation psychology. In I.B. Weiner & W. E. Craighead (Eds.), *The concise Corsini encyclopedia of psychology* (4th ed., Vol. 4., pp. 1444–1447). Hoboken, NJ: John Wiley & Sons, Inc.

Schuller, I., van Brakel, W., I, Beise, K., Wardhani, L., Silwana, S., van Elteren M., Hasibuan, Y., & Asapa, A. (2010). The way women experience disabilities and especially disabilities related to leprosy in rural areas in south Sulawesi, Indonesia. *Asia Pacific Disability Rehabilitation Journal, 21,* 60–70. Retrieved from EBSCO*host.*

Sharma, M., & Deepak, S. (2002). A case study of the community based rehabilitation programme in Mongolia. *Asia Pacific Disability Rehabilitation Journal, 13,* 11–18. Retrieved from EBSCO*host.*

Shontz, F. C., & Wright, B. A. (1980). The distinctiveness of rehabilitation psychology. *Professional Psychology: Research and Practice, 11,* 919–924.

Shurka, E. (1984). Attitudes towards disability and rehabilitation among political and professional leaders in Israeli development towns. *International Social work, 27,* 10–18.

Spanish Psychological Association (2011). *Working and applied fields in Clinical and Health Psychology. Retrieved from* http://www.cop.es/English/docs/working.htm

Stiers, W., Perry, K., Kennedy, P., & Scherer, M. (2011). Rehabilitation psychology. In P. Martin, F. Cheung, M. Kyrios, L. Littlefield, M. Knowles, B. Overmier, & J. Prieto (Eds.), *IAAP handbook of applied psychology* (pp. 537–587). Oxford, England: Wiley-Blackwell.

Stiers, W., & Stucky, K. (2008). A survey of training in rehabilitation psychology practice in the United States and Canada: 2007. *Rehabilitation Psychology, 53,* 536–543. doi: 10.1037/a0013827.

Stubbins, J. (1989). The interdisciplinary status of rehabilitation psychology. *Rehabilitation Psychology, 34*, 207–215.

Szymanski, E. (1985). Rehabilitation counseling: A profession with a vision, an identity, and a future. *Rehabilitation Counseling Bulletin, 29*, 2–5.

Tasiemski, T., Nielsen, S., & Wilski, M. (2010). Quality of life in people with spinal cord injury—earthquake survivors from Sichuan province in China. *Asia Pacific Disability Rehabilitation Journal, 21*, 28–36. Retrieved from EBSCO*host*.

Tate, D. G., & Pledger, C. (2003). An integrative conceptual framework of disability. *American Psychologist, 58*, 289–295. doi: 10.1037/0003–066X.58.4.289.

Thomas, K. R. (2004). Old wine in a slightly cracked new bottle. *American Psychologist, 59*, 274–275. doi: 10.1037/0003-066X.59.4.275.

Thomas, K. R., & Chan, F. (2000). On becoming a rehabilitation psychologist: Many roads lead to Rome. *Rehabilitation Psychology, 45*, 65–73. doi: 10.1037/0090-5550.45.1.65.

Thomas, K. R., Gottlieb, A. B., & Kravetz, S. P. (1974). Congruence and attributes of meaning: Community mental health Center and vocational rehabilitation personnel. *Community Mental Health Journal, 10*, 402–408.

Thomas, M., & Thomas, M. (2002). Status of women with disabilities in South Asia. *Asia Pacific Disability Rehabilitation Journal*, 27–34. Retrieved from EBSCO*host*.

Thurer, S. L. (1982). Women and rehabilitation. *Rehabilitation Literature, 43*, 194–197.

Turner, M., & Andrewes, D. (2010). Assessing the cognitive regulation of emotion in depressed stroke patients. *International Journal of Rehabilitation Research. [Internationale Zeitschrift Für Rehabilitationsforschung. Revue Internationale De Recherches De Réadaptation], 33*, 180–182. Retrieved from EBSCO*host*.

Turmusani, M. (2002). Disability and development in Kosovo: The case for community based rehabilitation. *Asia Pacific Disability Rehabilitation Journal 13*, 19–28.

UNT department receives grant to bring master's program to Mexico. Retrieved April 21, 2011, from http://www.unt.edu/president/insider/oct06/mexico.htm.

Vakil, E. (1994). Clinical neuropsychology and brain injury rehabilitation in Israel: A twenty-year perspective. *Neuropsychology Review, 4*, 271–278.

van Kampen, M., van Zijverden, I. M., & Emmett, T. (2008). Reflections on poverty and disability: A review of literature. *Asia Pacific Rehabilitation Journal, 19*, 1–16.

Vik, K., Lilja, M., & Nygard, L. (2007). The influence of the environment on participation subsequent to rehabilitation as experienced by elderly people in Norway. *Scandinavia Journal of Occupational Therapy, 14*, 86–95.

Wade, S. L., & Wolfe, C. R. (2005). Telehealth interventions in rehabilitation psychology: Postcards from the edge. *Rehabilitation Psychology, 50, 323–324*. doi: 10.1037/0090-5550.50.4.323.

Wales, C., Matthews, L., & Donelly, M. (2010). Medically unexplained chronic pain in Australia: Difficulties for rehabilitation providers and workers in pain. *Work (Reading, Mass.), 36*, 167–179. Retrieved from EBSCO*host*.

Wegener, S. T., Elliott, T. R., & Hagglund, K. J. (2000). On psychological identity and training: A reply to Thomas and Chan (2000). *Rehabilitation Psychology, 45*, 74–80. doi: 10.1037/0090-5550.45.1.74.

Wegener, S. T., Hagglund, K. J., & Elliott, T. R. (1998). On psychological identity and training: Boulder is better for rehabilitation psychology. *Rehabilitation Psychology, 43*, 17–29.

Whitehouse, F. A. (1975). Rehabilitation clinician., *Journal of Rehabilitation, 41*, 24–26. Retrieved from EBSCO*host*.

Working and applied fields in clinical and health psychology. Retrieved April 21, 2011, from http://www.cop.es/English/docs/working.htm.

Wright, B. (Ed.). (1959). *Psychology and rehabilitation*. Washington DC: American Psychological Association. doi:10.1037/10539–000.

Wright, B. A. (1960). *Physical disability: A psychological approach*. New York: Harper & Row.

Wright, B. A. (1972). Value-laden beliefs and principles for rehabilitation psychology. *Rehabilitation Psychology, 19*, 38–45.

Wright, B. A. (1983). *Physical disability: A psychosocial approach* (2nd ed.). New York: Harper & Row.

Wright, B. A. (1989). Extension of Heider's ideas to rehabilitation psychology. *American Psychologist, 44*, 525–528.

Wright, B. A. (1993). Division of rehabilitation psychology: Roots, guiding principle, and a persistent concern. *Rehabilitation Psychology, 38*, 63–65.

Wright, G. N. (1989). Rehabilitation counseling: International professional preparation and practice. *Rehabilitation Education, 3*, 233–237.

Wright, R. K., Wright B. A. & Dembo, T. (1948). Studies in Adjustment to visible injuries: Evaluation of curiosity by the injured. *Journal of Abnormal and Social Psychology, 43*, 13–28. doi:10.1037/h0057775

Zangwill, O. L. (1945). A review of psychological work at the brain injuries unit, Edinburgh, 1941–1945. *British Medical Journal, 2*, 248–251.

Psychological Models in Rehabilitation Psychology

Joseph F. Rath *and* Timothy R. Elliott

Abstract

Rehabilitation psychology depends upon a broad theoretical base incorporating frameworks, theories, models, and methodologies from many different areas of psychology, as well as from other professions invested in the health and rehabilitation of persons living with disabilities and chronic health conditions. This chapter considers some illustrative models that have been influential in rehabilitation psychology—both historically and in the present—including the biopsychosocial model, and psychological models derived from learning theory and behavior modification, psychoanalytic theory, social psychology, neuropsychology, and cognitive-behavioral theory. The current status of these models, their impact on current clinical practice, and future directions—including the role of dynamic models sensitive to differential trajectories of growth, adjustment, and development over time—will be discussed.

Key Words: Rehabilitation psychology, psychological models, disability, chronic illness, health care, assessment and intervention

Models are organizing tools that can help understand, explain, and predict related phenomena (Reel & Feaver, 2006). As aptly noted by Wilson (2002), psychological models vary in detail and complexity, ranging from simple analogies, such as comparing memory encoding to storing information on a computer's hard drive (Baddeley, 1998), to stage models of cognitive development (Flavell, 1971), to complex multivariate frameworks for explaining resilience following traumatic injury (deRoon-Cassini, Mancini, Rusch, & Bonanno, 2010).

In rehabilitation psychology, psychological models are necessary for facilitating treatment planning, explaining impairments and treatments to patients and caregivers, and allowing clinicians and interdisciplinary team members to conceptualize outcomes. As a field steeped in interdisciplinary endeavors, rehabilitation psychology depends upon a broad theoretical base incorporating frameworks, theories, models, and methodologies from many different areas of psychology, as well as from other professions invested in the health and rehabilitation of persons living with disabilities and chronic health conditions. Consistent with the historical background of the field (see, e.g., Elliott & Rath, 2011), rehabilitation psychologists routinely provide services informed by other academic and practice areas of psychology including, but not limited to, clinical, counseling, educational, and social psychology, behavioral neuroscience, and neuropsychology. Indeed, rehabilitation psychology has excelled in practical applications of otherwise esoteric, "academic" theories to the understanding and alleviation of problems encountered in the clinical setting (Elliott, 2002), including applications of Lewian field theory (Dembo, Leviton, & Wright, 1956) and operant conditioning principles (Fordyce, 1976).

The wide array of circumstances confronting individuals living with potentially disabling conditions demands a broad skill set and flexibility in the rehabilitation psychologist's approach. No one psychological model or group of models in the extant literature is sufficient to fully address all aspects of the diverse problems facing individuals with disabilities and chronic health concerns. This chapter considers some illustrative models that have been influential in rehabilitation psychology—both historically and in the present—including the biopsychosocial model, and psychological models derived from learning theory and behavior modification, psychoanalytic theory, social psychology, neuropsychology, and cognitive-behavioral theory. The current status of these models, their impact on current clinical practice, and future directions will be discussed.

Biopsychosocial Model

Although not a psychological model per se, the biopsychosocial model is considered here because this perspective permeates the psychological literature and is consistent with contemporary rehabilitation practice and processes (Frank & Elliott, 2000; Parker, Szymanski, & Patterson, 2005). The biopsychosocial model of disability considers the interactive effects of disease, psychosocial stressors, and personal and environmental factors that account for varying degrees of adaptation (Peterson & Elliott, 2008). Rehabilitation psychologists long have acknowledged the role of environmental and attitudinal barriers in society, and have advocated for their mitigation to improve life conditions for individuals living with disabilities and chronic health conditions (Scherer et. al, 2004). Biopsychosocial models—typically developed to study adjustment associated with specific diagnostic conditions (e.g., traumatic brain injury [TBI], multiple sclerosis, spinal cord injury [SCI])—have proliferated in the rehabilitation psychology literature (e.g., see Frank & Elliott, 2000). These models commonly attempt to integrate medical aspects of a given disability diagnosis with important psychological (e.g., coping abilities, personality traits) and social (e.g., social support, stressors) variables and their various interactions in the prediction of optimal adjustment.

Emanating from the biopsychosocial model, the *International Classification of Functioning, Disability, and Health* (ICF; World Health Organization [WHO], 2001) is based on an integration of earlier medical and social models of disability and addresses biological, individual, and societal perspectives on health (Peterson, 2005). The ICF's interactive conceptual framework illustrates how facilitators and barriers in the environment are key factors in understanding disability and how advocacy occurs through social change (Hurst, 2003). Most important to rehabilitation psychology, individuals' appraisals of environmental assets and liabilities, personal body functions, and their ability to participate in desired personal and social activities, are important considerations in classifying functioning, disability, and health with the ICF (Peterson & Elliott, 2008). In contrast to earlier medical models, specific medical conditions or physical disabilities are an insufficient means of explaining, understanding, anticipating, or rehabilitating any aspect of disability experienced by an individual.

The promise of the biopsychosocial model for rehabilitation psychology is that it is a stimulus for significant developments in theory, research, policy, and practice applications (Bruyère & Peterson, 2005), the results of which can be used to help identify, mitigate, or remove societal hindrances to the full participation of people with disabilities in mainstream society (Peterson & Rosenthal, 2005). Nonetheless, the biopsychosocial model is not a psychological model of adjustment; it does not provide explicit and testable hypotheses to advance understanding of behavioral processes among people living with chronic health problems and disabilities (Elliott & Warren, 2007). More recent psychological models, informed by social psychological theory (discussed below), emphasize the primacy of subjective, phenomenological appraisals of resources, stressors, and contextual issues across diagnostic conditions (Elliott, Kurylo, & Rivera, 2002). This shift is based partly on evidence that (a) individual differences and other psychological characteristics usually account for greater variance in the prediction of adjustment among persons with disability than does any condition-specific variable, and (b) stressors appear to vary as a function of psychological and social characteristics rather than being due to specific diagnostic conditions, with a few exceptions occurring among conditions that impose severe disruptions in brain–behavior relations (Peterson & Elliott, 2008).

Learning Theory and Behavior Modification

Psychological models stemming from learning theory and behavior modification have informed rehabilitation psychology research and practice for many years. Learning principles have been applied to identify environmental contingencies that reinforce and shape "disabled" behaviors and produce impairment that is beyond what can be attributed directly to a physical condition. These models also supply rehabilitation psychologists with many potential intervention strategies, such as shaping, modeling, desensitization, chaining, extinction, and reinforcement, any of which can be adapted or modified to suit particular individuals, purposes, and problems.

Wilbert E. Fordyce's application of operant conditioning theory to understanding the dynamics and contingencies that shape and reinforce "pain behavior" (Fordyce, 1971) and suffering following disability (Fordyce, 1988) had a broad, sweeping impact on rehabilitation psychology research, practice, and policy. His 1976 book, *Behavioral Methods for Chronic Pain and Illness*, is a classic in the rehabilitation and health psychology literature (Elliott & Byrd, 1986; Patterson, 2005). In his model, pain behaviors are conditioned by a patient's interpersonal and social environment, and these environmental reactions serve to maintain or increase pain behaviors. Applying operant learning theory, Fordyce also argued persuasively about the dangers of "as needed" medication schedules and advocated use of time-contingent schedules to prevent acquisition of maladaptive behavioral patterns, with the additional benefit of maintaining steady medication levels in the patient (Patterson, 2005). This model also was central in illuminating the value of exercise and activity at regular intervals by taking into account the initial "punishing" aspects of this activity in terms of increased pain, which may contribute to faulty learning patterns and decreased activity levels that reward pain behavior over time.

Similarly, Neal Miller, Bernard Brucker, and Lawrence Ince applied classical and operant conditioning theory to the study of visceral, reflex, and motor responses in the "clinical laboratory" of the rehabilitation hospital (Brucker & Ince, 1977; Ince, Brucker, & Alba, 1978; Miller & Brucker, 1979). In a series of creative, yet rigorous, single-case designs, this research team obtained sufficient evidence to establish biofeedback as an empirically based technique for use with persons with disabling conditions and cultivate a great appreciation for using behavioral strategies to augment rehabilitation therapies, enhance adjustment, and condition responses previously thought to be autonomic (Ince, 1980).

A contemporary extension of this work, grounded in state-of-the-art behavioral neuroscience, is evident in Edward Taub's model of learned nonuse of motor behavior (Taub & Uswatte, 2000), which stems directly from animal models of learning and behavior. In this model, organic damage results in an initial inability to use a body part, so that an animal is punished (through failure) for attempts to use that part of the body and rewarded for use of other parts of the body. The conditioned suppression of use that develops in the acute phase continues after the animal recovers the physical ability to use that body part (Uswatte & Taub, 2005).

This model has clear relevance for rehabilitation of motor impairments in humans following central nervous system (CNS) damage and other injuries (Taub, 1980; Taub & Uswatte, 2000). Among the implications for rehabilitation is that a portion of the impairment may be associated with a learning process that potentially can be reversed long after the initial injury. This reversal may be attained through the application of appropriate interventions so that substantial improvement in the use of the extremity can be effected (the signature technique involves restricting the contralateral arm in a sling, while training the affected arm; Taub, Crago, & Uswatte, 1998). This resulting family of intervention techniques—*constraint-induced movement therapy* (CIMT; Uswatte & Taub, 2005)—includes treatments for (a) upper extremity weakness in adults with brain injury and stroke, as well as children with cerebral palsy (Taub, Uswatte, & Pidikiti, 1999); impaired ambulation in individuals with SCI, stroke, and hip fracture (Taub et al., 1999); and aphasia in persons with stroke (Pulvermuller et al., 2001). Extensions of this model have been applied to the treatment of phantom limb pain (Weiss, Miltner, Adler, Buckner, & Taub, 1999) and focal hand dystonia (Candia et al., 1999).

Taub's model of learned nonuse of motor behavior has had enormous implications for researchers' understanding of brain–behavior relationships and neuroplasticity that extend far beyond the walls of the rehabilitation setting. Although stemming from learning theory, the model also is consistent with and informed by neuroscience research over the past two decades that has demonstrated that the adult CNS has capacity for substantial plasticity (e.g., see review by Taub, Uswatte, & Elbert, 2002). Notably, the intervention strategy—like the model developed by Fordyce for chronic pain rehabilitation programs—is implemented by the multidisciplinary treatment team and not by the psychologist per se in face-to-face interactions.

Today, a variety of interventions derived from learning theory and behavior-modification models routinely are used in many areas relevant to rehabilitation psychology (Elliott & Jackson, 2005). In rehabilitation settings, one of the most important applications of these models is to help patients optimize therapy participation by increasing the frequency of therapeutically on-task behaviors, while decreasing the frequency of therapy-competing behaviors. Contemporary behavioral interventions eschew use of aversive stimuli and punishment. Instead, focus is now on differential reinforcement of other (DRO) behavior, in which reinforcement is provided when the individual refrains from performing a problematic behavior during a specific time interval. The Premack principle also is applicable, wherein naturally occurring high-frequency responses (e.g., resting on exercise mat) reinforce lower frequency target responses (e.g., participating in uncomfortable range-of-motion exercises).

In the case of cognitive rehabilitation, Goodkin (1966) was among the first to apply interventions derived from learning theory to the rehabilitation of adults with brain injury, using operant conditioning techniques to improve language skills (Wilson, 2002). These approaches were later applied to cognitive impairments (Diller, 1980; Ince, 1980; Wilson, 1981). Today, approaches drawn from learning theory and behavior modification are widely used in cognitive rehabilitation. For example, interventions derived from behavioral models can be particularly useful for individuals with severe behavior problems that impede participation in traditional rehabilitative therapies. Such patients often can be engaged in therapy within highly structured behavioral programs. Similarly, agitated patients may be more successfully managed in acute hospital settings when behavior management techniques are employed (Wilson, 2002).

Initiation deficits may impede achievement of cognitive rehabilitation goals as much as behaviors typically perceived as socially unacceptable or inappropriate. Patients with such deficits may be engaged successfully using behavioral techniques, whereas similar behavioral strategies can be taught to family member caregivers. McGlynn (1990) offered a comprehensive review of interventions derived from behavioral models, pertaining to six categories of target behavior relevant to cognitive rehabilitation: inappropriate social behavior, attention and motivation, unawareness of deficits, memory, language and speech, and motor disturbance.

Across diagnostic categories and treatment settings, a key target for rehabilitation psychologists is helping patients maintain gains once they are discharged from rehabilitation programs or transitioned to less intensive programs. Individuals with SCI, for example, typically must follow a detailed

regimen if they are to prevent pressure sores following discharge. Prevention of pressure sores is just one example in which patient compliance is crucial; the application of interventions derived from behavioral models may reduce the need for patients to return to more restrictive and less cost-effective settings.

As with interventions derived from other psychological models, rehabilitation psychologists do not use behavioral techniques in isolation, but supplement them with theories, models, technologies, and interventions from other areas of psychology. In this context, behavior modification may best be conceptualized as discovering what produces the most effective results for specific individuals and then applying that approach throughout their rehabilitation (cf. Wilson, 2002).

Psychoanalytic Models

For many years, the prevailing models of adjustment to disability were based on Freudian views in which individuals were presumed to pass through predictable stages in reaction to severe loss (Grzesiak & Hicock, 1994). For example, Jerome Siller, a pioneering figure in rehabilitation psychology, extrapolated many of his ideas from psychoanalytic theory. Leaning on logic and clinical experience, Siller refined existing "stage models" of adjustment to enlighten understanding of acceptance and adjustment following the acute onset of severe disability (Siller, 1969, 1988). Certain specific features of stage models would vary, but to a considerable extent, many of these Freudian-based extrapolations posited that the ego would likely feel a sense of "castration" at the loss of a limb or motor function. According to these models, losses accompanying disability would deal a severe blow to the individual's inherent narcissism, and most individuals would use denial to defend against the anxiety precipitated by the loss. As the ego became able to permit experience of the loss, denial would be replaced by depression. Presumably, for individuals with strong enough egos, optimal adjustment would be attained when depression eventually was replaced by acceptance of the reality of their permanent disability.

Siller's stage model of adjustment to disability has been revisited and reworked over the years by others in rehabilitation psychology (Cubbage & Thomas, 1989; Grzesiak & Hicock, 1994). He expanded his thinking to incorporate contemporary ideas from object relations theory (Thomas & Siller, 1999). Unfortunately, these theoretical models generated very little empirical research. Recent evidence, however, indicates that certain constructs from self-psychology models can account for significant variance in clinical outcomes following acquired disability (Elliott, Uswatte, Lewis, & Palmatier, 2000). Siller and his colleagues also developed measures of attitudes toward disability and adaptation to disability based on models derived from classical psychoanalytic theory (Siller, Chipman, Ferguson, & Vann, 1967), but this work, too, failed to stimulate rigorous, sustained empirical scrutiny. Nonetheless, the intuitive, clinical appeal of psychoanalytic stage models influenced—and continues to influence—many clinical conceptualizations of adjustment following disability, and analytic psychotherapy approaches routinely are used in rehabilitation psychology practice. In cognitive rehabilitation, Prigatano (1999) is a leading advocate of adapting psychodynamic approaches for use with individuals with acquired brain injury.

Social Psychology

Beatrice Wright, one of the enduring pioneers of rehabilitation psychology, studied with scholars noted for their outstanding contributions to social psychology (Kurt Lewin, Tamara Dembo, Solomon Asch) and with others recognized for their contributions to clinical psychology (Kenneth Spence, Carl Rogers, Abraham Maslow; Dunn & Elliott, 2005). In 1960, Wright published the seminal *Physical Disability: A Psychological Approach*, the first theory-driven psychological statement from rehabilitation psychology, grounded in the best scholarly traditions, informed by the extant literature, and enriched with applications and illustrations to inform both academicians and clinicians.

In her somatopsychological model, Wright (1960) persuasively argued for appreciating disability within context, relying heavily on Lewinian field theory to depict disability as a social psychological phenomenon in which any atypical appearance, physique, or behavior attracts the attention of, and stimulates inferences from, observers. According to the Lewinian equation, $B = f(P, E)$, observed behavior following disability (e.g., passivity, aggression, well-being, search for meaning) is a function of the person *and* the environment (Wright, 1983). A cardinal tenet of social psychology is that behavior is erroneously presumed to disclose one's personality or character, or even skills (Heider, 1958; cf. Gilbert & Malone, 1995; Ross, 1977). As applied to disability, Wright's model posits that concerned, curious perceivers usually presume that the appearance of

physical deviation points to psychological or other deficits. Furthermore, Wright reminded readers that the environments where people with disabilities live can either promote or hinder adjustment. To be sure, characteristics of persons with disabilities affect coping, but following Lewin (1935), such interpretations were predicated on the interaction of the person and the situation (Ross & Nisbett, 1991). Wright's somatopsychological model extended her previous work with Tamara Dembo (Dembo et al., 1956) to draw explicit ramifications for understanding issues and behaviors presented by individuals with disabilities in clinical settings.

The direct influence of Wright's model on rehabilitation psychology may have waned in recent years (see Ryan & Tree, 2004). Nonetheless, the somatopsychological model and other aspects of Wright's work have remained influential in the emerging area of positive psychology (see Elliott et al., 2002, for a review). According to Wright (1983), persons who have developed greater acceptance of disability will demonstrate a sense of meaning in their circumstances, value their selfhood, and maintain positive beliefs about themselves. Such changes may be construed as both process and outcome and may be reflected in a heightened sense of priorities, a greater appreciation of the preciousness of life, and an inner strength and meaning that permeates daily decisions and activities (Tedeschi, Park, & Calhoun, 1998). Thus, individuals who incur physical disabilities may do more than survive their conditions; their resilience and clarity of purpose may result in a greater resolve for pursuing personal goals (Snyder, 1998) and an attainment of psychological adjustment and spiritual awareness that surpasses their previous level of adaptation (Wright, 1983).

Current interest in positive psychology may serve to regenerate application of social psychological models in rehabilitation psychology for a number of reasons. In particular, theoretical models concerning growth, happiness, life satisfaction, and well-being often are tested and refined in rigorous, real-world applications; therefore, empirical tests of these models often are conducted among persons who have sustained disabling injuries or live with severe chronic health conditions (e.g., Emmons & McCullough, 2003, study 4; Lucas, 2007; for integrative summaries, see Dunn, Uswatte, & Elliott, 2009; Elliott et al., 2002).

Current perspectives on subjective well-being following disability using sophisticated prospective methodologies now inform psychological models of adjustment to disability over time. One example of such a model of adjustment is the dynamic model for understanding positive growth following disability (Elliott et al., 2002). In this model, adjustment following disability is conceptualized as a dynamic and fluid process in which characteristics of the person and the injury, the social and interpersonal world, the environment in general, and the historical and temporal context interact to influence physical and psychological health.

This model conceptualizes several broad-based domains, each of which has considerable influence on two areas of adjustment: psychological well-being and physical health. The primary components involve enduring individual characteristics (i.e., demographic characteristics, disability-specific characteristics, predisability behavioral patterns, preinjury psychopathology, and personality constructs) and the immediate social and interpersonal environment (i.e., social supports and societal barriers, family relationships and caregiver–care recipient interactions, and environmental factors that promote or impede independence, mobility, and integration). These influence the phenomenological and appraisal processes that constitute elements of positive growth (e.g., personal meaning and purpose, positive side benefits and growth, and value shifts) and, in turn, predict psychological well-being and physical health outcomes.

The dynamic continuum encompasses changes in any of the five components of the model (i.e., individual characteristics, social and interpersonal environment, phenomenological and appraisal processes, psychological well-being, and physical health) as people age, technologies advance, relationships shift, and health and public policies evolve. This continuum reflects the ongoing process of growth, adaptation, and development in the person and the environment, and the subsequent alterations in interactions among these entities. The model therefore acknowledges the dynamic continuum in which behavior occurs, in terms of changes that follow in the wake of legislative and market trends, and in terms of changes that may be associated with age, family relationships, acquired abilities, and income. The model concedes that individuals vary considerably in the environmental conditions in which they live, which in turn may pose unique impediments to their adjustment, or conversely, unique supports that facilitate it.

Notably, the model emphasizes elements of positive adjustment, and its focus is not confined to matters of pathology. This point is of crucial importance to rehabilitation psychologists because optimal adjustment among persons with disability is the ultimate outcome goal in rehabilitation. Optimal adjustment is characterized by subjective well-being, meaningful activities, satisfying relationships, and good health; it also may be associated with fewer psychological problems such as depression, anxiety, social isolation, and loneliness. Because individuals who attain a greater degree of positive growth following disability are presumed to be more likely to engage in behaviors conducive to general well-being and optimal physical health, positive growth also may be associated with a decreased risk of secondary complications relevant to rehabilitation (e.g., urinary tract infections, pressure sore occurrence, respiratory problems).

Neuropsychology

In recent decades, neuropsychological approaches have grown in importance to rehabilitation psychology. Brain injuries and stroke are among the most frequent disabilities in society (Faul, Xu, Wald, & Coronado, 2010; National Institute of Neurological Disorders and Stroke, 2004), so it is not surprising that many rehabilitation psychologists encounter some form of neurological deficit in clinical practice. In rehabilitation, assessment must focus on impaired functional abilities in order to be relevant. However, the most prominent early neuropsychological assessment approaches consisted of fixed batteries designed to localize specific lesions. Popularized for English-speaking readers by the writings of Christensen, Majovski, and others (e.g., Christensen, 1974; Luria & Majovski, 1977; Majovski & Jacques, 1980), Alexander Luria's work provided a data-based theoretical model of brain functioning on which process-oriented neuropsychological assessments could be based. This hypothesis-testing or "process" model allows identification of an individual's cognitive strengths and deficits by successively formulating, testing, and accepting or rejecting hypotheses about the patient's cognitive functioning (Wilson, 2002). In Luria's model, the goal is to determine which components of a functional process are compromised—and which are intact—as the basis for treatment planning. Identifying which cognitive elements are disrupting a functional activity may allow for a more focused and shorter course of rehabilitation, with improved outcome.

The hypothesis-testing process approach is particularly important in cognitive rehabilitation. Based on an initial neuropsychological assessment—and on assessment data gathered by the other members of the interdisciplinary team—specific treatment recommendations are made. As with interventions based on other models noted above, often these treatment recommendations are integrated into other disciplines' regimens and not delivered directly by the rehabilitation psychologist in face-to-face interactions.

Luria's process model is just one of many models relevant to cognitive rehabilitation. Leonard Diller, founder of scientifically based cognitive rehabilitation (Goldstein, 2009), recognized that rehabilitation cannot be confined by one theoretical model, stating, "While current accounts of remediation have been criticized as lacking a theoretical base, it might be more accurate to state that remediation must take into account several theoretical bases" (Diller, 1987, p. 9). As Wilson (2002) aptly noted, other models are useful in cognitive rehabilitation, including models of premorbid personality and emotional behavior, and neurological, physical, and biochemical models.

Cognitive-Behavioral Theory

Psychological models stemming from cognitive-behavioral theory have great potential in promoting adjustment, well-being, and personal health among persons with disabling conditions. Interventions derived from these models are among the most promising and widely accepted treatments in rehabilitation psychology (Elliott & Jackson, 2005). As with interventions derived from the other psychological models discussed above, interventions derived from cognitive-behavioral models are more likely to be successful when they are designed or adapted to meet the needs and problems as perceived and experienced by the individual with the disability or chronic health problem. In this regard, Hibbard, Grober, Gordon, and Aletta (1990) offered a set of practical adaptations of cognitive-behavioral interventions to help compensate for cognitive deficits, whereas Radnitz (2000) discussed adaptations of cognitive behavior interventions for individuals with a variety of specific physical disabilities.

Over the past 25 years, D'Zurilla and Goldfried's (1971) seminal problem-solving model has had a significant impact on rehabilitation psychology theory and practice. With clear relevance to the adjustment of individuals with disabilities, problem-solving is defined as a conscious, rational, effortful, and purposeful coping process that can facilitate a person's ability to deal effectively with a wide range of problematic situations (D'Zurilla & Chang, 1995). In contrast to interventions arising from cognitive-behavioral social skills models, problem-solving interventions are aimed at the level of covert thinking processes; individuals are taught a generic sequence of problem-solving steps, which they then learn to apply to a variety of problematic situations (Coleman, Wheeler, & Webber, 1993).

In this model, problem solving is conceptualized as comprising two separate, but interacting, components, problem orientation and problem-solving skills. *Problem-solving skills* are the cognitive-behavioral skills or goal-directed tasks that, if successfully implemented, would enable a person to resolve a particular problem successfully. As defined by D'Zurilla and Goldfried (1971), the major problem-solving skills are problem definition and formulation (identifying the conditions and constraints of problematic situations and setting realistic goals), generation of alternatives (brainstorming a range of possible solutions), decision-making (examining potential consequences of options and selecting an optimal one, given the conditions and constraints of the problem), and solution implementation and verification (enacting a solution, monitoring its effectiveness, and making modifications as necessary).

In contrast, *problem orientation* focuses on the individual's immediate cognitive-behavioral-affective reactions when first confronted with a problematic situation. These orienting responses include a set of beliefs, assumptions, appraisals, and expectations concerning real-life problems and one's own general problem-solving ability. Problem-orientation processes include problem perception (recognizing problems as they occur, rather than avoiding, ignoring, or denying them), problem attribution (accepting problems as normal and inevitable, rather than a source of shame and guilt), problem appraisal (appraising problems as challenges, rather than as threatening or harmful), perceived control (belief that one is capable of solving problems and implementing effective solutions), and time/effort commitment (willingness to devote the required time and effort necessary to resolve a problem; D'Zurilla & Nezu, 2001).

According to this model, impaired problem orientation can lead to negative affect and avoidance, which can inhibit or disrupt implementation of problem-solving skills. Thus, through the articulation of the concept of problem orientation, the model extends the concept of problem solving beyond cognitive skills to emphasize motivational, attitudinal, and affective factors that may disrupt intent, motivation, and focus, and thereby interfere with effective problem resolution. In research with direct relevance to rehabilitation psychology, significant empirical support has accumulated for the premise that effective problem solving (with an adaptive problem orientation playing a key role) is an important coping strategy that has significant impact on psychological well-being and adjustment for individuals with and without disabilities.

Problem-solving abilities have been linked to a variety of adjustment criteria in medical and rehabilitation populations (see Elliot & Hurst, 2008, for an integrative review). For example, problem-solving ability is related to health expectancies and complications in surgical patients (see Heppner & Baker, 1997), regimen adherence in diabetics (Toobert & Glasgow, 1991), community integration in adults with brain injury (Rath, Hennessy, & Diller, 2003), and to levels of depression, psychosocial impairment, and assertiveness in adults with SCI (Elliott, Godshall, Herrick, Witty, & Spruell, 1991). Individuals with severe disabilities living with family caregivers who have impulsive and careless ways of solving problems were more likely to develop a pressure sore within the first year of acquired disability than were other individuals (Elliott, Shewchuk, & Richards, 1999). Caregiver dysfunctional styles also have been implicated in the distress and decreased life satisfaction reported by patients with congestive heart failure (Kurylo, Elliott, DeVivo, & Dreer, 2004).

Problem-solving therapy (or training; PST) has been promulgated as an attractive therapeutic option in many multidisciplinary health care settings. Indeed, the broader concept of "problem-solving" is considered an essential element in chronic disease education and self-management programs (Hill-Briggs, 2003). Problem solving training grounded explicitly in the principles espoused by D'Zurilla and Goldfried (i.e., incorporating both problem orientation and problem-solving skills) has been applied with notable success in alleviating distress among persons with cancer (Nezu, Felgoise, McClure, & Houts, 2003; Nezu, Nezu, Friedman, & Faddis, 1998) and in improving coping and emotional self-regulation skills among persons with acquired brain injury (Rath, Simon, Langenbahn, Sherr, & Diller, 2003).

Although the empirically driven specifics of problem-solving model may have evolved over time (see Elliott & Hurst, 2008, for a review), PST typically consists of didactics and practice in each of the five steps of the D'Zurilla and Goldfried (1971) model, followed by applied integration of the model and continued practice of the component steps.

Once the sequence is learned, it is applicable to the diverse problematic situations that arise in everyday life. Thus, as an intervention method, instruction in problem solving has important implications for rehabilitation psychologists in terms of treatment generalization and maintenance.

Problem-solving interventions have documented success in individual sessions provided in primary care settings (Mynors-Wallis, Garth, Lloyd-Thomas, & Tomlinson, 1995), structured group therapy (Rath, Simon, et al., 2003), telephone sessions with community-residing adults (Grant, Elliott, Weaver, Bartolucci, & Giger, 2002), in-home sessions with family caregivers of individuals with TBI (Rivera, Elliott, Berry, & Grant, 2008), and in internet-based online sessions for parents of children with TBI (Wade, Carey, & Wolfe, 2006a; and with observed benefits on child functioning, Wade, Carey, & Wolfe, 2006b).

Conceptualizations drawing on the problem-solving model also are relevant to family caregivers. Because individuals who acquire physical disabilities with considerable life expectancies (e.g., spinal cord and acquired brain injuries) often require life-long commitments from a family member to perform caregiving duties (Lollar & Crews, 2003), attending to the health and well-being of family caregivers—and the subsequent ability to assist their care recipients—is a significant concern for rehabilitation psychologists (Chwalisz & Clancy-Dollinger, 2009). In this regard, an effective problem-solving style has been associated with greater relationship satisfaction among family caregivers of stroke survivors (Shanmugham, Cano, Elliott, & Davis, 2009). Related research suggests that children of families that rely on problem-solving coping fare better over time than those from families who rely less on these strategies (Kinsella, Ong, Murtagh, Prior, & Sawyer, 1999; Rivara et al., 1996). Caregiver dysfunctional problem-solving styles also have been implicated in the distress and decreased life satisfaction reported by patients with congestive heart failure (Kurylo et al., 2004).

As applied to cognitive rehabilitation, D'Zurilla and Goldfried's model has been influential in assessment (Rath, Simon, Sherr, Langenbahn, & Diller, 2000), conceptualization and formulation (Gordon, Cantor, Ashman, & Brown, 2006; Rath, Hennessy, et al., 2003; Rath et al, 2004) and intervention (Rath, Simon, et al., 2003; von Cramon, Matthes-von Cramon, & Mai, 1991) for individuals with acquired brain injury. Due to decreased attentional and emotional self-regulatory resources, individuals with brain injury may be especially vulnerable to problem-orientation deficits, hypothesized to disrupt attention and focus on target tasks and subsequent implementation of problem-solving skills (see Rath, Litke, & Diller, 2011). Current empirically evaluated cognitive rehabilitative approaches informed by this model include improving emotional self-regulation skills and addressing problem-orientation factors in order to improve focus and attention on target tasks before engaging in rehabilitation of problem-solving skills per se (see Rath, Simon, et al., 2003; cf. Gordon et al., 2006). The two-component problem-solving model allows for the possibility of targeted interventions for specific populations; recent evidence suggests that individuals with milder cognitive impairments may have greater limitations in problem orientation, whereas those with more significant cognitive impairments may have greater limitations in problem-solving skills (Kim, 2011).

Informed by the problem-solving model, contemporary treatment recommendations now typically recommend incorporating interventions to address motivational, attitudinal, and affective factors in cognitive rehabilitation (Cicerone, Levin, Malec, Stuss, & Whyte, 2006; Kennedy et al., 2008). Such interventions commonly include identifying and counteracting impediments (e.g., emotional over-reactions, cognitive distortions, misattributions) to sustained focus and attention on target tasks, facilitating the individual's motivation to apply problem-solving skills to problematic situations, and teaching the person to feel self-efficacious in so doing (Rath et al., 2011; Rath, Simon, et al., 2003). Due to the emphasis on both emotional (i.e., problem orientation) and cognitive (i.e., problem-solving skills) aspects of real-life functional problem-solving abilities, cognitive rehabilitative interventions based on this model are anticipated to have broad applications in the treatment of the emotional and cognitive sequelae of combat-related mild TBI (Helmick, 2010), although this has not yet been evaluated empirically.

Other psychological models derived from cognitive-behavioral theory that have had broad influence in rehabilitation psychology include Lazarus and Folkman's (1984) *transactional model of stress and coping*, a framework for evaluating the process of coping with stressful life events. Focusing on the "transaction" between individuals' appraisals of stressors and the social and cultural resources at their disposal, the model posits that stress is not a direct response to stressful events. Instead, individuals' appraisals of events and their resources and coping skills mediate the stress response. Within this model, primary appraisal involves individuals' beliefs about events (e.g., threatening, positive, controllable, challenging, or irrelevant), whereas secondary appraisal involves individuals' assessments of their own coping resources and options.

Stress and coping models have been extended by others to inform rehabilitation psychology research and practice. For example, Kennedy, Duff, Evans, and Beedie (2003) found that *coping effectiveness training* (CET; King & Kennedy, 1999) reduced depression and anxiety in individuals with SCI, in part by changing participants' negative appraisals about the manageability of the consequences of SCI. In individuals with newly acquired SCI, Kennedy, Evans, and Sandu (2009) found that appraisals, in particular primary appraisals of threat, were the best predictors of anxiety and depression.

The final model considered here is Schwarzer's (2008) *health action process approach* (HAPA). Emphasizing the particular role of self-efficacy at different stages of health behavior change, HAPA comprises an open framework model of motivational and volitional constructs intended to explain and predict changes in various health-related behaviors (e.g., losing weight, quitting smoking, adhering to diet, medication, or exercise regimens). Within this model, the adoption, initiation, and maintenance of healthy behavior is conceived of as a process consisting of both motivation and volition phases. Analogous in many ways to the problem orientation and problem-solving skills components of the social problem-solving model described above, the *motivation phase* involves forming the intention to act, while the *volition phase* involves the planning and behavioral implementation of "good intentions." Once a healthy behavior has been initiated, it must be maintained through the use of self-regulatory skills and strategies. By explicitly incorporating postintentional factors, the HAPA model provides a framework for addressing the frequent failure of intention to predict behavior.

The HAPA model has direct implications for the development of phase-based interventions to address the needs of specific target groups (Schüz, Sniehotta, & Schwarzer, 2007). Individuals in the volitional phase can be subdivided into those who actually perform healthy behaviors ("actors") and those who only intend to perform them ("intenders"); thus, for intervention purposes, classification of individuals within the HAPA model yields three meaningful target groups: *nonintenders, intenders,* and *actors* (Luszczynska, Tryburcy, & Schwarzer, 2007). Nonintenders may benefit from some level of risk communication and learning that the new behavior has positive outcomes as opposed to the negative outcomes that accompany the current behavior (Schwarzer, Cao, & Lippke, 2010). In contrast, intenders would not be anticipated to benefit from such an intervention; instead, they should benefit from help in planning the steps necessary to translate their intentions into action (Wiedemann, Schüz, Sniehotta, Scholz, & Schwarzer, 2009). Finally, those already in the actor phase should be helped to prepare for specific high-risk situations in which lapses are imminent (Luszczynska, Mazurkiewicz, Ziegelman, & Schwarzer, 2007). The basic principle is that individuals pass through different mindsets on the way to behavior change, and interventions may be most efficient when tailored to these particular mindsets. A number of randomized controlled trials have examined the notion of stage-matched interventions based on HAPA; for example, in the context of dietary behaviors (Wiedemann et al., 2009) and physical activity (Lippke, Schwarzer, Ziegelmann, Scholz, & Schüz, 2010). Despite the model's clear relevance, HAPA has received remarkably little attention or integration into rehabilitation psychology practice in the United States. However, a few studies have appeared in the rehabilitation psychology literature demonstrating the theoretical and clinical relevance of the model in orthopedic (Reuter, Ziegelmann, Lippke, & Schwarzer, 2009) and cardiac rehabilitation (Luszczynska, & Sutton, 2006).

Conclusion

As we have seen, psychological models informed by a variety of academic and practice areas of psychology all have been influential in allowing rehabilitation psychologists to explain phenomena, predict strengths and weaknesses, and plan treatment for people living with disabilities and chronic health conditions. We also have seen that no one model or group of models in the extant literature is sufficient to fully address all aspects of the diverse and complex problems facing individuals with disabilities and chronic health concerns.

Notably, several of the most influential and long-lasting models reviewed tend to emphasize interventions that allow multidisciplinary team members (including nurses, physiatrists, and physical therapists) to work collaboratively to modify patient behavior to promote skill acquisition, health, and adjustment (rather than relying on face-to-face delivery by psychologists).

Reasonably enough, different psychological models appear to have different strengths, depending on their intended focus. For example, models derived from cognitive-behavioral theory, such as D'Zurilla and Goldfried's problem-solving model, demonstrate clear utility in providing meaningful interventional strategies for emotional and psychosocial adjustment concerns. Similarly, models stemming from learning theory, such as Taub's model of learned nonuse of motor behaviors, have led to a suite of effective interventions for individuals with a variety of motor impairments.

Other models have broader perspectives. By definition, the biopsychosocial model attempts to integrate medical aspects of a given disability diagnosis with important psychological (e.g., coping abilities, personality traits) and social (e.g., social support, stressors) variables and their various interactions in the prediction of optimal adjustment. The shortcoming here is that although the *ICF* (based on the biopsychosocial model) acknowledges the importance of psychological well-being and personal independence in everyday routines, it is not a psychological model of adjustment: It does not provide explicit and testable hypotheses to advance understanding of behavioral processes among people living with chronic health problems and disabilities (Elliott & Warren, 2007).

Informed by Wright's social psychological approach, the most comprehensive model considered is Elliott, Kurylo, and Rivera's dynamic model for understanding positive growth following disability. This model encompasses all aspects of the biopsychosocial model, but also emphasizes the primacy of subjective, phenomenological appraisals of resources, stressors, and contextual issues across diagnostic conditions.

Future Directions

Phenomenological and appraisal processes are the centerpiece of the dynamic model, yet this component remains the proverbial "black box" in which constructs and variables enter and exit on the other side significantly correlated with indices of adjustment (Elliott et al., 2002). Rehabilitation psychologists have yet to determine what kinds of value shifts occur following disability, how and why these occur, and their relationship to a sense of acceptance and well-being (Keany & Glueckauf, 1993). Consequently, when positive changes occur for an individual, the reasons are unknown.

Incorporating insights, methods, and interventions derived from other psychological models into the dynamic model may be helpful in illuminating the black box of subjective, phenomenological appraisal processes. For example, to understand the cognitive-behavioral mechanisms underlying optimal adjustment—and the precursors of such processes—models from cognitive-behavioral approaches, including the social problem-solving model and other models, such as the transactional model of stress and coping might prove useful. Similarly, psychoanalytic approaches might be adapted to provide useful tools for exploring the perceptions and beliefs through which people find meaning rather than despair following disability.

In the past, our theoretical advancements may have outpaced the ability of existing tools to adequately test hypotheses about change and responses to therapy and interventions. Consequently, much of our understanding of response to interventions (including rehabilitation and psychological treatments) is grounded in a linear model of behavioral change that relies on tests of means and standard deviations collected at Point A and again at Point B. Randomized clinical trials explicitly assume a linear model of change, and thus this design is ideal for relatively simple tests of drug-induced change over a short time interval (Ramkumar & Elliott, 2010; Tucker & Reed, 2008). But from an expanded perspective, complex behavior patterns over an extended period of time are influenced by an array of genetic, character-related, environmental, and cultural factors (Glass & McAtee, 2006). We already know that behavioral responses to psychotherapy are not conveniently linear; perhaps more times than not these responses are nonlinear and discontinuous (Hayes, Laurenceau, Feldman, Strauss, & Cardaciotto, 2007), and as such, true effects are obfuscated in tests that assume linear change (Laurenceau, Hayes, & Feldman, 2007). Very few theories explicate these kinds of nonlinear change in an a priori fashion, and practically none of the routine methods for analyzing outcomes over time during and following rehabilitation examine what kind of change occurs.

We hope that the next generation of rehabilitation psychology outcome research will be enriched by a dynamic perspective that will take a more sophisticated, informed approach, sensitive to differential trajectories of growth, adjustment, and development over time as we have seen in other literatures (e.g., personality, West, Ryu, Kwok, & Cham, 2011; developmental psychology, Holmbeck et al., 2010; school psychology, Wu, West, & Hughes, 2008). It is essential for our theories and our tools to work together and in a reciprocal manner if we are to reach the next level of insight about the behavioral and social mechanisms that influence responses to interventions and services (cf., Collins, 2006).

References

Baddeley, A. D. (1998). *Human memory: Theory and practice* (rev ed.). Boston: Allyn & Bacon.

Brucker, B. S., & Ince, L. P. (1977). Biofeedback as an experimental treatment for postural hypotension in a patient with a spinal cord lesion. *Archives of Physical Medicine and Rehabilitation, 58,* 49–53.

Bruyère, S. M., & Peterson, D. B. (2005). Introduction to the special section on the International Classification of Functioning, Disability and Health (*ICF*): Implications for rehabilitation psychology. *Rehabilitation Psychology, 50,* 103–104.

Candia, V., Elbert, T., Altenmuller, E., Rau, H., Schafer, T., & Taub, E. (1999). Constraint-induced movement therapy for focal hand dystonia in musicians [Research letter]. *The Lancet, 353,* 42.

Christensen, A. L. (1974). *Luria's neuropsychological investigation.* Copenhagen, Denmark: Munksgaard.

Chwalisz, K., & Clancy-Dollinger, S. (2009). Evidence-based practice with family caregivers: Decision-making strategies based on research and clinical data. In R. G. Frank, M. Rosenthal, & B. R. Caplan (Eds.), *Handbook of rehabilitation psychology* (2nd ed., pp. 301–312). Washington, DC: American Psychological Association.

Cicerone, K., Levin, H., Malec, J., Stuss, D. & Whyte, J. (2006). Cognitive rehabilitation interventions for executive function: Moving from bench to bedside in patients with traumatic brain injury. *Journal of Cognitive Neuroscience, 18,* 1212–1222.

Coleman, M., Wheeler, L., & Webber, J. (1993). Research on interpersonal problem-solving training: A review. *Remedial and Special Education, 14,* 25–37.

Collins, L. M. (2006). Analysis of longitudinal data: The integration of theoretical model, temporal design, and statistical model. *Annual Review of Psychology, 57,* 505–528.

Cubbage, M. E., & Thomas, K. R. (1989). Freud and disability. *Rehabilitation Psychology, 34,* 161–173.

Dembo, T., Leviton, G. L., & Wright, B. A. (1956). Adjustment to misfortune: A problem of social-psychological rehabilitation. *Artificial Limbs, 3,* 4–62.

deRoon-Cassini, T. A., Mancini, A. D., Rusch, M. D., & Bonanno, G. A. (2010). Psychopathology and resilience following traumatic injury: A latent growth mixture model analysis. *Rehabilitation Psychology, 55,* 1–11.

Diller, L. (1980). The development of a perceptual remediation program in hemiplegia. In L. P. Ince (Ed.), *Behavioral psychology in rehabilitation medicine: Clinical applications* (pp. 64–86). New York: Williams & Wilkins.

Diller, L. (1987). Neuropsychological rehabilitation. In M. J. Meier, A. L. Benton, & L. Diller (Eds.), *Neuropsychological rehabilitation* (pp. 3–17). New York: Guilford.

Dunn, D. S., & Elliott, T. R. (2005). Revisiting a constructive classic: Wright's "Physical Disability: A Psychosocial Approach." *Rehabilitation Psychology, 50,* 183–189.

Dunn, D. S., Uswatte, G., & Elliott, T. R. (2009). Happiness, resilience, and positive growth following disability: Issues for understanding, research, and therapeutic intervention. In

S. J. Lopez (Ed.), *The Oxford handbook of positive psychology* (2nd ed., pp. 651–664). New York: Oxford University Press.

D'Zurilla T. J., & Chang, E. C. (1995). The relations between social problem solving and coping. *Cognitive Therapy and Research, 19,* 547–562.

D'Zurilla, T. J., & Goldfried, M. R. (1971). Problem solving and behavior modification. *Journal of Abnormal Psychology, 78,* 107–126.

D'Zurilla, T. J., & Nezu, A. M. (2001). Problem-solving therapies. In K. S. Dobson (Ed.), *Handbook of cognitive-behavioral therapies* (2nd ed., pp. 211–245). New York: Guilford.

Elliott, T. R. (2002). Presidential address: Defining our common ground to reach new horizons. *Rehabilitation Psychology, 47,* 131–143.

Elliott, T. R., & Byrd, E. K. (1986). Frequently cited works, authors, and sources of research in *Rehabilitation Psychology. Rehabilitation Psychology, 31,* 112–115.

Elliott, T. R., Godshall, F., Herrick, S., Witty, T., & Spruell, M. (1991). Problem-solving appraisal and psychological adjustment following spinal cord injury. *Cognitive Therapy and Research, 15,* 387–398.

Elliott, T. R., & Hurst, M. (2008). Social problem solving and health. In B. Walsh (Ed.), *Biennial review of counseling psychology* (pp. 295–314). New York: Lawrence Erlbaum Press.

Elliott, T. R., & Jackson, W. T. (2005). Cognitive-behavioral therapy in rehabilitation psychology. In A. Freeman (Ed.), *Encyclopedia of cognitive behavior therapy* (pp. 324–327). New York: Springer Science + Business Media.

Elliott, T. R., Kurylo, M., & Rivera, P. A. (2002). Positive growth following acquired physical disability. In C. R. Snyder & S. J. Lopez (Eds.), *Handbook of positive psychology* (pp. 687–699). New York: Oxford University Press.

Elliott, T. R., & Rath, J. F. (2011). Rehabilitation psychology. In E. M. Altmaier & J. I. Hansen (Eds.), *Oxford handbook of counseling psychology* (pp. 679–702). New York: Oxford University Press.

Elliott, T. R., Shewchuk, R., & Richards, J. S. (1999). Caregiver social problem-solving abilities and family member adjustment to recent-onset physical disability. *Rehabilitation Psychology, 44,* 104–123.

Elliott, T. R., Uswatte, G., Lewis, L., & Palmatier, A. (2000). Goal instability and adjustment to physical disability. *Journal of Counseling Psychology, 47,* 251–265.

Elliott, T. R., & Warren, A. M. (2007). Why psychological issues are important. In P. Kennedy (Ed.), *Psychological management of physical disabilities: A practitioner's guide* (pp. 16–39). London: Brunner-Rutledge Press.

Emmons, R. A., & McCullough, M. E. (2003). Counting blessings versus burdens: An experimental investigation of gratitude and subjective well-being in daily life. *Journal of Personality and Social Psychology, 84,* 377–389.

Faul, M., Xu, L., Wald, M. M., & Coronado, V. (2010). *Traumatic brain injury in the United States: Emergency department visits, hospitalizations and deaths, 2002–2006.* Atlanta, GA: Centers for Disease Control and Prevention, National Center for Injury Prevention and Control.

Flavell, J. H. (1971). Stage-related properties of cognitive development. *Cognitive Psychology, 2,* 421–453.

Fordyce, W. E. (1971). Behavioral methods in rehabilitation. In W. S. Neff (Ed.), *Rehabilitation psychology* (pp. 74–108). Washington, DC: American Psychological Association.

Fordyce, W. E. (1976). *Behavioral methods for chronic pain and illness.* Saint Louis, MO: C. V. Mosby.

Fordyce, W. E. (1988). Pain and suffering. *American Psychologist, 43,* 276–283.

Frank, R. G., & Elliott, T. R. (Eds.). (2000). *Handbook of rehabilitation psychology.* Washington, DC: American Psychological Association.

Gilbert, D. T., & Malone, P. S. (1995). The correspondence bias. *Psychological Bulletin, 117,* 21–38.

Glass, T. A., & McAtee, M. (2006). Behavioral science at the crossroads in public health: Extending horizons, envisioning the future. *Social Science and Medicine, 62,* 1650–1671.

Goldstein, G. (2009). Neuropsychology in New York City (1930–1960). *Archives of Clinical Neuropsychology, 5,* 251–264.

Goodkin, R. (1966). Case studies in behavioral research in rehabilitation. *Perceptual and Motor Skills, 23,* 171–182.

Gordon, W. A., Cantor, J., Ashman T., & Brown, M. (2006). Treatment of post-TBI executive dysfunction: Application of theory to clinical practice. *Journal of Head Trauma Rehabilitation, 21,* 156–167.

Grant, J., Elliott, T. R., Weaver, M., Bartolucci, A., & Giger, J. (2002). A telephone intervention with family caregivers of stroke survivors after hospital discharge. *Stroke, 33,* 2060–2065.

Grzesiak, R. C., & Hicock, D. A. (1994). A brief history of psychotherapy in physical disability. *American Journal of Psychotherapy, 48,* 240–250.

Hayes, A. M., Laurenceau, J. P., Feldman, G. C., Strauss, J. L., & Cardaciotto, L. A. (2007). Change is not always linear: The study of nonlinear and discontinuous patterns of change in psychotherapy. *Clinical Psychology Review, 27,* 715–723.

Heider, F. (1958). *The psychology of interpersonal relations.* New York: John Wiley & Sons.

Helmick, K. and members of Consensus Conference. (2010). Cognitive rehabilitation for military personnel with mild traumatic brain injury and chronic post-concussional disorder: Results of April 2009 consensus conference. *NeuroRehabilitation, 26,* 239–255.

Heppner, P. P., & Baker, C. E. (1997). Applications of the problem solving inventory. *Measurement and Evaluation in Counseling and Development, 29,* 229–241.

Hibbard, M., Grober, S., Gordon, W., & Aletta, E. (1990). Modification of cognitive psychotherapy for the treatment of post-stroke depression. *The Behavior Therapist, 13*(1), 15–17.

Hill-Briggs, F. (2003). Problem solving in diabetes self-management: A model of chronic illness self-management behaviors. *Annals of Behavioral Medicine, 25,* 182–193.

Holmbeck, G. N., DeLucia, C., Essner, B., Kelly, L., Zebracki, K., Friedman, D., & Jandasek, B. (2010). Trajectories of psychosocial adjustment in adolescents with spinal bifida: A 6-year, four-wave longitudinal follow-up. *Journal of Consulting and Clinical Psychology, 78,* 511–525.

Hurst, R. (2003). The international disability rights movement and the *ICF. Disability and Rehabilitation, 25,* 572–576.

Ince, L. P. (1980). *Behavioral psychology in rehabilitation medicine.* Baltimore: Williams & Wilkins.

Ince, L. P., Brucker, B. S., & Alba, A. (1978). Reflex conditioning in a spinal man. *Journal of Comparative and Physiological Psychology, 92,* 796–802.

Keany, C. M.-H., & Glueckauf, R. L. (1993). Disability and value change: An overview and reanalysis of acceptance of loss theory. *Rehabilitation Psychology, 38,* 199–210.

Kennedy, M. R. T., Coelho, C., Turkstra, L., Ylvisaker, M., Moore Sohlberg, M., Yorkston, K., et al. (2008). Intervention for executive functions after traumatic brain injury: A systematic review, meta-analysis, and clinical recommendations. *Neuropsychological Rehabilitation, 18,* 257–299.

Kennedy P., Duff, J., Evans, M., & Beedie, A. (2003). Coping effectiveness training reduces depression and anxiety following traumatic spinal cord injuries. *British Journal of Clinical Psychology, 42,* 41–52.

Kennedy, P., Evans, M., & Sandhu, N. (2009). Psychological adjustment to spinal cord injury: The contribution of coping, hope, and cognitive appraisals. *Psychology, Health and Medicine, 14,* 17–33.

Kim, S. (2011). Heart rate variability biofeedback and executive functioning in individuals with chronic traumatic brain injury. Unpublished raw data, Yeshiva University.

King C., & Kennedy P. (1999). Coping effectiveness training for people with spinal cord injury: Preliminary results of a controlled trial. *British Journal of Clinical Psychology, 38,* 5–14.

Kinsella, G., Ong, B., Murtagh, D., Prior, M., & Sawyer, M. (1999). The role of the family for behavioral outcomes in children and adolescents following traumatic brain injury. *Journal of Consulting and Clinical Psychology, 67,* 116–123.

Kurylo, M., Elliott, T. R., DeVivo, L., & Dreer, L. (2004). Caregiver social problem solving abilities and family member adjustment following congestive heart failure. *Journal of Clinical Psychology in Medical Settings, 11,* 151–157.

Laurenceau, J. P., Hayes, A. M., & Feldman, G. C. (2007). Some methodological and statistical issues in the study of change processes in psychotherapy. *Clinical Psychological Review, 27,* 682–695.

Lazarus, R. S., & Folkman, S. (1984). *Stress, appraisal, and coping.* New York: Springer.

Lewin, K. (1935). *A dynamic theory of personality.* New York: McGraw-Hill.

Lippke, S., Schwarzer, R., Ziegelmann, J. P., Scholz, U., & Schüz, B. (2010). Testing stage-specific effects of a stage-matched intervention: A randomized controlled trial targeting physical exercise and its predictors. *Health Education and Behavior, 37,* 533–546.

Lollar, D. J., & Crews, J. E. (2003). Redefining the role of public health in disability. *Annual Reviews in Public Health, 24,* 95–208.

Lucas, R. E. (2007). Long-term disability is associated with lasting changes in subjective well-being: Evidence from two nationally representative longitudinal studies. *Journal of Personality and Social Psychology, 92,* 717–730

Luria, A. R., & Majovski, L. V. (1977). Basic approaches used in American and Soviet clinical neuropsychology. *American Psychologist, 32,* 959–968.

Luszczynska, A., Mazurkiewicz, M., Ziegelman J. P., & Schwarzer, R. (2007). Recovery self-efficacy and intention as predictors of running or jogging behavior: A cross-lagged panel analysis over a two-year period. *Psychology of Sport and Exercise, 8,* 247–260.

Luszczynska, A., & Sutton, S. (2006). Physical activity after cardiac rehabilitation: Evidence that different types of self-efficacy are important in maintainers and relapsers. *Rehabilitation Psychology, 51,* 314–321.

Luszczynska, A., Tryburcy, M., & Schwarzer, R. (2007). Improving fruit and vegetable consumption: A self-efficacy intervention compared to a combined self-efficacy and planning intervention. *Health Education Research, 22,* 630–638.

Majovski, L. V., & Jacques, S. (1980). Current neuropsychological approaches in assessment, rehabilitation, and clinical research of central nervous system disorders. *Neurosurgery, 7,* 182–186.

McGlynn, S. M. (1990). Behavioral approaches to neuropsychological rehabilitation. *Psychological Bulletin, 108,* 420–441.

Miller, N. E., & Brucker, B. S. (1979). A learned visceral response apparently independent of skeletal ones in patients paralyzed by spinal lesions. In N. Birbaumer & H. D. Kimmel (Eds.), *Biofeedback and self-regulation* (pp. 287–304). Hillside, NJ: Erlbaum.

Mynors-Wallis, L. M., Gath, D. H., Lloyd-Thomas, A. R., & Tomlinson, D. (1995). Randomised controlled trial comparing problem-solving treatment with amitriptyline and placebo for major depression in primary care. *British Medical Journal, 310,* 441–445.

National Institute of Neurological Disorders and Stroke (2004). *Stroke: Hope through research.* Bethesda, MD: National Institutes of Health.

Nezu, A. M., Felgoise, S. H., McClure, K. S., & Houts, P. (2003). Project Genesis: Assessing the efficacy of problem-solving therapy for distressed adult cancer patients. *Journal of Consulting and Clinical Psychology, 71,* 1036–1048.

Nezu, A. M., Nezu, C. M., Friedman, S., & Faddis, S. (1998). *Helping cancer patients cope: A problem-solving approach.* Washington, DC: American Psychological Association.

Parker, R., Szymanski, E., & Patterson, J. (Eds.). (2005). *Rehabilitation counseling: Basics and beyond* (4th ed.). Austin, TX: Pro-Ed.

Patterson, D. R. (2005). Behavioral methods for chronic pain and illness: A reconsideration and appreciation. *Rehabilitation Psychology, 50,* 312–315.

Peterson, D. B. (2005). International Classification of Functioning, Disability and Health (*ICF*): An introduction for rehabilitation psychologists. *Rehabilitation Psychology, 50,* 105–112.

Peterson, D. B., & Elliott, T. R. (2008). Advances in conceptualizing and studying disability. In R. Lent & S. Brown (Eds.), *Handbook of counseling psychology* (4th ed., pp. 212–230). New York: Sage

Peterson, D. B., & Rosenthal, D. R. (2005). The International Classification of Functioning, Disability, and Health (*ICF*) as an allegory for history and systems in rehabilitation education. *Rehabilitation Education, 19,* 75–80.

Prigatano, G. P. (1999). Psychotherapy and psychotherapeutic interventions in brain injury rehabilitation. In M. Rosenthal, E. R. Griffith, J. S. Kreutzer, & B. Pentland (Eds.), *Rehabilitation of the adult and child with traumatic brain injury* (3rd ed., pp. 275–283). Philadelphia: F. A. Davis.

Pulvermuller, F. B., Neininger, B., Elbert, T., Mohr, B., Rockstroh, B., Koebbel, P., & Taub, E. (2001). Constraint-induced therapy of chronic aphasia after stroke. *Stroke, 32,* 1621–1626.

Radnitz, C. L. (Ed.) (2000). *Cognitive-behavioral interventions for persons with disabilities.* Northvale, NJ: Jason Aronson, Inc.

Ramkumar, N., & Elliott, T. R. (2010). Family caregiving of persons following neurotrauma: Issues in research, service, and policy. *NeuroRehabilitation, 27,* 105–112.

Rath, J. F., Hennessy, J. J., & Diller, L. (2003). Social problem solving and community integration in post-acute rehabilitation outpatients with traumatic brain injury. *Rehabilitation Psychology, 48,* 137–144.

Rath, J. F., Hradil, A. L., Litke, D. R., & Diller, L. (2011). Clinical applications of problem-solving research in neuro-psychological rehabilitation: Addressing the subjective experience of cognitive deficits in outpatients with acquired brain injury. *Rehabilitation Psychology, 56,* 320–328.

Rath, J. F., Langenbahn, D. M., Simon, D., Sherr, R. L., Fletcher, J., & Diller, L. (2004). The construct of problem solving in higher level neuropsychological assessment and rehabilitation. *Archives of Clinical Neuropsychology, 19,* 613–635.

Rath, J. F., Simon, D., Langenbahn, D. M., Sherr, R. L., & Diller, L. (2000). Measurement of problem-solving deficits in adults with acquired brain damage. *Journal of Head Trauma Rehabilitation, 15,* 724–733.

Rath, J. F., Simon, D., Langenbahn, D. M., Sherr, R. L., & Diller, L. (2003). Group treatment of problem-solving deficits in outpatients with traumatic brain injury: A randomized outcome study. *Neuropsychological Rehabilitation, 13,* 461–488.

Reel, K., & Feaver, S. (2006). Models: Terminology and usefulness. In S. Davis (Ed.), *Rehabilitation: The use of theories and models in practice* (pp. 49–62). New York: Elsevier.

Reuter, T., Ziegelmann, J. P., Lippke, S., & Schwarzer, R. (2009). Long-term relations between intentions, planning, and exercise: A 3-year longitudinal study after orthopedic rehabilitation. *Rehabilitation Psychology, 54,* 363–371.

Rivera, P. A., Elliott, T. R., Berry, I., & Grant, J. (2008). Problem-solving training for family caregivers of persons with traumatic brain injuries: A randomized controlled trial. *Archives of Physical Medicine and Rehabilitation, 89,* 931–941.

Rivara, J., Jaffe, K., Polissar, N., Fay, G., Liao, S., & Martin, K. (1996). Predictors of family functioning and change 3 years after traumatic brain injury in children. *Archives of Physical Medicine and Rehabilitation, 77,* 754–764.

Ross, L. (1977). The intuitive psychologist and his shortcomings: Distortions in the attribution process. In L. Berkowitz (Ed.), *Advances in experimental social psychology* (vol. 10, pp. 173–220). New York: Academic Press.

Ross, L., & Nisbett, R. E. (1991). *The person and the situation: Perspectives of social psychology.* New York: McGraw-Hill.

Ryan, J. J., & Tree, H. A. (2004). Essential readings in rehabilitation psychology. *Teaching of Psychology, 31,* 138–140.

Shanmugham, K., Cano, M., Elliott, T. R., & Davis, M. J. (2009). Social problem solving abilities, relationship satisfaction, and distress among family caregivers of stroke survivors. *Brain Injury, 23,* 92–100.

Scherer, M. J., Blair, K. L., Banks, M. E., Brucker, B., Corrigan, J., & Wegener, S. H. (2004). Rehabilitation psychology. In W. E. Craighead & C. B. Nemeroff (Eds.), *The concise Corsini encyclopedia of psychology and behavioral science* (3rd ed., pp. 801–802). Hoboken, NJ: Wiley .

Schüz, B., Sniehotta, F. F., & Schwarzer, R. (2007). Stage-specific effects of an action control intervention on dental flossing. *Health Education Research, 22,* 332–341

Schwarzer, R. (2008). Modeling health behavior change: How to predict and modify the adoption and maintenance of health behaviors. *Applied Psychology: An International Review, 57,* 1–29.

Schwarzer, R., Cao, D. S., & Lippke, S. (2010). Stage-matched minimal interventions to enhance physical activity in Chinese adolescents. *Journal of Adolescent Health, 47,* 533–539.

Siller, J. (1969). Psychological situation of the disabled with spinal cord injuries. *Rehabilitation Literature, 30,* 290–296.

Siller, J. (1988). Intrapsychic aspects of attitudes toward persons with disabilities. In H. E. Yuker (Ed.), *Attitudes toward persons with disabilities* (pp. 58–67). Springer: New York.

Siller, J., Chipman, A., Ferguson, L. T., & Vann, D. H. (1967). *Attitudes of the nondisabled toward the physically disabled.* New York: New York University School of Education.

Snyder, C. R. (1998). *A case for hope in pain, loss, and suffering.* New York: Brunner Mazel.

Taub, E. (1980). Somatosensory deafferentation research with monkeys: Implications for rehabilitation medicine. In L. P. Ince (Ed.), *Behavioral psychology in rehabilitation medicine: Clinical applications* (pp. 371–401). New York: Williams & Wilkins.

Taub, E., Crago, J. E., & Uswatte, G. (1998). Constraint-induced movement therapy: A new approach to treatment in physical rehabilitation. *Rehabilitation Psychology, 43,* 152–170.

Taub, E., & Uswatte, G. (2000). Constraint-induced movement therapy based on behavioral neuroscience. In R. G. Frank & T. R. Elliott (Eds.), *Handbook of rehabilitation psychology* (pp. 475–496). Washington, DC: American Psychological Association.

Taub, E., Uswatte, G., & Elbert, T. (2002). New treatments in neurorehabilitation founded on basic research [Review]. *Nature Reviews Neuroscience, 3,* 228–236.

Taub, E., Uswatte, G., & Pidikiti, R. (1999). Constraint-induced movement therapy: A new family of techniques with broad application to physical rehabilitation—a clinical review. *Journal of Rehabilitation Research and Development, 36,* 237–251.

Tedeschi, R. G., Park, C. L., & Calhoun L. G. (1998). Posttraumatic growth; Conceptual issues. In R. G. Tedeschi, C. L. Park, & L. G. Calhoun (Eds.), *Posttraumatic growth: Positive changes in the aftermath of crisis* (pp. 1–22). Mahwah, NJ: Lawrence Erlbaum.

Thomas, K. R., & Siller, J. (1999). Object loss, mourning, and adjustment to disability. *Psychoanalytic Psychology, 16,* 179–197.

Toobert, D. J., & Glasgow, R. E. (1991). Problem solving and diabetes self-care. *Journal of Behavioral Medicine, 14,* 71–86.

Tucker, J. A., & Reed, G. (2008). Evidentiary pluralism as a strategy for research and evidence-based practice in rehabilitation psychology. *Rehabilitation Psychology, 53,* 279–293.

Uswatte, G., & Taub, E. (2005). Implications of the learned nonuse formulation for measuring rehabilitation outcomes: Lessons from constraint-induced movement therapy. *Rehabilitation Psychology, 50,* 34–42.

von Cramon, D., Matthes-von Cramon, G., & Mai, N. (1991). Problem-solving deficits in brain injured patients: A therapeutic approach. *Neuropsychological Rehabilitation, 1,* 45–64.

Wade, S. L., Carey, J., & Wolfe, C. R. (2006a). An online family intervention to reduce parental distress following pediatric brain injury. *Journal of Consulting and Clinical Psychology, 74,* 445–454.

Wade, S. L., Carey, J. & Wolfe, C. R. (2006b). The efficacy of an online cognitive behavioral family intervention in improving child behavior and social competence in pediatric brain injury. *Rehabilitation Psychology, 51,* 179–189.

Weiss, T., Miltner, W. H. R., Adler, T., Bruckner, L., & Taub, E. (1999). Decrease in phantom limb pain associated with prosthesis-induced increased use of an amputation stump. *Neuroscience Letters, 272,* 131–134.

West, S. G., Ryu, E., Kwok, O.-M., & Cham, H. (2011). Multilevel modeling: Current and future applications in personality research. *Journal of Personality, 79,* 2–50.

Wiedemann, A. U., Schüz, B., Sniehotta, F. F., Scholz, U., & Schwarzer, R. (2009). Disentangling the relation between intentions, planning, and behaviour: A moderated mediation analysis. *Psychology and Health, 24,* 67–79.

Wiedemann, A. U., Lippke, S., Reuter, T., Schüz, B., Ziegelmann, J. P., & Schwarzer, R. (2009). Prediction of stage transitions in fruit and vegetable intake. *Health Education Research, 24,* 596–607.

Wilson, B. A. (1981). A survey of behavioural treatments carried out at a rehabilitation centre. In G. E. Powell (Ed.), *Brain function therapy* (pp. 256–275). Aldershot, England: Gower Press.

Wilson, B. A. (2002). Towards a comprehensive model of cognitive rehabilitation, *Neuropsychological Rehabilitation, 12,* 97–110

World Health Organization. (2001). *ICF: International Classification of Functioning, Disability, and Health.* Geneva, Switzerland: Author.

Wright, B. A. (1960). *Physical disability: A psychological approach.* New York: Harper & Row.

Wright, B. A. (1983). *Physical disability: A psychosocial approach* (2nd ed.). New York: Harper & Row.

Wu, W., West, S. G., & Hughes, J. N. (2008). Effect of retention in first grade on children's achievement trajectories over four years: A piecewise growth analysis using propensity score matching. *Journal of Educational Psychology, 100,* 727–740.

Adjustment to Chronic Illness and Disabilities: Theoretical Perspectives, Empirical Findings, and Unresolved Issues

Hanoch Livneh *and* Erin Martz

Abstract

Chronic illnesses and disabilities (CID) are integral parts of life, and their likelihood of occurrence increases with one's age. The experience of CID invariably necessitates personal adaptation to both the individual's diminished functional capacities and their altered interactions with the physical and social environments. The field of psychosocial adaptation (PA) to CID has exponentially grown during the past 30 years and can be conveniently collapsed into two broad domains, namely, conceptual and empirical approaches to the study of PA to CID. The conceptual approach is mostly rooted in extensive clinical observations of individuals following the aftermath of CID onset and has led to the development of numerous theoretical frameworks of PA to CID and coping with CID. Here, we provide a review of the most influential conceptual models of PA to CID. The empirical literature is examined in this chapter by focusing on those studies that have directly sought to investigate the relationships (albeit not necessarily causal in nature) among a wide range of sociodemographic characteristics, CID-linked factors, personality attributes and coping strategies, and environmental influences (these four classes of variables are typically considered as predictors, mediators or moderators), and measures of PA to CID (the latter commonly regarded as outcomes). Due to space restrictions, our review of the empirical literature only focuses on certain types of CIDs, namely, spinal cord injuries, cancer, and multiple sclerosis. This chapter concludes with a discussion of those issues that need to be addressed by future researchers in the field of adaptation to CID.

Key Words: Psychosocial adaptation, models of adaptation, biopsychosocial, coping, engagement coping, disengagement coping, depression, anxiety, social support, perceptions of control, self-efficacy, hope, optimism, quality of life, well-being, life satisfaction.

Chronic illnesses and disabilities (CID) are integral parts of life, and their likelihood of occurrence increases with age (Fries, 2002; Murray & Lopez, 1997a, 1997b). The experience of CID invariably necessitates personal adaptation to both the individual's diminished functional capacities and the altered interactions with the physical and social environments. Clinicians and researchers in the field of rehabilitation psychology have made remarkable strides that have resulted in better understanding of the experiences a person undergoes following the onset of CID. Moreover, extant theoretical models

and empirical findings have emerged over the past decades that successfully place many of these experiences within a scientifically based context, linking the various components and processes of psychosocial adaptation to CID with measurable outcomes. Indeed, over the past half-century, rehabilitation psychologists have amassed a body of knowledge that rivals that produced by any other established psychological specialties.

The exponential growth of the field of psychosocial adaptation (PA) to CID during the past 30 years has been solidly documented in areas such as the development of both clinically driven and empirically validated models of adaptation; the investigation of numerous predictors, mediators, and moderators of PA to CID; and the study of various outcome criteria and measures of success that reflect PA to CID. In fact, the existing literature on adaptation to CID can be conveniently collapsed into two broad domains; namely, conceptual and empirical approaches to the study of PA to CID. The conceptual approach is mostly rooted in extensive clinical observations of individuals following the aftermath of CID onset. These mostly longitudinal observations then spawn theoretical models of the nature, progression, and variability of adaptation to CID. The empirical approach, although often derived from theoretical models, reflects more squarely the post-positivistic framework that shoulders the search for those correlates and predictive variables that elucidate the conditions under which people with CID best adapt to their conditions. To this end, the proponents of the latter approach also strive to construct, or thoughtfully adopt, psychometrically sound instruments that measure both disability-related and psychosocial (e.g., personality attributes, coping modes) predictors, as well as specific and global outcomes that best capture successful PA to CID. The wealth of theoretical models and empirical findings on adaptation to CID has, invariably, resulted in competing models of PA and conflicting findings on the nature of the relationships between many of the examined predictors and the various PA outcomes.

In this chapter, therefore, we first review the most influential theoretical frameworks of PA to CID. In view of space constraints, not all theoretical perspectives are included in our review. We then turn our attention to the empirical literature and to those studies that have directly sought to examine the relationships (albeit not necessarily causal in nature) among a wide range of sociodemographic characteristics, CID-linked factors, personality attributes, environmental influences (typically considered as predictors, mediators, or moderators), and measures of PA to CID (the latter commonly regarded as outcomes). Again, due to space restrictions, our review of the empirical literature, by necessity, can only focus on certain types of CIDs. Our review, therefore, is mostly restricted to findings obtained from studies of people with spinal cord injuries (SCI), cancer, and multiple sclerosis (MS). (*Note:* Bolded references in this chapter indicate that the research involved a longitudinal study.)

Theoretical Models of Psychosocial Adaptation to Chronic Illness and Disability

Conceptual frameworks of adaptation to CID have been part of the field of rehabilitation psychology for over half a century and span a wide spectrum of views. Naturally, these models differ with regard to the essential components, processes, dynamics, and temporal relationships among the proposed ingredients of the model. Although virtually all share certain perspectives on the nature of human adaptation to adversity, or more specifically the onset of CID (e.g., PA as a dynamic, continuously evolving process; PA as an integrated homeostatic phenomenon of intrapersonal, interpersonal, and environmental elements; PA as a fine amalgam of both idiosyncratic and universal life experiences), they do differ in their philosophical-theoretical underpinnings and the complexities of the proposed systems. In this section, we offer a review of those proposed models of PA that have kindled the most interest among researchers and clinicians.

Unidimensional, Linear Models of Adaptation

Earlier models of PA to CID were noted mostly by their rather rigid adherence to the concept of linearity (Cohn, 1961; Dunn, 1975; Falek & Britton, 1974; Fink, 1967; Matson & Brooks, 1977; Shontz, 1965). Proponents of these models maintained that, following the onset of CID, the human psyche typically followed a somewhat predictable, indeed almost universal, sequence of psychological experiences or reactions (also termed stages or phases). These experiences were viewed as largely internally driven. Although certain structural discrepancies existed among these models regarding the purported nature, number, and sequencing of these psychic reactions, they nevertheless most often included such reactions as shock, anxiety, denial, depression, anger, and some form of acceptance/reintegration (Livneh & Parker, 2005). A shared assumption by all these models was that reactions observed at a later time (more distal to CID onset) can only be experienced after certain earlier reactions (more proximal to CID onset) have been experienced and successfully resolved. Although enviously parsimonious in nature, these early models failed to consider the complexity of the human experience and the continuously interactive power of external influences—both environmental and sociocultural—and lacked empirical support.

Pendular Models of Adaptation

Proponents of the notion that PA to CID and related human losses (Charmaz, 1983, 1993, 1995; Kendall & Buys, 1998; Stroebe & Schut, 1999; Yoshida, 1993) posit that the process of adaptation consists of alternation (often referred to as "swings") between pre-CID and post-CID identities. Put differently, the person with sudden-onset CID oscillates between perceptions of health or normalcy (past orientation) and realization of existing illness or disability (present orientation). These alternating perceptions are portrayed as pendular motions or trajectories. The process of adaptation, accordingly, follows a gradual progression through which an altered identity (self with CID) is reconstructed. This newly emerging identity now incorporates the incurred physical losses and changes in functional abilities (Charmaz, 1983, 1995; Yoshida, 1993). Adaptation, in line with this conceptual framework, does not follow a linear trajectory but, instead, is composed of repeated experiences and efforts to accommodate and assimilate perceived losses and limitations. In a related vein, Paterson and her colleagues (Paterson, 2001; Thorne & Paterson, 1998), based on their meta-synthesis of qualitative research findings, arrived at a similar model they term the "shifting perspectives" model of CID. They posit that, following the onset of CID, the individual lives in a dual world in which both wellness and illness exist. Moreover, in their dual world, people with CID shift perspectives in accordance with their viewing the CID as being a foreground versus background factor. To wit, following the onset of CID, personal perspectives often shift from adaptive (wellness in foreground) to nonadaptive (illness in foreground). These shifts are likely to be influenced by both internal and external life events. As with the previously reviewed linear model, the pendular model, despite its clinical appeal and reliance on only a few essential elements, is lacking empirical support. Also, the role played by external factors is only tangentially addressed. Finally, these models are mostly silent on how the experience and duration of the CID contribute to the proposed shifts.

Interactive Models of Adaptation

The roots of interactive models of PA to CID could be traced to the seminal work of Kurt Lewin (Lewin, 1997; Lewin, Heider, & Heider, 1936) and his followers in the fields of social psychology and somatopsychology. These researchers (L. Meyerson, T. Dembo, R. Barker, G. Leviton, and B. Wright) viewed adaptation as a reciprocal, iterative process that emphasized that human behavior is best determined by two sets of interactive variables. The first set is comprised of intraindividual variables that include both physical determinants (e.g., nature and severity of the CID) and psychological aspects (e.g., self-concept, belief system). The second set is made up of external variables that are part of the environment or life space in which the person operates, and refers to the physical, social, and vocational domains of one's environment. The interaction between these two sets of variables, then, determines the person's behavior, or more specifically, the level of PA to CID (Livneh, 2001; Shontz, 1975; Smedema, Bakken-Gillen, & Dalton, 2009; Wright, 1983). In Lewin's formulaic notation—$B = f(P, E)$—that is, behavior (or adaptive functioning) is a function of the interaction between the person and his or her environment. In the context of the field of somatopsychology, Barker, Wright, and their colleagues (Barker, Wright, Meyerson, & Gonick, 1953; Dembo, Leviton, & Wright, 1956; Wright, 1960, 1983) argued that the meaning of, and attitudes toward, CID, as well as the success of this adaptation, is best understood as the product of the interaction between the person's internal needs, wishes, and motives and the external influences (both mitigating and repressive) exerted by the individual's overall life context. The strengths of the somatopsychological interactive model stem from its clinically intuitive approach to human behavior, its attention to contextual factors, and the body of research findings it has generated over the past few decades. An area that has not been fully addressed by proponents of this model is the role that the passage of time plays in this interactive model, namely, $B = f(P, E, T)$.

Ecological Models

Ecological models of adaptation to life crises (Moos & Schaefer, 1984), life transitions (Schlossberg, 1981), and CID span a wide range of life conditions and, by necessity, vary along several dimensions, including their complexity, the nature and type of crisis (e.g., sudden onset vs. gradual, unexpected vs. expected), experienced symptoms, incurred functional limitations, duration of presenting problem(s), developmental stage, predictability and controllability of medical manifestations, and temporal unfolding of experienced reactions (for overview of several of these earlier ecological models the reader is referred to Livneh and Antonak (1997, chapter 23) and Smedema et al. (2009). In this section, we focus on four of these models, namely Moos and colleagues' *crisis and coping model* (Moos & Holahan, 2007; Moos & Schaefer, 1984, 1986); Livneh and Antonak's *adaptation to CID model* (Livneh, 2001; Livneh & Antonak, 1997); Devins' *illness intrusiveness model* (Devins, 1989; Devins, Edworthy, Guthrie, & Martin, 1992; Devins, Seland, Klein, Edworthy, & Saary, 1993); and Bishop's *disability centrality model* (Bishop, 2005a, 2005b; Bishop, Smedema, & Lee, 2009; Bishop, Stenhoff, & Shepard, 2007).

MOOS' CRISIS AND COPING MODEL

Moos and his colleagues' model of coping with life crises and CID has undergone several changes and refinements over the past 25 years. In reviewing this model, we focus on its most recent version (Moos & Holahan, 2007). Broadly speaking, this biopsychosocial model (Figure 4.1) consists of three sets of components. The first component addresses three interacting factors (panels); namely, personal resources, health-related factors, and the person's social-physical environment. The panel of personal resources includes two subsets of resources. The first is made up of sociodemographic characteristics (age, gender, education), while the second refers to personal (intellectual and affective) characteristics, such as cognitive ability, ego strength, belief system, self-concept, and perceived locus of control. The second panel, that of health-related factors, refers to those CID-related characteristics that are inherent in the nature, severity, and duration of the condition (e.g., body part/function affected, progression of condition, stage and severity of CID), as well as the nature of the health care environment and

availability of therapeutic modalities. The third and final panel of the first component is composed of the person's physical and social environments. The former refers to the individual's social network, whereas the latter addresses the physical features of the environment, including the accessibility of one's community, home, and work settings.

These three panels of the first model's component influence in concert the second component, which is made up of three linearly related panels; namely, cognitive appraisal, adaptive tasks, and coping skills. Cognitive appraisal acts as a kind of filtering device for the previous three panels and, in turn, influences the next two panels—adaptive tasks and coping skills. The cognitive appraisal panel, reminiscent of Lazarus' (Lazarus, 1966; Lazarus & Folkman, 1984) conception of primary coping, refers to the perceived meaning that the person associates with the existence of CID. It also includes those perceptions regarding the condition's controllability, predictability, and changeability. Cognitive appraisals precede and partially determine the adaptive tasks (next panel) that the person adopts to manage the CID. Adaptive tasks include a wide range of CID-generated tasks, such as those that focus on managing symptoms of discomfort and pain; managing the hospital environment, treatment procedures, and relationships with health care providers; sustaining positive relationships with family members and social network; and managing and balancing one's emotions.

The third and final panel of the second component is that of coping skills. In their most recent work, Moos and Holahan (2007) described eight categories

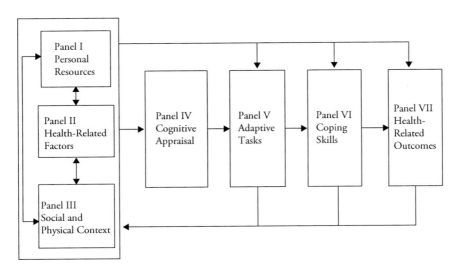

Figure 4.1 Conceptual model of the deteminants of health-related outcomes of chronic illness and disability.

of coping classified along to a 2 × 2 (approach vs. avoidance × cognitive vs. behavioral) grid. Examples of these coping modes include logical analysis (cognitive/approach), seeking support (behavioral/approach), avoidance-denial (cognitive/avoidance), and emotional venting (behavioral/avoidance).

The third and final component of this model consists of a single panel: health-related outcomes. This panel addresses the end product of the interactions among and progression of the earlier six panels. Although health-related outcomes are viewed as the final component of the model, Moos and Holahan (2007, p. 109) maintain that "in a mutual feedback cycle, health-related outcomes may alter the preceding sets of factors and consequently change longer-term health outcomes."

The strengths of Moos and colleagues' model are its continuous growth from extensive review of earlier theoretical analyses and empirical research findings. In fact, it could be argued that it combines a "rehabilitation-derived" approach of grounded theory with accumulated empirical findings to the understanding PA to crisis and CID. The model is clinically useful and offers rehabilitation psychologists fertile ground for working with diverse populations of people with CID. Also, the heuristic value of the model is evident from its carefully orchestrated structure and the continuous efforts to refine its applicability to people with CID. An area that has not been fully explored evolves around the nature and scope of the health-related outcomes as framed by Moos' model, and their relationships to the more encompassing concept of quality of life.

LIVNEH AND ANTONAK'S ADAPTATION TO THE CID MODEL

Livneh and Antonak's (Livneh, 2001; Livneh & Antonak, 1997) model bears certain similarities to that of Moos and his colleagues and may even be considered an outgrowth of it (Figure 4.2). It consists of three main components; namely, antecedents, processes, and outcomes of adaptation. The first component (antecedents) includes two interacting sets of variables: CID-triggering events (e.g., genetics, injury, chronic illness, and ageing processes) and contextual variables (existing biological, psychosocial, and environmental conditions). The latter are those mostly stable situational conditions that prevailed at the time of CID onset and include, among others, the person's health status, age, gender, and ethnicity (biological status); cognitive and emotional developmental phase, personal and social identities (psychosocial status); and physical, socioeconomic, and attitudinal contexts (environmental status).

These two sets of background variables exert considerable influence upon the next two sets of interacting factors, categorized under the "process" component. These include, first, unfolding psychosocial reactions to the onset of CID and, second, contextual influences that exist (and often shift) during the period following CID onset. The former set (experienced reactions) refers to those reactions often reported by people following the onset of CID (e.g., anxiety, depression, anger). The latter set of existing contextual influences refers to those dynamic and interacting forces that, directly or indirectly, affect the nature, valence, and progression of the adaptation process. These continuously evolving external and internal forces commonly refer to the personal, interpersonal, and environmental influences that undergo constant, even if subtle, changes during the process of adaptation. They normally stem from changes in functional capacities, course of the CID, the individual's self-concept, perceived control, sense of coherence, and coping modalities, as well as encountered architectural barriers and available social support.

The two interacting process sets, in turn (and with the added influence of the previously described antecedent sets), determine to a large extent the outcomes of the person's level of PA to CID. The third and final set, named "outcomes," is viewed conceptually as the end product of the adaptation process. It is further equated with the concept of quality of life (QOL), the overarching outcome criterion of PA to CID. Quality of life is normally regarded as a multidimensional concept (Bishop, 2005a; Diener, Suh, Lucas, & Smith, 1999; Kinney, Burfitt, Stullenbarger, Rees, & DeBolt, 1996) and, in the current model, it is depicted as consisting of three broad domains. These are intrapersonal functioning (subjective well-being, life satisfaction, perceived health), interpersonal functioning (satisfaction with family life, peer relations, and social activities), and extrapersonal functioning (performance of work activities and/or recreational pursuits, living arrangements, financial status). The person's adaptation to CID is, accordingly, determined by his or her QOL across these life domains.

As was observed with Moos' model of coping with crisis, the Livneh and Antonak model is based on theoretical formulations and clinical observations, as well as a growing body of empirical data derived from the rehabilitation psychology and disability studies literatures of the past half-century. As such,

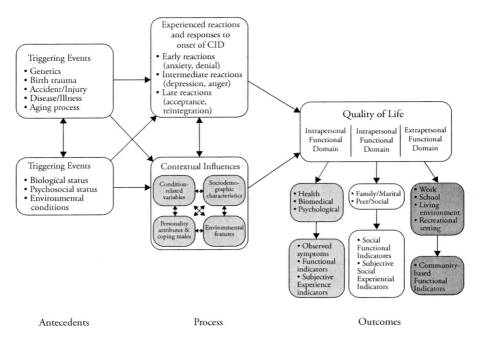

Antecedents　　　　　　　Process　　　　　　　Outcomes

Figure 4.2 A model depicting the structure, content, and process of psychosocial adaptation to CID.

the model may also be regarded as a loose derivative of the grounded theory framework, honed by recent empirical research findings. Because of its inherent complexity and reliance on a large number of interacting components, the model may defy traditional validation procedures and may require a segmented approach to examining its various components and the proposed interactions among them.

DEVINS' ILLNESS INTRUSIVENESS MODEL

Devins' model of PA to CID mostly grew out of the author's and his colleagues' research in the areas of end-stage renal disease (Devins et al., 1983, 1990) and MS (Devins et al., 1993). Illness intrusiveness (II) is defined by the author as "illness-induced disruptions to valued activities and interests" (Devins & Binik, 1996, p. 642). As such, II is regarded as a set of events that is experienced frequently by people with CID. These CID-triggered interruptions stem from both internally induced characteristics (e.g., severity of symptoms, functional limitations, discomfort, pain, fatigue), as well as from externally derived influences. The latter are mostly associated with treatment-linked factors, such as the nature of the therapeutic modalities, the time required for treatment, and the stress engendered by treatment (Devins, 1989; Devins et al., 1992; Devins et al., 1993). Although the model has assumed slightly different versions over the years, it

can best be depicted as follows: Burden of Illness → Functional Deficits → Physical Disability → Illness Intrusiveness → Personal Control → Psychosocial Well-Being (Devins et al., 1992; Devins et al., 1993).

The first three of these components (burden of illness, functional deficits, physical disability) focus on CID-triggered anatomical, physiological, and biochemical changes in the person's body (burden of illness); the functional implications that follow these changes, as expressed in diminished physical capacity (functional deficits); and the progression of impairments—discrete, organ-specific limitations to more complex, integrative body systems (physical disability). The next two hypothesized components (II and personal control) reflect the cumulative contributions of the first three components to more global lifestyle disruptions. These disruptions can be found in diminished participation in valued activities (II), as well as in perceptions of decreased capacity to influence positive outcomes in one's life (personal control). Put differently, CID-induced lifestyle disruptions exert their harmful impact through two main mechanisms that operate to limit the availability of positive experiences that stem from reduced accessibility to personally valued activities and interests, and/or minimize the ability to exert personal control over valued life interests and experiences.

The final component of the model targets the impact of II and diminished perceptions of personal control on PA to CID, here indicated by measures of psychosocial well-being and its complementary concept of emotional distress (Devins et al., 1983, 1992, 1993). In a later model, Devins, apparently realizing an earlier omission of the direct and moderating roles played by psychosocial factors in the II model, offered a slightly expanded version of the model that now included these factors. These psychological (e.g., personality attributes) and social (e.g., stigma) factors are regarded in the revised model as forces that either directly or indirectly influence each of the model's existing components, including II and the psychosocial well-being outcomes. Furthermore, psychosocial well-being and emotional distress were now portrayed as two facets of a global outcome component of quality of life, according to the work of Devins and Shnek (2000). One additional modification of the revised model includes the parceling out of the treatment factors from the II component and inserting them as precursors to the II factor.

Devins' model is one of the most empirically researched models of PA to CID and has been consistently validated with various groups of people with CID. When compared to the earlier models of Moos, and Livneh and Antonak, the II model appears as a streamlined version of the two, incorporating a far smaller number of overall variables while paying particular attention to one important moderating variable—II. Indeed, according to Devins' model, II is that crucial link among the antecedent components of sociodemographic variables, CID-liked factors, and existing personality attributes, and the outcome component of psychosocial well-being. As such, the II model can also be regarded as a "carved out," empirically supported model within the larger contextual framework offered by the previously discussed models. Moreover, the concept of II, which carries certain theoretical affinity to concepts such as perceived personal control (Partridge & Johnston, 1989) and perceived health locus of control (Christensen, Wiebe, Benotsch, & Lawton, 1996), could also be viewed as a form of appraisal coping, as suggested by the work of Lazarus and his colleagues (Folkman & Lazarus, 1990; Lazarus, 1966; Lazarus & Folkman, 1984). The II model's minimal attention of the role played by other coping modalities is one area that may suggest some deficiency in this otherwise well conceived and empirically sound model.

BISHOP'S DISABILITY CENTRALITY MODEL

Bishop's model (Bishop, 2005a, 2005b; Bishop et al., 2009) has been described by its author as an extension of the II model. The disability centrality (DC) model, however, differs from its predecessor in several aspects, among them: its more fully developed conceptualization of QOL and its integrated domains; its broader theoretical underpinnings, which were established by a thorough synthesis of several existing frameworks derived from reviews of both the rehabilitation psychology and counseling literature, and leading QOL models; and the introduction of two new and promising constructs that are conceptually and temporally linked to QOL, namely, domain centrality and domain control.

Bishop (2005a, 2005b) describes his model in terms of three broad underlying components. The first focuses on the ultimate outcome criterion of adaptation to CID, that of QOL. He views QOL as a dynamic and balanced summative evaluation of well-being and life satisfaction construed by the individual with regard to those life domains invested with greater personal importance. Quality of life, therefore, is best understood by Bishop as a subjective overall perception of the person's PA to life, including life with CID. The second component incorporates Devins' II model. As such, the concept of II is regarded as a prime moderator of the impact of CID-related factors on PA to CID (i.e., QOL). Finally, Bishop's model further suggests the existence of two additional psychosocial mechanisms that link the impact of CID to QOL; namely, domain satisfaction and domain control. Domain satisfaction is seen as "a dynamic process of maintaining satisfaction in central domains and reprioritizing domain centrality to close perceived gaps between the presently experienced QOL and the desired or expected level of QOL" (Bishop et al., 2009, p. 537). Domain satisfaction is, therefore, a concept parallel to Frisch's (1999) concept of domain importance, as both suggest that people value certain personal life domains and, accordingly, regard these as more influential on their overall QOL. Domain control, in contrast, refers to the perceived impact that CID exerts on the individual's ability to control changing life conditions (e.g., social, vocational, environmental) and pursued outcomes.

Bishop argues that, following the onset of CID, the individual experiences appreciable impact on his or her perceived QOL. He further posits that three possible outcomes typically follow. First, the person could de-emphasize the importance of certain previously held beliefs as central life domains so that they now become marginalized to the overall QOL (importance change). This outcome also suggests that hitherto more peripheral domains may now be elevated in their ability to satisfy QOL and gradually occupy a more central role in the perception of QOL. Second, the person could seek to increase personal control over his or her life conditions and outcomes (control change). Typically, the assuming of increased control is manifested through self-management, medical or psychosocial interventions, or environmental accommodations. Finally, the individual adopts neither of the two venues and the overall diminished QOL continues unmitigated.

The DC model, as posited by Bishop (Bishop, 2005a, 2005b; Bishop et al., 2009), should be assessed within the contexts of the earlier reviewed models, especially Devins' II model. Also, it draws on concepts introduced by other CID-linked, psychodynamic-driven models such as Beatrice Wright's somatopsychological model (Wright, 1983) and Shontz's (1975) principles of subjectively interpreted reality (i.e., individually perceived QOL) and the person as a dynamically integrated unit (i.e., QOL domains shift and are reprioritized following the onset of CID). Within these contexts, Bishop's model can be regarded as a further extension and refinement of Devins' model. In fact, it can also be viewed as a conceptually sound effort to link Devins' model to a broader understanding of the concept of QOL and its multidimensional structure. In a similar vein to the II model, the DC model explores the moderating role of domain importance/satisfaction and domain control on PA to CID (or, more accurately, perceived QOL following the onset of CID). In addition to incorporating the theoretical framework and the supportive findings generated by Devins' model, the DC model also draws on the strengths inherent in Wright's (1983) clinical insights on the necessitated value changes following the onset of CID. That is, the shift in the importance and prioritizing of QOL domains posited by Bishop is reminiscent of Wright's views on the significance of value changes, following the onset of CID, such as subordinating physique and enlarging the scope of values.

Bishop's model is one of the newest to join the field of PA to CID. As such, empirical support for its two main concepts of domain centrality and domain control has only recently begun to accumulate (Bishop, 2005a, 2005b; Bishop et al., 2009).

The model's generalizability across diverse rehabilitation settings must await further studies.

Summary

The models of adaptation to CID reviewed in this section do not, by any means, offer a complete picture of all existing models. They do, however, offer a rather balanced view of those models encountered more frequently in both the historical and extant literatures on adaptation to CID. The recent growth of ecological models of adaptation to CID suggests that the new generation of rehabilitation theoreticians, researchers, and clinicians is striving to expand our understanding of the adaptation process through the development of robust, heuristic, and evidence-based models that more accurately portray the intricacy of human adaptation to stressful life conditions, such as those engendered by the onset of CID.

In the next section, we report on empirical research efforts that have sought to examine the relationships among several frequently studied predictive variables and outcomes of psychosocial adaptation, as suggested by these ecological models. We focus on findings obtained from three commonly researched conditions in the rehabilitation psychology field. When appropriate, we also document contradictory findings. Possible reasons for discrepant results are further discussed in the final section of the chapter.

Empirical Findings—Predicting Psychosocial Adaptation to Chronic Illness and Disability

The findings reported in this section are loosely derived from research efforts that have followed, to some extent, the previously sketched ecological models of PA to CID. They therefore provide somewhat unique interpretations of these models and their various components. To wit, these empirical applications have largely followed a rather prescribed yet selective course of research in which sets of variables have been chosen in such a manner as to examine their predictive contributions to traditional outcome measures that reflect PA to CID. Foremost among these commonly investigated predictors of adaptation are sociodemographic variables (e.g., present age, age of onset, gender); CID- (or medically) related factors (e.g., degree of severity, extent of functional limitations, time since disability onset/duration); and personality- (psychologically) linked attributes (e.g., coping modalities, self-efficacy, optimism/pessimism, hope, perceived level of control). Another predictor often considered is that of social support. The latter has been viewed from several vantage points, among them: a coping strategy (e.g., seeking social support), a personality attribute (e.g., social interest in others), and an environmental (contextual) feature (e.g., the availability of a social network or support system). Obviously, the relative importance (predictive power) of each of these variables to PA to CID is a function of numerous factors, among them the clinical nature of the condition, type of onset (sudden vs. gradual), course (static vs. variable), affected life domains, degree of life threat, and personal meaning of the CID.

In this section, we review the literature on PA obtained from three types of CID. These were selected based on two primary criteria; namely, the total number of content-related publications obtained from PsychInfo and Medline database searches, and the representativeness of these medical conditions (the nature of their functional implications, type of onset, course, and impact on life) in the field of rehabilitation psychology. Searches of PsychInfo and Medline databases for approximately 20 medical conditions under the keywords (psychosocial) adaptation, (psychosocial) adjustment, and coping indicated that, of those conditions searched, six were most frequently researched. These included cancer, diabetes, heart diseases, MS, SCI, and traumatic brain/head injuries (TBI). Available literature on two of the conditions exceeded the scope of this chapter; namely, adaptation, adjustment, or coping among children and adolescents (diabetes), and within the context of cognitive deficits and neuropsychological functioning (TBI). Because of space restrictions we decided to focus on three of the remaining four medical conditions. The three conditions and their relevant defining features are:

• SCI, which typically represents conditions of sudden onset; of mostly stable course; having functional implications that impact physical performance, such as mobility (paraplegia) and manipulation (added to tetraplegia); and that normally do not pose life threat.

• Cancer, which typically involves gradual onset (but "sudden" diagnosis); an unpredictable course that may undergo remissions, exacerbation periods, and extended normalcy; functional limitations that are body site-determined, including experiences of pain, and severe and fluctuating side effects; and that poses a threat to life.

• MS, which commonly is of gradual onset; has an extended diagnostic period; has an unpredictable course marked by periods of remission and exacerbation with a general deteriorating trend; features varied functional limitations that often include mobility, sensory, endurance, fatigue, and cognitive aspects; and typically not life-threatening.

The predictors chosen for the review include those that were found to be among the most commonly discussed among the previously addressed ecological models of PA and those most researched and cited in the relevant literature. Accordingly, we selected for our review gender; age of onset/diagnosis (both representing sociodemographic variables); duration of CID; severity and functionality[1] of condition (both representing CID-associated variables); coping strategies; perceived and received social support; and perceptions of control, self-efficacy, hope, and optimism representing personality- or psychological-linked variables.

In our discussion of personality-linked predictors, we have adopted the following practices. First, the wide spectrum of coping strategies has been divided into two broad categories, following the pioneering theoretical and empirical work of Lazarus and Folkman (1984), Krohne (1993), Tobin, Holroyd, Reynolds, and Wigal (1989), and Moos and Schaefer (1993), namely: *engagement* that includes approach-based and problem-focused coping efforts, and *disengagement* that includes avoidance-type and mostly emotion-focused efforts. A third class of coping efforts has also been considered in the extant literature and includes seeking/using social support (Amirkhan, 1990; Carver, Scheier, & Weintraub, 1989; Parker & Endler, 1992; Pierce, Sarason, & Sarason, 1996). This category, however, is frequently used interchangeably with the availability of social resources or network and will, therefore, be discussed under a separate heading. Second, the multifaceted constructs of self-schema and self-perception have been further stretched in our discussion to include other partially overlapping, self-related terms such as perceived locus of control (both health-related and more generally of environmental contingencies), self-efficacy, hope, and optimism. We do, however, address each of these concepts individually during our review of the empirical literature.

Finally, we have considered a wide scope of psychosocial indicators of adaptation to CID. Foremost among these outcome indicators are measures of (a) depression: the Beck Depression Inventory

(BDI; Beck, Ward, Mendelson, Mock, & Erbaugh, 1961), the Center for Epidemiological Studies-Depression scale (CES-D; Radloff, 1977), and the Hospital Anxiety and Depression Scale (HADS; Zigmond & Snaith, 1983); (b) anxiety: the Beck Anxiety Inventory (BAI; Beck, Epstein, Brown, & Steer, 1988), State-Trait Anxiety Inventory (STAI; Spielberger, Gorsuch, & Lushene , 1970), and the HADS; (c) generic measures of psychological distress or impairment: the Psychosocial Adjustment to Illness Scale (PAIS-PD subscale; Derogatis, 1986), Profile of Mood States (POMS; McNair, Lorr, & Droppleman, 1971), Sickness Impact Profile (SIP; Bergner, Bobbitt, Carter, & Gilson, 1981), and Symptom Checklist (SCL-90-R; Derogatis, 1977); (d) measures of life-satisfaction, well-being, and perceived quality of life: the Life Satisfaction Survey (LSS; Chubon, 1987), Life Satisfaction Index (LSI; Decker & Schulz, 1985), Life Situation Questionnaire (Crewe & Krause, 1990), Diener's Satisfaction With Life Scale (SWLS; Diener, Emmons, Larsen, & Griffin, 1985); (e) measures of (successful) psychosocial adjustment: the Acceptance of Disability Scale (ADS; Linkowski, 1971), the Reactions to Impairment and Disability Inventory (RIDI; Livneh & Antonak, 1990), the Post-Traumatic Growth Inventory (PTGI; Tedeschi & Calhoun, 1996); and (f) measures of combined positive and negative affectivity, such as the Positive Affect and Negative Affect Scale (PANAS; Watson, Clark, & Tellegen, 1988).

In the next section, we discuss the contributions of each of the predictors to PA of CID. The review is obviously selective because of space constraints and is organized according to the three CIDs:, SCI, cancer, and MS.

Sociodemographic Predictors of Psychosocial Adaptation to Chronic Illness and Disability

GENDER

Studies examining the predictive power of the person's gender on PA to CID largely report that gender, in and of itself, does not appear to be a successful predictor of adaptation, as indicated by measures of depression, anxiety, life satisfaction, well-being, or quality of life (QOL) following the onset of CID. Such findings have been documented among people with SCI (Bracken & Bernstein, 1980; Curran, Ponsford, & Crowe, 2000; Fuhrer, Rintala, Hart, Clearman, & Young, 1992; Kennedy, Evans, & Sandhu, 2009; Krause,

1998; Krause & Anson, 1997; Krause, Kemp, & Coker, 2000; Kreuter, Sullivan, Dahllöf, & Siösteen, 1998; McNett, 1987), survivors of cancer (Gotay, 1985; Osowiecki & Compas, 1998; Parle, Jones, & Maguire, 1996; Sneed, Edlund, & Dias, 1992), and individuals diagnosed with MS (Minden, Orav, & Reich, 1987).

However, a small number of discrepant findings have also been reported. For example, Judd, Brown, and Burrows (1991) found that women with SCI scored higher on psychological adjustment (i.e., using the PAIS) than men with SCI, and Tate, Forchheimer, Maynard, and Dijkers (1994), in a similar vein, reported that females showed less psychological distress than males with SCI. Finally, Woodrich and Patterson (1983) found that women were more accepting of their disability (using the AD Scale) than were men with SCI. In contrast, Woolrich, Kennedy, and Tasiemski (2006) and Kennedy and colleagues (Kennedy et al., 2009) found that women reported higher levels of anxiety than did men with SCI. Among people with MS, Chalk (2007) reported higher levels of anxiety among women than men diagnosed with the condition, while Montel and Bungener (2007) found no gender differences in either levels of anxiety or depression. In sum, therefore, gender is a poor predictor of PA to CID. Available data suggest that, with the exception of a decidedly small number of studies, adaptation to SCI, cancer, and MS is not determined by respondents' gender.

AGE OF CID ONSET

The literature on the role that age of CID onset plays in PA to CID yields mixed results. The available findings also appear to be partially determined by the nature of the CID and the outcome measures used. Among people who sustained SCI, age of injury onset was found to be independent of acceptance of disability (Mazzulla, 1984) and psychological maladjustment, using the SIP scale (McColl & Rosenthal, 1994). Other researchers, however, found age of onset to be negatively correlated with perceived well-being (Decker & Schulz, 1985), psychological distress (Wu & Chan, 2007), QOL (Elfström, Rydén, Kreuter, Taft, & Sullivan, 2005; Kreuter et al., 1998), and life satisfaction (McColl & Rosenthal, 1994), yet positively related to psychological dysfunction (Alfano, Neilson, & Fink, 1993). In contrast, Krause, Kemp, and Coker (2000) reported that symptoms of depression correlated positively with age of injury.

Among cancer survivors and people diagnosed with MS, the existing literature on the relationships between age of diagnosis and PA suggests that age of diagnosis was moderately associated with adaptation (as tapped by measures of depression, anxiety, and positive affect). However, McCabe, McKern, and McDonald (2004), McCabe, Stokes, and McDonald (2009), and Pakenham and Cox (2009), in samples of people with MS, found the two to be unrelated. Park, Edmondson, Fenster, and Blank (2008), in a sample of cancer survivors; and McNulty, Livneh, and Wilson (2004) and Montel and Bungener (2007), in a sample of people with MS, reported that advanced age was associated with better psychological well-being and lower levels of depression and distress. An often unresolved issue, however, in many of the existing studies is the treatment of the variables of age at cancer or MS diagnosis versus present (chronological) age. The two, despite addressing two distinct and separate variables, are often used interchangeably, a fact that limits any efforts to examine the differential effect of the former on PA. Although some evidence suggests that present age (at the time of the data collection stage of the study but not necessarily at CID onset) may be positively associated with PA to cancer (younger people diagnosed with cancer show more psychological distress than older ones; Beckham, Burker, Feldman, & Costakis, 1997; Edlund & Sneed, 1989; Ell, Mantell, Hamovitch, & Nishimoto, 1989; Friedman et al., 2006; Kornblith et al., 2007; Manne et al., 2008; Parker, Baile, Moor, & Cohen, 2003; Shelby et al., 2008; Vinokur, Threatt, Caplan, & Zimmerman, 1989), and negatively with PA to SCI (younger people with SCI adapt better to SCI than older; Craig, Hancock, Dickson, Martin, & Chang, 1990; North, 1999; Pollard & Kennedy, 2007), teasing out findings on the unique impact of age of onset on PA is marred by the confound of present (at study time) age. In conclusion, only a marginal trend exists regarding the relationship between age of onset for the three reviewed CIDs and PA. This finding, however, suggests different trends for people with SCI and cancer. The weak empirical support for this trend, however, should be regarded cautiously because of measurement confounds inherent in reporting age of condition-onset and present age of respondents.

SEVERITY LEVEL, FUNCTIONALITY, AND COMMUNITY PARTICIPATION

In this section, we review results from three conceptually independent, yet at times empirically overlapping types of measures: First, degree or level of condition severity (these are typically viewed from the World Health Organization [WHO] definition of impairments or problems with bodily physiological functions and anatomical parts and organs). Second, (in)ability to execute various activities, such as an action (behavior) or a task (these are regarded by the WHO as disabilities or functional limitations). Third, participation restrictions in getting successfully involved in various life situations (these are the former "handicaps" in fulfilling one's social and vocational roles). For example, in the context of SCI, impairments or anatomical/physiological involvement would refer mostly to problems with movement, use of hands, and strength, whereas for people with cancer, they would indicate problems triggered by specific cancer-site involvement and metastatic progression (problems with movement, breathing, and ensuing pain). Disabilities or activity restrictions for both survivors of SCI and cancer would refer to interference with performing activities of daily living (ADLs), performing specific work activities, and completing household chores. Finally, participation restrictions would extend the disability-triggered restrictions to include interference with involvement in various life situations, such as employment, social relationships, educational pursuits, and leisure activities. In actuality, however, these distinctions have not always been adopted by researchers and, accordingly, findings obtained from several of the measures used to predict PA to CID are tainted by lack of conceptual clarity and often marred by instrument shortcomings.

Among survivors of SCI, findings obtained from studies that focused mainly on measuring level of medical injury (largely referring to degree of impairment) as a predictor of PA have typically reported that degree of severity alone did not successfully predict adaptation, as indicated by measures of emotional distress, acceptance of disability, well-being, and QOL (Alfano et al., 1993; Chase, Cornille, & English, 2000; Craig, Hancock, & Dickson, 1994; Decker & Schulz, 1985; deRoon-Cassini, de St. Aubin, Valvano, Hastings, & Horn, 2009; Fuhrer, 1996; Fuhrer et al., 1992; Kennedy et al., 2009; Kennedy, Lowe, Grey, & Short, 1995; Kishi, Robinson, & Forrester, 1994; Krause & Crewe, 1990; Kreuter et al., 1998; Lundqvist, Siosteen, Blomstrand, Lind, & Sullivan, 1991; Malec & Neimeyer, 1983; Martz, Livneh, Priebe, Wuermser, & Ottomanelli, 2005; Matheis, Tulsky, & Matheis, 2006; McColl & Rosenthal, 1994; McMillen & Cook, 2003; Post, de Witte, van Asbeck, van Dijk, & Schrijvers, 1998; Shanmugham, Elliott, & Palmatier, 2004; Stensman, 1994; Thompson, Coker, Krause, & Henry, 2003; Woodrich & Patterson, 1983). In contrast, studies that addressed how functional impact on participation in life activities is associated with PA to SCI, using such measures as the Craig Handicap Assessment and Reporting Technique (CHART; Whiteneck et al., 1992), have yielded different findings. These studies have mostly indicated that higher levels of community participation (lower handicap) are negatively correlated with measures of depression and anxiety (Curran et al., 2000; Fuhrer et al., 1992; Tate et al., 1994).

Similar results have also been reported in the PA to cancer literature. Severity of cancer, as generally indicated by stage of illness, degree of physical impairment, and extent of metastasis, has been found to be mostly independent of such measures of psychological distress as depression, anxiety, and mood disturbance or measures of adaptation such as well-being and QOL (Andrykowski et al., 1996; Ell, Mantell et al., 1989; Ell, Nishimoto, Morvay, Mantell, & Hamovitch, 1989; Epping-Jordan et al., 1999; Ferrero, Barreto, & Toledo, 1994; Friedman, Nelson, Baer, Lane, & Smith, 1990; Gotay, 1985; Schnoll, Harlow, Stolbach, & Brandt, 1998; Shelby et al., 2008). Exceptions to these findings, however, have also been noted in which greater degree of physical and functional impairments have been found to predict increased levels of depression and psychological distress (Bukberg, Penman, & Holland, 1984; Cella et al., 1987; Manne et al., 2008; Marks, Richardson, Graham, & Levine, 1986; Mendelsohn, 1991; Vinokur et al., 1989; Vinokur, Threatt, Vinokur-Kaplan, & Satariano, 1990). In a study by Andrykowski and Brady (1994), perceived disease severity was found to moderate the relationship between locus of control and psychological distress such that disease severity was positively correlated with distress only for those cancer survivors with high perceptions of internal locus of control.

Findings on the relationships between severity of condition and PA among people diagnosed with MS present a mixed picture. Whereas several researchers obtained findings indicating that disability status (severity of neuromuscular symptoms, as typically measured by the Expanded Disability Status Scale [EDSS]; Kurtzke, 1983), is not directly associated with indicators of psychosocial functioning such as depression and anxiety (**Aikens, Fischer, Namey, & Rudick, 1997**; Chalk, 2007; Devins et al., 1996; Macleod & Macleod, 1998; Minden et al., 1987; Mohr, Goodkin, Gatto, & Van Der Wende, 1997; **Pakenham, 1999**; Shnek et al., 1997; Shnek, Foley, LaRocca, Smith, & Halper, 1995), other researchers reported that degree of physical impairment or extent of disability was positively related to higher levels of depression (Barnwell & Kavanagh, 1997; Lynch, Kroencke, & Denney, 2001; McIvor, Riklan, & Reznikoff, 1984).

In sum, therefore, medical severity of injury, as expressed via measures of degree of impairment and extent of disability, appears to be a poor predictor of PA to CID. On the other hand, the impact of the resultant functional limitations on the ability or willingness to participate in community activities suggests a different pathway to adaptation. Although findings are available exclusively for samples of people with SCI, and are scarce, they do suggest a possible positive trend between extent of community participation (lower perceived handicap) and better adaptation.

TIME SINCE INJURY/DIAGNOSIS (DURATION OF CID)

The investigation of the relationships between time since injury/diagnosis (TSI) and PA outcomes has spawned one of the most controversial and very likely heated discussions in the field of rehabilitation psychology (Buckelew, Frank, Elliott, Chaney, & Hewett, 1991; Duff & Kennedy, 2003; Heinemann, 1995; Livneh & Antonak, 1997; Trieschmann, 1988; Wortman & Silver, 1987, 1989). Indeed, the concept of TSI has often been equated with "stage" models of adaptation to CID. From this perspective, findings from either cross-sectional or longitudinal studies that failed to demonstrate an appreciable trend of improved PA over time have been regarded as conclusive evidence that adaptation by stages (or clinically defined increments) does not exist, and/or the passage of time itself is independent of adaptation to sudden- or gradual-onset medical conditions. Although the bulk of longitudinal empirical research, unlike some clinical observations, has failed to support any of the proposed stage (or phase) models of PA, research on the relationships between TSI and PA outcomes has yielded a much more complex and often inconclusive picture on these relationships. For example, careful scrutiny of the literature on PA to SCI, cancer, and MS suggests that the relationships between condition duration and PA may be determined by a complex set of interactions of moderating variables, including the nature, suddenness, and impact of the condition on the person's life, the context of injury (civilian vs.

combat), its stability over time, pre-CID personality attributes, coping modes used, span of examined years since injury/diagnosis, and outcome measures adopted, among others.

More specifically, among survivors of SCI, a large body of empirical data indicate that TSI was not found to be associated with such measures as psychological/emotional distress (Alfano et al., 1993; Buckelew, Baumstark, Frank, & Hewett, 1990; Buckelew et al., 1991; Krause & Crewe, 1990; McColl & Rosenthal, 1994; Tate et al., 1994; Wineman, Durand, & Steiner, 1994), depression (Crisp, 1992; Hammell, 2004; Kennedy et al., 2009; McColl & Rosenthal, 1994), anxiety (Hammell, 1994; Kennedy et al., 2009), life satisfaction (Crisp, 1992), psychological well-being (de Roon-Cassini, Aubin, Valvano, Hastings; Horn, 2009), acceptance of disability (Mazzulla, 1984), quality of life (Kreuter et al., 1998; Martz et al., 2005; Matheis et al., 2006), and psychosocial adjustment (Martz et al., 2005).

Yet, a considerable body of literature also exists that suggests that the relationships between TSI and PA following the onset of SCI, although not necessarily indicative of stages of adaptation, do follow some clinical trajectory of improved adaption over time. Put differently, with the passage of TSI, survivors of SCI reported increased life satisfaction (Chase et al., 2000; McColl & Rosenthal, 1994) and showed more acceptance of their condition (Elfström, Kennedy, Lude, & Taylor, 2007; Elfström, Kreuter, Rydén, Persson, & Sullivan, 2002; Elfström, Rydén, Kreuter, Persson, & Sullivan, 2002; Heinemann, Bulka, & Smetak, 1988; Woodrich & Patterson, 1983). TSI was also correlated negatively with depression (Elliott, Herrick, Witty, Godshall, & Spruell, 1992b; Macleod & Macleod, 1998; Woolrich et al., 2006), emotional/psychological distress (Elliott et al., 1992b; Livneh & Martz, 2003; Shadish, Hickman, & Arrick, 1981), and post-traumatic stress disorder (PTSD; Hatcher, Whitaker, & Karl, 2009; Nielsen, 2003). Finally, TSI predicted indirectly (through its influence on perceptions of health) higher reported QOL (McColl et al., 2003). The complexity of studying the relationships between TSI and PA to CID was further evidenced by findings reported by Krause, Kemp, and Coker (2000). These authors found that the relationship between the two may not be captured by a simple linear trend but may follow a more complex trend. In their study, Krause and his colleagues reported a quadratic trend such that those with the least (shortest TSI) and the most (longest TSI) years since injury experienced higher levels of depression, whereas those in the middle range of duration since disability onset reported the lowest levels of depression.

Findings obtained from the literature on PA to cancer further support the intricate nature of the relationships between TSD (time since diagnosis; at times measured as time since cancer surgery) and adaptation. Again, a solid body of literature suggests that duration of cancer and adaptation to it may be unrelated. These findings were obtained from measures of depression (Osowiecki & Compas, 1998; Parker et al., 2003; Santos, Kozasa, Chauffaille, Colleoni, & Leite, 2006), anxiety (Lewis, 1989; Osowiecki & Compas, 1998; Parker et al., 2003; Rodrigue, Boggs, Weiner, & Behen, 1993; Rodrigue, Behen, & Tumlin, 1994; Santos, Kozasa, Chauffaille et al., 2006), emotional/psychiatric distress (Friedman, Baer, Lewy, Lane, & Smith, 1988; Friedman et al., 1990; Merluzzi & Martinez Sanchez, 1997a), and general psychosocial adjustment (Schnoll, Knowles, & Harlow, 2002). The veracity of these findings is, however, compromised by contradictory reports that showed TSD to be negatively linked to anxiety (Kaczorowski, 1989) and psychological distress (Carver et al., 2005; McCaul et al., 1999; Meyerowitz, 1983), as well as to improved psychological adjustment (Lowery, Jacobsen, & DuCette, 1993), better psychological well-being (Park et al., 2008), and higher scores on post-traumatic growth (Sears, Stanton, & Danoff-Burg, 2003). Still other research findings linked TSD with decreased psychological well-being and increased distress (Ell, Mantell et al., 1989; Vinokur et al., 1989). In other words, the findings from the cancer literature portray a mixture of results, suggesting that the relationships between TSD and PA may be moderated or mediated by a host of possible medical, psychological, experiential, and environmental variables not directly addressed by most authors. Because of the relatively small numbers of these studies, the various types of cancer studied, and the heterogeneous outcome measures adopted, it is presently impossible to tease out those influencing factors (e.g., type of cancer, degree of threat to life, present age of survivor, available social support, prediagnosis personality factors, outcome measures used) that may have contributed to the nature and scope of these conflicting findings.

Findings from the literature on PA to MS further document the contradictory nature of the relationships between TSD and adaptation. For example, several researchers have reported findings suggesting that TSD among people with MS is independent of degree of psychosocial outcomes. These findings were documented for depression (Arnett & Randolph, 2006; Devins et al., 1996; Lynch et al., 2001; McCabe et al., 2004; Pakenham, 2007; Pakenham & Cox, 2009), anxiety (Pakenham, 2007; Pakenham & Cox, 2009), psychological/emotional distress (McNulty et al., 2004; Pakenham, 2005; Wineman et al., 1994), life satisfaction (Pakenham, 2005, 2007), and QOL (McCabe, Firth, & O'Connor, 2009). However, conflicting findings were reported as well and mostly suggested a negative association between length of TSD and depression (Barnwell & Kavanagh, 1997; Pakenham, 1999). TSD was also found to be positively related to personal growth (Pakenham, 2005). Indeed, Pakenham and Cox (2009) found that benefit-finding, which is a tendency to identify personal benefits following adversity and a concept closely aligned with post-traumatic growth, hope, and optimism (see later review), was found to correlate positively with positive affect and lower levels of anxiety and depression, and is nonlinearly associated with TSD of MS. In fact, it appeared to have only substantially emerged in that study years after diagnosis.

To summarize the findings related to MS, it appears that, despite the paucity of research, it could be argued that the relationships between duration and PA to MS could be partially a function of an intricate interaction among several variables including the specific constructs (and measures) of adaptation used, phase-related symptoms experienced by the person with MS (stable, deteriorating, fluctuating), certain pre-MS personality attributes that failed to be addressed by researchers, and the effect of certain moderating variables (benefit-finding, coping strategies). An intriguing insight could be extracted from a finding by MacLeod and MacLeod (1998), in which the correlation between DSI/D measures of depression and anxiety was reported for both samples of survivors of SCI and for people with MS. For the former group, TSI was *negatively* correlated with both measures of depression (significantly) and anxiety (approaching statistical significance). In contrast, for the latter group, these relationships were not statistically significant, but anxiety was *positively* correlated with TSD (again, approaching statistical significance), thus suggesting a reversed trend to that revealed among people with SCI. Although obviously speculative, it is possible that the nature of the TSI/D (among several other variables indicated earlier) may exert an influence on PA, such that for relatively stable and more predictable courses of CID (e.g., SCI), adaptation does follow a general trend of improvement over time; whereas for deteriorating (or fluctuating) and mostly unpredictable conditions (e.g., MS, cancer), adaptation may be more strongly influenced by other factors, such as personality attributes, coping strategies, and the availability of social support.

Psychosocial predictors of Psychosocial Adaptation to Chronic Illness and Disability

Undoubtedly, the largest body of literature linking psychosocial and personality-type predictors and PA to CID has been generated by research in the field of coping. To bring some sense of semblance into this voluminous literature, we elected to adopt the oft-cited tripartite classificatory model of coping strategies that includes engagement, or approach-based, problem-focused, task-oriented strategies; disengagement or avoidance, emotion-focused strategies[2]; and seeking and using social support. The first two coping groups have been theoretically conceptualized and empirically supported by the work of Suls and Fletcher (1985), Tobin el al. (1989), Lazarus and Folkman (1984), and Moos and Schaefer (1993), while the third group has been often regarded as a separate coping mode following the work of Amirkhan (1990) and (with some discrepancies) that of Stone and Neal (1984), Feifel and Strack (1989), and, more recently, Folkman and Moskowitz (2004) and Litman (2006).

In the following paragraphs we have, therefore, collapsed coping strategies under one of the three overarching coping groups:

• *Engagement/approach coping*: (Planned) problem-solving/focused, active, confrontive, acceptance/accepting responsibility, positive reappraisal/restructuring, and fighting spirit.
• *Disengagement/avoidance coping*: Emotion-focused, distancing, escape, avoidance, denial, wishful thinking, self-blame/criticism, resignation, fatalistic outlook, behavioral and mental disengagement, and substance use.
• *Social-support coping*: Seeking and using social support (for emotional, cognitive, or instrumental purposes).

Engagement or approach-based coping normally addresses those efforts that are task-oriented and seek to problem-solve, change, reduce the impact of, or nullify the stressful situation. Disengagement or emotion-based coping commonly refers to those efforts that seek to manage negative emotions engendered by the stressful situation. Finally, seeking and using social support addresses those coping strategies that are directed at securing emotional (e.g., sharing painful experiences), cognitive (e.g., requesting medical advice), or instrumental (e.g., seeking financial assistance) support from other people, including family members, peers, co-workers, and professional staff members.

Engagement Coping and Psychosocial Adaptation to Chronic Illness and Disability

SPINAL CORD INJURY

A large body of empirical work supports earlier clinical anecdotes of the link between engagement coping (EC) and better psychosocial outcomes (increased psychological well-being and life satisfaction and lower psychological distress) following the onset of SCI (Martz & Livneh, 2007b). For example, the use of active, problem-solving coping was found to be positively associated with lower levels of anxiety (Curran et al., 2000) and depression (Elliott, Godshall, Herrick, Witty, & Spruell, 1991), and also successfully predicted, in a longitudinal study, future post-traumatic growth (**Pollard & Kennedy, 2007**). Individuals who used problem-focused coping were also found to score significantly lower on depression than were users of emotion-focused coping, as determined by a cluster-analytic study (Moore, Bombardier, Brown, & Patterson, 1994).

Another form of EC—acceptance—was found to positively relate to personal growth and negatively to feelings of helplessness (Elfström, Kreuter et al., 2002; Elfström, Rydén et al., 2002), depression (Elfström et al., 2005; Kennedy et al., 2009; Kennedy et al., 1995; **Kennedy et al., 2000**; McMillen & Cook, 2003), and anxiety (Kennedy et al., 2009; Kennedy et al., 1995; McMillen & Cook, 2003). It was also positively associated with psychological well-being (McMillen & Cook, 2003) and QOL (Elfström & Kreuter, 2006). Positive interpretation and cognitive restructuring, two similar coping strategies that focus on reframing perspectives of events, were also found to be consistently linked to better PA, including lower depression (**Pollard & Kennedy, 2007**), and acceptance of disability (**Buckelew & Hanson, 1992; Hanson, Buckelew, Hewett, & O'Neal, 1993**). Finally, spiritual coping, a form of engagement-based coping that seeks to draw strength from spiritual perspectives on life was also found to be positively correlated with higher levels of perceived QOL (Matheis et al., 2006).

CANCER

Findings from the cancer literature on the relationships between engagement-type coping and PA further support the trend depicted earlier among SCI survivors. Direct, active, problem-focused, task-oriented, confrontive coping, including the more cancer-specific "fighting spirit" coping modality, which was derived from the Mental Adjustment to Cancer Scale (MAC; Watson, Greer, Young, & Inayat, 1988), which purports to measure cancer survivors' positive attitude, optimistic outlook, and determination to overcome the disease, have been shown to relate to better indices of PA. These include lower levels of psychological distress (Bloom, 1982; Chen, David, Thompson, Smith et al., 1996; Classen, Koopman, Angell, & Spiegel, 1996; Ferrero et al., 1994; Friedman et al., 1988; Friedman et al., 1990; Kim, Yeom, Seo, Kim, & Yoo, 2002; Matthews & Cook, 2009; Nelson, Friedman, Baer, Lane, & Smith, 1994; Schnoll et al., 1998), depression (Burgess, Morris, & Pettingale, 1988; **Epping-Jordan et al., 1999**; Osborne, Elsworth, Kissane, Burke, & Hopper, 1999; **Osowiecki & Compas**, 1998, **1999**; Rodrigue et al., 1994; Schnoll, Mackinnon, Stolbach, & Lorman, 1995; Schwartz, Daltroy, Brandt, Friedman, & Stolbach, 1992; Watson, Greer, Rowden, & Gorman, 1991; Watson et al., 1994a), and anxiety (Burgess et al., 1988; **Epping-Jordan et al., 1999**; Osborne et al., 1999; **Osowiecki & Compas**, 1998, **1999**; Schwartz et al., 1992; Watson et al., 1994b). A dissenting finding was reported by Mytko, Knight, Chastain, Mumby, Siston, and Williams (1996) in a sample of cancer patients awaiting bone-marrow transplant, in which problem-solving and positive reappraisal coping were not associated with measures of depression, anxiety, and generic psychological distress.

Echoing a similar trend, cancer survivors who have relied on positive reframing/reappraisal and cognitive restructuring coping (Carver et al., 1993; Chen, David, Thompson, Smith et al., 1996; Ell, Mantell et al., 1989; Filipp, Klauer, Freudenberg, & Ferring, 1990; Manne et al., 2008; Manne et al., 1994; Mishel & Sorenson, 1993; Sears et al., 2003; Stanton et al., 2000; Stanton, Danoff-Burg, & Huggins, 2002), as well as acceptance coping (**Carver et al., 1993**; Merluzzi & Martinez Sanchez, 1997b), also reported lower levels of psychological distress and higher levels of psychological well-being and perceived QOL. A final engagement-based coping, namely information seeking, was similarly found to be positively related to better psychological adjustment (Lavery & Clarke, 1996; Merluzzi & Martinez Sanchez, 1997a).

A finding of intriguing clinical implications was reported by **Fang, Daly, Miller, Zerr, Malick, and Engstrom (2006)**. In this prospective study of women with breast cancer, problem-focused coping was positively linked to distress (POMS), yet was moderated by perceived control such that, under conditions of high perceived control (but not low perceived control), problem-focused coping was associated with higher future experienced distress. This finding attests to the multifaceted and interactive nature of several of the predictors of adaptation to CID.

MULTIPLE SCLEROSIS

Empirical findings on the relationships between EC and adaptation among people with MS paint a similar portrait. Research indicates that those who have adopted plan-based, active, problem-solving coping modes experience lower overall psychological distress (Pakenham, 2001), as well as lower levels of depression (**Arnett & Randolph, 2006**; Chalk, 2007; Mohr et al., 1997; **Pakenham, 1999**, 2001; Pakenham, Stewart, & Rogers, 1997), higher life satisfaction (Chalk, 2007), and positive affect (**Pakenham, 2006**). Yet, research suggests that the influence of problem-solving coping on psychological distress may be moderated by degree of physical impairment among people with MS (Mohr et al., 1997). Acceptance was also found to be correlated with lower levels of depression and anxiety (**Pakenham, 2006, 2007**). In a similar vein, positive reappraisal and cognitive reframing coping were also linked to lower levels of depression (**Aikens et al., 1997**; Arnett, Higginson, Voss, Randolph, & Grandey, 2002; Mohr et al., 1997) and to higher levels of psychological well-being (**McCabe, 2006**). Finally, benefit finding, a more recently conceptualized and explored form of positive reappraisal, was also found to be related to higher reports of life satisfaction and positive affectivity (**Pakenham, 2005, 2007; Pakenham & Cox, 2009**). A handful of dissenting voices have also been reported. For example, Jean, Paul, and Beatty (1999), Lynch et al. (2001), and **Pakenham (1999, 2006)**, reported that, in their studies, problem-focused coping was not significantly correlated with measures of psychological distress or depression. Other researchers (McCabe et al., 2004) found gender-related differences in

relationships between problem-focused coping and depression, such that a negative association between the two variables existed only among men. Similarly, focus on the positive was negatively correlated with depression in men only, suggesting that, under certain conditions, coping modes may be moderated by gender to influence PA to MS.

In sum, therefore, and consistent with Stanton et al.'s (2007) conclusions regarding PA to chronic illnesses (e.g., arthritis, cardiovascular disease), we have observed from our review of the literature trends in research among the three selected disabilities that strongly suggest that the use of engagement-type coping is associated with lower levels of psychological distress indicators and higher levels of adaptive psychological outcomes (e.g., well-being, perceived QOL, adjustment, post-traumatic growth).

Disengagement Coping and Psychosocial Adaptation to Chronic Illness and Disability

SPINAL CORD INJURY

Research on the relationships between DC and adaptation to SCI has conclusively established that virtually all forms of DC are associated with poorer levels of adaptation, including higher levels of depression, anxiety, and generic psychological distress. For example, studies have linked the use of wish-fulfilling fantasy (wishful thinking) with increased depression (Curran et al., 2000), anxiety (Curran et al., 2000), and psychological distress (Buckelew et al., 1990), and with lower levels of disability acceptance (Buckelew & Hanson, 1992; Hanson et al., 1993). Similarly, coping efforts that reflect behavioral and mental disengagement (e.g., avoidance, escapism, drug and alcohol use) have been documented to correlate with higher psychological distress (Buckelew et al., 1990; Meyer, O'Leary, & Hagglund, 1999; Shanmugham et al., 2004) and depression (Kemp & Krause, 1999; Kennedy et al., 1995; **Kennedy et al., 2000**; **Pollard & Kennedy, 2007**) and lower levels of disability acceptance (Heinemann et al., 1988) and life satisfaction (Kemp & Krause, 1999).

Self-blaming is considered another form of disengagement coping. It was found to relate to higher levels of psychological distress and, in general, poor adjustment (Buckelew et al., 1990; Nielson & MacDonald, 1988), as well as to increased levels of depression and anxiety (Curran et al., 2000; Reidy & Caplan, 1994). Another often-cited DC strategy, namely, emotional venting/expression has been associated likewise with higher levels of psychological distress, depression, and anxiety (Buckelew et al., 1990; Kennedy et al., 1995; **Kennedy et al., 2000**).

Finally, the literature on the relationships between denial, another DC-linked coping strategy, and PA to SCI indicates that denial might be associated with either negative or positive outcomes depending on several factors, including the nature of the measuring instrument, time since SCI onset, and its overall duration. Denial was associated with lower levels of depression, anxiety, and generic psychological distress in some studies (**Elliott & Richards, 1999**), but also with higher level of psychological distress indices (**Kennedy et al., 2000**; Martz et al., 2005; McMillen & Cook, 2003).

CANCER

Data regarding the association of DC use and adaptation among cancer survivors mirror those highlighted earlier for people with SCI. The use of DC appears to be solidly correlated with poorer PA. These findings have been observed for wishful thinking coping, such that greater reliance on this coping strategy was found to be related to greater psychological distress (Chen, David, Thompson, & Smith, 1996; Mishel, Padilla, Grant, & Sorenson, 1991; Mishel & Sorenson, 1993; Quinn, Fontana, & Reznikoff, 1986). Another type of DC, namely generalized avoidance (both cognitive and behavioral) coping, which frequently includes such related terms as resignation, escapism, fatalistic outlook, and social withdrawal, has been consistently linked to generic emotional/psychological distress, depression, and anxiety (**Behen & Rodrigue, 1994**; Dunkel-Schetter, Feinstein, Taylor, & Falke, 1992; **Epping-Jordan et al., 1999**; Ferrero et al., 1994; Friedman et al., 1988; Friedman et al., 1990; Heim, Valach, & Schaffner, 1997; Keyes, Bisno, Richardson, & Marston, 1987; Manne et al., 1994; **McCaul et al., 1999**; **Miller, Manne, Taylor, Keates, & Dougherty, 1996**; Mytko et al., 1996; Nelson et al., 1994; **Osowiecki & Compas**, 1998, **1999**; Parle et al., 1996; Rodrigue et al., 1993; Rodrigue et al., 1994; Schnoll et al., 2002; Schnoll et al., 1998; **Stanton et al., 2000**; Stanton & Snider, 1993; Watson et al., 1991).

Findings on the relationships between denial and PA again suggest a complex and nonuniform trend. Whereas some research suggests that the use of denial is linked to higher levels of psychological distress (**Carver et al., 1993**; Ferrero et al., 1994) and lower reported psychosocial adjustment (Schnoll et al., 2002), contradictory findings suggest that the use of denial may be unrelated to reported psychosocial adjustment (**Classen et al., 1996**; **Heim et al., 1997**), and possibly even to lower psychological distress (Meyerowitz, 1983). Finally, coping via self-blame was found to be related to poor PA, including higher levels of psychological distress (**Malcarne, Compas, Epping-Jordan, & Howell, 1995**; Quinn et al., 1986), but was independent of depression in another study (**Newsom, Knapp, & Schulz, 1996**). A small number of contradictory findings have also been reported. For instance, Watson et al. (1988), Schwartz et al. (1992), and Schnoll et al. (1995) found that avoidance and fatalistic-type coping were not correlated with measures of depression and anxiety in their studies.

MULTIPLE SCLEROSIS

Although less voluminous in size, the literature on the relationships between DC and adaptation to MS indicates that most forms of avoidance/escape-type coping are associated with higher levels of depression and generic psychological distress (**Aikens et al., 1997**; Arnett et al., 2002; Goretti et al., 2009; Jean et al., 1999; Lynch et al., 2001; Mohr et al., 1997; Montel & Bungener, 2007; **Pakenham, 1999**, 2001, **2006**). In other studies, wishful thinking was similarly associated with higher levels of depression (McCabe et al., 2004), global psychological distress (**Pakenham, 1999**), and lower levels of psychological well-being (**McCabe, 2006**). In a recent longitudinal study, **Rabinowitz and Arnett** (**2009**) reported that the use of avoidant coping did not predict future depression, yet a composite index (a combined score on a set of active coping strategies minus a combined score on a set of avoidant coping strategies) did successfully predict, as well as moderate, the relationship between cognitive dysfunction and depression. We will return to the implications of this study later in the chapter.

To summarize the findings on DC and adaptation, most research indicates that usage of DC is associated with poorer levels of adaptation (i.e., nonadaptive outcomes such as depression, anxiety, and generic psychological distress). Denial is one form of DC that has exhibited contradictory findings, such that, depending on the circumstances surrounding its presence, it might be associated with either negative or positive psychosocial outcomes.

Perceived and Received Social Support and Psychosocial Adaptation to Chronic Illness and Disability

Social support is typically viewed as a multifaceted construct. It has been broadly portrayed as including one or more of the following components: a coping mode (seeking support), a measure of the availability of community resources, an indicator of the amount and density of social ties, or the belief that one can turn to others for emotional, informational, or material support when stressful events necessitate their help (alternatively referred to as receiving support or functional support). Each of these components can influence PA outcomes in a number of ways, including physiological (reducing reactivity to stress and distress), cognitive (improving understanding of the stressful situation and ways of nullifying its impact), and affective approaches (minimizing fears and concerns by using a supportive interpersonal network) (Wills & Fegan, 2001).

However, definitions of social support, as commonly adopted in research on PA to CID, demonstrate the wide range and at times the different interpretations applied by researchers. These views span the spectrum, ranging from (a) perceived (subjective) support to received (generally objective) support, (b) internally anchored coping efforts (seeking social support) to externally based resources (availability of social support), (c) actively oriented efforts (e.g., seeking social support when faced with stressful situations) to more passively determined efforts (e.g., being aware of available social resources), (d) instrumental or practical support to emotional or spiritual support, (e) structural views of support (e.g., size of available social network) or functional views of support (e.g., the actual "flow" of support through emotional or informational avenues), and (f) quantitative (e.g., number of social activities participated in, number of friends/family members in one's social network) to qualitative (e.g., strength, depth of, satisfaction with, reliance upon members of social network) measures. Unfortunately, much of the available research has largely failed to clearly differentiate among these interpretations (as typically inherent in the many measures used by researchers) and, as a result, the findings linking social support coping with PA to CID are often fraught with both conceptual and psychometric limitations. In this section, when feasible, we try to match the researchers' adopted definitional formula of social support with the reported empirical findings. In other words,

we attempt to separate the differential influences of types of social support on adaptation to SCI, cancer, and MS. This task, however, is at times compromised by the absence of a clear conceptualization and/or description of social support measures used in some of the studies.

SPINAL CORD INJURY

The primacy of social support (perceived and received, sought and available) in influencing adaptation to SCI has been documented consistently throughout the available literature. Indeed, a compelling body of evidence has been aggregated to show that most forms of social support are associated with better adaptation outcomes. Subjective perceptions of social support that include satisfaction with social contacts and the immediate social network—both in quality and quantity—have been consistently been linked to lower levels of psychological distress, depression, and anxiety (Crisp, 1992; Decker & Schulz, 1985; Kemp & Krause, 1999; Kennedy et al., 1995; **Kennedy et al., 2000**; **Kennedy & Rogers, 2000**; Pollard & Kennedy, 2007; Rintala, Young, Hart, Clearman, & Fuhrer, 1992; Schulz & Decker, 1985), as well as to higher life satisfaction (Crisp, 1992; Kemp & Krause, 1999; Rintala et al., 1992).

Other indicators of social support, including measures of perception of belongingness, social integration, tangible or instrumental support, and emotional support, were also found to be generally linked with better PA, as demonstrated by higher reported life satisfaction (Elfström et al., 2005; Fuhrer et al., 1992; McColl & Rosenthal, 1994; Post et al., 1998) and well-being (Schulz & Decker, 1985), and lower levels of anxiety (including PTSD) and depression (Elliott, Herrick, Patti, & Witty, 1991; Elliott et al., 1992b; **McColl, Lei, & Skinner, 1995**; McColl & Rosenthal, 1994; McMillen & Cook, 2003; Nielsen, 2003). These findings on the influence of social support on PA were, however, contradicted by research that showed social support be unrelated for measures of depression (Craig et al., 1994) and perceived adequacy of social interactions and depression (Hammell, 1994).

The relationships between objective, quantitative measures of social support and PA to SCI, such as number of social activities, present a more diluted picture. Although some researchers reported that a larger number of such activities correlated with better perceived QOL (Clayton & Chubon, 1994), lower level of psychological distress (Elliott & Richards, 1999), and higher life satisfaction and perceived well-being (Rintala et al., 1992), findings from other researchers (Kennedy et al., 1995; **Kennedy & Rogers, 2000**), failed to lend support to these findings. Additionally, research findings on social reliance or coping via reliance on others have been shown to relate to indices of poor adaptation, including increased helplessness (Elfström, Kreuter et al., 2002; Elfström, Rydén et al., 2002; Elfström et al., 2005) or to be independent of psychological distress measures (Kennedy et al., 2009). A parallel trend was observed for a similar social support measure, that of nurturance, whose use was found to correlate with higher levels of depression and psychosocial impairment (Elliott, Herrick, Witty, Godshall, & Spruell, 1992a). These findings suggest that oversolicitous responses by others and assuming a passive recipient role may actually be associated with poorer adaptation to SCI.

CANCER

Findings on the relationships between measures of received and perceived social support and adaptation to cancer generally mirror those reported among survivors of SCI. In an earlier review article, Irvine, Brown, Crooks, Roberts, and Browne (1991) concluded from the available findings prior to 1989 that social support is positively correlated with PA among cancer survivors. Later, Helgeson and Cohen (1996), in their review of the literature on social support and cancer, reached similar conclusions, positing that social support, mostly in the form of perceived emotional support, is strongly associated with PA to cancer. This trend was also evident in more recent studies as measures of perceived social support, satisfaction with social support, and social integration were found to be correlated with better PA and psychological well-being (Ell, Mantell et al., 1989; Ell, Nishimoto et al., 1989; Friedman et al., 2006; **Heim et al., 1997**; Matthews & Cook, 2009; Shelby et al., 2008), perceived QOL (Parker et al., 2003; Vinokur et al., 1990), lower levels of depression and anxiety (Grassi, Rosti, Albertazzi, & Marangolo, 1996; Heidrich, Forsthoff, & Ward, 1994; Jones & Reznikoff, 1989; Parker et al., 2003; Rodrigue et al., 1994; Santos, Kozasa, Chauffaille Mde, Colleoni, & Leite, 2006), and lower psychological distress (Dunkel-Schetter et al., 1992; Merluzzi & Martinez Sanchez, 1997b; Shelby et al., 2008; **Trunzo & Pinto, 2003**). Other indicators of social support have yielded mostly parallel findings. For example, family cohesiveness and satisfaction with family reactions to the disease were found to relate to lower levels of psychological distress (Bloom, 1982; Friedman et al., 1988). Schnoll et al. (2002) reported in their study of breast and prostate cancer survivors that all of their assessed social support indicators (instrumental, informational, companionship, and emotional) successfully predicted psychosocial adjustment to cancer as depicted by scores on the PAIS. A study by Norton et al. (2005) provides further support to the nature of the relationships between social support and PD by demonstrating that perceived unsupportive (critical) behaviors by family and friends are positively associated with experienced psychological distress. This finding, then, attests to the dual nature of the perceived quality of social support and its relationship with PA to CID.

Dissenting findings were also reported. **Carver et al.'s** study (**1993**) indicated that the use of social support did not predict psychological distress in their study of breast cancer survivors. In another longitudinal study, **Sears et al.** (**2003**) reported that perceptions of emotional-social support failed to predict post-traumatic growth among women with breast cancer. And more recently, **Manne et al.** (**2008**) reported that both positive social support from friends and family, as well as unsupportive responses from these groups, were predictive of depression in women with gynecological cancers. The unexpected findings from these three longitudinal studies may reflect those situations in which continuous psychological distress may necessitate seeking social support to alleviate difficult life situations (Barrera, 1986; Penninx et al., 1998).

MULTIPLE SCLEROSIS

The positive effect that perceived and received social support has on PA is further documented in the literature on MS. Perceived social support was found to correlate negatively with depression (McIvor et al., 1984). More generic measures of social support were also reported to be associated with lower levels of depression in both men and women with MS (Chalk, 2007; Wineman, 1990), and in women only (McCabe et al., 2004). Similarly, social support was reported to be positively linked to better perceived QOL and life satisfaction (Chalk, 2007; Goretti et al., 2009; Motl, McAuley, & Snook, 2007). Social activity, as performed by the respondent, was also found to be beneficial as indicated by its relationship with lower reported depression (Barnwell & Kavanagh, 1997). In contrast, **Pakenham** (**1999**) found social support to be unrelated, both concurrently and at a 12-month follow-up, to measures of global distress and depression.

To summarize, findings on social support as a predictor of PA to the three conditions of SCI, cancer, and MS indicate compellingly its beneficial effects.

Personality Attributes and Psychosocial Adaptation to Chronic Illness and Disability

A considerable body of work has been devoted to examining the influence that psychological (personality) attributes, alternatively referred to as *personal resources* (**Helgeson, Snyder, & Seltman, 2004**), has on PA among people with CID. In this section, we focus on studies that sought to investigate the predictive utility of four such personality attributes that are typically associated with the field of positive psychology: self perceptions of control (including perceived health control), self-efficacy, optimism, and hope, on PA to CID.

The constructs of locus of control (LOC; Rotter, 1966) and health locus of control (HLOC; Levenson, 1974; Wallston & Wallston, 1978) have been extensively researched within the context of PA to CID. In a similar vein, the influence of positive psychology–derived constructs, such as self-efficacy (Bandura, 1977), optimism (Scheier & Carver, 1985), and hope (Snyder, 1994), on adaptation to CID has been receiving growing attention in the rehabilitation and health psychology literatures. Briefly, perceived control indicates a person's belief that he or she can influence the immediate environment, resulting in a desired personal outcome. In a related fashion, perceived health control reflects personal beliefs regarding what party most influences outcomes associated with one's health status; namely, the individual (internality), powerful others (medical personnel and the like), or chance.

A large number of salutary personal attributes were implicated as predictors of successful PA to CID. We review two clusters of these attributes: self-efficacy, optimism, and hope. Self-efficacy, as promulgated by Bandura, is viewed as the individual's appraisal of his or her ability to manage future situations. The partially overlapping constructs of hope (a cognitive-motivational tendency that integrates personal goals, pathways to reach them, and personal agency) and optimism (a dispositional tendency to expect successful achievement of personal goals and positive future outcomes) have also been explored more recently as potential predictors of PA to CID.

SPINAL CORD INJURY

Perceived personal control or perceptions of LOC are typically regarded as falling on a continuum, extending from internal LOC (a generalized expectancy that personal attributes and actions will cause future reinforcements or outcomes) to external LOC (the belief that outside, impersonal forces, including other people or plain luck, are responsible for future outcomes). The available literature on perceived control and adaptation to SCI indicates that higher levels of externality are both concurrently associated with and also predict future poorer adaptation, as manifested by increased levels of depression and emotional distress. In contrast, higher levels of internality, or perceived personal control, are linked to better present and prospective adaptation indicators, such as higher life satisfaction, perceived well-being, and acceptance of disability (Bracken, Shepard, & Webb, 1981; Chan, Lee, & Lieh-Mak, 2000; Craig et al., 1994; Decker & Schulz, 1985; Elfström & Kreuter, 2006; Ferington, 1986; Mazzulla, 1984; Schulz & Decker, 1985; Shadish et al., 1981). In a similar vein, Dean and Kennedy (2009) reported that the use of "personal agency" and "determined resolve" (both reflecting internality) were associated with lower levels of anxiety. Exceptions to these findings, however, were noted in an early study by Bracken and Bernstein (1980) and more recently by MacLeod and MacLeod (1998). Recent research also suggests that the association of LOC and well-being may be mediated by the use of coping, such that those with ILOC who report using more acceptance and fighting-spirit coping experience higher levels of well-being (Elfström & Kreuter, 2006).

Findings with regard to perceptions over personal health generally echo the earlier findings. Internal health LOC was found to correlate with lower avoidance tendencies (a defining symptom of depression) and emotional distress, and with better adjustment (Chung, Preveza, Papandreou, & Prevezas, 2006; Krause, Stanwyck, & Maides, 1998; Thompson et al., 2003), whereas perceptions of external/chance health LOC were related to higher reported anxiety, depression, and general psychological distress (Chung et al., 2006; Frank & Elliott, 1989; Frank et al., 1987; Shanmugham et al., 2004) and with lower overall life satisfaction (Krause et al., 1998) and psychological adjustment (Thompson et al., 2003). Thompson et al.'s findings further suggest that the relationship between health LOC and PA among people with SCI may be mediated by a construct they termed "purpose in life" (a Viktor Franklian–derived concept depicting the need to find meaning in and fulfillment of life).

CANCER

Among cancer survivors, an appreciable body of work suggests that internal perceptions of personal control are associated with lower levels of psychological distress, depression, and anxiety, and with higher levels of adaptive experiences (Burgess et al., 1988; **Edgar, Rosberger, & Nowlis, 1992**; Ell, Mantell et al., 1989; Taylor, Lichtman, & Wood, 1984). In contrast, external perceptions of control were found to relate to higher levels of depression and anxiety (**Grassi et al., 1996**; Watson, Greer, Pruyn, & Van den Borne, 1990). Contradictory findings, however, were also reported by Berckman and Austin (1993) and Osowiecki and Campos (1998), in which control perceptions were independent of levels of depression and psychological distress.

Data on the relationships between perceived health control and adaptation to cancer indicate, in contrast to earlier reviewed findings from SCI samples, that perceptions of health control (either internal or external) may not be predictive of psychological distress (Andrykowski & Brady, 1994; Friedman et al., 1988), anxiety (Lewis, 1989; **Osowiecki & Compas, 1999**), or depression (Marks et al., 1986; **Osowiecki & Compas, 1999**). Lowery, Jacobsen, and DuCette (1993) and Norton et al. (2005), however, did report that perceived loss of personal control over personal health (or perceived control of the illness) was related to psychological distress (or to reduced PD) in their studies of breast and ovarian cancer survivors, respectively. In the latter study (Norton et al.), perceived control over cancer also mediated the relationship between physical impairment and psychological distress. Andrykowski and Brady (1994) further showed that perceptions of health control (both of internal and external nature) may be moderated by contextual factors, such as perceived disease severity and treatment history. It could be argued that perceptions of health control for mostly an unpredictable and only partially controllable condition by one's own efforts may be a poor predictor of PA because assuming control over the unfolding course of cancer is often seen as beyond personal control and only partially controllable by medical staff. Indeed, Lowery et al. (1993) reported that 55% of their cancer survivors

believed that they had "no" or "only little" personal control of the course of their cancer, whereas 44% believed others had "no" or "only little" control of the disease.

MULTIPLE SCLEROSIS

Only three studies were located that addressed the relationships between generalized perception of control and adaptation to MS. In two of these studies (Devins et al., 1993; Halligan & Reznikoff, 1985), internal (personal) perceptions of control were linked to lower levels of depression and psychological distress. In contrast, the third study (Macleod & Macleod, 1998) found no relationship between internality and either depression or anxiety. In two studies that addressed perceptions of health control and adaptation to MS, no relationships were discovered between these two variables (Hickey & Greene, 1989; Marks & Millard, 1990). As was speculated earlier for cancer survivors, these findings may suggest that perceptions of control over personal health are weak predictors of adaptation because of the mounting realization that personal efforts to maintain health in the face of mostly uncontrollable and unpredictable conditions are generally doomed to fail, or at best are of little utility.

Salutary Attributes and Psychosocial Adaptation
SPINAL CORD INJURY

Self-efficacy, or the belief in one's ability to successfully perform certain behaviors in various situations, has been found to be correlated with positive perceptions of QOL (Hampton, 2000), psychological well-being (McMillen & Cook, 2003), lower depression (**Middleton, Tate, & Geraghty, 2003**; Shnek et al., 1997), and lower anxiety (**Middleton et al., 2003**). However, perceived self-efficacy also failed to predict depression and anxiety in McMillen and Cook's study. Hope, or holding positive expectations for oneself about the future, has been reported to be associated with lower levels of depression, anxiety, and psychological impairment (Elliott, Witty, Herrick, & Hoffman, 1991; Kennedy et al., 2009), as well as greater life satisfaction and QOL (Kortte, Gilbert, Gorman, & Wegener, 2010; Smedema, Catalano, & Ebener, 2010).

CANCER

Research on the influence of self-efficacy on adaptation to early-stage breast cancer indicated positive effects of self-efficacy on a variety of outcomes, such as higher relationship satisfaction, less functional impairment, and higher self-esteem over 1 year (Manne et al., 2006). Similarly, Beckham, Burker, Feldman, and Costakis (1997) found that, in men with cancer, self-efficacy was positively correlated with better overall psychological adjustment, as well as specific measures of depression and negative affect. Higher reported dispositional hope was found to be associated with lower levels of negative affect and higher levels of positive affect, as measured by the PANAS among college women with cancer (Irving, Snyder, & Crowson, 1998). In contrast, hope was unrelated to post-traumatic growth in a sample of breast cancer survivors (**Sears et al., 2003**) and also to psychological distress (Stanton et al., 2002).

Research on the salutary effect of dispositional optimism on adaptation to cancer has yielded a rather consistent picture. Optimism was found to be linked to lower levels of depression, anxiety, and generalized psychological distress (**Carver et al., 1993**; **Carver et al., 2005**; **Epping-Jordan et al., 1999**; Miller et al., 1996; Mishel, Hostetter, King, & Graham, 1984; Stanton & Snider, 1993; **Trunzo & Pinto, 2003**) and higher perceived well-being (**Carver et al., 1994**; Friedman et al., 2006; Matthews & Cook, 2009; **Miller et al., 1996**). Similarly, optimism was also linked to better psychological adjustment following cancer diagnosis (Carver et al., 2005; Friedman et al., 2006; Schnoll et al., 2002). On the other hand, findings by **Sears et al.** (**2003**) showed that optimism was unrelated to post-traumatic growth among women with breast cancer. Optimism was also found to predict subjective well-being and perceived QOL through the mediating role of both engagement-type (acceptance) and disengagement-type coping (behavioral disengagement) coping (**Carver et al., 1993**; **Schou, Ekeberg, Sandvik, Hjermstad, & Ruland, 2005**), demonstrating, once again, the need to examine more complex predictive models of PA.

Two additional studies provide further insight into the intricacy inherent in the interrelationships among predictor variables and the relative roles of optimism and perceived social support among women with breast cancer (Shelby et al., 2008; **Trunzo & Pinto, 2003**). In the first study, social support was found to *mediate* the relationship between optimism and better PA, while the latter study demonstrated a *moderating* (buffering) effect, such that a high level of social support was positively associated with PA only in women reporting low levels of optimism but not in those with high levels of optimism. The findings from these studies

thus suggest that social support may be a more useful resource only when levels of optimism are low.

MULTIPLE SCLEROSIS

Self-efficacious beliefs for general problematic life situations among people with MS were found to be linked to a number of positive PA indicators, including lower levels of depression and anxiety (Airlie, Baker, Smith, & Young, 2001; **Barnwell & Kavanagh, 1997**; Shnek et al., 1997; Shnek et al., 1995), higher levels of perceived QOL (Motl et al., 2007; Stuifbergen, 1995; Stuifbergen, Seraphine, & Roberts, 2000), and better psychological adjustment (Wassem, 1992). Optimistic views of the future were also found to be associated with lower levels of depression and anxiety and better psychological adjustment (de Ridder, Fournier, & Bensing, 2004; de Ridder, Schreurs, & Bensing, 2000; Fournier, de Ridder, & Bensing, 1999, 2002), suggesting that positive future-oriented expectations may indeed play a beneficial role in adaptation to MS. Finally, research on the relationships between hope and adaptation to MS, although sporadic in nature, generally testifies to the salutary consequences that hope confers on mood, as indicated by lower levels of depression (Hickey & Greene, 1989; Lynch et al., 2001; Patten & Metz, 2002).

In summary, the empirical findings across the three disability groups suggest strong trends in the predictive value of the three salutary attributes considered (self-efficacy, optimism, and hope) on PA to CID. The findings generally indicate that all three of the salutary attributes predict lower negative affect (i.e., depression, anxiety, and generalized psychological distress) and higher positive affect (i.e., well-being, QOL, psychosocial adjustment).

Issues Associated with Psychosocial Adaptation to Chronic Illness and Disability

In the final section of this chapter we highlight several unresolved issues that still prevail in the field of PA to CID and need to be addressed by rehabilitation psychologists. We discuss these issues under four broad headings: coping and PA, conceptualization and measurement of outcomes, predictors of PA, and blurring of personality attributes and outcomes of PA.

Issues Associated with Coping and Psychosocial Adaptation

First, coping strategies are largely seen by rehabilitation researchers and clinicians as precursors to and causative factors of adaptation to CID. Therefore, they are typically studied as predictors of PA, the latter indicated by either negatively valenced measures, such as global psychological distress, depression and anxiety, or positively valenced measures, such perceived life satisfaction or psychological well-being. The relationships between coping and adaptation, however, may be better conceptualized as reciprocal since stress-induced coping does influence psychological distress/adaptation outcomes but the latter, in turn, triggers the use of additional coping efforts to mitigate the impact of ongoing levels of distress (Bolger, 1990; Folkman & Moskowitz, 2004; Penley, Tomaka, & Wiebe, 2002). Longitudinal research could, in part, elucidate the nature of such a recursive set of relationships, but even well-designed prospective longitudinal research that controls for prior levels of adaptation (Aldwin & Revenson, 1987) is limited in its capacity to unravel the continually interactive nature of these relationships. The reason for this limitation is inherent in the nature of longitudinal research and the typically wide time gaps (often extending over months and even years) between two adjacent measurement periods. The in-between, wide measurement gaps invite a host of unrelated experiential and environmental life events that could very likely interfere with, interact with, or bolster the assumed interaction between coping and adaptation. Indeed, it is an ill-conceived assumption that merely because coping (or for that matter, any other intrapersonal psychological attribute), envisioned as preceding in time PA outcomes and measured earlier than these assumed outcomes, will prove sufficient (statistically and logically) to be indicative of a causal relationship between coping and PA outcomes. It would, therefore, behoove researchers to temper their claims of causative proof even when derived from well-designed longitudinal research because of the uncontrolled conditions that permeate most of these studies. The many personal, interpersonal, and environmental factors that intercede between adjacent measurement periods render the findings obtained from such predictive models tenuous, even if statistically significant, and limited in their generalizability. Furthermore, these types of designs often fail to detect the possible presence of discontinuous and qualitative changes (Slife, 1993). Anchored within the classical three-tier paradigm promulgated by of David Hume (see, for example, Cook & Campbell, 1979), causal relationships can only be inferred when: (a) cause and effect are proximal in time, (b) temporal precedence of cause to effect has been established, and (c) presumed cause

must be *continuously* present whenever the effect is observed. Examining available longitudinal research findings through this empirical lens convincingly indicates that the first and third conditions have not been met thus far. To bolster arguments of casual relationships between coping efforts and PA outcomes, future research should seek to obtain more frequent assessments of both types of measures and, as importantly, ascertain that study participants clearly realize that in their responses they are to assess how their coping efforts directly seek to manage CID-triggered stress and how these efforts are linked to their subsequent perceptions of distress or well-being. Finally, meta-analytic research could prove invaluable in this respect. Aggregating results from several longitudinal studies could add credence to detecting causal relationships by both increasing statistical power and including a wider range of measurement points of coping strategies and PA outcomes.

Second, research findings on the comparative benefits of engagement (problem-focused) and disengagement (emotion-focused and avoidance) coping to adaptation to CID, are fraught with unresolved conceptual and empirical obstacles. These include the theoretical underpinnings of the concept of coping; the nature of coping (coping as an enduring personality trait vs. coping as an environmentally triggered response to stressful events); the scope of measured coping strategies (ranging from two to about 20; Martz & Livneh, 2007a; Schwarzer & Schwarzer, 1996); the life stresses addressed by the measure (generic vs. CID-specific); and the psychometric soundness of the measure and its initial sample-obtained statistics, which range from narrowly defined, homogeneous groups of respondents to highly heterogeneous groups. It is no surprise, therefore, that findings on the relationships between coping and adaptation yield an inconsistent, indeed often contradictory picture. Future work, then, must be directed at both further elucidation of the construct of coping and its various functions, mechanisms, and processes, as well as at its empirical correlates and psychometric properties.

Third, empirical findings linking coping (engagement vs. disengagement) to adaptation to CID have convincingly shown that factors such as controllability and manageability of CID-engendered stressful experiences play an important role in determining these relationships (Chronister & Chan, 2007; Penley et al., 2002; Zeidner & Saklofske, 1996). Other research has suggested that the earlier benefits (or failures to benefit) accrued from the initial use of either engagement or disengagement coping may determine their use during later stressful encounters. For example, the employment of emotion-focused or avoidance coping may be relied upon more frequently if efforts to manage stress first via problem-solving efforts have failed to yield reduction in stress levels (Tennen, Affleck, Armeli, & Carney, 2000). Further epistemological complications of the coping–PA link arise from the oft-neglected necessity to specify to respondents which phase of the CID-triggered stressful encounter should considered when completing the coping measure. The available literature compellingly indicates that coping efforts are differentially applied, depending upon how stress is temporally perceived. Preparatory or anticipatory coping occurs when stress is anticipated in the near future (e.g., prior to surgery, intense medical regimen). On the other hand, dynamic or crisis-related coping is employed during ongoing acute, stressful encounters (e.g., when injury occurs, when experiencing acute pain). Finally, reactive and residual coping are typically applied following the experienced stressful episode or the recovery period, such as dealing with the aftermath of the accident, living with the long-lasting implications of disability (Aspinwall & Taylor, 1997; Folkman & Moskowitz, 2004; Livneh & Martz, 2007; Penley et al., 2002). Future research needs to further examine the specific conditions and time frames under which engagement and disengagement coping are adopted by people with CID, and how the relative merits of these two groups of strategies are determined by the stress-inducing event. Put differently, researchers should focus more squarely on untangling the moderating and mediating roles of coping, and their time references to the injury or diagnosis, in influencing the relationships between demographic, medical, personal, and interpersonal variables and adaptation to CID.

Fourth, efforts to investigate the role played by coping strategies in predicting PA to CID have commonly taken the form of examining separate and unique contributions by the various strategies (e.g., planning, wishful thinking) or their aggregated value (i.e., engagement or disengagement, problem-focused or emotion-focused). Very rarely have researchers in the field of PA to CID sought to examine the combined or differential (net) composite yielded by the totality of these coping efforts; that is, obtaining a single composite that depicts the relative or proportional values of engagement and disengagement coping. (See also Rabinowitz and Arnett [2009] and Zeidner and Saklofske [1996].) The latter may portray a more realistic, accurate, and useful global coping predictor of adaptation and should be included in future research (see, for example, discussion on the effects of coping on stress by several authors [Conway & Terry, 1992; Vitaliano, DeWolfe, Maiuro, Russo, & Katon, 1990; Vitaliano, Maiuro, Russo, & Becker, 1987]).

Issues Related to the Conceptualization and Measurement of Outcomes of Psychosocial Adaptation

First, PA—conceptually and psychometrically—is a multifaceted construct, spanning a wide spectrum of components and domains (affective, cognitive, motivational, behavioral, physical, and spiritual). It also has been measured by numerous instruments and assigned many indicators, both positive and negative in nature (Dennison, Moss-Morris, & Chalder, 2009; Livneh & Antonak, 1997; Stanton et al., 2007). Earlier efforts to study adaptation in the context of CID focused almost exclusively on negative indicators. Only more recently has the importance of including positive indicators of adaptation been recognized. This is not to suggest that the measurement of indicators of psychological distress should no longer be a concern among rehabilitation psychologists. It does, however, afford researchers a more balanced view of PA outcomes, ensuring a broader and more realistic perspective of adaptation to CID. The inclusion of positive outcomes is also likely to broaden the recognition that the human experience following the onset of CID is not exclusively that of psychological distress, or worse, the domain of psychopathological processes but does, indeed, offer the potential for growth, benefit, and meaning finding; the pursuit of lifestyles and behaviors conducive to better mental health; the improvement of interpersonal relations; and a deepening the individual's spiritual connectedness to the world around (Folkman & Moskowitz, 2000; Stanton et al., 2007; Tedeschi & Calhoun, 1995). Moreover, the experience of personal growth and benefit finding is not necessarily the antithesis of psychological distress and negative affectivity but, in fact, often coexists with the latter following the onset of traumatic experiences (Calhoun & Tedeschi, 1999; Manne et al., 2004; **Pakenham, 2006**). Research, therefore, would benefit from considering a wider view of the spectrum of human adaptation to traumatic experiences and more specifically to the onset and diagnosis of CID.

Second, a plethora of constructs and measures has been used to indicate PA to CID. Even a cursory glance at the large body of available literature on adaptation to CID strongly indicates that a large number of predictors, and more recently, moderators and mediators, may be differentially associated with each type of the many outcome measures. Undertaking a series of meta-analytical studies to bring some semblance of order into this continuously growing literature by examining the unique and combined contributions of the many implicated predictors (demographic, medical, personal, social) to each of these outcome measures (e.g., depression, anxiety, well-being, life-satisfaction, QOL) and anchoring these findings within CID-specific groups may be an important next step for rehabilitation researchers to consider.

Issues Related to Predictors of Psychosocial Adaptation to Chronic Illness and Disability

First, one of the most thoroughly studied groups of predictors of adaptation is that of social support. Despite the compelling evidence that most forms of perceived and received social support are linked to better adaptation to CID, several unanswered issues still remain. Foremost among these is the poorly defined concept of social support. Review of item content and breadth, as included in instruments available to measure social support, indicates that despite the aggregated research thus far little is known about the specific mechanisms of social support that facilitate better PA to CID. It is still unclear whether the salutary ingredients of social support stem from: the specific composition of the provider group (family, friends, medical personnel); the type of support extended (physical, social, emotional, instrumental); the duration of the provided support; the intensity of the effort; the structural aspects of the social network or the functionality (i.e., actual support provision) associated with these social ties; and/or the unidirectionality or bidirectionality of the supportive efforts (see also Berkman & Glass, 1999; Chronister, 2009; Dennison et al., 2009; Kosciulek, 2007; Pierce et al., 1996). The comparative benefits of each of these aspects of social support in predicting adaptation to CID need to be addressed by future research.

Second, the assumption often made of an ostensible distinction between hope/optimism and wishful thinking/denial, although taken for granted by most rehabilitation researchers and clinicians, is conceptually blurred at best. It is also of interest to note that although the two are periodically viewed as two poles of a single continuum, the former is more often aligned with positively valenced personality attributes while the latter is seen as a form of non-adaptive coping modalities. Indeed, unrealistic hope and unfounded optimism are often equated with signs of denial and wishful thinking (Aspinwall & Brunhart, 1996; Livneh, 2009; Wright, 1983). The field of rehabilitation psychology would benefit from concerted empirical efforts to investigate if hope and denial, following the onset of CID, present two distinct categories or if they occupy opposing poles of a single continuum.

Third, as was pointed out earlier, recent research has demonstrated that the relationships between some predictors (e.g., time since injury, benefit finding) and outcomes of adaptation to CID (e.g., depression) may not be strictly linear but may, in fact, demonstrate a curvilinear (quadratic) trend (Krause et al., 2000; Lechner, Carver, Antoni, Weaver, & Phillips, 2006; Manne et al., 2008). Most of the literature to date has focused squarely on testing linear predictive models of adaptation to CID, as demonstrated by such procedures as multiple regression analysis and path analysis. The complexity inherent in studying the differential contributions of demographic, medical, functional, psychological, and interpersonal attributes to PA, however, may require that future research be directed at exploring nonlinear trends as suggested by quadratic, cubic, or more complex models of adaptation. For example, recent nonlinear dynamic models generated by chaos and complexity theory (Gleick, 1987; Prigogine & Stengers, 1984) suggest that understanding complex human behaviors is better approximated by viewing these behaviors as part of an open, nonlinear, non-equilibrium, and self-organizing system, capable of modeling more accurately phase transitions, as are often observed during the process of PA to CID (Livneh & Parker, 2005).

Fourth, although several well-conducted longitudinal studies have tracked levels of depression, anxiety, and general psychological adjustment since onset of SCI, and several of these have reported only minor fluctuations over time in these symptoms (**Craig et al., 1994**; **Kennedy et al., 1995**; **Pollard & Kennedy, 2007**), other studies have found that experienced levels of anxiety and in particular depression do gradually decrease over time (**Krause & Crewe, 1991**; **Richards, 1986**; **Tate, Forchheimer, Kirsch, Maynard, & Roller, 1993**). One of reasons for these apparent discrepancies stems from the fact that invariably all longitudinal research relies on occasional "snapshots" (typically measured monthly or annually and linked to specific transitions, such as entry into a rehabilitation facility, beginning of treatment, discharge into the community, etc.) of the measured psychological distress indicators and cannot accurately address possible continuous (e.g., daily) fluctuations of the experiences. In other words, the obtained sporadic assessments of psychosocial distress and well-being indicators, along their longitudinal trajectories can, at best, provide merely a rough estimate of how these indicators of distress co-vary with truncated temporal trends. They cannot, however, account for any detailed variations that may occur between these measurement points and environmental transitions. Findings from longitudinal studies conducted with other groups of people with CID, such as in cancer and MS patients, have demonstrated a decrease in reported levels of depression over time (**Carver et al., 1993**; Edgar et al., 1992; McCabe, Stokes et al., 2009; Miller et al., 1996). Based on these conflicting results, it may be speculated that longitudinal indicators of psychological distress and well-being may be outcome-specific (e.g., depression, anxiety, adjustment), CID-specific, and influenced by a condition's implications (e.g., degree of life threat invoked, experienced pain, degree of functional limitations). Furthermore, the reported longitudinal trends may follow complex nonlinear trends, and equally important recent research among cancer survivors has even suggested that, regardless of longitudinal depression mean slopes, score variability may very likely vary significantly around the mean over time, indicating a strong within-subject variability in experienced levels of depression (Manne et al., 2008). Further support to the nonlinearity of the adaptation process among breast cancer survivors was also provide by **Helgeson, Snyder, and Seltman (2004)**. In their longitudinal investigation of mental health–related QOL extending over a period of 4.5 years and including seven distinct time measures, these researchers found that four distinct and separate trajectories of adaptation were evident among respondents. These trajectories not only revealed different trends of adaptation (although most suggested psychosocial improvement) but as importantly, indicated differential and nonlinear trends (both quadratic and cubic). Future research, then, must devote more time to investigating CID-specific adaptation trends and the factors that might influence these trends, as well as exploring more thoroughly nonlinear relationships that might exist between predictors and the many indicators of psychosocial adaptation to CID.

Fifth, one of the most stultifying issues that research on PA to CID has yet to grapple with stems from the universal practice of adopting measures of psychological distress—typically depression and anxiety—as the prima facie indicators of adaptation. The extensive reliance on these outcome indicators, however, is fraught with a dauntingly logical inconsistency. If, as has been widely reported in the literature, depression is only experienced by about 25–35% of people with SCI (**Craig et al., 1994**; **Kennedy & Rogers, 2000**), 20–50% of cancer survivors (Grassi et al., 1996; Parle et al., 1996), and 15–60% in people with MS (Chalfant, Bryant, & Fulcher, 2004; Goretti et al., 2009; Mohr & Cox, 2001), whereas anxiety is reported in about 20–35% of those with SCI (**Kennedy et al., 2000**; North, 1999), 20–45% of cancer survivors (Jenkins, May, & Hughes, 1991; Parle et al., 1996), and 15–40% of individuals diagnosed with MS (Chalfant et al., 2004; Goretti et al., 2009; Mohr & Cox, 2001), then how are these indicators to be justified as measures of adaptation?[3] By definition, outcome measures should be selected to denote dynamic characteristics that change over time. That is, in the context of adaptation to CID, outcomes are clinically conceptualized at distal "phases" of a continuous process (see earlier discussion of ecological models of adaptation) that commences following a traumatic event (Trieschmann, 1988; Wright, 1983). However, if anywhere from one-half to over three-quarters of the sampled clinical population have never experienced these targeted reactions, it then stands to reason that they cannot be ontologically and formally measured on these ostensible outcomes since they have never been a part of their adaptation process. How, then, can their unmitigated use by researchers be justified in light of their failure to cogently and validly sample the domain of PA? Put succinctly, how can a nonexisting indicator of adaptation (for most respondents) be justifiably used as practically a universal outcome measure? The problem inherent in the adoption of anxiety and depression as the sine qua non outcome measures of adaptation stems, to a large extent, from the unsupported assumption that these are dichotomous constructs, a view favored by most diagnostic systems including the *Diagnostic and Statistical Manual of Mental Disorders* (DSM-IV-TR; APA, 2000) and International Classification of Functioning, Disability, and Health (ICD; WHO, 2004). The reliance on these medical models serves to dilute the complexity of these and other measures of psychological distress by reducing them to an "all or nothing" human experience (Widiger, 2001; Widiger & Trull, 1991). Although such a practice may be defensible in the medical field when decisions are based on a "treat vs. no-treat" philosophy and are further fueled by insurance companies' demands for diagnostic-based fiduciary efficiency, they have little merit when studying the entire spectrum of human experiences and behaviors following traumatic events, such as the onset of CID, where many shades of distress are possible and often may go unnoticed. Indeed, other outcome measures of PA, such as QOL, life satisfaction, well-being, and positive affectivity are commonly perceived as continuous in nature and as delving into a broader range of human experiences under stressful and nonstressful life conditions. Moreover, these outcomes are more commensurate with the concepts of hardiness (Kobasa, Maddi, & Courington, 1981) and more recently resilience (Bonanno, 2004) that have been shown to be soundly linked to better adaptation to a host of traumatic life experiences. Indeed, the literature on resilience in the aftermath of traumatic injuries suggests that resilience is comprised not merely of the absence of symptoms of psychological distress but, as importantly, incorporates healthy manifestations of psychosocial functioning, including positive affect. It may be that, as rehabilitation psychologists and researchers, we need to take a fresh look at our current practices that often equate PA outcomes with indicators of psychological distress when a plethora of available statistics indicate that these experiences only infrequently play a role in the lives of many people with CID.

Issues Related to Blurring of Personality Attributes and Psychosocial Adaptation

First, one of the thorniest issues that have failed to be fully addressed by researchers of adaptation to CID is the conceptual blurring of certain personality (psychological) attributes, such as self-concept (self-esteem) and acceptance, and outcomes of psychosocial adaptation to CID. If, indeed, self-concept and acceptance are viewed as personality attributes that either interact with other demographic, medical, and environmental variables, or are moderated by coping strategies to influence adaptation to CID, then they must not be employed as an outcome measure. The lack of appropriate and consensual anchoring point for self-concept in the hierarchical process of adaptation is of continuing concern and requires careful attention. Self-concept, acceptance,

and similar constructs should be studied as either predictors (or moderators) of PA or as outcome measures. They cannot, however, be conceived as conveniently belonging to both categories (see also Curbow, Somerfield, Legro, & Sonnega, 1990; Livneh, 2001).

Second, a related issue that requires attention stems from the construct and content blurring (or overlap) of certain predictors and outcomes of adaptation to CID. Mostly, this predictor–outcome overlap can be found in studies that examine the influence of optimism or hope on PA, as depicted by measures of depression. Measures of depression typically include items that denote both cognitive and affective indicators of pessimism, hopelessness, helplessness, and the like (e.g., "I look forward with enjoyment to things," "I am discouraged about the future," "I feel hopeful about the future"). In a conceptually reversed fashion, measures of optimism (such as the Life Orientation Test; LOT) and hope (such as the Hope Scale) invariably include items (e.g., "I usually expect the best," "I energetically pursue my life goals," "I'm always optimistic about my future") that are of opposite nature to depression, as broadly defined by most depression scales such as the BDI, HADS, the CES-D, and more. In other words, the negative relationship between measures of optimism and hope with depression is a reflection of contrasting two opposing poles of the same construct. Empirically, therefore, demonstrating a negative relationship between optimism or hope and depression could be a mere artifact of the measuring instruments and their item content rather than a cogent argument for the predictive power of the former when depression is chosen as the sole outcome indicator of adaptation.

Third, an appreciable amount of theoretical and thematic overlap, common statistical variance, and clinical interpretations exist among such personality attributes as hope, optimism, personal growth, personal agency, resolve, fighting spirit, benefit finding, meaning finding/making, sense of coherence, hardiness, mastery, resilience, self-efficacy, post-traumatic growth, and purpose in life (Almedom, 2005; Folkman & Moskowitz, 2000; Tedeschi & Calhoun, 1995). All of these interrelated constructs reflect various facets and are derivatives of what Antonovsky (1979) referred to as the "salutogenic framework" (a perspective that originates from health) and more recently the "Appraisals of Disability" (Dean & Kennedy, 2009). These positive views on human endurance and transformation in the face of adversity reflect, in part, developments in different disciplines (e.g., rehabilitation psychology, health psychology, social psychology, clinical psychology). Their unique contributions as personality attributes or paths to adaptation undertaken by people facing major life crises including that of CID onset must be further examined, differentiated, and clarified.

Conclusion

Psychosocial adaptation to CID, which typically encompasses the study of the nature, process, dynamics, correlates, and predictors of adaptation, inarguably constitutes one of the most researched topics in rehabilitation psychology. Yet, review of the growing body of clinical evidence, research findings, and theoretical frameworks strongly indicates that it is also one of the most controversial and least agreed upon domains of the field. In this chapter, we focused on reviewing three primary topics; namely, theoretical frameworks of adaptation to CID, empirical findings gleaned from studies of three widely researched conditions (SCI, cancer, and MS), and finally unresolved issues inherent in conceptualizing and examining adaptation. The first section was devoted to an overview of leading theoretical models of PA to CID. Reviewed were linear (stage, phase) models, pendular models, interactive models, and finally ecological models, the latter offering a broader and more heuristic, as well as better empirically derived and supported frameworks of adaptation to the onset and diagnosis of CID. Although no consensus exists on the relative merits of these ecological models, their empirical soundness, or their clinical utility, they do share several process or predictor components (e.g., personal, functional, social, and environmental resources; psychological attributes such as cognitive appraisals, coping skills and strategies, personality characteristics) and several outcome or adaptation indicators (e.g., physical and mental health, QOL, perceptions of life satisfaction and well-being, vocational performance) that suggest that future, multicomponent frameworks of adaptation derived from these models might further bolster our understanding of the complexity inherent in studying the processes and outcomes of adaptation to CID.

The chapter's second section offered a review of empirical findings linking three of the ecological models' most prominent components—demographic, CID-related, and psychological correlates and predictors—with various indices of PA to CID. Focusing on findings from three representative medical conditions, the aggregated data suggest that although some consistency exists as to the predictive power of certain psychosocial variables (e.g., type of coping, perceived social support, perceived level of control, self-efficacy, hope, optimism), most demographic and CID-related variables examined (e.g., gender, age of condition onset or diagnosis, level of severity, time since onset or diagnosis) have been found to be poor predictors of adaptation or, at best, condition-specific. The chapter concludes with a review of 14 yet to be fully addressed and resolved issues in the field of PA to CID. These issues were discussed under four broad headings: (a) issues with coping and PA (for example, the reciprocal rather than the recursive nature of coping and adaptation; the comparative, contextually specific, temporally based, and medical condition–associated merits of various coping modalities; examining the relationships between specific coping strategies vs. composites of strategies and adaptation); (b) issues with conceptualization and measurement of adaptation outcomes (for example, the many indicators and multidimensionality of adaptation to CID, the need for aggregated findings across the many outcome measures used); (c) issues related to the prediction of adaptation (for example, the complexity and often inconsistency inherent in using measures of social support; the fallacy of relying mostly on linear models of prediction while excluding no less valid nonlinear models; the overreliance on two, three, or four time interval points in longitudinal studies to reach decisions of irrefutable causal relationships among sets of interacting predictors and outcomes of adaptation; and the use of depression and anxiety as the prototypical indicators of adaptation to CID despite emerging evidence of their apparent far-from-universal occurrence or unchanging nature over time); and (d) the blurring of mostly stable personality attributes and indicators of adaptation to CID (e.g., the role of self-concept, self-esteem, and acceptance as either predictors, moderators/mediators, or outcomes of adaptation; and the weak theoretical and empirical evidence of discriminant validity for several of the constructs and indicators typically employed to assess positive outcomes of adaptation).

We, therefore, conclude from the presence of these unresolved issues that although the field of PA to CID has made tremendous strides in its conceptual underpinnings, sophisticated research methodologies and statistical acumen, and clinical applications, there is still much more that we need attend to as we seek to better understand the many psychosocial vicissitudes that follow the onset of CID and subsequently to use this knowledge to improve the QOL of people with CID.

Future Directions
TREATMENT IMPLICATIONS

Because most demographic and CID-related factors are seldom changeable, this section explores those potentially alterable psychosocial and personality-type attributes that empirically exhibited strong associations with PA to CID and that, therefore, may be responsive to treatment interventions. This section summarizes five major empirical findings obtained from the research on the three selected CIDs discussed in this chapter, followed by a brief description of possible treatment interventions:

(1) *Findings:* For engagement, or approach-based, problem-focused, task-oriented coping strategies, research trends strongly suggest that the use of engagement-type coping is associated with lower levels of psychological distress and higher levels of adaptive psychological outcomes (e.g., perceived well-being and quality of life, adjustment, post-traumatic growth).

Intervention suggestions: Cognitive-behavior interventions often involve teaching stress-management skills, (progressive) relaxation and meditation, cognitive restructuring skills (i.e., challenging irrational beliefs/thoughts), and cognitive reframing. Teaching specific problem-solving skills (e.g., decision-making, time management, conflict resolution, money management) can also serve to bolster engagement coping abilities.

A limited number of clinical interventions (Eng et al., 2007) indicate that both cognitive-behavioral therapy (CBT) and affective counseling interventions have demonstrated positive impact on psychosocial outcomes after SCI. Several resources exist that describe the use of CBT-based interventions for individuals with CID, including those by Radnitz (2000) and Taylor (2006). Sperry's (2006) book explicates CID-related interventions based on a biopsychosocial model. Further, Chan, Berven, and Thomas' (2004) book contains descriptions of a broad range of psychosocial theories and their possible applications for successful coping among individuals with a wide range of CIDs.

A specific approach to teaching and fostering problem-solving skills was developed by D'Zurilla and Nezu (1999). This strategy involves five steps: identifying/defining the problem, assessing the consequences of the problem, generating a list of possible solutions, making a decision/choosing the most appropriate solution, and evaluating the success of the choice.

A *coping effectiveness training* (CET) program was created by Kennedy and his co-workers (Kennedy, 2008; Kennedy & Duff, 2001; Kennedy, Duff, Evans, & Beedie, 2003; Kennedy, Taylor, & Hindson, 2006). CET outlines psychosocial interventions tailored to help individuals with SCI cope with their disabilities, and the training approaches coping skill development in multiple ways. One CET-based intervention focuses on developing skills for appraising a stressful situation, such as identifying cause(s) of stress, becoming aware of signs/indicators of stress (i.e., emotional, cognitive, physiological, and behavioral reactions), and breaking down complex/global stressors into specific stressors.

Cognitive coping therapy (CCT) by Sharoff (2004) is based on CBT. It uses a therapeutic perspective that trains individuals not to take their thoughts as facts, but rather, to view thoughts as hypotheses that need to be tested and validated. Sharoff's CCT is based on a holistic model that utilizes cognitive, emotional, perceptual, physical, and behavioral abilities. Some of Sharoff's techniques or strategies to promote coping include cognitive rehearsal (i.e., practicing self-statements), values clarification (i.e., helping a person let go of activities based on no longer attainable goals belonging to one's "old self"), and acceptance training (i.e., recognizing that certain actions are a more reasonable fit within one's CID-related limitations). Other techniques mentioned by Sharoff include the psychological strategies of thought-stopping (i.e., commanding oneself to stop distressing thoughts) and time projection (i.e., projecting thoughts 6 months to 1 year ahead, to a time when the individual becomes more aware of the CID and has acquired better coping/problem-solving skills).

(2) *Findings:* For disengagement coping (i.e., avoidance, wishful thinking, emotion-focused coping strategies), most research indicates that usage of such coping strategies is associated with poorer levels of adaptation outcomes (e.g., depression, anxiety, psychological distress), with the exception of denial, which is one form of DC that may be associated with either negative or positive psychosocial outcomes, depending on the circumstances surrounding its presence.

Intervention suggestions: Psychotherapeutic-related interventions (including psychodynamic,

Gestalt, and Rogerian approaches) can be used to explore and validate feelings. Generally speaking, for unchangeable CID-related stressors, the adoption of an emotion-focused approach (e.g., regulating emotions or thoughts about the situation) is regarded as justifiable.

Kennedy and Duff's (2001) CET program can be used to bolster emotion regulation strategies for an "unchangeable" situation. These strategies include a range of strategies, such as participating in pleasant social activities, finding competency (goal-achievement) activities, engaging in activities incompatible with emotional distress, learning relaxation techniques, focusing on acceptance of the reality of the CID, reframing/challenging negative thinking, using spirituality to transcend the restrictions imposed the CID, using humor, and seeking social support in order to vent emotions/concerns.

Sharoff (2004) suggests a variety of techniques that can be used in a therapeutic setting to reduce the impact of disengagement coping and bolster more adaptive forms of coping. These include self-instruction training (i.e., setting up self-dialogue to be used when CID-related issues trigger emotional suffering from one's illness) and creating positive self-talk (i.e., creating one's own responses to be used when CID-related frustration is experienced). Use of predetermined/preselected imagery or symbolic gesturing can be implemented by the individual with CID when suffering occurs, in order to facilitate coping. Other strategies to minimize disengagement coping and bolster positive coping with CID, as described by Sharoff and that also may be found in the broader field of psychological interventions, include self-monitoring of autonomic arousal (i.e., a strategy to help an individual understand what is triggering the reactions), relaxation exercises (e.g., deep breathing, muscle relaxation), systematic desensitization (i.e., individualized categorization and prioritization of anxiety-producing stimuli followed by pairing of these imagined stimuli with resulting anxiety while in a state of relaxation), and worry management training (i.e., instructing the individual to worry *only* at a specific times, such as from 6 to 8 PM, in order to learn control over the worrying). Finally, techniques such as mindfulness could be beneficial for those who rely heavily on negative self-perceptions and ruminative appraisals (Dean & Kennedy, 2009).

(3) *Findings:* For coping strategies that involved seeking and using social support, research findings demonstrate compelling evidence of the beneficial effects of requesting and utilizing proper social support.

Intervention suggestions: Social support systems can be accessed for emotional support, tangible support, and informational support (Kleinke, 1998). Psychotherapeutic-related interventions can be used to facilitate proper use of interpersonal support. These interventions involve the engagement of interpersonal components, such as marital, family, and group counseling, to help facilitate CID-related coping and adaptation.

(4) *Findings:* Generalized LOC and HLOC research indicated that having an internal LOC or internal HLOC was associated with lower levels of avoidance and emotional distress and with better adjustment. There were, however, some contradictory empirical findings, especially related to perceived control over health, suggesting that relying on an internal HLOC may be related to poorer levels of adaptation. These findings could be explained as reflecting personal efforts of little utility to manage health in the face of mostly uncontrollable and unpredictable conditions.

Intervention suggestions: The fact that certain aspects of CID are immutable and beyond personal control can create a sense of helplessness, frustration, and even anger for people with CID. Sharoff (2004) proposed several strategies that could be used to manage LOC/HLOC-related issues, although these strategies are yet untested. Sharoff's ideas include area thinking (i.e., encouraging an individual with a CID to select goals that are mostly under the individual's control and that are also realistic as far as their modifiability) and surrendering versus non-surrendering strategy (i.e., knowing "when to surrender, when not to surrender, or when surrender is inevitable"; Sharoff, 2004, p. 73).

(5) *Findings:* The use of salutary attributes of self-efficacy, hope, and optimism generally demonstrated a trend that indicated their association with a variety of psychosocial outcomes, such as better overall psychological adjustment and lower levels of depression, anxiety, and negative affectivity.

Intervention suggestions: Psychotherapeutic-related interventions (e.g., psychodynamic, Gestalt, and Rogerian therapeutic approaches) can be used to validate positive self-perceptions and encourage individuals to maintain optimism and hope (see Chan et al., 2004, for applications of these theories to CID). Marks and Allegrante (2005) briefly summarized clinical interventions that were specifically targeted to promote self-efficacy among individuals with CID (see Table 2, p. 152, in their article). They noted the importance of the role of self-efficacy in encouraging the self-management of CID and CID-related issues.

Sharoff (2004) suggested several strategies that could be used to bolster self-efficacy, hope, and optimism. These include identity coalescing (i.e., designing a new and positive identity that incorporates the presence of CID), blending one's old and new identities (i.e., "weighting" or balancing the power of the new self with a CID with old images of oneself, so that one does not focus only on negative images), avoiding value judgments by changing to descriptive judgments (i.e., recording one's actions and experiences but not condemning or criticizing them), acting without comparing oneself to norms/standards (i.e., working to suspend standards and instead, setting one's own personal goals), and self-booster training (i.e., overemphasizing one's abilities and underemphasizing the negative aspects/shortcomings of one's life, in order to stress the positive and counteract negative thinking triggered by the CID).

Notes

1. Although we conveniently collapsed severity of CID, functionality, and community integration/participation into a single broad category, in what follows, we were careful to separately discuss findings that were obtained from measures of medical severity (mostly addressing impairment and disability) and those derived from measures of participation in various life activities (handicap).

2. It should be mentioned, however, that emotion-focused and avoidance coping have been, occasionally, viewed as two separate groups of coping strategies (Billings & Moos, 1981; Endler & Parker, 1994; Roth & Cohen, 1986).

3. If one considers the figures available on the prevalence of anxiety and depressive disorders in the general population, estimated to be approximately 10–15% (Barlow & Durand, 2009), then removing these "preexisting" or independent clinical diagnoses from the reported findings further reduces the figures associated with the prevalence of depression and anxiety triggered by the onset of CID.

References

Aikens, J. E., Fischer, J. S., Namey, M., & Rudick, R. A. (1997). A replicated prospective investigation of life stress, coping, and depressive symptoms in multiple sclerosis. *Journal of Behavioral Medicine, 20*(5), 433–445.

Airlie, J., Baker, G., Smith, S., & Young, C. (2001). Measuring the impact of multiple sclerosis on psychosocial functioning: the development of a new self-efficacy scale. *Clinical rehabilitation, 15*(3), 259–265.

Aldwin, C., & Revenson, T. (1987). Does coping help? A reexamination of the relation between coping and mental health. *Journal of Personality and Social Psychology, 53*(2), 337–348.

Alfano, D., Neilson, P., & Fink, M. (1993). Long-term psychosocial adjustment following head or spinal cord injury. *Neuropsychiatry, Neuropsychology, and Behavioral Neurology, 6,* 117–117.

Almedom, A. (2005). Resilience, hardiness, sense of coherence, and posttraumatic growth: All paths leading to "light at the end of the tunnel"? *Journal of Loss and Trauma, 10*(3), 253–265.

Amirkhan, J. (1990). A factor analytically derived measure of coping: The coping strategy indicator. *Journal of Personality and Social Psychology, 59*(5), 1066–1074.

Andrykowski, M., & Brady, M. (1994). Health locus of control and psychological distress in cancer patients: Interactive effects of context. *Journal of Behavioral Medicine, 17*(5), 439–458.

Andrykowski, M., Curran, S., Studts, J., Cunningham, L., Carpenter, J., McGrath, P., et al. (1996). Psychosocial adjustment and quality of life in women with breast cancer and benign breast problems: A controlled comparison. *Journal of Clinical Epidemiology, 49*(8), 827–834.

Antonovsky, A. (1979). *Health, stress, and coping: New perspectives on mental and physical well-being.* New York: Jossey-Bass.

APA (2000). *Diagnostic and Statistical Manual of Mental Disorders: DSM-IV, 4th ed., text revision.* Washington, DC: American Psychiatric Association.

Arnett, P., Higginson, C., Voss, W., Randolph, J., & Grandey, A. (2002). Relationship between coping, cognitive dysfunction and depression in multiple sclerosis. *The Clinical Neuropsychologist, 16*(3), 341–355.

Arnett, P. A., & Randolph, J. J. (2006). Longitudinal course of depression symptoms in multiple sclerosis. *Journal of Neurology, Neurosurgery, and Psychiatry, 77*(5), 606–610.

Aspinwall, L., & Brunhart, S. (1996). Distinguishing optimism from denial: Optimistic beliefs predict attention to health threats. *Personality and Social Psychology Bulletin, 22*(10), 993–1003.

Aspinwall, L., & Taylor, S. (1997). A stitch in time: Self-regulation and proactive coping. *Psychological bulletin, 121,* 417–436.

Bandura, A. (1977). Self-efficacy: Toward a unifying theory of behavioral change. *Psychological Review, 84*(2), 191–215.

Barker, R., Wright, B., Meyerson, L., & Gonick, M. (1953). *Adjustment to physical handicap and illness: A survey of the social psychology of physique and disability (Bulletin 55).* New York: Social Science Research Council.

Barlow, D., & Durand, V. (2009). *Abnormal psychology: An integrative approach* (5th ed.). Belmont, CA: Wadsworth.

Barnwell, A., & Kavanagh, D. (1997). Prediction of psychological adjustment to multiple sclerosis. *Social Science and Medicine, 45*(3), 411–418.

Barrera, M. (1986). Distinctions between social support concepts, measures, and models. *American Journal of Community Psychology, 14*(4), 413–445.

Beck, A., Epstein, N., Brown, G., & Steer, R. (1988). An inventory for measuring clinical anxiety: psychometric properties. *Journal of Consulting and Clinical Psychology, 56*(6), 893–897.

Beck, A., Ward, C., Mendelson, M., Mock, J., & Erbaugh, J. (1961). An inventory for measuring depression. *Archives of General Psychiatry, 4,* 561–571.

Beckham, J., Burker, E., Feldman, M., & Costakis, M. (1997). Self-efficacy and adjustment in cancer patients: a preliminary report. *Behavioral Medicine, 23*(3), 138–142.

Behen, J. M., & Rodrigue, J. R. (1994). Predictors of coping strategies among adults with cancer. *Psychological Reports, 74*(1), 43–48.

Berckman, K., & Austin, J. (1993). Causal attribution, perceived control, and adjustment in patients with lung cancer. *Oncology Nursing Forum 20*(1), 23–30.

Bergner, M., Bobbitt, R., Carter, W., & Gilson, B. (1981). The Sickness Impact Profile: development and final revision of a health status measure. *Medical Care, 19*(8), 787–805.

Berkman, L., & Glass, T. (1999). Social integration, social networks, social support, and health. In L. F. B. T. Glass (Ed.), *Social epidemiology* (pp. 137–173). New York: Oxford University Press.

Billings, A., & Moos, R. (1981). The role of coping responses and social resources in attenuating the stress of life events. *Journal of Behavioral Medicine, 4*(2), 139–157.

Bishop, M. (2005a). Quality of life and psychosocial adaptation to chronic illness and acquired disability: A conceptual and theoretical synthesis. *The Journal of Rehabilitation, 71*(2), 5–14.

Bishop, M. (2005b). Quality of life and psychosocial adaptation to chronic illness and disability: Preliminary analysis of a conceptual and theoretical synthesis. *Rehabilitation Counseling Bulletin, 48*(4), 219–231.

Bishop, M., Smedema, S., & Lee, E. (2009). Quality of life and psychosocial adaptation to chronic illness and disability. In F. Chan, E. da Silva Cardoso, & J. Chronister (Eds.), *Understanding psychosocial adjustment to chronic illness and disability: a handbook for evidence-based practitioners in rehabilitation* (pp. 521–550).New York: Springer.

Bishop, M., Stenhoff, D., & Shepard, L. (2007). Psychosocial adaptation and quality of life in multiple sclerosis: Assessment of the disability centrality model. *Journal of Rehabilitation, 73*(1), 3–12.

Bloom, J. (1982). Social support, accommodation to stress and adjustment to breast cancer. *Social Science and Medicine, 16*(14), 1329–1338.

Bolger, N. (1990). Coping as a personality process: A prospective study. *Journal of Personality and Social Psychology, 59*(3), 525–537.

Bonanno, G. (2004). Loss, trauma, and human resilience. *American Psychologist, 59*(1), 20–28.

Bracken, M., & Bernstein, M. (1980). Adaptation to and coping with disability one year after spinal cord injury: An epidemiological study. *Social Psychiatry and Psychiatric Epidemiology, 15*(1), 33–41.

Bracken, M., Shepard, M., & Webb, S. (1981). Psychological response to acute spinal cord injury: An epidemiological study. *Paraplegia, 19*, 271–283.

Buckelew, S., Baumstark, K., Frank, R., & Hewett, J. (1990). Adjustment following spinal cord injury. *Rehabilitation Psychology, 35*(2), 101–109.

Buckelew, S., Frank, R., Elliott, T., Chaney, J., & Hewett, J. (1991). Adjustment to spinal cord injury: stage theory revisited. *Paraplegia, 29*(2), 125–130.

Buckelew, S., & Hanson, S. (1992). Coping and adjustment following spinal cord injury. *Spinal Cord Injury Psychosocial Process, 5*, 99–103.

Bukberg, J., Penman, D., & Holland, J. (1984). Depression in hospitalized cancer patients. *Psychosomatic Medicine, 46*(3), 199–212.

Burgess, C., Morris, T., & Pettingale, K. (1988). Psychological response to cancer diagnosis—II. Evidence for coping styles (coping styles and cancer diagnosis). *Journal of Psychosomatic Research, 32*(3), 263–272.

Calhoun, L., & Tedeschi, R. (1999). *Facilitating posttraumatic growth: A clinician's guide.* New York: Lawrence Erlbaum Associates.

Carver, C., Pozo, C., Harris, S., Noriega, V., Scheier, M., Robinson, D., et al. (1993). How coping mediates the effect of optimism on distress: A study of women with early stage breast cancer. *Journal of Personality and Social Psychology, 65*, 375–375.

Carver, C., Scheier, M., & Weintraub, J. (1989). Assessing coping strategies: A theoretically based approach. *Journal of Personality and Social Psychology, 56*(2), 267–283.

Carver, C., Smith, R., Antoni, M., Petronis, V., Weiss, S., & Derhagopian, R. (2005). Optimistic personality and psychosocial well-being during treatment predict psychosocial well-being among long-term survivors of breast cancer. *Health Psychology, 24*, 508–516.

Carver, C. S., Pozo-Kaderman, C., Harris, S. D., Noriega, V., Scheier, M. F., Robinson, D. S., et al. (1994). Optimism versus pessimism predicts the quality of women's adjustment to early stage breast cancer. *Cancer, 73*(4), 1213–1220.

Cella, D. F., Orofiamma, B., Holland, J. C., Silberfarb, P. M., Tross, S., Feldstein, M., et al. (1987). The relationship of psychological distress, extent of disease, and performance status in patients with lung cancer. *Cancer, 60*(7), 1661–1667.

Chalfant, A., Bryant, R., & Fulcher, G. (2004). Posttraumatic stress disorder following diagnosis of multiple sclerosis. *Journal of Traumatic Stress, 17*(5), 423–428.

Chalk, H. (2007). Mind over matter: Cognitive-behavioral determinants of emotional distress in multiple sclerosis patients. *Psychology, Health and Medicine, 12*(5), 556–566.

Chan, F., Berven, N., & Thomas, K. (2004). *Counseling theories and techniques for rehabilitation health professionals.* New York: Springer.

Chan, R. C., Lee, P. W., & Lieh-Mak, F. (2000). The pattern of coping in persons with spinal cord injuries. *Disability and Rehabilitation, 22*(11), 501–507.

Charmaz, K. (1983). Loss of self: A fundamental form of suffering in the chronically ill. *Sociology of Health and Illness, 5*(2), 168–195.

Charmaz, K. (1993). *Good days, bad days: The self in chronic illness and time.* Piscataway, NJ: Rutgers University Press.

Charmaz, K. (1995). The body, identity, and self: Adapting to impairment. *Sociological Quarterly*, 657–680.

Chase, B., Cornille, T., & English, R. (2000). Life Satisfaction among Persons with Spinal Cord Injuries. *Journal of Rehabilitation, 66*(3), 14–20.

Chen, C., David, A., Thompson, K., & Smith, C. (1996). Coping strategies and psychiatric morbidity in women attending breast assessment clinics. *Journal of Psychosomatic Research, 40*(3), 265–270.

Chen, C. C., David, A., Thompson, K., Smith, C., Lea, S., & Fahy, T. (1996). Coping strategies and psychiatric morbidity in women attending breast assessment clinics. *Journal of Psychosomatic Research, 40*(3), 265–270.

Christensen, A., Wiebe, J., Benotsch, E., & Lawton, W. (1996). Perceived health competence, health locus of control, and patient adherence in renal dialysis. *Cognitive Therapy and Research, 20*(4), 411–421.

Chronister, J. (2009). Social support and rehabilitation: Theory, research and measurement. In F.Chan, E. da Silva Cardoso, and J. A. Chronister (Eds.), *Understanding psychosocial adjustment to chronic illness and disability: a handbook for evidence-based practitioners in rehabilitation* (pp. 149–183). New York: Springer.

Chronister, J., & Chan, F. (2007). Hierarchical coping: A conceptual framework for understanding coping within the context of chronic illness and disability. In E. Martz and H. Livneh (Eds.), *Coping with chronic illness and disability: Theoretical, empirical, and clinical aspects*, (pp. 49–71). New York: Springer.

Chubon, R. A. (1987). Development of a quality-of-life rating scale for use in health-care evaluation. *Evaluation and the Health Professions, 10*(2), 186–200.

Chung, M., Preveza, E., Papandreou, K., & Prevezas, N. (2006). Spinal cord injury, posttraumatic stress, and locus of control among the elderly: A comparison with young and middle–aged patients. *Psychiatry: Interpersonal and Biological Processes, 69*(1), 69–80.

Classen, C., Koopman, C., Angell, K., & Spiegel, D. (1996). Coping styles associated with psychological adjustment to advanced breast cancer. *Health Psychology, 15*, 434–437.

Clayton, K., & Chubon, R. (1994). Factors associated with the quality of life of long-term spinal cord injured persons. *Archives of Physical Medicine and Rehabilitation, 75*(6), 633–638.

Cohn, N. (1961). Understanding the process of adjustment to disability. *Journal of rehabilitation, 27*, 16–18.

Conway, V., & Terry, D. (1992). Appraised controllability as a moderator of the effectiveness of different coping strategies: A test of the goodness of fit hypothesis. *Australian Journal of Psychology, 44*(1), 1–7.

Cook, T., & Campbell, D. (1979). *Quasi-experimentation: Design and analysis for field settings*. Chicago: Rand McNally

Craig, A., Hancock, K., & Dickson, H. (1994). Spinal cord injury: A search for determinants of depression two years after the event. *British Journal of Clinical Psychology, 33*(2), 221–230.

Craig, A., Hancock, K., Dickson, H., Martin, J., & Chang, E. (1990). Psychological consequences of spinal injury: A review of the literature. *Australasian Psychiatry, 24*(3), 418–425.

Crewe, N., & Krause, J. (1990). An eleven-year follow-up of adjustment to spinal cord injury. *Rehabilitation Psychology, 35*(4), 205–210.

Crisp, R. (1992). The long-term adjustment of 60 persons with spinal cord injury. *Australian Psychologist, 27*(1), 43–47.

Curbow, B., Somerfield, M., Legro, M., & Sonnega, J. (1990). Self-concept and cancer in adults: Theoretical and method-ological issues. *Social Science and Medicine, 31*(2), 115–128.

Curran, C., Ponsford, J., & Crowe, S. (2000). Coping strategies and emotional outcome following traumatic brain injury: A comparison with orthopedic patients. *Journal of Head Trauma Rehabilitation, 15*(6), 1256–1274.

D'Zurilla, T., & Nezu, A. (1999). *Problem-solving therapy: A social competence approach to clinical intervention.* New York: Springer.

de Ridder, D., Fournier, M., & Bensing, J. (2004). Does optimism affect symptom report in chronic disease? What are its consequences for self-care behaviour and physical functioning? *Journal of Psychosomatic Research, 56*(3), 341–350.

de Ridder, D., Schreurs, K., & Bensing, J. (2000). The relative benefits of being optimistic: Optimism as a coping resource in multiple sclerosis and Parkinson's disease. *British Journal of Health Psychology, 5*(2), 141–155.

De Roon-Cassini, T., Aubin, E., Valvano, A., Hastings, J., & Horn, P. (2009). Psychological well-being after spinal cord injury: Perception of loss and meaning making. *Rehabilitation Psychology, 54*(3), 306–314.

Dean, R. E., & Kennedy, P. (2009). Measuring appraisals following acquired spinal cord injury: A preliminary psychometric analysis of the appraisals of disability. *Rehabilitation Psychology, 54*(2), 222–231.

Decker, S., & Schulz, R. (1985). Correlates of life satisfaction and depression in middle-aged and elderly spinal cord-injured persons. *American Journal of Occupational Therapy, 39*(11), 740–745.

Dembo, T., Leviton, G. L., &, & Wright, B. A. (1956). Adjustment to misfortune—a problem of social-psychological rehabilitation. *Artificial Limbs, 3*, 4–62.

Dennison, L., Moss-Morris, R., & Chalder, T. (2009). A review of psychological correlates of adjustment in patients with multiple sclerosis. *Clinical Psychology Review, 29*(2), 141–153.

Derogatis, L. (1977). *SCL-90-R (revised version) manual I.* Baltimore: Johns Hopkins University School of Medicine.

Derogatis, L. (1986). The psychosocial adjustment to illness scale (PAIS). *Journal of Psychosomatic Research, 30*(1), 77–91.

deRoon-Cassini, T. A., de St. Aubin, E., Valvano, A., Hastings, J., & Horn, P. (2009). Psychological well-being after spinal cord injury: Perception of loss and meaning making. *Rehabilitation Psychology, 54*(3), 306–314.

Devins, G. (1989). Enhancing personal control and minimizing illness intrusiveness. In N.G. Kutner, D.O. Cardenas. and J.D. Bower (Eds.), *Maximizing rehabilitation in chronic renal disease* (pp.109–136). New York: PMA Publishing Corp.

Devins, G., & Binik, Y. (1996). Facilitating coping with chronic physical illness. In M. Zeidner and N. S. Endler (Eds.), *Handbook of coping: Theory, research, applications* (pp. 640–696). Oxford, England: John Wiley & Sons Inc.

Devins, G., Binik, Y., Hutchinson, T., Hollomby, D., Barre, P., & Guttmann, R. (1983). The emotional impact of end-stage renal disease: Importance of patients' perceptions of intrusiveness and control. *International Journal of Psychiatry and Medicine, 13*(4), 327–343.

Devins, G., Edworthy, S., Guthrie, N., & Martin, L. (1992). Illness intrusiveness in rheumatoid arthritis: Differential impact on depressive symptoms over the adult lifespan. *Journal of Rheumatology, 19*(5), 709–715.

Devins, G., Seland, T., Klein, G., Edworthy, S., & Saary, M. (1993). Stability and determinants of psychosocial well-being in multiple sclerosis. *Rehabilitation Psychology, 38*(1), 11–26.

Devins, G., & Shnek, Z. (2000). Multiple sclerosis. In R. Frank & T. Elliott (Eds.), *Handbook of rehabilitation psychology* (pp. 163–184). Washington, DC: American Psychological Association.

Devins, G., Styra, R., O'Connor, P., Gray, T., Seland, T., Klein, G., et al. (1996). Psychosocial impact of illness intrusiveness moderated by age in multiple sclerosis. *Psychology, Health and Medicine, 1*(2), 179–191.

Devins, G. M., Mandin, H., Hons, R. B., Burgess, E. D., Klassen, J., Taub, K., et al. (1990). Illness intrusiveness and quality of life in end-stage renal disease: comparison and stability across treatment modalities. *Health Psychology, 9*(2), 117–142.

Diener, E., Emmons, R., Larsen, R., & Griffin, S. (1985). The satisfaction with life scale. *Journal of Personality Assessment, 49*(1), 71–75.

Diener, E., Suh, E., Lucas, R., & Smith, H. (1999). Subjective well-being: Three decades of progress. *Psychological Bulletin, 125*, 276–302.

Duff, J., & Kennedy, P. (2003). Spinal cord injury. In S. Llewelyn and P. Kennedy (Eds.), *Handbook of clinical health psychology* (pp. 251–275). Chichester, UK: John Wiley & Sons, Ltd.

Dunkel-Schetter, C., Feinstein, L., Taylor, S., & Falke, R. (1992). Patterns of coping with cancer. *Health Psychology*, *11*(2), 79–87.

Dunn, M. E. (1975). Psychological intervention in a spinal cord injury center: An introduction. *Rehabilitation Psychology*, *22*(4), 165–178.

Edgar, L., Rosberger, Z., & Nowlis, D. (1992). Coping with cancer during the first year after diagnosis. Assessment and intervention. *Cancer*, *69*(3), 817–828.

Edlund, B., & Sneed, N. (1989). Emotional responses to the diagnosis of cancer: Age-related comparisons. *Oncology Nursing Forum*, *16*(5), 691–697

Elfström, M., Kennedy, P., Lude, P., & Taylor, N. (2007). Condition-related coping strategies in persons with spinal cord lesion: A cross-national validation of the Spinal Cord Lesion-related Coping Strategies Questionnaire in four community samples. *Spinal Cord*, *45*(6), 420–428.

Elfström, M., & Kreuter, M. (2006). Relationships between locus of control, coping strategies and emotional well-being in persons with spinal cord lesion. *Journal of Clinical Psychology in Medical Settings*, *13*(1), 89–100.

Elfström, M., Kreuter, M., Rydén, A., Persson, L., & Sullivan, M. (2002). Effects of coping on psychological outcome when controlling for background variables: A study of traumatically spinal cord lesioned persons. *Spinal Cord*, *40*(8), 408–415.

Elfström, M., Rydén, A., Kreuter, M., Persson, L., & Sullivan, M. (2002). Linkages between coping and psychological outcome in the spinal cord lesioned: Development of SCL-related measures. *Spinal Cord*, *40*(1), 23.

Elfström, M., Rydén, A., Kreuter, M., Taft, C., & Sullivan, M. (2005). Relations between coping strategies and health-related quality of life in patients with spinal cord lesion. *Journal of Rehabilitation Medicine*, *37*(1), 9–16.

Ell, K., Mantell, J., Hamovitch, M., & Nishimoto, R. (1989). Social support, sense of control, and coping among patients with breast, lung, or colorectal cancer. *Journal of Psychosocial Oncology*, *7*(3), 63–89.

Ell, K., Nishimoto, R., Morvay, T., Mantell, J., & Hamovitch, M. (1989). A longitudinal analysis of psychological adaptation among survivors of cancer. *Cancer*, *63*(2), 406–413.

Elliott, T., Godshall, F., Herrick, S., Witty, T., & Spruell, M. (1991). Problem-solving appraisal and psychological adjustment following spinal cord injury. *Cognitive Therapy and Research*, *15*(5), 387–398.

Elliott, T., Herrick, S., Patti, A., & Witty, T. (1991). Assertiveness, social support, and psychological adjustment following spinal cord injury. *Behaviour Research and Therapy*, *29*(5), 485–493.

Elliott, T., Herrick, S., Witty, T., Godshall, F., & Spruell, M. (1992a). Social relationships and psychosocial impairment of persons with spinal cord injury. *Psychology and Health*, *7*(1), 55–67.

Elliott, T., Herrick, S., Witty, T., Godshall, F., & Spruell, M. (1992b). Social support and depression following spinal cord injury. *Rehabilitation Psychology*, *37*(1), 37–48.

Elliott, T., & Richards, J. (1999). Living with the facts, negotiating the terms: Unrealistic beliefs, denial, and adjustment in the first year of acquired physical disability. *Journal of Loss and Trauma*, *4*(4), 361–381.

Elliott, T. R., Witty, T. E., Herrick, S., & Hoffman, J. T. (1991). Negotiating reality after physical loss: hope, depression, and disability. *Journal of Personality and Social Psychology*, *61*(4), 608–613.

Endler, N., & Parker, J. (1994). Assessment of multidimensional coping: Task, emotion, and avoidance strategies. *Psychological Assessment*, *6*, 50–60.

Eng J, Teasell R, Miller W, Wolfe D, Townson A, Aubut J, et al. (2007). Spinal Cord Injury Rehabilitation Evidence: Methods of the SCIRE Systematic Review. *Topics in Spinal Cord Injury Rehabilitation Summer 2007*, *13*(1), 1–10.

Epping-Jordan, J., Compas, B., Osowiecki, D., Oppedisano, G., Gerhardt, C., Primo, K., et al. (1999). Psychological adjustment in breast cancer: processes of emotional distress. *Health Psychology*, *18*, 315–326.

Falek, A., & Britton, S. (1974). Phases in coping: The hypothesis and its implications. *Social Biology*, *21*(1), 1–7.

Fang, C., Daly, M., Miller, S., Zerr, T., Malick, J., & Engstrom, P. (2006). Coping with ovarian cancer risk: The moderating effects of perceived control on coping and adjustment. *British Journal of Health Psychology*, *11*(4), 561–580.

Feifel, H., & Strack, S. (1989). Coping with conflict situations: Middle-aged and elderly men. *Psychology and Aging*, *4*(1), 26–33.

Ferington, F. (1986). Effectiveness in spinal cord injured persons. *Research in Nursing and Health*, *9*, 257–265.

Ferrero, J., Barreto, M., & Toledo, M. (1994). Mental adjustment to cancer and quality of life in breast cancer patients: An exploratory study. *Psycho-Oncology*, *3*(3), 223–232.

Filipp, S., Klauer, T., Freudenberg, E., & Ferring, D. (1990). The regulation of subjective well-being in cancer patients: An analysis of coping effectiveness. *Psychology and Health*, *4*(4), 305–317.

Fink, S. (1967). Crisis and motivation: A theoretical model. *Archives of Physical Medicine and Rehabilitation*, *48*, 592–597.

Folkman, S., & Lazarus, R. (1990). Coping and emotion. In N. L. Stein, B. Leventhal, and T. Trabasso (Eds.), *Psychological and biological approaches to emotion*, (pp. 313–332). Hillsdale, NJ: Lawrence Erlbaum Associates, Inc.

Folkman, S., & Moskowitz, J. (2000). Positive affect and the other side of coping. *American Psychologist*, *55*(6), 647–654.

Folkman, S., & Moskowitz, J. (2004). Coping: Pitfalls and promise. *Annual Review of Psychology*, *55*, 745–774.

Fournier, M., de Ridder, D., & Bensing, J. (1999). Optimism and adaptation to multiple sclerosis: What does optimism mean? *Journal of Behavioral Medicine*, *22*(4), 303–326.

Fournier, M., De Ridder, D., & Bensing, J. (2002). Optimism and adaptation to chronic disease: The role of optimism in relation to self-care options of type 1 diabetes mellitus, rheumatoid arthritis and multiple sclerosis. *British Journal of Health Psychology*, *7*(4), 409–432.

Frank, R., & Elliott, T. (1989). Spinal cord injury and health locus of control beliefs. *Paraplegia*, *27*(4), 250–256.

Frank, R., Umlauf, R., Wonderlich, S., Askanazi, G., Buckelew, S., & Elliott, T. (1987). Differences in coping styles among persons with spinal cord injury: A cluster-analytic approach. *Journal of Consulting and Clinical Psychology*, *55*(5), 727–731.

Friedman, L., Baer, P., Lewy, A., Lane, M., & Smith, F. (1988). Predictors of psychosocial adjustment to breast cancer. *Journal of Psychosocial Oncology*, *6*(1), 75—94.

Friedman, L., Kalidas, M., Elledge, R., Chang, J., Romero, C., Husain, I., et al. (2006). Optimism, social support and psychosocial functioning among women with breast cancer. *Psycho-Oncology*, *15*(7), 595.

Friedman, L., Nelson, D., Baer, P., Lane, M., & Smith, F. (1990). Adjustment to breast cancer: A replication study. *Journal of Psychosocial Oncology, 8*(4), 27–40.

Fries, J. F. (2002). Reducing disability in older age. *JAMA: The Journal of the American Medical Association, 288*(24), 3164–3166.

Frisch, M. B. (Ed.). (1999). *Quality of life assessment/intervention and the Quality of Life Inventory.* Mahwah, NJ: Erlbaum.

Fuhrer, M. (1996). The subjective well-being of people with spinal cord injury: relationships to impairment, disability, and handicap. *Top Spinal Cord Injury Rehabilitation, 1*(4), 56–71.

Fuhrer, M., Rintala, D., Hart, K., Clearman, R., & Young, M. (1992). Relationship of life satisfaction to impairment, disability, and handicap among persons with spinal cord injury living in the community. *Archives of Physical Medicine and Rehabilitation, 73*(6), 552–557.

Gleick, J. (1987). *Chaos: Making a new science* (p. 8). New York: Viking Penguin.

Goretti, B., Portaccio, E., Zipoli, V., Hakiki, B., Siracusa, G., Sorbi, S., et al. (2009). Coping strategies, psychological variables and their relationship with quality of life in multiple sclerosis. *Neurological Sciences, 30*(1), 15–20.

Gotay, C. (1985). Why me? Attributions and adjustment by cancer patients and their mates at two stages in the disease process. *Social Science and Medicine, 20*(8), 825–831.

Grassi, L., Rosti, G., Albertazzi, L., & Marangolo, M. (1996). Depressive symptoms in autologous bone marrow transplant (ABMT) patients with cancer: An exploratory study. *Psychological Oncology, 5*(4), 305–310.

Halligan, F., & Reznikoff, M. (1985). Personality factors and change with multiple sclerosis. *Journal of Consulting and Clinical Psychology, 53*(4), 547–548.

Hammell, K. (1994). Psychosocial outcome following spinal cord injury. *Paraplegia, 32*(11), 771–779.

Hammell, K. (2004). Quality of life among people with high spinal cord injury living in the community. *Spinal Cord, 42*(11), 607–620.

Hampton, Z. (2000). Self-efficacy and quality of life in people with spinal cord injuries in China. *Rehabilitation Counseling Bulletin, 43*(2), 66–74

Hanson, S., Buckelew, S., Hewett, J., & O'Neal, G. (1993). The relationship between coping and adjustment after spinal cord injury: A 5-year follow-up study. *Rehabilitation Psychology, 38*(1), 41–52.

Hatcher, M., Whitaker, C., & Karl, A. (2009). What predicts post-traumatic stress following spinal cord injury? *British Journal of Health Psychology, 14*(3), 541–561.

Heidrich, S., Forsthoff, C., & Ward, S. (1994). Psychological adjustment in adults with cancer: The self as mediator. *Health Psychology, 13*, 346–346.

Heim, E., Valach, L., & Schaffner, L. (1997). Coping and psychosocial adaptation: longitudinal effects over time and stages in breast cancer. *Psychosomatic Medicine, 59*(4), 408–418.

Heinemann, A. (1995). Spinal cord injury. In A. J. Goreczny (Ed.), *Handbook of health and rehabilitation psychology* (pp. 341–360). New York: Plenum Press.

Heinemann, A., Bulka, M., & Smetak, S. (1988). Attributions and disability acceptance following traumatic injury: A replication and extension. *Rehabilitation Psychology, 33*(4), 195–206.

Helgeson, V., & Cohen, S. (1996). Social support and adjustment to cancer: Reconciling descriptive, correlational, and intervention research. *Health Psychology, 15*(2), 135–148.

Helgeson, V., Snyder, P., & Seltman, H. (2004). Psychological and physical adjustment to breast cancer over 4 years: Identifying distinct trajectories of change. *Health Psychology, 23*, 3–15.

Hickey, A., & Greene, S. (1989). Coping with multiple sclerosis. *Irish Journal of Psychological Medicine, 6*, 118–124.

Irvine, D., Brown, B., Crooks, D., Roberts, J., & Browne, G. (1991). Psychosocial adjustment in women with breast cancer. *Cancer, 67*(4), 1097–1117.

Irving, L., Snyder, C., & Crowson, J. (1998). Hope and coping with cancer by college women. *Journal of Personality, 66*, 195–214.

Jean, V., Paul, R., & Beatty, W. (1999). Psychological and neuropsychological predictors of coping patterns by patients with multiple sclerosis. *Journal of Clinical Psychology, 55*(1), 21–26.

Jenkins, P., May, V., & Hughes, L. (1991). Psychological morbidity associated with local recurrence of breast cancer. *International Journal of Psychiatry in Medicine, 21*(2), 149.

Jones, D., & Reznikoff, M. (1989). Psychosocial adjustment to a mastectomy. *The Journal of Nervous and Mental Disease, 177*(10), 624–631.

Judd, F., Brown, D., & Burrows, G. (1991). Depression, disease and disability: application to patients with traumatic spinal cord injury. *Paraplegia, 29*(2), 91.

Kaczorowski, J. M. (1989). Spiritual well-being and anxiety in adults diagnosed with cancer. *Hospital Journal, 5*(3–4), 105–116.

Kemp, B., & Krause, J. (1999). Depression and life satisfaction among people ageing with post-polio and spinal cord injury. *Disability and Rehabilitation, 21*(5–6), 241–249.

Kendall, E., & Buys, N. (1998). An integrated model of psychosocial adjustment following acquired disability. *Journal of Rehabilitation, 64*(3), 16–20.

Kennedy, P. (2008). *Coping effectively with spinal cord injury: Therapist guide.* New York: Oxford University Press.

Kennedy, P., & Duff, J. (2001). Posttraumatic stress disorder and spinal cord injuries. *Spinal Cord, 39*(1), 1–10.

Kennedy, P., Duff, J., Evans, M., & Beedie, A. (2003). Coping effectiveness training reduces depression and anxiety following traumatic spinal cord injuries. *British Journal of Clinical Psychology, 42*(1), 41–52.

Kennedy, P., Evans, M., & Sandhu, N. (2009). Psychological adjustment to spinal cord injury: The contribution of coping, hope and cognitive appraisals. *Psychology, Health and Medicine, 14*, 17–33.

Kennedy, P., Lowe, R., Grey, N., & Short, E. (1995). Traumatic spinal cord injury and psychological impact: A cross-sectional analysis of coping strategies. *British Journal of Clinical Psychology, 34*(4), 627–640.

Kennedy, P., Marsh, N., Lowe, R., Grey, N., Short, E., & Rogers, B. (2000). A longitudinal analysis of psychological impact and coping strategies following spinal cord injury. *British Journal of Health Psychology, 5*(2), 157–172.

Kennedy, P., & Rogers, B. (2000). Anxiety and depression after spinal cord injury: A longitudinal analysis. *Archives of Physical Medicine and Rehabilitation, 81*(7), 932–937.

Kennedy, P., Taylor, N., & Hindson, L. (2006). A pilot investigation of a psychosocial activity course for people with spinal cord injuries. *Psychological Health Medicine, 11*(1), 91–99.

Keyes, K., Bisno, B., Richardson, J., & Marston, A. (1987). Age differences in coping, behavioral dysfunction and depression following colostomy surgery. *The Gerontologist, 27*(2), 182–184.

Kim, H., Yeom, H., Seo, Y., Kim, N., & Yoo, Y. (2002). Stress and coping strategies of patients with cancer: a Korean study. *Cancer Nursing, 25*(6), 425–431.

Kinney, M., Burfitt, S., Stullenbarger, E., Rees, B., & DeBolt, M. (1996). Quality of life in cardiac patient research: A meta-analysis. *Nursing Research, 45*(3), 173–180.

Kishi, Y., Robinson, R., & Forrester, A. (1994). Prospective longitudinal study of depression following spinal cord injury. *Journal of Neuropsychiatry and Clinical Neurosciences, 6*(3), 237–244

Kleinke, C. L. (1998). *Coping with life challenges* (2nd ed.). Prospect Heights, IL: Waveland Press.

Kobasa, S., Maddi, S., & Courington, S. (1981). Personality and constitution as mediators in the stress-illness relationship. *Journal of Health and Social Behavior, 22*(4), 368–378.

Kornblith, A. B., Powell, M., Regan, M. M., Bennett, S., Krasner, C., Moy, B., et al. (2007). Long-term psychosocial adjustment of older vs younger survivors of breast and endometrial cancer. *Psycho-oncology, 16*(10), 895–903.

Kortte, K., Gilbert, M., Gorman, P., & Wegener, S. (2010). Positive psychological variables in the prediction of life satisfaction after spinal cord injury. *Rehabilitation Psychology, 55*(1), 40.

Kosciulek, J. (2007). The social context of coping. In E. M. H. Livneh (Ed.), *Coping with chronic illness and disability: Theoretical, empirical, and clinical aspects* (pp. 73–88). New York: Springer.

Krause, J. (1998). Subjective well-being after spinal cord injury: relationship to gender, race-ethnicity, and chronologic age. *Rehabilitation Psychology, 43*, 282–296.

Krause, J., & Anson, C. (1997). Adjustment after spinal cord injury: Relationship to gender and race. *Rehabilitation Psychology, 42*(1), 31–46.

Krause, J., & Crewe, N. (1990). Concurrent and long-term prediction of self-reported problems following spinal cord injury. *International Journal of Paraplegia, 28*, 186–202.

Krause, J., & Crewe, N. (1991). Chronologic age, time since injury, and time of measurement: effect on adjustment after spinal cord injury. *Archives of Physical Medicine and Rehabilitation, 72*(2), 91–100.

Krause, J., Kemp, B., & Coker, J. (2000). Depression after spinal cord injury: Relation to gender, ethnicity, aging, and socioeconomic indicators. *Archives of Physical Medicine and Rehabilitation, 81*(8), 1099–1109.

Krause, J., Stanwyck, C., & Maides, J. (1998). Locus of control and life adjustment: Relationship among people with spinal cord injury. *Rehabilitation Counseling Bulletin, 41*(3), 162–172.

Kreuter, M., Sullivan, M., Dahllöf, A., & Siösteen, A. (1998). Partner relationships, functioning, mood and global quality of life in persons with spinal cord injury and traumatic brain injury. *Spinal Cord, 36*(4), 252–261.

Krohne, H. (1993). *Attention and avoidance: Strategies in coping with aversiveness*: Cambridge, MA: Hogrefe & Huber.

Kurtzke, J. (1983). Rating neurologic impairment in multiple sclerosis: an expanded disability status scale (EDSS). *Neurology, 33*(11), 1444–1152.

Lavery, J. F., & Clarke, V. A. (1996). Causal attributions, coping strategies, and adjustment to breast cancer. *Cancer Nursing, 19*(1), 20–28.

Lazarus, R. (1966). *Psychological stress and the coping process*: New York: McGraw-Hill.

Lazarus, R., & Folkman, S. (1984). *Stress, appraisal, and coping.* New York: Springer.

Lechner, S., Carver, C., Antoni, M., Weaver, K., & Phillips, K. (2006). Curvilinear associations between benefit finding and psychosocial adjustment to breast cancer. *Journal of Consulting and Clinical Psychology, 74*(5), 828–840.

Levenson, H. (1974). Activism and powerful others: Distinctions within the concept of internal-external control. *Journal of Personality assessment, 38*(4), 377–383.

Lewin, K. (1997). Psycho-Sociological Problems of a Minority Group (1935). In *Resolving social conflicts and field theory in social science* (pp. 107–115). Washington, DC: American Psychological Association.

Lewin, K., Heider, F., & Heider, G. M. (1936). *Principles of topological psychology*: New York: McGraw-Hill.

Lewis, F. (1989). Attributions of control, experienced meaning, and psychosocial well-being in patients with advanced cancer. *Journal of Psychosocial Oncology, 7*(1–2), 105–119.

Linkowski, D. (1971). A scale to measure acceptance of disability. *Rehabilitation Counseling Bulletin, 14*(4), 236–244.

Litman, J. (2006). The COPE Inventory: Dimensionality and relationships with approach-and avoidance-motives and positive and negative traits. *Personality and Individual Differences, 41*(2), 273–284.

Livneh, H. (2001). Psychosocial adaptation to chronic illness and disability: A conceptual framework. *Rehabilitation Counseling Bulletin, 44*(3), 151–160.

Livneh, H. (2009). Denial of chronic illness and disability: Part I. Theoretical, functional, and dynamic perspectives. *Rehabilitation Counseling Bulletin, 52*(4), 225–236.

Livneh, H., & Antonak, R. (1990). Reactions to disability: An empirical investigation of their nature and structure. *Journal of Applied Rehabilitation Counseling, 21*(4), 13–21.

Livneh, H., & Antonak, R. F. (1997). *Psychosocial adaptation to chronic illness and disability.* Gaithersburg, MD: Aspen Publishers.

Livneh, H., & Martz, E. (2003). Psychosocial adaptation to spinal cord injury as a function of time since injury. *International Journal of Rehabilitation Research, 26*(3), 191–200.

Livneh, H., & Martz, E. (Eds.). (2007). An introduction to coping theory and research. In E. Martz and H. Livneh, *Coping with chronic illness and disability: Theoretical, empirical, and clinical aspects* (pp. 3–27). New York: Springer

Livneh, H., & Parker, R. M. (2005). Psychological adaptation to disability: Perspectives from chaos and complexity theory. *Rehabilitation Counseling Bulletin, 49*(1), 17–28.

McNair, D., Lorr, M., & Droppleman, L. (1971). *Manual for the POMS.* San Diego, CA: Educational and Industrial Testing Service.

Lowery, B., Jacobsen, B., & DuCette, J. (1993). Causal attribution, control, and adjustment to breast cancer. *Journal of Psychosocial Oncology, 10*(4), 37–53.

Lundqvist, C., Siosteen, A., Blomstrand, C., Lind, B., & Sullivan, M. (1991). Spinal cord injuries. Clinical, functional, and emotional status. *Spine, 16*(1), 78–83.

Lynch, S., Kroencke, D., & Denney, D. (2001). The relationship between disability and depression in multiple sclerosis: The role of uncertainty, coping, and hope. *Multiple Sclerosis, 7*(6), 411–416.

Macleod, L., & Macleod, G. (1998). Control cognitions and psychological disturbance in people with contrasting physically disabling conditions. *Disability and Rehabilitation, 20*(12), 448–456.

Malcarne, V., Compas, B., Epping-Jordan, J., & Howell, D. (1995). Cognitive factors in adjustment to cancer: Attributions of self-blame and perceptions of control. *Journal of Behavioral Medicine, 18*(5), 401–417.

Malec, J., & Neimeyer, R. (1983). Psychologic prediction of duration of inpatient spinal cord injury rehabilitation and performance of self-care. *Archives of Physical Medicine and Rehabilitation, 64*(8), 359–363.

Manne, S., Ostroff, J., Winkel, G., Goldstein, L., Fox, K., & Grana, G. (2004). Posttraumatic growth after breast cancer: Patient, partner, and couple perspectives. *Psychosomatic Medicine, 66*(3), 442–454.

Manne, S., Rini, C., Rubin, S., Rosenblum, N., Bergman, C., Edelson, M., et al. (2008). Long-term trajectories of psychological adaptation among women diagnosed with gynecological cancers. *Psychosomatic Medicine, 70*(6), 677–687.

Manne, S. L., Ostroff, J. S., Norton, T. R., Fox, K., Grana, G., & Goldstein, L. (2006). Cancer-specific self-efficacy and psychosocial and functional adaptation to early stage breast cancer. *Annals of Behavioral Medicine, 31*(2), 145–154.

Manne, S. L., Sabbioni, M., Bovbjerg, D. H., Jacobsen, P. B., Taylor, K. L., & Redd, W. H. (1994). Coping with chemotherapy for breast cancer. *Journal of Behavioral Medicine, 17*(1), 41–55.

Marks, G., Richardson, J., Graham, J., & Levine, A. (1986). Role of health locus of control beliefs and expectations of treatment efficacy in adjustment to cancer. *Journal of Personality and Social Psychology, 51*(2), 443–450.

Marks, R., & Allegrante, J. (2005). A review and synthesis of research evidence for self-efficacy-enhancing interventions for reducing chronic disability: Implications for health education practice (part II). *Health Promotion Practice, 6*(2), 148–156.

Marks, S. F., & Millard, R. W. (1990). Nursing assessment of positive adjustment for individuals with multiple sclerosis. *Rehabilitation Nursing, 15*(3), 147–151.

Martz, E., & Livneh, H. (2007a)(Eds.). *Coping with chronic illness and disability: theoretical, empirical, and clinical aspects.* New York: Springer.

Martz, E., & Livneh, H. (2007b). Coping with spinal cord injuries: Wholeness is a state of mind. In E. Martz and H. Livneh (Eds.)., *Coping with chronic illness and disability: Theoretical, empirical, and clinical aspects* (pp. 363–387). New York: Springer

Martz, E., Livneh, H., Priebe, M., Wuermser, L. A., & Ottomanelli, L. (2005). Predictors of psychosocial adaptation among people with spinal cord injury or disorder. *Archives of Physical Medicine Rehabilitation, 86*(6), 1182–1192.

Matheis, E., Tulsky, D., & Matheis, R. (2006). The relation between spirituality and quality of life among individuals with spinal cord injury. *Rehabilitation Psychology, 51*(3), 265–271.

Matson, R. R., & Brooks, N. A. (1977). Adjusting to multiple sclerosis: An exploratory study. *Social Science and Medicine, 11*(4), 245–250.

Matthews, E. E., & Cook, P. F. (2009). Relationships among optimism, well-being, self-transcendence, coping, and social support in women during treatment for breast cancer. *Psychooncology, 18*(7), 716–726.

Mazzulla, J. (1984). The relationship between locus of control expectancy and acceptance of acquired traumatic spinal cord injury. *American Archives of Rehabilitation Therapy, 1*(Winter), 10–13.

McCabe, M. (2006). A longitudinal study of coping strategies and quality of life among people with multiple sclerosis. *Journal of Clinical Psychology in Medical Settings, 13*(4), 367–377.

McCabe, M., Firth, L., & O'Connor, E. (2009). A comparison of mood and quality of life among people with progressive neurological illnesses and their caregivers. *Journal of Clinical Psychology in Medical Settings, 16*(4), 355–362.

McCabe, M., McKern, S., & McDonald, E. (2004). Coping and psychological adjustment among people with multiple sclerosis. *Journal of Psychosomatic Research, 56*(3), 355–361.

McCabe, M., Stokes, M., & McDonald, E. (2009). Changes in quality of life and coping among people with multiple sclerosis over a 2 year period. *Psychology, Health, and Medicine, 14*(1), 86–96.

McCaul, K., Sandgren, A., King, B., O'Donnell, S., Branstetter, A., & Foreman, G. (1999). Coping and adjustment to breast cancer. *Psycho-Oncology, 8*(3), 230–236.

McColl, M., Arnold, R., Charlifue, S., Glass, C., Savic, G., & Frankel, H. (2003). Aging, spinal cord injury, and quality of life: structural relationships. *Archives of Physical Medicine and Rehabilitation, 84*(8), 1137–1144.

McColl, M., Lei, H., & Skinner, H. (1995). Structural relationships between social support and coping. *Social Science and Medicine, 41*(3), 395–407.

McColl, M. A., & Rosenthal, C. (1994). A model of resource needs of aging spinal cord injured men. *Paraplegia, 32*(4), 261–270.

McIvor, G., Riklan, M., & Reznikoff, M. (1984). Depression in multiple sclerosis as a function of length and severity of illness, age, remissions, and perceived social support. *Journal of Clinical Psychology, 40*(4), 1028–1033.

McMillen, J., & Cook, C. (2003). The positive by-products of spinal cord injury and their correlates. *Rehabilitation Psychology, 48*(2), 77–85.

McNett, S. (1987). Social support, threat, and coping responses and effectiveness in the functionally disabled. *Nursing Research, 36*(2), 98–103.

McNulty, K., Livneh, H., & Wilson, L. (2004). Perceived uncertainty, spiritual well-being, and psychosocial adaptation in individuals with multiple sclerosis. *Rehabilitation Psychology, 49*(2), 91–99.

Mendelsohn, G. A. (1991). Psychosocial adaptation to illness by women with breast cancer and women with cancer at other sites. *Journal of Psychosocial Oncology, 8*(4), 1–25.

Merluzzi, T., & Martinez Sanchez, M. (1997a). Assessment of self-efficacy and coping with cancer: Development and validation of the Cancer Behavior Inventory. *Health Psychology, 16*, 163–170.

Merluzzi, T., & Martinez Sanchez, M. (1997b). Factor structure of the Psychosocial Adjustment to Illness Scale (Self-Report) for persons with cancer. *Psychological Assessment, 9*(3), 269–276.

Meyer, T., O'Leary, V., & Hagglund, K. (1999). *Coping and adjustment during acute rehabilitation for spinal cord injury.* Paper presented at the APA annual convention, Boston, Massachusetts.

Meyerowitz, B. (1983). Postmastectomy coping strategies and quality of life. *Health Psychology, 2*(2), 117–132.

Middleton, J., Tate, R., & Geraghty, T. (2003). Self-efficacy and spinal cord injury: psychometric properties of a new scale. *Rehabilitation Psychology, 48*, 281–288.

Miller, D., Manne, S., Taylor, K., Keates, J., & Dougherty, J. (1996). Psychological distress and well-being in advanced cancer: The effects of optimism and coping. *Journal of Clinical Psychology in Medical Settings, 3*(2), 115–130.

Minden, S., Orav, J., & Reich, P. (1987). Depression in multiple sclerosis. *General Hospital Psychiatry, 9*(6), 426–434.

Mishel, M., Padilla, G., Grant, M., & Sorenson, D. (1991). Uncertainty in illness theory: A replication of the mediating effects of mastery and coping. *Nursing Research, 40*(4), 236–240.

Mishel, M., & Sorenson, D. (1993). Revision of the ways of coping checklist for a clinical population. *Western Journal of Nursing Research, 15*(1), 59–76.

Mishel, M. H., Hostetter, T., King, B., & Graham, V. (1984). Predictors of psychosocial adjustment in patients newly diagnosed with gynecological cancer. *Cancer Nursing, 7*(4), 291–299.

Mohr, D., & Cox, D. (2001). Multiple sclerosis: Empirical literature for the clinical health psychologist. *Journal of Clinical Psychology, 57*(4), 479–499.

Mohr, D., Goodkin, D., Gatto, N., & Van Der Wende, J. (1997). Depression, coping and level of neurological impairment in multiple sclerosis. *Multiple Sclerosis, 3*(4), 254–258.

Montel, S., & Bungener, C. (2007). Coping and quality of life in one hundred and thirty five subjects with multiple sclerosis. *Multiple Sclerosis, 13*(3), 393.

Moore, A., Bombardier, C., Brown, P., & Patterson, D. (1994). Coping and emotional attributions following spinal cord injury. *International Journal of Rehabilitation Research, 17*(1), 39–48.

Moos, R., & Holahan, C. (2007). Adaptive tasks and methods of coping with illness and disability. In E. Martz and H. Livneh (Eds.), *Coping with chronic illness and disability: Theoretical, empirical, and clinical aspects*, (pp. 107–126). New York: Springer.

Moos, R., & Schaefer, J. (1984). The crisis of physical illness. *Coping with physical Illness, 2*, 3–25.

Moos, R., & Schaefer, J. (1986). *Coping with life crises: An integrated approach.* New York: Plenum Press.

Moos, R., & Schaefer, J. (1993). Coping resources and processes: Current concepts and measures. In L. Goldberger & S. Breznitz (Eds.), *Handbook of stress: Theoretical and clinical aspects* (Vol. 2, pp. 234–257). New York: Free Press.

Motl, R., McAuley, E., & Snook, E. (2007). Physical activity and quality of life in multiple sclerosis: Possible roles of social support, self-efficacy, and functional limitations. *Rehabilitation Psychology, 52*(2), 143–151.

Murray, C. J. L., & Lopez, A. D. (1997a). Global mortality, disability, and the contribution of risk factors: Global Burden of Disease Study. *The Lancet, 349*(9063), 1436–1442.

Murray, C. J. L., & Lopez, A. D. (1997b). Regional patterns of disability-free life expectancy and disability-adjusted life expectancy: Global Burden of Disease Study. *The Lancet, 349*(9062), 1347–1352.

Mytko, J., Knight, S., Chastain, D., Mumby, P., Siston, A., & Williams, S. (1996). Coping strategies and psychological distress in cancer patients before autologous bone marrow transplant. *Journal of Clinical Psychology in Medical Settings, 3*(4), 355–366.

Nelson, D., Friedman, L., Baer, P., Lane, M., & Smith, F. (1994). Subtypes of psychosocial adjustment to breast cancer. *Journal of Behavioral Medicine, 17*(2), 127–141.

Newsom, J., Knapp, J., & Schulz, R. (1996). Longitudinal analysis of specific domains of internal control and depressive symptoms in patients with recurrent cancer. *Health Psychology, 15*, 323–331.

Nielsen, M. (2003). Prevalence of posttraumatic stress disorder in persons with spinal cord injuries: The mediating effect of social support. *Rehabilitation Psychology, 48*, 289–295.

Nielson, W., & MacDonald, M. (1988). Attributions of blame and coping following spinal cord injury: Is self-blame adaptive. *Journal of Social and Clinical Psychology, 7*, 163–175.

North, N. T. (1999). The psychological effects of spinal cord injury: a review. *Spinal Cord, 37*(10), 671–679.

Norton, T., Manne, S., Rubin, S., Hernandez, E., Carlson, J., Bergman, C., et al. (2005). Ovarian cancer patients' psychological distress: the role of physical impairment, perceived unsupportive family and friend behaviors, perceived control, and self-esteem. *Health Psychology, 24*, 143–152.

Osborne, R. H., Elsworth, G. R., Kissane, D. W., Burke, S. A., & Hopper, J. L. (1999). The Mental Adjustment to Cancer (MAC) scale: Replication and refinement in 632 breast cancer patients. *Psychological Medicine, 29*(6), 1335–1345.

Osowiecki, D., & Compas, B. (1998). Psychological adjustment to cancer: Control beliefs and coping in adult cancer patients. *Cognitive Therapy and Research, 22*(5), 483–499.

Osowiecki, D., & Compas, B. (1999). A prospective study of coping, perceived control, and psychological adaptation to breast cancer. *Cognitive Therapy and Research, 23*(2), 169–180.

Pakenham, K. (1999). Adjustment to multiple sclerosis: Application of a stress and coping model. *Health Psychology, 18*, 383–392.

Pakenham, K. (2001). Application of a stress and coping model to caregiving in multiple sclerosis. *Psychology, Health and Medicine, 6*(1), 13–27.

Pakenham, K. (2005). Benefit finding in multiple sclerosis and associations with positive and negative outcomes. *Health Psychology, 24*, 123–132.

Pakenham, K. (2006). Investigation of the coping antecedents to positive outcomes and distress in multiple sclerosis (MS). *Psychology and Health, 21*(5), 633–649.

Pakenham, K. (2007). Making sense of multiple sclerosis. *Rehabilitation Psychology, 52*(4), 380–389.

Pakenham, K., & Cox, S. (2009). The dimensional structure of benefit finding in multiple sclerosis and relations with positive and negative adjustment: A longitudinal study. *Psychology and Health, 24*(4), 373–393.

Pakenham, K., Stewart, C., & Rogers, A. (1997). The role of coping in adjustment to multiple sclerosis-related adaptive demands. *Psychology, Health and Medicine, 2*(3), 197–211.

Park, C., Edmondson, D., Fenster, J., & Blank, T. (2008). Meaning making and psychological adjustment following cancer: The mediating roles of growth, life meaning, and restored just-world beliefs. *Journal of Consulting and Clinical Psychology, 76*(5), 863–875.

Parker, J., & Endler, N. (1992). Coping with coping assessment: A critical review. *European Journal of Personality, 6*, 321–344.

Parker, P., Baile, W., Moor, C., & Cohen, L. (2003). Psychosocial and demographic predictors of quality of life in a large sample of cancer patients. *Psycho-Oncology, 12*(2), 183–193.

Parle, M., Jones, B., & Maguire, P. (1996). Maladaptive coping and affective disorders among cancer patients. *Psychological Medicine, 26*(4), 735–744.

Partridge, C., & Johnston, M. (1989). Perceived control of recovery from physical disability: measurement and prediction. *British Journal of Clinical Psychology, 28*(1), 53–59.

Paterson, B. L. (2001). The shifting perspectives model of chronic illness. *Journal of Nursing Scholarship, 33*(1), 21–26.

Patten, S., & Metz, L. (2002). Interferon ß1a and depression in secondary progressive MS: Data from the SPECTRIMS Trial. *Neurology, 59*(5), 744–746.

Penley, J., Tomaka, J., & Wiebe, J. (2002). The association of coping to physical and psychological health outcomes: A meta-analytic review. *Journal of Behavioral Medicine, 25*(6), 551–603.

Penninx, B., van Tilburg, T., Boeke, A., Deeg, D., Kriegsman, D., & van Eijk, J. (1998). Effects of social support and personal coping resources on depressive symptoms: Different for various chronic diseases? *Health Psychology, 17*(6), 551–558.

Pierce, G., Sarason, I., & Sarason, B. (1996). Coping and social support. In M. Zeidner and N. S. Endler (Eds.), *Handbook of coping: Theory, research, applications* (pp. 434–451). Oxford, England: John Wiley & Sons Inc.,.

Pollard, C., & Kennedy, P. (2007). A longitudinal analysis of emotional impact, coping strategies and post-traumatic psychological growth following spinal cord injury: a 10-year review. *British Journal of Health Psychology, 12*(Pt 3), 347–362.

Post, M., de Witte, L., van Asbeck, F., van Dijk, A., & Schrijvers, A. (1998). Predictors of health status and life satisfaction in spinal cord injury. *Archives of Physical Medicine and Rehabilitation, 79*(4), 395–401.

Prigogine, I., & Stengers, I. (1984). *Order out of chaos: Man's new dialogue with nature.* New York: Bantam Books.

Quinn, M., Fontana, A., & Reznikoff, M. (1986). Psychological distress in reaction to lung cancer as a function of spousal support and coping strategy. *Journal of Psychosocial Oncology, 4,* 79–90.

Rabinowitz, A. R., & Arnett, P. A. (2009). A longitudinal analysis of cognitive dysfunction, coping, and depression in multiple sclerosis. *Neuropsychology, 23*(5), 581–591.

Radloff, L. S. (1977). The CES-D Scale: A Self-Report Depression Scale for Research in the General Population. *Applied Psychological Measurement, 1*(3), 385–401.

Radnitz, C. (2000). *Cognitive-behavioral therapy for persons with disabilities.* Lanham, MD: Jason Aronson Inc.

Reidy, K., & Caplan, B. (1994). Causal factors in spinal cord injury: Patients' evolving perceptions and association with depression. *Archives of Physical Medicine and Rehabilitation, 75*(8), 837–842.

Richards, J. S. (1986). Psychologic adjustment to spinal cord injury during first post-discharge year. *Archives of Physical Medicine and Rehabilitation, 67*(6), 362–365.

Rintala, D., Young, M., Hart, K., Clearman, R., & Fuhrer, M. (1992). Social support and the well-being of persons with spinal cord injury living in the community. *Rehabilitation Psychology, 37*(3), 155–163.

Rodrigue, J., Boggs, S., Weiner, R., & Behen, J. (1993). Mood, coping style, and personality functioning among adult bone marrow transplant candidates. *Psychosomatics, 34*(2), 159–165

Rodrigue, J. R., Behen, J. M., & Tumlin, T. (1994). Multidimensional determinants of psychological adjustment to cancer. *Psycho-Oncology, 3*(3), 205–214.

Roth, S., & Cohen, L. (1986). Approach, avoidance, and coping with stress. *American Psychologist, 41*(7), 813–819.

Rotter, J. (1966). *Generalized expectancies for internal versus external control of reinforcement.* Washington, DC: American Psychological Association.

Santos, F. R., Kozasa, E. H., Chauffaille Mde, L., Colleoni, G. W., & Leite, J. R. (2006). Psychosocial adaptation and quality of life among Brazilian patients with different hematological malignancies. *Journal of Psychosomatic Research, 60*(5), 505–511.

Scheier, M., & Carver, C. (1985). Optimism, coping, and health: Assessment and implications of generalized outcome expectancies. *Health Psychology, 4*(3), 219–247.

Schlossberg, N. (1981). A model for analyzing human adaptation to transition. *Counseling Psychologist, 9*(2), 2–18.

Schnoll, R., Knowles, J., & Harlow, L. (2002). Correlates of adjustment among cancer survivors. *Journal of Psychosocial Oncology, 20*(1), 37–59.

Schnoll, R., Mackinnon, J., Stolbach, L., & Lorman, C. (1995). The relationship between emotional adjustment and two factor structures of the Mental Adjustment to Cancer (MAC) scale. *Psychooncology, 4,* 265–272.

Schnoll, R. A., Harlow, L. L., Stolbach, L. L., & Brandt, U. (1998). A structural model of the relationships among stage of disease, age, coping, and psychological adjustment in women with breast cancer. *Psycho-Oncology, 7*(2), 69–77.

Schou, I., Ekeberg, Ø., Sandvik, L., Hjermstad, M., & Ruland, C. (2005). Multiple predictors of health-related quality of life in early stage breast cancer. Data from a year follow-up study compared with the general population. *Quality of Life Research, 14*(8), 1813–1823.

Schulz, R., & Decker, S. (1985). Long-term adjustment to physical disability: The role of social support, perceived control, and self-blame. *Journal of Personality and Social Psychology, 48*(5), 1162–1172.

Schwartz, C. E., Daltroy, L. H., Brandt, U., Friedman, R., & Stolbach, L. (1992). A psychometric analysis of the Mental Adjustment to Cancer scale. *Psychological Medicine, 22*(1), 203–210.

Schwarzer, R., & Schwarzer, C. (1996). A critical survey of coping instruments In M. Zeidner and N. S. Endler (Eds.), *Handbook of coping: Theory, research, applications* (pp. 107–132). Oxford, England: John Wiley & Sons Inc.

Sears, S., Stanton, A., & Danoff-Burg, S. (2003). The yellow brick road and the emerald city: Benefit finding, positive reappraisal coping, and posttraumatic growth in women with early-stage breast cancer. *Health Psychology, 22*(5), 487–497.

Shadish, W., Hickman, D., & Arrick, M. (1981). Psychological problems of spinal cord injury patients: Emotional distress as a function of time and locus of control. *Journal of Consulting and Clinical Psychology, 49*(2), 297.

Shanmugham, K., Elliott, T., & Palmatier, A. (2004). Social problem solving abilities and psychosocial impairment among individuals recuperating from surgical repair for severe pressure sores. *NeuroRehabilitation, 19*(3), 259–269.

Sharoff, K. (2004). *Coping skills therapy for managing chronic and terminal illness.* New York: Springer.

Shelby, R. A., Crespin, T. R., Wells-Di Gregorio, S. M., Lamdan, R. M., Siegel, J. E., & Taylor, K. L. (2008). Optimism, social support, and adjustment in African American women with breast cancer. *Journal of Behavioral Medicine, 31*(5), 433–444.

Shnek, Z., Foley, F., LaRocca, N., Gordon, W., DeLuca, J., Schwartzman, H., et al. (1997). Helplessness, self-efficacy, cognitive distortions, and depression in multiple sclerosis and spinal cord injury. *Annals of Behavioral Medicine, 19*(3), 287–294.

Shnek, Z., Foley, F., LaRocca, N., Smith, C., & Halper, J. (1995). Psychological predictors of depression in multiple sclerosis. *Neuro-rehabilitation and Neural Repair, 9*(1), 15–23

Shontz, F. C. (1965). Reactions to crisis. *The Volta Review, 67,* 364–370.

Shontz, F. (1975). *The psychological aspects of physical illness and disability*: New York: MacMillan.

Slife, B. (1993). *Time and psychological explanation.* Albany, NY: State University of New York Press.

Smedema, S., Bakken-Gillen, S., & Dalton, J. (2009). Chronic illness and disability: models and measurement. In F. Chan, E. da Silva Cardoso, & J. Chronister (Eds.), *Understanding psychosocial adjustment to chronic illness and disability: a handbook for evidence-based practitioners in rehabilitation* (pp. 51–74). New York: Springer.

Smedema, S., Catalano, D., & Ebener, D. (2010). The relationship of coping, self-worth, and subjective well-being: A structural equation model. *Rehabilitation Counseling Bulletin, 53,* 131–142.

Sneed, N. V., Edlund, B., & Dias, J. K. (1992). Adjustment of gynecological and breast cancer patients to the cancer diagnosis: Comparisons with males and females having other cancer sites. *Health Care Women International, 13*(1), 11–22.

Snyder, C. (1994). *The psychology of hope: You can get there from here.* New York: Free Press

Sperry, L. (2006). *Psychological treatment of chronic illness: The biopsychosocial therapy approach.* Washington, DC: American Psychological Association.

Spielberger, C., Gorsuch, R.L, & Lushene, R.E. (1970). *STAI manual for the State-trait anxiety inventory.* Palo Alto, CA: Consulting Psychologists Press.

Stanton, A., Danoff-Burg, S., Cameron, C., Bishop, M., Collins, C., Kirk, S., et al. (2000). Emotionally expressive coping predicts psychological and physical adjustment to breast cancer. *Journal of Consulting and Clinical Psychology, 68*(5), 875–882.

Stanton, A., Danoff-Burg, S., & Huggins, M. (2002). The first year after breast cancer diagnosis: hope and coping strategies as predictors of adjustment. *Psycho-Oncology, 11*(2), 93–102.

Stanton, A., Revenson, T., & Tennen, H. (2007). Health psychology: psychological adjustment to chronic disease. *Annual Review of Psychology, 58,* 565–592.

Stanton, A. L., & Snider, P. R. (1993). Coping with a breast cancer diagnosis: A prospective study. *Health Psychology, 12*(1), 16–23.

Stensman, R. (1994). Adjustment to traumatic spinal cord injury. A longitudinal study of self-reported quality of life. *Paraplegia, 32*(6), 416–422.

Stone, A., & Neale, J. (1984). New measure of daily coping: Development and preliminary results. *Journal of Personality and Social Psychology, 46*(4), 892–906.

Stroebe, M., & Schut, H. (1999). The dual process model of coping with bereavement: Rationale and description. *Death Studies, 23*(3), 197–224.

Stuifbergen, A. (1995). Health-promoting behaviors and quality of life among individuals with multiple sclerosis. *Scholarly Inquiry for Nursing Practice, 9*(1), 31–50; discussion 51–35.

Stuifbergen, A., Seraphine, A., & Roberts, G. (2000). An explanatory model of health promotion and quality of life in chronic disabling conditions. *Nursing Research, 49*(3), 122–129.

Suls, J., & Fletcher, B. (1985). The relative efficacy of avoidant and non-avoidant coping strategies: A meta-analysis. *Health Psychology, 4*(3), 249–288.

Tate, D., Forchheimer, M., Kirsch, N., Maynard, F., & Roller, A. (1993). Prevalence and associated features of depression and psychological distress in polio survivors. *Archives of Physical Medicine and Rehabilitation, 74*(10), 1056–1060.

Tate, D., Forchheimer, M., Maynard, F., & Dijkers, M. (1994). Predicting depression and psychological distress in persons with spinal cord injury based on indicators of handicap. *American Journal of Physical Medicine and Rehabilitation, 73*(3), 175–183.

Taylor, R. (2006). *Cognitive behavioral therapy for chronic illness and disability*: New York: Springer Verlag.

Taylor, S., Lichtman, R., & Wood, J. (1984). Attributions, beliefs about control, and adjustment to breast cancer. *Journal of Personality and Social Psychology, 46*(3), 489–502.

Tedeschi, R., & Calhoun, L. (1995). *Trauma and transformation: Growing in the aftermath of suffering*: Thousand Oaks, CA: Sage.

Tedeschi, R., & Calhoun, L. (1996). The Posttraumatic Growth Inventory: Measuring the positive legacy of trauma. *Journal of Traumatic Stress, 9*(3), 455–471.

Tennen, H., Affleck, G., Armeli, S., & Carney, M. (2000). A daily process approach to coping: Linking theory, research, and practice. *American Psychologist, 55*(6), 626–636.

Thompson, N., Coker, J., Krause, J., & Henry, E. (2003). Purpose in life as a mediator of adjustment after spinal cord injury. *Rehabilitation Psychology, 48*(2), 100–107.

Thorne, S., & Paterson, B. (1998). Shifting images of chronic illness. *Journal of Nursing Scholarship, 30*(2), 173–178.

Tobin, D., Holroyd, K., Reynolds, R., & Wigal, J. (1989). The hierarchical factor structure of the Coping Strategies Inventory. *Cognitive Therapy and Research, 13*(4), 343–361.

Trieschmann, R. (1988). *Spinal cord injuries: Psychological, social and vocational rehabilitation.* New York: Demos Medical Publishers.

Trunzo, J., & Pinto, B. (2003). Social support as a mediator of optimism and distress in breast cancer survivors. *Journal of Consulting and Clinical Psychology, 71*(4), 805–811.

Vinokur, A. D., Threatt, B. A., Caplan, R. D., & Zimmerman, B. L. (1989). Physical and psychosocial functioning and adjustment to breast cancer. Long-term follow-up of a screening population. *Cancer, 63*(2), 394–405.

Vinokur, A. D., Threatt, B. A., Vinokur-Kaplan, D., & Satariano, W. A. (1990). The process of recovery from breast cancer for younger and older patients. Changes during the first year. *Cancer, 65*(5), 1242–1254.

Vitaliano, P., DeWolfe, D., Maiuro, R., Russo, J., & Katon, W. (1990). Appraised changeability of a stressor as a modifier of the relationship between coping and depression: A test of the hypothesis of fit. *Journal of Personality and Social Psychology, 59*(3), 582–592.

Vitaliano, P., Maiuro, R., Russo, J., & Becker, J. (1987). Raw versus relative scores in the assessment of coping strategies. *Journal of Behavioral Medicine, 10*(1), 1–18.

Wallston, K., & Wallston, S. (1978). Development of the multidimensional health locus of control (MHLC) scales. *Health Education and Behavior, 6*(1), 160–170.

Wassem, R. (1992). Self-efficacy as a predictor of adjustment to multiple sclerosis. *Journal of Neuroscience Nursing, 24*(4), 224–229.

Watson, D., Clark, L. A., & Tellegen, A. (1988). Development and validation of brief measures of positive and negative affect: the PANAS scales. *Journal of Personality and Social Psychology, 54*(6), 1063–1070.

Watson, M., Greer, S., Pruyn, J., & Van den Borne, B. (1990). Locus of control and adjustment to cancer. *Psychological Reports, 66*(1), 39–48.

Watson, M., Greer, S., Rowden, L., & Gorman, C. (1991). Relationships between emotional control, adjustment to cancer and depression and anxiety in breast cancer patients. *Psychological Medicine, 21*(1), 51–57.

Watson, M., Greer, S., Young, J., & Inayat, Q. (1988). Development of a questionnaire measure of adjustment to cancer: The MAC scale. *Psychological Medicine, 18*(1), 203–209.

Watson, M., Law, M., Santos, M., Greer, S., Baruch, J., & Bliss, J. (1994a). The Mini-MAC. *Journal of Psychosocial Oncology, 12*(3), 33–46.

Watson, M., Law, M., Santos, M., Greer, S., Baruch, J., & Bliss, J. (1994b). The Mini-MAC—Further Development of the Mental Adjustment to Cancer Scale. *Journal of Psychosocial Oncology, 12*(3), 33–46.

Whiteneck, G., Brooks, C., Charlifue, S., Gerhart, K., Mellick, D., Overholser, D., et al. (1992). *Guide for use of the CHART: Craig handicap assessment and reporting technique.* Englewood, CO: Craig Hospital.

WHO. (2004). *International Statistical Classification of Diseases, Injuries and Causes of Death.* Geneva: World Health Organization.

Widiger, T. (2001). Official classification systems. *Handbook of personality disorders. Theory, research, and treatment* (pp. 60–83). New York: Guilford.

Widiger, T., & Trull, T. (1991). Diagnosis and clinical assessment. *Annual Review of Psychology, 42*(1), 109–133.

Wills, T., & Fegan, M. (2001). Social networks and social support. In T. A. R. A. Baum, & J. E. Singer (Eds.), *Handbook of health psychology* (pp. 139–173). Mahwah, NJ: Erlbaum.

Wineman, N. (1990). Adaptation to multiple sclerosis: The role of social support, functional disability, and perceived uncertainty. *Nursing Research, 39*(5), 294–299.

Wineman, N., Durand, E., & Steiner, R. (1994). A comparative analysis of coping behaviors in persons with multiple sclerosis or a spinal cord injury. *Research in Nursing and Health, 17*(3), 185–194.

Woodrich, F., & Patterson, J. (1983). Variables related to acceptance of disability in persons with spinal cord injuries. *Journal of Rehabilitation, 49*(3), 26–30.

Woolrich, R., Kennedy, P., & Tasiemski, T. (2006). A preliminary psychometric evaluation of the Hospital Anxiety and Depression Scale (HADS) in 963 people living with a spinal cord injury. *Psychology, Health and Medicine, 11*, 80–90.

Wortman, C., & Silver, R. (1987). Coping with irrevocable loss. *Cataclysms, crises, catastrophes: Psychology in action.* Washington, DC: American Psychological Association.

Wortman, C., & Silver, R. (1989). The myths of coping with loss. *Journal of Consulting and Clinical Psychology, 57*(3), 349–357.

Wright, B. (1960). *Physical disability—a psychological approach.* New York: Harper & Brothers.

Wright, B. (1983). *Physical disability—a psychosocial approach* (2nd ed.). New York: HarperCollins Publishers.

Wu, M. Y., & Chan, F. (2007). Psychosocial adjustment patterns of persons with spinal cord injury in Taiwan. *Disability and Rehabilitation, 29*(24), 1847–1857.

Yoshida, K. (1993). Reshaping of self: A pendular reconstruction of self and identity among adults with traumatic spinal cord injury. *Sociology of Health and Illness, 15*(2), 217–245.

Zeidner, M., & Saklofske, D. (1996). Adaptive and maladaptive coping. In M. Zeidner and N. S. Endler (Eds.), *Handbook of coping: Theory, research, applications* (pp. 505–531). Oxford, England: John Wiley & Sons Inc.

Zigmond, A., & Snaith, R. (1983). The Hospital Anxiety and Depression Scale. *Acta Psychiatrica Scandinavica, 67*(6), 361–370.

Epidemiological Context and Concerns

Yuying Chen *and* Yue Cao

Abstract

As the basic science of public health, epidemiology has been an important approach in public health and also in clinical practice. Epidemiology is now used together with measurement scales and instruments developed by psychologists to assess the subjective well-being of the target population and to identify psychosocial determinants of diseases and outcomes. As rehabilitation psychologists are becoming more involved in the effort to improve patients' quality of life, epidemiologic data are valuable in guiding the establishment of viable goals for rehabilitation psychology and the health care endeavor more broadly. This chapter provides background information about epidemiology: working definitions, types of epidemiology and epidemiologic studies, measures of disease occurrence and potential sources of errors, how to critically evaluate epidemiologic statistics, and sources of data for use in epidemiology. The practice of epidemiology is also illustrated, along with numerous applications to rehabilitation.

Key Words: Epidemiology, incidence, prevalence, mortality, relative risk, odds ratio, bias, confounding factor, causality, rehabilitation.

Rehabilitation psychology is enriched by epidemiology in several ways. The knowledge of health and disease at the population level established by the epidemiology helps set viable goals for rehabilitation and for the health care endeavor more broadly. The quantitative tools and methodology provided by epidemiology also aid in the identification of long-term rehabilitation outcomes and their determinants. Moreover, epidemiology has been used together with measurement scales and instruments developed by health psychologists to assess psychosocial functioning and quality of life of individuals with chronic conditions. This chapter is an introduction to epidemiology and epidemiologic approaches to problems of health and disease. Basic principles and methods will be presented, together with examples of applications to rehabilitation psychology.

What Is Epidemiology?

Epidemiology is conventionally defined as a study of the distribution and determinants of disease frequency in human populations (MacMahon & Pugh, 1970). *Distribution* refers to the frequency or quantification of disease occurrence that often varies from one population to another. *Determinants* are factors or events that potentially change an individual's health, including biologic agents (i.e., bacteria) and even lifestyle factors (i.e., smoking). More importantly, epidemiology is population-based medicine. For example, epidemiologists gain knowledge of health and disease by collecting data about an entire population through surveillance systems or descriptive studies. In contrast, clinicians, including rehabilitation psychologists, typically collect information on an individual patient basis by taking a medical history and conducting an assessment.

A broader definition of epidemiology, which has also been widely used, is "the study of distribution and determinants of health-related states in specified populations, and the application of this study to control of health problems" (Last, 2001). This definition includes both the description of the content and the purpose or application of this discipline. It further points out that epidemiology is not only concerned with disease but also with overall health and well-being.

Epidemiology is commonly classified into two broad categories: descriptive epidemiology and analytic epidemiology. *Descriptive epidemiology* measures the occurrence of a disease over the disease spectrum and over time to understand the natural history of a disease and to project future trends. This information helps determine the extent and burden of a disease in the community currently and in the future, which is critical for planning health services and facilities and for training health professions for future needs. Descriptive epidemiology also characterizes the distribution of a disease within a population; for instance, who gets sick and who does not, where the disease occurs, and when it happens. Based on patterns identified, research hypotheses can be generated concerning preventive or therapeutic factors for a disease. Furthermore, the process of case ascertainment facilitates and coordinates the provision of various clinical and support services to needed individuals.

Whereas descriptive epidemiology tries to answer the questions of who, where, and when, *analytic epidemiology* tries to answer how and why questions by investigating the association between exposure and disease to identify factors that are responsible for the increase or decrease of disease risk. With this knowledge, strategies can be developed to prevent a disease and to promote and restore health.

In addition to a traditional role as an analytic tool for studying diseases and their determinants, epidemiology has been applied to evaluate rehabilitation services provided to patients and to document outcomes and the cost-effectiveness of care systems (Bushnik, 2008; Chen et al., 2011; Patterson, 2007). For example, the Spinal Cord Injury Model Systems Program, established in 1970s with original funding from the Rehabilitation Services Administration, U.S. Department of Education, created a database and maintained sufficient records to document the efficiency of a comprehensive system approach in the management of persons with spinal cord injury (SCI), including optimal rehabilitation outcomes and cost-effectiveness (Stover, DeVivo, &

Go, 1999). Moreover, epidemiology serves an active role in steering public health decision-making and aiding in developing and evaluating interventions to control and prevent health problems, as well as in setting research priorities.

Measures of Disease Occurrence

A central task of epidemiology is to quantify health and disease in populations. This chapter discusses three basic measures of disease occurrence. *Incidence* measures the occurrence of a new disease or event. *Mortality* is the incidence of death from a disease. *Prevalence* is a measure of status, rather than of a newly occurring disease. There are three requirements for construction of these measures: number of persons affected by a particular disease, expressed as the numerator; population within which the affected individuals are observed, expressed as the denominator; and a specified period of time.

Incidence, Mortality, and Prevalence

The numerator of incidence has to be new cases of the disease—those people who develop the disease during a specified period of time and who did not have the disease previously. The denominator represents the number of people who are at risk for developing the disease. In other words, the denominator should not include those who are not susceptible to the disease. For example, for uterine cancer rate, women who had hysterectomies should not be included in the denominator because they are not at risk for developing uterine cancer. Occasionally, correction to the denominator sometimes is not made when the disease is of low frequency and is being measured in a large population where this correction would make little statistical difference.

Another important note about the denominator is the issue of time. The units of time and population may be selected by the investigator to suit his or her own purposes, but they must be specified. *Annual incidence*, for instance, is based on observation made during a 1-year interval. Because the size of the population (or denominator) could change over time through birth, death, migration, and other reasons, the number of persons in the population at midyear is usually selected as a denominator for calculating annual incidence. For example, there were 74 new cases of SCI identified in 1980 through the SCI surveillance program in Arkansas. Given a population size of 2.35 million in Arkansas, according to the 1980 U.S. Census, the annual incidence rate of SCI would be 31.4 cases per million population in Arkansas, in 1980 (Acton et al., 1993).

Cumulative incidence is a measure of disease risk or probability (i.e., transition from nondiseased to diseased state) during a specified period of time. To calculate cumulative incidence requires all of the individuals represented by the denominator to be followed for that specified time interval; for instance, during a 1-month period (1-month cumulative incidence) and in 5 years (5-year cumulative incidence). Consider a follow-up study beginning with 16,240 individuals with SCI who were free of venous thromboembolism. After 91 days' follow-up, 883 of them developed venous thromboembolism, corresponding to a 3-month cumulative incidence rate of 5.4% (Jones, Ugalde, Franks, Zhou, & White, 2005).

Because of the problems of attrition and also because individuals may come under observation at different points after a study is initiated, persons included in the denominator may be observed for different lengths of time, which makes the calculation of cumulative incidence difficult. A person–time unit that equals the sum of the different lengths of time that each individual was at risk is thus created for the denominator in order to construct *incidence density*. Incidence density is often expressed in terms of person-years and used to measure the instantaneous rate of development of disease in a population and how fast the new cases are occurring in the population. For example, the overall incidence density of kidney stones after SCI was estimated to be approximately 12 cases per 1,000 person-years. This figure was based on a study of 7,784 persons who sustained an SCI between 1986 and 1999 and were evaluated on a regular basis until they developed kidney stones, were deceased or lost to follow-up, or until the conclusion of the study in December 1999, whichever came first. Because of the dynamic nature of entry into the study, maximum follow-up varied by individuals from several months to 13 years. The person-years approach was thus utilized to calculate incidence density, with a total of 24,492 person-years of follow-up accumulated and 286 new cases with kidney stones identified (Chen, Roseman, DeVivo, & Huang, 2000).

Mortality is an index of the severity of a disease and can be used to assess whether the treatment for a disease has become more effective over time. It can also serve as a surrogate for incidence when the disease being studied is severe and fatal. The same principles of denominator correction mentioned in the discussion of incidence apply to mortality. The numerator of mortality, however, is

new deaths—people who died from the disease during a specified period of time.

Prevalence is a snapshot of disease status in a population at a specific point or period in time. The numerator for calculating prevalence is the number of existing cases of a disease, regardless of the duration of the disease. The denominator is the total number of persons in the population at that specific point in time. For example, reviewing records of 3,678 veterans with traumatic and non-traumatic SCI who received health care at the Department of Veterans Affairs facilities between fiscal years 1999 and 2001 found that 22% of them had a depression diagnosis. As the time of the diagnosis was not clear (new or existing), the measure of depression occurrence (22%) is the prevalence or, more appropriately, period prevalence as it covered a 3-year period (Smith, Weaver, & Ullrich, 2007).

Interrelation of Incidence, Mortality, and Prevalence

Each new incident case enters a prevalence pool and remains there until either recovery or death. As incidence is a direct measure of risk, prevalence is determined by incidence and disease duration. In a steady-state situation, in which the rates are not changing and immigration equals emigration, prevalence is the product of the incidence and duration of the disease. For example, it was estimated that the prevalence of SCI was 906 cases per million population in 1980 in the United States, based on an annual incidence of 30 new cases per million and an average 30.2 years of life expectancy after SCI (DeVivo, Fine, Maetz, & Stover, 1980). A high prevalence does not necessarily signify a high incidence of the disease; it may merely reflect a decrease in mortality and the chronic nature of a disease. In contrast, low prevalence may reflect a rapidly fatal process or rapid cure of disease, as well as low incidence.

Incidence is useful for studying etiological factors and evaluating primary prevention programs. Prevalence is quantified as the burden of disease and is useful for planning for health services delivery. Prevalence also suits to identify groups of people who should be targeted for control measures and for studying determinants of survival.

Major Sources of Errors

Like all other scientific endeavors, there are potential errors in measuring disease occurrence. Epidemiologic statistics, therefore, have to be interpreted with caution. Completeness of the ascertainment of cases for the numerator could be a concern. For example, the diagnosis of cases sometimes is not explicit, and where to find cases is not always straightforward. Diagnostic practices and adequacy can vary from one clinician to another. To minimize this type of variation and error, a number of approaches have been proposed, including but not limited to a common protocol, precise definition used for cases, standardization of methods for data collection, and training of personnel to carry out procedures and record observations.

For a rate to make sense, the total group or a representative sample of the target population should be included in the investigation. However, much of our epidemiologic information comes from convenient, but not random, samples of the population. The nonparticipation of members of the target group is a problem when making inferences about a population. At a minimum, study participants should be evaluated to see whether they differ in demographic characteristics and health status from nonparticipants and the target population to provide an insight on potential errors and biases.

Crude, Specific, and Adjusted Rates

Disease frequency can be expressed for a total population (crude or adjusted rates) or for a population subgroup (specific rates). A *crude rate* is based on the actual number of diseases or events in a total population over a specified time period, without consideration of the heterogeneity of the population regarding age, sex, race, and other characteristics. We may not always be interested in a rate for the entire population; perhaps we are interested in a certain age group, in one sex, or in one racial group. When specification is placed on rates, they are called *specific rates*. Examination of specific rates gives in-depth information about populations. For example, age-specific incidence rates provide a comprehensive view of the incidence of a condition for subgroups of the population stratified by age. In this case, the numerator and denominator for the calculation of each age-specific rate are restricted to a specific age group. Consider the age-specific incidence rates of SCI in the state of Oklahoma as an example. The highest annual incidence is among persons aged 15–19 years (94 cases per million population). It declines gradually to 85 cases per million for those of aged 20–24 years, 71 cases per million for those of aged 25–29 years, 47 cases per million for those of aged 30–44 years, 32 cases per million for those of aged

45–59 years, and 26 cases per million for those aged 60 or older (Price, Makintubee, Herndon, & Istre, 1994).

Specific rates are more homogeneous than crude rates and therefore can be more accurately compared across populations. However, they are cumbersome to calculate and compare, particularly across more than two specific categories and/or populations. It is desirable to have one single summary measure of disease occurrence, such as the *adjusted or standardized rate*, that allows a fair comparison of disease occurrence between populations of different characteristics. There are two methods for standardization or adjustment of rates: direct and indirect. Both of these methods utilize a standard population to eliminate demographic differences between groups or populations. Although it is somewhat arbitrary, the standard population selected for adjustment should not be markedly different from the groups or populations that are being compared regarding age or whatever other variable for which the adjustment is being made. For example, the 1940 U.S. population was regularly used as the standard population for age adjustment for most purposes for more than 5 decades until recently. Beginning in the 1999 mortality statistics, the National Center for Health Statistics was required to use the 2000 U.S. population as a standard population for adjustment to reflect the changing age and race structure of the United States. Discussion of the direct and indirect methods of adjustment and their computational requirements is beyond the scope of this chapter, but can be found in previous publications (Friis & Sellers, 2008; Woodward, 2004).

PROBLEMS WITH ADJUSTED RATES

Although adjusted rates can be very useful in making comparisons, the first step in examining and analyzing comparative morbidity or mortality data should always be to carefully examine the specific rates for any interesting differences or changes that may be hidden by the adjusted rates. Adjusted rates are hypothetical because they involve applying actual specific rates of the study group to a hypothetical standard population, for instance, in the direct adjustment. They do not reflect the true risk of the populations because the numerical value of the adjusted rate depends on the standard population used.

Epidemiologic Studies

The purpose of analytic epidemiology is to discover and quantify the relationship between an exposure or risk factor and a health outcome, attempting to answer the how and why questions. Epidemiologic studies can be classified as either experimental or observational. In an experimental or intervention study, investigators have control over the circumstances from the start—for instance, who gets the experimental treatment and who does not, determined by the randomization procedure but not by the self-selection of study participants. In contrast, the allocation into groups on the basis of exposure to a factor (i.e., cigarette smoking) is not under the control of the investigators in observational studies. While experimentation can establish the causal association of a factor with a health outcome more conclusively, observational studies have provided and continue to provide major contribution to our understanding of many diseases and outcomes. Observational epidemiologic studies can be further subdivided into four major designs: ecologic, cross-sectional, cohort, and case–control.

Ecologic Study

Ecologic studies utilize the group (i.e., geographic region) rather than an individual person, as the unit of analysis. These studies compare the rate of a disease or outcome across groups and relate the disease or outcome to the group profile (i.e., community socioeconomic status) rather than personal characteristics. As ecologic studies are typically based on data from existing databases, they are easy and inexpensive to conduct and can suggest areas for further investigation of causal relationships. Nevertheless, it is not always clear whether the observed relationship between exposure and disease assessed at the group level would hold true at the individual level since no account is taken of variability between individuals within the group. This problem is called the *ecologic fallacy*, which exists when the group members possess characteristics that they do not possess as individuals.

Cross-sectional Study

A cross-sectional study, such as a population survey, collects information from members of the group about their health status and experiences along with the exposure or risk factor simultaneously. The data represent a snapshot of the population at a certain point in time and can be suggestive of possible causal association. Nevertheless, given the fact that both factor and health outcome are determined at the same time in each subject, it is often impossible to establish a temporal sequence of the exposure and health outcome. As a result, cross-sectional studies

cannot be conclusive in examining cause-and-effect relationships.

Cohort Study

A cohort study has different alternative names, such as *follow-up study* and *longitudinal study*. It is "the archetype for all epidemiologic studies" (Rothman, 2002). Cohort studies typically begin with a disease-free group, called a cohort, and follow the members of the group over time to determine the health outcomes and compare them on the basis of the individuals' exposure to the factors in question. An example will be dividing a group of patients with SCI on the basis of their methods of bladder management and following them for 20 years to see how many of them develop bladder cancer. Because of the follow-up nature, the temporal sequence of the exposure (bladder management) and health outcome (bladder cancer) can be logically established, and the incidence rates can directly be calculated.

In a cohort study, the investigator can select the study population according to its members' experiences with the factor of interest, which makes a cohort study useful in examining rare exposures. Multiple outcomes for a single exposure can also be examined. The disadvantage is that cohort studies are costly in time and resources, which is particularly true when studying rare diseases that need a large number of subjects to ensure that enough cases develop by the end of the study period to permit valid analysis and conclusion. For health outcomes that take many years to develop, it may involve a long period of follow-up of the cohort and considerate logistical difficulty. Subject attrition is also virtually inevitable.

Case–Control Study

Case–control studies begin with the identification of individuals with the health outcome of interest (cases), and then a group of individuals without the health outcome (controls) for comparison. In a case–control study, epidemiologists work backward, from the effect to the suspected cause, to identify factors that mark cases as being different from controls. For this reason, the selection of controls is critical for a valid conclusion of the association between exposure and disease. Ideally, the controls should be similar to the cases in all respects other than having the disease in question.

Case–control studies are well suited for studying rare diseases and those illness that require a long interval between exposure and development of disease, since it is often possible to identify cases for study from disease registries and hospital records. Case–control studies allow one to examine multiple exposures for a single disease or outcome and are less expensive to conduct than cohort studies. Case–control studies, however, are subject to bias because of the method used to select controls and to recall past exposures. It is impossible to calculate the incidence of disease or outcome in case–control studies. They are not ideal for studying rare exposures. Finally, because they look backward, the temporal sequence between exposure and disease in the case–control studies is sometimes uncertain.

Measures of Association

Regardless of designs, epidemiologic studies aim at determining the extent of the association between exposure to a factor and development of a health outcome. Consider a cohort study of indwelling catheterization after SCI and the development of bladder cancer. The association can be measured as the ratio of the incidence of bladder cancer among SCI individuals who used indwelling catheterization to the incidence of bladder cancer among those who used other methods for urinary drainage. This ratio is called the *incidence rate ratio* or *relative risk*. If the rate ratio equals 1, there is no evidence for an association between indwelling catheterization after SCI and bladder cancer. If the rate ratio is greater than 1, it suggests an increased risk of bladder cancer for indwelling catheterization. If the rate ratio is less than 1, the risk of bladders cancer is lowered in indwelling catheterization users than in nonusers.

For studies in which the calculation of incidence rates is impossible, an alternative measure of association is *odds ratio*, the ratio of two odds. What are odds? The odds of an event can be described as the chance of the event happening against the chance of the event not happening. Suppose we administered a psychological assessment to 100 persons with SCI who had pressure ulcers (cases) and found that 30 of them had an alcohol abuse history. The odds of alcohol problems in the pressure ulcers group can be estimated as 30% (probability of the event) divided by 70% (probability of no event), which equals 0.43. Suppose we also administered a psychological evaluation to 100 persons with SCI who were free of pressure ulcers (controls) and found that 15 of them had an alcohol abuse history. The odds of alcohol problems in the control group would be 15% divided by 85%, equal to 0.18. We can then calculate the odds ratio, which in a case–control study, is defined as the ratio of the odds that the cases were exposed to the odds that the controls were exposed. In this example, the odds ratio of 2.39 (= 0.43/0.18) suggests that alcohol abuse is positively associated with pressure ulcers.

When an association between exposure and health outcome is identified, we must always ask ourselves: Is the association valid (do the study findings reflect the truth)? And, is the association causal (is there sufficient evidence to infer a cause-and-effect relationship between exposure and disease?

Is the Association Valid?

In addition to a true relationship, there are at least three possible explanations for an observed association: bias, confounding, and chance (random error).

Bias is defined as any systematic error that leads to an incorrect estimate of association between exposure and disease. It can occur at any stage of the study from design and conduct to analysis. Inappropriate selection of study participants can lead to *selection bias*. Inappropriate acquisition of information from study participants and inappropriate data management and analysis can cause *information bias*. For example, studies of immigrants' health may yield different results from similar studies of the general population because of the selective nature of immigration; immigrants are generally healthier. In a case–control study, cases (i.e., mothers of children with congenital malformations) may report past exposures (i.e., infections during pregnancy) differently than controls (i.e., mothers of children without malformations), which is called *recall bias*.

Confounding is the term that describes the distortion of an estimate of the association between exposure and disease because of a third variable, known as a confounder. By definition, the confounder must be associated with both the exposure and disease in question and must not be an intermediate factor in the causal pathway between exposure and disease. A classic example is the confounding effect of smoking on the assessment of the association between coffee consumption and pancreatic cancer, as smoking is highly related to coffee drinking and smoking is a well-known risk factor for pancreatic cancer. An uncontrolled study may mistakenly conclude that coffee consumption increases the risk of pancreatic cancer. Confounding can be controlled and minimized in the design and analysis process, such as by randomization, restriction, matching, stratified analysis, and multivariable analysis.

An observed association can also be caused by *random variation or chance,* the luck of the draw.

Statistical significance testing is a procedure used to quantitatively measure the role of chance as an explanation for an observed association. It answers the question "How much of the observed association could be due to chance?" By convention, the *p*-value of a statistical test of less than 0.05 suggests that the association between exposure and disease is considered to be statistically significant, and chance is an improbable explanation for the finding. The problem of random variation or chance can be minimized by a sufficient study size (i.e., number of study participants) that provides appropriate statistical power to detect the association, if it exists.

Is the Association Causal?

A valid association does not necessarily and sufficiently infer causality. The judgment of causality must be made in the presence of all available information and reevaluated with each new finding. To establish causation between exposure and disease, different criteria and philosophical views have been proposed. One of the seminal articles on causality was published in 1965, by Sir Austin Bradford Hill, then professor emeritus of medical statistics at the University of London (Hill, 1965). "Hill's Criteria for Causation" includes:

- *Strength of association*: The stronger the association, the more likely it is causal.
- *Consistency*: The observed association must be repeatable in different populations at different times.
- *Temporal relationship*: The cause must precede the effect.
- *Biological gradient*: There must be a dose–response relationship.
- *Plausibility*: The association must make sense biologically.
- *Coherence*: The observation should not conflict with existing knowledge about the disease.
- *Experimental evidence*: A controlled experiment provides the strongest support for causation.
- *Specificity*: When a certain exposure is associated with only one disease, it provides additional support for causal inference.
- *Analogy*: An existing evidence can be applied to similar exposure or outcome.

The criteria commonly used by health psychologists for judging whether an association is causal include co-variation, temporal precedence, and elimination of plausible alternative explanation, which is a similar concept to the Hill's criteria (Moon, Gould, et al., 2000). Although it is not always possible that all these lines of evidence be presented to support a cause-and-effect relationship, the more that are supported, the more the case of causality is strengthened.

Sources of Data for Use in Epidemiology and Rehabilitation

Secondary analysis using large datasets plays an important role in epidemiologic research. It has been applied in descriptive and analytic epidemiology, as well as in different designs of ecologic, cross-sectional, case–control, and even cohort studies. Common sources of data include, but are not limited to, demographic data (i.e., U.S. census, www.census.gov), vital statistics registrations (i.e., National Center for Health Statistics, www.cdc.gov/nchs/VitalStats.htm), population surveillance (i.e., National Health Interview Survey, www.cdc.gov/nchs/nhis.htm; Behavioral Risk Factor Surveillance System, www.cdc.gov/brfss), specific disease registries (i.e., cancer registries), utilization data (i.e., Centers for Medicare and Medicaid Services claims records), and numerous large-scale research databases (Friis et al., 2008).

For rehabilitation research, exceptional efforts have been made by federal and nonfederal agencies in collecting and archiving large amounts of information related to disability and rehabilitation, as well as in standardizing the methods of data collection and reporting to improve comparability across research findings. Advances in statistical methodology, information technology, and the internet have also facilitated the development of high-quality databases and easier access. For example, the SCI Model Systems Database sponsored by the National Institute on Disability and Rehabilitation Research contains baseline and follow-up data on more than 27,000 individuals with SCI, including information on demographics, clinical characteristics, and psychosocial outcomes (Chen et al., 2011). The Traumatic Brain Injury Model Systems Database (Bushnik, 2008) and the Burn Injury Model Systems Database (Patterson, 2007) were also created by similar collaborative efforts.

The International SCI Data Standards and Data Sets is an example of the international collaboration in the development of recommendations to standardize the way that data is collected and reported for SCI studies (Biering-Sorensen et al., 2006). The

Common Data Element project (www.commonda-taelements.ninds.nih.gov) initiated by the National Institute of Neurological Disorders and Stroke is also undertaken to facilitate the development of neurological data standards and tools that allow data to be collected and stored in a uniform way to promote data sharing across the research community. In addition to the General Common Data Element Standards, recommendations have been established for epilepsy, Parkinson disease, SCI, stroke, and traumatic brain injury as of April 2011.

Conclusion

This chapter aims to provide the reader with a basic understanding of epidemiologic methods and the use of epidemiology in rehabilitation medicine. It is anticipated that, after finishing this chapter, the reader will be able to interpret the epidemiologic statistics that are commonly reported in published articles and to critically assess the validity of the conclusions reached in those studies. It is also hoped that this chapter will convey to the reader the excitement of epidemiology and its application in rehabilitation, as well as an appreciation of the potential role of epidemiology in enriching rehabilitation psychology through interdisciplinary collaboration and quantitative research.

Future Directions

Epidemiology is an invaluable tool for providing the rational basis for conducting rigid clinical trials that contribute to the control of disease and the improvement of health outcomes. Recent unprecedented efforts by federal and nonfederal agencies in the creation and maintenance of large administrative and research databases, as well as in the standardization of data collection and reporting, provide an exceptional opportunity for epidemiologic research in rehabilitation outcomes. With advances in informational technology and the application of modern epidemiologic methodology, there is no doubt that the quantity and quality of rehabilitation outcomes research will be substantially improved through the analysis of these large datasets. It is the hope of the authors that our knowledge in rehabilitation science and the contribution to evidence-based rehabilitation practice will be significantly advanced through interdisciplinary collaboration.

References

Acton, P. A., Farley, T., Freni, L. W., Ilegbodu, V. A., Sniezek, J. E., & Wohlleb, J. C. (1993). Traumatic spinal cord injury in Arkansas, 1980 to 1989. *Archives of Physical Medicine and Rehabilitation, 74*, 1035–1040.

Biering-Sorensen, F., Charlifue, S., DeVivo, M., Noonan, V., Post, M., Stripling, T. et al. (2006). International Spinal Cord Injury Data Sets. *Spinal Cord, 44*, 530–534.

Bushnik, T. (2008). Traumatic Brain Injury Model Systems of Care 2002–2007. *Archives of Physical Medicine and Rehabilitation, 89*, 894–895.

Chen, Y., Deutsch, A., DeVivo, M. J., Johnson, K., Kalpakjian, C. Z., Nemunaitis, G. et al. (2011). Current research outcomes from the spinal cord injury model systems. *Archives of Physical Medicine and Rehabilitation, 92*, 329–331.

Chen, Y., Roseman, J. M., DeVivo, M. J., & Huang, C. T. (2000). Geographic variation and environmental risk factors for the incidence of initial kidney stones in patients with spinal cord injury. *Journal of Urology, 164*, 21–26.

DeVivo, M. J., Fine, P. R., Maetz, H. M., & Stover, S. L. (1980). Prevalence of spinal cord injury: A reestimation employing life table techniques. *Archives of Neurology, 37*, 707–708.

Friis, R. H. & Sellers, T. A. (2008). *Epidemiology for public health practice* (4th ed.). Sudbury: Jones & Bartlett Publishers.

Hill, A. B. (1965). The environment and disease: Association or causation? *Proceedings of the Royal Society of Medicine, 58*, 295–300.

Jones, T., Ugalde, V., Franks, P., Zhou, H., & White, R. H. (2005). Venous thromboembolism after spinal cord injury: Incidence, time course, and associated risk factors in 16,240 adults and children. *Archives of Physical Medicine and Rehabilitation, 86*, 2240–2247.

Last, J. M. (2001). *A dictionary of epidemiology* (4th ed.). New York: Oxford University Press.

MacMahon, B., & Pugh, T. F. (1970). *Epidemiology: principles and methods*. Boston: Little, Brown.

Moon, G., Gould, M., Brown, T., Duncan, C., Iggulden, P., Jones, K., et al. (2000). *Epidemiology: An introduction*. Milton Keynes: Open University Press.

Patterson, D. R. (2007). The NIDRR burn injury rehabilitation model system program: Selected findings. *Archives of Physical Medicine and Rehabilitation, 88*, S1–S2.

Price, C., Makintubee, S., Herndon, W., & Istre, G. R. (1994). Epidemiology of traumatic spinal cord injury and acute hospitalization and rehabilitation charges for spinal cord injuries in Oklahoma, 1988–1990. *American Journal of Epidemiology, 139*, 37–47.

Rothman, K. J. (2002). *Epidemiology: An introduction*. New York: Oxford University Press.

Smith, B. M., Weaver, F. M., & Ullrich, P. M. (2007). Prevalence of depression diagnoses and use of antidepressant medications by veterans with spinal cord injury. *American Journal of Physical Medicine and Rehabilitation, 86*, 662–671.

Stover, S. L., DeVivo, M. J., & Go, B. K. (1999). History, implementation, and current status of the National Spinal Cord Injury Database. *Archives of Physical Medicine and Rehabilitation, 80*, 1365–1371.

Woodward, M. (2004). *Epidemiology: Study design and data analysis* (2nd ed.). Boca Raton: Chapman and Hall/CRC.

Rehabilitation Outcomes and Assessment: Toward a Model of Complex Adaptive Rehabilitation

Nancy Hansen Merbitz, Charles T. Merbitz, *and* Judy P. Ripsch

Abstract

Vigorous international debate continues regarding standards of evidence in rehabilitation and guidelines for evidence reviews, as these impact reimbursement and drive scientific and clinical practices. A large portion of rehabilitation research funding in the United States goes toward the development of standardized rating scales and taxonomies of treatments. Another trend—quality improvement—is increasingly evident in the study of services in medicine, nursing, and psychotherapy, and is just beginning to enter the rehabilitation literature. Among many contributions, international communities collaborating in quality improvement have promoted greater awareness of the challenges and opportunities posed by complex adaptive systems. In this chapter, after reviewing dominant trends, we describe how methods of research from the quality improvement tradition and other methods compatible with it may transform processes and outcomes in rehabilitation.

Key Words: Complex adaptive systems, quality improvement, single-case experimental designs, Precision Teaching, selectionism, rehabilitation outcomes, process measures, patient-centered rehabilitation, Standard Celeration Chart.

When reviewing the rehabilitation outcomes research literature, it is possible to go back many years and see recommendations that sound as fresh and relevant—and urgent—as anything that could have been written this year and findings that could still beneficially shape policy and practice today (see Meyerson & Kerr [1979] and Johnston et al. [1992] as just two examples). This growing sense of urgency could be detected even a decade ago:

It is imperative that we initiate collaborative partnerships with consumers to develop relevant supports and health care programs.... In reality, inpatients have very little choice about the therapeutic goals set in the negotiations between administration and third-party payers, and local labor market opportunities and declining and variable state budgets typically dictate vocational options. (Elliott, 2002, p. 139)

The Committee on Disability, writing for the Institute of Medicine (IOM) on "The Future of Disability in America" (Institute of Medicine [IOM], 2007), stated:

Disability research is a miniscule item in the federal government's research budget; and the federal government's funding for disability research is not in line with the current and, particularly, the future projected impact of disability on individuals, families, and American society. This committee reiterates the call in the 1997 IOM report for increased funding for disability research, which is becoming increasingly urgent in light of the approaching large increase in the numbers of people at highest risk of disability.... [T]he overall federal funding picture remains as muddled and murky as it was in 1997. (p. 288)

If defined by numbers of good-quality randomized controlled trials (RCTs), the evidence base for comprehensive rehabilitation programs, although slowly growing, remains thin. For instance, Geurtsen and colleagues (2010) conducted a systematic review of the effectiveness of comprehensive rehabilitation programs for adults in the chronic phase following severe acquired brain injury, including studies from 1990 to 2008. They identified only 13 studies, including twoRCTs. They concluded that "clear-cut clinical recommendations cannot yet be set out due to limited methodological quality and poor description of patient and intervention characteristics" (p. 97). In a recent Cochrane Review by Turner-Stokes et al. (2011) of studies published before April 2008, on multidisciplinary rehabilitation for acquired brain injury in adults of working age, 16 trials were included, including eight single-blinded RCTs. The authors concluded that there was strong evidence of benefit for formal intervention following moderate to severe injuries, but only limited evidence that specialist inpatient rehabilitation and specialist multidisciplinary community rehabilitation may provide additional functional gains. They stated,

> Not all questions in rehabilitation can be addressed by randomized controlled trials or other experimental approaches. Some questions include which treatments work best for which patients over the long term, and which models of service represent value for money in the context of life-long care. (p. 2)

The struggles over what gets to count as evidence can evoke some cynicism when one realizes that observational studies statistically "controlling for" confounds are accepted as evidence for some purposes. Such statistical control of potential confounds is seen in the RAND study (Buntin et al., 2005), whose data were used in support of the Medicare "75% rule" (now the "60% rule") regarding post-acute care (PAC); however, RCT data are demanded for other purposes, as in the 2009 ECRI review of brain injury research on cognitive rehabilitation, whose findings were used to support the TRICARE insurance company's decision to deny services to veterans and military personnel (report available at www.propublica.org via the Freedom of Information Act).

The RAND study (Buntin et al., 2005) is instructive for its authors' detailed description of the limitations they encountered and the suggestions they make, because it captures honestly the types of current problems in research that hinder an informed allocation of resources for Medicare patients and others:

• It is important in evaluating these findings to understand a key limitation of studies of health outcomes based on observational data: ... *No risk adjustment approach* can control for every factor affecting outcomes of care.

• In addition, our outcome measures do *not capture other dimensions of quality of life*.

• Ultimately, in order to fully assess the impact of the 75% rule, we would need three additional types of information. First, we would ideally measure *real resource use across sites* of care rather than measuring only Medicare payments. Second, we would need a method for evaluating the trade-off between better outcomes and higher costs. Finally, we would need *better measures of outcomes, including a measure of functional status that was captured consistently across all discharge settings.* (p. 3, emphasis added).

The research and health policy recommendations developed by participants at the symposium "State-of-the-Science on Post-Acute Rehabilitation: Setting a Research Agenda and Developing an Evidence Base for Practice and Public Policy" (Clohan et al., 2007) address many of these limitations. A diverse group of participants represented federal government agencies, private insurers, professional organizations, providers of rehabilitation services, patients and their advocates, and health researchers. They called for a greater focus on understanding those elements of rehabilitation treatment (the "active ingredients") that are critical to patient success. They noted that although researchers have taken initial steps to measure rehabilitation processes, there is much to learn about those processes of care that are critical to outcomes.

Rehabilitation psychologists have been and will continue to be involved in research efforts with a range of other health professionals, and even topics that may not seem to directly involve psychologists' clinical efforts nevertheless are relevant in the development of research questions, measures, methods, and projects to which rehabilitation psychologists contribute (Brown, DeLeon, Loftis, & Scherer, 2008; DeLeon & Kazdin, 2010; Dunn & Elliott, 2008). However, rehabilitation psychology researchers have many pressing demands competing for their energy and limited resources. The frenetic activities of various agencies and entities operating under the contingencies of cost controls and "pay for performance," joined with the laudable efforts toward producing international definitions and metrics in function and disability (World Health Organization (WHO), 2001), are producing a dizzying array of measures, item banks, and patented systems for gathering and reporting outcomes data to payers.

In this chapter, we review several of the obstacles and challenges within rehabilitation research. We highlight some promising developments while underscoring an unfortunate fact: political and financial pressures and incentives notwithstanding, the goal of rapidly producing standardized outcomes data on a large scale that fairly discriminates among settings and providers, while driving improvement in knowledge and knowledge translation, not only exceeds the capacity of the rehabilitation research infrastructure to develop *within a process of scientific consensus*, but may be a distraction from the real work that lies ahead. If rehabilitation is to achieve stunning outcomes, attention must be paid to the processes—idiosyncratic as well as standardized—by which organizations, teams, providers, and patients set goals, learn about their progress in real time, and adjust what they are doing. It is as simple, and as complex, as that.

We have chosen to summarize a broad, although not exhaustive, selection of current efforts in rehabilitation outcomes research. The choice of clinical examples reflects the happenstance of our own clinical experiences, certainly not the relative importance of other conditions. We draw connections with other efforts from psychology, especially concerning the study of process and outcomes in psychotherapy, as well as quality improvement efforts under way in a variety of medical settings. We are fascinated by the rise of complexity science as an explanatory theme within the Continuous Quality Improvement (CQI) movement, and we point to how the concepts of fractals, attractors, and complex adaptive systems (CAS) can be applied in analyzing processes observable in the therapeutic dyad, the team, the hospital, and beyond. We sketch the beginnings of a model of CQI for CAS of rehabilitation, and argue that, although it may appear to be a luxury in these times, gathering data that are applicable to the improvement of rehabilitation processes in real time for individual clients should be prioritized, and the efforts already under way by individual providers, organizations, and formal and informal nonprofit collaboratives should be nurtured.

The Evidence Hierarchy

The dominant evidence hierarchy, as typified by the Cochrane Collaboration, was developed for trials of medical interventions, such as pharmaceutical agents, and has continued to present obstacles to rehabilitation research. A recent controversy on the evidence base for and reimbursement of cognitive rehabilitation can serve as an example. The decision of TRICARE insurance company not to reimburse cognitive rehabilitation for soldiers and veterans with brain injury was based in part on a commissioned study by the ECRI Institute, a nonprofit research center best known for evaluating the safety of medical devices. ECRI concluded there was insufficient evidence to support its use. ECRI relied on 18 RCTs selected as meeting its criteria of acceptable quality. This led to considerable outcry among rehabilitation professionals and Congressional members. Leading researchers in neurological rehabilitation—Keith Cicerone, Wayne Gordon, and James Malec—were each given access to ECRI's full report and each of them wrote letters to the medical director of TRICARE (Cicerone, 2009; Gordon, 2009a; Malec, 2009; accessed from ProPublica.org). Addressing some of the "flaws" that led ECRI to exclude hundreds of published studies, they pointed to the absurdity of requirements for "double blinding" and "sham interventions," and the bias inherent in imposing such requirements on cognitive rehabilitation while not restricting reimbursement for standard rehabilitation therapies, which also lack this type of evidence base (as do many practices within routine medical care). They also pointed to ECRI's apparent lack of awareness regarding, for example, the rigorous methodologies used for small-sample research with single-case experimental designs, which are accepted and widespread within neuropsychological research. Apparently, at least partly in response to TRICARE's decision, the IOM is working to determine the efficacy and effectiveness of cognitive rehabilitation for TBI. The presentations to the Committee by a number of prominent clinical researchers have been excellent (see Appendix for website).

In addition to these cogent arguments and others (e.g., Giles, 2010; Gordon, 2009b; Tucker & Reed, 2008; Whyte, 2009), all rehabilitation professionals—not simply rehabilitation psychologists—will benefit by sampling from the ongoing and spirited debate within clinical and counseling psychology regarding evidence-based treatments and RCTs. Many (including Westen, Novotny, & Thompson-Brenner, 2004, and Tucker & Reed, 2008) have noted limitations to RCTs for psychotherapy treatments quite parallel to those noted for rehabilitation. Westen and colleagues (2004) suggest a shift from validating treatment packages to testing intervention strategies and theories of change that clinicians can integrate into empirically informed therapies. At times, the arguments have become polarized (e.g., Levant, 2004), some have voiced concern about a widening rift between science and practice (e.g., Beutler, 2004), and some believe that criticisms of RCTs in psychotherapy research are overstated (e.g., Crits-Christoph, Wilson, & Hollon, 2005; Weisz, Weersin, & Henggeler, 2005). In the meantime, there appears to be a growing number of scientist-practitioners in psychotherapy research whose work joins rigor and frontline relevancy.

Even within the Cochrane Collaboration, there is indication of some changes under way as more discussion is engendered regarding the evaluation of complex interventions. A fascinating example (Shepperd et al., 2009) can be found at PLoS Medicine, a peer-reviewed, open-access journal published by the Public Library of Science. In 2009, several people affiliated with the Cochrane Collaboration, as well as two of their un-affiliated colleagues, published a dialog on the question, "Can we systematically review studies that evaluate complex interventions?" They note important difficulties, including defining the intervention, locating relevant evidence, standardizing the selection of studies for a review, and synthesizing data. They suggest that, to improve the description and conceptual understanding of the content of a complex intervention, reviewers may use typologies to guide classification and supplementary evidence, such as qualitative or descriptive data, as well as theory regarding how and why a complex intervention worked (or didn't) in particular contexts. In additional commentary within the PLoS dialog, one of the authors (Wong) not affiliated with the Cochran Collaboration stated that the results of complex health interventions (CHIs) are not ultimately deterministic:

[T]he greatest progress is likely to be made by focusing on theories that can explain and "predict" how certain contexts influence individuals to act in certain ways to produce certain outcomes. Pawson [2006] and colleagues have already made some progress towards such explanation and "prediction" using the "realist review" method of systematic review.... [seeking] not so much to answer the question of "If" a CHI works, but "How," "Why," "In what circumstances," "For whom," and "To what extent" it works. (p. 4–5)

The other non-Cochrane affiliate in the PLoS dialog (Sheikh) adds a further point of particular interest to our discussion here:

[It] is important that researchers...capture and describe how *the intervention may have evolved* during the course of delivering it.... [S]uch modifications should not be seen as compromising the fidelity of the intervention...but recorded and described as fully as possible in order to allow readers to make sense of what modifications were considered necessary and why. (pp. 6–7, emphasis added)

In the United Kingdom, the Medical Research Council (Craig et al., 2008) has developed and updated a set of guidelines for conducting and reviewing CHIs. We note that the Council's guidelines actually prescribe rather than penalize adaptation of an intervention to local settings and recommend using individual or subgroup variations to develop, refine, or modify theory regarding the active ingredients of change.

In a recent meta-review, Hoffmann et al. (2010), following current Cochrane guidelines, asked the question whether cognitive rehabilitation is effective for cognitive impairment after stroke and concluded that there is insufficient evidence to support it. Imagine a similar review asking "Is diabetes treatment helpful for diabetes?" or "Does surgery help people with tumors?" There have been several other recent reviews of rehabilitation for brain injury, notable for the rather general questions being asked, the search for group comparison RCTs addressing those general questions, and the ubiquitous call for better quality research before conclusions can be drawn (e.g., Cattelani, Zettin, & Zoccolotti, 2010; Cernich, Kurtz, Mordecai, & Ryan, 2010; Geurtsen et al., 2010; Teasell et al., 2007). We are reminded of Smith and Pell's (2003) comment, pointing out that no statisticians are likely to volunteer for "a double blind, randomised, placebo controlled, crossover trial" of parachute usage. As has been pointed out repeatedly by others, the RCT is simply one form of design that has a useful place in the research toolkit, but it is not the only sharp chisel in the kit. Compare this to the ongoing work of Cicerone and colleagues (most recently updated in 2011), who combined methods of review established by the American Congress of Rehabilitation Medicine (ACRM) and the European Federation of Neurological Societies (EFNS) and found a wealth of acceptable evidence supporting holistic cognitive rehabilitation and specific methods within cognitive rehabilitation. We also note findings by Cappa et al. (2005) for the EFNS Task Force indicating benefits of specific interventions for specific deficits.

Research Challenges Posed by Treatment Variables

Increasing dissatisfaction regarding lack of knowledge about treatments and benefits has led to interest in the Clinical Practice Improvement methodology developed by Susan Horn and her company, International Severity Info Systems, Inc., for the purpose of building practice-based evidence (e.g., DeJong, Horn, Gassaway, Slavin, & Dijkers, 2004; Gassaway & Horn, 2007; Horn et al., 2005a; Rhodes, Sharkey, & Horn, 1995). These collaborative efforts among rehabilitation researchers and Horn have included National Institute on Disability and Rehabilitation Research (NIDRR)-funded projects in stroke rehabilitation (Gassaway et al., 2005; Horn et al., 2005b) and spinal cord injury (SCI) rehabilitation (Gassaway & Whiteneck, 2010; Gassaway, Whiteneck, & Dijkers, 2009), as well as a new National Institutes of Health (NIH)-funded project in acute TBI rehabilitation (NIH-NCMRR, 5R01HD050439, Improving Outcomes in Acute Rehabilitation for TBI).

Horn's methodology includes a phase of taxonomy specification to standardize the variables related to treatment, heretofore referred to as "the black box of rehabilitation." DeJong et al. (2005), in describing the rationale for developing a taxonomy of stroke rehabilitation interventions, wrote:

> [Much of stroke rehabilitation] remains a trial-and-error matter that is difficult to characterize. Rehabilitation practitioners, it is said, customize their interventions to each individual patient. One result is that stroke rehabilitation practice varies from one patient to another and from one rehabilitation center to another and thus often lacks the standardization that is being demanded in other areas of medical practice, as evidenced by the development of practice guidelines and standardized protocols.... (p. S-1)

Here, we note that the implementation of practice guidelines and standardized protocols in medical practice is very far from realized, and vigorous debate continues while efforts are being made to better understand the processes of medical decision-making by health care providers and patients and to personalize medicine. Patient-centered medicine is a response not only to the variation in patient values and preferences, but also to the increasing evidence of individual physiological response to different medications and of individual factors affecting disease manifestations (IOM, 2001). When it comes to humans, variation *is* the norm. While we in rehabilitation chase the elusive standards supposedly driving research in medical settings, the latter is meanwhile advancing toward a more sophisticated understanding of variability not as error but as a fundamental phenomenon.

Publication of results from Horn's seven-site Post-Stroke Rehabilitation Outcomes Project (PSROP) began in 2005, in a supplement to the *Archives of Physical Medicine and Rehabilitation*, and a host of publications followed (15 as of this writing), presenting results of various analyses from the original large sample. Starting in 2006, the SCIRehab Project began at six SCI clinical treatment facilities, including five NIDRR Model SCI System Centers. As with PSROP, the stated plan is for center-to-center practice differences (as indicated by usage within the taxonomies) to be analyzed as treatment variables using Horn's proprietary system of severity adjustment to statistically control for differences across sites in variables related to patient needs or other patient characteristics, thus enabling determination of which SCI rehabilitation interventions were associated with positive outcomes.

By 2008 (as reported by Gassaway et al., 2009), seven discipline-specific taxonomies, including for psychology, were developed, as well as a system for data collection via personal digital assistants. With apologies to its members, the taxonomy developed by the committee for psychological interventions (Wilson et al., 2009) brings to mind the old description of the camel as a horse that was assembled by a committee (except that a camel only looks ungainly). Several items within this taxonomy conflate goals or targets with actions of the psychologist; that is, *they are not interventions* e.g. "emotional adjustment," "family functioning or coping," "building rapport/engagement," "locus of control issues," "pain management." Whiteneck and colleagues (2011) are now reporting on initial results, looking at basic data regarding hours and timing of service by various disciplines; no data are yet reported regarding associations between specific taxonomic intervention categories and outcomes.

Efforts to categorize and quantify interventions also can be seen internationally; for example, a list of occupational therapy categories in vocational rehabilitation was described by Phillips and colleagues (2010), and work is under way in the

Netherlands (van Langeveld et al., 2009) on an SCI-interventions classification system (SCI_ICS). As with the PSROP and SCIRehab projects, the categories in these projects (e.g., "work preparation," "self-care exercises") look very broad.

Although hoping that these efforts prove fruitful, we have reservations about the utility of a static taxonomy of broad categories of rehabilitation provider behaviors for studying and predicting rehabilitation outcomes. Considering the mounting evidence on therapeutic alliance (e.g., Baldwin et al., 2007; Elkin et al., 2006; Evans et al., 2007; Schönberger, Humle, & Teasdale, 2006, 2007) and the body of work regarding variation in placebo effects based on something as "objective" as the instructions given with a pill, the present enormous efforts going into developing these treatment categories would seem better spent in studying how variations in treatment delivery and treatment matching (at a granular level) affect the course of therapy for individual cases.

Efforts under way to open the black box of rehabilitation for stroke, SCI, and TBI must evolve past the development of static taxonomies. These efforts must look not simply at which of a long list of activities were encouraged via which of a long list of potential interventions to lead to various outcomes, but must consider how this process unfolded over time. They must study the quality of and details about how those activities and interventions were chosen; the sequence of interactions between therapist and patient; how ongoing data were used to adjust those goals, activities, and interventions; and what was revealed by snapshot views of outcomes at various points in time. Whyte (2009) described the rationale for (and obstacles to) defining the "active ingredients" of rehabilitation:

> Similar to psychotherapy—whose efficacy has also been challenging to study—most rehabilitation treatments are delivered through some form of interpersonal interaction between rehabilitation therapist and patient/client, may be tailored to the goals, strengths, and weaknesses of the individual, and may incorporate multiple active ingredients.... Because of these complexities, many attempts at clinical rehabilitation research have resorted to defining the treatments merely as numbers of hours of physical, occupational, speech, and other therapies; length of stay in a particular type of institution; or the goal of the treatment (e.g., "attention training"), as though the actual services delivered by clinicians and institutions during the treatment time are unimportant. Although numbers

of sessions or hours may certainly be relevant, just as the dose of a medication is important, the dose does nothing to define the active ingredients of the treatment. (p. 14)

Likewise, Tucker and Reed (2008) also note that rehabilitation as an enterprise shares many of the characteristics that make psychotherapy difficult to study using RCTs. First, rehabilitation is generally *not of fixed duration*, whereas in an RCT the treatment typically stops after a certain interval or number of sessions, regardless of progress or lack thereof. Second, rehabilitation is *self-correcting*, such that if one technique is not working, then another technique or modality is tried; conversely, treatment within an RCT is confined to specified techniques, administered in a standardized manner. Ahn and Wampold (2001) wrote that strict adherence to a treatment manual can lead to "ruptures in the alliance and, consequently, poorer outcomes," as well as thwart the therapist's ability to adapt treatment to the "attitudes, values, and culture of the client" (p. 255, cited in L. Seligman & Reichenberg, 2007).

Are We Missing Key Variables Related to Treatment?

If reimbursement will some day depend on measures of treatment quality and effectiveness to generate data for payers, what will happen if those measures are seriously deficient for tracking individual clinical progress or miss key relevant features of treatment and outcome? Linda Seligman and Lourie Reichenberg (2007) summarized the body of research on determinants of treatment outcome in psychotherapy: although the absolute and relative effect sizes are still subject to debate, little question remains that the therapist (or provider) as a variable must be reckoned with in any investigation of treatment outcome differences (e.g., Lutz, Leon, Martinovich, Lyons, & Stiles, 2007; Wampold & Brown, 2005). This leads us to question what exactly makes for that difference, and then leads to another variable typically missing in rehabilitation research but exhaustively studied in psychotherapy research: the therapeutic alliance. Sparks and colleagues (2008) point out that the alliance is one of the most researched variables in all psychotherapy outcome literature, reflecting over 1,000 findings and counting. Hart (2009) and Vong et al. (2011) have encouraged the consideration of common factors, including therapeutic alliance, in rehabilitation research.

If, as psychotherapy research strongly suggests, the person delivering the intervention has at least as much impact on success as the type of intervention, then attention should be paid to the effects of consistent staffing. Nursing research has demonstrated the impact of nurse and nurse aide assignment on important quality and outcomes indicators (e.g., Bowers, 2003; Bowers, Fibich, & Jacobson, 2001; Goldman, 1998; Mueller, 2000; Patchner, 1989). Research by Begley et al. (2004) on factors affecting patients' participation in rehabilitation focuses attention on therapist factors. A rehabilitation team is more than a collection of fungible clinicians. Studies of the effects of rehabilitation treatments must include information on *who* (i.e., which provider, not only which type of provider) provided a given treatment or service, so that provider can be studied as a variable in its own right. Rehabilitation comes down to physical modalities (heat, surgery, exercises, etc.), *and* person-mediated modalities, thus what a physical therapist does is not separate from who the physical therapist is. Maybe it's time for us to acknowledge this point in research designs.

Challenges of Measurement Within and Across Studies

The number of different variables and scales in use has not been decreasing, but many national and international efforts are under way to reduce the heterogeneity of measurement across studies, as through the development of item banks, common data elements, and Computerized Adaptive Testing (CAT). Here, we very briefly describe some of the challenges of measurement in rehabilitation, some of the ongoing efforts toward standardization, and the challenges we believe will remain.

Sensitivity to Differences and Change

The importance of a measure's sensitivity varies according to the purpose of its use. Measures or observations used to make real-time clinical decisions for individuals must be sensitive indeed and their use informed by knowledge of the person and his or her context, as well as the natural course of his or her condition (e.g., stroke recovery). As an example, back in the days of the first author's (NHM) clinical training (in the 1980s, the "golden age" of rehabilitation), an elderly but formerly very independent woman, Betty, was placed in a post-acute hospital rehabilitation program. She had dense hemiplegia of her left upper extremity; she had begun ambulating but still needed more assistance than could be provided by her frail husband. After about 30 days, with no sign of any arm or hand function, discharge for further care in a nursing home was scheduled. The morning of the day of that scheduled discharge, she and her nurse discovered that Betty was able to move a finger. The celebration was great (Betty was very popular), and her stay was extended while more function returned, until she was able to discharge to home. Knowing the natural history of recovery for her pattern of stroke enabled that one "measure"—finger movement—to accurately predict her ability to benefit from more rehabilitation. Betty might have gotten better in a nursing home, too, but then again, every change in continuity of care, especially for an older person, risks complications and additional expense.

If the standardization of measurement is going to proceed (as several converging efforts suggest it may) and item banks become widely applied, used not only to indicate gross level outcomes but to aid in clinical decision-making, they will need specificity and sensitivity sufficient for that purpose; for example, we will need an item bank that includes items developed specifically for stroke, and with its potential recovery trajectory characteristics included (i.e., first signs of recovery from hemiplegia). Otherwise, individual clinical observations of idiographic data will be overruled by uniformly applied rating scales to determine length of stay and discharge destination.

A study by Rintala et al. (2008) illustrates the clarity possible when the dependent (outcome) variable is well-defined, observable, and highly relevant for the condition being studied, in this case SCI and the occurrence of pressure ulcer. Each of three randomly assigned groups received follow-up contacts regarding skin status, but the groups varied by frequency and intensity of education and encouragement. A lovely dose–response effect was noted in pressure ulcer incidence or recurrence over 2 years' time. Conversely, a study by Walker and Pickett (2007) nicely illustrates the shortcomings of the Functional Independence Measure (FIM) in vocational rehabilitation after TBI, since persons with severe TBI attained "full independence" on FIM motor ratings in spite of persisting deficits of ataxia and imbalance. Because of the ceiling effects of the FIM (particular insensitivity near the top of the measure), features were missed that could be critical for job placement and sustained performance, as well as for safety. Johnston and colleagues (1992) noted that the floor and ceiling effects of widely used measures such as the FIM serve to limit who gets into rehabilitation because facilities are incentivized to admit people in the middle range who will show change. Detecting ceiling and floor effects becomes a critical issue as measures are developed and applied across settings to assess function and health from hospital to community (Johnston, Graves, & Greene, 2007).

The timing of a measurement also can affect its ability to detect meaningful differences between people receiving different types of rehabilitation or between people in different rehabilitation settings. Duncan and Velozo (2007) and Clohan et al. (2007) point out the obvious but nevertheless ubiquitous problems of variation in the timing of assessments, which introduces a large confound into comparative studies of treatments and/or treatment settings for people with new-onset disabling conditions. As Duncan and Velozo (2007) frankly assess, pressure to get data to the payers (e.g., for comparative studies of PAC) does not yet lead to good science or practice.

The Selection of What to Measure

Responding to the oft-lamented heterogeneity among measures that bedevils meta-reviews and meta-analyses, Duncan and Velozo (2007) say that first we must ask if we are measuring the most appropriate outcomes to influence policy: "The suggestion that a uniform measure could meet the purposes of care planning, risk adjustment, quality assessments, serve as a basis for Medicare reimbursement, and establish most cost-effective sites of care may be overly optimistic" (p. 1482). Conflicts exist regarding what is most important to measure, as opposed to what is most convenient or familiar. Buntin (2007) and Clohan et al. (2007) noted inadequacies in variables selected for measurement after PAC; long-term outcomes and premorbid status have not been measured systematically, although both are keys to judging the effectiveness of what is often a sequence of post-acute services. Elliott (2002) argues for measuring the kinds of information that will require multiple avenues (e.g., qualitative methods). As he notes, we have yet to determine what kinds of value shifts occur following disability, how and why these occur, and their relationship to a sense of acceptance and well-being.

Full participation in society is viewed as the ultimate goal of rehabilitation, but development of measures is complicated by the fact that participation outcomes evolve long after specific rehabilitation interventions. Nevertheless, it is essential for research to address the outcomes that individuals with disability say are most important to their lives (Heinemann, 2005). Collection of data on these domains will require new resources and incentives lacking thus far in PAC.

Compared to What? The Natural Course of Recovery (or Decline)

Research needs to be informed by the "natural course" of various disabling conditions and on variation within that course. To study the natural course, information must come from both qualitative and quantitative sources. Yet, there are very limited data of either kind to help guide theory development, clinical and organizational decision-making, and the formation of policy regarding resources. Although we need a more in-depth understanding of natural course and trajectories of recovery and/or adaptation or decline, studies often lack even basic, readily available natural history data on individual participants (e.g., type and severity of stroke or SCI, time since onset), even though time frames of natural recovery and intervening markers of longer term adjustment and outcomes could serve as benchmarks against which to assess further benefits due to rehabilitation (Tucker & Reed, 2008). For example, the most valuable information in predicting long-term outcome after TBI unfolds during the first minutes and hours after onset, yet hospitals generally have no process in place by which emergency medical technicians and emergency room staff can routinely record basic behavioral information. This impedes research to refine the classification of brain injury, which in turn muddles conclusions about the effectiveness of and necessity for treatment after "mild" TBI. Clinically, this loss of data impedes delivery of good information and care to families and patients and also leads to many cases lacking any follow-up whatsoever.

A ubiquitous problem in studying interventions is the question of how to distinguish between natural recovery curves (or natural decline curves) and effects of rehabilitation. Johnston and colleagues (1992) noted the need for repeated functional measurement over time and the need for aggregated data across populations of people with similar conditions and impairments in order to "model chronicity" and get data on expected curves over time. "If we had such standard models or curves, research could focus on finding factors that improve accuracy of prediction beyond this basis" (p. 89). They recommended that rehabilitation prediction models routinely use longitudinal functional measures. Although initial functional impairment is a strong predictor of later impairment, variability exists: some patients do continue recovery from stroke, for example, long after the more typical plateau; thus, "prediction is not sufficiently accurate to deny a patient a try at rehab simply because someone labels the stroke 'severe'" (p. 88). Individual improvement curves vary substantially from group averages. "Both time and function are continuous variables, so categorical approaches inevitably are unsatisfactory, as many patients do not fit neatly into extant categories" (p. 88).

Wilson and Cockburn (1997) also note the paucity of information regarding recovery and long-term outcomes of people who have experienced a severe neurological insult, in that they have found substantial improvements among some. These results remind us that, for each severely impaired individual patient, we should not assume no progress is possible after the first year or some other arbitrary point in time.

Common Data Elements, Core Sets, and Computerized Adaptive Testing

The development of measures and the awarding of federal grants for large research teams, as well as the awarding of federal grants, contracts, and patents to developers of proprietary data management systems, is proceeding very quickly; thus, what follows is but a snapshot and inevitably is neither comprehensive nor completely up to date. Only time will tell if a semipermanent system of selected outcome measures takes hold or if political contingencies shift and new demands arise, followed by another scramble.

COMPUTERIZED ADAPTIVE TESTING

When completing a scale using CAT, the respondent begins by answering a small set of items given to everyone, then subsequent items are automatically selected and presented based on some algorithm (typically Rasch analysis). Thus, each person may take a slightly different test, but the entire set of questions has already been completed by a large sample whose answers have been used to calibrate each item's difficulty. Items for an individual are selected based on an estimate of which items will yield the most information about that person on the dimension the test is intended to measure, while sparing him or her from answering questions that are too hard or too easy (see Hobart & Cano's excellent 2009 monograph on Rasch analysis and applications in neurorehabilitation). Examples of CAT measures being developed include the Patient Reported Outcomes Measurement Information System (PROMIS; Cella et al., 2007; Hahn et al., 2010), the Activity Measure for Post-Acute Care (AM-PAC; Haley et al., 2004, 2009; Jette et al., 2007), and measures developed using Ware and colleagues' proprietary system, QualityMetric Incorporated (2005).

Duncan and Velozo (2007) have concluded that item response theory (IRT) and CAT are promising methodologies for advancing outcomes measurement in health care, yet they also encourage their readers to consider Fayers' review (2007), in which he voiced concern over the rush to embrace these methods. Fayer offers suggestions, such as the need for differential item functioning (DIF) analysis, for examining whether the likelihood of item (category) endorsement is equal across subgroups that are matched on the state or trait measured. He cautions that IRT does not supplant the need for rigorous instrument development using qualitative methods.

COMMON DATA ELEMENTS

Efforts are also under way to identify or develop measures and sets of patient variables to use in a consistent way, so that studies can be compared and meta-analyses are facilitated. Thurmond et al. (2010) describe the growing interest among those serving civilian, military, and veteran populations in identifying core data elements (CDEs) related to TBI and psychological health. Whyte, Vasterling, and Manley (2010) are among those who have been involved with CDE projects; not surprisingly, the participants in this endeavor have had their hands full:

> Across all of the working groups, there were challenges in striking a balance between specificity in recommendations to researchers and the need to tailor the selection of variables to specific study aims. The domains addressed by the different working groups varied in the research available to guide the selection of important content areas to be measured and the specific tools for measuring them. The working groups also addressed this challenge in somewhat different ways. The CDE effort must enhance consensus among researchers with similar interests while not stifling innovation and scientific rigor. This will require regular updating of the recommendations and may benefit from more standardized criteria for the selection of important content areas and measurement tools across domains. (p. 1692)

INTERNATIONAL EFFORTS: THE INTERNATIONAL CLASSIFICATION OF DISABILITY AND CORE SETS

Related work on core sets of measures is extending internationally, as exemplified by teams involved with the World Health Organization's International Classification of Disability, Functioning, and Health (ICF; WHO, 2001). The ICF domains of Body, Activity and Participation, and Environmental Contextual Factors each have a large number of categories to be rated; ICF Core Sets are selections of category subsets identified as relevant for assessment of individuals who are affected by specific diseases or conditions. The ICF provides only a framework for understanding and does not identify the methods or technology required to conduct assessments in the domains specified (Grill & Stucki, 2011). Jette (2008) has provided a succinct summary of the rationale and scoring process for categories and Core Sets. Efforts are under way to develop measures or apply existing measures to ICF categories or to Core Sets of categories. Velozo (2005), as cited in Peterson, Mpofu, & Oakland (2010), states that IRT and CAT hold great promise for converting the ICF into measurement systems that individualize the assessment process, reduce respondent burden, and increase measurement precision. Likewise, Jette (2008) promotes the development of CAT scales that incorporate the categories of ICF Core Sets to generate total scores.

As currently conceived, the Core Sets are permeable collections of categories, adjustable according to the individual and any concomitant comorbidities; conversely, a CAT measure from a Core Set cannot be adjusted for an individual by adding categories not in that Core Set. Furthermore, as currently conceived, each category can be accompanied by information about Environmental Contextual Factors that hinder or facilitate functioning in that category. This richness, although cumbersome, would presumably be lost in a summary score from a CAT measure. Teams who have experimented with flexibly applying permeable Core Sets to inform communication and guide rehabilitation include Rentsch et al. (2003) and Rauch et al. (2008).

As Core Sets have been developed, surveys and focus groups that include providers and people living with health conditions have elicited examples of important aspects to include. Typically, many identified aspects fit only within the undeveloped Personal Contextual Factors component (e.g., Finger, Cieza, Stoll, Stucki, & Huber, 2006; Glaessel, A., Kirchberger, I., Stucki, G., & Cieza, A., 2011), thus suggesting an unfortunate vacuum. The utility of the ICF for rehabilitation research on process and outcomes will not approach realization until Personal Contextual Factors are defined and explicated. A growing number of voices within rehabilitation and disability research (e.g., Badley, 2008; Geyh, 2008; Huber, Sillick, & Skarakis-Doyle, 2010; IOM, 2007; Peterson, Mfopu, & Oakland, 2010; Wang, Badley, & Gignac, 2006) have begun that process.

Patient-Centered Rehabilitation and Single-Case/Single-Subject Designs

Mark Ozer is a seminal figure in patient-centered rehabilitation. He and his colleagues (Ozer, 1999; Ozer & Kroll, 2002; Ozer, Payton, & Nelson, 2000) developed methods to guide providers in eliciting personally relevant problems and goals from people in rehabilitation even when they had significant impairments in cognition and communication. These methods led to better engagement and participation, and better outcomes relevant to independent living (Ozer, 1999). Patient-centered rehabilitation, as practiced by Ozer and his team, involves a three-part plan: setting goals with the patient after he or she has identified the most salient problems, applying methods to reach those goals, and reviewing the plan with respect to progress and the patient's satisfaction. "At each iteration, the patient can be expected to contribute to a greater degree in making these plans and evaluating them" (p. 275).

Ozer and Kroll (2002) describe and recommend several other patient-centered methods of assessment and progress-monitoring in rehabilitation, including goal attainment scaling (GAS), which is a method for aggregating achievement scores in several individually set goals into a single score, thus providing an outcome measure focused on that person's priorities (Kiresuk & Sherman, 1968). The application of GAS in rehabilitation settings has increased (e.g., see Bouwens, VanHeugten, & Verhey, 2009; Hale, 2010; Malec, 1999; Turner-Stokes, Williams, & Johnson, 2009), reflecting the rising emphasis on patient-centered care. Difficulties have been noted as providers develop their skills for eliciting goals from their patients; Hale (2010) notes this among physical therapists trying GAS in home-based rehabilitation. Ozer's methods could be a very useful addition here, as he provides detailed guidance regarding the very first conversations between provider and patient, starting with identification of those problems most salient to the patient.

For methods of progress monitoring and outcomes measurement that are consistent with their participatory planning system, Ozer and Kroll (2002) encourage the consideration of single-subject experimental designs, suggesting that the multiple-baseline variant is particularly well-suited for use in rehabilitation because of its rigor and flexibility in adaptation.

Single-Case/Single-Subject Experimental Designs

Single-case experimental designs (SCEDs) (or single-subject experimental designs; the terms are used more or less interchangeably) utilize methods that maximize the amount of clearly interpretable information gained from working with an individual or small numbers of people. They are well-suited for small-scale clinical research. Kratochwill, Hitchcock, Horner, Levin, Odom, Rindskopf and Shadish (2010) have provided a good, detailed summary of SCEDs for the What Works Clearinghouse. Single-case experimental designs are identified by the following features (p. 2):

- An individual "case" is the unit of intervention and unit of data analysis.... A case may be a single participant or a cluster of participants (e.g., a classroom or a community).
- Within the design, the case provides its own control for purposes of comparison. For example, the case's series of outcome variables are measured prior to the intervention and compared with measurements taken during (and after) the intervention.
- The outcome variable is measured repeatedly within and across different conditions or levels of the independent variable. These different conditions are referred to as phases (e.g., baseline phase, intervention phase).

Experimental control involves replication of the intervention in the experiment through one of the following (p. 3):

- Introduction and withdrawal (i.e., reversal) of the independent variable (e.g., ABAB design)
- Iterative manipulation of the independent variable across different observational phases (e.g., alternating treatments design)
- Staggered introduction of the independent variable across different points in time (e.g., multiple baseline design)

There are also instances of AB only (pre–post) designs that, in particular circumstances, may provide supportive evidence of an intervention effect; a common example is when an intervention is initiated for a person with stable deficits of long-standing duration (e.g., a person with TBI who is several years post injury and has persisting problems in everyday memory). ABA or ABAB designs can provide strong evidence of intervention effects, but are limited in applicability to those interventions that can be withdrawn without leaving persisting treatment effects, and to those interventions for which no ethical dilemma is associated with their termination.

Multiple baseline designs are highly flexible, as "multiple" can refer to having interventions introduced in a staggered fashion: as with one person working on two or more different goals; or with one person, for whom interventional strategies with respect to the same goal are sequentially introduced, looking for additive or contrasting effects; or with different people working on the same or very similar goal. Strong evidence for an intervention effect can be provided when a change from baseline occurs across people (or across goals) only when and not before each intervention begins.

Zhan and Ottenbacher (2001) argue that SCEDs have particular advantages for clinicians studying their own treatment effectiveness. Rassafiani and Sahaf (2010) provide an excellent introduction and detailed critique of SCED and encourage its wider use internationally and among various health and rehabilitation professions. Single-case experimental designs have long been used in research and clinical work in neurorehabilitation, particularly for TBI. In a recent survey by Wilson (2008) of 54 neuropsychologists working in TBI rehabilitation in the United Kingdom, 72% reported using SCEDs to evaluate their rehabilitation programs. Just a few examples of TBI rehabilitation applications of SCEDs include vocational rehabilitation (Ownsworth, Fleming, Desbois, Strong, & Kuipers, 2006); independent living (Kelly & Nikopoulos, 2010), smartphone technologies for memory deficits (Svoboda & Richards, 2009), and web-based assistive technology use (Kirsch et al., 2004). Mateer (2009) provides SCED examples from memory rehabilitation, but also describes the advantages of this form of design for clinical research more generally. Other applications have included studying the benefits of errorless learning in memory rehabilitation for patients with Alzheimer disease (Clare et al., 2000), evaluating precision teaching for aphasia (Cherney, Merbitz, & Grip, 1986), and applying interventions to reduce self-injurious behaviors (Rizvi & Nock, 2008). Janosky (2005) recommends that physicians use SCEDs to study treatment effectiveness and quality improvement in primary care. Ottenbacher (1990) and Michaud (1995) recommend single-subject research in rehabilitation and medical settings. Schlosser (2009) discusses the usefulness and appropriateness of SCEDs across several phases of research, as described by Robey (2004); likewise, Whyte et al. (2009) have noted that progress in research requires a phased approach drawing on a variety of methods, such as the use of SCEDs.

Barlow and Nock (2009) argue for much more widespread use of SCEDs in psychotherapy research:

> Scientifically, relying on a relatively small group of researchers requiring enormous amounts of time and resources to perform a single treatment trial [RCT] can be seen as an inefficient method of advancing knowledge.... The flexibility and efficiency of these designs [SCEDs] make them ideally suited for use by psychological scientists, clinicians, and students alike, given that they require relatively little time and few resources and subjects and yet they can provide strong evidence of causal relations between variables. (p. 20)

Beeson and Robey (2006) describe the long history of SCED applications in aphasia treatment and report that of 620 published articles on interventions in aphasiology over the past five decades, 252 (41%) were single-case experimental designs. They provide ideas for calculating effect sizes to help establish evidence-based practices. Callahan and Barissa (2005) provide a persuasive account of why and how to use simple statistical process control charts to display and analyze SCED data:

> [The] scientist–practitioner model's... original intent was that the diagnosis and treatment of each individual case was to be regarded as a single and well-controlled experiment. Executing this ideal in rehabilitation has been problematic owing to practical, ethical, and technical concerns. Statistical process control (SPC), a robust, graphical analytic strategy developed in industry, is offered as a means to deploy single-subject designs on the front lines of rehabilitation. (p. 24)

For descriptions of other statistical methods of analysis applied to SCEDs, also see Brossart et al. (2008), Kratochwill and Levin (2010), and Zhan and Ottenbacher (2001).

Tate et al. (2008) and Perdices and Tate (2009) have worked to improve standards of quality for conducting, reporting, and reviewing SCED research, and they have developed the SCED Scale to assist reviewers in rating levels of evidence. The American Academy for Cerebral Palsy and Developmental Medicine (AACPDM) Treatment Outcomes Committee (TOC) updated their systematic review process in 2008 with the addition of Levels of Evidence and conduct ratings for single-subject design studies. However, we also note that the Cochrane guidelines still do not (as of this writing) include any recognition of single-subject/single-case experimental designs. Other research classification systems are making progress in this regard, including those of the EFNS (Cappa et al., 2005) and the Quality Standards Subcommittee of the American Academy of Neurology (Miller et al., 1999), whose guidelines were later adopted by the Academy of Neurologic Communication Disorders and Sciences.

Ylvisaker et al. (2007) agree with Perdices and Tate (2009) regarding the place of single-subject methods in research, stating that:

> [A] rigorous, well-designed SS experiment may yield scientifically more solid evidence for its specific conclusion (i.e., that the intervention caused improved performance in the studied individual) than a randomized controlled trial yields for its conclusion (i.e., that the intervention causes an average improvement in performance across a sub-group of members of the studied population) (p. 781).... Indeed, the strongest evidence (reason) for a specific clinical decision is *experimental validation with that individual* (i.e., trial therapy, diagnostic teaching, experimental behaviour assessment or dynamic, hypothesis-testing assessment). (p. 782, emphasis added)

Read what Strauss (2010) wrote in an article entitled "Exploiting Single Cell Variation for New Antibiotics" and think about its implications for all we have yet to learn about people and rehabilitation, and how we have been going about it so far:

> Much of what we do as chemical biologists rests on an often unstated but widely accepted supposition that the results of our studies of populations—of cells, proteins or any particular enzyme—are equally applicable and relevant to each member of that particular population.... Variations between single members of a bacterial population can lead to antibiotic resistance that is not gene based. The future of effective infectious disease management might depend on a better understanding of this phenomenon. (p. 873)

Now, here is where it gets interesting. As an illustration, Strauss cites the work of Balaban et al. (2004). To test a decades-old theory (Bigger, 1944) of antibiotic resistance among a genetically identical bacterial population (his theory being that the subset of resistant bacteria were those who stayed longest in a nongrowth phase, during which they were not susceptible to the effects of the antibiotic on their cell walls), Balaban's team developed a method to hold on to individual bacteria, *one at a time*.

> In an innovative approach, the authors of the study [trapped] individual bacterial cells in the channels of a microfluidic device, which allowed the growth of each cell to be monitored both before and after antibiotic treatment. In this manner it could be clearly shown that persisters are subpopulations of slow-dividing or non-dividing bacteria that exist before the addition of the antibiotic agent—just as Bigger predicted. (p. 874)

We suggest that it is perhaps misaligned contingencies (e.g., the money going into and flowing out from pharmaceutical research) and the relative status of "soft" (behavioral) versus "hard" (chemical biological) sciences that makes a study of individual bacteria via a single-cell experimental design warrant publication in *Nature*, whereas the study of individual people in medical care or rehabilitation remains unrecognized within the dominant evidence hierarchies of medical science.

Quality Improvement

As we explored the literature on outcomes research within rehabilitation and health care more generally, frankly looking for any work using close-up data and real-time research, we found compelling efforts under way in somewhat unexpected places. Quality improvement in its varied manifestations has drawn together impassioned and pragmatic people from all over the globe, sharing a keen interest in science and service in many areas of health care, including rehabilitation.

Quality Improvement in Health Care

Donald Berwick, one of the leading figures in U.S. and international efforts for quality improvement in health care (and currently head of the Centers for Medicare and Medicaid Services) has long argued that quality improvement is a profound endeavor requiring nothing less than a new epistemology of evidence-based practice (Berwick, 2005, 2009). We particularly enjoy Berwick's unapologetic

depiction (2005) of quality improvement as a compelling science:

> Broadly framed, much of human learning relies wisely on effective approaches to problem solving, learning, growth, and development that are different from the types of formal science so well explicated and defended by the scions of evidence-based medicine. Although they are far from RCTs in design, some of those approaches offer good defenses against misinterpretation, bias, and confounding.... The methods of observation and reflection on the basis of which most human learning occurs and, frankly, on the basis of which many modern industries and enterprises are building their futures, are systematic, theoretically grounded, often quantitative, and powerful. (pp. 315–316)

Berwick goes on to summarize key elements of pragmatic science (Brock, Nolan, & Nolan, 1998; Langley et al., 1996), including the following:

- *Tracking effects over time, especially with graphs* (rather than summarizing with statistics that do not retain the information involved in sequences);
- *using local knowledge—the knowledge of local workers—in measurement* (rather than relegating measurement to people least familiar with the subject matter and work);
- *integrating detailed process knowledge into the work of interpretation* (inviting observers to comment on what they notice rather than "blinding" them to protect them against what they know);
- *using small samples and short experimental cycles to learn quickly* (rather than overpowering studies and delaying new theories with samples larger than needed at the time). (Berwick, 2005, p. 316, emphasis added)

Drawing upon methods developed within various subfields of quality improvement, Berwick (1998) started the Institute for Healthcare Improvement (IHI) in 1998, an independent not-for-profit organization that has a growing international network of partnerships and research collaboratives (Berwick, James, & Coye, 2003; Brandrud et al., 2011). He says with understandable pride that "Pragmatic science...is alive and well. It thrives in the halls of continual improvement of care now engaging the energies of thousands of healthcare leaders worldwide" (Berwick, 2005, p. 316).

Among its many efforts, the IHI initiated IMPACT Learning and Innovation Communities:

groups of member organizations that work together, along with IHI, on solutions to improve care. Compelling examples include the work of MacDavitt et al. (2011), who report on the work of their hospital in the Learning and Innovation Community of "Transforming Medical/Surgical Care" and describe their use of Plan-Do-Study-Act (PDSA) cycles: planning a change, trying it, studying the results, acting on what is learned, and then moving into the next "small cycle" in an iterative process. Similarly, Davis and Huska (2009) from ImpactBC (British Columbia) have described the Model for Improvement used by their teams in collaboration with the IHI:

1. *What are we trying to accomplish? (Aim)* Here, participants determine which specific outcomes they are trying to change through their work.

2. *How will we know that a change is an improvement? (Measures)* Here, team members identify appropriate measures to track their success.

3. *What changes can we make that will result in improvement? (Changes)* Here, teams identify key changes that they will actually test. Key changes are then implemented in a cyclical fashion: teams thoroughly plan to test the change, taking into account cultural and organizational characteristics.

This process continues serially over time, and refinement is added with each PDSA cycle. Measurement is integrated into daily routines. Data are plotted for the measures over time on a simple "run chart," which is annotated to indicate when a process change is implemented. (See Table 6.1 for characteristics of data that are well suited for this type of application.)

Interest in methods of CQI that Deming developed for industry (presented in Walton, 1986) has generated applications by a number of health care teams within and external to the IHI. A vigorous, long-established and growing movement exists among physicians and other providers for quality improvement among primary care practices (e.g., Nelson, Splaine, Batalden, & Plume, 1998; Ruhe, Carter, Litaker, & Stange, 2009). Needham and Korupolu (2010) concluded from their work that a structured CQI model can be applied to implementation of early rehabilitation in the intensive care unit. Callahan and Griffen (2003) and colleagues (Barenfanger et al., 2008) have used statistical process control techniques from CQI (specifically the average moving range individual control chart) to improve processes and outcomes in emergency departments.

Many have called for use of Donabedian's model of structure, process, and outcomes (1981, 1988) in the design and analysis of health care research, recognizing that research focusing on processes of care can better guide the translation of knowledge into practice than can RCT research on outcomes that controls for process variations via randomization (see Duncan & Velozo, 2007; Hoenig et al., 2002; Duncan et al., 2002; Asch et al., 2004). As described by Schiff and Rucker (2001), Donabedian contributed far more than the structure-process-outcome elements to a framework of quality improvement. Beyond system design, he advocated quality monitoring, or "the process by which performance is periodically or continuous reviewed and when found to be deficient, first modified and then monitored once again." To his triad of elements, Donabedian added elements of access, technical quality, affect/relationship quality, and continuity of care, and he argued that responsibility for quality can be relatively dispersed, vested in persons (professionals and others) who are closest to where care is provided. These persons coordinate to identify processes needing to be changed, redesign the processes, and continue monitoring through mutual participation that is self-evaluating and self-motivating. Clearly, the methods in use today by the IHI and others are rooted in his insights.

Quality Improvement in Psychotherapy

In recognition of the inability of any model, no matter the evidence from RCTs, to predict success for the individual client, the American Psychological Association (APA) Task Force on evidence-based practice (APA Task Force, 2006) suggested that "ongoing monitoring of patient progress and adjustment of treatment as needed are essential." Of direct relevance to rehabilitation psychologists are CQI practices that are being used by many to adjust the delivery of counseling and psychotherapy in response to ongoing feedback. For example, Bickman and Mulvaney (2005) called for service organizations to collect data for expanding common factors research in underrepresented community treatment settings, particularly among those that work with children and adolescents. Many collaborative research programs have been and are being developed with the goal of aggregating process and outcomes data collected by psychologists and other mental health providers dispersed across settings and countries. Common elements of these programs include brief measures completed regularly by clients, guidance/coordination led by a team of researchers, the use of principles of patient-focused research, and extensions into larger service delivery systems, in addition to applications within private practices (see Lueger & Barkham, 2010, for a review of these programs). One particular benefit of such systems is in helping to prevent treatment failure; Lambert and colleagues point to research indicating that without regular, formalized client feedback, such as with their Outcome Questionnaire-45 (OQ-45) system or other similar systems, clinicians generally do quite poorly at detecting and preventing treatment failures (defined as premature drop-outs or clients who become worse by the end of therapy).

We found particularly noteworthy Lambert and colleagues' work with the OQ-45 (Lambert, Hansen, & Harmon, 2010; Lambert et al., 2002) and the CORE measures system (Barkham, Mellor-Clark et al., 2010), as well as the body of work known as client-directed, outcome-informed (CDOI) service delivery (Duncan, Miller, & Sparks, 2004; Knaup, Koesters, Schoefer, Becker, & Puschner, 2009; Miller, Duncan, Sorrell, Brown, & Chalk, 2006; Miller, Mee-Lee, Plum, & Hubble, 2005). Information about the development and practice of CDOI is very accessible thanks to the websites developed by its founders (see Appendix A). Client-directed, outcome-informed (CDOI) service delivery provides a method to combine evidence-based practice (EBP) with practice-based evidence (PBE) to empower success at the individual client level, and it helps identify clients at risk for treatment failure based on predictors of outcome and retention that have been developed from prior analyses of aggregated data on client factors and responses to the short questionnaires administered at each session.

In these and other systems springing up to provide flexible guidance to and collaboration among therapists in real-world settings, the aim is not to advocate or train in particular models of therapy, but rather to harness the potential for learning and growth in each therapeutic dyad. This approach represents a logical development of the ideas first expounded by the earliest common factors theorists (Sparks et al., 2008).

Complexity Science and Complex Adaptive Systems

It is a truism that the longer a person or organization is followed after an intervention, the greater the likelihood for any previously detected treatment effects to dissipate and become undetectable. This prompts an apt comparison with complex systems, such as the weather: proximal predictions may be accurate, but the further out in time one looks, prediction becomes much fuzzier: too many nonlinear variables are at play. Our patients or clients will have innumerable interactions with other systems long after our work with them is done; these interactions affect long-term outcomes via the quality and continuity of supports, or lack thereof.

According to Brown (2006), the U.K.'s National Health Service is promoting understanding of complexity science and CAS theory through educational efforts aimed at its leaders in quality improvement, and the *British Medical Journal* has made freely available on its website a series of articles about health care and complexity science (see Appendix). As summarized by Wilson and Holt (2001), CAS uses a collection of individual agents with freedom to act in ways that are not always totally predictable and whose actions are interconnected, so that the action of one part changes the context for other agents. In relation to human health and illness, several levels of such systems exist:

• The human body is composed of multiple interacting and self-regulating physiological systems including biochemical and neuroendocrine feedback loops.

• The behaviour of any individual is determined partly by an internal set of rules based on past experience and partly by unique and adaptive responses to new stimuli from the environment.

• Individuals and their immediate social relationships are further embedded within wider social, political, and cultural systems which can influence outcomes in entirely novel and unpredictable ways.

• A small change in one part of this web of interacting systems may lead to a much larger change in another part through amplification [nonlinear] effects.

• For all these reasons neither illness nor human behavior is predictable and neither can safely be "modeled" in a simple cause and effect system. (p. 685)

In his "Crossing the Quality Chasm," Plsek (2001) presented to the IOM committee a set of features characterizing CAS as applicable to humans, nonhuman organisms, and natural phenomena including health care organizations, thus demonstrating the poor fit of a machine model to quality improvement in health care. In addition to the characteristics also noted by Wilson and Holt (above), he described the following (p. 313):

- *Adaptable elements.* The elements of the system can change themselves. Examples include antibiotic-resistant organisms and anyone who learns. In machines, change must be imposed, whereas under the right conditions in CAS, change can happen from within.
- *Simple rules.* Complex outcomes can emerge from a few simple rules that are locally applied.
- *Emergent behavior, novelty.* Continual creativity is a natural state of the system....
- *Not predictable in detail.* For example, in weather forecasting, the fundamental laws governing pressure and temperature in gases are nonlinear. For this reason, despite reams of data and very powerful supercomputers, detailed, accurate long-range weather forecasting is fundamentally not possible....
- *Inherent order.* Systems can be orderly even without central control. Self-organization is the key idea in complexity science. For example, termites build the largest structures on earth when compared with the height of the builders, yet there is no CEO termite.
- *Co-evolution.* A CAS moves forward through constant tension and balance. Fires, though destructive, are essential to a healthy, mature forest....Tension, paradox, uncertainty, and anxiety are healthy things in a CAS. In machine thinking, they are to be avoided.

David Labby, medical director for CareOregon, a nonprofit health plan serving Medicaid and Medicare recipients in Oregon, presented an example of nonlinear effects in his report to the Oregon Health Policy Board regarding the results of participation in a collaborative with the IHI (Labby, 2010). Consistent with the "small cycles of change" philosophy of IHI, Labby interspersed examples of individual interventions throughout his report of large-scale changes and very large cost-savings because the efforts of his organization rest upon finding those small-scale opportunities that have the potential to produce a big impact; that is, he focused on those nonlinear effects in which small perturbations to an entrenched situation can produce large and even surprising effects. He related how the provision of a bus pass dropped the emergency room visits of a woman with heroin addiction from more than 20 per month to zero because, by using public transportation, she could access regular, cheaper,

and more effective care. This example was entitled: "Bus Pass $23 versus ED $1,400."

Using the concepts of CAS, Plsek (2001) addressed the IOM's concerns for improvement on a very large scale (i.e., health care organizations and the U.S. health care system), and Brown (2006) and Wilson and Holt (2001) have sought to inform the individual work of rehabilitation therapists and physicians in primary care, respectively. However, it is possible to discern levels of complexity in a single individual organism—even in a single cell—that appear hardly less complex than a department, office, or hospital. This is the "fractal" quality often noted in complexity science—patterns appear and repeat at different levels of observation, like the branching patterns of capillaries, leaf veins, and tree branches. In chemical biological research, investigators (e.g., Wong & Bodovitz, 2010) are trying to determine why response to pharmaceuticals is so varied across individuals. Fine-grained observations and modeling of the work of enzymes *within individual cells* are revealing that genetically identical cells vary in supply and location of enzymes and substrates that can substantially affect rates of metabolic and other processes. These findings have implications for pharmaceutical research, as well as for basic science in systems biology. If investigators in chemistry, biology, and genetics have to adjust their investigations to take into account the varied responses of individual cells, why should not the adaptation of rehabilitation to individuals likewise be recognized as a scientific quest?

As changes are attempted within CAS, we are informed by complexity science about the phenomena of "attractors": patterns through which a system returns to a sometimes idiosyncratic but persistent equilibrium or "set-point." Within a health care system, an example might be consciously expressed (e.g., "This is the way we have always done things") or implicit, denied or unconscious, but nevertheless powerfully persistent, such as Rintala's finding (Rintala et al., 1986) that observational data from a rehabilitation team ostensibly dedicated to interdisciplinary functioning revealed a large majority of physician-generated questions and directives in team meetings. The history of a person or organization leads nonlinearly to the development of attractors that cannot be predicted in detail, although some kinds of patterns are broadly predictable (e.g., policies that emphasize punishment for mistakes will likely be associated with patterns of behavior reflecting concealment, because human functioning seems to be organized around the attractors of "avoidance of punishment" and "preservation of personal status and esteem").

When viewed through the lens of complexity science and CAS, Carl Rogers' nondirective, person-centered therapy (1986; Brazier, 1996) seems specifically designed for the reality of human attractors, especially the near-universal "resistance to taking obvious directions from other people." It also fits well with the recognition of nonlinearity of effects, whereby the therapist might have much more impact via small variations in how she responds to the client, within a zone defined by positive regard and genuineness, than she will by lecturing and pushing in a particular direction. In a working alliance, the therapeutic relationship becomes its own attractor, resisting and healing from disruptions in communication and returning to an equilibrium that is robust but subtly altered over time.

Applying Complexity Science to Rehabilitation

Awareness of the challenges posed by CAS should not deter efforts to improve rehabilitation. Rather, this knowledge points to approaches and strategies that, taken together, make for more powerful effects. It means paying attention to the details of individuals and the relationships among individuals and departments within an organization. It means that engaging others' efforts toward goals may require involving them in identifying and defining those goals, thus working with typical attractors such as "self image" and "resistance," and in the process benefitting in real ways from their up-close knowledge of their own portion of the system that is targeted for change. Among the factors Labby (2010) identified as impeding quality improvement in health care is "misalignment of incentives." Attempts to improve the functioning of a patient or a team must include a focus on common as well as idiosyncratic incentives—activities and goals that make it "worth their while," interesting, and rewarding to share information, keep working, be constructive, try again, and so forth. These efforts must also include frequent data regarding progress toward identified goals; otherwise, incentives can be misaligned because of missing feedback. When this happens, focus and energy are misplaced toward irrelevant features and ineffective actions.

The following study serves as an example of the power of interactive feedback in rehabilitation on a small but intensely data-rich scale. In a fascinating collaborative effort, a team of researchers at Arizona State University (Duff et al., 2010a, 2010b) and students from the School of Biological and Health Systems Engineering and the School of Arts, Media, and Engineering joined together to study applications of "mixed reality" to stroke rehabilitation, specifically to help the person with upper extremity hemiparesis relearn reaching and grasping skills. Central to those efforts has been the development of a two-way feedback system that adapts the presented stimuli according to what the patient is doing, moment-to-moment, and in turn provides immediate feedback to the patient regarding accuracy and speed of movements. Because somatosensory inputs are altered in hemiparesis, the use of visual and auditory feedback appears to play a critical role in the success of this mixed reality method. For example, in one portion of the treatment protocol, the real object the patient reaches for also appears projected as an image on a screen just beyond the object; the image is partially occluded, only coming into focus as the patient comes closer to grasping it, and all the while a rhythmic musical score changes tempo to match the patient's speed of movement. The system also collects highly detailed data regarding patients' movements so that the therapist can adjust the intervention; graphs of these data for a pilot sample of eight people with chronic hemiparesis show promising results of the mixed reality feedback system. This study is exciting in its own right, but also reminds us again of fractals: scaled up to team level and beyond, interactive feedback data could help everybody in rehabilitation improve their reach.

An Integrative Model for Complex Adaptive Rehabilitation

In this section, we present a synthesis of some of the possibilities for progress that can be found in the literature on outcomes and process measurement described above. As we consider data in complex adaptive rehabilitation (CAR), we will focus on process data about the behavior of individuals in rehabilitation that may be used by clinicians to improve outcomes, as well as contextual data, specifically with respect to *clinician* actions. For example, there is every reason to believe that measures of interpersonal interactions, such as the alliance between patient and clinician or the quality of team dynamics, especially if formulated as counts of relevant indicator variables (e.g., count of physician statements vs. therapist statements in team meetings, Rintala et al., 1986), could be examined to inform rehabilitation processes in real time. Space prevents comment on some other very important types of data that are also useful in judging outcomes. For example, the incidence of skin breakdown as a complication of SCI is an important outcome, but here we consider behaviors germane to the prevention of breakdown, such as pressure relief lift-offs. Similarly, following Rintala and Willems (1987), our focus here will be on data that have the potential to change over time, as opposed to demographics or characteristics that do not change (e.g., we are not modeling risk or case mix adjustors). The methods we describe are within the SCED tradition, thus each person (client or patient, clinician, etc.) serves as his or her own control.

It is important to consider the purposes for which the data are collected and analyzed, and the direct implications that flow from those purposes. For example, governmental entities may use "outcomes" data to evaluate the cost-effectiveness of service providers. For this purpose, the "cost" data come during the rehabilitation treatment as one aggregate amount of money, and the "effectiveness" part may be assessed at the end of treatment or at some point post-treatment. It seems obvious that the total calculation is eased considerably if "effectiveness" can be assigned one number as well, in spite of the logical and practical hazards involved (Merbitz, Morris, & Grip, 1989); the goals of rehabilitation may encompass so much of human life that the reduction of assessment of effectiveness to one number seems breathtaking in its hubris.

A level of sophistication above the single point of "outcome" measure may demand "effectiveness" data in the form of a change score that reflects the extent to which the client improved coincident to the rehabilitation, perhaps even adjusted by the predicted difficulty of achieving that level of change, given all variables documented for that case. For a change score, measures are often taken at two points in time to enable the comparison of data across time, with additional data points to fill out the course or path of the rehabilitation. As we add data points, the outcomes measures may become useful also as process measures to clinicians interested in adapting current treatments in the interest of improving the outcome scores (see Chapman, Ewing, & Mozzoni, 2005; Halstead, 1976; Patrick, Mozzoni, & Patrick, 2000).

Rehabilitation of individuals takes place over time, and the relative success of any case may involve progress and change in many arenas of functioning, social interaction, communication, behavior, and so forth. Ideally, the actions and interventions of the clinicians are "tuned" to the individual such that great progress is made and the desired outcome(s) are achieved. Note here the transition between a process and an outcome measurement system. The former should inform clinicians about how well a given patient is progressing and signal the need for tuning or changes in the type, quality, number, or intensity of interventions to keep progress on track. However, "outcome" implies an assessment at a point in time appropriate to make the judgment of the extent to which the process has resulted in a known and desirable outcome. We focus on the former in this section because the ideal process measure(s) seamlessly scale up into and predict the outcomes while there are still resources and time to change if they are not being approached. The unspoken holy grail of a measurement system would allow a *scalable focus*, from the minutia of interactions during treatment to an assessment of all of an individual's behavioral, personality, social, repertoires and how well they fit the discharge environment and the remainder of the individual's life. (We may note that some hubris exists here, too!)

We generally assume that data reflecting progress or increased functionality rely upon learning or gaining strength as underlying constructs, and goals of this type are quite common in rehabilitation (Bleiberg & Merbitz, 1983). Whyte (2009) notes that most intervention in rehabilitation is literally the behavior of clinicians. One implication is that clinicians must measure their behavior (the treatment) with sufficient precision to replicate it as needed, to report it in the literature, and to train others to apply it. Otherwise, the treatment producing the outcome is unknown and can't be reapplied with any degree of certainty. The difference here from the taxonomic efforts described earlier is the recognition that defining a treatment means defining the circumstances (and microcircumstances) within which it unfolds and to which it adjusts.

Evidence-based practice (EPB) is here taken to mean that evidence (typically research articles) supports the clinician's choice of procedures, assessments, interventions, and so forth used within each case. Beyond evidence provided by the RCT and analysis of between-group designs lies information from the SCED. However, the SCED makes another and very desirable level of EBP possible. Using a SCED clinically would be ideal if an inexpensive, ongoing data collection system were in place that provided the clinician with up-to-date evidence that the procedures and interventions in place for each client were producing as much change as detailed in the supporting literature; such data would simultaneously serve to validate the fidelity of the treatment to the practices in the literature. Any discrepancy (for better or worse) would then serve to signal the clinician to investigate the fit of the client to the classic literature and/or the fidelity of the treatment applied. Such data would also support the clinician in search of better effects to systematically vary the procedures given in the literature and provide a seamless transition to practice-based evidence (PBE), as such data would then form the basis for further research and development.

Following the ICF, we see each individual behaving within a complex context that includes at least social, economic, political, and physical dimensions, both during rehabilitation and afterward. Here, we frame this interplay between individual and environment as a selectionist process in order to uncover some of its fundamental and useful implications for measurement and treatment in rehabilitation.

In the selectionist view, as in the ICF view, the individual acts and the environment reacts—or perhaps does not react. (The latter case, *operant extinction* is not discussed further as its behavioral effects are well-known: frustration, disengagement, and burn-out, and/or superstitious behaviors). When the environment reacts or changes in some way, the individual is now living in a changed environment. Note that the change may accelerate, maintain, or decelerate whatever action the individual performed; in this way, the environment selects actions (or "behaviors," broadly defined; Baum, 1994; Skinner, 1953). With selectionism enters the notion of biological and behavioral variability; the environment may demand variations of any given action, and hence select variants that may in time morph (see also Tawfik, 2010) into completely different appearing actions. (Harbourne & Stergiou, 2009, discuss how this variability may be exploited within physical therapy.) This model of behavior being selected by the environment has the advantage of requiring analysis at the level of the behavior while supporting analysis at other useful levels (e.g., we surmise that pharmacological intervention is effective only when its behavioral effects are detected).

A second implication is that rehabilitation is a process that occurs with individuals over time. Time is, of course, a ubiquitous substrate of life, and therefore one may model any life as a time series. The time series view is fundamental. It implies that whatever other views of rehabilitation one chooses, all interventions involve the individual in a way that can be modeled (or at least plotted) as a time series.

In practice, the interventions with any given client may be hopelessly confounded, data may be missing, measures may be taken at irregular intervals, and so forth, but, despite these problems and confounds, a surprising amount of information may be revealed when data are plotted as a time series. Given multiple clinicians and other actors in a client's life, the client's rehabilitation most closely resembles a multiple baseline design, and clinicians may also use it to schedule and adjust the treatments, both to maintain individual progress and to preserve the greatest possibility of detecting effects. An additional level of complexity to be recognized here is that, although the clinician serves as part of the environment in which a client may change, conversely, the client serves as part of the environment in which the clinician may change; both improve in functioning under the influence of the other.

The replicated time series seems particularly suited to the development of useful clinical measures and better clinical decisions simply because all treatments are applied in time and all effects (if any) are seen after treatments are initiated. The time series also encourages us to view clinician behavior with the same temporal lens; the interaction of client and clinician may be seen as possibilities for accelerating some behaviors, maintaining some, and decelerating other behaviors of both participants. The clinician may adjust treatment for maximum progress only by learning what adjustments work for which individuals; empowering the individual in rehabilitation thus springs from empowering the clinician and individual with data.

A note here is that the basic time series is plotted over continuous time units—minutes, days, weeks, months or years, whatever units are relevant—to ensure the clearest possible interpretations. Plotting by "sessions," a common but unfortunate practice, trades interval data (time units) for ordinal data (session number). This choice may work under some circumstances, but may mislead in others as it calls into question the mathematical basis for assessing trends over time. Because ordinal data always involve a greater risk of misinference, here we will focus on the continuous time series as opposed to ordinal (sessions) data.

It may be useful at this juncture to consider what properties of data may make different types of data more or less useful in CAR. Functionally, the data are used to help the clinician tune the environment to help the client change at an optimum pace (e.g., before he is bored, tired, or runs out of insurance). Table 6.1 (van der Ploeg & Merbitz, 1998) lists

Table 6.1 Characteristics of best data

Simple	Concrete	Visible	Discrete
Shared, public	Self-correcting	Countable (ratio-level)	Relevant (valid)
Sensitive	Achievable	Predictive	Consistent
Important	Interpretable	Robust	Reliable
Comparable	Cheap	In-the-stream	Replicable
Resistant to misinference	High signal-to-noise ratio	No ceiling, no floor	Time-conserving

Table shows characteristics or attributes of data that make them particularly useful and economical for the purpose of process control. The ease, accuracy, and utility of the data for process control may increase as the data collection, storage, and analysis process approximates these features. Note that these are adapted for collaborative human decisions and activity. Adapted from van der Ploeg, A., & Merbitz, C. Data Driven Decisions. A presentation at the American Educational Research Association, Chicago, IL, 1998.

properties that make data more useful in process control and hence for steering the CAR toward progress. One sophisticated system that meets these criteria is human behavioral frequency data displayed on the *Celeration Chart* (developed by Lindsley, 1992, for Precision Teaching). Note that Callahan and Barisa (2005) present an argument for using statistical process control (SPC) methods, another alternative, in much the same way.

In Precision Teaching, as in complexity science, each client is viewed as a perfect sample of him- or herself, and how each individual responds to the treatment is the effect of that treatment modulated by the full complexity of his or her life circumstances, economic and physical resources, social environment, and so forth. We know that these individual differences make for lower statistical homogeneity, complicate RCTs, bedevil statistical analyses, and call into question the applicability of RCT data in cases that do not match the statistical profile of the RCT participants. We know that patients have lives and that their life circumstances may overwhelm our clinical interventions. These facts challenge us as scientists to take advantage of the strengths of many types of research designs, in addition to RCTs, to inform clinical practice and make such practice a CAR. Variation in the responses of each individual over time is the basic index that may be used to understand how contextual variables impact that individual. A time series permits individual variability to become a *critically important source of inference* about effects engendered by the clinician and environment. When data are tied to specific points in time, contextual factors can be examined and may be highly instructive for that and future cases (see Kubina, Ward, & Mozzoni, 2000).

For example, Figure 6.1 shows 24/7 time-series data (Merbitz, King, Bleiberg, & Grip, 1985) of daily frequency (count over time) of pressure-relief behaviors for Patient B, who consented to provide data while in rehabilitation for SCI (monitored via an electronic device). His chart shows dramatic drops in frequency associated with home visits and excessive drinking at Christmas and New Years, an example of how good data can reveal more than planned. The cited article presents a measure of behavior and a process control model via the Celeration Chart that can and should be extended. This case also shows the advantages of inexpensive and rapid analysis: one glance, and the two weekends in question stand out dramatically. There is no need for a separate statistical analysis to see the huge effect and its clinical (and statistical) significance. The dialog prompted by mutual examination of such data could lead to further discussion of substance use and abuse. Note also that the interpretation of these data would be complicated if plotted by sessions instead of plotting by the calendar date on which they were collected. Both the patterning of days of the week and any days with missing data can be seen in this data set.

This case also suggests another ideal: What if wheelchairs of all consenting patients in SCI rehabilitation were instrumented as in the studied case? Then, these data could flow into a computerized, internet-based database. If appropriate privacy controls were in place, an authorized clinician with access to the database could see immediately where his or her client was with respect to the population and to the goal of one lift every 20 minutes (or any other goal that emerged from the data set as adequate and safe). Modern electronics may make such a data collection system trivial from an engineering

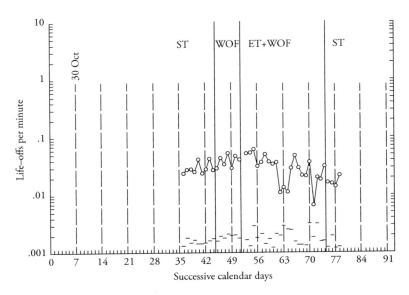

Figure 6.1 Pressure-Reliefs by Individual with Spinal Cord Injury (SCI). Patient B from Merbitz, King, Bleiberg, & Grip (1985). Dotted vertical lines denote Sundays. Dots are lifts per minute, dashes are the reciprocal of the number of minutes in the wheelchair that day. Day 0 is the Sunday before admission. Note the lift-off frequencies on the weekends at Days 62–64 (Christmas) and Day 71 (New Years). Originally presented as Fig. 3 in Merbitz, C. T., King, R. B., Bleiberg, J., & & Grip, J. C. (1985). Wheelchair push-ups: Measuring pressure relief frequency. *Archives of Physical Medicine and Rehabilitation, 66,* 433–438. Reprinted by permission.

perspective, but with a history of over three decades of development of similar devices (for example, see Malament, Dunn, & Davis, 1975, through Guenther, 1999), no one has attracted sufficient venture capital to support the needed engineering research and development to make such data collection and utilization routine.

Other possibilities for data use are illustrated by Merbitz, Miller, and Hansen (2000), who reported the course of a speech-language–based treatment for a young man with TBI. In this case, correct logical inferences per minute by the patient and cues per minute by the clinician were among the measured variables. A line of best fit (a celeration line or slope indicating change in count/minute/day/week) through the data points for each person's actions provides a convenient and robust measure of progress by the dyad (see Figure 6.2). One major and unexpected finding was an inverse relation between the celeration of the patient's correct inferences and the celeration of the clinician's cueing, clearly revealed when lines of best fit were superimposed on local reversals of trends within the data points. One possible explanation for this variability in the patient's responses could involve changes in medication and other life events, such as the effects of alcohol consumption, which were discussed in the studied case of SCI above. However, during these sessions, the speech-language pathologist

also collected frequency data on a number of other exercises that did not show any similar fluctuations. Hence, the data formed a simultaneous multiple baseline. The lack of synchronized changes across all of the behaviors was compelling evidence that the patterning in logical inferences per minute was due to the clinician's cueing and *not* to changes in medication, life circumstances, or other variables, just as the pattern of variability seen in the pressure-relief dataset was evidence *for* the effects of such variables. When the clinician held her cueing constant, the patient's correct inferences per minute eventually rose. Prior to that, one could speculate, if he waited long enough, another cue was forthcoming, then eventually the clinician caught herself over-cueing and cut back, the patient produced more inferences, but then the pattern recurred, until examination of the data lead to a strategic change in the intervention. That a patient with severe brain injury could lead such a subtle and complex social dance was completely unexpected.

Note also that these data and the logic of CAR make it possible to measure and quantify change (count/time/time), and hence it can be used to compare treatment environments directly in terms of the amount of change that was engendered by each, even though the clients had different diagnoses and the behaviors in question were vastly different. It is impossible to overstate the potential

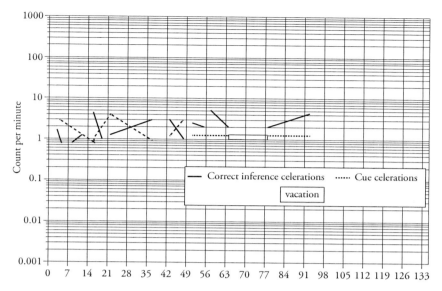

Figure 6.2 Clinician and Client Behaviors in Traumatic Brain Injury Cognitive Rehabilitation. Celerations (trends) of patient correct inferences and clinician cues. Note the inverse relationship prior to Day 49. Appeared originally as Figure 5 in Merbitz, C. T., Miller, T. K., & Hansen, N. K. (2000). Cueing and logical problem solving in brain trauma rehabilitation: Frequency patterns in clinician and patient behaviors. *Behavioral Interventions, 15,* 169–187. Reprinted by permission.

of this statistic. The possibility of using celeration as a direct measure of change allows the clinician to see immediately the extent to which the desired goals are being reached and the effects of any variation in clinical process.

A related point is that the same data display can be used and interpreted across all frequency measures of human behavior, and the particular display of calendar time against a base-ten multiple scale (as seen in Figure 6.2) provides many advantages. The particular scale and display chosen was developed by Lindsley and associates over a period of several decades (Lindsley, 1992) to support very rapid and accurate decisions about changing behavior. Without trivializing the effort required to learn to use this system or the research required to add it to current practice, we offer it here as an ideal because it offers so many conceptual and pragmatic advantages over other available systems we have seen, including statistical process control. (See the Appendix for links to research communities using celeration charts and precision teaching.)

Briefly, a very wide range of behavior frequencies can be displayed on a celeration chart because the base of the scale is one per day and the top is 1,000 per minute. The minimum frequency seen is one per day; since a waking day is 1,000 minutes long, the frequency is .001. Figure 6.3 shows an intervention for a client with dementia whose undesired behaviors

(e.g., yelling) were occurring up to 20 times per day, or at a frequency of .02/min. Note that this case was not designed for research but simply illustrates some possibilities for using the chart in local quality improvement projects. Counts of patient behavior were collected by staff members on the unit. Having staff count desired behaviors (e.g., eating most of a meal, participating cooperatively in getting dressed) can be a deliberate intervention as well as a measurement procedure; notice that the frequency of desired behaviors reported by staff (*indicated by dots*) increase and undesired (*indicated by x's*) behavior decrease in an orderly way over days, as a set of changes (including psychoactive medication reduction) was pragmatically implemented. With moderate training, any rehabilitation professional on any unit may use this simple technique to plot frequencies and determine behavioral influences, regardless of patient diagnoses, age, or other variables.

The conceptual roots of this system have been discussed elsewhere (Baum, 1994; Chiesia, 1992; Glenn & Madden, 1995; Merbitz, 1996; Palmer & Donahoe, 1992; Skinner, 1953). Because data can be entered directly onto a celeration chart by a clinician (or sometimes a client), because the display of those data is specifically designed to be sensitive to small changes at the lower end of performance, and because variability can be examined separately from frequency and celeration, the clinician may

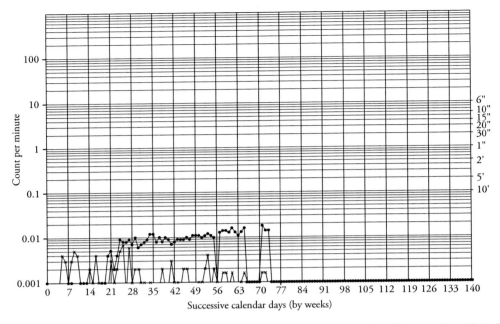

Figure 6.3 Nursing Home Resident Showing Improvement. Data reflecting staff counts of undesired behaviors (*x*) and desired behaviors (*dots*) per day of an elderly man residing in a nursing home. Note how the chart shows the orderly acceleration of desired behaviors recorded by staff after the second week of counting, and rapid deceleration of undesired behaviors. Data and graph from Nancy Hansen Merbitz's clinical database.

avoid either holding the client in ineffective treatment after gains stop or switching out of effective treatment simply because gains proceed slowly from a low baseline.

Although many systems attempt to measure a latent trait or construct (Wright & Linacre, 1989), frequency explicitly marks the intersection of the person with a specific environment during a specific time. Therefore, the variability seen as one changes the environment informs us as to the effects of that changed environment. So, for example, we may consider ambulation by a healthy average adult and measure her performance as 20 meters per minute for 6 minutes on a level surface. Now let us arrange a treadmill tilted at a 30-degree angle and have her ambulate again. We can describe "handicap" for her as the increased time she will take to travel the 120 meters as we tilt the treadmill; at some angle, she will be unable to move across it. Similarly, if the substrate for ambulation changes from a hard, level, nonskid surface to a tilted, slippery surface, there will be a drop in safe ambulation speed, and we can relate these speeds to the surface characteristics. However, the reverse is also true; we can detect and describe the effects of any variation in conditions that causes variability in frequency, and exploit that variance by repeating those conditions under which better frequencies are seen and avoiding those that

produce the reverse. Thus, the variability becomes information to the clinician and it signals promising directions to explore with each client, instead of interfering with inference.

Note that this conceptual framework up-ends the ICF's problematic system of rating performance versus capacity; instead, an *environment* is measured in terms of what the individual does within its context, compared to what the individual does within another environmental context. A house with a ramp could be measured in terms of how many times its wheelchair-using occupant leaves home per week, compared to the same house before the ramp. What the individual does in an environment becomes a metric for measuring that environment. A therapeutic environment could be measured in terms of number of goal-oriented and/or self-disclosing statements by the client in a session, comparing different approaches by the therapist (or comparing one therapist to another).

The discussion here is oversimplified, truncated, and abbreviated; it is intended only to sketch the possibilities found within a view of rehabilitation as a CAS. However, we believe that an approach using selectionism and behavior frequencies does offer great promise and that the possibilities now for automated and simplified data acquisition and display can bring these benefits within reach in a cost-effective way.

Conclusion

Although we have been enthusiastically engaged in reviewing obstacles to and progress in the rehabilitation research enterprise, it is still sobering to reflect on the larger context, in which seemingly no amount of data in the absence of political force can suffice to change the practices and policies of hospitals, providers, payers, or governments. As one example, although it is now well-established that quicker entry into rehabilitation after onset of a potentially disabling event (e.g., stroke, TBI) is associated with better outcomes, and there is indication that consistent staffing and therapeutic alliance may play a large role in rehabilitation effectiveness, observations by the authors in central rural Illinois reveal substantial inadequacies and fragmentation in services. It appears that many, if not most, people who could benefit from rehabilitation get very little, and they receive it from various therapists (even within one discipline) whose efforts are not coordinated with each other or with referring physicians. Or, they do not get referred at all, or only after complications have become obvious. We believe this is likely typical for many regions, nationally and internationally, that are far from university teaching hospitals.

Time will tell if current market forces push the evolution of better science and better care, but we are reminded of Stephen Jay Gould (1990) writing that evolution is a directionless process, with no systematic bias toward any particular kind of fitness; by chance, evolution also produces the survival of the lucky, the already well-positioned, the "happened to be at the right place at the right time." Occasionally, these forces operate to produce something beautiful and efficient, but sometimes the surviving organisms are simply big and able to crowd others out. And when contingencies shift, the dinosaurs may be at a disadvantage while the mammals, carrying on all the while, may come to the fore. In the final analysis, practitioners and organizations will have to act, individually and in concert with one or more of the research collaboratives and practice research networks that have been springing up to carry on a kind of vigilante research with or without the support of traditional grant funding or salaried, dedicated research time.

Future Directions

An investigation into processes of rehabilitation can be organized along multiple paths, and asking productive questions leads to stronger rehabilitation effects.

- The benefits of existing rehabilitation efforts could be studied and compared in the context of variation in environmental or "nonspecific" process factors. Pertinent questions may include: "Is a change in staffing pattern, such as primary nursing or consistent therapist assignment, related to improvement in patient functioning, such as quicker gains toward independent dressing? Does patient performance on similar tasks vary by therapist? Is a quality improvement project that focuses on team functioning associated with reduced length of stay and fewer rehospitalizations? Is a quality improvement project focused on patient-centered skills in listening and goal-setting associated with reduced refusals of therapy appointments?"

- Other kinds of investigation blur the boundary between quality improvement and intervention, looking at how changes in process, particularly with respect to data—its availability, specificity, and interpretability—lead to improvements in effectiveness organizationally and at the level of individual patients. Here, it may be particularly advisable to track proximal (i.e., today, for this patient, this provider, this department, etc.) as well as organization-wide data over longer periods of time. Single-case designs can be particularly powerful for accumulating immediately useful information for a given patient, provider, or department. A set of research questions at this level could be, for example: "Does daily sharing of visually displayed performance data on mutually selected targets help this patient persist longer with tasks? Does it help me decide when to change a strategy, modify a target, or check on the patient's current priorities and perhaps change the goal to something else? Does the record of these data on a celeration chart (or even a simple run chart), with annotation of any changes in strategy or other conditions, support a multiple baseline study that reduces the likelihood of competing explanations for rate of progress? Are these efforts having a larger impact on my patients (e.g., length of stay) compared to before I started using data in this way?"

- Accumulating data (e.g., Binder, 1996) relate the successful teaching of independent performance on complex tasks (e.g., dressing) to prior achievement of particular frequencies on simpler component skills (e.g., buttoning, grasp-release). This "fluency" relation has also been seen in reading comprehension and other cognitive tasks. Could a taxonomy of component behaviors arranged by frequency help clinicians more efficiently select and sequence target behaviors?

• Routine data collection could represent a kind of "universal design," one done for a particular purpose, yet benefitting other efforts in unforeseen ways. A "just-in-time" data supply for research, similar to inventory that is stocked and ready when needed, means that baseline data are always available for studying natural experiments as they occur, as well as planned changes.

Appendix: Research Resources

The British Medical Journal has made freely available a series of articles about health care and complexity science on its website: http://www.bmj.com/search?fulltext=complexity+science&submit=yes

Burn Injury Model Systems: http://msktc.washington.edu/burn/findms.asp#datacenter

Center for Outcomes Measurement in Brain Injury (COMBI): http://www.tbims.org/combi/

This is an online resource for those needing detailed information and support in regards to outcome measures for brain injuries. The measures included in the COMBI are commonly used in the field of brain injury rehabilitation and assessment. The COMBI is a collaborative project of 16 brain injury facilities or centers, most of them Traumatic Brain Injury Model Systems.

CORE System (Clinical Outcomes for Routine Evaluation) (Barkham et al.):
http://www.coreims.co.uk/

Division 22 page linking to resources: http://www.div22.org/links.php

Heart and Soul of Change Project (Duncan et al.): http://heartandsoulofchange.com/

International Center for Clinical Excellence (Miller, et al.): http://www.centerforclinicalexcellence.com/site.php?page=home.php

Institute for Healthcare Improvement (Berwick et al.): http://www.ihi.org/ihi

The Institute for the Study of Therapeutic Change (Miller, Duncan, & Hubble):
http://www.talkingcure.com/reference.asp?id=66

IOM Committee on Cognitive Rehabilitation Therapy for Traumatic Brain Injury:
http://www.iom.edu/Activities/SelectPops/RehabBrainInjury/2011-MAR-16.aspx

This site features free PowerPoint downloads of excellent presentations to the committee.

Model Systems Knowledge Translation Center (MSKTC):
www.msktc.washington.edu

Nursing Home Quality Campaign—Advancing Excellence in America's Nursing Homes:
http://www.nhqualitycampaign.org/star_index.aspx?controls=welcome

A password-protected website created for nursing home quality improvement data. Quality management targets can be set and data entered; monitoring tools are available for Staff Turnover, Consistent Assignment, Restraints, Pressure Ulcers, Pain, Depression, and Advance Care Planning.

Outcome Questionnaire System, including OQ-45 (Lambert et al.): http://www.oqmeasures.com/

Precision Teaching Wiki, with links to multiple articles and learning communities using the Celeration Chart:
http://precisionteaching.pbworks.com/w/page/18240978/FrontPage

PsycBITE collaborative for evidence reviews:
http://www.psy.unsw.edu.au/research/resources/psycbite.html

PsycBITE™ is a database cataloging studies of cognitive, behavioral, and other treatments for psychological problems and issues occurring as a consequence of acquired brain impairment. The types of studies contained on this database are systematic reviews, randomized controlled trials, nonrandomized controlled trials, case series, and single-subject design. These studies are rated for their methodological quality, evaluating various aspects of scientific rigor.

The Rehabilitation Research and Training Center (RRTC) on Community Integration of Persons with Traumatic Brain Injury (TBI): http://www.tbicommunity.org/

Spinal Cord Injury Model Systems: https://www.nscisc.uab.edu/public_content/sci_model_systems.aspx

Spinal Cord Injury Rehabilitation Evidence (SCIRE) project: http://www.scireproject.com/

Traumatic Brain Injury (TBI) National Data and Statistical Center:
www.tbindsc.org

Veterans Administration Center for the Study of Healthcare Provider Behavior: http://www.providerbehavior.research.va.gov/

http://www.spinalcord.uab.edu/show.asp?durki=21392

References

Ahn, H., & Wampold, B. (2001). Where oh where are the specific ingredients? A meta-analysis of component studies in counseling and psychotherapy. *Journal of Counseling Psychology, 38,* 251–257.

APA Presidential Task Force on Evidence-Based Practice. (2006). Evidence-based practice in psychology. *American Psychologist, 61,* 271–285.

Asch, S. M., McGlynn, E. A., Hogan, M. M., Hayward, R. A., Shekelle, P., Rubenstein L., et al. (2004). Comparison of quality of care for patients in the Veterans Health Administration and patients in a national sample. Annals of Internal Medicine, 141, 938–945.

Badley, E. M. (2008). Enhancing the conceptual clarity of the activity and participation components of the International Classification of Functioning, Disability, and Health. *Social Science and Medicine, 66,* 2335–2345.

Baldwin, S.A., Imel, Z.E., & Wampold, B.E. (2007). Untangling the alliance-outcome correlation: Exploring the relative importance of therapist and patient variability in the alliance. *Journal of Consulting and Clinical Psychology, 75*(6), 842–852.

Barkham, M., Mellor-Clark, J., Connell, J., Evans, C., Evans, R., & Margison, F. (2010). Clinical Outcomes in Routine Evaluation (CORE) -The CORE measures system: Measuring, monitoring and managing quality evaluation in the psychological therapies. In M. Barkham, G.E. Hardy, & J. Mellor-Clark (eds.), (2010). *Developing and delivering practice-based evidence: A guide for the psychological therapies.* Sussex, UK: Wiley-Blackwell.

Barenfanger, J., Graham, D. R., Kolluri, L., Sangwan, G., Lawhorn, J., Drake, C. A., et al. (2008). Decreased mortality associated with prompt gram staining of blood cultures. *American Journal of Clinical Pathology, 130*(6), 870–887.

Balaban, N. Q., Merrin, J., Chait, R., Kowalik, L., & Leibler, S. (2004). Bacterial persistence as a phenotypic switch. *Science, 305*(5690),1622–1625.

Barlow, D. H., & Nock, M. K. (2009). Why can't we be more idiographic in our research? *The Journal of the Association for Psychological Science, 4*(1), 19–21.

Baum, W. M. (1994). *Understanding behaviorism: Science, behavior, and culture.* New York: HarperCollins.

Beeson, P. M., & Robey, R. R. (2006). Evaluating single-subject treatment research: Lessons learned from the aphasia literature. *Neuropsychology Review, 16*(4), 161–169.

Begley, A.E., Dew, M.A., Lenze, E.J., Munin, M.C., Quear, T., Reynolds, C.F., et. al. (2004). Significance of poor patient participation in physical and occupational therapy for functional outcome and length of stay. *Archives of Physical Medicine and Rehabilitation*, 85(10), 1599–1601.

Berwick, D. M. (1998). Developing and testing changes in delivery of care. *Annals of Internal Medicine, 128,* 651–656.

Berwick, D. M. (2005). Broadening the view of evidence-based medicine. *Quality Safe Health Care, 14,* 315–316.

Berwick, D. M. (2009). What 'patient-centered' should mean: Confessions of an extremist. *Health Affairs, 28*(4), w555–w565.

Berwick, D. M., James, B., & Coye, M. J. (2003). Connections between quality measurement and improvement. *Medical Care, 41*(1), i30–i38.

Beutler, L. (2004). The empirically supported treatments movement: A scientist-practitioner's response. *Clinical Psychology: Science and Practice, 11*(3), 225–229.

Bickman, L., & S. Mulvaney. (2005). Large scale evaluations of children's mental health services: The Ft. Bragg and Stark County studies. In R. Steele & M. Roberts (Eds.), *Handbook of mental health services for children, adolescents, and families*

(pp. 371–386). New York: Kluwer Academic/Plenum Publishers.

Bigger, J. W. (1944). Treatment of staphylococcal infections with penicillin by intermittent sterilization. *Lancet, 244,* 497–500.

Binder, C. (1996). Fluency: Evolution of a new paradigm. *The Behavior Analyst, 19*(2), 163–197.

Bleiberg, J., & Merbitz, C. (1983). Learning goals during initial rehabilitation hospitalization. *Archives of Physical Medicine and Rehabilitation, 64*(10), 445–450.

Bouwens, S. F. M., VanHeugten, C. M., & Verhey, F. R. J. (2009). The practical use of goal attainment scaling for people with acquired brain injury who receive cognitive rehabilitation. *Clinical Rehabilitation, 23,* 310–320.

Bowers, B. J. (March 2003). Turnover reinterpreted: CNAs talk about why they leave. *Journal of Gerontological Nursing, 29*(3), 36–44.

Bowers, B. J., Fibich, B., & Jacobson, N. (2001). Care-as-service, care-as-relating, care-as-comfort: Understanding nursing home residents' definitions of quality. *The Gerontologist, 41*(4), 539–545.

Brandrud, A. S., Schreiner, A., Hjortdahl, P., Helljesen, G. S., Nyen, B., & Nelson, E. C. (2011). Three success factors for continual improvement in healthcare: An analysis of the reports of improvement team members. *British Medical Journal Quality and Safety, 20,* 251–259.

Brazier, Dh. D. J. (1996). Post Rogerian therapy of Robert Carkhuff. Amida trust papers. Retrieved from http://www.amidatrust.com/article_carkhuff.html

Brock, W. A., Nolan, K. M., & Nolan, T. W. (1998). Pragmatic science: Accelerating the improvement of critical care. *New Horizons, 6,* 61–68.

Brossart, D. F., Meythaler, J. M., Parker, R. I., McNamara, J., & Elliott, T. R. (2008). Advanced regression methods for single-case designs: Studying propranolol in the treatment for agitation associated with traumatic brain injury. *Rehabilitation Psychology, 53*(3), 357–369.

Brown, C. A. (2006). The application of complex adaptive systems theory to clinical practice in rehabilitation. *Disability and Rehabilitation, 28*(9), 587–593.

Brown, K. S., DeLeon, P. H., Loftis, C. W., & Scherer, M. J. (2008). Rehabilitation psychology: Realizing the true potential. *Rehabilitation Psychology, 53*(2), 11–121.

Buntin, M. B. (2007). Access to postacute rehabilitation. *Archives of Physical Medicine Rehabilitation, 88,* 1488–1493.

Buntin, M. B., Deb, P., Escarce, J., Hoverman, C., Paddock, S., & Sood, N. (2005). Comparison of Medicare Spending and Outcomes for Beneficiaries with Lower Extremity Joint Replacements. Working Paper, RAND Health. Retrieved from http://works.bepress.com/cgi/viewcontent.cgi?article=1006&context=melinda_buntin&sei-redir=1#search="joint+replacement+JOINTS+rehabilitation+study+research+cms+pac+irf+snf"

Callahan, C. D., & Barisa, M. T. (2005). Statistical process control and rehabilitation outcome: The single-subject design reconsidered. *Rehabilitation Psychology, 50*(1), 24–33.

Callahan, C. D., & Griffen, D. L. (2003). Advanced statistics: Applying statistical process control techniques to emergency medicine: A primer for providers. *Academic Emergency Medicine, 10*(8), 883–890.

Cappa, S. F., Benke, T., Clarke, S., Rossi, B., Stemmer, B., & van Heugten, C. M. (2005). EFNS guidelines on cognitive rehabilitation: Report of an EFNS task force. *European Journal of Neurology, 12,* 665–680.

Cattelani, R., Zettin, M., & Zoccolotti, P. (2010). Rehabilitation treatments for adults with behavioral and psychosocial disorders following acquired brain injury: A systematic review. *Neuropsychology Review, 20*(1), 52–85.

Cella, D., Yount, S., Rothrock, N., Gershon, R., Cook, K., Reeve, B., et al. (2007). The Patient Reported Outcomes Measurement Information System (PROMIS): Progress of an NIH Roadmap Cooperative Group during its first two years. *Medical Care, 45*(5), S3–11.

Cernich, A. N., Kurtz, S. M., Mordecai, K. L., & Ryan, P. B. (2010). Cognitive rehabilitation in traumatic brain injury. *Current Treatment Options in Neurology, 12*, 412–423.

Chapman, S. S., Ewing, C. B., & Mozzoni, M. P. (2005). Precision teaching and fluency training across cognitive, physical, and academic tasks in children with traumatic brain injury: A multiple baseline study. *Behavioral Interventions, 20*(1), 37–49.

Cherney, L. R., Merbitz, C. T., & Grip, J. C. (1986). Efficacy of oral reading in aphasia treatment outcome. *Rehabilitation Literature, 47*(5–6), 112–118.

Chiesia, M. (1992). Radical behaviorism and scientific frameworks: From mechanistic to relational accounts. *American Psychologist, 47*(11), 1287–1299.

Cicerone, K. D. (November 30, 2009). Letter to TriCare. Retrieved from http://www.propublica.org/article/pentagon-health-plan-wont-cover-brain-damage-therapy-for-troops/single

Cicerone, K. D., Langenbahn, D. M., Braden, C., Malec, J. F., Kalmar, K., Fraas, M., et al. (2011). Evidence-based cognitive rehabilitation: Updated review of the literature from 2003 through 2008. *Archives of Physical Medicine and Rehabilitation, 92*(4), 519–530.

Clare, L., Wilson, B. A., Carter, G., Breen, K., Gosses, A., & Hodges, J. R. (2010). Intervening with everyday memory problems in dementia of Alzheimer type: An errorless learning approach. *Journal of Clinical and Experimental Neuropsychology, 22*(1), 132–146.

Clohan, D. B., Durkin, E. M., Hammel, J., Murray, P., Whyte, J., Dijkers, M., et al. (2007). Postacute rehabilitation research and policy recommendations. *Archives of Physical Medicine and Rehabilitation, 88*(11), 1535–1541.

Craig, P., Dieppe, P., Macintyre, S., Michie, S., Nazareth, I., & Petticrew, M. (2008). Developing and evaluating complex interventions: The new Medical Research Council guidance. *British Medical Journal, 337*, 979–983. Retrieved from http://eprints.gla.ac.uk/42736/1/42736.pdf

Crits-Christoph, P., Wilson, G. T., & Hollon, S. D. (2005). Empirically supported psychotherapies: Comment on Westen, Novotny, and Thompson-Brenner (2004). *Psychology Bulletin, 131*(3):412–417, discussion 427–433.

Davis, C., & Huska, D. (February 5, 2009). The model for improvement. ImpactBC. Retrieved February 27, 2011, from http://www.impactbc.ca/search/apachesolr_search?filters=type%3Aresource%20tid%3A156

DeJong, G., Horn, S. D., Conroy, B., Nichols, D., & Healton, E. B. (2005). Opening the black box of post stroke rehabilitation: Stroke rehabilitation patients, processes, and outcome. *Archives of Physical Medicine and Rehabilitation, 86*(12), S1–S7.

DeJong, G., Horn, S. D., Gassaway, J. A., Slavin, M. D., & Dijkers, M. P. (2004). Toward a taxonomy of rehabilitation interventions: Using an inductive approach to examine the "Black Box" of rehabilitation. *Archives of Physical Medicine and Rehabilitation, 85*, 678–686.

DeLeon, P. H., & Kazdin, A. E. (2010). Public policy: Extending psychology's contributions to national priorities. *Rehabilitation Psychology, 55*(3), 311–319.

Donabedian, A. (1981). Criteria, norms and standards of quality: What do they mean? *American Journal of Public Health, 71*(4), 49–412.

Donabedian, A. (1988). The quality of care. How can it be assessed? *Journal of the American Medical Association, 260*, 1743–1748.

Duff, M., Chen, Y., Attygalle, S., Herman, J. Sundaram, H., Qian, G., et al. (2010b). An Adaptive Mixed Reality Training System for Stroke Rehabilitation. *Rehabilitation Engineering, IEEE Transactions, 18*(5), 531–541.

Duff, M., Chen, Y., Attygale, S., Sundaram, H., & Rikakis, T. (2010a). Mixed Reality Rehabilitation for Stroke Survivors Promotes Generalized Motor Improvements. EMBC 2010, Buenos Aires, Argentina, September 2010. Retrieved from http://ame2.asu.edu/faculty/thanassis/papers.html and http:// www.igert.org/highlights/410.

Duncan, B., Miller, S. D., & Sparks, J. (2004). *The heroic client: A revolutionary way to improve effectiveness through client-directed, outcome-informed therapy.* San Francisco: Jossey-Bass.

Duncan, P. W., Horner, R. D., Reker, D. M., Samsa, G. P., Hoenig, H. M., Hamilton, B. B., et al. (2002). Adherence to post acute rehabilitation guidelines is associated with functional recovery in stroke. *Stroke, 33*, 167–177.

Duncan, P. W., & Velozo, C. A. (2007). State-of-the-science on post acute rehabilitation: Measurement and methodologies for assessing quality and establishing policy for post acute care. *Archives of Physical Medicine and Rehabilitation, 88*(11), 1482–1487.

Dunn, D. S., & Elliott, T. R. (2008). The place and promise of theory in rehabilitation psychology research. *Rehabilitation Psychology, 53*(3), 254–267.

Elkin, I., Krupnick, J. L., Moyer, J., Pilkonis, P. A., Simmens, S., Sotsky, S. M., & Watkins, J. (2006). The role of the therapeutic alliance in psychotherapy and pharmacotherapy outcome: Findings in the national institute of mental health treatment of depression collaborative research program. *The Journal of Lifelong Learning of Psychiatry, 4*(2), 269–277.

Elliott, T. R. (2002). Defining our common ground to reach new horizons. *Rehabilitation Psychology, 47*(2), 131–143.

Evans, C. C., Irby, J. W. J., Lee J. E., Leverenz, J., Sherer, M., Stouter, J., & Yablon, S. A. (2007). Therapeutic alliance in post-acute brain injury rehabilitation: Predictors of strength of alliance and impact of alliance on outcome. *Brain Injury, 21*(7), 663–672.

Fayers, P. M. (2007). Applying item response theory and computer adaptive testing: The challenges for health outcomes assessment. *Quality Life Research, 16*, 187–194.

Finger, M. E., Cieza, A., Stoll, J., Stucki, G., & Huber, E. O. (2006). Identification of intervention categories for physical therapy, based on the International Classification of Functioning, Disability and Health: A Delphi exercise. *Physical Therapy, 86*(9), 1203–1220.

Gassaway, J., & Horn, S. D. (2007). Practice-based evidence study design for comparative effectiveness research. *Medical Care, 45*(10), S50–S57.

Gassaway, J., Horn, S. D., DeJong, G., Smout, R. J., Clark, C., & James, R. (2005). Applying the clinical practice improvement approach to stroke rehabilitation: Methods used and baseline results. *Archives of Physical Medicine and Rehabilitation, 86*(Suppl 2), S16–S33.

Gassaway, J., & Whiteneck, G. G. (2010). SCIrehab: A model for rehabilitation research using comprehensive person, process and outcome data. *Disability and Rehabilitation, 32*(12), 1035–1042.

Gassaway, J., Whiteneck, G., & Dijkers, M. (2009). Classification of SCI rehabilitation treatments clinical taxonomy development and application in spinal cord injury research: The SCI rehab project. *Journal of Spinal Cord Medicine, 32*(3), 260–269.

Geurtsen, G. J., van Heugten, C. M., Martina, J. D., & Geurts, A. C. H. (2010). Comprehensive rehabilitation programs in the chronic phase after severe brain injury: A systematic review. *Journal of Rehabilitation Medicine, 42,* 97–110.

Geyh, S. (August, 2008). ICF Linking Rules: Identifying Personal Factors. Presentation at the 14th Annual North American Collaborating Center Conference on ICF "Evaluating Social Participation: Applications of ICF & ICF-CY" in Quebec City, Quebec, Canada. Retrieved from http://www.cihiconferences.ca/icfconference/ataglance.html

Giles, G. M. (2010). Cognitive versus functional approaches to rehabilitation after traumatic brain injury: Commentary on a randomized controlled trial. *American Journal of Occupational Therapy, 64,* 182–185.

Glaessel, A., Kirchberger, I., Stucki, G., & Cieza, A. (2011). Does the comprehensive international classification of functioning, disability and health (ICF) core set of breast cancer capture the problems in functioning treated by physiotherapists in women with breast cancer? *Physical Therapy, 97*(1), 33–46.

Glenn, S. S., & Madden, G. J. (1995). Units of interaction, evolution, and replication: Organic and behavioral parallels. *The Behavior Analyst, 18,* 237–251.

Goldman, B. D. (1998). Nontraditional staffing models in long-term care. *Journal of Gerontological Nursing, 24,* 29–34.

Gordon, W. A. (November 30, 2009a). Letter to TriCare. Retrieved from http://www.propublica.org/article/pentagon-health-plan-wont-cover-brain-damage-therapy-for-troops/single

Gordon, W. A. (2009b). Clinical trials in rehabilitation research: Balancing rigor and relevance. *Archives of Physical Medicine and Rehabilitation, 90*(11), sppl1–sppl2.

Gould, S. J. (1990). *Wonderful life.* New York: Norton.

Grill, E., & Stucki, G. (2011). Criteria for validating comprehensive ICF core sets and developing brief ICF core set versions. *Journal of Rehabilitation Medicine, 43,* 87–91.

Guenther, R. (1999, September). Development and application of a microprocessor-based pressure relief monitor. Las Vegas, Nevada: Paper presented at the annual conference of the American Association of Spinal Cord Injury Psychologists and Social Workers.

Hahn, E. A., DeVellis, R. F., Bode, R. K., Garcia, S. F., Castel, L. D., Eisen, S. V., et al. (2010). Measuring social health in the patient-reported outcomes measurement information system (PROMIS): Item bank development and testing. *Quality of Life Research, 19*(7), 1035–1044.

Hale, L. A. (2010). Using goal attainment scaling in physiotherapeutic home-based stroke rehabilitation. *Advances in Physiotherapy, 12,* 142–149.

Haley, S. M., Coster, W. J., Andres, P. L., Ludlow, L. H., Ni, P., Bond, T. L. Y., et al. (2004). Activity outcome measurement for postacute care. *Medical Care, 42*(Suppl. 1), I49–I61.

Haley, S. M., Ni, P., Jette, A. M., Tao, W., Moed, R., Meyers, D., & Ludlow, L. H. (2009). Replenishing a computerized adaptive test of patient-reported daily activity functioning. *Quality Life Research, 18,* 461–471.

Halstead, L. S. (1976). Longitudinal unobtrusive measurements in rehabilitation. *Archives of Physical Medicine and Rehabilitation, 57*(4), 189–193.

Harbourne, R. T., & Stergiou, N. (2009). Movement variability and the use of nonlinear tools: Principles to guide physical therapist practice. *Physical Therapy, 89*(3), 267–282. doi:10.2522/ptj.20080130

Hart, T. (2009). Treatment definition in complex rehabilitation interventions. *Neuropsychological Rehabilitation, 19*(6), 824–840.

Heinemann, A. W. (2005). Putting outcome measurement in context: A rehabilitation psychology perspective. *Rehabilitation Psychology, 50*(1), 6–14.

Hobart, J., & Cano, S. (2009). Improving the evaluation of therapeutic interventions in multiple sclerosis: The role of new psychometric methods. *Health Technology Assessment, 13*(12), iii, ix–x, 1–177.

Hoenig, H., Duncan, P. W., Horner, R. D., Reker, D. M., Samsa, G. P., Dudley, T. K., et al. (2002). Structure, process, and outcomes in stroke rehabilitation. *Medical Care, 40,* 1036–1047.

Hoffmann, T., Bennett, S., Koh, C. L., & McKenna, K. (Mar-Apr 2010). A systematic review of cognitive interventions to improve functional ability in people who have cognitive impairment following stroke. *Topics in Stroke Rehabilitation, 17*(2), 99–107.

Horn, S. D., Dejong, G., Ryser, D. K., Veazie, P. J., & Teraoka, J. (2005a). Another look at observational studies in rehabilitation research: Going beyond the holy grail of the randomized controlled trial. *Archives of Physical Medicine and Rehabilitation, 86*(12 Suppl 2), S8–S15.

Horn, S. D., DeJong, G., Smout, R. J., Gassaway, J., James, R., & Conroy, B. (2005b). Stroke rehabilitation patients, practice, and outcomes: Is earlier and more aggressive therapy better? *Archives of Physical Medicine and Rehabilitation, 86,* 101–114.

Huber, J. G., Sillick, J., & Skarakis-Doyle, E. (2010). Personal perception and personal factors: Incorporating health-related quality of life into the international classification of functioning, disability and health. *Disability and Rehabilitation, 32*(23), 1955–1965.

Institute of Medicine (IOM). (2001). *Crossing the quality chasm: A new health system for the 21st century.* Washington, DC: National Academy Press.

Institute of Medicine, Committee on Disability in America. (2007). *The future of disability in America.* Field, M. J. and Jette, A. M. (Eds.). Washington, DC: National Academies Press.

Janosky, J. E. (2005). Use of the single subject design for practice based primary care research. *Postgraduate Medicine, 81,* 549–551.

Jette, A. (2008). Invited commentary. *Physical Therapy, 88*(7), 851–853.

Jette, A. M., Haley, S. M., Tao, W., Ni, P., Moed, R., Meyers, D., & Zurek, M. (2007). Prospective evaluation of the AM-PAC-CAT in outpatient rehabilitation settings. *Physical Therapy, 87*(4), 385–398.

Johnston, M. V., Graves, D., & Greene, M. (2007). The uniform postacute assessment tool: Systematically evaluating the quality of measurement evidence. *Archives of Physical Medicine and Rehabilitation, 88*(11), 1505–1512.

Johnston, M. V., Kirshblum, S., Zorowitz, R., & Shiflett, S. C. (1992). Prediction of outcomes following rehabilitation of stroke patients. *Neurorehabilitation, 2*(4), 72–97.

Kelly, F., & Nikopoulos. (2010). Facilitating independence in personal activities of daily living after a severe traumatic brain injury. *International Journal of Therapy and Rehabilitation, 17*(9), 474–482.

Kiresuk, T., & Sherman, R. (1968). Goal attainment scaling: A general method of evaluating comprehensive mental health programmes. *Community Mental Health Journal, 4,* 443–453.

Kirsch, N. L., Lopresti, E. F., Schreckenghost, D., Shenton, M., Simpson, R., & Spirl, E. (2004). Web-based assistive technology interventions for cognitive impairments after traumatic brain injury: A selective review and two case studies. *Rehabilitation Psychology, 49*(3), 200–212.

Knaup, C., Koesters, M., Schoefer, D., Becker, T., & Puschner, B. (2009). Effect of feedback of treatment outcome in specialist mental healthcare: Meta-analysis. *The British Journal of Psychiatry, 195,* 15–22.

Kratochwill, T. R., Hitchcock, J., Horner, R. H., Levin, J. R., Odom, S. L., Rindskopf, D. M., & Shadish, W. R. (2010). Single-case designs technical documentation. What Works Clearinghouse website. Retrieved from http://ies.ed.gov/ncee/wwc/pdf/wwc_scd.pdf.

Kratochwill, T. R., & Levin, J. R. (2010). Enhancing the scientific credibility of single-case intervention research: Randomization to the rescue. *Psychological Methods, 15*(2), 124–144.

Kubina, R. M., Ward, M. C., & Mozzoni, M. P. (2000). Helping one person at a time: Precision teaching and traumatic brain injury rehabilitation. *Behavioral Interventions, 15,* 189–203.

Labby, D. (May, 2010). Achieving the triple aim: The simultaneous pursuit of population health, enhanced individual care and controlled costs. Presentation to the Oregon Health Policy Board. Retrieved from http://www.oregon.gov/OHA/OHPB/meetings/2010/100511-lab.ppt

Lambert, M. J., Hansen, N. B., & Harmon, S. C. (2010). Outcome Questionnaire System (The OQ System): Development and practical applications in healthcare settings. In M. Barkham, G. E. Hardy, & J. Mellor-Clark (Eds.), *Developing and delivering practice-based evidence: A guide for the psychological therapies* (pp. 141–154). Sussex, UK: Wiley-Blackwell.

Lambert, M. J., Whipple, J. L. O., Vermersch, D. A., Smart, D. W., Hawkins, E. J., Nielsen, S. L., et al. (2002). Enhancing psychotherapy outcomes via providing feedback on client progress: A replication. *Clinical Psychology and Psychotherapy, 9,* 91–103.

Langley, G. J., Moen, R. D., Nolan, K. M., Nolan, T. W., Norman, C. L., & Provost, L. P. (1996). *The improvement guide, 2nd edition: A practical approach to enhancing organizational performance.* San Francisco: Jossey-Bass.

Levant, R. F. (2004). The empirically-validated treatments movement: A practitioner/educator perspective. *Clinical Psychology: Science and Practice, 11,* 219–224.

Lindsley, O. R. (1992). Precision teaching: Discoveries and effects. *Journal of Applied Behavior Analysis, 25*(1), 51–57.

Lueger, R. J., & Barkham, M. (2010). Using benchmarks and benchmarking to improve quality of practice and services. In M. Barkham, G. E. Hardy, & J. Mellor-Clark (Eds.), *Developing and delivering practice-based evidence: A guide for the psychological therapies* (pp. 223–256). Sussex, UK: Wiley-Blackwell.

Lutz, W., Leon, S. C., Martinovich, Z., Lyons, J. S., & Stiles, W. B. (2007). Therapist effects in outpatient psychotherapy: A three-level growth curve approach. *Journal of Counseling Psychology 54*(1), 32–39.

MacDavitt, K., Cieplinski, J. A., & Walker, V. (January 2011). Implementing small tests of change to improve patient satisfaction. *Journal of Nursing Administration, 41*(1), 5–9.

Malament, I. B., Dunn, M. E., & Davis, R. (1975). Pressure sores: Operant conditioning approach to prevention. *Archives of Physical Medicine and Rehabilitation, 56,* 161–165.

Malec, J.F. (1999). Goal attainment scaling in rehabilitation. *Neuropsychological Rehabilitation, 9*(3–4), 253–275.

Malec, J. F. (November 24, 2009). Letter to TriCare. Retrieved from http://www.propublica.org/article/pentagon-health-plan-wont-cover-brain-damage-therapy-for-troops/single

Mateer, C. (2009). Neuropsychological interventions for memory impairment and the role of single-case design methodologies. *Journal of the International Neuropsychological Society, 15*(4), 623–628.

Merbitz, C. (1996). Frequency measures of behavior for assistive technology and rehabilitation. *Assistive Technology, 8,* 121–130.

Merbitz, C. T., King, R. B., Bleiberg, J., & Grip, J. C. (1985). Wheelchair push-ups: Measuring pressure relief frequency. *Archives of Physical Medicine and Rehabilitation, 66,* 433–438.

Merbitz, C. T., Miller, T. K., & Hansen, N. K. (2000). Cueing and logical problem solving in brain trauma rehabilitation: Frequency patterns in clinician and patient behaviors. *Behavioral Interventions, 15,* 169–187.

Merbitz, C. T., Morris, J., & Grip, J. C. (1989). Ordinal scales and foundations of misinference. *Archives of Physical Medicine and Rehabilitation, 70,* 308–312.

Meyerson, L., & Kerr, N. (1979). Research strategies for meaningful rehabilitation research. *Rehabilitation Psychology, 26*(4), 228–238.

Michaud, L. J. (1995). Evaluating efficacy of rehabilitation after pediatric traumatic brain injury. In S. Broman & M. Michel (Eds.), *Traumatic head injury in children* (pp. 247–257). New York: Oxford Press.

Miller, R. G., Rosenberg, J. A., Gelinas, D. F., Mitsumoto, H., Newman, D., Sufit, R., et al. (1999). Practice parameter: The care of the patient with amyotrophic lateral sclerosis (an evidence-based review): Report of the Quality Standards Subcommittee of the American Academy of Neurology: ALS Practice Parameters Task Force. *Neurology, 52,* 1311–1323.

Miller, S. D., Duncan, B. L., Sorrell, R., Brown, G. S., & Chalk, M. B. (2006). Using outcome to inform therapy practice. *Journal of Brief Therapy, 5*(1), 5–22.

Miller, S. D., Mee-Lee, D., Plum, B., & Hubble, M. A. (2005). Making treatment count: Client-directed, outcome-informed clinical work with problem drinkers. *Psychotherapy in Australia, 11*(4), 32–56.

Mueller, C.(2000) A framework for nurse staffing in long-term care facilities. *Geriatric Nursing, 21*(5), 262–267.

Needham, D. M., & Korupolu, R. (2010). Rehabilitation quality improvement in an intensive care unit setting: Implementation of a quality improvement model. *Topics in Stroke Rehabilitation, 17*(4), 271–281.

Nelson, E. C., Splaine, M. E., Batalden, P. B., & Plume, S. K. (1998). Building measurement and data collection into medical practice. *Annals of Internal Medicine, 128*(6), 460–466.

Ottenbacher, K. (1990). Clinically relevant designs for rehabilitation research: The idiographic model. *American Journal of Physical Medicine and Rehabilitation, 70*(1Suppl), S144–S150.

Ownsworth, T., Fleming, J., Desbois, J., Strong, J., & Kuipers, P. (2006). A metacognitive contextual intervention to enhance error awareness and functional outcome following traumatic brain injury: A single-case experimental design. *Journal of the International Neuropsychological Society, 12*, 54–63.

Ozer, M. N. (1999). Patient participation in the management of stroke re Turner-Stokes habilitation. *Topics in Stroke Rehabilitation, 6*, 43–59.

Ozer, M. N., & Kroll, T. (2002). Patient-centered rehabilitation: Problems and opportunities. *Critical Reviews in Physical and Rehabilitation Medicine, 14*, 273–289.

Ozer, M. N., Payton, O., & Nelson, C. E. (2000). *Treatment planning for rehabilitation: A patient-centered approach.* New York: McGraw-Hill.

Palmer, D. C., & Donohoe, J. W. (1992). Essentialism and selectionism in cognitive science and behavior analysis. *American Psychologist, 47*(11), 1344–1358.

Patchner, M. A. (1989). Permanent assignment: A better recipe for the staffing of aides. *Successful nurse aide management in nursing homes* (pp. 66–75). Phoenix, AZ: Oryx Press.

Patrick, P. D., Mozzoni, M., & Patrick, S. T. (2000). Evidence-based care and the single-subject design. *Infants and Young Children, 13*(1) 60–73.

Pawson, R. (2006). *Evidence-based policy. A realist perspective.* London: Sage.

Perdices, M., & Tate, R. L. (2009). Single-subject designs as a tool for evidence-based clinical practice: Are they unrecognized and undervalued? *Neuropsychological Rehabilitation, 19*(6), 904–927.

Peterson, D. B., Mpofu, E., & Oakland, T. (2010). Concepts and models in disability, functioning, and health. In E. Mpofu & T. Oakland, T. (Eds.), *Rehabilitation and health assessment: Applying ICF guidelines* (pp. 18–40). New York: Springer.

Phillips, J., Drummond, A., Radford, K., & Tyerman, A. (2010). Return to work after traumatic brain injury: Recording, measuring and describing occupational therapy intervention. *The British Journal of Occupational Therapy, 73*(9), 422–430.

Plsek, P. (2001). Redesigning health care with insights from the science of complex adaptive systems. In *Crossing the quality chasm: A new health system for the 21st century* (Appendix B). National Academies Press. Retrieved from http://www.nap.edu/openbook.php?record_id=10027&page=309

Rassafiani, M., & Sahaf, R. (2010). Single case experimental design: An overview. *International Journal of Therapy and Rehabilitation, 17*(6), 285–289.

Rauch, A., Cieza, A., & Stucki, G. (2008). How to apply the International Classification of Functioning, Disability and Health (ICF) for rehabilitation management in clinical practice. *European Journal of Physical Rehabilitation Medicine, 44*, 329–343.

Rentsch, H. P., Bucher, P., Dommen Nyffeler, I, Wolf, C. Hefti, H., Fluri, E., et al. (2003). The implementation of the 'International Classification of Functioning, Disability and Health' (ICF) in daily practice of neurorehabilitation: An interdisciplinary project at the Kantonsspital of Lucerne, Switzerland. *Disability And Rehabilitation, 25*(8), 411–421.

Rhodes, R. S., Sharkey, P. D., & Horn, S. D. (1995). Effect of patient factors on hospital costs for major bowel surgery: Implications for managed health care. *Surgery, 117,* 443–450.

Rintala, D. H., Garber, S. L., Friedman, J. D., & Holmes, S. A. (2008). Preventing recurrent pressure ulcers in veterans with spinal cord injury: Impact of a structured education and follow-up intervention. *Archives of Physical Medicine & Rehabilitation, 89,* 1429–1441.

Rintala, D. H., Hanover, D., Alexander, J. L., Sanson-Fisher, R. W., Willems, E. P., & Halstead, L. S. (1986). Team care: An analysis of verbal behavior during patient rounds in a rehabilitation hospital. *Archives of Physician Medicine and Rehabilitation, 67*(2), 188–122.

Rintala, D. H., & Willems, E. P. (1987). Behavioral and demographic predictors of postdischarge outcomes in spinal cord injury. *Archives of Physical Medicine and Rehabilitation, 68*(6), 357–362.

Rizvi, S. L., & Nock, M. K. (2008). Single-case experimental designs for the evaluation of treatments for self-injurious and suicidal behaviors. *The American Association of Suicidology, 38*(5), 498–510.

Robey, R. R. (2004). A five-phase model for clinical-outcome research. *Journal of Communication Disorders, 37*(5), 401–411.

Rogers, C. R. (1986). On the development of the person-centered approach. *Person-Centered Review, 1*(3), 257–259.

Ruhe, M. C., Carter, C., Litaker, D., & Stange, K. C. (2009). A systematic approach to practice assessment and quality improvement intervention tailoring. *Quality Management in Health Care, 18*(4), 268–277.

Schiff, G. D., & Rucker, T. D. (2001). Beyond structure-process-outcome: Donabedian's seven pillars and eleven buttresses of quality. *The Joint Commission Journal on Quality Improvement, 27*(3), 169–174.

Schlosser, R. (2009). The Role of single-subject experimental designs in evidence-based practice times. *FOCUS Technical Brief, 22,* Washington, D.C: National Center for the Dissemination of Rehabilitation Research.

Schönberger, M., Humle, F., & Teasdale, T. W. (2006). The development of the therapeutic working alliance, patients' awareness and their compliance during the process of brain injury rehabilitation. *Brain Injury, 20*(4), 445–454.

Schönberger, M., Humle, F., & Teasdale, T. W. (2007). The relationship between clients' cognitive functioning and the therapeutic working alliance in post-acute brain injury rehabilitation. *Brain Injury 21*(8), 825–836.

Seligman, L., & Reichenberg, L. W. (2007). *Selecting effective treatments: A comprehensive, systematic guide to treating mental disorders,* (3rd ed.). New York: John Wiley & Sons.

Shepperd, S., Lewin S, Straus S, Clarke M, Eccles MP, Fitzpatrick, R., & Wong, G. (2009). Can we systematically review studies that evaluate complex interventions? *PLoS Med 6*(8): e1000086. doi:10.1371/journal.pmed.1000086.

Skinner, B. F. (1953). *Science and human behavior.* New York: Free Press.

Smith, G. C. S., & Pell, J. P. (2003). Parachute use to prevent death and major trauma related to gravitational challenge: Systematic review of randomised controlled trials. *British Medical Journal, 327*(7429), 1459–1461.

Sparks, J. A., Duncan, B. L., & Miller, S. D. (2008). Common factors in psychotherapy. In J. L. Lebow (Ed.), *Twenty-first century psychotherapies: Contemporary approaches to theory and practice* (pp. 453–498). Hoboken, NJ: John Wiley & Sons.

Strauss, E. (2010). Grand Challenge Commentary: Exploiting single cell variation for new antibiotics. *Nature Chemical Biology, 6,* 873–875.

Svoboda, E., & Richards, R. (2009). Compensating for anterograde amnesia: A new training method that capitalizes on emerging smartphone technologies. *Journal of the International Neuropsychological Society, 15*(4), 629–638.

Tate, R. L., Mcdonald, S., Perdices, M., Togher, L., Schultz, R., & Savage, S. (2008). Rating the methodological quality of single-subject designs and *n*-of-1 trials: Introducing the Single-Case Experimental Design (SCED) Scale. *Neuropsychological Rehabilitation: An International Journal, 18*(4), 385–401.

Tawfik, D. S. (October 2010). Messy biology and the origins of evolutionary innovations. *Nature Chemical Biology, 6,* 692–696.

Teasell, R., Bayona, N., Marshall, S., Cullen, N., Bayley, M., Chundamala, J., et al. (2007). A systematic review of the rehabilitation of moderate to severe acquired brain injuries. *Brain Injury 21*(2), 107–112.

Thurmond, V. A., Hicks, R., Gleason, T., Miller, C. A., Szuflita, N., Orman, J., & Schwab, K. (2010). Advancing integrated research in psychological health and traumatic brain injury: Common data elements. *Archives of Physical Medicine and Rehabilitation, 91,* 1633–1636.

Treatment Outcomes Committee. (2008). *Methodology to Develop Systematic Reviews of Treatment Interventions.* (Revision 1.2). The American Academy for Cerebral Palsy and Developmental Medicine (AACPDM). Retrieved from http://www.aacpdm.org/publications/outcome/resources/systematicReviewsMethodology.pdf

Tucker, J. A., & Reed, G. M. (2008). Evidentiary pluralism as a strategy for research and evidence-based practice in rehabilitation psychology. *Rehabilitation Psychology, 53*(3), 279–293.

Turner-Stokes, L., Nair, A., Sedki, I., Disler, P. B., & Wade, D. T. (2011). Multi-disciplinary rehabilitation for acquired brain injury in adults of working age. *Cochrane Database of Systematic Reviews, 3,* CD004170. doi: 10.1002/14651858.CD004170.pub2.

Turner-Stokes, L., Williams, H., & Johnson, J. (2009). Goal attainment scaling: Does it provide added value as a person-centered measure for evaluation of outcome in neurorehabilitation following acquired brain injury? *Journal of Rehabilitation Medicine, 41,* 528–535.

van der Ploeg, A., & Merbitz, C. (1998). *Data driven decisions.* Chicago, IL: Paper presented at American Educational Research Association.

van Langeveld, S. A., Post, M. W., van Asbeck, F. W., ter Horst, P., Leenders, J., Postma, K., & Lindeman, E. (2009). Reliability of a new classification system for mobility and self-care in spinal cord injury rehabilitation: The spinal cord injury-interventions classification system. *Archives of Physical Medicine and Rehabilitation, 90*(1), 229–236.

Vong, S. K., Cheing, G. L., Chan, F., So, E. M., & Chan, C. C. (2011). Motivational enhancement therapy in addition to physical therapy improves motivational factors and treatment outcomes in people with low back pain: A randomized controlled trial. *Archives of Physical Medicine and Rehabilitation, 92*(2), 176–183.

Walker, W. C., & Pickett, T. C. (2007). Motor impairment after severe traumatic brain injury: A longitudinal multicenter study. *Journal of Rehabilitation Research and Development, 44*(7), 975–982.

Walton, M. (1986). *The Deming management method.* New York: Perigee Books.

Wampold, B. E., & Brown, G. S. (October 2005). Estimating variability in outcomes attributable to therapists: A naturalistic study of outcomes in managed care. *Journal of Consulting and Clinical Psychology, 73*(5), 914–923.

Wang, P. P., Badley, E. M., & Gignac, M. (2006). Exploring the role of contextual factors in disability models. *Disability and Rehabilitation, 28*(2), 135–140.

Ware, J. E., Gandek, B., Sinclair, S. J., & Bjorner, J. B. (2005). Item response theory and computerized adaptive testing: Implications for outcomes measurement in rehabilitation. *Rehabilitation Psychology, 50*(1), 71–78.

Weisz, J. R., Weersing, V. R., & Henggeler, S. W. (2005). Jousting with straw men: Comment on Westen, Novotny, and Thompson-Brenner (2004). *Psychology Bulletin, 131*(3), 418–420, discussion 427–433.

Westen, D., Novotny, C. M., & Thompson-Brenner, H. (2004). The empirical status of empirically supported psychotherapies: Assumptions, findings, and reporting in controlled clinical trials. *Psychology Bulletin, 130*(4), 131–163.

Whiteneck, G. G., Gassaway, J., Dijkers, M. P., Lammertse, D. P., Hammond, F., Heinemann, A. W., et al. (2011). Inpatient and postdischarge rehabilitation services provided in the first year after spinal cord injury: Findings from the SCIRehab study. *Archives of Physical Medicine and Rehabilitation, 92*(3), 361–368.

Whyte, J. (2009). Defining the active ingredients of rehabilitation. *Health Policy Newsletter, 22*(4), 13.

Whyte, J., Gordon, W. J., Nash, J., & Rothi, L. J. (2009). A phased developmental approach to neurorehabilitation research: The science of knowledge building. *Archives of Physical Medicine and Rehabilitation, 90*(11), S3–S10.

Whyte, J., Vasterling, J., & Manley, G. T. (2010). Common data elements for research on traumatic brain injury and psychological health: Current status and future development. *Archives of Physical Medicine and Rehabilitation, 91*(11), 1692–1696.

Wilson, B. (2008). The current practice of neuropsychological rehabilitation in the United Kingdom. *Applied Neuropsychology, 15,* 229–240.

Wilson, B. A., & Cockburn, J. (1997). A seven- to fourteen-year follow-up study of adults with very severe intellectual impairment following a neurological insult. *Journal of Rehabilitation Outcomes Measurement, 1*(2), 60–66.

Wilson, C., Huston, T., Koval, J., Gordon, S. A., Schwebel, A., & Gassaway, J. (2009). Classification of SCI rehabilitation treatments SCIRehab project series: The psychology taxonomy. *Journal of Spinal Cord Medicine, 32*(3), 319–328.

Wilson, T., & Holt, T. (2001). Complexity science: Complexity and clinical care. *British Medical Journal, 323,* 685–688.

Wong, D., & Bodovitz, S. (2010). Single cell analysis: The new frontier in 'omics.' *Trends in Biotechnology, 28*(6) 281–290.

Summarized in Grossman, L. (July 17, 2010). Enzymes exposed. *Science News, 178*(2), 22–26.

World Health Organization. (2001). International Classification of Functioning, Disability and Health (ICF). Geneva: Author.

Wright, B. D., & Linacre, J. M. (1989). Observations are always ordinal; measurements, however, must be interval. *Archives of Physical Medicine and Rehabilitation, 70*(12), 857–867.

Ylvisaker, M., Turkstra, L., Coehlo, C., Yorkston, K., Kennedy, M., Sohlberg, M. M., & Avery, J. (2007). Behavioural interventions for children and adults with behaviour disorders after TBI: A systematic review of the evidence. *Brain Injury, 21*(8), 769–805.

Zhan, S., & Ottenbacher, K. J. (2001). Single subject research designs for disability research. *Disability and Rehabilitation, 23*(1), 1–8.

Organization and Planning in Person-Centered Hospital-Based Rehabilitation Services

Emilie F. Smithson *and* Paul Kennedy

Abstract

Improvements in medical care, advanced methods of detection, and innovations in pharmacological treatment have led to decreased mortality rates following traumatic injury and increased life expectancies for people living with long-term health conditions. Recent years have seen a conversion of views from the medical and social fields as a growing body of research highlighted links among biological, psychological, and social aspects of chronic illness. In a step back from the medical model that dominated hospital care for so long, clinicians began to consider how individual differences inherent to the patient can impact on treatment, adherence, and motivation. Psychological theory has provided an ideal framework on which to structure the provision of person-centered rehabilitation and to engage the patient in taking responsibility and ownership of treatment plans under the guidance of specialists in the field.

This chapter discusses issues pertinent to the organization and delivery of person-centered rehabilitation services, the theories underlying the approach, the challenges faced by hospital-based rehabilitation services, and future directions through which the provision of rehabilitation care can continue to improve.

Key Words: Person-centered care, goal setting, needs assessment, rehabilitation, empowerment.

Hospital rehabilitation aims to support the individual toward re-engaging in those activities, interests, and pursuits enjoyed prior to injury or illness; to provide essential education and skills for the long-term management of health; to minimize disablement; and to maximize societal participation. Rehabilitation professionals strive to promote the acquisition of relevant knowledge and skills so that the patient remains autonomous in the decision-making process, and to provide them with the transferrable skills they will require for the future.

Rehabilitation services, in comparison to other tertiary-care providers, are required to consider multiple organ systems and complex issues when planning the provision of care for service users. In recent years, health services have begun to acknowledge the importance of empowering the patient with essential knowledge about his or her health condition. More than ever before, services are encouraging patient involvement in the process of planning how relevant skills and knowledge can be attained. The Commission on Accreditation of Rehabilitation Facilities (CARF), founded in 1966, seeks to endorse rehabilitation services according to internationally recognized standards of care. These standards include inclusion of patients and the public in decision-making and service delivery, individual-centered planning, and respect for the patient's dignity and rights. Such approaches to rehabilitation policy can be found internationally. In Canada, disability rehabilitation services are structured around models of participation that focus on full citizenship, return to work, and societal participation. The values integral to this approach are based on person-centered approaches such as community rehabilitation (Browne et al., 1994) and independent living (Boschen & Krane, 1992).

Research has found that the management of long-term medical conditions and chronic illness is dependent on the active behavioral involvement of the patient (Department of Health, 2001; Holman & Long, 2000). In most cases, the amount of time spent on rehabilitation in a hospital environment is outweighed by the duration of time that the individual manages a long-term condition in the community. Therefore, for the period of time that the person is hospitalized, it is imperative that he or she should feel equipped with the skills and knowledge to manage his or her condition effectively in the community.

In 1973, the United States Rehabilitation Act promoted consumer involvement in constructing rehabilitation plans and established the National Institute for Disability and Rehabilitation Research, which would work toward improving health care services based on sound empirical evidence. Following a survey conducted in the United Kingdom, it was found that patients did not feel involved in the decision-making process regarding their care; patients were found to report that they received little clear information about medical procedures that had been carried out, insufficient information was provided to family and friends, and insufficient information was provided about future prognosis and recovery. The report also suggested that patients felt they had no one to talk to about their concerns, anxieties, and fears regarding their health care treatment (Coulter, Picker Institute, 2001, cited in Department of Health, 2001). Through emerging research in the area, the U.K. government recognized that, with proper support, patients were able to take the lead in managing their chronic conditions. These self-management programs were found to improve health, quality of life, and adherence to medical regimes, and also helped to minimize the patient's incapacity from chronic pain, social isolation, and unemployment. This method of health care was adopted as a new approach to the management of chronic diseases and became known as the Expert Patient Programme (Department of Health, 2001).

However, the laying down of standards and policies and publication of research evidence to promote effective models of care is not enough to reform service provision. Implementing person-centered rehabilitation services in hospital-based settings involves consideration of multiple factors intrinsic to both the individual and to the organization, and from this recognition of psychosocial variables developed a more person-centered approach to medical and physical rehabilitation.

The Person-Centered Approach to Rehabilitation

For the provision of effective rehabilitation, it is important to acknowledge that each individual will cope and adjust to injury or illness in a different way, and that this diversity should inform the way in which health care is structured. Furthermore, in order to achieve optimum engagement and motivation from the patient in the rehabilitation process, and to ensure that the patient is sufficiently equipped to manage his own long-term health care needs after discharge, the planning of rehabilitation should be both patient-focused and collaborative.

The person-centered approach, originally developed from the work of psychologist Carl Rogers (1902–1987), advocated the view that the therapist should not be seen as the "expert." Instead, Rogers suggested that the patient should be encouraged to fulfil his own potential; that the patient is the best authority on his own experience and thus is fully capable of achieving growth through self-discovery and self-directed behavior. He acknowledged that the more the patient's hospital experience revolved around illness and associated medical facts, the more the patient would come to rely on the clinician as a "healer." The result of this reliance, Rogers proposed, was that the patient then becomes dependent on medical decisions and passive in the decision-making process regarding his care. Through empowering the patient by providing information, skills, and goals, this balance of power can be shifted. Rather than perceiving the clinician as being in control of his health, the patient begins to view them as a source of information and education—someone to facilitate a responsible and independent attitude to self–health care management.

An integral element of this approach is through communicating an open, trusting, and compassionate psychological environment in which the patient can feel unthreatened, valued, understood, and empowered. Although initially developed for use in psychotherapy, the underlying assumptions and philosophy of this approach have been easily transferred into other areas of health care provision.

Person-centered planning (PCP) was originally developed in the 1960s as a back-lash against the institutionalization of people with learning difficulties; it supported the transition to community-living through collaborative construction of plans and goals for the future. It takes into consideration the physical, social, and environmental factors important in optimizing participation, independence, and quality of life, and is now widely used in services for people with disabilities or chronic health conditions. Prior to the introduction of PCP, traditional provision of care was service-oriented and tended to operate around the individual being cared for in terms of the services he or she was provided; doctors, nurses, and social workers would more often make decisions on behalf of the patient in their care, with little consultation about what was important to the person from his or her perspective. Conversely, the person-centered approach focuses on managing the impact of the long term condition on the individual's level of activity and functioning, in the context of his or her own unique environment and with consideration of personal and social factors. It requires a creative approach to care planning—tailoring resources to help an individual to live the way she wants to—rather than fitting the individual into a preordained service structure. The person-centered approach takes into account all aspects of the individual's life; putting the patient at the center of care and at the heart of goals for rehabilitation.

In addition to providing both the patient and the care team with clear and definable aims for rehabilitation and provision of care, the person-centered approach also allows the patient an opportunity to express her views and feelings and have her wishes acknowledged by the treating team. Not only does this empower the patient with the feeling of being in control of her own care, but it also allows the team to gain a deeper understanding of the patient as an individual and establish those goals that are personally relevant to her. Houts and Scott (1975) state that rehabilitation should be organized around client need rather than being therapist-led, and that the goals of rehabilitation should build on the strengths and personal routine of the individual to ensure that any new skills and knowledge acquired can be generalized into the everyday natural environment. They theorize that, through collaborative discussion and mutual agreement on meaningful and personally relevant goals, the individual becomes motivated to engage in rehabilitation and thus achieve optimum outcomes.

Standards for rehabilitation services set out by the British Society of Rehabilitation Medicine (BSRM; 2009) and CARF have identified the need for interdisciplinary involvement in conducting assessments, making decisions, and setting and reviewing short- and long-term rehabilitation goals. In concordance with Houts and Scott (1975), these guidelines also underscore the importance of including the patient and his or her family in this process. Patient involvement in decision-making and planning is essential to the person-centered approach and provides the individual with a sense of inclusion and responsibility for his own care. Through collaborative discussion with the clinical team, the patient is able to construct personally relevant and meaningful goals that he will be motivated to pursue during rehabilitation. This provision of knowledge increases the patient's sense of ownership over care plans and enhances his coping skills, in turn increasing commitment to mutually agreed-upon goals. Involvement and inclusion of patients in rehabilitation planning has not only been linked to successful treatment outcomes, but is also found to facilitate adjustment through maintenance of knowledge and through the extrapolation of newly learned skills to individual lifestyles outside of hospital settings (Norris-Baker, Stephens, Rintala, & Willems, 1981).

However, it is not enough for each professional to simply apply the principles of the person-centered approach in isolation to his or her own areas of work. Patients admitted into a rehabilitation environment will present a multifaceted combination of difficulties and problems that stretch far beyond the actual nature of their diagnoses—problems that will be influenced or exacerbated by the idiosyncrasies of their personal and social lives. Therefore, as no one professional discipline would be able to meet all the complex needs of the patient, a comprehensive multidisciplinary team will be found at the heart of every effective rehabilitation service. An interdisciplinary approach to working within rehabilitation settings ensures that actions carried out by each member of the team contribute to a common goal, and it reduces the risk that other important actions are not overlooked (Wade, 2009). For instance, in physical rehabilitation after spinal cord injury (SCI) the relearning of dressing tasks would involve the coordination and integration of specialist skills across different disciplines—a physiotherapist may work with the patient to increase his strength and improve balance, while an occupational therapist would provide information on new techniques and skills to compensate for mobility limitations and assess the need for any assistive aides. The patient would then be supported by the nursing staff in practising these skills and contextualizing knowledge to everyday settings.

Communication is essential if the patient is to integrate knowledge in everyday practice, and this is also true for the continued assessment and monitoring of progress. If this does not take place, each team member will see the patient on the basis of his or her own expertise and without forming a comprehensive understanding of how the patient may integrate her skills into an overall problem-solving framework.

At the Pamela Youde Nethersol Easton Hospital in Hong Kong, hospital managers sought to redevelop their pediatric rehabilitation center to improve interunit communication between the different professionals working within the center. Prior to the redevelopment, these professionals operated independently and in different areas of the hospital; appointments were rarely synchronized and medical notes were duplicated or not integrated. Patients would be treated by each discipline separately, and each professional group would act without consulting other team members involved in the patient's care. After reviewing current practice, the service was remodelled to a patient-focused mold. Joint-held assessment clinics reduced the number of separate visits made by the patient's families, and therapies were integrated to maximize rehabilitation outcomes. For example, the former gym was converted into functional areas in which patients could be assisted by more than one therapist at a time. Surveys conducted with both patients and staff following the changes expressed a high degree of satisfaction with the new model and highlighted markedly improved interdisciplinary communication (Gilleard & Tarcisius, 2003).

Implementing Patient-Centered Approaches in Hospital-Based Rehabilitation Services

In 1988, Kennedy, Fisher, and Pearson employed a behavioral mapping procedure to investigate patient rehabilitation in a specialist SCI center. Rather than finding patients to be actively participating in rehabilitation for a large proportion of the day, the study revealed that only a small amount of time was being spent in active treatment. In fact, the results of the study revealed very little difference in the activity levels of patients by day or by evening— patients were spending prolonged periods of time in the ward areas during the day rather than engaging in active rehabilitation or treatment. Furthermore, Kennedy and colleagues found very little evidence of patient involvement in the planning of their rehabilitation or in the decision-making process regarding their care. The authors concluded that the there was a need for institutional changes based on the goal planning strategies discussed by Houts and Scott (1975). These were outlined as defining a problem, setting identifiable goals toward managing the problem, implementing change, and evaluating progress.

Goal planning is an effective psychological intervention that can affect change both at an individual and at a service level. Incorporating psychological principles such as self-efficacy (Bandura, 1986) and developed through the work of Locke and Latham (1990), the process of goal planning has been championed as an integral key to successful rehabilitation. Goal planning involves the care team, the patient (and family where appropriate) in discussing and negotiating a set of mutually agreed-upon aims or "goals" to work toward during rehabilitation. Compared to the typical hospital-based model of care, in which professionals often treat the patient without explicit explanation or rationale for their decision-making, the goal planning approach provides the patient with a clear action plan and with the reasons underlying these chosen actions. By the nature of its process, the introduction of this approach into hospital-based rehabilitation facilitates a person-centered service.

With many admissions to hospital-based rehabilitation services requiring extended or frequent periods of acute care, the service must ensure that measures are put in place to minimize institutionalization and dependency. Goal planning encourages active participation and autonomy within a supportive and encouraging environment by utilizing the essential elements of an effective therapeutic relationship—a collaborative approach to goal-setting, the timely provision of information, and support for the individual in regaining a sense of control. Two of the main elements of the goal planning approach are self-management and empowerment. In equipping the patient with the knowledge and confidence to apply his coping skills across a variety of situations, the individual's internal attributions of self-efficacy, competence, and mastery are nurtured. Furthermore, an efficient goal planning system can help the clinical team in structuring rehabilitation and the provision of education at a pace to suit the needs of the individual, and it can increase psychological awareness within the multidisciplinary team.

The theory of goal planning was developed from the basic assertion that human behavior is affected by plans and intentions (Ryan, 1970, cited in Locke and Latham 2002). Locke and Latham (1990) describe a goal as being the ultimate aim of a given action or behavior, and suggest that a number of personal and extrinsic factors can influence goal performance and attainment. Although originally developed in the context of industrial organization psychology, it is evident how these factors—attention and effort, persistence, learning new task-relevant skills and knowledge—could be integrated into theories of goal-directed behavior in health care and rehabilitation settings. Additional variables, such as the importance and relevance of the goal to the individual, the difficulty of the tasks required in order to achieve the goal, the amount of feedback that the individual receives about his performance, and the individual's beliefs of self-efficacy, have also been found to moderate goal performance. Furthermore, and most pertinent to the translation of the theory into a rehabilitation context, the research found the *specificity* and *difficulty* of goals to have a great influence on performance levels during set tasks. Specifically, Locke and Latham (1990) suggested that when specific, challenging goals are set, it will more likely result in a greater degree of effort than when general "do your best" instructions are given.

Implementing the goal planning approach in practice involves four key principles: client involvement, an interdisciplinary team, holistic assessment of the strengths and needs of the client, and the setting of specific targets or goals. Locke and Latham (2002) suggest that the relationship between goals and performance is strongest when an individual is committed to the goals that are set. User involvement in setting and planning goals, the first principle of goal planning, ensures that goals are personally relevant. This in turn enhances commitment to and performance in achieving goals, and by building on existing skills and setting goals that are applicable to their everyday routine, new skills are easily transferred to novel situations outside of the rehabilitation environment. Locke and Latham (2002) furthermore suggest there be a cognitive benefit to patients when they are involved in the decision-making process, as such involvement facilitates information exchange and formulation of problem-solving strategies. Deci and Ryan (1985) found that the internally meaningful rewards reaped by intrinsic goals were more inspiring to patients than were those gleaned by extrinsic, externally imposed goals, whereas Emmons (1996) suggested that emotion-driven goals provide a stronger internal motivation

and therefore a more successful outcome. There is a substantial body of evidence to advocate patient involvement when setting rehabilitation goals. Wade (1999) reviewed the evidence from stroke rehabilitation settings and concluded that personally relevant goals—set after collaborative discussion and involvement from the patient—were more effective in achieving the desired outcome, reducing handicap, and enhancing the maintenance of new skills. Positive results have also been found in patients recovering from heart failure, from patients with rheumatic disease, those with schizophrenia, older adults, and in with patients with acquired brain injury (see Levack et al., 2006, for a review). A further major benefit to collaborative goal setting is to prevent the risk of rehabilitation professionals setting goals that are based purely on the patient's diagnosis (McClain, 2005).

Second, as discussed earlier, rehabilitation often involves the relearning of complex tasks for which a number of professionals can provide support. In the example discussed earlier, the patient's physiotherapist, occupational therapist, and named nurse provided individual professional knowledge and skills toward helping a patient with SCI achieve a needs-led goal. This interdisciplinary approach to rehabilitation may even involve holding joint therapy sessions between two disciplines to contextualize specific skills. Without effective communication within the patient's team, each profession is in danger of working within its own discipline and without a global perspective of what the patient can realistically achieve in other areas of functioning. For example, an occupational therapist beginning to practice dressing skills with a spinal cord injured patient will need to ensure that the patient has built up the required strength and balance during physiotherapy sessions that will be required to begin dressing practice. Without effective communication between team members, such information is not available and may impact on the patient's progress by reducing the likelihood of goal achievement. For the patient concerned, this experience may be perceived as a personal "failure," thereby reducing self-belief, motivation, and commitment to pursuing the set goals. Practically, an interdisciplinary approach involves setting goals jointly between professional disciplines at prearranged and well-coordinated meetings, and requires an open and collaborative approach to teamwork. McGrath and Adams (1999) suggest that two major difficulties with goal selection and goal planning arise due to incompatibility of goals, either between professional disciplines or between the client's and professional's views. They point out that if such discrepancies are left unaddressed, they can lead to problems with motivation and compliance, both on the part of the patient and between team members. Their discussion provides a clear example of how user involvement is integral to the goal planning process and its relationship to interdisciplinary teamwork.

The third component to goal planning is through a structured, multidisciplinary, and holistic assessment of the patient's needs, capabilities, and personal goals. Wade (1998) cites evidence to suggest that assessment by a single profession can lead to a failure to identify problems, and that a structured assessment may lead to a better outcome than using a clinical approach. He suggests that a rehabilitation assessment that focuses specifically on the individual's specific health care issues is effective in reducing disability, but that this benefit is dependent on a number of factors: first, that experienced assessors covering a number of areas in depth is more likely to achieve a significant benefit; and second, that structured assessment leads to better results in identifying all the complex needs of the patient. In addition to ensuring that all the physical, psychological, and social needs of the patient are met, a multidisciplinary approach to assessment also allows the professionals working with the patient to identify common goals. After these goals have been established, the team can then work toward prioritizing goals in relation to the skills that will be required throughout the rehabilitation process. Again, this ensures that team members are working consistently toward a shared objective and providing a structured and consistent approach when guiding the patient through rehabilitation.

One consideration to be made when using assessment in rehabilitation is what type of assessment tool will be used. Primarily, the service must consider the nature of the patients being rehabilitated and whether it is more suitable to use a generic measure developed for use across a range of populations or one that has been designed specifically to the population group in question. Glueckauf (1993) argues that the development of an assessment tool itself can be person-centered through consultation and collaboration with consumers in the design and evaluation of the measure. When designing an assessment measure for use in rehabilitation settings, it is necessary to ensure that small increments of change can be detected, in addition to obtaining a more global impression of the amount of assistance and support that the patient requires to perform a given task.

Wade and de Jong (2000) also point to the need for the assessment measure to include current participation and the individual's own perception of his or her current needs and abilities.

An example of a comprehensive and multidisciplinary assessment measure used within a specific population group is the Needs Assessment Checklist, developed by Kennedy and colleagues (NAC; Kennedy & Hamilton, 1999) at the National Spinal Injuries Centre (NSIC), in the United Kingdom. The NAC provides a holistic view of the individual's need that not only identifies the physical and functional changes relating to his injury but incorporates the personal, social, and psychological areas affected by SCI. The multidisciplinary subsections of the NAC (e.g., physical health care, mobility, skin care, bladder and bowel, discharge coordination) allow the clinical team to monitor patients' progress through rehabilitation by highlighting areas of need still to be addressed and those targets that have been achieved. What differentiates the NAC from other clinical outcome measures and makes it particularly relevant to the SCI population is that it acknowledges the potential for *verbal* independence. This allows those patients with high lesions or considerable physical disability to achieve rehabilitation targets through their knowledge and ability to instruct others in an autonomous and self-directed manner.

At the NSIC, NACs are administered when the patient begins active rehabilitation and repeated when the patient is nearing the end of his or her rehabilitation stay. Scores from the NAC are translated into charts to illustrate the percentage of NAC targets achieved within each subsection, and a summary report is provided to give an overview of the patient's current strengths and needs. This summary can then be utilized during multidisciplinary goal planning meetings to facilitate the setting of clear and identifiable goals in collaboration with the patient. The strategic incorporation of such tools into routine clinical care not only provides staff and services users with a clear framework around which rehabilitation can be structured, but the collection of data such as this can also provide services with an opportunity to evaluate patient rehabilitation outcomes. Data from NACs completed at the NSIC over the course of 9 years allowed clinicians to review rehabilitation effectiveness by comparing the average percentage of rehabilitation targets achieved at the first and second NAC (see Figure 7.1). The generated graph demonstrates improvement across all NAC domains between the two time points.

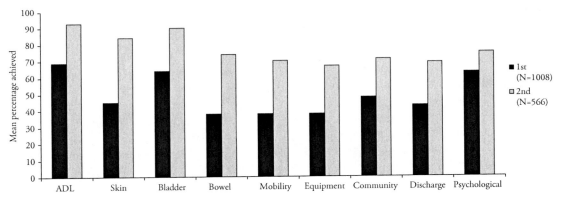

Figure 7.1 Mean percentage of Needs Assessment Checklist (NAC) targets achieved in each domain at first and second NAC.

The NAC has also been subject to psychometric analysis (Berry & Kennedy, 2002) and has received a favorable evaluation in a review of SCI-specific outcome measures (Dawson, Shamley, & Jamous, 2008). This review acknowledged the benefit of patient involvement in functional assessment when the assessment is used in the construction of rehabilitation goals and found the NAC to cover the full range of condition-specific, multidimensional measurements required when assessing outcomes in this patient group. Recently, the NAC has been further evaluated as a reliable measure of SCI rehabilitation progress, and the findings reiterated the importance of having a comprehensive and person-centered measure of assessment (Kennedy & Smithson, 2010). The study found a significant relationship between pain severity and mood, and that those who were reporting interference from pain early in their rehabilitation had significantly lower mobility scores later in their rehabilitation. Furthermore, earlier scores on measures of mood, perceived manageability, and adjustment were significantly related to subsequent scores on attainment in activities of daily living, skin care, and mobility. This investigation highlights the need for assessments to take into consideration factors that, although not directly related to injury or illness, may impact on the way in which the patient engages with the rehabilitation process or impedes his or her ability to act on intentions.

The fourth stage of the approach is the setting of specific goals. As previously mentioned, research has found that performance is best when specific, challenging, but achievable goals are set (Locke & Latham, 1990). Wade (2009) points out that a goal is by definition the "intended consequence of actions undertaken by the rehabilitation team... [and] the

intended result of some intervention(s)." Again, the importance of a team- and user-involved approach to goal setting is underscored, as this ensures that each individual's involvement in the process is contributing to an overall aim, and also that no important actions are omitted. Furthermore, aside from providing a structure and objectives for rehabilitation, the goal setting process may also improve the patient's insight and understanding of his health care needs and encourage acceptance where limited recovery is expected. Duff (2008) cites evidence to suggest that the goal setting process can facilitate adjustment through helping the patient reevaluate his priorities in light of his current health care needs in situations where previous life goals could be unrealistic or unachievable. Duff also argues that the goal planning approach can be beneficial in supporting the patient's family through difficult and emotional times, helping them adjust to change and cope with stress and anxiety. Furthermore, the family is encouraged to accept clear and realistic feedback from the clinical team regarding the patient's progress, with the aim of encouraging them to engage in realistic planning for the future.

Across time, the use of a formal goal setting process ensures that the effectiveness of therapeutic interventions can be monitored, introducing new strategies or terminating those strategies that are not eliciting the expected result. In practice, the setting of clear goals involves three stages. First, the process involves identification of an overall need within a particular area of rehabilitation that has been identified from the needs assessment. Second, the team and patient work together to establish objectives or goals through which this need will be meet. At this stage, it is important to specify a particular behavior that is to be carried out, what is to be learned, and how this will be done. Based upon theoretical findings, providing a specific time frame within which the target is to be achieved enhances motivation and commitment. It is therefore important to also ensure that objectives include a clear and specific time frame, where appropriate. The third level involves setting precise targets that explain how the overall goal will be achieved. This stage includes the details of who, why, and what, and several targets may be set when planning how an overall goal is to be achieved. An example of the type of goals and targets set within an SCI setting is shown in Figure 7.2.

Although the regularity with which goal planning meetings take place may depend on the nature of the service user, maintaining structure through regular and prearranged meetings ensures that the patient and the team have clear time frames within which to achieve the set targets. Over the course of the rehabilitation period, the regular goal planning meetings allow the patient's progress and goals to be reviewed and targets reset as required. An example of how targets may develop throughout rehabilitation is displayed in Figure 7.3.

Locke and Latham (1990) acknowledge Bandura's social-cognitive theory (1986) in the application of goal setting. They describe role modeling as having a great influence on behavioral action and acknowledge the impact of self-efficacy on goal choice, commitment, and performance. Self-efficacy describes the degree to which an individual feels confident that she has the abilities and resources to achieve a goal in the face of perceived barriers or facilitators, and interacts with the individual's beliefs about what the outcome of an action would be. The relationship of self-efficacy to health behaviors is through its influence on an individual's incentive and motivation to pursue a goal, and through her resilience in the presence of impediments to goal attainment. Locke and Latham (1990) have found a clear relationship between self-efficacy, goal setting, and task performance, with self-efficacy found to impede or increase an individual's motivations to act; those with high self-efficacy were found to choose more challenging tasks and stick to them. Self-efficacy is also found to affect an individual's persistence and commitment to set goals. Those with high efficacy will recover more quickly following setbacks, exploring new options for tackling the task (Latham, Winters & Locke, 1994) and investing more effort (Schwarzer & Fuch, 1994).

The nature of chronic health conditions or injury can also mean exposure to a multitude of unfamiliar terminology, the learning of new or alternate strategies for daily living activities, and often dealing with major changes to everyday life. In addition to living with or adjusting to health changes, the patient could easily become overwhelmed and left with the sense that she is not able to manage her illness or injury. Another psychological theory that has influenced the goal planning approach for chronic health problems is Lazarus and Folkman's (1984) *cognitive model of stress and coping*. A major component of this theory is the appraisal process. *Appraisals* refer to the way in which an individual interprets a problem or "stressor," and Lazarus and Folkman (1984) suggest there are two different types of appraisal process: primary and secondary. Primary appraisals involve an initial assessment of the stressor, whether it is a threat, a challenge, or benign, appraisals of which lead to further evaluations of certainty, predictability, and novelty. Secondary appraisals are the

NAC DOMAIN	GOAL	TARGET & DATE
SKIN CARE	To be independent in performing pressure relief by the next meeting	• To practice pushing up for pressure relief in the gym (daily) and in OT (3 times a week) • To attend patient education on skin management • To attend the seating and posture clinic in the next two weeks
	To be knowledgeable about skin management and skin checks by the next meeting	• For JP to arrange for a relative to bring in a mirror in the next week • For nursing staff to teach JP what to look for on his skin and where to check
ACTIVITIES OF DAILY LIVING (ADLs)	To be able to pick up a cup and drink independently	• To practise balance in short sitting during physiotherapy to enable right hand to be lifted to mouth without wobbling by next week • To have practised drinking sessions in OT each week by next meeting

Figure 7.2 Goals and targets within a spinal cord injury setting.

GPM	NAC DOMAIN	GOAL	TARGET & DATE
FIRST	ACTIVITIES OF DAILY LIVING (ADLs)	To be able to pick up a cup and drink independently	• To practise balance in short sitting during physiotherapy to enable right hand to be lifted to mouth without wobbling by next week • To have practised drinking sessions in OT each week by next meeting
SECOND	ACTIVITIES OF DAILY LIVING (ADLs)	To be able to pick up a cup and drink independently	• To be able to lift a half filled cup when in reach each time JP wants a drink • For nursing staff to support JP by refilling and positioning cup if required
THIRD	ACTIVITIES OF DAILY LIVING (ADLs)	To be able to drink independently	• To practice maintaining balance in physiotherapy whilst lifting a jug and drinking from a water bottle over the next week. • To practice picking up and throwing bean bags while maintaining balance in physio sessions over the next week. • To drink from a full cup and practise pouring a drink from a jug in OT the following week. • To drink independently from a drinking bottle in wheelchair and without a table by the next meeting.

Figure 7.3 Development of targets through rehabilitation.

individual's assessment of his own coping resources; whether these resources are adequate and sufficient to manage the stressor, and the likelihood that these coping resources will be effective if applied.

The use of the goal planning approach in rehabilitation directly impacts on the appraisal processes of the individual by encouraging challenge-based appraisals rather than cognitions based on threat and loss (Duff & Kennedy, 2003). The system is constructed to communicate to the patient that his situation is manageable, and the setting of realistic and achievable goals conveys to the patient that he has the resources and skills to be able to cope with the challenges that he faces. The support and encouragement of the clinical team during the goal setting process provides the patient with behavioral reinforcement of practical skills and knowledge. Furthermore, goal planning has also been found to be an effective psychological tool with which to reduce anxiety (McGrath & Adams, 1999), which in turn can enhance the patient's problem-solving skills and help him to cope with the changes arising from his health problem or injury.

Assessing needs and implementing goal planning strategies provides the patient with a clear framework and direction for his rehabilitation. Including the patient in the process helps to focus his attention on his own personal objectives and aims and also facilitates motivation and commitment. Through feedback and guidance during the goal planning process, the individual will gain valuable

insight as to his capabilities, the strengths he can utilize to compensate for changes arising from illness/injury, and an understanding of how best to utilize these qualities when managing his condition in his home environment. The process of goal planning encourages patients to think about strategies with which to overcome obstacles; being involved in this process increases the individual's capacity to problem-solve—skills that can be transferrable to everyday life.

More recently, this theoretical connection between goal planning and problem-solving has been developed for clinical application, and the two approaches combined as "action planning and coping planning." Sniehotta, Scholz, and Schwarzer (2006) investigated the comparative benefits of action planning (when, where, how to act) versus action planning plus coping planning (how to deal with anticipated barriers to implementing actions) on adhering to prescribed physical exercise recommendations in a sample of cardiac rehabilitation patients. They suggest that planning can be broken down into the specification of intended actions and the identification of coping strategies that will prioritize the intended action in favor of habitual responses in the face of challenges and setbacks. In practice, the approach utilized techniques found in cognitive-behavioural therapy in that the patients were encouraged to pair anticipated risk situations with predefined coping responses. The results of the study found that, when compared to the control group, both groups reported more exercise activity, and that those in the combined coping group also engaged in significantly more exercise than did those who completed the action planning only. However, although the action planning alone did lead participants to engage in more physical activity than those in the control group, this difference was not statistically significant, leading the researchers to conclude that action planning alone may not be sufficient to produce behavioural change. Instead, the authors suggest that action planning should be augmented by additional support interventions that increase patient self-efficacy and develop personal coping strategies based on existing knowledge and past experience.

After the introduction of a goal planning system, Kennedy, Walker, and White (1991) conducted a follow-up study of activity levels in a specialist spinal injuries center (the NSIC, UK). They found that patients were now spending more time interacting with each other and with staff, that significantly less time was being spent on the ward during the therapy day, and that a significantly smaller proportion of time was spent in disengaged behaviors. They concluded that goal planning was an effective way of increasing patient engagement and activity and reducing disengagement in SCI rehabilitation settings.

In addition to the objective benefits that were observed following the introduction of goal planning at the NSIC, qualitative reports from service users suggested that patients were likewise satisfied with the approach. Duff and colleagues (Duff, Kennedy, & Swalwell, 1999) carried out an audit of patient views regarding goal planning and found the majority of patients considered the process useful in helping them to plan rehabilitation and that they felt involved in the planning process. The most important aspect of the process was felt by patients to be the clarity of goals that were set. Macleod and Macleod (1996) also looked at patient satisfaction after the introduction of goal planning and found patients to report an increased sense of control from participating in the goal planning process, and that this sense of control was positively associated with perceived informativeness.

Although the goal planning process is built around a structured framework, it is an individualized and flexible approach that can be tailored to suit the needs of the individual. In two studies evaluating the rehabilitation gains of patient groups who may have additional or complex needs, there is evidence that the needs assessment and goal planning approach is beneficial to older patients (Kennedy, Evans, Berry, & Mullin, 2003) and people with preexisting mental health difficulties (Kennedy, Sherlock, & Sandhu, 2008) as these population groups show comparable rehabilitation gains and draw equal benefit from the program as those patients without additional needs. Similarly, the basic structure of goal planning theory can be modified to suit the needs of the service users.

The utility and effectiveness of implementing goal planning approaches in other clinical settings has been evaluated across a number of different populations. One of the main concerns with the use of goal setting is that it may be affected by the patient's cognitive ability to identify, plan, and act on specific goals, an ability that can very frequently be compromised following acquired brain injury.

Doig and colleagues (Doig, Fleming, Cornwell, & Kuipers, 2009) conducted a qualitative investigation of patient, family, and therapist perspectives on the goal planning process when implemented with those who were undergoing rehabilitation following a traumatic brain injury (TBI). They found that not only was the approach considered effective and beneficial, but that the setting of goals provided them with a structure for rehabilitation and made the aims and expected outcomes clear and understandable. The patients also found that setting goals increased their motivation and gave them a sense of ownership of and control over the plans for their treatment and care. A further theme that emerged in the study was that the structure of goal planning also provided patients with an objective record of their progress, which further increased their motivation and persistence. Family involvement was also highlighted as an important element in enhancing motivation through the encouragement and shared understanding of goals. With regards to the cognitive impairments that may impede engagement with the goal planning approach, memory problems and diminished self-awareness arising as a result of the injury were found to create barriers to the generation of realistic goals. However, for these cases, therapists reported that the goal planning process allowed more realistic goals to be set in light of these barriers, and that with appropriate support, the setting of goals was actually found to increase self-awareness in some cases.

In a systematic review conducted by Levack and colleagues (2006), the results of 19 studies suggested that goal planning could increase patient adherence to treatment regimes and that "prescribed, specific and challenging goals can improve immediate patient performance in some specific clinical contexts." Included in this review was one study that investigated the effect of goal planning on self-regulation strategies in patients with TBI with positive results. However, the review did highlight that the studies included in the analysis did not provide a reliable estimation as to how the effects of goal planning during rehabilitation translated to long-term outcomes.

The utilization of goal planning in hospital-based rehabilitation settings is not only found to be beneficial in terms of facilitating patient engagement in rehabilitation, but also advantageous to the clinical service. Goal planning can also provide a means of evaluating the effectiveness of the services being provided and a way to develop care pathways based on the needs of specific client groups. Evaluating the effectiveness of goal planning for older adults with SCI, Kennedy and colleagues (Kennedy et al., 2003) were able to identify specific areas of need in this population compared with younger adults. These findings led to the introduction of enhanced patient education and support for older adults in the self-management of skin integrity.

Similarly, goal planning has been utilized by rehabilitation services to develop evidence-based "process maps" of rehabilitation for specific services. Process maps describe a process of plan of care by identifying milestones within a specific time frame. These can be used by services to provide a generic picture of what achievements patients may make during their rehabilitation and at what point. The development of process maps not only facilitates clinical planning but offers managers a description of the way in which the organization delivers its services and facilitates discharge planning. With the complex array of impairment severity arising from variances in level and completeness of SCI, Goodwin-Wilson and colleagues (Goodwin-Wilson, Watkins, & Gardner-Elahi, 2010) drew on data from the Needs Assessment and Goal Planning records of 280 patients when developing process maps of rehabilitation for different lesion categories. They structured the map according to the domains within the NAC and then identified patient progress during rehabilitation through reviewing the goals that were set in response to the results of the NAC. Time scales were set according to average length of time between setting a particular goal and goal achievement, and the authors suggest that the inclusion of such time scales may act as an "early warning system" for patients falling behind in their rehabilitation, in addition to auditing service performance.

CHALLENGES IN IMPLEMENTING HOSPITAL-BASED PERSON-CENTERED REHABILITATION SERVICES

Goal setting is underpinned by a number of psychological theories, and its success in facilitating rehabilitation is underscored in the literature. However, as previously mentioned, the utility and generalizability of using a generic approach with people who have cognitive impairments may be compromised by the intrinsic requirements underpinning the theory. The challenges in implementing a person-centered goal-oriented approach to rehabilitation after TBI have been well documented. One such complication of working within a generic goal-setting process is that the client's diminished self-awareness may prevent him or her from selecting appropriate long-term goals. As discussed earlier, patient involvement and engagement in the goal planning process is integral to its success; the cognitive and motivational impairments associated with TBI could therefore limit the potential for assessing achievement when using traditional goal planning approaches in this patient group.

Goal attainment scaling (GAS) is a method of quantifying the achievement of goals set during the course of rehabilitation, one which offers more discrimination of achievement than simply recording performance as a "pass" or "fail." The approach is commonly used in brain injury rehabilitation, where heterogeneity of deficits means standardized measures are difficult to apply. In addition to the benefits of goal setting discussed in this chapter, GAS is also suggested to be more sensitive to change than other standardized measures. The approach involves establishing criteria with both patients and their families as to the "success" of the goal outcome. Each goal is rated on a 5-point scale, with 0 meaning achievement at the expected level, −2 a much less than the expected level, and +2 a much higher level than expected. An additional feature is that goals can be weighted to take account of the importance, relevance, and likelihood of attainment, and by any difficulties anticipated by the rehabilitation team. Although this flexible approach to measuring outcome allows reflection of outcomes that are of importance to patients and their families in the context of their own lives, it is not suggested that this method should replace existing standardized outcome measures. Instead, it is suggested that GAS should be used to complement and augment existing instruments (Turner-Stokes, 2009). The feasibility of using GAS in a rehabilitation center for people with TBI was evaluated by Bouwens, van

Heugten, and Verhey (2009) in terms of the number of goals set, how realistic the goals set were, the time taken to set goals, the number of domains in which a goal was set, the progress of attainment over a 6-month period, and the clinical experiences of patient involvement. The study found that it proved possible to set three goals within an acceptable time frame, that it was possible to involve patients in the goal setting process, and that the goals set were both realistic and reached across a number of different domains. They concluded that not only is GAS suitable for use in clinical rehabilitation settings, but that the individualized and inclusive approach can also prove beneficial to the patient's mood and quality of life.

Another approach that would lend itself to working within TBI settings is self-regulation theory. Self-regulation theory approaches the concept of goal orientation and attainment armed with a wider perspective, describing goal management as an inter-relationship of multiple personal and external factors rather than the attainment of a specific goal. In this respect, constructing rehabilitation based upon self-regulation theory can help to minimize the risk of the negative consequences of TBI—such as low mood and motivation—being exacerbated by a "failure" to achieve a set goal (McPherson, Kayes, & Weatherall, 2009). Implementing goal setting in this patient group and facilitating goal attainment may require an element of behavioural therapy in its delivery. *Goal management training* (GMT), developed by Levine et al. (2000), aims to prevent goal failure through repeated verbal rehearsal of a set task prior to the physical activity taking place. The approach involves identifying discreet areas of activity in which goal failure may occur, such as omitting a crucial step in an everyday activity (e.g., pouring milk and hot water into a mug without putting a tea bag in) or an error in the order of steps required (e.g., putting on shoes before socks). The patient and the practitioner then work together on developing a structured intervention in which each step is recorded in detail and rehearsed before the activity is performed, in order to eliminate the chance of goal failure and increase awareness of where difficulties may arise. In this respect, we can see a link between GMT and the coping planning introduced by Sniehotta and colleagues (2006).

A clear and comprehensible service philosophy provides a strategy for setting objectives, clarifying roles, and assessing performance (Madge & Khair, 2000). Recognition of the contribution of each discipline to rehabilitation and showing a willingness to work together and share responsibilities toward a common goal both integrates and enhances the team. Where services do not have a shared understanding of purpose and a common vision, it can lead to friction and consequently impacts on the provision of care to service users. Many professionals will receive training in their own discipline, but very few will be given opportunity to learn or experience how they can integrate their own work with others' or how to function as part of a team (Dunn, Sommer, & Gambina, 1992). Unrealistic expectations and demands can be minimized through understanding and clarifying each member's role and contribution, and an awareness of workload distribution minimizes the potential for staff friction and work-related illness. With a clear strategy and service philosophy, provision of care can be reviewed and evaluated against these objectives, then assessed, adjusted, and enhanced toward an efficient and effective rehabilitation service for the patient group.

Rehabilitation services are often separated from general hospital wards. Health care professionals work with specific client groups for which a certain degree of specialist knowledge will be required. However, for many new staff, it may be the first time that they have worked with patients with chronic illness or disability, and it is important for professionals working in rehabilitation to be aware of how their own attitudes toward disability and chronic conditions may affect the way in which they work and interact with patients. Basic-level training regarding the medical needs of the patient group can be enriched through providing education to also increase awareness of emotional needs and concerns of the patient group, with additional support and advice for managing their own emotional reactions. Such methods of role induction would not only be beneficial in increasing staff confidence in the workplace and integration into the team, but would also enhance the quality of care provided to patients and families.

There is also a need to increase staff awareness of the theoretical underpinnings of needs assessment goal planning. McClain (2005) suggests that the process of collaborative goal setting in health care would be improved through incorporating patient involvement and person-centered approaches into the educational training of health care professionals, including the advantages of patient participation in the goal setting process. She also suggests that education should include advice on how to overcome communicative or cognitive barriers to patient involvement through involving family members, interpreters, communication devices, or other resources to maximize their inclusion in the planning of care. Similarly, McClain argues that patients are not always made aware of their roles in the goal setting process, and providing education for patients on how to evaluate, analyze, and communicate their needs effectively would also prove beneficial to collaborative goal setting in health care services.

Despite modern-day perspectives on interdisciplinary rehabilitation and the importance of empowering the patient through involvement in decision-making, studies have found that nursing staff often don't have the confidence in their knowledge and skills to contribute to such methods of rehabilitation. Using a grounded theory method, Pryer and colleagues (Pryer, Walker, O'Connell, & Worrall-Carter, 2009) found that staff without formal preparation for the role of the rehabilitation nurse tended to "opt in" or "opt out" of contributing to inpatient rehabilitation. "Opting in" was described as actively accepting responsibility to learn about the role, thus facilitating self-care and independence, helping with coping and adjustment, and preventing re-admissions. They found that factors that contributed to role ambiguity and the segregation of nursing staff from allied health professionals led to nursing staff distancing themselves from systemic practice in order to focus solely on direct patient care. Ultimately, even if services have a clear and well-defined philosophy of care, interdisciplinary segregation compromises nurses' contribution to patient rehabilitation. Through providing nurses with clear objectives, role clarification, and skills in supporting and encouraging patient autonomy, their potential in facilitating patient self-care can be enhanced.

Currently, one of the major shortcomings of our understanding about goal planning and the beneficial impact of its use in rehabilitation is the lack of a standard terminology used in relation to goal setting (Scobbie, Wyke, & Dixon, 2009). Not only does this pose difficulty in the evaluation of the efficacy of goal planning, it also leads to major variation in how goal planning is implemented between services. Scobbie and colleagues (Scobbie et al., 2009) suggest that goal setting practice is too frequently implemented within a commonsense approach rather than one that is practice-based and driven by sound theoretical underpinnings. They argue that without clear understandings as to the purpose of goal setting, the evaluation of its success

is difficult to ascertain, whereas Wade (2005) points out that it is essential to base evaluation and analysis on a clear theory or explanatory model in order to reliably evaluate a situation, define concepts, and arrive at a clear action plan. Furthermore, this absence of a clear theoretical basis may contribute to difficulties experienced in clinical practice in the process of setting goals. Scobbie, Wyke, and Dixon discuss a number of psychologically based theories that can be used to structure goal planning in rehabilitation, and their discussion reiterates those theories discussed here; self-efficacy, goal setting, coping, self-regulation, and planning. Through focusing on clear theoretical perspectives, it is hoped that the process of goal setting theory can be unified, thus allowing a more individualized intervention for patients and one that can be subject to empirical evaluation and development.

Conclusion

This chapter has presented a psychologically informed approach to the planning and provision of person-centered hospital-based rehabilitation services. The development of rehabilitation plans that have been constructed around the individuals' needs and interests and that are personally relevant to their lives can take a considerable amount of commitment and involvement from the clinical team, patients, and their families.

It is not the plan that is suggested to be the central objective of the rehabilitation, but the real, positive differences that a well-constructed plan can bring not only to an individual's current quality of life but in increasing confidence in long-term health care management.

Future Directions

The beneficial impact, both to the patient and to the service, of establishing a goal setting structure within hospital-based rehabilitation is evidenced throughout this chapter. However, to allow reliable empirical evaluation and theory development, work should continue to establish a unified framework for goal setting based on clear theoretical underpinnings and explore the long-term benefits of goal setting beyond the initial rehabilitation period. A clear consensus is required on how goal setting strategies are implemented and how achievement is assessed, in order to provide both clinicians and service users with a structured framework in which to plan the provision of care. Similarly, those specific components of goal setting that could potentially enhance or impede the beneficial effect of the process, such as the inclusion of self-regulation or coping planning strategies, should be subject to further investigation and thereafter utilized in the development of the approach. Future research should continue to identify the unique patterns of appraisal and coping strategies that are associated with positive and negative outcomes, and those findings integrated into the organizational framework.

Currently, there is limited evidence of how goal setting translates across diverse population groups; further research is required to investigate how the goal theories discussed in this chapter can be adapted across rehabilitation contexts and patients with complex needs, and how we can facilitate patient involvement, engagement, and collaboration with the goal setting process in populations that are cognitively or communicatively impaired. With this in mind, we should continue to explore research that illuminates the factors involved with engagement, reducing social reliance and maximizing patient autonomy, determination, and adjustment.

References

Bandura, A. (1986). *Social foundations of thought and action: A social-cognitive theory.* Englewood Cliffs, NJ: Prentice-Hall.

Berry, C., & Kennedy, P. (2002). A psychometric analysis of the Needs Assessment Checklist (NAC). *Spinal Cord, 41,* 490–501.

Boschen, K. A., & Krane, N. (1992). A history of independent living in Canada. *Canadian Journal of Rehabilitation, 6*(2), 79–88.

Bouwens, S.F.M., van Heugten, C.M., & Verhey, F.R.J. (2009). The practical use of goal attainment scaling for people with acquired brain injury who receive cognitive rehabilitation. *Clinical Rehabilitation, 23*(4), 310–320.

British Society of Rehabilitation Medicine. (2009). *BSRM standards for rehabilitation services, mapped on to the National Service framework for long-term conditions.* London: BSRM.

Browne, G., Roberts, J., Watt, S., Gafni, A., Stockwell, M., & Alcork, S. (1994). Community Rehabilitation: Strategies, outcomes, expenditures. *Canadian Journal of Rehabilitation, 8*(1), 9–22.

Coulter, A., & Picker Institute. Cited in Department of Health. (2001). *The Expert Patient: A new approach to chronic disease management for the 21st century.* London: Department of Health.

Dawson, J., Shamley, D., & Jamous, M.A. (2008). A structured review of outcome measures used for the assessment of rehabilitation interventions for spinal cord injury. *Spinal Cord, 46,* 768–780.

Deci, E., & Ryan, R (1985). *Intrinsic motivation and self-determination in human behaviour.* New York: Plenum

Department of Health. (2001). *The expert patient: A new approach to chronic disease management for the 21st century.* London: Department of Health.

Doig, E., Fleming, J., Cornwell, P. L., & Kuipers, P. (2009). Qualitative exploration of a client-centered, goal-directed approach to community-based occupational therapy for adults with traumatic brain injury. *American Journal of Occupational Therapy, 63*(5), 559–568.

Duff, J. (2008). Rehabilitation and goal planning approaches following spinal cord injury: Facilitating adjustment. In A. Craig & Y. Tran (Eds.), *Psychological aspects associated with spinal cord injury: New directions and best evidence.* New York: Nova.

Duff, J., & Kennedy, P. (2003). Spinal cord injury. In S. Llewelyn & P. Kennedy (Eds.), *Handbook of clinical health psychology* (pp. 251–278). Chichester: John-Wiley & Sons.

Duff, J., Kennedy, P., & Swalwell, E. (1999). Clinical audit of physical rehabilitation: patients' views of goal planning. *Clinical Psychology Forum, 129,* 34–38.

Dunn, M., Sommer, R.N., & Gambina, H. (1992). A practical guide to team functioning in spinal cord injury rehabilitation. In C. Perry Zejdlik (Ed.), *Managing spinal cord injury.* Boston, MA: Jones & Barlett.

Emmons, R. A. (1996). Striving and feeling: Personal goals and subjective well-being. In P. M. Gollwitzer & J. A. Bargh (Eds.), *The psychology of action linking cognition and motivation to behavior* (pp. 313–337). New York: Guilford Press.

Gilleard, J. D., & Tarcisius, L. C. (2003). Improving the delivery of patient services: Alternative workplace strategies in action. *Facilities, 21*(1/2), 20–27.

Goodwin-Wilson, C., Watkins, M., & Gardner-Elahi, C. (2010). Developing evidence based process maps for spinal cord injury rehabilitation. *Spinal Cord, 48,* 122–127.

Glueckauf, R. L. (1993). Use and misuse of assessment in rehabilitation. In R. L. Glueckauf, L. B. Secrest, G. R. Bond, & E. C. McDonel (Eds.), *Improving assessment in rehabilitation and health* (pp. 33–60). Newbury Park, CA: Sage

Holman, H., & Long, K. (2000). Patients as partners in managing chronic disease. *British Medical Journal, 320,* 520–527.

Houts P., & Scott, R. (1975). *Goal planning with developmentally disabled persons: Procedures for developing an individualized client plan.* Hershey, PA: Department of Behavioural Science, Pennsylvania State University College of Medicine.

Kennedy, P., Evans, M. J., Berry, C., & Mullin, J. (2003). Comparative analysis of goal achievement during rehabilitation for older and younger adults with spinal cord injury. *Spinal Cord, 41,* 44–51.

Kennedy, P., Fisher, K., & Pearson, E. (1988). Ecological evaluation of a rehabilitation environment for spinal cord injured people: Behavioural mapping and feedback. *British Journal of Clinical Psychology, 27,* 239–246.

Kennedy, P., & Hamilton, L. R. (1999). The Needs Assessment Checklist: A clinical approach to measuring outcome. *Spinal Cord, 37*(2), 136–139.

Kennedy, P., Sherlock, O., & Sandhu, N. (2008). Rehabilitation outcomes in people with pre-morbid mental health disorders following spinal cord injury. *Spinal Cord, 47,* 290–294.

Kennedy, P Smithson, E., & Blakey. L. (in press). Planning and Structuring Spinal Cord Injury Rehabilitation. Topics in Spinal Cord Injury.

Kennedy, P., Walker, L., & White, D. (1991). Ecological evaluation of goal planning and advocacy in a rehabilitation environment for spinal cord injured people. *Paraplegia, 29,* 197–202

Latham, G. P., Winters, D., & Locke, E. (1994). Cognitive and motivational effects of participation: a mediator study. *Journal of Organisational Behaviour, 15,* 49–63.

Lazarus, R. S., & Folkman, S. (1984). *Stress, appraisal and coping.* New York: Springer.

Levack, W. M. M., Taylor, K., Siegart, R. J., Dean, S. G., McPherson, K. M., & Weatherall, M. (2006). Is goal planning in rehabilitation effective? A systematic review. *Clinical Rehabilitation, 20*, 739–755.

Levine, B., Robertson, I. H., Clare, L., Carter, G., Hong, J., Wilson B.A., Duncan, J., and Stuss, D.T. (2000). Rehabilitation of executive functioning: An experimental-clinical validation of Goal Management Training. *Journal Of the International Neuropsychological Society, 6*, 299–312.

Locke, E., & Latham, G. (1990). *A theory of goal setting and task performance.* Englewood Cliffs, NJ: Prentice-Hall.

Locke, E. A., & Latham, G. P. (2002). Building a practically useful theory of goal setting and task motivation. *American Psychologist, 57*(9), 705–717.

Macleod, G. M., & Macleod L. (1996). Evaluation of client and staff satisfaction with a goal planning project implemented with people with spinal cord injuries. *Spinal Cord, 34*, 525–530.

Madge, S., & Khair, K. (2000). Multidisciplinary teams in the United Kingdom: Problems and Solutions. *Journal of Paediatric Nursing, 15*(2), 131–135.

McClain, C. (2005). Collaborative rehabilitation goal setting. *Topics in Stroke Rehabilitation, 12*(4), 56–60.

McGrath, J. R., & Adams, L. (1999). Patient-centered goal planning: A systematic psychological therapy? *Topics in Stroke Rehabilitation, 6*(2), 43–50.

McPherson, K. M., Kayes, N., & Weatherall, M. (2009). A pilot study of self-regulation informed goal setting in people with traumatic brain injury. *Clinical Rehabilitation, 23*, 296–309.

Norris-Baker, C., Stephens, M. A., Rintala, D. H., & Willems, E. P. (1981). Patient Behavior as a predictor of outcomes in spinal cord injury. *Archives of Physical Medicine and Rehabilitation, 62*(12), 602–608.

Pryer, J., Walker, A., O'Connell, B., & Worrall-Carter, L. (2009). Opting in and opting out: A grounded theory of nursing contribution to inpatient rehabilitation. *Clinical Rehabilitation, 20*, 1124–1135.

Ryan T.A. (1970). Intentional Behavior. New York: Ronald Press

Scobbie, L., Wyke, S., & Dixon, D. (2009). Identifying and applying psychological theory to setting and achieving rehabilitation goals. *Clinical Rehabilitation, 23*, 321–333.

Schwarzer, R., & Fuchs, R. (1994). Self-efficacy and health behaviours. In M. Conner & P. Norman (Eds.), *Predicting health behaviour.* Philadelphia: Open University Press.

Sniehotta, F. F., Scholz, U., & Schwarzer, R. (2006). Action plans and coping plans for physical exercise: A longitudinal intervention study in cardiac rehabilitation. *British Journal of Social Psychology, 11*, 23–37.

Turner-Stokes, L. (2009). Goal attainment scaling (GAS) in rehabilitation: A practical guide. *Clinical Rehabilitation, 23*, 362–370.

Wade, D. T. (1998). Evidence relating to assessment in rehabilitation. *Clinical Rehabilitation, 12*, 183–186.

Wade, D. T. (1999). Goal planning in stroke rehabilitation: Evidence. *Topics in Stroke Rehabilitation, 6*(2), 37–42.

Wade, D. T. (2005). Describing rehabilitation interventions. *Clinical Rehabilitation, 19*, 811–818.

Wade, D. T. (2009). Goal setting in rehabilitation: An overview of what, why and how. *Clinical Rehabilitation, 23*, 291–295.

Wade, D. T., & de Jong, B. A. (2000). Recent advances in rehabilitation. *British Medical Journal, 320*, 1385–1388.

An Emerging Role for the Rehabilitation Psychologist in Community Rehabilitation Service Delivery

Craig Ravesloot *and* Tom Seekins

Abstract

Most people with disabilities have used community services to meet their needs as they engage the community for work and leisure. These services include independent living, vocational, health care and educational services. Some individuals depend on these services to participate as full citizens in the community, and, without them, would be institutionalized. As rehabilitation evolves toward an ecological model that recognizes participation as the ultimate goal, the rehabilitation psychologist is uniquely positioned to maximize these outcomes. Working in a traditional role, the rehabilitation psychologist can make knowledgeable referrals to community services that improve participation outcomes. Working in a new role that we label "community rehabilitation psychologist," psychologists may use community psychology concepts and methods to deliver "treatments" at the community level, to make the local community accessible to the full participation of all people with disabilities.

Key Words: Independent living, vocational rehabilitation, health care, transition services, community psychology, ecological disability model.

People with disabilities face all the same challenges to community living that everyone does, including acquiring education, training and health care; making a living; and finding ways to engage in social and civic life. For many, community services are essential to their participation as full citizens.

Rehabilitation psychology has a long history of recognizing the value of community participation and the influence of community structures on the lives of people with disabilities. Indeed, rehabilitation psychology has long recognized the dynamic interplay of the person and the environment (Wright, 1983). Today, an ecological view of disability is pervasive, and rehabilitation outcomes are considered complex derivatives of personal and environmental factors.

The goal of rehabilitation generally, and rehabilitation psychology more specifically, is quality of life (QOL) for the people served. As we consider the role of the community and community services in QOL outcomes, a case can be made that rehabilitation psychologists may expand their role to incorporate more community psychology. In the role of *community rehabilitation psychologist* (CRP), psychologists will find their skills are valuable not only to individuals, but also to the community in helping facilitate the change process that makes communities accessible to people with disabilities.

Driven by a long history of policy that pays to reimburse services to individuals, it has been difficult for researchers and practitioners to find funding to shift their attention to community issues. However, even with the limitations imposed by health care reimbursement, changes in preferred outcomes may create opportunities for rehabilitation psychology. The past decade has witnessed a shift in preferred rehabilitation outcomes, with community participation becoming the gold standard (Gobelet, Luthi, Al-Khodairy, & Chamberlain, 2007; U.S. Department of Education, 2007). With this shift in outcomes, the role of the rehabilitation psychologist may expand to further support and develop community services.

In this chapter, we examine the conceptual and social policy underpinnings for organizing community rehabilitation services using a community development framework. We describe an emerging role for rehabilitation psychologists that incorporates principles of community psychology into practice to affect community change that improves participation for people of all ages with disabilities. Then, having laid the groundwork for understanding the conceptual linkages between community services and outcomes, we will describe the state of practice in community rehabilitation services, highlighting the role of the rehabilitation psychologist in community-based rehabilitation. Specifically, we will review educational and vocational services, independent living services, and, finally, health care, rehabilitation, and health promotion services.

Rehabilitation Psychology and Community Participation

The International Classification of Function, Disability, and Health (ICD) was a revision to the International Classification of Impairment, Disability, and Handicap (World Health Organization [WHO], 2001). One of the significant changes in this revision was the replacement of the word "handicap" with "activities and participation." The ICF breaks out eight major areas in which to classify activities and participation; these range from "learning and applying knowledge" to "community, social, and civic life."

The ICF defines participation as the outcome of an interaction between an individual and environmental factors. Although not fully embraced by all countries (e.g., the United States), the ICF clearly suggests that successful rehabilitation outcomes that increase community participation are multimodal. These developments have created opportunities for rehabilitation psychologists to more fully realize the biopsychosocial perspective. We might envision interventions to achieve successful participation at three different levels, including medical rehabilitation that maximizes functional ability, psychotherapy to change malleable personal factors (e.g., self-efficacy), and social change to reduce environmental barriers.

The Ecology of Disability

Ecological models of human development have a long history. For example, Charles Darwin is often credited with placing humans back into the environment in order to understand behavior (e.g., Bolles, 1993). In Russia, in the 1920s, Lev Vygotsky, a developmental psychologist, articulated a theory of child development that described the interaction of a child with her environment as the causal mechanism for change (Wertsch & Tulviste, 1992). In the United States, Urie Bronfenbrenner began developing his model of social influence on child development in the 1950s and 1960s. In the 1960s and 1970s, Roger Barker and his colleagues developed an ecological psychology in which they argued that behavior could not be understood outside of context (Barker, 1968).

By the 1970s, disability rights advocates were articulating a "new paradigm" of disability in which the cause of disability shifted from impairment to environment (DeJong, 1979). As this perspective evolved in the 1980s and 1990s, it became more dynamic and is often now referred to as the *ecological model of disability*. Concepts such as reasonable accommodation and least restrictive environment cannot be judged without considering a specific individual, with all of his or her strengths and weaknesses, interacting with specific environmental arrangements.

Within the field of disability and rehabilitation, the environment is understood to be the community in which we all live. Models such as this suggest that the best rehabilitation outcomes with regard to participation will result from a combination of individually and community focused interventions. For example, cognitive-behavior therapy may prepare an individual with skills to integrate back into the community, but if that community lacks accessibility, the level of participation the patient achieves will be limited. As with the traditional rehabilitation model that focuses on remediating impairment, this ecological model assumes that the environment is infinitely malleable and that it can be organized (treated) to accommodate individuals with various impairments. Figure 8.1 depicts participation outcome as the interaction between individual and environmental factors. This model suggests that a person with many vulnerable characteristics can experience a good outcome if engaged in a robust, supportive environment.

In the ecological model the environment is the community in which people live. However, the concept of community is deceptively simple. In fact,

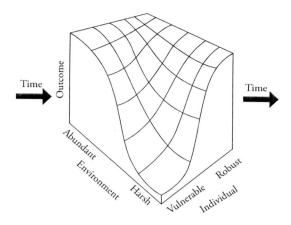

Figure 8.1 Ecological model of disability.

it is vast and complex and varies across important dimension like urban versus rural environments. It includes physical infrastructure—roads, sidewalks, public places, telecommunications, and the like, as well as social policy, social capital, and community functions such as medical services, health programs, housing, education, employment supports, and opportunities, and much more. The density of these community services, which varies dramatically across urban and rural areas can have a dramatic effect on rehabilitation and participation outcomes (Seekins et al., 2011).

The World Health Organization's (WHO) Community-Based Rehabilitation matrix lists five major community functions, including health, education, livelihood, social, and empowerment (WHO, 2010). Major service systems are then organized under these functions. For example, under the function of health, the matrix lists medical care, health promotion, disease prevention, rehabilitation, and access to assistive devices. An emerging challenge for rehabilitation psychology is to understand the processes of community change and to engage change in such a way as to support the achievement of their patient's participation in community.

Rehabilitation Psychology and Community Development

The fields of community development and community psychology focus on the process for promoting change within communities (Chavis & Wandersman, 1990) and on creating new settings (e.g., Sarason, 1972). The focus of the process is on aspects of the structure of a community, including the ways in which a community arranges, delivers, and maintains its members. These community functions reflect the features of environment targeted by

the ICF as environmental features that influence disability outcome. A crucial feature of community structure for people who experience disability involves various community supports for independent living, health, education, and employment.

Communities vary considerably in how they organize and deliver services, and in how they provide supports to maintain their members. Some nations operate a more centralized system in which a wide range of social and health services are linked together. This facilitates efficient planning, delivery, and evaluation. Others, such as the United States, rely on a more decentralized system in which programs are loosely or contingently linked. In the decentralized context, where programs are independent, coordination and collaboration become important objectives. So, linking disability groups advocating for accessible community environments with programs and services that rely on accommodating environments for success becomes an important mediating role.

Community psychologists are one group of professionals with a skill set to manage the community development process. As the importance of the environment becomes more salient to the outcome of rehabilitation, rehabilitation psychologists may find themselves drawn further away from treatment centers that focus on restoration and further into the community, where the effects of the environment must be managed to achieve participation goals. Community psychology has employed an ecological framework for research and practice since its beginning (Sarason, 1972). This framework is consistent with the ICF and may offer resources and examples for rehabilitation psychologists.

Rehabilitation psychologists cannot be expected to be solely responsible for community development. They can, however, work with and through those organizations and agencies with community development responsibilities. In addition, rehabilitation psychologists might offer their unique knowledge and skills to help facilitate community processes. This might include team building work with human service agencies, organizational development for community groups, training for support groups, and advocacy and empowerment consultation for disability rights organizations. At that point, the rehabilitation psychologist might engage colleagues who are community psychologists in a discussion about the intersection of these two specialty groups because they share considerable overlap of interest in both research and practice.

COMMUNITY REHABILITATION PSYCHOLOGICAL RESEARCH

Rehabilitation psychologists must focus research to build new treatment approaches or interventions to develop arrangements of community environments that enhance the impact and utility of individual rehabilitation. Community psychologists are expert in working with communities to design and conduct such research. Rehabilitation psychologists might collaborate with community psychologists to develop "community treatments" to address disability issues. One line of potential research might involve building innovative rehabilitation approaches that anticipate variations and changes in community environments. Similarly, rehabilitation psychologists are involved in conducting research regarding the Livable Communities and Healthy Communities programs. Community planners are incorporating design features of the environment to promote greater engagement with and function for people with mobility, sensory, and cognitive impairments. These include but are not limited to the evaluation of the effects of urban design that incorporates paved walkways on community interactions, as well as the benefits of exercise in their use. Others have worked to establish the measurement of visitable homes as part of the Healthy People 2020 agenda (Centers for Disease Control and Prevention, 2010). Still others are exploring the effects of accessible public transportation on participation (Gonzales, Stombaugh, Seekins, & Kasnitz, 2006; Perenboom & Chorusa, 2003).

One research strategy that may be particularly useful to the CRP is *community-based participatory research* (CBPR; Whyte, 1991). This community research strategy engages community stakeholders in the development of research questions, design, data collection, and interpretation of results. Although this strategy has been used in circumscribed areas, such as disability research, more recently it has been widely adopted in public health. Advantages to CBPR include the social validity and effectiveness of interventions developed and implemented. For people with disabilities, CBPR may incorporate both individual and environmental factors in the ecological model that lead to robust participation outcomes.

COMMUNITY REHABILITATION PSYCHOLOGIST PRACTICE

As with research, rehabilitation psychologists must focus some of their treatment approaches or interventions on developing community environments that enhance the impact and utility of individual rehabilitation. In this effort, psychologists often encounter barriers to building more accommodating environments. These barriers may include public resistance to change, public ambivalence toward disability, habits and traditions, lack of awareness/knowledge, competing interests, authoritarian hierarchies, and simple fear of change. Psychologists are skilled in addressing such barriers to focus on rational planning. For example, psychologists have skills that might be applied to address these problems, including facilitation and negotiation skills, cognitive and behavioral strategies, stages of change knowledge, empowerment and support of grass roots efforts, and skills in CBPR. In addition, psychologists can offer skills for evaluating change and its impacts to develop evidence about the impact of CRP services on community participation.

We have noted that practice is driven by reimbursement, which requires a focus on individual functional outcomes (e.g., Khan, Ng, & Turner-Stokes, 2009). If the rehabilitation psychologist is to take on more community development research and practice, funding mechanisms must support these activities. First, rehabilitation psychologists may advocate for changes in reimbursement policy to support community development activities. It is in the best interest of all parties, including clients, payers, and providers, to create community environments that foster full participation of all citizens. Second, many hospitals have community health initiatives to provide services that improve and maintain the health of all citizens in the community. If these programs employed a CRP, they would be more effective at improving the health of all citizens, including those with disabilities.

Community-Based Rehabilitation Services

We have suggested that, historically, the role of the rehabilitation psychologist has evolved along with our understanding of disability and rehabilitation. Further, we have outlined how emphasizing the methods of community psychology may expand the rehabilitation psychologist's role to support and help develop community-based services. In this section, we will briefly review four community-based services that reflect the WHO's community-based rehabilitation components (WHO, 2010), discuss how rehabilitation psychologist have traditionally interfaced with these services, and examine how their role may be expanded in light of current ecological models of disability.

Independent Living Services

Centers for independent living (CILs) are community-based service and advocacy agencies that were early adopters of the community development framework. These agencies first developed in the United States but have been implemented in communities around the world (Doe, 1999; Fisher & Jing, 2008; Hayashi & Okuhira, 2008; Holland, 2008; Kim, 2008). They are community-based, nonprofit, consumer-directed, nonresidential organizations designed to both advocate for and provide support services to people with disabilities to help them live independently in their community. These grassroots service organizations have developed into a national network that has over 600 offices in the United States and additional programs around the world (Usiak, Moffat, & Wehmeyer, 2004).

Historically, the values and philosophy of independent living were based on traditions of consumer sovereignty, self-reliance, and political and economic civil rights (DeJong, 1983). They grew out of the disability rights movement, which embraced the ecological disability model with its emphasis on aspects of the environment as the source of disability. Hence, the emphasis of these agencies has been on systems change at the local and national levels to reduce barriers and increase opportunities for people with disabilities. Centers for independent living advance this systems change agenda with a core set of independent living services, including information and referral, independent living skills training, peer counseling, and advocacy (i.e., individual and systems). These services provide a two-pronged approach to advancing civil rights: empowerment of the individual and changing social policy.

The clients of CIL services are individuals who experience disability, but often have had little or no rehabilitation services. Hence, they have not had the benefit of a rehabilitation team that would include a rehabilitation psychologist. Even for individuals who go through inpatient rehabilitation, transition back to the local community following relatively brief length of stays limits the services rehabilitation centers can provide for community integration (Seekins et al., 2010). In the absence of professional services, the four core CIL services function to help individuals adapt to living with a disability in the community and change community environments to increase opportunities for participation. To this end, CILs deliver the four core services using methods that reflect independent living philosophy. Central to this philosophy is consumer choice and consumer control (Batavia, 2002; Independent Living Research Utilization, 2005; Rehabilitation Services Administration, 2003).

New CIL service recipients (referred to as "consumers") often initially require information and referral to acquire basic needs such as food, shelter, and safety. Where needed, independent living skills training, as in self-advocacy, communication/social skills, money management, and using transportation services, is provided to begin building self-efficacy for community living (Independent Living Research Utilization, 2005). Peer support is provided during this process to develop insight into community participation possibilities and to further develop the individual's personal independent living philosophy. Some consumers go on to participate in local, state, and national advocacy efforts to affect social policy and protect civil rights (Jones & Brooks, 2010). Hence, CIL services are designed to increase the quality of participation of *individual* consumers, as well as to stimulate social and community change to accommodate all individuals with disabilities.

TRADITIONAL REHABILITATION PSYCHOLOGIST ROLE IN INDEPENDENT LIVING SERVICES

The typical interface that rehabilitation psychologists have with CILs would be through referral of clients to those service agencies. Although no data are available regarding referral sources for CILs, we suspect referral rates from rehabilitation psychologists are very low because it would be unlikely for psychologists working in inpatient settings to have any contact with CILs. It may be more likely for community-based psychologists to be aware of CIL services, but here again, there is little documented practice of these agencies working closely or even consistently with rehabilitation psychologists. This may be due in part to each party emphasizing different aspects of the ecological model: CILs focus more on environmental factors, and rehabilitation psychologists focus more on personal factors. Nonetheless, rehabilitation clients would benefit substantially from referrals to a CIL for reasons already described.

Unlike the other three community services we will review, CILs have no academic training program, thus limiting the research and training available to support their programmatic mission. For example, there is little academic research to support their effectiveness, despite the fact that anecdotal evidence abounds (O'Day, 2005; O'Day, Wilson, Killeen, & Ficke, 2004). Nonetheless, as the pressure mounts to demonstrate the effectiveness of government-funded programs, CILs would benefit from the research and program evaluation skills of rehabilitation psychologists.

Rehabilitation psychologists and CILs have worked as community change agents on a number of common social policy changes, including the U.S. Rehabilitation Act and the Americans with Disabilities Act (Cox, Hess, Hibbard, Layman, & Stewart, 2010). This history provides a good starting place for rehabilitation psychologists to become more active in working with CILs to increase community participation for people with disabilities. For example, peer support is a core CIL service that would benefit from further development. We surveyed all CILs in the United States about their peer support services. Although 90% of CILs provide peer support services, only 45% indicated that they use a formal training program to train peer counselors. Clearly, there is room for program development in this area. Within rehabilitation research, there are studies about using peer support in rehabilitation settings (e.g., Bally & Bakke, 2007; Davidson et al., 2005; Mohr, Burke, Beckner, & Merluzzi, 2005; Rogers et al., 2007; Schwartz & Sendor, 2000). These studies review well-developed training programs and even results from randomized experimental designs. The management of centers for independent living would benefit from consultation on developing and evaluating peer training curricula specific to their mission.

COMMUNITY REHABILITATION PSYCHOLOGIST ROLE IN INDEPENDENT LIVING SERVICES

As noted, CILs are deeply invested in social change. A CRP working with a CIL would form a powerful team for decreasing barriers and increasing opportunities for community participation. Applying his or her skills in the community, the CRP could work with CILs to identify barriers and opportunities of interest to people with disabilities living in the community; facilitate communication with other community agencies, such as housing and transportation providers; and use effective communication and advocacy skills with community leaders to assure that communities build out accessible infrastructure and develop accessible programs (e.g., recreation and fitness centers).

Last, the CRP could partner with CILs to conduct community-based participatory research. The CRP could work with community members to identify relevant topics for research, collect data and report results that could be used by disability advocates in their systems change initiatives. For example, research on the effects of housing and transportation accessibility on the health status of people with disabilities could be used to influence social policy on the provision of home modifications and transportation services.

Vocational Rehabilitation and Employment

From the perspective of a rehabilitation psychologist working in a rehabilitation hospital, vocational rehabilitation (VR) may start as part of the inpatient treatment process, and vocational goals may be incorporated into a treatment plan. At discharge, a patient may be referred to community VR to help retain current employment or to find other employment.

Individuals with disabilities experience higher rates of unemployment compared to their counterparts without disability (U.S. Census Bureau, 2006; U.S. Department of Labor, 2010). In the United States, a system of VR programs has evolved since the end of World War I to provide a wide range of services and supports aimed at assisting individuals with disabilities to acquire and maintain employment. This system evolved into a national federal–state partnership in which the federal government provides 80% of the funding while the states administer the program and provide 20% of the funding. The Rehabilitation Services Administration (2006) served approximately 981,054 individuals, including 346,835 (35%) individuals whose cases were closed after receiving services. Of those individuals with closed cases, 205,448 (59.6%) achieved an employment outcome.

Vocational rehabilitation offers a wide range of services designed to help individuals with disabilities prepare for and engage in gainful employment (e.g., Frank, Rosenthal, & Caplan, 2010). Eligible individuals are those who have a physical or mental impairment that results in a substantial impediment to employment, who can benefit from VR services for employment, and who require VR services. Priority must be given to serving individuals with the most significant disabilities if a state is unable to serve all eligible individuals. Overall, the public VR system serves clients who experience intellectual and developmental disabilities, mental illness, sensory impairments, cognitive impairments from injury and stoke, and mobility impairments from injury and chronic disease.

The standard model of VR involves five broad phases: initial intake (e.g., conducting client interviews and intake assessments to determine legibility), developing individual plans for employment (IPEs; e.g., developing goals, formulating plans, etc.), organizing and providing services to implement the IPE's objectives (e.g., purchasing training services, conducting client follow-ups, making referrals, etc.), providing counseling and guidance (i.e. therapeutic counseling), and providing job-related services (e.g., completing resumes, job searches, etc.; Holmes, 2007).

Although the VR process varies from country to country, and even from state to state within countries, the basic structure and process of the public program is universal (Gard & Larsson, 2006; Holmes, 2007; Tompa, de Oliveira, Dolinschi, & Irvin, 2008). After establishing eligibility based on disability, a VR counselor provides counseling to the client. This counseling may address issues ranging from adjustment to disability to exploring employment goals. As part of the counseling process, the VR counselor works with a client to develop an IPE. This plan states an employment goal and outlines the steps a client needs to take to achieve the goal. The counselor arranges services designed to achieve the client's employment goal. In most cases, the VR counselor contracts with other community service providers for those services.

Despite decades of service, the unemployment rate among people with disabilities has remained stubbornly high (Dutta, Gervey, Chan, Chih-Chin Chou, & Ditchman, 2008). Recently, some analysts have redefined the problem. They pointed out that many people with disabilities counted in these high estimates of unemployment are technically not in the labor force (U.S. Department of Labor, 2010). These analysts argue that the "true" rate of unemployment is calculated only for those in the labor force; approximately 14%. This estimate comes from excluding those who are "out of the labor force" from the calculation and including only those who are actively seeking employment. Of course, this tends to produce an underestimate of the rate of employment of those who would like to work but who have given up searching for a job.

Others continue to search for new strategies for promoting economic self-sufficiency for people with disabilities—regardless of the rate of unemployment. Surprisingly, little experimental research has been conducted to establish an evidence base for VR practice. Still, new models are going beyond traditional VR counseling to develop community models that emerge from the environmental model that forms the foundation for the ICF (Chan, Tarvydas, Blalock, Strauser, & Atkins, 2009). In developing countries, these approaches may come as little surprise. For example, self-employment has been identified as a viable employment option for many, and support for business ownership from VR has grown (Arnold & Ipsen, 2005; Kendall, Buys, Charker, & MacMillan, 2006). Research has also demonstrated the feasibility of community economic development programs led by people with disabilities that create new business that are either owned by or employ people with disabilities (Ipsen, Seekins, Arnold, & Kraync, 2006). Similarly, researchers have explored the potential involvement of worker cooperatives (Lorenzo, van Niekerk, & Mdlokolo, 2007; Sperry & Brusin, 2001).

TRADITIONAL REHABILITATION PSYCHOLOGIST ROLE EMPLOYMENT SERVICES

Vocational rehabilitation may contract with a rehabilitation psychologist for specific services in support of achieving an employment goal. These services may include individual- and group-oriented therapies that help individuals prepare for work (e.g., stress management). They also may address specific psychiatric conditions that are interfering with the VR process (e.g., depression, anxiety, post-traumatic stress disorder [PTSD]). They also may contribute to the ongoing physical rehabilitation process by addressing motivation and adaptation to disability issues. These functions are similar to those observed in support of inpatient rehabilitation services.

COMMUNITY REHABILITATION PSYCHOLOGIST ROLE IN EMPLOYMENT SERVICES

For individuals who are ready for employment, employers are the key to their success. As with many community members, employers often lack understanding and awareness about disability, and this limits their willingness to hire people with disabilities. The CRP may be an effective community advocate on behalf of people with disabilities who helps employers change attitudes and learn the value of including people with disabilities in their businesses. This work could come through collaboration with employer membership organizations (e.g., chambers of commerce), public employment programs for the general population, and business development groups working to attract business for local economic development. A CRP is uniquely qualified to move this agenda forward and create employment opportunities where none currently exists. Because employment and business development are cornerstones of the community development process, working for inclusion of people with disabilities increases the likelihood that new community infrastructure will be accessible to all. Increasing employment opportunities may be the single most important activity undertaken by the CRP to improve the full participation of people with disabilities.

Community-Based Health Services

People with disabilities use many of the same community health care services as the general population, only at much higher rates (LaPlante, Rice, & Wenger, 1995; Lustig, Strauser, & Donnell, 2003; Neri & Kroll, 2003; Rice & Trupin, 1996). This is in part due to disability that results from chronic health conditions (Drum, Horner-Johnson, & Krahn, 2008). The full array of community health services includes acute, rehabilitative, and health promoting services. Figure 8.2 depicts a conceptual continuum of health services that encompasses interventions at both the individual and environmental levels. It begins with acute medical services and shows linkages through rehabilitation to health promotion. The line drawn from left to right shows how a patient might progress through these health services to result in a good quality of life.

Reading the diagram from left to right, acute medical care treats acute conditions that may either be primarily or secondarily disabling. The outcome of acute medical procedures is a function of patient characteristics, such as existing health conditions and demographic population (e.g., age, gender, race). When acute medical interventions are 100% effective, individuals are returned to a priori and preintervention levels of participation and QOL. Of course, not all medical procedures lead to 100% recovery or cure.

When acute medical outcomes do not lead to full recovery, medical rehabilitation interventions may be used to improve functional outcome for accessing the community. People with disabilities use community-based rehabilitation services intermittently (Batt-Rawden & Tellness, 2005). People with degenerative conditions that cause functional loss over time may use physical, occupational, speech, and psychological services at various stages. Similarly, individuals who are aging with traditionally static functional loss (e.g., spinal cord injury) may use rehabilitation services during the aging process. These interventions range from increasing the function of particular body structures (e.g., vocal cords via speech therapy) through the use of assistive technology like wheelchairs. Again, the outcome from medical rehabilitation procedures is considered a function of patient characteristics (i.e., post-acute residual function and age).

When medical rehabilitation outcomes are 100% effective, the patient will have gained the ability to fully participate in his or her community. Using the best available rehabilitation technology, full participation could be a common rehabilitation outcome.

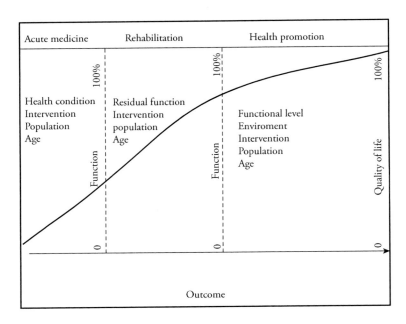

Figure 8.2 Continuum of community-based health services.

However, the cost of providing assistive technology for accessing the environment is often prohibitive. This can be viewed as either a technological or an environmental problem. Accessible environments require less expensive rehabilitation equipment for participation. For example, the Ibot, an expensive wheelchair that can climb stairs, is unnecessary in ramp- and lift-equipped environments.

People spend most of their lives in the last part of the framework, which represents the goal of all health services: regaining and maintaining health-related QOL through health promotion and health maintenance. Ultimately, the translation of acute medical and rehabilitative procedures into QOL depends on the behavioral choices available to the individual. These choices occur at the intersection of the individual and his or her environment; the richer and more accessible the environment, the greater the opportunity to participate in community life, including health promoting activities (Masala & Petretto, 2008). Traditionally, health promotion interventions aim to reduce health risk factors and increase health protective factors to reduce morbidity and mortality. When considering health promotion for people with functional loss, interventions also must include features of the environment that facilitate or impede participation. For example, a health promotion intervention might target the establishment of programs or policies that increase the accessibility of the built environment (i.e., trails or public places) or address social environments (i.e., modifying negative attitudes; Antle, Mills, Steele, Kalnins, & Rossen, 2008). From this perspective, the absence of participation opportunities is a health risk factor (Ravesloot et al., 2011).

Health promotion programs for people with disabilities are relatively recent innovations. They have used both generic and novel health behavior change strategies, such as increasing self-efficacy for health behaviors (Becker, Stuifbergen, Oh, & Hall, 1993), increasing physical activity (Rimmer, Nicola, Riley, & Creviston, 2002), and altering health beliefs about the utility of health behavior in the context of one's disability (Ravesloot, Seekins, & Young, 1998). Most interventions have focused on specific impairments, such as multiple sclerosis (Stuifbergen, 1995), cerebral palsy (Lollar, 1994), and post-polio syndrome (Zemper et al., 2003), to name a few. Alternatively, to accommodate the needs of rural people, cross-disability approaches have emerged. For example, we used participatory research methods to develop a health promotion program for people with disabilities in conjunction with centers for independent living titled, "Living Well with a Disability" (www.livingandworkingwell. org). This intervention uses concepts from the stress and illness (Antonovsky, 1987), positive psychology (Seligman, 1990), and rehabilitation (Ravesloot et al., 1998) literature to affect health behavior change. Participants engage in a 10-week workshop to develop QOL goals, confidence to reach those goals, and exploration of health behavior that supports goal attainment. Results indicate health behavior and secondary condition improvements that are maintained over 12 months. Additionally, reductions in health care utilization translate into overall cost savings after accounting for the costs of program implementation (Ravesloot, Seekins, & White, 2005).

Last, complementary medicine is a family of services often included in community health discussions. Although psychotherapy is sometimes grouped with complementary medicine, the field also includes disciplines like acupuncture, massage, homeopathy, and energy medicine (Trieschmann, 1995). The rehabilitation psychologist working in the community settings will benefit from a working knowledge of complementary medicine, if for no other reason than the popularity of these services among clients. However, many of these modalities have shown effectiveness clinically (Trieschmann, 1995), as well as in clinical research trials (Chapman, Weintraub, Milburn, Pirozzi, & Woo, 1999; Molsberger, Mau, Pawelec, & Winkler, 2002; Moyer, Rounds, & Hannum, 2004).

TRADITIONAL ROLE OF THE REHABILITATION PSYCHOLOGIST IN HEALTH SERVICES

Rehabilitation psychologists have played an important role in each of the health service areas in Figure 8.2. With regard to acute medical care, rehabilitation psychologists make referrals when they detect the potential need for acute services that the client may not be aware of or acknowledge (e.g., diabetes screening). For clients with disability related to chronic health conditions, regular communication with primary care providers can facilitate common treatment goals between clients and providers. Additionally, motivation for self-management of chronic conditions is commonly addressed by rehabilitation psychologists. Unfortunately, most of the chronic disease self-management research has been conducted by health psychologists who understand issues related to health behavior change, but have less familiarity with the impact disability may have on self-management. For people with disabilities, the rehabilitation psychologist may be a better source for learning to management chronic conditions within the disability context (Ravesloot et al., 2011).

Rehabilitation psychologists work with community-based rehabilitation providers to help clients meet their participation goals by making efficient use of physical, occupational, and speech therapies. Traditionally, this role has used referral and consultation with these allied health providers.

Finally, with regard to health promotion, health psychologists working in community settings promote both the physical and mental health of clients. Rehabilitation psychologists may add the provision of health promotion services to traditional practice. In the United States, these individual and group services are reimbursable through Health Behavior Assessment and Intervention clinical procedure codes (e.g., 96150–96154).

COMMUNITY REHABILITATION PSYCHOLOGIST ROLE IN HEALTH SERVICES

The community psychologist role has potential functions in each of the three health service areas in Figure 8.2. In acute medical care, the CRP may play an important role in access to care. Although people with disabilities use health care services at a higher rate, they actually have poorer access to care than the general population (Lustig & Strauser, 2010; McColl, Jarzynowska, & Shortt, 2010). For example, access to basic primary care can be limited by physical accessibility, as well as by communication inaccessibility. Physical inaccessibility often relates to accessibility of medical equipment, including exam tables and diagnostic equipment (e.g., mammogram machines). Communication inaccessibility occurs when health care professionals do not provide access to interpreter services for people who are deaf or self-help materials in alternative formats for people with visual impairments. The rehabilitation psychologist may work with community health service providers to improve health care infrastructure and access to care. This may be easier in countries with socialized medicine, where the government plays a central role in health care service delivery.

Working with community rehabilitation service providers, the CRP may be instrumental in coordinating services to meet the participation goals of clients. For example, the CRP may work with physical therapists and transportation providers to meet transportation needs of clients with goals that require regular transportation services. Using a broader community perspective, the CRP may work with local transportation providers to use the most accessible transportation options available, communicate with the physical therapist regarding the physical demands of available transportation, and work with the client to develop self-efficacy for using those services.

Last, community-based health promotion may provide the greatest opportunities for the rehabilitation psychologist to go beyond clinical practice to address community change that leads to improved health outcomes (Letcher & Perlow, 2009). Many studies have indicated health and QOL are related to the level of participation of people with disabilities (e.g., Batt-Rawden & Tellnes, 2005; Huang, Chou, Lin, & Chao, 2007; Jette, Keysor, Coster, Ni, & Haley, 2005). While clinical practice may address the individual factors that limit participation, it is the consultation, training and education, and research of the CRP that can move the community participation agenda forward at the national and local levels.

Education

Schools are one of the most prolific community-based services used by people with disabilities. Although not traditionally included within the scope of rehabilitation psychology, transition from schools to community living is an evolving topic in special education that needs the skills of rehabilitation psychologists (Frank, Gluck, & Buckelew, 1990). Consistent with the theme of this chapter, the purpose of education as specified by the U.S. Department of Education includes preparing students "to hold desired employment and to participate actively and wisely in the nation's civic affairs" p. 6 (U.S. Department of Education, 2007). As agents of systems and community change, engaging schools in the community transition process may be a very productive strategy for creating equal access to improved participation for all individuals with disabilities. In this section, we will briefly review the current state of transition practice to highlight the contributions rehabilitation psychologists can make to maximize the participation and QOL of young adults.

The International Labour Office (1998) defined transition as:

> [A] process of social orientation that implies status and role change (e.g., from student to trainee, from trainee to worker and from dependence to independence), and is central to integration into society.... Transition requires a change in

relationships, routines and self-image. In order to guarantee a smoother transition from school to the workplace, young people with disabilities need to develop goals and identify the role they want to play in society.

Similarly, in a report regarding transitions, the European Agency for Development in Special Needs Education suggests " 'A good life for all', as well as 'a good job for all' are the ultimate goals of a successful overall transition process." In the United States, amendments to the Individuals with Disabilities Education Act (IDEA; PL-105–17) in 1997 mandated that, starting at age 14, all individualized education programs (IEP) include transition plan statements (Individuals with Disabilities Education Act of 1997).

Although many students with disabilities have learning and psychiatric impairments, a sizeable proportion has physical and sensory impairments. According to the Office of Special Education Programs (OSEP; 2002), 9% of all U.S. students attending public school between the ages of 3 and 21 were served by the Individuals with Disabilities Education Act. Of these, 1.2% of the students had hearing impairments, 1.3% had orthopedic impairments, and 0.4% had visual impairments. 0.4% had traumatic brain injury, 18.6% had speech and language impairments, 2.2% had multiple disabilities, and 5.8% were classified as "other health impaired." In the United Kingdom, 1,656,000, or approximately 21% of students, were served by special education. Of these students, 5% had speech language and communication difficulties, 3% had hearing/visual/multi-sensory impairments, 2% had physical disabilities, and 8% had other difficulties/disabilities (Department of Children, Schools and Families, 2009).

The number of special education students has increased in recent years; however, the ability of schools to prepare students to participate has improved only marginally (Test et al., 2009). The most recent data from the United States indicated that 72.6% of youth with disabilities lived with parents after high school, 7.7% attended 4-year college, 12.8% attended 2-year community college, and 9.9% lived alone (Test et al., 2009). These statistics clearly show that it has been difficult for schools to transition students into communities that often are neither environmentally or socially accessible to people with disabilities.

Transition from special education to community living is a common problem internationally.

The European Agency for Development in Special Needs Education analyzed policies and practices from 16 countries and identified eight issues and difficulties for moving the transition agenda forward, including lack of data, poor completion rates, poor access to education and training, limited vocational preparation, high unemployment rates, low expectations and attitudes, poor workplace accessibility, and problems with implementing existing legislation. (European Agency for Development in Special Needs Education/Soriano, V., 2006).

Consistent with social models of disability, recommendations for transition planning commonly include both individually focused and community collaboration elements. For example, the European Agency Transition from School to Employment Report (European Agency for Development in Special Needs Education/Soriano, V. 2006) made recommendations based on the issues cited above, taken together with testimony from 80 young people (14 to 20 years old) with disabilities, their parents, and employers representing 22 countries at the European Parliament, in Brussels, in 2003. Recommendations from this process included specifying transition planning as a separate component of the IEP that includes active participation of the student and families, interagency cooperation, and flexibility that is responsive to the student's changing values and experiences. Others have identified a variety of evidence-based components to transition best practice including interagency and interdisciplinary collaboration; integrated schools, classrooms, and employment; functional life-skills curriculum and community-based instruction; social and personal skills development and training; career and vocational assessment and education; business and industry linkages with schools; development of effective IEP planning documents; processes addressing IDEA 1997 transition services language requirements; student self-determination, advocacy, and input in transition planning; and parent or family involvement in transition planning (Zhang, Ivester, Chen, & Katsiyannis, 2005).

A recent systematic review of the transition literature suggests the relative contributions of community-focused and individually focused interventions (Test et al., 2009). This review of 22 studies involving over 24,000 participations identified 16 predictor variables associated with improved transition outcomes. Of these, 11 were correlated with post-secondary education, five with independent living, and all 16 with post-school employment. Those predictors with the greatest effect sizes are malleable to individually focused interventions, including empowerment, self-realization, and self-regulation. This is in contrast to the emphasis of most current transition programs that emphasize interagency coordination. The National Longitudinal Study-2, conducted over 10 years and involving 9,000 students in the United States, reported that only 58% of students provided some input into their transition planning, while only 12% took a leadership role (Cameto, Levine, & Wagner, 2004).

REHABILITATION PSYCHOLOGIST TRADITIONAL ROLES IN SCHOOL TRANSITIONS

Traditionally, rehabilitation psychologists have not played a significant role in transition from school to community living despite the clear overlap in student needs and the rehabilitation psychologist's skills. As noted earlier, this may be largely due to work settings and reimbursement policy that impact practice. However, as we have suggested, current values guiding rehabilitation outcomes that create more opportunities for community practice may also create opportunities for improving transition practice.

In contrast to the experience of adults living in community, students in schools have a lot of support. For example, schools are usually accessible. Accommodations for a disability are common and protected by laws that are watched carefully by parents. There typically are multiple safety nets that help students progress through school, with multiple adults monitoring the educational process. In fact, special education may be "too special," in that students learn to depend on the school at the expense of developing self-confidence and empowerment (Kochhar-Bryant & Izzo, 2006). When they graduate, many of these students struggle to transition to adult roles, including community resident and employee. Rehabilitation psychologists are well equipped to help individuals adapt to community living with a disability, which is the challenge that students with disabilities face.

Rehabilitation psychologists are skilled at helping individuals new to disability to develop self-confidence for community engagement. Students with disabilities are not new to disability, but instead may be considered "new" to community. Becoming confident to fully participate in community has been described as a process with 12 distinct components: choice-making; decision-making; problem-solving; goal setting and attainment; independence, risk-taking, and safety skills; self-observation, evaluation, and reinforcement skills; self-instruction; self-advocacy and leadership skills; internal locus of control; positive attributes of efficacy and outcome expectancy; self -awareness; and self-knowledge (Wehmeyer, Agran, & Hughes, 1998). A retrospective study of college students asked how they became empowered. The most common response was "trial and error" (Thoma & Getzel, 2005). Clearly, the expertise of the rehabilitation psychologist would benefit the transition process.

Schools have worked to improve transitions by using "person-centered planning" that puts the needs of the student at the center of the transition process. This approach has been criticized because the student can be central yet uninvolved in the planning process (Wehman, 2006). Putting students first and empowering them to lead the transition process requires planning and implementing transition in a student-driven manner, thereby empowering the student, and the significant people in his or her life, to actualize individual specific goals for adulthood (Carter et al., 2009; Wehman 2006; Williams, Westmorland, Lin, Schmuck, & Creen, 2006). This approach, although effective, may require changes in family dynamics that allow emancipation of the student with a disability. The rehabilitation psychologist who commonly works with family members has important skills that can help schools realize student-driven transition planning.

COMMUNITY REHABILITATION PSYCHOLOGIST ROLE IN SCHOOL TRANSITIONS

The CRP could also improve community transition outcomes by working in community development. Negative attitudes toward people with disabilities in the community have been cited as one of the most problematic aspects of successful transitions (Schwartz, Mactavish, & Lutfiyya, 2006). Working in communities to improve the education and understanding of employers regarding the needs of transitioning students would also benefit the transitions process. Further, working with VR counselors to better understand the empowerment needs of the transitioning student would be beneficial. (Luecking, 2003, 2008). Last, communities that are truly open to the needs of people with disabilities will facilitate better transitions for students.

Other Community Services
GOVERNMENT SERVICES

Other community services used frequently by people with disabilities are government services such as basic subsistence payments, subsidized housing, and public transportation. Although these services vary enormously by governing body, they are essential to the community participation of individuals. Access to these services is generally tightly controlled through determination criteria. Even these criteria can vary significantly based on which services are being accessed. For example, the U.S. government has 50 different definitions of disability depending on the department providing services. Seekins et al. (2010) reported that support service fragmentation is among the top 10 barriers individuals face when transitioning from a skilled nursing facility back to community living. Unfortunately, in countries with decentralized service systems, this kind of fragmentation is the rule rather than the exception and is well known to those who conduct discharge planning from rehabilitation hospitals back to community living (Chan et al., 2009; Chavis & Wandersman, 1990). The rehabilitation psychologist needs to be sensitive to the difficulties people face in accessing government services and must recognize the sense of helplessness and stress accompanying accessing these services. Here again, the rehabilitation psychologist can play an important role in working with communities to implement systems that work for people with disabilities.

PERSONAL ASSISTANT SERVICES

People with severe disabilities often rely on personal assistant services (PAS). These services may be provided by community nursing agencies, CILs, or other service agencies. The availability of these services is often the difference between living in the community versus institutionalization. Recent years have witnessed a shift in PAS from agency to consumer-directed services (Usiak, Stone, House, & Montgomery, 2004). With consumer-directed services, the person with a disability hires, trains, manages, and pays the personal assistant with funds passed through an agency such as a CIL. This approach is in contrast to PAS provided through an agency that accomplishes each of these tasks. Self-directed PAS has developed to address problems with personal assistants being responsive to the agency, rather than the consumer. As self-directed PAS becomes more widely available, teaching consumers communication and management skills becomes increasingly important. This is another need that the rehabilitation psychologist is well suited to meet, whether it be through curriculum development, program evaluation, or direct service provision to individuals using PAS. Finally, because the vast majority of community services and supports used by individuals are provided by informal supports (Thompson, 2004), the rehabilitation psychologist may use family therapies to address the role changes and caregiver stress that are common difficulties in these informal arrangements.

DURABLE MEDICAL EQUIPMENT VENDORS

People with disabilities are often in need of durable medical equipment (DME). Equipment vendors typically supply equipment that rehabilitation professionals have determined is necessary to maximize community participation by the individual. These needs are not static. Changes in functional level due to health condition progression and changes related to the aging process itself affect needs for DME. The individual's needs for DME are best determined by his or her goals to function in specific environments. For example, an individual who can use a manual wheelchair may need a power wheelchair to go long distances. In this instance, the person will need to have good communication skills to convince medical providers to approve the equipment and for DME providers to get the best possible equipment. Fostering this communication through skills training, as well as through direct advocacy represents yet another role the rehabilitation psychologist may play.

Conclusion

Changes in community hold great promise for improving rehabilitation outcomes that include participation of people with disabilities. The rehabilitation psychologist is uniquely qualified to support the individual's adaptation to community and the community's adaption to the individual. From an ecological perspective, both are necessary to maximize outcomes. The CRP may work with community service providers to better meet the needs of individual clients and join forces with these providers to continue the work of community change. Through this combined effort, the promise of full participation for all citizens will one day be realized.

Future Directions

The role of community services is becoming increasingly important to the experience of people with disabilities. These changes are creating further opportunities for the rehabilitation psychologist, and this raises important questions about roles and responsibilities:

• Who is responsible for representing disability issues in the ongoing routine of community development and planning?

- What is the role of rehabilitation psychologists in community development?
- What is the role of rehabilitation psychologists in shaping social policies that affect rehabilitation outcome in the community?

The answers to these questions will evolve over time as the rehabilitation psychologist engages the community to define and establish a CRP role that compliments the roles taken by other community members. Ideally, they will come from a dialog established between rehabilitation psychologists and the communities they serve. If participation is in fact, the ultimate rehabilitation outcome, then rehabilitation psychologists have much more to offer this dynamic and changing field by engaging communities to accelerate social change.

Acknowledgments

This chapter was supported in part by a grant from the U.S. Department of Education (H133B080023). The authors wish to thank Lauri Lindquist for background research she contributed to the project.

References

Antle, B. J., Mills, W., Steele, C., Kalnins, I., & Rossen, B. (2008). An exploratory study of parents' approaches to health promotion in families of adolescents with physical disabilities. *Child: Care, Health and Development, 34*(2), 185–193.

Antonovsky, A. (1987). *Unraveling the mystery of health.* San Francisco: Jossey-Bass.

Arnold, N. L., & Ipsen, C. (2005). Self-employment policies: Changes through the decade. *Journal of Disability Policy Studies, 16*(2), 115–122.

Bally, S. J., & Bakke, M. H. (2007). A peer mentor training program for aural rehabilitation. *Trends in Amplification, 11*(2), 125–131.

Barker, R. (1968). *Ecological psychology: Concepts and methods for studying the environment of human behavior.* Stanford, CA: Stanford University Press.

Batavia, A. I. (2002). Consumer direction, consumer choice, and the future of long-term care. *Journal of Disability Policy Studies. Special Issue: Self-Determination, 13*(2), 67–73.

Batt-Rawden, K. B., & Tellnes, G. (2005). Nature-culture-health activities as a method of rehabilitation: An evaluation of participants' health, quality of life and function. *International Journal of Rehabilitation Research, 28*(2), 175–180.

Becker, H., Stuifbergen, A., Oh, H. S., & Hall, S. (1993). Self-rated abilities for health practices: A health self-efficacy measure. *Health Values: The Journal of Health Behavior, Education and Promotion, 17*(5), 42–50.

Bolles, R. C. (Ed.). (1993). *The story of psychology: A thematic history.* Pacific Grove, CA: Brooks/Cole Publishing Company.

Cameto, R., Levine, P., & Wagner, M. (2004). *Transition planning for students with disabilities: A special topic report of findings from the national longitudinal transition study-2 (NLTS2).* Washington, DC: National Center for Special Education Research.

Carter, E. W., Trainor, A. A., Cakiroglu, O., Cole, O., Swedeen, B., Ditchman, N., et al. (2009). Exploring school-employer partnerships to expand career development and early work experiences for youth with disabilities. *Career Development for Exceptional Individuals, 32*(3), 145–159.

Centers for Disease Control and Prevention. (2010). *Healthy people 2020: The road ahead.* Retrieved August 8, 2010, from http://healthypeople.gov/HP2020/

Chan, F., Tarvydas, V., Blalock, K., Strauser, D., & Atkins, B. J. (2009). Unifying and elevating rehabilitation counseling through model-driven, diversity-sensitive evidence-based practice. *Rehabilitation Counseling Bulletin, 52*(2), 114–119.

Chapman, E. H., Weintraub, R. J., Milburn, M. A., Pirozzi, T. O., & Woo, E. (1999). Homeopathic treatment of mild traumatic brain injury: A randomized, double-blind, placebo-controlled clinical trial. *The Journal of Head Trauma Rehabilitation, 14*(6), 521–542.

Chavis, D. M., & Wandersman, A. (1990). Sense of community in the urban environment: A catalyst for participation and community development. *American Journal of Community Psychology, 18*(1), 55–81.

Cox, D. R., Hess, D. W., Hibbard, M. R., Layman, D. E., & Stewart, R. K., Jr. (2010). Specialty practice in rehabilitation psychology. *Professional Psychology: Research and Practice, 41*(1), 82–88.

Davidson, L., Chinman, M. J., Kloos, B., Weingarten, R., Stayner, D. A., & Tebes, J. K. (2005). *Peer support among individuals with severe mental illness: A review of the evidence.* Boston, MA: Center for Psychiatric Rehabilitation/Boston U.

DeJong, G. (1979). Independent living: From social movement to analytic paradigm. *Archives of Physical Medicine and Rehabilitation, 60,* 435–446.

DeJong, G. (1983). Defining and implementing the independent living concept. *Independent living for physically disabled people* (pp. 4–27). San Francisco: Jossey-Bass Publishers.

Department of Children, Schools and Families. (2009). *Chapter 1: Prevalence of pupils with special education needs.* Retrieved July 22, 2010, from http://www.dcsf.gov.uk/rsgateway/DB/STA/t000851/index.shtml

Doe, T. (1999). *Definitions of independent living worldwide.* Retrieved July 28, 2010, from http://www.ilru.org/html/projects/international/23-definitions.htm

Drum, C. E., Horner-Johnson, W., & Krahn, G. L. (2008). Self-rated health and healthy days: Examining the "disability paradox." *Disability and Health Journal, 1*(2), 71–78.

Dutta, A., Gervey, R., Chan, F., Chih-Chin Chou, & Ditchman, N. (2008). Vocational rehabilitation services and employment outcomes for people with disabilities: A united states study. *Journal of Occupational Rehabilitation, 18*(4), 326–334.

European Agency for Development in Special Needs Education/ Soriano, V. (Ed.). (2006). *Transition from school to employment. Main issues and options faced by students with special educational needs in 16 European countries.* European Agency for Development in Special Needs Education: Middelfart.

Fisher, K., & Jing, L. (2008). Chinese disability independent living policy. *Disability and Society, 23*(2), 171–185.

Frank, R. G., Gluck, J. P., & Buckelew, S. P. (1990). Rehabilitation: Psychology's greatest opportunity? *American Psychologist, 45*(6), 757–761.

Frank, R. G., Rosenthal, M., & Caplan, B. (2010). *Handbook of rehabilitation psychology* (2nd ed.). Washington, DC: American Psychological Association.

Gard, G., & Larsson, A. (2006). How can cooperation between rehabilitation professionals in rehabilitation planning be improved? A qualitative study from the employer's perspective. *Work: Journal of Prevention, Assessment and Rehabilitation, 26*(2), 191–196.

Gobelet, C., Luthi, F., Al-Khodairy, A. T., & Chamberlain, M. A. (2007). Vocational rehabilitation: A multidisciplinary intervention. *Disability and Rehabilitation: An International, Multidisciplinary Journal. Special Issue: Return to Work (RTW) in Selected Disabilities, 29*(17), 1405–1410.

Gonzales, L., Stombaugh, D., Seekins, T., & Kasnitz, D. (2006). Accessible rural transportation: An evaluation of the travelers cheque voucher program. *Community Development: Journal of the Community, 37*(3), 106–115.

Hayashi, R., & Okuhira, M. (2008). The independent living movement in Asia: Solidarity from Japan. *Disability and Society, 23*(5), 417–429.

Holland, D. (2008). The current status of disability activism and non-governmental organizations in post-communist Europe: Preliminary findings based on reports from the field. *Disability and Society, 23*(6), 543–555.

Holmes, J. (Ed.). (2007). *Vocational rehabilitation* (8th ed.). Oxford, UK: Blackwell Publishing.

Huang, H., Chou, C., Lin, K., & Chao, Y. C. (2007). The relationships between disability level, health-promoting lifestyle, and quality of life in outpatients with systemic lupus erythematosus. *The Journal of Nursing Research: JNR, 15*(1), 21–32.

Independent Living Research Utilization. (2005). *An orientation to independent living centers.* Retrieved July 12, 2010, from http://www.ilru.org/html/publications/ilru/general_orientation_to_IL.pdf

Individuals with Disabilities Education Act, 20 U.S.C. 1400 et seq. U.S.C. §601 (1997); amended.

Ipsen, C., Seekins, T., Arnold, N., & Kraync, K. (2006). A citizen led program for rural community economic development: Two case studies. *Community Development: Journal of the Community Development Society, 37*(3), 53–69.

International Labour Office. (1998). *Education, employment and training policies and programmes for youth with disabilities in four European countries.* Geneva: International Labour Office.

Jette, A. M., Keysor, J., Coster, W., Ni, P., & Haley, S. (2005). Beyond function: Predicting participation in a rehabilitation cohort. *Archives of Physical Medicine and Rehabilitation, 86*(11), 2087–2094.

Jones, G., & Brooks, B. (2010). *Get to the core of it: Individual advocacy.* Retrieved July 13, 2010, from http://www.ilru.org/html/training/webcasts/archive/2010/06–09-CIL-NET.html

Kendall, E., Buys, N., Charker, J., & MacMillan, S. (2006). Self-employment: An under-utilised vocational rehabilitation strategy. *Journal of Vocational Rehabilitation, 25*(3), 197–205.

Khan, F., Ng, L., & Turner-Stokes, L. (2009). Effectiveness of vocational rehabilitation intervention on the return to work and employment of persons with multiple sclerosis. *Cochrane Database of Systematic Reviews (Online), 1,* CD007256–CD007256.

Kim, K. M. (2008). The current status and future of centers for independent living in Korea. *Disability and Society, 23*(1), 67–76.

Kochhar-Bryant, C. A., & Izzo, M. V. (2006). Access to post-high school services: Transition assessment and the summary of performance. *Career Development for Exceptional Individuals, 29*(2), 70–89.

LaPlante, M. P., Rice, D. P., & Wenger, B. L. (1995). Medical care use, health insurance, and disability in the united states. *Disability Statistics Abstracts, 8,* 1–4.

Letcher, A. S., & Perlow, K. M. (2009). Community-based participatory research shows how a community initiative creates networks to improve well-being. *American Journal of Preventive Medicine, 37*(6 Suppl 1), S292–S299.

Lollar, D. J. (1994). *Preventing secondary conditions associated with spina bifida or cerebral palsy.* Proceedings and recommendations of a symposium. Washington, DC: Spina Bifida Association of America.

Lorenzo, T., van Niekerk, L., & Mdlokolo, P. (2007). Economic empowerment and black disabled entrepreneurs: Negotiating partnerships in Cape Town, South Africa. *Disability and Rehabilitation, 29*(5), 429–436.

Luecking, R. G. (2003). Employer perspectives on hiring and accommodating youth in transition. *Journal of Special Education Technology, 18*(4), 65–72.

Luecking, R. G. (2008). Emerging employer views of people with disabilities and the future of job development. *Journal of Vocational Rehabilitation, 29*(1), 3–13.

Lustig, D. C., & Strauser, D. R. (2010). Health benefits for vocational rehabilitation consumers: Comparison of access rates with workers in the general population. *Rehabilitation Counseling Bulletin, 53*(2), 87–95.

Lustig, D. C., Strauser, D. R., & Donnell, C. (2003). Quality employment outcomes: Benefits for individuals with disabilities. *Rehabilitation Counseling Bulletin, 47*(1), 5–14.

Masala, C., & Petretto, D. R. (2008). From disablement to enablement: Conceptual models of disability in the 20th century. *Disability and Rehabilitation: An International, Multidisciplinary Journal, 30*(17), 1233–1244.

McColl, M. A., Jarzynowska, A., & Shortt, S. E. D. (2010). Unmet health care needs of people with disabilities: Population level evidence. *Disability and Society, 25*(2), 205–218.

Mohr, D. C., Burke, H., Beckner, V., & Merluzzi, N. (2005). A preliminary report on a skills-based telephone-administered peer support programme for patients with multiple sclerosis. *Multiple Sclerosis (Houndmills, Basingstoke, England), 11*(2), 222–226.

Molsberger, A. F., Mau, J., Pawelec, D. B., & Winkler, J. (2002). Does acupuncture improve the orthopedic management of chronic low back pain: A randomized, blinded, controlled trial with 3 months follow up. *Pain, 99*(3), 579–587.

Moyer, C. A., Rounds, J., & Hannum, J. W. (2004). A meta-analysis of massage therapy research. *Psychological Bulletin, 130*(1), 3–18.

Neri, M. T., & Kroll, T. (2003). Understanding the consequences of access barriers to health care: Experiences of adults with disabilities. *Disability and Rehabilitation, 25*(2), 85.

O'Day, B. (2005). *Independence and the transition to community living: The role of the independent living center.* Retrieved July 28, 2010, from http://www.ilru.org/html/publications/ilru/issues_transition_community1.htm

O'Day, B., Wilson, J., Killeen, M., & Ficke, R. (2004). Consumer outcomes of centers for independent living program. *Journal of Vocational Rehabilitation. Special Issue: Independent Living Management/Rehabilitation Counseling, 20*(2), 83–89.

Office of Special Education Programs (OSEP). (2002). *Table AA6. Number of children served under IDEA, Part B by disability and age group during the 2000–01 school year.* Available at http://www.Ideadata.org/arc_toc2.html#partbCC

Perenboom, R. J. M., & Chorusa, A. M. J. (2003). Measuring participation according the international classification of functioning, disability and health (ICF). *Disability and Rehabilitation, 25*(11), 577–587.

Ravesloot, C., Seekins, T., & White, G. (2005). Living well with a disability health promotion intervention: Improved health status for consumers and lower costs for policy makers. *Rehabilitation Psychology, 50*(3), 239–245.

Ravesloot, C., Seekins, T., & Young, Q. (1998). Health promotion for people with chronic illness and physical disabilities: The connection between health psychology and disability prevention. *Clinical Psychology and Psychotherapy, 5*(2), 76–85.

Ravesloot, C., Ruggiero, C., Ipsen, C., Traci, M., Seekins, T., Boehm, T., et al. (2011). Disability and health behavior change. *Disability and Health Journal, 4,* 19–23.

Rehabilitation Services Administration. (2003). *Evaluation of the centers for independent living program.* Retrieved July 29, 2010, from http://www2.ed.gov/rschstat/eval/rehab/2003-il-final-report.pdf

Rehabilitation Services Administration. (2006). *Rehabilitation services administration case service report (RSA 911)* No. PD-09–01. Washington, DC: Rehabilitation Services Administration.

Rice, M. W., & Trupin, L. (1996). Medical expenditures for people with disabilities. *Disability Statistical Abstracts, 12,* 1–4.

Rimmer, J. H., Nicola, T., Riley, B., & Creviston, T. (2002). Exercise training for African Americans with disabilities residing in difficult social environments. *American Journal of Preventive Medicine, 23*(4), 290–295.

Rogers, E. S., Teague, G. B., Lichenstein, C., Campbell, J., Lyass, A., Chen, R., et al. (2007). Effects of participation in consumer-operated service programs on both personal and organizationally mediated empowerment: Results of multisite study. *Journal of Rehabilitation Research and Development, 44*(6), 785–799.

Sarason, S. B. (1972). *The creation of settings and the future societies.* San Francisco: Jossey-Bass Inc. Publishing.

Schwartz, C. E., & Sendor, M. (Eds.). (2000). *Helping others helps oneself: Response shift effects in peer support.* Washington, DC: American Psychological Association.

Schwartz, K., Mactavish, J., & Lutfiyya, Z. M. (2006). Making community connections: Educator perspectives on transition planning for students with intellectual disabilities. *Exceptionality Education Canada, 16*(2–3), 73–100.

Seekins, T., Ravesloot, C., Oxford, M., Altom, B., White, G., Petty, R. E., et al. (2010). *Nursing home emancipation: A community-based participatory research study.* Missoula, MT: University of Montana Research and Training Center on Disability in Rural Communities.

Seekins, T., Ravesloot, C., Rigles, B., Enders, A., Arnold, N., Ipsen, C., et al. (2011). The Future of Disability and Rehabilitation in Rural Communities: Rural Futures Lab Foundation Paper No. 3. Rural Futures Lab of the Rural Research Policy Institute, http://www.ruralfutureslab.org/docs/The_Future_of_Disability_073111.pdf.

Seligman, M. E. (1990). *Learned optimism.* New York: Pocket Books.

Sperry, C., & Brusin, J. (2001). *Worker cooperatives and employment of people with disabilities.* Missoula: The University of Montana Rural Institute.

Stuifbergen, A. (1995). Health-promoting behaviors and quality of life among individuals with multiple sclerosis. *Scholarly Inquiry for Nursing Practice, 9(1),* 31–50.

Test, D. W., Mazzotti, V. L., Mustian, A. L., Fowler, C. H., Kortering, L., & Kohler, P. (2009). Evidence-based secondary transition predictors for improving postschool outcomes for students with disabilities. *Career Development for Exceptional Individuals, 32*(3), 160–181.

Thoma, C. A., & Getzel, E. E. (2005). "Self-determination is what it's all about": What post-secondary students with disabilities tell us are important considerations for success. *Education and Training in Developmental Disabilities, 40*(3), 234–242.

Thompson, L. (2004). *Long-term care: Support for family caregivers.* Retrieved August 5, 2010, from http://ltc.georgetown.edu/pdfs/caregivers.pdf

Tompa, E., de Oliveira, C., Dolinschi, R., & Irvin, E. (2008). A systematic review of disability management interventions with economic evaluations. *Journal of Occupational Rehabilitation, 18*(1), 16–26.

Trieschmann, R. B. (1995). The energy model: A new approach to rehabilitation. *Rehabilitation Education. Special Double Issue: Spirituality, Disability, and Rehabilitation, 9*(2–3), 217–227.

U.S. Census Bureau. (2006). *Statistical abstract of the united states.* Retrieved August 6, 2010, from http://www.census.gov/compendia/statab/2006/labor_force_employment_earnings/labor.pdf

U.S. Department of Education. (2007). *Strategic plan for fiscal years 2007–12.* Washington, DC: U.S. Department of Education.

U.S. Department of Labor. (2010). *Labor force statistics from the current population survey.* Retrieved August 6, 2010, from http://data.bls.gov/PDQ/servlet/SurveyOutputServlet

Usiak, D. J., Moffat, J., & Wehmeyer, M. L. (2004). Independent living management. *Journal of Vocational Rehabilitation. Special Issue: Independent Living Management, 20*(1), 1–3.

Usiak, D. J., Stone, V. I., House, R. B., & Montgomery, M. E. (2004). Stakeholder perceptions of an effective CIL. *Journal of Vocational Rehabilitation. Special Issue: Independent Living Management, 20*(1), 35–43.

Wehman, P. (2006). Individualized transition planning: Putting self-determination into action. In P. Wehman (Ed.), *Life beyond the classroom: Transition strategies for young people with disabilities* (4th ed., pp. 71–96). Baltimore, MD: Paul H Brookes Publishing.

Wehmeyer, M. L., Agran, M., & Hughes, C. (1998). *Teaching self-determination to students with disabilities: Basic skills for successful transition.* Baltimore, MD: Paul H Brookes Publishing.

Wertsch, J. V., & Tulviste, P. (1992). L. S. Vygotsky and contemporary developmental psychology. *Developmental Psychology, 28*(4), 548–557.

Whyte, W. F. (1991). *Participatory action research.* Newbury Park, CA: Sage Publication.

Williams, R. M., Westmorland, M. G., Lin, C., Schmuck, G., & Creen, M. (2006). A systematic review of workplace rehabilitation interventions for work-related low back pain. *The International Journal of Disability Management Research, 1*(1), 21–30.

World Health Organization (2001). *International classification of functioning, disability, and health.* Geneva: World Health Organization.

World Health Organization (2010). *About the community based rehabilitation matrix*. Retrieved August 8, 2010, from http://www.who.int/disabilities/cbr/matrix/en/index.html

Wright, B. A. (1983). *Circumscribing the problem*. New York: HarperCollins Publishers.

Zemper, E. D., Tate, D. G., Roller, S., Forchheimer, M., Chiodo, A., Nelson, V. S., et al. (2003). Assessment of a holistic wellness program for persons with spinal cord injury. *American Journal of Physical Medicine and Rehabilitation/Association of Academic Physiatrists, 82*(12), 957–968.

Zhang, D., Ivester, J. G., Chen, L., & Katsiyannis, A. (2005). Perspectives on transition practices. *Career Development for Exceptional Individuals, 28*(1), 15–25.

Families in Rehabilitation

Patricia A. Rivera

Abstract

Traditional models of chronic care management have failed to consider the involvement of family members in patient care. Systemic, socio-economic, and cultural factors demand continued care from family members during and following rehabilitation. The financial and emotional burdens incurred by care providers of a family member living with a disability increase caregiver risk for distress, depression, and physical health problems. Current approaches to the efficacious management of caregiver distress emphasize the importance of identifying the reasons and mechanisms behind positive treatment results. Organizational shifts in thinking about the role of families in rehabilitation, as well as refinements in national health care policy will require recognition of the differing care needs of persons with varying disabilities and the impact these have on approaches to effective managing of caregiver stress. It is proposed that interventions including psychotherapy, education, and supportive services to families as they begin their caregiver roles become a "standard of care" and that continued research focus on development of technologically driven devices to increase availability or tools to enhance quality of life while maintaining lower costs. Culturally appropriate services to meet the needs of diverse, underserved populations will result in huge dividends for consumers and providers of health care services.

Key Words: Caregivers, distress, coping, rehabilitation, quality of life

[D]isease affects single individuals but illness incorporates his social circle.
—*Kleinman*, 1988

The health care landscape is changing. Factors including rising medical costs, competition for health care dollars from public and private entities, and decreasing length of hospitalizations, along with an aging population with increased prevalence of chronic illnesses and disability are reasons to pause and re-evaluate current delivery processes. In spite of evidence of the need for greater attention to management of chronic conditions, acute care continues to be the main focus of today's health care models.

The consequence of this targeted approach is the increased demands that the care of chronic health problems places on family members. The financial and emotional burdens incurred by the informal care providers of a family member living with a disability have been well documented and collectively paint a grim picture of the increased risks for distress, depression, and physical health problems incurred by the caregiver. Also indicated in the literature is the importance of considering the care recipient's social context, including the caregiver, throughout the treatment process. Families differ in the ways that they perceive their role in treatment, disability, and medical settings, and they may actually have goals for the patient that diverge from those of the rehabilitation staff. This chapter discusses the experience of individuals who care for a family member with a chronic illness or disability.

Demographics

Demographic trends from the past several decades have shown cause for continued interest and concern regarding the welfare and quality of life (QOL) of the increasing elderly and disabled population. More than 65 million community-dwelling Americans have long-lasting disabilities or conditions requiring assistance with basic health care needs such as bathing, dressing, and toileting, and it is generally up to their family members to provide this care in addition to the emotional and financial support required (National Alliance for Caregiving and American Association for Retired Persons [NAC & AARP] 2010). In most Western countries, the confluence of increased chronic health problems in people living longer and severely limited long-term care services has all but demanded that family members assume greater responsibility in the care and adjustment of the aging and disabled (Kleinman, 1988). In addition, the firm establishment of managed care mechanisms has demanded increased family responsibility as health care options diminish and health care needs increase.

One-third of American households report having at least one adult serve as an informal caregiver. Most caregivers are related to the care recipient (86%), and 36% care for an aging parent (NAC & AARP, 2010). The average age of caregivers is 49 years, and the majority consists of women (66%), who often provide 20 or more hours per week of care. In the absence of a spouse, the responsibility of care typically falls on the adult daughter or daughter-in-law in closest geographic proximity and with the fewest competing family or work obligations, followed by sons or other male family members (Cantor & Little, 1985). When parents of adult children with mental illness are no longer available to provide care, siblings are most likely to step in and assume primary care roles (Lohrer, Lukens, & Thorning, 2007). Cultural differences exist the hierarchical role assignment of care, with males of Asian heritage taking on equal caregiving responsibilities with females, African Americans reporting lower household incomes, and Hispanic family members

providing care at a younger age compared to their white counterparts (NAC & AARP, 2010).

Costs of Caregiving

The financial consequences of providing care to a family member when the caregiver is employed include reduced hours in the workforce or change in status from full- to part-time employment because of the competing care demands. The average caregiver provides the equivalent of a part time job (20.4 hours) in uncompensated care in addition to working a full-time job. Two-thirds of employed caregivers (66%) report being forced to change work schedules, such as going in late, leaving early, or taking extended breaks during the day for caregiving responsibilities. Employed caregivers are also more likely to experience stress-related illness, take more sick-leave, and use company-provided health services more often than their non-caregiving counterparts. Other work-related changes include decreased productivity, taking a leave of absence, or leaving the workforce altogether by termination or taking early retirement. Additional consequences that are not immediately evident include negatively impacted promotional prospects, training, or other opportunities for advancement, and monetary reduction in retirement contributions (U.S. Department of Labor, 2010). A recent survey (NAC & AARP, 2010) revealed that half of caregivers caring for someone 50 years or older spent an average of $5,531 per year on caregiving, and one-third of caregivers reported having used a portion of their savings to cover caregiving costs. Global economic changes have resulted in additional stress and financial concerns for family caregivers in the form of unemployment, weak housing markets that prevent the sale of caregiver or care recipient's homes, and regional budget cuts resulting in fewer community resources for respite (Jones, Harper, Pantuliano, & Pavanelo, 2009).

Financial Support for Caregiving

In August 1993, the U.S. federal government enacted the Family and Medical Leave Act (FMLA). This legislation allows employees to take protected, unpaid leave from work for the purpose of caring for a spouse, parent, or child with a serious health condition. Caregivers, for example, may be eligible to take up to 12 weeks of work without pay during a 12-month period. This provision also allows employee health benefits to be maintained during that time off work. In 2008, military entitlements were added to the law, and in 2009, revisions were added to reflect a national need to care for wounded war veterans. This update allows a spouse, adult child, parent, or next of kin to take up to 26 work weeks of unpaid leave to care for a member of the Armed Forces who is undergoing treatment, recuperating, or otherwise disabled.

In 2006, the Lifespan Respite Care Act was established to assist individual states in creating affordable respite care for caregivers of all persons, regardless of age, requiring assistance with activities of daily living and who require supervision in order to prevent injury to themselves or others. More recently, creative measures are being considered as means of financial support to family caregivers. Tax credits, increased funding for respite, and employer-based programs such as flex-time options, telecommuting, job sharing, and educational and self-care programs are proposed means of assistance. Because maintained employment is a goal for most caregivers, employers, and society as a whole, corporate eldercare programs and other services are targeted for further development.

Cultural Elements in Caregiving

The rehabilitation paradigm has historically been based on the medical model, with the concept of disability being viewed as a deficiency in an individual's functioning within society and therefore requiring corrective action. Within the past 30 years, social trends focusing on consumer satisfaction have increasingly recognized the social and family elements that mediate improved functioning. As family members demand greater inclusion in the rehabilitation process, changes in rehabilitation policy and legislation have resulted. Nevertheless, the importance of a family's experience in and perspective of rehabilitation does not appear to be adequately addressed in practice (Accordino & Hunt, 2001; Ehrmann & Herbert, 2005), and in addition, relatively little is known about how culture influences rehabilitation outcomes. Cultural elements include age, race and ethnicity, sexual orientation, relationship to the care recipient, and socioeconomic status.

In the United States, ethnic minorities have significantly higher rates of physical disability than do non-Hispanic Whites, and this inequality is further demarcated by poverty (U.S. Census Bureau, 2000). Ethnic minorities are also likely to experience discrimination, language barriers, health disparities, and stigma related to their own inexperience with and cultural beliefs about illness and disability (Chwalisz & Clancy Dollinger, 2009). Women

from paternalistic cultures that foster dependence may experience distress when required to show initiative and creative problem-solving in the care of their loved one (Rivera & Marlo, 1999), whereas domestic partners seeking to engage in active caregiving may be overlooked or purposely discounted (Gallantis, 2002) in the rehabilitation partnership.

Rehabilitation services have traditionally been developed to address the well-documented needs of the largely white, heterosexual, middle-class health care consuming population. It is not surprising, therefore, that caregivers of varied cultural backgrounds underutilize existing services (Gallagher-Thompson, Coon, Rivera, Powers, & Zeiss, 1998). Valle (1992) proposed that to best address the needs of minority caregivers, misconceptions that surround the utilization of services must be addressed, including the belief that culturally diverse caregivers lack psychological insight and experience stress in the same way, and that only culturally similar health care providers can be effective interventionists. Marshall (2008) proposes that seemingly different populations often share values of family, religion, and lack of access to health care or educational opportunities, often resulting in more similarities than actual differences within the rehabilitation setting. Feist-Price and Ford-Harris (1994) identified fear of being disrespected or shamed, the perceived threat of family destabilization secondary to acknowledgment of change, and differing problem-solving styles as factors that prevent African-American family members from participation in the rehabilitation process. Similarly, fears of discrimination, intolerance, absence of legal protection, and social stigma affect lesbian, gay, bisexual, and transgender caregivers from seeking or obtaining suitable care (Coon & Zeiss, 2003) and may result in withholding of critical health care information or prevent help-seeking behavior itself.

Results from a survey of training needs (Chan, Leahy, Saunders, Tarvydas, Ferrin, & Lee, 2003) found that counselors in proprietary rehabilitation settings reported no relevance for understanding disability within a family framework and self-reported high perceived competence requiring no further education. Culturally competent rehabilitation providers recognize their own limitations, embrace understanding and appreciation of cultures different from their own, acknowledge their own biases, provide services in a manner that is appropriately respectful to the culture at hand, and embrace principles and ethics of multicultural counseling (Baruth & Manning, 1999). These behaviors can best be reflected in three stages: developing a relationship of trust and respect with the patient and family; assessing the strengths, weaknesses, and available resources of the family system; and providing support and/or services, which may include knowledge such as problem-solving skills, information and referral services, and practical skills training (Ehrmann & Herbert, 2005; McKenna & Power, 2000).

Competing Roles and Expectations

The relationship between the caregiver and the care recipient plays a significant role in the experiences of all involved. The provision of care to an older adult suffering the effects of stroke or a progressive, dementing condition may be an expected, albeit stressful, sequence in the developmental trajectory of a family (Maslow, 1943). By comparison, disabling injuries that occur as a result of accidents are unforeseen, often producing catastrophic reactions to the abrupt and life-changing event. For example, when a child or young adult acquires a disability that necessitates a parent, sibling, or spouse to assume care, a disruption in expectations of that individual's development can be particularly difficult to accept. Reactions such as denial and inability to acknowledge the implications of the disability are fairly common during the initial period of adjustment. Caregivers who report no problems with role adaptation during their family member's initial inpatient hospitalization are likely to report continued adjustment and positive growth over that first year of caregiving (Shewchuk, Richards, & Elliott, 1998); thus, in many cases, the continued positive rehabilitation upon hospital discharge may be more dependent on caregiver characteristics than on those of the care recipient (Meijer et al., 2004).

Premorbid relationship history refers to the quality of interactions within a family system prior to the onset of conditions requiring care. Numerous studies show that relationships characterized as nurturing are more protective for the care recipient while adult children caring for a parent benefitted most from interventions aimed at reducing stress and burden (Sorensen, Pinquart, & Duberstein, 2002). Indeed, most female caregivers view their role in the process of rehabilitation and healing as offering instrumental support, encouraging rest for the patient, and providing company and social support (Sturkenboom, Dekker, Scheppers, Dongen, & Dekker, 2007). Some caregivers may not recognize the benefit of functioning as a coach or guide to help their family member obtain the greatest return

to independence in daily activities. As a result, caregivers who solely serve to offer comfort, take over in self-care activities, and respond to solicitous behaviors may be inadvertently reinforcing dependence (Fitzgerald, 2004). In general, studies have shown that family communication patterns, problem-solving skills, and role recognition are important for adjustment, although the mechanisms by which these supportive factors operate are not well understood. In fact, more is known about the family factors and characteristics that have a negative impact on adaptation. Although the occurrence of trauma is known to result in a sudden, initial mobilization of support that predictably fades with time and leaves family members to cope alone, more experienced family caregivers have reported greater adaptability via an evolution of their values and expectations. This experience facilitates the reconsideration of previous goals and are reflective of a stress-related growth process (King & Patterson, 2000; King, Scollon, Ramsey, & Williams, 2000). These psychological processes are of the kind that result in the health and emotional benefits some caregivers enjoy from providing care to a loved one (Beach, Schulz, Yee, & Jackson, 2000).

Caregiver-Guided Research

Qualitative research designs, such as case studies or interviews, assist researchers in obtaining in-depth understanding of human behavior. These analytical methodologies investigate the *why* and *how* of caregivers' experiences and provide valuable insights into the family process. Observations made via these techniques may not always parallel assumptions obtained from empirical research or professionals' opinions, which typically drive the development of services and programs. Thus, consultation with the "experts" who manage chronic health conditions on a regular basis becomes of particular importance (Shewchuk & Elliott, 2000). The use of complementary medicine, spiritual healing, and traditional Chinese medicine in rehabilitation settings illustrates the concept of recognizing and working with patients' and families' pluralistic health practices to achieve optimal outcomes (Chang & Wang, 2009). Existing theoretically grounded psychometric tools that do not consider the experience of caregivers who live with the day-to-day responsibility of care to a family member with a chronic health condition are phenomenologically unsound.

Severe disabilities requiring dependence on others for basic self-care, such as eating, dressing, or toileting, force families to manage a vast number of objective problems and challenges that professionals assume constitute the greatest source of burden. Qualitative assessment methodologies are varied in the means by which they obtain information from caregivers about their experiences, opinions, and goals. Thematic analyses of essays (Chwalisz & Stark-Wroblenski, 1996) and structured interviewing (Long, Glueckauf, & Rasmussen 1998) have been utilized to gain understanding of the unique perspectives and concerns about interpersonal relationships, QOL, and emotional commitments in the caregiving relationship. These approaches obtain information that is unique to each individual's experience. Case studies such as Gillian and Rose's (2005) report of a 12-year-old child with unexplained chronic pain revealed the parents' belief that a purely organic cause was to blame for their child's pain. The caregivers consequently developed a pattern of help-seeking behaviors characterized by repeated medical evaluations, emergency room visits, and hospitalizations. Problem-solving interventions (D'Zurilla & Nezu, 1999) with the family, who exhibited anxious coping styles, were developed and implemented to focus on enhanced patient functioning rather than symptoms.

In contrast, focus groups facilitate the identification of shared experiences within specific populations represented in the group. It is not uncommon for caregivers to initially respond with denial of problems. Focus groups allow information to be gathered in the language used by the individuals, and the interactive nature of this strategy often solicits information that other approaches cannot. When focus groups were conducted with caregiving consumers in the United States, the problems identified primarily reflected concerns over the caregiver–care recipient relationship, the physical versus emotional demands of caregiving, and temporal versus emotional limitations, thus revealing vastly different concerns from those assumed to cause the greatest distress (Shewchuk, Rivera, Elliott, & Adams, 2004). Participants in a focus group of caregivers for persons with spinal cord injury (SCI) ranked problems concerning interpersonal and familial stress significantly higher than instrumental activities associated with self-care regimens such as bathing or transferring. Specifically, caregivers rated problems reflecting the care recipient's negative, demanding, and unappreciative attitude toward the caregiver; feelings of guilt and obligation; keeping the care recipient occupied and stimulated; and lack of time. Out of the 18 problems ranked by these caregivers, only one specifically concerned self-care activities (Elliott & Shewchuk, 2002).

Differing methodologies, cultural differences as they regard familial obligations, and disease processes may have led to opposing findings from a sample of Chinese spouses who reported health concerns as producing greater stress than interpersonal or relationship matters (Chan, 2000) and Turkish parents of children with neurodevelopmental conditions who identified behavior problems during the initial years of care as most problematic (Sipal, Schuengel, Voorman, Van Eck, & Becher, 2010). Neurological conditions that impair cognition as well as cause physical limitations can be particularly distressing for family members who must cope with multiple aspects of disability. Such deteriorative changes often affect behavioral expression, memory, and self-regulation in ways that result in interpersonal distress for the caregiver. Williams and her colleagues (2009) reported on the emotional experience of family caregivers of people with Huntington disease who acknowledged anticipating the time of death for their care recipient and grief over the loss of relationship. These caregivers dealt with the distress by disregarding their care recipient as an intimate partner. Some evidence exists that chronic and manageable disease processes may result in vastly differing coping processes compared to more mobility-impacted impairments or disabilities such as spinal cord or brain injuries. Bambara et al. (2008) reported that 35% of caregivers of visually impaired adults experienced distress and suggested that these caregivers undergo routine screening and treatment. Miller, Shewchuk, Elliott, and Richards (2000) reported that once their caregivers' confidence with the instrumental tasks of insulin dosing stabilized, the interpersonal aspects of the relationship increased in salience.

Caregiver Burden and the Physical Consequences of Chronic Stress

The term "caregiver burden" (Poulshock & Deimling, 1984) was coined to reflect the psychological toll experienced by family care providers. Although each caregiving situation is unique, issues often contributing to the perceived distress are the physical and psychological demands from the care recipient, the limitations on time, the economic costs, the legal concerns, and the role conflicts experienced by the caregiver. Caregiver stress has been implicated in a variety of physical and mental health concerns. The chronic stress experienced by individuals caring for a loved one for extended periods of time results in impaired physical and emotional well-being.

Caregiver Interventions

Caregiver interventions must be designed to meet the differing needs of today's health care–driven consumers. Not all individuals begin their caregiving careers with the same degree of knowledge, experience, skills, or support. The most helpful programs are those that begin with a formal assessment of the caregiving situation. Structured interviews that evaluate the current as well as premorbid functioning of the caregiver–care recipient dyad will facilitate understanding of the interpersonal dynamics at work in the relationship. Additional evaluation of caregiver practical skills or abilities, such as comfort with use of medical equipment or behavioral management and problem-solving skills, will direct the focus of education. Finally, an assessment of family resources, such as the availability and willingness of other family members to provide care or financial support, will help guide the caregiver toward supplemental, fee-based services. It is important to engage caregivers in some form of intervention as early in the process as possible to prevent the negative impact that can lead to burnout and result in chronic management problems or institutional placement of the care recipient (Parks & Novielli, 2000).

Information and Referral

Information and referral is usually the first intervention received by newly identified caregivers. Information provided must go beyond the definition of care services and how to obtain such, and must include knowledge regarding the care recipient's disease process, expected challenges, and potential solutions. However, studies of programs offering information and referral reveal increased caregiver knowledge without the desired positive outcomes (Kennett, Burgio, & Schulz, 2000). Additional yet critical features of knowledge provision include the availability and accessibility of services within the community, practical and cultural appropriateness of service for the need of the caregiver, and affordability. In a study examining the effectiveness of case management services in the reduction of burden in caregivers, Weave, Boult, and Morishita (2000) found that individuals who were provided with a care plan and linked directly to the needed services reported less burden than did those caregivers who were only provided a generic list of services.

Respite Care

Respite care refers to the service of care by an individual other than the primary caregiver(s). Respite services include in-home attendants, adult day care programs, or overnight stays in a health care facility. The relief offered to the caregiver allows for the completion of other responsibilities or tasks, including self-care. Although respite has been shown to boost morale and subjective stress, it has not been found to relieve caregiver depression (Lyons & Zarit, 1999; Zarit, Gaugler, & Jarrot, 1999). The preferences and behavior of 950 Dutch caregivers revealed that although close to 80% of the respondents reported a desire for support or respite care in general, 42–47% actually preferred more communication with other caregivers or more information about professional attendants (Koopmanschap, van Exel, van den Bos, van den Berg, & Brouwer, 2004). Toseland and her colleagues (2001) found that regular use of respite services early on in the caregiving career reduced the experience of burden and increased psychological well-being. Few studies have been conducted on the effects of respite on the care recipient or the benefits of overnight respite. The absence of these studies may reflect the practical, real-life situations that necessitate consideration of the ethical and practical factors that prevent randomization with distressed caregivers who find themselves in need of help and enroll in research studies. The absence of true randomized controlled studies has prevented the identification of evidence-based findings in the caregiver literature (Nathan & Gorman, 2002).

Counseling and Support Groups

Programs of a supportive nature are designed to increase caregivers' emotional and experiential connection with others in order to decrease isolation. Group interventions not only help participants understand the disease or disability process of their loved one, but may also help with identification of community resources, coping skills, and learning stress management strategies. By definition, support groups facilitate the expression of frustration and other negative affect, and encourages affirmation of experiences among participants. Jones-Cannon and Davis (2005) reported that their African-American caregivers reported group benefits in maintaining a positive attitude and religious faith that helped sustain them in their caregiving duties. Whitlach, Judge, Zarit, and Femia (2006) conducted a study designed to address the needs of both the caregiver and care recipient in recognition of the care recipients' progressive cognitive deficits and eventual aphasia. The authors hypothesized that if emotional issues were addressed while the dementing elder was able to communicate, and long-term care plans were made collaboratively, caregiver stress related to care and end-of-life decisions would be significantly reduced. Trained counselors held sessions with the caregiver and care recipient to improve communication, knowledge of the disease and its course, and planning for the future. Individual sessions were also held between client and counselor to address personal issues and concerns regarding care options. Although results showed that both participants reported benefit from the intervention, counselor variables, such as comfort with and knowledge about the population and their needs, must be considered. Individual counseling can be helpful to address topics such as the emotional responses surrounding illness, problem-solving and behavioral management skills, family relationship problems, and case management skills (Toseland, Smith, & McCallion, 2001).

Family Factors

In a review of empirical studies in the rehabilitation literature that focused on family factors in the adjustment to chronic illness and disability, Kelley and Lambert (1992) concluded that several serious shortcomings exist and must be resolved in order for the support mechanisms in family functioning to be elucidated. First, the authors point to the inadequate conceptualization of support and further add that, although social support is understood to be a process of reciprocity, none of the studies appeared to have acknowledged or addressed this exchange. Indeed, studies have shown the potentially negative aspect of social support due to absence of reciprocity (Rivera, Rose, Futterman, Lovett, & Gallagher-Thompson, 1991). Second, valid indicators of social support are elusive and are replete with confounding variables. Third, the specialization to populations of psychometrically validated questionnaires requires adaptability of items for use with persons with disabilities. Because different sources of support offer differential degrees of impact, more attention is needed to the conditions under which different types of support do or do not impact outcomes in rehabilitation. Sander, Caroselli, High, Becker, Neese, and Scheibel (2002) approached their definition of support to include the entire family environment during the process of rehabilitation of 37 persons with traumatic brain injury (TBI). Because successful rehabilitation has the goal of achieving maximum independence, family distress or conflict may hinder cooperation with treatment or sabotage progress by fostering dependence. Sanders et al.'s findings supported previous observation that TBI patients with supportive families do better in rehabilitation than those who do not have such support (Braga, Da Paz Junior, & Ylvisaker, 2005). Unfortunately, many family systems report unhealthy family functioning that may have be due to a variety of premorbid factors including behavioral problems, substance abuse in the patient, or psychiatric problems prior to the injury.

Psychological Interventions

Caregiver intervention programs have produced varied outcomes over the past decades. Sorensen, Pinquart, and Duberstein (2002) performed a meta-analysis composed of 78 different studies of caregiver interventions. The majority of the participants in the evaluated studies were caregivers to dementia patients, as well as those who had cancer or strokes. The interventions included psychoeducational, supportive, educational, and multicomponent approaches. The psychoeducational interventions revealed a significant effect on the entire group of caregiver outcome variables studied: burden, depression, perception of well-being, satisfaction with caregiving, and coping ability. Supportive interventions were helpful in improving caregiver burden and caregiver knowledge. Multicomponent, year-long problem-solving training and telephone support with caregivers of women with disabilities and persons with TBI revealed significant results on burden, well-being, and coping ability (Rivera, Elliott, Berry, Shewchuk, Oswald, & Grant, 2006), as well as depression (Rivera, Elliott, Berry, & Grant, 2008; Rivera, Elliott, Berry, Grant, & Oswald, 2007). A systematic review of English-language journals for randomized controlled trials of interventions for adult caregivers of individuals post-stroke concluded that more high-quality research to address the needs of stroke caregivers is needed (Brereton, Carroll, & Barnston, 2007). The authors recommended that interventions be based upon theoretical frameworks, so that potential confounds can be adequately predicted and addressed, and so that appropriate interventions can be developed and tested with the necessary outcome measures. The argument was made to include members of the population targeted for the intervention in its development, as they are the primary stakeholders. Persons with disability can also become active participants in the development of interventions and family process events (Fronek, 2005). Treatment intervention studies based on observation, individual cases, and exploratory approaches (Rothi & Barrett, 2006) that document effectiveness and refinement to targeted audiences can augment randomized clinical trials to expand our knowledge base and add to the growing repertoire of beneficial interventions.

Technological Applications

Advances in technology have allowed for the increased availability of information and services to information-seeking individuals. Video-conferencing, webinars, telephone-based interventions, internet-based groups, and list-serves are some of the ways technology has helped to improve communication and accessibility to services by persons living in rural communities or who are simply unable to leave their care recipient (Toseland, Smith, & McCallion, 2001). Basic tools, such as websites that offer "fact sheets" or topic-focused pamphlets, and referrals to local services and resources, are easily available on the internet. Most major public institutions such as hospitals, libraries, and educational facilities often allow the general public use of computers and other technological tools for information-gathering purposes.

Creative uses of technology are limited only by the vision of its users. Prior to the availability of internet, web-based video, or picture phones, the use of land-line telephony was a method of monitoring progress and treatment delivery to caregivers (Grant, Elliott, Weaver, Bartolucci, & Giger, 2002; Wisniewski et al., 2003). Now obsolete, videophone technology was successfully used as a platform to provide problem-solving training to rural caregivers of persons with SCI (Rivera, Shewchuk, & Elliott, 2003), and practical difficulties related to connectivity and comfort with visual media were documented.

Internet-based applications, such as real-time support groups (Gustafson et al., 2005; Rochette, Korner-Bitensky, Tremblay, & Kloda, 2008) have been well received by health care consumers. Studies examining the receptivity to wearable technology by physically or cognitively impaired individuals have revealed a welcoming approach to tools that are designed to assist and provide care, although none available is without identified flaws (Mahoney & Mahoney, 2010). Multi-touch technologies have proven valuable as tools to increase social interaction between patients and therapists in rehabilitation programs (Annett, Anderson, & Bischof, 2010). The value of technology-based applications is that they can be adapted or adjusted to meet the individual needs of patients, caregivers, or situations with relative ease and low cost, thus promising potentially limitless uses.

Conclusion
Future Directions

Traditional models of chronic care management have failed to consider the involvement of family members. As populations of older and disabled individuals increase globally, a more family-centered perspective in health and long-term care must take place. A paradigm shift toward inclusion of family systems thinking and caregiver assessments will be required to best meet the needs of these consumers while maintaining cost-effectiveness. The variability in efficacy of current approaches to the management of caregiver distress emphasizes the importance of identifying the reasons and mechanisms behind positive treatment results. Refinement of existing theoretical models is one way to begin to increase our understanding of such desired change processes. For example, Berry and his colleagues (2007) examined personality characteristics of individuals with SCI to identify those individuals with definite, positive problem-solving capacities and better adjustment. Such findings have important implications for targeted interventions in rehabilitation settings as these characteristics have protective factors that are involved in preventing secondary complications (e.g., decubitus ulcers).

In addition to organizational shifts in thinking about the role of the family in rehabilitation, refinement of national health policies regarding practice and research are recommended. Such changes include the recognition of differential care needs of persons with different disabilities and degrees of impairment and the impact these have on continued systematic attempts to identify innovative approaches to reduce distress. The inclusion of psychotherapy, counseling, and education-based supportive services to families as they begin their caregiver roles must become a "standard of care" that would benefit not only consumers but health care providers as well. Continued research and development of technologically driven devices will capitalize on decreased cost and increased availability of tools that enhance QOL. Finally, efforts to increase the availability of culturally competent services to meet the needs of diverse, underserved populations will pay huge dividends for health care consumers and well-prepared providers of quality health services.

References

Accordino, M. P., & Hunt, B. (2001). Family counseling training in rehabilitation counseling programs. *Rehabilitation Education, 15*, 225–264.

Annett, M., Anderson, F., & Bischof, W. F. (2010). Hands, tables and groups make rehabilitation awesome! *Studies in Health Technology Informatics, 154*, 3–8.

Bambara, J. K., Owsley, C., Wadley, V., Martin, R., Porter, C., & Dreer, L. E. (2008). Family caregiver social problem-solving abilities and adjustment to caring for a relative with vision loss. *Investigative Ophthalmology and Visual Science, 50*, 1585–1592.

Baruth, L. G., & Manning, M. L. (1999). *Multicultural counseling and psychotherapy: A lifespan perspective* (2nd ed.). Columbus, OH: Merrill.

Beach, S. R., Schulz, R., Yee, J., & Jackson, S. (2000). Negative and positive health effects of caring for a disabled spouse: Longitudinal findings from the carer health effects study. *Psychology and Aging, 15*, 259–271.

Berry, J. W., Elliott, T. R., & Rivera, P. (2007). Resilient, undercontrolled, and overcontrolled personality prototypes among persons with spinal cord injury. *Journal of Personality Assessment, 89*(3), 292–302.

Braga, L. W., Da Paz Junior, A. C., & Ylvisaker, M. (2005). Direct clinician-delivered versus indirect family-supported rehabilitation of children with traumatic brain injury: A randomized controlled trial. *Brain Injury, 19*(10), 819–831.

Brereton, L., Carroll, C., & Barnston, S. (2007). Interventions for adult family carers of people who have had a stroke: a systematic review. *Clinical Rehabilitation, 21*, 867–884.

Cantor, M. H., & Little, V. (1985). Aging and social care. In R. H. Binstock & E. Shanas (Eds.), *Handbook of aging and the social sciences* (2nd ed., pp. 745–781). New York: Van Nostrand Reinhold.

Chan, C. K. (2000). Stress and coping in spouses of persons with spinal cord injuries. *Clinical Rehabilitation, 14*, 137–144.

Chan, F., Leahy, M. J., Saunders, J. L., Tarvydas, V., Ferrin, J. M., & Lee, G. (2003). Training needs of certified rehabilitation counselors for contemporary practice. *Rehabilitation Counseling Bulletin, 46*, 82–91.

Chang, L., & Wang, J. (2009). Integration of complementary medical treatments with rehabilitation from the perspective of patients and their caregivers: A qualitative inquiry. *Clinical Rehabilitation, 23*, 730–740.

Chwalisz, K., & Stark-Wroblewski, K. (1996). The subjective experiences of spouse carers of persons with brain injuries: A qualitative analysis. *Applied Neuropsychology, 3*, 28–40.

Chwalisz, K., & Clancy Dollinger, S. M. (2009). Evidence-based practice with family caregivers. In R. G. Frank, B. R. Caplan, & M. Rosenthal (Eds.), *Handbook of rehabilitation psychology*. Washington DC: American Psychological Association.

Coon, D. W., & Zeiss, L. M. (2003). The families we choose: Intervention issues with LGBT caregivers. In D. W. Coon, D. Gallagher-Thompson, & L. Thompson (Eds.), *Innovative interventions to reduce dementia caregiver distress: A clinical guide* (pp. 267–295). New York: Springer.

D'Zurilla, T. J., & Nezu, A. (1999). *Problem-solving therapy: A social competence approach to clinical intervention.* New York: Springer.

Ehrmann, L. A., & Herbert, J. T. (2005). Family intervention training: A course proposal for rehabilitation counselor education. *Rehabilitation Education, 19*(4), 235–244.

Elliott, T., & Rivera, P. (2003). The experience of families and their carers in health care. In S. Llewelyn and P. Kennedy (Eds.), *Handbook of clinical health psychology* (pp. 61–77). Oxford: Wiley & Sons, Ltd.

Elliott, T., & Shewchuk, R. M. (2002). Using the nominal group technique to identify the problems experienced by persons living with severe physical disabilities. *Journal of Clinical Psychology in Medical Settings, 9*(2), 65–76.

Elliott, T., & Shewchuk, R. M. (2003). Social problem-solving abilities and distress among family members assuming a caregiving role. *British Journal of Health Psychology, 8*(2), 149–163.

Feist-Price, S., & Ford-Harris, D. (1994). Rehabilitation counseling: Issues specific to providing services to African-American clients. *Journal of Rehabilitation, 60*(4), 13–19.

Fitzgerald, M. H. (2004). A dialogue on occupational therapy, culture, and families. *American Journal of Occupational Therapy, 58*(5), 489–498.

Fronek, P. (2005). Insights from the family conference: Observations in rehabilitation. *Australian Social Work, 59*(4), 395–406.

Gallagher-Thompson, D., Coon, D. W., Rivera, P., Powers, D., & Zeiss, A. (1998). Family caregiving: Stress, coping and intervention. In M. Hersen & V. B. Van Hasselt (Eds.), *Handbook of clinical geropsychology* (pp. 469–493). New York: Plenum Press.

Gallantis, T. P. (2002). Aging and the nontraditional family. The University of Memphis Law Review. FindArticles.com. Retrieved July 29, 2010, from http://findarticles.com/p/articles/mi_qa3843/is_200204/ai_n9035403/

Gillian, K., & Rose, G. (2005). Family-oriented rehabilitation for unexplained chronic pain. *Canadian Journal of Psychiatry. Canadian Psychiatric Association.* Retrieved January 10, 2012 from HighBeam Research: http://www.highbeam.com/doc/1P3-791450041.html

Grant, J. S., Elliott, T., Weaver, M., Bartolucci, A., & Giger, J. (2002). A telephone intervention with family caregivers of stroke survivors after hospital rehabilitation. *Stroke, 33*, 2060–2065.

Gustafson, D. H., McTavish, F. M., Stengle, W., Ballard, D., Hawkins, R., Shaw, B., et al. (2005). Use and impact of eHealth system by low-income women with breast cancer. *Journal of Health Communication, 10*, 195–218.

Jones-Cannon, S., & Davis, B. L. (2005). Coping among African-American daughters caring for aging parents. *Association of Black Nursing Faculty Journal, 16*(6). 118–123.

Jones, N., Harper, C., Pantuliano, S., & Pavanello, S. (2009). The global economic crisis and impacts on children and caregivers: Emerging evidence and possible policy responses in the Middle East and North Africa, ODI Background Notes. Retrieved July 29, 2010, from http://www.odi.org.uk/resources/download/4412.pdf

Kelley, S. D. D., & Lambert, S. S. (1992). Family support in rehabilitation: A review of research, 1980–1990. *Rehabilitation Counseling Bulletin, 36*(2), 98. Retrieved from EBSCO, March 31, 2010.

Kennet, J., Burgio, L., & Schulz, R. (2000). Interventions for in-home caregivers: A review of research 1990 to present. In R. Schulz (Ed.), *Handbook of dementia caregiving* (pp. 61–125). New York: Springer.

King, L. A., & Patterson, C. (2000). Reconstructing life goals after the birth of a child with Down's syndrome: Finding happiness and growing. *International Journal of Rehabilitation and Health, 5*, 17–30.

King, L. A., Scollon, C., Ramsey, C., & Williams, T. (2000). Stories of life transition: subjective well-being and ego development in parents of children with Down's syndrome. *Journal of Research in Personality, 34*, 509–536.

Kleinman, A. (1988). *The illness narratives: Suffering, healing, and the human condition.* New York: Basic Books Publishers.

Koopmanschap, M. A., van Exel, N. J., van den Bos, G. A., van den Berg, B., & Brouwer, W. B. (2004). The desire for support and respite care: preferences of Dutch informal caregivers. *Health Policy. 68*(3), 309–20.

Lohrer, S. P., Lukens, E. P., & Thorning, H. (2007). Economic expenditures associated with instrumental caregiving roles of adult siblings of persons with severe mental illness. *Community Health Journal, 43*(2), 129–151.

Long, M. P. Glueckauf, R. L., & Rasmussen, J. (1998). Developing family counseling interventions for adults with episodic neurological disabilities: Presenting problems, persons involved, and problem severity. *Rehabilitation Psychology, 43*, 101–117.

Lyons, K., & Zarit, S. (1999). Formal and informal support: The great divide. *International Journal of Geriatric Psychiatry, 14*, 183–196.

Mahoney, E. L., & Mahoney, D. F. (2010). Acceptance of wearable technology by people with Alzheimer's Disease: Issues and accommodations. *American Journal of Alzheimer's Disease and Other Dementias.* [Epub ahead of print]. Retrieved August 20, 2010, http://www.ncbi.nlm.nih.gov/pubmed

Marshall, C. A. (2008). Family and culture: Using autoethnography to inform rehabilitation practice with cancer survivors. *Journal of Applied Rehabilitation Counseling, 39*(1), 9–19.

Maslow, A. H. (1943). A theory of human motivation. *Psychological Review, 50*, 370.

McKenna, M. A., & Power, P. A. (2000). Engaging the African American family in the rehabilitation process: An intervention model for rehabilitation counselors. *Journal of Applied Rehabilitation Counseling, 31*(1), 12–18.

Meijer, R., van Limbeek, J., Kriek, B., Ihnenfeldt, D., Vermeulen, M., & de Haan, R. (2004). Prognostic social factors in the subacute phase after a stroke for the discharge destination from the hospital stroke unit: A systematic review of the literature. *Disability Rehabilitation, 26*, 191–197.

Miller, D., Shewchuk, R., Elliott, T., & Richards, J. S. (2000). Nominal group technique: A process for identifying diabetes self-care issues among patients and carers. *The Diabetes Educator, 26*, 305–314.

Nathan, P., & Gorman, J. M. (Eds.). (2002). *A guide to treatments that work* (2nd ed.). New York: Oxford University Press.

National Alliance for Caregiving & The American Association of Retired Persons. (2010). *Caregiving in the United States.* Retrieved July 27, 2010, from http://www.caregiving.org/data/Emblem_CfC10_Final2.pdf

National Alliance for Caregiving (NAC), in collaboration with AARP, funded by MetLife Foundation. (November 2009). Caregiving in the U.S. Executive Summary; November 2009. Retrieved July 27, 2010, from http://www.caregiving.org/data/CaregivingUSAllAgesExecSum.pdf

Parks, S. M., & Novielli, K. D. (2000). A practical guide to caring for caregivers. *American Family Physician, 62*, 2613–2620.

Poulshock, S. W., & Deimling, G. T. (1984). Families caring for elders in residence: Issues in the measurement of burden. *Journal of Gerontology, 39*, 230–239.

Rivera, P., Elliott, T., Berry, J., Shewchuk, R., Oswald K., & Grant J. (2006). Family caregivers of women with physical disabilities. *Journal of Clinical Psychology in Medical Settings, 13*, 431–440.

Rivera, P., Elliott, T., Berry, J., & Grant, J. (2008). Problem-solving training for family caregivers of persons with traumatic brain injuries: A randomized controlled trial. *Archives of Physical Medicine and Rehabilitation, 89*, 931–941.

Rivera, P., Elliott, T. R., Berry, J, Grant, J. S., & Oswald, K. (2007). Predictors of caregiver depression among community-residing families living with traumatic brain injury. *NeuroRehabilitation, 22*(1), 3–8.

Rivera, P. A., & Marlo, H. (1999). Cultural, interpersonal and psychodynamic factors in caregiving: Toward a greater understanding of treatment non-compliance. *Clinical Psychology and Psychotherapy, 6*, 63–68.

Rivera, P. A., Rose, J. M., Futterman, A., Lovett, S. B., & Gallagher-Thompson, D. (1991). Dimensions of perceived social support in clinically depressed and non-depressed female caregivers. *Psychology and Aging, 6*, 232–237.

Rivera, P. A., Shewchuk, R., & Elliott, T. R. (2003). Project FOCUS: Using videophones to provide problem-solving training to family caregivers of persons with spinal cord injury. *Topics in Spinal Cord Injury Rehabilitation, 9*(1), 53–62.

Rochette, A., Korner-Bitensky, N., Tremblay, V., & Kloda, L. (2008). Stroke rehabilitation information for clients and families: Assessing the quality of the StrokEngine-Family website. *Disability and Rehabilitation, 30*(19), 1506–1512.

Rothi, L. J. G., & Barrett, A. M. (2006). The changing view of neurorehabilitation: A new era of optimism. *Journal of the International Neuropsychological Society, 12*, 812–815.

Sander, A. M., Caroselli, J. S., High, Jr., W. M., Becker, C., Neese, L., & Scheibel, R. (2002). Relationship of family functioning to progress in a post-acute rehabilitation programme following traumatic brain injury. *Brain Injury, 16*(8), 649–657.

Shewchuk, R., & Elliott, T. (2000). Family caregiving in chronic disease and disability: Implications for rehabilitation psychology. In R. G. Frank & T. Elliott (Eds.), *Handbook of Rehabilitation Psychology* (pp. 553–563). Washington, DC: American Psychological Association Press.

Shewchuk, R., Richards, J. S., & Elliott, T. (1998). Dynamic processes in health outcomes among caregivers of patients with spinal cord injuries. *Health Psychology, 17*, 125–129.

Shewchuk, R., Rivera, P. A., Elliott, T., & Adams, A. M. (2004). Using cognitive mapping to understand problems experienced by family caregivers of persons with severe physical disabilities. *Journal of Clinical Psychology in Medical Settings, 11*(3), 141–150.

Sipal, R. F., Schuengel, C., Voorman, J. M., Van Eck, M., & Becher, J. G. (2010). Course of behaviour problems of children with cerebral palsy: The role of parental stress and support. *Child Care Health Development, 36*(1), 74–84.

Sorensen, S., Pinquart, M., & Duberstein, P. (2002). How effective are interventions with caregivers? An updated meta-analysis. *The Gerontologist, 42*, 356–372.

Sturkenboom, I., Dekker, J., Scheppers, E., Dongen, E. V., & Dekker, J. (2007). Healing care? Rehabilitation of female immigrant patients with chronic pain from a family perspective. *Disability and Rehabilitation, 29*(4), 323–332.

Toseland, R., Smith, G., & McCallion, P. (2001). Family caregivers of the frail elderly. In Gutterman (Ed.), *Handbook of social work practice with vulnerable and resilient populations* (pp. 548–581). New York: Columbia University Press.

U.S. Census Bureau. (2000). Disability. American FactFinder. Retrieved July 29, 2010, from http://factfinder.census.gov

U.S. Department of Labor Website. Wage and Hour Division (WHD). Family and Medical Leave Act. Retrieved July 29, 2010, from http://www.dol.gov/whd/fmla/index.htm

Valle, R. (1992). *Culture & caregiving*. Aging. FindArticles.com. Retrieved July 29, 2010, from http://findarticles.com/p/articles/mi_m1000/is_n363–64/ai_12519940/

Weave, J., Boult, C., & Morishita, L. (2000).The effects of outpatient geriatric evaluation and management on caregiver burden. *The Gerontologist, 40*, 429–436.

Whitlach, C., Judge, K., Zarit, S. H., & Femia, E. (2006). Dyadic intervention for family caregivers and care receivers in early-stage dementia. *The Gerontologist, 46*, 688–694.

Williams, J. K., Skirton, H., Paulsen, J. S., Tripp-Reimer, T., Jarmon, L., McGonigal Kenney, M., et al. (2009). The emotional experiences of family carers in Huntington disease. *Journal of Advanced Nursing, 65*(4), 789–798.

Wisniewski, S. R., Belle, S. H., Marcus, S. M., Burgio, L. D., Coon, D. W., Ory, M, et al. (2003). The Resources for Enhancing Alzheimer's Caregiver Health (REACH): Project design and baseline characteristics. *Psychology and Aging, 18*(3), 375–384.

Zarit, S., Gaugler, J., & Jarrot, S. (1999). Useful services for families: Research findings and directions. *International Journal of Geriatric Psychiatry, 14*, 165–181.

Children with Chronic Health Conditions

Kathleen K. M. Deidrick *and* Elena Harlan Drewel

Abstract

Children with chronic health conditions form a heterogeneous group at increased risk for cognitive and emotional difficulties that may lead to difficulties in academic and social environments. Rehabilitation psychologists are in a unique position to provide support to children with chronic health conditions due to their expertise in neuropsychology, mental health, and psychological aspects of illness and disability. However, research in pediatric rehabilitation psychology is limited by small sample sizes, cross-sectional research designs, and a lack of empirically supported interventions that are population and domain specific. In the future, research in these areas will provide a rich literature to guide work in pediatric rehabilitation psychology.

Key Words: Pediatrics, chronic health condition, neurodevelopmental, rehabilitation, epilepsy, cerebral palsy.

Pediatric rehabilitation psychology is a relatively new specialty with an emerging literature that highlights the unique aspects of caring for children with chronic health conditions. The experience of children during an illness or following an injury differs from that of adults because physical, cognitive, and psychosocial development is occurring at the same time that children are trying to adjust to their condition (Farmer, Kanne, Grissom, & Kemp, 2010; Spevack, 2007). In addition to depending on their parents to meet basic needs and facilitate normal development, children must rely on their families to access and fully participate in treatment (Wade & Walz, 2010). When children are not with their families, they typically spend their time in school and with peers, where they may experience opportunities for support (e.g., specialized instruction) as well as stigma and misunderstanding (Nowicki, 2006). Children may experience medical conditions that place them at risk for frank neurological deficits (e.g., low birthweight, treatment for leukemia, sickle cell anemia) (Farmer & Deidrick, 2006; Halfon & Newacheck, 2010). Observers may not recognize these risks and perceive children as defiant or unmotivated when they are struggling with "invisible" neurologically based weaknesses in learning and self-regulation. Children may have more difficulty communicating than adults, leading those working with them to underestimate the presence and impact of physical factors such as pain and fatigue.

Professionals working with children must be able to identify and address these developmental and contextual factors during assessment and treatment. Learning about children with chronic illness and acquiring the skills necessary to work with them can be challenging, as this information exists in a fragmented research literature extending across more than one discipline (e.g., education, psychology, medicine, occupational and physical therapy, speech-language pathology, developmental disabilities, public health) (Deidrick, Grissom, &

Farmer, 2009). The purpose of this chapter is to provide an introduction to the complex set of factors that psychologists must address when working with children who have chronic health conditions.

Overview

Children with chronic health conditions form a heterogeneous group that is defined in the research literature in one of three ways: by medical diagnosis, eligibility criteria for social programs, or broad definitions that encompass a cross-categorical group of children (Farmer & Deidrick, 2006). In a recent review, van der Lee and colleagues (2007) reported that the following terms are used most often to describe this group: *chronic conditions, chronic health conditions, chronic illness,* and *children with special health care needs* (CSHCN). Operational definitions for these terms vary, with most definitions requiring the presence of a medical condition that is persistent and impairing. Some definitions are broader, including conditions that are developmental, cognitive, or behavioral/emotional. Impairment is commonly defined by functional limitations (e.g., reduction in a child's ability to participate in age-typical activities like play or school) and/or elevated use of medical, educational, or mental health services and supports. The term CSHCN has the broadest definition: "Children who have or are at increased risk of a chronic physical, developmental, behavioral, or emotional condition and who also require health care and related services of a type or amount beyond that required by children generally" (McPherson et al., 1998).

Due to variable methods of defining chronic health conditions and a tendency for researchers to study health conditions in isolation from one another the calculation of reliable prevalence rates can be challenging. As a result, prevalence rates vary widely across research studies and rates calculated in different countries cannot be reliably compared to one another (van der Lee et al., 2007). Difficulties in comparing rates across countries may be compounded by cultural factors that impact key definitions. For example, Mung'ala-Odera and Newton (2007), note that definitions of impairment may be quite different in developing countries due to cultural, economic, and societal factors.

Recent national datasets collected through telephone interviews of parents in the United States provide estimates that are based on clear and comprehensive operational definitions of chronic health conditions, despite some concerns about informant bias and methodology (e.g., types of questions asked,

uniformity in the way questions are asked across multiple years of the survey). For example, a recent review of three national telephone surveys designed to gather information about CSHCN suggested that prevalence rates ranged from 13% to 20% (Bethell, Read, Blumberg, & Newacheck, 2008). Although special education data in the United States is also an imperfect source for prevalence rates, it provides information about a relatively representative group of children that is carefully defined. National data about children receiving special education services indicate that 9.2% of children aged 6–12, 5.9% of children aged 3–5, and 2.3% of children aged 0–2 qualified for special education services in 2004 (U.S. Department of Education, 2009).

Variable prevalence rates of children with chronic health conditions are not just reported in the United States, but in other developed countries as well (Blackburn, Read, & Spencer, 2006; van der Lee et al., 2007). For example, 30% of parents who responded to the National Longitudinal Survey of Children in Canada reported that their child exhibited at least one of a list of chronic conditions (duration of 6 months). Parents identified a smaller number of children (3.6% of the total sample) as experiencing limits in their ability to participate in age-appropriate activities as a result of their health condition (McDougall et al., 2004). In the Family Resources Survey (FRS) conducted in the United Kingdom, parents were asked to identify whether their child had a chronic health condition lasting 12 months or longer or would have such a condition if he or she was not treated with medication; 7.3% of children met this definition per parent report (Blackburn, Spencer, & Read, 2010). In another contemporary study, a subgroup of parents were surveyed as part of the 2001 U.K. census, 5% of whom reported that their child experienced a chronic health condition that interfered with their functioning (Spencer, Blackburn, & Read, 2009). In developing countries, the task of obtaining reliable prevalence rates for children with chronic health conditions is more daunting. Sophisticated datasets associated with government services or departments and/or high-quality research studies are less common because these countries have fewer resources (Mung'ala-Odera & Newton, 2007). However, regardless of the definition and methodology used or the country in which the study is conducted, current research suggests that there is a sizable group of children who have chronic health conditions worldwide.

Comparison of prevalence rates in developed countries over time suggests that the number of affected children is growing (Van Cleave,

Gortmaker, & Perrin, 2010). Advances in medical care may impact prevalence rates by improving our ability to identify children who are at risk or who have "invisible" conditions (e.g., problems with learning due to injury or disease) and improving treatments so that children with certain medical conditions (e.g., low birthweight, traumatic brain injury [TBI]) are more likely to survive and go on to display neurodevelopmental sequela related to their condition (Halfon & Newacheck, 2010). Alternately, increases in prevalence could reflect changes in research methodology, including new definitions of chronic health conditions and changes in methods of data collection and measurement. Finally, increasing shared societal risk factors (e.g., changes in family compositions, increased television watching and video game use) could result in an increased risk for multiple health conditions simultaneously, such as obesity, attention deficit-hyperactivity disorder (ADHD), and asthma (Perrin Bloom, & Gortmaker, 2007).

Information about the types of chronic health conditions that rehabilitation psychologists are likely to encounter in their practices is more difficult to obtain than are overall prevalence rates. Data from the National Survey of Children's Health, which provides parent report of specific conditions for a representative sample of children in the United States, is provided in Table 10.1 (U.S. Department of Health and Human Services, 2009). Data from the 2005–2006 National Survey of CSHCN identifies the proportion of CSHCN whose parents reported a specific condition (U.S. Department of Health and Human Services, 2008). This data suggest that rehabilitation psychologists are most likely to encounter children who are diagnosed with behavioral and mental health conditions (30% ADHD, 21% depression/anxiety/emotional), select medical conditions (15% migraine/frequent headaches, 4% joint problems, 4% seizure problems, 4% heart problems), and developmental concerns (11% intellectual disability, 5% autism or autism spectrum disorder). Additional information from the Department of Education (U.S. Department of Education, 2009) indicates that among children aged 6–12, small numbers of children receive special education services under categories that suggest the presence of a chronic health condition (<0.05% TBI, 0.1% orthopedic impairments, 0.2% multiple disabilities, 0.4% sensory impairments, 0.8% other health impairments). It should be noted that these statistics may underestimate the number of children with chronic health conditions who are receiving

Table 10.1 Percent of children with parent-reported chronic conditions per the National Survey of Children's Health (2007)

	Percent
Asthma	9.0
Learning disabilities	7.8
Attention deficit-hyperactivity disorder	6.4
Speech problems	3.7
Developmental delay	3.2
Bone, joint, or muscle problems	2.2
Hearing problems	1.4
Vision problems	1.3
Autism spectrum disorder	1.1
Epilepsy or seizure disorder	0.6
Diabetes	0.4
Brain injury	0.3
Any chronic condition	22.3%

special education services, as children who qualify for services under categories of learning disability or intellectual disability may also have an underlying health condition (e.g., learning problems in a child with sickle cell disease). Taken together, these data indicate that pediatric rehabilitation psychologists are likely to encounter children with a diverse set of diagnoses in their practices.

Models for Understanding Chronic Health Conditions and Service Provision in Children

To understand the complex interaction of factors that impact children with chronic health conditions, conceptual models can be useful. The most comprehensive available model is posed by the International Classification of Functioning, Disability, and Health (ICF), illustrating the impact of the interaction between chronic health conditions and contextual factors (characteristics of the child and characteristics of the child's environment) on a child's functioning (body structures and functions) and the child's ability to participate in daily activities and be active (World Health Organization, 2001). A version of the ICF that is tailored to pediatrics provides a comprehensive overview of important factors that are related to the functioning of children with chronic health conditions (ICF-CY; World Health Organization, 2007). Narrower models of specific interactions within the domains outlined in the ICF-CY are available throughout the pediatric psychology, neuropsychology, and rehabilitation literatures. Examples include models of risk and resilience factors that predict psychological outcomes for children with health conditions and their caregivers (Wallander, Thompson, & Alriksson-Schmidt, 2003); the relation between cognitive, psychological factors, and social functioning in children with chronic physical conditions (Warschausky, 2006); adherence to medical treatment (La Greca & Mackey, 2009); and development in children with central nervous system (CNS) compromise (Baron, 2010).

Although the ICF-CY links functioning to appropriate levels of health care, the model is conceptual and is focused on the classification of children with chronic health conditions. Of practical consequence for pediatric rehabilitation psychologists are emerging models of service delivery. Models that focus on family-centered care are influential in the field, repositioning the structure of multidisciplinary teams to place families at the forefront of treatment planning and implementation (Naar-King & Donders, 2006). In addition, a model of comprehensive service is emerging that reflects the ICF-CY by addressing the needs of the child (support, information, training in foundational and applied skills), his or her family (support, information, skills training), and community (information and education) during important transitions throughout the child's development (King et al., 2002). This model is practical and focuses the reader on the logistics of providing comprehensive and life-long services for children with chronic health conditions.

In summary, an overview of the literature suggests that chronic health conditions occur in a sizable subsample of children, and the number of affected children is growing. To help rehabilitation psychologists become familiar with how chronic health conditions interact with developmental and contextual factors to impact child well-being, this chapter examines two contexts that heavily influence child development: peer relationships and school. In addition, two of the most common childhood chronic health conditions are used as examples: epilepsy and cerebral palsy. These two particular conditions were selected because they vary on dimensions that are of interest to rehabilitation psychologists, including visibility to others, degree of physical impairment, and neurocognitive impairment.

Peer Interactions and Children with Chronic Health Conditions: Epilepsy as an Example
Prevalence and Definition

Epilepsy is the most common neurological disorder to affect children and adolescents. According to recent estimates, 7 out of every 1,000 children and adolescents have epilepsy, and roughly 45,000 children under the age of 15 develop the disorder each year (Epilepsy Foundation, 2010; Williams & Sharp, 2000). Epilepsy is defined as having multiple, unprovoked, nonfebrile seizures (e.g., staring, loss of consciousness, odd behaviors, convulsions), which are sudden, excessive discharges of electrical energy in the brain (Epilepsy Foundation, 2010; Thompson & Trimble, 1996). Children with epilepsy can have more than one type of seizure. There are several epilepsy syndromes characterized by certain seizure types and prognoses. A more extensive discussion of these syndromes can be found in Williams and Sharp (2000) and Hamiwka and Wirrell (2009). A seizure is classified as either primary generalized or partial (Epilepsy Foundation, 2010; Thompson & Trimble, 1996). Primary generalized seizures involve electrical epileptic discharges in both hemispheres of the brain, have an abrupt onset, and usually create a sudden loss of consciousness. They include convulsive seizures (i.e., loss of consciousness followed by tonic and/or clonic movements of the trunk and/or extremities), absence seizures (i.e., brief staring episodes involving sudden cessation of activity and momentary loss of consciousness), atonic seizures (i.e., extremely abrupt loss of muscle tone that produce a sudden fall), and myoclonic seizures (i.e., brief, single, symmetrical jerks of the head and upper extremities that occur in a series or cluster). Partial seizures involve electrical epileptic discharges in a localized region of the brain and are frequently preceded by an aura or warning (e.g., strange feeling of fear, nausea, foul odor or taste, dizziness, déjà vu). The clinical presentation of the aura and seizure typically reflect the function of the neurons involved. They include simple partial seizures, which do not result in a loss of consciousness, and complex partial seizures, which cause an alteration of consciousness, during which the child may appear confused and exhibit automatisms (e.g., lip smacking, facial grimacing, mumbling, picking at clothing). It is possible for both simple and complex partial seizures to spread from the local region to involve both hemispheres of the brain, resulting in a secondary generalized convulsion (Epilepsy Foundation, 2010; Thompson & Trimble, 1996; Williams & Sharp, 2000).

The course of epilepsy is highly variable and depends on the seizure type, syndrome, and underlying brain pathology (Thompson & Trimble, 1996). Seizures are controlled in approximately 70–80% of children who are treated with antiepileptic medications (i.e., AEDs). There is a slightly higher mortality rate for children with epilepsy compared to children in the general population. Experiencing status epilepticus (i.e., a seizure or many short seizures lasting over 30 minutes) poses a higher risk, but mortality is usually due to underlying brain pathology rather than to the prolonged seizure activity (Thompson & Trimble, 1996; Williams & Sharp, 2000).

Approximately 70% of children with epilepsy have idiopathic or cryptogenic epilepsy, in which the cause of their seizures cannot be identified (Epilepsy Foundation, 2010). Of the remaining 30% who have symptomatic epilepsy, the etiology of the seizures is evident and may include structural brain abnormalities, birth anoxia, cerebrovascular insults, CNS infections, brain tumors, or moderate to severe head trauma (Williams & Sharp, 2000).

Social Functioning in Children with Epilepsy

Peer relationships are important for shaping children's social development and influencing their psychological well-being (Bierman, 2004; Hartup, 1983). Moreover, research shows that children who experience considerable peer difficulties, such as low peer acceptance, are at risk for later problems such as dropping out of school and psychopathology (Parker & Asher, 1987). Within the empirical literature, there is considerable evidence that children with epilepsy are at increased risk for social problems, such as peer difficulties, relative to other children (Harlan Drewel & Caplan, 2007). In particular, children with epilepsy experience less popularity and social acceptance (Hodes, Garralda, Rose, & Schwartz, 1999; Matthews, Barabas, & Ferrari, 1982), have lower levels of social competence (Austin, Smith, Risinger, & McNelis, 1994; Caplan et al., 2005; Rantanen et al., 2009; Schoenfeld et al., 1999), more social problems (Caplan et al., 2008; Dunn, Austin, & Perkins, 2008; Schoenfeld et al., 1999), experience more social isolation (Long & Moore, 1979; Stores, 1978), are bullied more frequently by their peers (Hamiwka et al., 2009), and have more peer difficulties in general (Davies, Heyman, & Goodman, 2003; Ferrari, Matthews, & Barabas, 1983; Sillanpaa, 1992) than do healthy children (Caplan et al., 2005, 2008; Davies et al., 2003; Dunn et al., 2008; Ferrari et al., 1983; Hodes et al.,

1999; Long & Moore, 1979; Matthews et al., 1982; Rantanen et al., 2009; Schoenfeld et al., 1999; Sillanpaa, 1992; Stores, 1978) or children with non-CNS health conditions (i.e., asthma, diabetes, chronic kidney disease; Austin et al., 1994; Davies et al., 2003; Ferrari et al., 1983; Hamiwka et al., 2009; Matthews et al., 1982). These results were after controlling for potential confounds such as age, sex, and socioeconomic status. Moreover, a fairly recent meta-analysis that examined the psychological adjustment of children with epilepsy (Rodenburg, Jan Stams, Meijer, Aldenkamp, & Deković, 2005) concluded that, compared to healthy children or children with other chronic health conditions, social problems were considerably greater in children with epilepsy. The differences between children with epilepsy and healthy or normative samples yielded large to medium effect sizes, and the differences between children with epilepsy and children with other chronic health conditions resulted in small to medium effect sizes. Hence, it appears that there is something specific to having a CNS condition such as epilepsy that places a child at risk for experiencing peer difficulties.

The Role of Emotional and Behavioral Functioning in Peer Relationships

Some researchers speculate that the unpredictable and unusual nature of seizures potentially increases the likelihood that children with epilepsy will be viewed negatively by their peers, thereby heightening their risk for peer relationship difficulties relative to other children (Kim, 1991; Williams, 2004). Within the developmental literature, a well-established association exists between behavioral and emotional functioning and the quality of children's peer relationships (Bierman, 2004). Coie (1990) explains that maladaptive social behaviors likely play a key role in perpetuating children's peer difficulties. For example, a child may have a certain condition or characteristic that triggers peer teasing and harassment (e.g., seizures), but it is the negative behavior that the child exhibits in response to peer provocation (e.g., avoiding or aggressing toward the peer group instead of reacting in a good-natured or skillful manner) that reinforces peers' initial dislike of the child (Coie, 1990). Several studies indicate that, relative to their peers, children with epilepsy exhibit more externalizing behaviors, such as inattention, hyperactivity, and aggression. In particular, a greater percentage of children with epilepsy have a diagnosis of ADHD, oppositional defiant disorder, and/or conduct disorder relative to normative samples (Caplan et al., 2008; Dunn et al., 2008). Children with epilepsy also score higher on parent-rated measures of inattention relative to their siblings (Schoenfeld et al., 1999) and healthy children (Caplan et al., 2008). A meta-analysis conducted by Rodenburg et al. (2005) concluded that children with epilepsy exhibit more inattentive behavior compared to healthy children and children with other chronic health conditions.

Children with epilepsy are also at greater risk for internalizing behaviors such as anxiety and depression compared to other children. Caplan and colleagues (2008) found that a greater percentage of children with epilepsy had affective and anxiety disorder diagnoses compared to healthy children. Dunn and colleagues (2008) also revealed that a greater percentage of children with epilepsy were at risk for phobias, posttraumatic stress disorder, panic attacks, and dysthymic disorder relative to normative samples. When compared to children with non-CNS health conditions, children with epilepsy rated themselves as more anxious than did children with asthma (Austin et al., 1994) and children with diabetes (Matthews et al., 1982).

Recent studies that have examined the association between emotional and behavioral functioning and social functioning in children with epilepsy indicated that externalizing behaviors such as inattention, hyperactivity, and aggression were significantly related to measures of social competence and peer difficulties (Caplan et al., 2005; Harlan Drewel, Bell, & Austin, 2009). Moreover, Harlan Drewel and colleagues also found that anxiety was significantly related to peer difficulties.

The Role of Cognitive Functioning and Seizure Variables in Peer Relationships

Researchers speculate that difficulties with memory, attention, and executive functioning (e.g., planning, problem-solving, multitasking) may adversely affect social interactions between children and their peers (Nassau & Drotar, 1997; Semrud-Clikeman & Wical, 1999). For example, a recent study found that, in children with TBI, inattention and executive dysfunction were related to generating fewer prosocial solutions in response to hypothetical peer group scenarios (Warschausky, Argento, Hurvitz, & Berg, 2003). Research on childhood epilepsy has found that affected children experience more difficulties with memory (Schoenfeld et al., 1999; Westerveld, 2010), attention (Schoenfeld et al., 1999; Semrud-Clikeman & Wical, 1999; Westerveld, 2010), and executive functioning (Hernandez et al., 2002;

Schoenfeld et al., 1999; Westerveld, 2010) compared to healthy children.

Along with neuropsychological deficits, researchers posit that seizures may have an adverse influence on children's social behaviors. For example, children with epilepsy may be anxious around their peers due to fear of having a seizure in their presence. Moreover, by reducing the exposure to positive peer group interactions, seizures may decrease the opportunity for children with epilepsy to develop prosocial behaviors (La Greca, 1990; Nassau & Drotar, 1997). Likewise, seizure characteristics (e.g., lapses in consciousness) may make children with epilepsy act inattentive or "spacey" around their peers (Coulter, 1982). Seizures may also contribute to other variables associated with peer difficulties. Studies that investigated if seizure characteristics were related to behavioral and cognitive variables found that children with epilepsy who had an active seizure status (i.e., had at least one seizure in the last year) had greater inattentive behaviors compared to children with epilepsy who had a controlled seizure status (i.e., had no seizures within the last year) (Austin et al., 2002; Williams & Sharp, 1996). Moreover, earlier age at epilepsy onset was related to greater deficits on several indicators of neuropsychological functioning, including verbal and nonverbal memory, processing speed and attention, and executive functioning (Schoenfeld et al., 1999).

A recent study by Harlan Drewel and colleagues (2009) examined the associations among neuropsychological functioning, seizure variables, and emotional and behavioral functioning in children with epilepsy. They found that seizure variables, such as age at epilepsy onset and active versus controlled seizures, and neuropsychological variables, such as executive functioning, memory, and attention, were related to peer difficulties in children with epilepsy. Caplan and colleagues (2005) also found an association between IQ and social competence in children with epilepsy. However, in the study by Harlan Drewel and colleagues, the association between seizure and neuropsychological variables and peer difficulties was mediated by behavioral functioning. In particular, the association between earlier age at epilepsy onset and peer difficulties was mediated by neuropsychological functioning and inattentive behavior. Likewise, the association between active seizure status and peer difficulties was mediated by anxiety. These findings suggested that, consistent with findings in the literature on healthy children (Bierman, 2004), behavioral and emotional functioning appears to have a direct correlation with peer difficulties in children with epilepsy. Moreover, variables such as seizure and neuropsychological functioning may play a more indirect role in their peer relationships by having a significant association with their emotional and behavioral functioning.

The Role of Psychologists in Addressing Peer Difficulties in Children with Epilepsy

Up to this point, research studies that have evaluated the efficacy of social skills interventions for children with epilepsy are sparse. Some research indicates that family-targeted interventions may have some use in improving social functioning in adolescents with epilepsy. For example, a study by Glueckauf et al. (2002) assessed the efficacy of *issue-specific family counseling model* (ICFM) in increasing social skills and other behaviors in adolescents with epilepsy. ICFM involves working with parents and the adolescent to tailor the intervention to specific issues identified by the family members. A behavioral-systemic analysis of the targeted issues is then conducted by the counselor and tentative intervention strategies are formulated and discussed with the family regarding their feasibility. The family members are then encouraged to set realistic and measurable treatment goals and required to track their progress over the course of treatment (i.e., six sessions for this study). Glueckauf and colleagues found that parents' ratings of their adolescents' prosocial behavior increased significantly from pre- to post-treatment. However, these gains were not evident at the 6-month follow-up, which may indicate a need for a longer course of family therapy. Moreover, it is uncertain if these findings were significantly different from those of a wait-list control group.

Pediatric rehabilitation psychologists may also find it useful to apply interventions that have been effective with children who have other health conditions. Considering that anxious and inattentive behaviors are directly associated with peer difficulties in children with epilepsy, these behaviors would be an important target for intervention. Maladaptive social behaviors are likely due, in part, to deficits in social-information processing (i.e., how an individual encodes, interprets, and responds to social information; Bierman, 2004; Coie, 1990). Therefore, employing social-cognitive skills training techniques that target how children with epilepsy process their social environment may be beneficial. Evidence indicates that this type of intervention, paired with instructing parents on how to reinforce positive behaviors and arrange exposures to social

situations, have yielded improvements in social competence and peer relationships for both healthy children (McFayden-Ketchum & Dodge, 1998) and children with CNS conditions such as brain tumors (Barakat et al., 2003). Social skills training techniques that promote the acquisition of social skills (e.g., teaching a child how to behave in social situations) and enhance the child's use of these skills through reinforcement strategies also have been shown to increase social competence in children with ADHD, learning disabilities, and/or intellectual impairment (Gresham, Sugai, & Horner, 2001). Moreover, cognitive-behavioral approaches, which involve balancing negative thoughts with more realistic ones and encouraging behaviors that would help disprove negative and/or catastrophic thinking, may be useful in helping children with epilepsy and their families manage feelings of anxiety and develop coping strategies for living with epilepsy (Wagner & Smith, 2007).

In addition to directly addressing maladaptive social behaviors and social skills, it may also be helpful for interventions to target variables indirectly associated with peer difficulties, such as neuropsychological deficits and seizure control. For example, pediatric rehabilitation psychologists may play a key role in evaluating neuropsychological functioning in children with epilepsy and, in turn, utilize this information to enhance social skills interventions in children with epilepsy to capitalize on their relative neuropsychological strengths (e.g., picture stories for children with stronger nonverbal skills). It may also be useful for interventions to address issues regarding treatment adherence in order to maximize seizure control. In particular, pediatric rehabilitation psychologists may be instrumental in educating both parents and children regarding the importance of medication adherence (La Greca & Mackey, 2009). Moreover, if a child has certain neuropsychological difficulties that could affect medication adherence, such as deficits in executive functioning and/or memory, providing clear reminders and external cues both to the child and family may also be beneficial. Certain AEDs are associated with undesirable side effects such as weight gain and clumsiness (Epilepsy Foundation, 2010), and children with epilepsy may feel especially self-conscious about the social impact of the side effects, as well as about explaining to their peers why they take medication (La Greca & Mackey, 2009). There is evidence that involving peers in medication management (e.g., educating children's friends regarding the disorder and how they can be supportive; teaching friends listening, problem-solving, and stress management skills) increases knowledge about the disorder and feelings of support in adolescents with chronic health conditions such as diabetes (La Greca & Mackey, 2009). Therefore, pediatric rehabilitation psychologists may play a key role in guiding children with epilepsy on how to skillfully educate their peers on the nature of the disorder and the effects of medication.

School and Children with Chronic Health Conditions: Cerebral Palsy as an Example
Prevalence and Definition

Cerebral palsy (CP) is one of the most common neurodevelopmental disorders in childhood, diagnosed in 1.3–3 out of every 1,000 children, with prevalence rates increasing in premature infants (Ancel et al., 2006) although remaining stable in full-term infants (Mukherjee & Gaebler-Spira, 2007). According to the International Workshop on the Definition and Classification of CP, CP is a nonprogressive and permanent condition caused by a cerebral event/injury occurring either before, during, or shortly after birth (e.g., intraventricular hemorrhage, stroke, malformation of the brain) that interferes with daily functioning by affecting movement and posture (Rosenbaum et al., 2007). CP in premature infants is typically caused by intraventricular hemorrhage and/or periventricular leukomalacia (Menkes & Sarnat, 2000). In full-term infants, CP can be caused by prenatal infections, anoxic or ischemic injuries, genetic syndromes, brain malformations, or stroke. Atypical CP with athetoid movements is most often caused by basal ganglia damage secondary to hyperbilirubinemia (Mukherjee & Gaebler-Spira, 2007).

Despite some disagreement about classification schemes for CP (Accardo & Hoon, 2008), classification is typically based on two dimensions: type of disturbance in muscle tone and affected limbs (Menkes & Sarnat, 2000). *Spastic CP* is the most common type of muscle tone disturbance, in which children exhibit increased muscle tone when they move. Children may also exhibit *dyskinetic CP*, with abnormal body movements and posturing (athetoid movements; dystonia) or *hypotonic CP*. Mixed forms of CP can also occur, including a combination of spasticity and extrapyramidal symptoms. One (hemiplegia) or both (diplegia) sides of the body may be involved, and the disorder may be confined to the lower or upper limbs or may affect the entire body (quadriplegia).

Recent studies using classification systems that quantify functional impairment suggest that about one-third of children with CP are unable to walk. Wide variability in ambulation is observed based on type of CP, age of child, and initial assessment of motor abilities during infancy. Furthermore, children may vary in their need for assistance with walking based on features in the environment, including the type of terrain, demands for movement, and available supports and accommodations (Palisano et al., 2009; Shevell, Dagenais, Hall, & Repacq, 2009). Children with spastic quadriplegia are the most likely to require wheelchair assistance in order to walk (Shevell et al., 2009), in contrast to children with spastic hemiplegia and diplegia, for whom wheelchair use is less likely. Even in children who are ambulatory, more subtle difficulties with apraxia, weakness, hemi-neglect, and motor overflow can be problematic (Stiles, Nass, Levine, Moses, & Reilly, 2010). Poor fine motor dexterity and visual motor integration skills are commonly reported in the literature and oral–motor problems may impede communication (Straub & Obrzut, 2009). Multiple comorbid physical conditions can be associated with CP, including problems with muscles and muscle movements, orthopedic issues (e.g., bone deformities), sensory impairments, trouble eating and digesting food, dental problems, and pain and fatigue (Menkes & Sarnat, 2000; Mukherjee & Gaebler-Spira, 2007). Pain can be life-limiting and may be overlooked in children with CP for multiple reasons, including the inability to communicate clearly using verbal or nonverbal means, greater experience with painful procedures, and a lack of sensitivity by providers to the experiences of children with cognitive disabilities (Houlihan, O'Donnell, Conaway, & Stevenson, 2004). Children with CP may get tired because it takes extra energy to complete daily tasks, which can interfere with functioning (Berrin et al., 2007). Ideally, children receive multidisciplinary treatment that includes medical and physical therapies designed to increase adaptive functioning, although many of these treatments are unproven (Braddom, 2007).

Children with Cerebral Palsy at School

Overall, children with neurodevelopmental disabilities are more likely than typically developing children and children with other chronic health conditions to exhibit difficulties with academics, as measured by receipt of special education services (Msall et al., 2003), reduced graduation rates (Blackorby & Wagner, 1996; Msall et al., 2003; Newman, Davies-Mercier, & Marder, 2003), and longer time spent in high school before graduation

(Keogh, Bernheimer, & Guthrie, 2004). Little specific information is available about how children with CP fare in school, but the available evidence is suggestive of academic concerns. Studies involving parent and child surveys that measure quality of life (QOL) indicate that children with CP and their parents report academic struggles (Arnaud et al., 2008). Some studies report higher rates of special education service use (Arnaud et al., 2008; Boulet, Boyle, & Schieve, 2009) and learning problems (Schenker, Coster, & Parush, 2005) for children with CP in comparison to typically developing children. In the only study to identify children with CP with learning disabilities using psychometric data, Frampton and colleagues (Frampton, Yude, & Goodman, 1998) found discrepancies between ability and achievement in 36% of children with CP who had IQs of 70 or higher (25% reading disability and 19% math disability).

The Role of Behavioral and Emotional Functioning in School

Emotional and behavioral disorders may interfere with a child's ability to participate in and benefit from academic instruction. Children with chronic health conditions are at increased risk for emotional and behavioral problems in comparison with healthy children (Wallander et al., 2003). Children with neurologically based disabilities are even more likely to exhibit behavioral and emotional problems of all types (Breslau, 1985; Howe, Feinstein, Reiss, Molock, & Berger, 1993). Multiple factors mediate the relation between neurological disability and behavioral and emotional difficulties, including difficulties with communication, brain-based problems with regulating attention and activity level, and the impact of cognitive difficulties on academic performance, peer relationships, and coping (Graham & Rutter, 1968; Witt et al., 2003).

The empirical literature regarding mental health in children with CP is sparse (Warschausky & Kaufman, 2010) but suggests increased rates of emotional and behavioral concerns similar to those seen in children with other neurologically based disabilities (Warschausky, 2006). Parents of children with CP report more problems on behavior questionnaires/interviews than do parents of typically developing children (Parkes et al., 2008) and children with other health conditions (McDermott et al., 1996). In these studies, approximately one-quarter of parents reported significant levels of overall emotional and behavioral problems, including difficulties with peer relationships, emotional

regulation, dependency, anxiety, overactivity, and conduct. In contrast to findings from studies on mental health in children with CP, studies of overall adjustment suggest that most children with CP fare well. Children with CP may show specific weaknesses in self-concept in areas directly impacted by physical disability (e.g., attractiveness, social interaction, athletics, academics; Miyahara & Cratty, 2004), particularly girls (Shields, Murdoch, Loy, Dodd, & Taylor, 2006). Studies looking at QOL suggest lower QOL for children with CP in similar domains, with poorer QOL reported for children with quadriplegia/more severe CP (Livingston, Rosenbaum, Russell, & Palisano, 2007). Risk factors for behavioral and emotional problems in children with CP may include the presence of seizures or intellectual disability and high levels of pain (Carlsso, Olsson, Hagberg, & Beckung, 2008; McDermott et al., 1996; Parkes et al., 2008). Findings on the relation between level of motor impairment and behavioral and emotional problems are mixed.

Family factors can increase the risk of emotional or behavioral concerns for children with chronic health conditions. Although most parents adjust positively to caring for a child with a chronic health condition (Hastings & Taunt, 2002), a subgroup of parents report a high level of stress related to caring for their child (Wallander et al., 2003). Caregivers of children with CP report difficulties that are similar to those of caregivers of children who have other chronic health conditions (Britner, Morog, Pianta, & Marvin, 2003). Although the research on caregivers of children with CP is sparse and findings are mixed, a recent review indicates that multiple child (e.g., functional status, behavior), parent (e.g., stressful life events, socioeconomic status, education, size of social support network, perceived level of social support, psychological factors), and systems (e.g., access to care) factors may interact to influence the psychological well-being of caregivers (Rentinck, Ketelaar, Jongmans, & Gorter, 2006). For example, in a study surveying mothers of children with CP, Manuel and colleagues (Manuel, Naughton, Balkrishnan, Smith, & Koman, 2003) found that 30% of the mothers endorsed clinically significant symptoms of depression. Disability severity and child functional status were not directly related to maternal depression, although level of social support was related. Although some factors may be more strongly related to psychological well-being in caregivers than others (e.g., child behavior problems, family functioning), the reasons for poor caregiver functioning vary widely by family.

For example, Glenn et al. (2008) noted that family adaptability, family needs, and child cognitive status were all related to maternal stress for 80 children with CP. However, the impact of these factors varied by family. Some families who were experiencing elevated levels of stress had a child with severe cognitive impairment but good family functioning. In contrast, other families experiencing elevated stress reported poor family functioning and a child with relatively mild cognitive impairment. High levels of stress and poor psychological well-being may be reflected in caregiver perceptions of their QOL. For example, some caregivers report social isolation, physical strain and fatigue; trouble getting away for family vacations; and difficulty accessing adequate supports (particularly for fathers) (Davis et al., 2009).

Parents of children with chronic health conditions often express concern about the well-being of other children in the household. In addition to the impact that caregiver stress may have on the unaffected sibling, parents often note that the intense needs of the affected child result in parental absences and reduced time spent with other children in the family. Other factors that can impact siblings include responsibilities for caregiving, which can sometimes be life-long realities (Cohen, 1999). Meta-analyses of research on the adjustment to a sibling with chronic illness (Sharpe & Rossiter, 2002) or intellectual disability (Rossiter & Sharpe, 2001) and qualitative review of research on the adjustment to a sibling with a physical disability (Dew, Balandin, & Lewellyn, 2008) suggest that parents of children with chronic health conditions are more likely to endorse difficulties with psychological well-being, participation in social activities, and cognitive functioning for the unaffected sibling than are parents whose children do not have any health concerns. This may be particularly true when the affected sibling requires more intensive care. In contrast to maternal report, unaffected siblings are more likely to endorse positive outcomes of their relationship with a sibling who has a chronic health condition, despite acknowledging specific areas of difficulty in some studies (e.g., feeling socially isolated, decreased self-esteem and adjustment in some domains, trouble interacting with their sibling, upset about the way their sibling is treated by others; Dew et al., 2008). Many of the same factors that impact the psychosocial well-being of the child with a chronic health condition also impact the well-being of the sibling (e.g., socioeconomic status, the well-being of the mother, family cohesion, knowledge and attitude regarding the sibling's health condition, social support; Williams et al., 2002). It should be noted that the available research on this topic is primarily focused on siblings who are younger than 18 years of age, rather than on adult siblings of persons with chronic health conditions. More information regarding sibling relationships during adulthood may be particularly important, as it may impact caregiving for the person with a chronic health condition after the death of the parents (Dew et al., 2008).

When family stress is high, it can exacerbate child behavioral or emotional difficulties for the child with CP and for the sibling. For example, a recent study presented information about behavior and family stress in cohorts of children with CP aged 9, 11, and 13 who were followed for 3 years (Sipal, Schuengel, Voorman, Van Eck, & Becher, 2009). Children with CP showed more problems with behavioral and emotional functioning than did children in a community control group. Children who were moderately limited in their motor functioning showed the most problem behaviors, with overall level of behavior problems decreasing as children got older. The more stress a family reported, the more behavioral and emotional problems were observed in the child. The reason for the link between stress and behavioral issues is unclear, but is likely due to the link between stress on parenting behavior observed in typically developing children. Little information exists about parenting behavior in families with children who have CP. A recent study suggests that children whose parents are rated by their children as nurturing and encouraging autonomy in their child functioned better psychologically and exhibited a higher QOL than did children whose parents were rated as using a controlling and harsh style (Aran, Shalev, Biran, & Gross-Tsur, 2007). Despite the connection between parental stress, parenting style, and child well-being, empirically supported treatments that target parenting are not yet available for this population (Whittingham, Wee, & Boyd, 2011).

The Role of Cognitive Functioning in Learning

Academic problems in children with CP likely have their origins in core neuropsychological deficits. Reviews of the literature on CP suggest that 30–50% of children with CP may have a diagnosis of intellectual disability, with higher rates for children who are more neurologically compromised (Menkes & Sarnat, 2000; Mukherjee & Gaebler-Spira, 2007;

Warschausky, 2006). However, as noted above, children with CP can exhibit deficits in basic cognitive and motor processes (e.g., trouble seeing, moving, or speaking) that limit output. Therefore, conclusions from traditional neuropsychological test measures that rely on children to show their knowledge through speaking or writing must be interpreted with caution (Fennell & Dikel, 2001).

For children with CP who do not meet criteria for a diagnosis of intellectual disability, a pattern of neuropsychological strengths and weaknesses is emerging from a fledgling research literature (Blondis, 2004; Bottcher, 2010; Straub & Obrzut, 2009; Warschausky, 2006). On tests of intellectual functioning, children with CP who have an intelligence quotient of higher than 70 often exhibit stronger performance on verbal subtests than on visual-spatial subtests (Bottcher, 2010). This pattern is not surprising, given research suggesting weaknesses in visual-spatial processing for children with CP that may be linked to cerebral white matter damage due to periventricular leukomalacia (Warschausky & Kaufman, 2010). Visual-motor integration deficits are also reported. However, it is difficult to determine whether weak performance on tests of visual-spatial and/or visual-motor skills are due to basic sensory or perceptual deficits, fine motor problems, or problems with motor planning (Bottcher, 2010; Warschausky, 2006).

The research literature on language in this population is mixed (Bottcher, 2010; Straub & Obrzut, 2009). Basic language skills appear to be spared, perhaps in some cases due to successful cerebral reorganization of language control. However, children with more severe forms of CP may exhibit deficits in expressive and receptive language that go beyond any difficulties with oral–motor apraxia (Straub & Obrzut, 2009). Furthermore, deficits in higher level language, such as social pragmatics, may be observed. In areas of higher level cognitive functioning, preliminary studies suggest difficulties with learning and memory, with deficits in attention and short-term/working memory, rather than in long-term memory (Pueyo, Junque, Vendrell, & Segarra, 2009; Straub & Obrzut, 2009). Emerging research is also suggestive of deficits in the area of executive functioning, including inhibitory control (White & Christ, 2005), sustained attention, and the use of efficient and organized strategies for learning (Bottcher, 2010; Christ, White, Brunstrom, & Abrams, 2003).

Emerging research linking neuropsychological deficits to academic weaknesses provides insight into the way that children with CP learn. In the area of math, Jenks and colleagues recently published a series of reports from a longitudinal study following children in the Netherlands with CP and verbal intellectual functioning estimates of more than 70. The sample included 57 children with CP, 41 of whom attended special education schools and 16 of whom were placed in mainstream classes with special education supports (Jenks et al., 2007). Children with CP who attended special schools showed early deficits in accurate addition and subtraction in comparison to age- and gender-matched controls. Problems with mathematics calculation persisted through the third grade (Jenks, de Moor, & van Lieshout, 2009; Jenks et al., 2007; Jenks, van Lieshout, & de Moor, 2009b). Group differences were not accounted for by intellectual ability, but were related to early weaknesses in numeracy (e.g., counting, understanding number concepts) and later deficits in automaticity of math facts. Children with CP who attended special schools compensated by using inefficient strategies for completing math tests, relying on counting rather than memory of facts (Jenks, de Moor et al., 2009; Jenks, van Lieshout, & de Moor, 2009a). In addition, weaknesses in executive functioning (auditory and visual working memory and shift) were associated with mathematics computation skills. Medical factors related to math learning problems included the presence of epilepsy, although motor impairment and type of CP were unrelated (Jenks, van Lieshout et al., 2009b).

Children with CP who were placed in mainstream classrooms showed weaknesses in numeracy at the beginning of first grade that were similar to those seen in children with CP who were placed in special schools. However, by the end of first grade, problems with numeracy had resolved in mainstreamed children, and they continued to be similar to controls in mathematics fluency and accuracy through the third grade. The authors noted marked differences in the time spent in math instruction across the groups, with children with CP receiving 103 fewer minutes/week of math instruction than controls if they were placed in a special education setting and 86 fewer minutes if they were placed in a mainstream classroom, presumably due to time spent in medical therapies (e.g., physical, occupational, speech-language) (Jenks et al., 2007). The authors speculate that time spent on math instruction may be a key factor, as instruction time was clearly related to math performance in statistical analyses.

Studies suggest that reading disorders in children with CP may emerge due to the same cognitive processing problems (e.g., phonological processing, receptive and expressive language level, intellectual ability) and environmental issues (e.g., environmental stimulation) observed among typically developing children (Asbell et al., 2010). However, the origin of these language based processing deficits may be somewhat different (Peeters, Verhoeven, van Balkom, & de Moor, 2008), with phonological processing weaknesses arising from speech articulation problems (Asbell et al., 2010; Peeters, Verhoeven, & de Moor, 2009; Peeters, Verhoeven, de Moor, & van Balkom, 2009). The higher prevalence of deficits in auditory comprehension and expressive language in children with CP may also place them at higher risk for reading disorders than children in the general population. In addition, there are some concerns about a lack of opportunity for children and parents to enjoy language together through interactions related to storybook reading, an activity that has been shown to be related to early reading level (Peeters, Verhoeven, de Moor, van Balkom, & van Leeuwe, 2009).

The Role of Psychologists in Helping Children to Thrive in the School Environment

Rehabilitation psychologists often collaborate with educational teams to help children perform their best at school. Sometimes, the relationship between the psychologist and the school begins when a child is reintegrated back into school after an absence due to hospitalization or medical treatment. Alternatively, the psychologist may become involved during outpatient psychological treatment for a child who is struggling at school. Because children with CP can exhibit a complex set of sensory, physical, communication, cognitive, and emotional and behavioral difficulties, thorough multidisciplinary evaluation can be an invaluable starting point for planning and intervention (Farmer et al., 2010). Initially, an evaluation that fully characterizes the child's basic sensory processing (hearing and vision), gross and fine motor deficits, functional communication skills, and any comorbid medical problems that may interfere with school performance (e.g., uncontrolled seizure activity) can be informative.

As part of this evaluation, the psychologist can provide the team with a specialized assessment of pain and fatigue. This can include evaluation of acute pain associated with medical treatments, as well as chronic pain, which is known to interfere with school performance in children with CP (Berrin

et al., 2007). The assessment of pain may be particularly challenging for children with CP who have difficulty communicating clearly to professionals and parents about their pain experiences due to oral–motor, language, and/or cognitive deficits. Simple adaptation of common self-report pain assessment scales may be effective. For example, enlarging and/or simplifying the scale (e.g., 3- or 5- point instead of 7-point scale), allowing a simple pointing response, or providing training in the use of the scale may be sufficient. In addition, several measures have been developed for children who have communication problems (Hadden & von Baeyer, 2005). For example, the Non-Communicating Children's Pain Checklist (NCCPC) was developed for use in children with cognitive disabilities that precluded accurate self-report of pain (Breau, McGrath, Camfield, Rosmus, & Finley, 2000). The checklist asks parents to rate behaviors in several domains: vocal, eating/sleeping, social, facial, activity, body/limb, and physiologic symptoms. Preliminary investigations suggest that a revised version of the NCCPC (NCCPC-R) exhibits acceptable internal consistency and external validity (Breau, McGrath, Camfield, & Finley, 2002). A briefer version of the checklist is under development, as is a version of the NCCPC specific to postoperative pain (Breau, Camfield, McGrath, Rosmus, & Finley, 2001; Breau, Finley, McGrath, & Camfield, 2002). Another strategy is to ask for caregivers to rate the child's facial expressions using a specialized scale. Research suggests that ratings of behavior, like the NCCPC-R, may be more useful in assessing pain than ratings of facial expression for children with more severe cognitive impairments, who may react to pain with a "freezing" response that is atypical among children with less severe cognitive impairments (Defrin, Lotan, & Pick, 2006).

Based on the information provided by the medical team, a more in-depth neuropsychological evaluation can be planned, with appropriate adaptations in place. These might include choosing measures that optimize the child's ability to participate by reducing demands for motor or verbal output (e.g., use of nonverbal tests of intelligence that minimize requirements for motor output), modifying materials to reduce the impact of sensory deficits (e.g., enlarging visual stimuli), and/or providing alternative communication methods (e.g. picture exchange systems, computerized devices, simple buttons to allow the child to make choices) (Fennell & Dikel, 2001). Regardless of whether accommodations are necessary, evaluations should focus on characterizing neuropsychological deficits (e.g., executive functioning, learning and memory, higher level language abilities, visual-spatial, and visual motor) and identifying neuropsychological strengths (e.g., basic verbal abilities) to help the psychologist and school develop a comprehensive intervention plan. Academic assessment including broad measures of achievement and examination of foundational skills, such as phonological processing and fluency, can be helpful. Assessment of psychological functioning can involve standardized behavioral questionnaires completed by multiple informants (e.g., child, parent, teacher), each of whom can offer a different perspective on child functioning. Psychologists should interpret questionnaires carefully and supplement them with information gathered through child and parent interview, as some questionnaire items may be inappropriate for children with marked motor and communication deficits (Shank, Kaufman, Leffard, & Warschausky, 2010).

Following a complete evaluation, the family, educational team, and psychologist can work together to create a plan for intervention that is individualized on the child's profile of strengths and weaknesses. Initial efforts may include medical and therapeutic strategies for improving functional motor and communication skills. Psychologists may assist the team in developing behavioral strategies for promoting adherence to physical, occupational, and speech-language therapy regimens (La Greca & Mackey, 2009) and developing medical and behavioral strategies for reducing pain and managing fatigue (Dahlquist & Nagel, 2009). Psychologists may also become involved with the team in planning for the implementation of constraint-induced movement therapy (CIT) for children with hemiplegic CP. Constraint-induced movement therapy uses behavioral techniques (e.g., antecedent controls, shaping, massed practice, scaffolding, and positive reinforcement) to help children learn to use the affected limb while the unaffected limb is immobilized for 2–3 weeks (Hoare, Wasiak, Imms, & Carey, 2007). Other behavioral treatments address problems with drooling (Van der Burg, Didden, Jongerius, & Rotteveel, 2007) and strategies for training children to communicate more effectively, sometimes while using an assistive communication device (Bambara, Dunlap, & Schwartz, 2004).

Many children with CP will benefit from special education supports. Parents, teachers, and treating professionals can work together to create an individualized education plan that outlines educational support services. The plan may include an individualized health plan to address medical care that must occur in the school setting. In addition, the plan can reflect physical accommodations to address motor and communication difficulties and fatigue (e.g., scheduled breaks, pacing). Plans for three types of strategies that are commonly used in pediatric rehabilitation populations can also be included: remediation of cognitive deficits, development of compensatory strategies, and accommodations to promote learning (Dawson & Guare, 2004; Deidrick et al., 2009; Farmer, Donders, & Warschausky, 2006; Hunter & Donders, 2007). If necessary, a behavior plan can be included that outlines antecedent- and consequence-based interventions to address disruptive behavior or to build positive social or adaptive skills (Bambara et al., 2004).

Conclusion
Future Directions

In summary, there is a burgeoning population of children with chronic health conditions that pediatric rehabilitation psychologists are uniquely equipped to support due to their expertise in neuropsychological functioning in children, psychosocial concerns in children with chronic health conditions and their families, and behavioral and emotional problems in children. At this point, the research literature provides information about children with chronic health conditions as a cross-categorical group. Information about specific diagnostic groups is also growing and is summarized in recent volumes (e.g., Peterson, Yeates, Ris, & Taylor, 2009; Roberts & Steele, 2010). Rehabilitation psychologists can rely on this research base as they evaluate children and their families and intervene to promote learning, mental health, and positive social functioning. However, several gaps are evident in the literature, and these limit psychologists' understanding and ability to apply existing knowledge.

First, studies often have small sample sizes, thus limiting researchers in their ability to examine the mediators and moderators of outcome in a thorough manner. For example, contextual factors that are unrelated to the child's medical condition and could impact social functioning have not been thoroughly investigated (e.g., parenting, mental health disorders in family members). Thorough evaluation of mediators and moderators might allow for the identification of subgroups of children who are more vulnerable to poor outcomes, so that psychologists could screen for risk and offer more targeted interventions. Given that pediatric rehabilitation psychologists have extensive access to children with chronic health conditions, they will be integral not only in selecting key variables to examine but also in subject recruitment. Pediatric rehabilitation psychologists may find it of great benefit to enhance subject recruitment through multisite collaboration with other pediatric rehabilitation psychologists and related health professionals. Additionally, efforts to identify issues that cut across chronic conditions allow for larger sample sizes and more sophisticated evaluations of mediators and moderators.

Second, although authors writing about pediatric rehabilitation psychology frequently caution providers to attend to developmental issues, research in this area tends to be cross-sectional in nature. This limits understanding of how children with neurodevelopmental disorders evolve over time and leads to minimal understanding of the causal relationships between risk factors and outcomes. Even more concerning is the relative lack of study regarding transition to adulthood for children with chronic health conditions. Lack of knowledge about lifespan developmental issues is reflected by a service system that is fragmented and provides poor support to adolescents and young adults.

Finally, rehabilitation psychologists will need to continue their efforts to develop manualized treatments for children with chronic health conditions and establish their efficacy. Although established treatments exist in some areas of pediatric psychology (Roberts & Steele, 2010), interventions for children with neurodevelopmental disorders are in their infancy. Recent volumes addressing treatment issues in this population cover issues that are relevant to treatment, but emphasize the need for ongoing research in this area (Farmer, Donders, & Warschausky, 2006; Hunter & Donders, 2007). Because there does not appear to be a body of literature that clearly establishes the efficacy of a given treatment for a given population (e.g., a specific social skills intervention for children with epilepsy), pediatric rehabilitation psychologists are often forced to piece together interventions in anticipation that they will lead to a significant improvement for a given group. Clearly, there is a continued need to establish empirically supported treatments for improving social functioning, academic learning, behavioral and emotional functioning, and family coping in children with chronic health conditions. In addition, development of clearly defined treatments will allow psychologists to investigate the practical worth of the services they provide, such as information about long-term outcomes and cost savings due to enhanced functioning.

References

Accardo, P. J., & Hoon, A. H., Jr. (2008). The challenge of cerebral palsy classification: The ELGAN study. *Journal of Pediatrics, 153,* 451–452.

Ancel, P. Y., Livinec, F., Larroque, B., Marret, S., Arnaud, C., Pierrat, V., et al. (2006). Cerebral palsy among very preterm children in relation to gestational age and neonatal ultrasound abnormalities: The EPIPAGE cohort study. *Pediatrics, 117,* 828–835.

Aran, A., Shalev, R. S., Biran, G., & Gross-Tsur, V. (2007). Parenting style impacts on quality of life in children with cerebral palsy. *The Journal of Pediatrics, 151,* 56–61.

Arnaud, C., White-Koning, M., Michelsen, S. I., Parkes, J., Parkinson, K., Thyen, U., et al. (2008). Parent-reported quality of life of children with cerebral palsy in Europe. *Pediatrics, 121,* 54–64.

Asbell, S., Donders, J., Van Tubbergen, M., & Warschausky, S. (2010). Predictors of reading comprehension in children with cerebral palsy and typically developing children. *Child Neuropsychology, 16,* 313–325.

Austin, J. K., Dunn, D. W., Caffrey, H. M., Perkins, S. M., Harezlak, J., & Rose, D. F. (2002). Recurrent seizures and behavior problems in children with first recognized seizures: A prospective study. *Epilepsia, 43,* 1564–1573.

Austin, J. K., Smith, S., Risinger, M. W., & McNelis, A. M. (1994). Childhood epilepsy and asthma: Comparison of quality of life. *Epilepsia, 35,* 608–615.

Bambara, L. M., Dunlap, G., & Schwartz, I. S. (Eds.). (2004). *Positive behavior support: Critical articles on improving practice for individuals with severe disability.* Austin, TX: PRO-ED and TASH.

Barakat, L. P., Hetzke, J. D., Foley, B., Carey, M. E., Gyato, K., Phillips, P. C. (2003). Evaluation of a social-skills training group intervention with children treated for brain tumors: A pilot study. *Journal of Pediatric Psychology, 28,* 299–307.

Baron, I. S. (2010). Maxims and a model for the practice of pediatric neuropsychology. In K. O. Yeates, M. D. Ris, H. G. Taylor, & B. F. Pennington (Eds.), *Pediatric neuropsychology: Research, theory, and practice* (2nd ed., pp. 473–498). New York: Guilford.

Berrin, S. J., Malcarne, V. L., Varni, J. W., Burwinkle, T. M., Sherman, S. A., Artavia, K., et al. (2007). Pain, fatigue, and school functioning in children with cerebral palsy: A path-analytic model. *Journal of Pediatric Psychology, 32,* 330–337.

Bethell, C. D., Read, D., Blumberg, S. J., & Newacheck, P. W. (2008). What is the prevalence of children with special health care needs? Toward an understanding of variations in findings and methods across three national surveys. *Maternal and Child Health Journal, 12,* 1–14.

Bierman, K. L. (2004). *Peer rejection: Developmental processes and intervention strategies.* New York: Guilford.

Blackburn, C., Read, J., & Spencer, N. (2006). Can we count them? Scoping data sources on disabled children and their households in the U.K. *Child: Care, Health, and Development, 33,* 291–295.

Blackburn, C. M., Spencer, N. J., & Read, J. M. (2010). Prevalence of childhood disability and the characteristics and circumstances of disabled children in the UK: Secondary analysis of the Family Resources Survey. *BMC Pediatrics, 10,* 1–12.

Blackorby, J., & Wagner, M. (1996). Longitudinal post-school outcomes of youth with disabilities: Findings from the National Longitudinal Transition Study. *Exceptional Children, 62,* 399–413.

Blondis, T. A. (2004). Neurodevelopmental Motor Disorders: Cerebral Palsy and Neuromuscular Diseases. In D. Dewey & D. E. Tupper (Eds.), *Developmental motor disorders: A neuropsychological perspective.* (pp. 113–136). New York: Guilford.

Bottcher, L. (2010). Children with spastic cerebral palsy, their cognitive functioning, and social participation: A review. *Child Neuropsychology, 16,* 209–228.

Boulet, S., Boyle, C. A., & Schieve, L. A. (2009). Health care use and health and functional impact of developmental disabilities among US children, 1997–2005. *Archives of Pediatrics and Adolescent Medicine, 163,* 19–26.

Braddom, R. L. (2007). *Physical medicine and rehabilitation* (3rd ed.). Philadelphia: Elsevier.

Breau, L. M., Camfield, C., McGrath, P. J., Rosmus, C., & Finley, G. A. (2001). Measuring pain accurately in children with cognitive impairments: Refinement of a caregiver scale. *Journal of Pediatrics, 138,* 721–727.

Breau, L. M., Finley, G. A., McGrath, P. J., & Camfield, C. S. (2002). Validation of the Non-communicating Children's Pain Checklist-Postoperative Version. *Anesthesiology, 96,* 528–535.

Breau, L. M., McGrath, P. J., Camfield, C. S., & Finley, G. (2002). Psychometric properties of the non-communicating children's pain checklist-revised. *Pain, 99,* 349–357.

Breau, L. M., McGrath, P. J., Camfield, C. S., Rosmus, C., & Finley, G. (2000). Preliminary validation of an observational pain checklist for persons with cognitive impairments and inability to communicate verbally. *Developmental Medicine and Child Neurology, 42,* 609–616.

Breslau, N. (1985). Psychiatric disorder in children with physical disabilities. *Journal of the American Academy of Child Psychiatry, 24,* 87–94.

Britner, P. A., Morog, M. C., Pianta, R. C., & Marvin, R. S. (2003). Measures of functioning in families of young children with Cerebral Palsy or no medical diagnosis. *Journal of Child and Family Studies, 12,* 335–348.

Caplan, R., Sagun, J., Siddarth, P., Gurbani, S., Koh, S., Gowrinathan, R., et al. (2005). Social competence in pediatric epilepsy: Insights into underlying mechanisms. *Epilepsy and Behavior, 6,* 218–228.

Caplan, R., Siddarth, P., Stahl, L., Lanphier, E., Vona, P., Gurbani, S., et al. (2008). Childhood absence epilepsy: Behavioral, cognitive, and linguistic comorbidities. *Epilepsia, 49,* 1838–1846.

Carlsso, M., Olsson, I., Hagberg, G., & Beckung, E. (2008). Behaviour in children with cerebral palsy with and without epilepsy. *Developmental Medicine and Child Neurology, 50,* 784–789.

Christ, S. E., White, D., Brunstrom, J. E., & Abrams, R. A. (2003). Inhibitory control following perinatal brain injury. *Neuropsychology, 17,* 171–178.

Cohen, M. S. (1999). Families coping with childhood chronic illness: A research review. *Families, Systems, and Health, 17,* 149–164.

Coie, J. D. (1990). Toward a theory of peer rejection. In S. R. Asher & J. D. Coie (Eds.), *Peer rejection in childhood* (pp. 365–401). Cambridge, UK: Cambridge University Press.

Coulter, D. L. (1982). The psychosocial impact of epilepsy in childhood. *Children's Health Care, 11,* 48–53.

Dahlquist, L. M. and Nagel, M. S. (2009). Chronic and recurrent pain. In M. C. Roberts & R. G. Steele (Eds.), *Handbook of pediatric psychology* (4th ed., pp. 153–171). New York: Guilford.

Davies, S., Heyman, I., & Goodman, R. (2003). A population survey of mental health problems in children with epilepsy. *Developmental Medicine and Child Neurology, 45,* 292–295.

Davis, E., Shelly, A., Waters, E., Boyd, R., Cook, K., & Davern, M. (2009). The impact of caring for a child with cerebral palsy: Quality of life for mothers and fathers. *Child: Care, Health and Development, 36,* 63–73.

Dawson, P., & Guare, R. (2004). *Executive skills in children and adolescents.* New York: Guilford.

Defrin, R., Lotan, M., & Pick, C. G. (2006). The evaluation of acute pain in individuals with cognitive impairment: A differential effect of the level of impairment. *Pain, 124,* 312–320.

Deidrick, K. K. M., Grissom, M. O., & Farmer, J. E. (2009). Central nervous system disorders: Epilepsy and spina bifida as exemplars. In M. C. Roberts & R. G. Steele (Eds.), *Handbook of pediatric psychology* (4th ed., pp. 350–365). New York: Guilford.

Dew, A., Balandin, S., & Lewellyn, G. (2008). The psychosocial impact on siblings of people with lifelong physical disability: A review of the literature. *Journal of Developmental and Physical Disability, 20,* 485–507.

Dunn, D. W., Austin, J. K., & Perkins, S. (2008). Prevalence of psychopathology in childhood epilepsy: Categorical and dimensional measures. *Developmental Medicine and Child Neurology, 51,* 364–372.

Epilepsy Foundation. (2010). Retrieved July 25, 2010, from http://www.epilepsy foundation.org

Farmer, J. E., & Deidrick, K. K. (2006). Introduction to childhood disability. In J. E. Farmer, J. Donders, & S. Warschausky (Eds.), *Treating neurodevelopmental disabilities: Clinical research and practice* (pp. 3–20). New York: Guilford.

Farmer, J. E., Donders, J., & Warschausky, S. (Eds.). (2006). *Treating neurodevelopmental disabilities: Clinical research and practice.* New York: Guilford.

Farmer, J. E., Kanne, S. M., Grissom, M. O., & Kemp, S. (2010). Pediatric neuropsychology in medical rehabilitation settings. In R. G. Frank, M. Rosenthal, & B. Caplan (Eds.), *Handbook of rehabilitation psychology* (2nd ed., pp. 315–328). Washington, DC: American Psychological Association.

Fennell, E. B., & Dikel, T. N. (2001). Cognitive and neuropsychological functioning in children with Cerebral Palsy. *Journal of Child Neurology, 16,* 58–63.

Ferrari, M., Matthews, W. S., & Barabas, G. (1983). The family and the child with epilepsy. *Family Process, 22,* 53–59.

Frampton, I., Yude, C., & Goodman, R. (1998). The prevalence and correlates of specific learning difficulties in a representative sample of children with hemiplegia. *British Journal of Educational Psychology, 68,* 39–51.

Glueckauf, R. L., Fritz, S. P., Ecklund-Johnson, E. P., Liss, H. J., Dages, P., & Karney, P. (2002). Videoconferencing-based family counseling for rural teenagers with epilepsy: Phase 1 findings. *Rehabilitation Psychology, 47,* 49–72.

Glenn, S, Cunningham, C., Poole, H., Reeves, D., & Weindling, M. (2008). Maternal parenting stress and its correlates in families with a young child with cerebral palsy. *Child: Care, Health and Development, 35,* 71–78.

Graham, P., & Rutter, M. (1968). Organic brain dysfunction and child psychiatric disorder. *British Medical Journal, 3,* 695–700.

Gresham, F. M., Sugai, G., & Horner, R. H. (2001). Interpreting outcomes of social skills training for students with high-incidence disabilities. *Learning Disabilities Research and Practice, 67,* 331–344.

Hadden, K. L., & von Baeyer, C. L. (2005). Global and specific behavioral measures of pain in children with Cerebral Palsy. *Clinical Journal of Pain, 21,* 140–146.

Halfon, N., & Newacheck, P. W. (2010). Evolving notions of childhood chronic illness. *JAMA, 303,* 665–666.

Hamiwka, L. D., & Wirrell, E. C. (2009). Comorbidities in pediatric epilepsy: Beyond "just" treating the seizures. *Journal of Child Neurology, 24,* 734–742.

Hamiwka, L. D., Yu, C. G., Hamiwka, L. A., Sherman, E. M. S., Anderson, B., & Wirrell, E. (2009). Are children with epilepsy at greater risk for bullying than their peers? *Epilepsy and Behavior, 15,* 500–505.

Harlan Drewel, E., Bell, D. J., & Austin, J. K. (2009). Peer difficulties in children with epilepsy: Association with seizure, neuropsychological, academic, and behavioral variables. *Child Neuropsychology, 15,* 305–320.

Harlan Drewel, E., & Caplan, R. (2007). Social difficulties in children with epilepsy: Review and treatment recommendations. *Neurotherapeutics, 7,* 865–873.

Hartup, W. W. (1983). Peer relations. In E. Mavis Hetherington (Ed.), *Handbook of child psychology* (vol. 4, pp. 104–196). New York: John Wiley & Sons.

Hastings, R. P., & Taunt, H. M. (2002). Positive perceptions in families of children with developmental disabilities. *American Journal on Mental Retardation, 107,* 116–127.

Hernandez, M. T., Sauerwein, H. C., Jambaque, I., De Guise, E., Lussier, F., Lortie, A., et al. (2002). Deficits in executive functions and motor coordination in children with frontal lobe epilepsy. *Neuropsychologica, 40,* 384–400.

Hoare, B. J., Wasiak, J., Imms, C., & Carey, L. (2007). Constraint-induced movement therapy in the treatment of the upper limb in children with hemiplegic cerebral palsy. *Cochrane Database of Systematic Reviews,* CD004149.

Hodes, M., Garralda, M. E., Rose, G., & Schwartz, R. (1999). Maternal expressed emotion and adjustment in children with epilepsy. *Journal of Child Psychology and Psychiatry, 40,* 1083–1093.

Houlihan, C. M., O'Donnell, M., Conaway, M., & Stevenson, R. D. (2004). Bodily pain and health-related quality of life in children with cerebral palsy. *Developmental Medicine and Child Neurology, 46,* 305–310.

Howe, G. W., Feinstein, C., Reiss, D., Molock, S., & Berger, K. (1993). Adolescent adjustment to chronic physical disorders: I. Comparing neurological and non-neurological conditions. *Journal of Child Psychology and Psychiatry, 34,* 1153–1171.

Hunter, S. J., & Donders, J. (Eds.). (2007). *Pediatric Neuropsychological Intervention.* Cambridge, NY: Cambridge University Press.

Jenks, K. M., de Moor, J., & van Lieshout, E. C. (2009). Arithmetic difficulties in children with cerebral palsy are related to executive function and working memory. *Journal of Child Psychology and Psychiatry, 50,* 824–833.

Jenks, K. M., de Moor, J., van Lieshout, E. C., Maathuis, K. G., Keus, I., & Gorter, J. W. (2007). The effect of cerebral palsy on arithmetic accuracy is mediated by working memory, intelligence, early numeracy, and instruction time. *Developmental Neuropsychology, 32,* 861–879.

Jenks, K. M., van Lieshout, E. C., & de Moor, J. (2009a). Arithmetic achievement in children with cerebral palsy or spina bifida meningomyelocele. *RASE: Remedial and Special Education, 30,* 323–329.

Jenks, K. M., van Lieshout, E. C., & de Moor, J. (2009b). The relationship between medical impairments and arithmetic development in children with cerebral palsy. *Journal of Child Neurology, 24,* 528–535.

Keogh, B. K., Bernheimer, L. P., & Guthrie, D. (2004). Children with developmental delays twenty years later: Where are they? How are they? *American Journal on Mental Retardation, 109,* 219–230.

Kim, W. J. (1991). Psychiatric aspects of epileptic children and adolescents. *Journal of the American Academy of Child and Adolescent Psychiatry, 30,* 874–886.

King, G., Tucker, M. A., Baldwin, P., Lowry, K., LaPorta, J., Martens, L., et al. (2002). A life needs model of pediatric service delivery: Services to support community participation and quality of life for children and youth with disabilities. *Physical and Occupational Therapy in Pediatrics, 22,* 53–77.

La Greca, A. M. (1990). Social consequences of pediatric conditions: Fertile area for future investigation and intervention? *Journal of Pediatric Psychology, 15,* 285–308.

La Greca, A. M., & Mackey, E. R. (2009). Adherence to pediatric treatment regimens. In M. C. Roberts & R. G. Steele (Eds.), *Handbook of pediatric psychology* (4th ed., pp. 130–152). New York: Guilford.

Livingston, M. H., Rosenbaum, P. L., Russell, D. J., & Palisano, R. J. (2007). Quality of life among adolescents with cerebral palsy: What does the literature tell us? *Developmental Medicine and Child Neurology, 49,* 225–231.

Long, C. G., & Moore, J. R. (1979). Parental expectations for their epileptic children. *Journal of Child Psychology and Psychiatry, 20,* 299–312.

Manuel, J., Naughton, M. J., Balkrishnan, R., Smith, B. P., & Koman, L. (2003). Stress and adaptation in mothers of children with cerebral palsy. *Journal of Pediatric Psychology, 28,* 197–201.

Matthews, W. S., Barabas, G., & Ferrari, M. (1982). Emotional concomitants of childhood epilepsy. *Epilepsia, 23,* 671–681.

McDermott, S., Coker, A. L., Mani, S., Krishnaswami, S., Nagle, R. J., Barnett-Queen, L. L., et al. (1996). A population-based analysis of behavior problems in children with cerebral palsy. *Journal of Pediatric Psychology, 21,* 447–463.

McDougall, J., King, G., de Wit, D. J., Miller, L. T., Hong, S., Offord, D. R., et al. (2004). Chronic physical health conditions and disability among Canadian school-aged children: A national profile. *Disability and Rehabilitation, 26,* 35–45.

McFadyen-Ketchum, S. A., & Dodge, K. A. (1998). Problems in social relationships. In E. J. Mash & R. A. Barkley (Eds.), *Treatment of childhood disorders* (pp. 338–365). New York: Guilford.

McPherson, M., Arango, P., Fox, H., Lauver, C., McManus, M., Newacheck, P. W., et al. (1998). A new definition of children with special health care needs. *Pediatrics, 102,* 137–140.

Menkes, J. H., & Sarnat, H. B. (2000). Perinatal asphyxia and trauma. In J. H. Menkes & H. B. Sarnat (Eds.), *Child neurology* (6th ed., pp. 401–466). Philadelphia: Lippincott Williams & Wilkins.

Miyahara, M., & Cratty, B. J. (2004). Psychosocial functions of children and adolescents with movement disorders. In D. Dewey & D. E. Tupper (Eds.), *Developmental motor disorders: A neuropsychological perspective* (pp. 427–442). New York: Guilford.

Msall, M. E., Avery, R. C., Tremont, M. R., Lima, J. C., Rogers, M. L., & Hogan, D. P. (2003). Functional disability and school activity limitations in 41,300 school-age children: Relationship to medical impairments. *Pediatrics, 111,* 548–553.

Mukherjee, S., & Gaebler-Spira, D. J. (2007). Cerebral palsy. In R. L. Braddom (Ed.), *Physical medicine and rehabilitation* (3rd ed., pp. 1243–1267). Philadelphia: Elsevier.

Mung'ala-Odera, V., & Newton, C. R. J. C. (2007). Identifying children with neurological impairment and disability in resource-poor countries. *Child: Care, Health, and Development, 33,* 249–256.

Naar-King, S., & Donders, J. (2006). Pediatric family-centered rehabilitation. In J. E. Farmer, J. Donders, & S. Warschausky (Eds.), *Treating neurodevelopmental disabilities: Clinical research and practice.* (pp. 149–169). New York: Guilford.

Nassau, J. H., & Drotar, D. (1997). Social competence in children with central nervous system-related chronic health conditions: A review. *Journal of Pediatric Psychology, 22,* 771–793.

Newman, L., Davies-Mercier, E., & Marder, C. (2003). School engagement of youth with disabilities. In M. Wagner, C. Marder, J. Blackorby, R. Cameto, L. Newman, P. Levine, & E. Davies-Mercier (Eds.), *The achievements of youth with disabilities during secondary school. A report from the National Longitudinal Transition Study-2 (NLTS2).* Menlo Park, CA: SRI International.

Nowicki, E. (2006). A cross-sectional multivariate analysis of children's attitudes towards disabilities. *Journal of Intellectual Disability Research, 50,* 335–348.

Palisano, R. J., Kang, L. J., Chiarello, L. A., Orlin, M., Oeffinger, D., Maggs, J., et al. (2009). Social and community participation of children and youth with cerebral palsy is associated with age and gross motor function classification. *Physical Therapy, 89,* 1304–1314.

Parker, J. G., & Asher, S. R. (1987). Peer relations and later personal development: Are low-accepted children "at risk"? *Psychological Bulletin, 102,* 357–389.

Parkes, J., White-Koning, M., Dickinson, H. O., Thyen, U., Arnaud, C., Beckung, E., et al. (2008). Psychological problems in children with cerebral palsy: A cross-sectional European study. *Journal of Child Psychology and Psychiatry, 49,* 405–413.

Peeters, M., Verhoeven, L., & de Moor, J. (2009). Predictors of verbal working memory in children with cerebral palsy. *Research in Developmental Disabilities, 30,* 1502–1511.

Peeters, M., Verhoeven, L., de Moor, J., & van Balkom, H. (2009). Importance of speech production for phonological awareness and word decoding: The case of children with cerebral palsy. *Research in Developmental Disabilities, 30,* 712–726.

Peeters, M., Verhoeven, L., de Moor, J., van Balkom, H., & van Leeuwe, J. (2009). Home literacy predictors of early reading development in children with cerebral palsy. *Research in Developmental Disabilities, 30,* 445–461.

Peeters, M., Verhoeven, L., van Balkom, H., & de Moor, J. (2008). Foundations of phonological awareness in preschool children with cerebral palsy: The impact of intellectual disability. *Journal of Intellectual Disability Research, 52,* 68–78.

Perrin, J. M., Bloom, S. R., & Gortmaker, S. L. (2007). The increase of childhood chronic conditions in the United States. *JAMA, 297,* 2755–2759.

Peterson, R. L., Yeates, K. O., Ris, M. D., & Taylor, H. G. (2009). *Pediatric Neuropsychology, Second Edition: Research, Theory, and Practice.* New York: Guilford.

Pueyo, R., Junque, C., Vendrell, P., Narberhaus, A., & Segarra, D. (2009). Neuropsychologic impairment in bilateral cerebral palsy. *Pediatric Neurology, 40,* 19–26.

Rantanen, K., Timonen, S., Hagstrom, K., Hamalainen, P., Eriksson, K., & Nieminen, P. (2009). Social competence of preschool children with epilepsy. *Epilepsy and Behavior, 14,* 338–343.

Rentinck, I. C. M., Ketelaar, M., Jongmans, M. J., & Gorter, J. W. (2006). Parents of children with cerebral palsy: A review of factors related to the process of adaptation. *Child: Care, Health and Development, 33,* 161–169.

Roberts, M., & Steele, R. (Eds.). (2010). *Handbook of pediatric psychology* (4th ed.). New York: Guilford.

Rodenburg, R., Jan Stams, G., Meijer, A. M., Aldenkamp, A. P., & Deković, M. (2005). Psychopathology in children with epilepsy: A meta-analysis. *Journal of Pediatric Psychology, 30,* 453–468.

Rosenbaum, P., Paneth, N., Leviton, A., Goldstein, M., Bax, M., Damiano, D., et al. (2007). A report: The definition and classification of cerebral palsy April 2006. *Developmental Medicine and Child Neurology—Supplementum, 109,* 8–14.

Rossiter, L., & Sharpe, D. (2001). The siblings of individuals with mental retardation: A quantitative integration of the literature. *Journal of Child and Family Studies, 10,* 65–84.

Schenker, R., Coster, W. J., & Parush, S. (2005). Neuroimpairments, activity performance, and participation in children with cerebral palsy mainstreamed in elementary schools. *Developmental Medicine and Child Neurology, 47,* 808–814.

Schoenfeld, J., Seidenberg, M., Woodard, A., Hecox, K., Inglese, C., Mack, K., et al. (1999). Neuropsychological and behavioral status of children with complex partial seizures. *Developmental Medicine and Child Neurology, 41,* 724–731.

Semrud-Clikeman, M., & Wical, B. (1999). Components of attention in children with complex partial seizures with and without ADHD. *Epilepsia, 40,* 211–215.

Shank, L. K., Kaufman, J., Leffard, S., and Warschausky, S. (2010). Inspection time and attention-deficit/hyperactivity disorder symptoms in children with cerebral palsy. *Rehabilitation Psychology, 55,* 188–193.

Sharpe, D., & Rossiter, L. (2002). Siblings of children with a chronic illness: A meta-analysis. *Journal of Pediatric Psychology, 27,* 599–710.

Shevell, M. I., Dagenais, L., Hall, N., & Repacq, C. (2009). The relationship of cerebral palsy subtype and functional motor impairment: A population-based study. *Developmental Medicine and Child Neurology, 51,* 872–877.

Shields, N., Murdoch, A., Loy, Y., Dodd, K. J., & Taylor, N. F. (2006). A systematic review of the self-concept of children with cerebral palsy compared with children without disability. *Developmental Medicine and Child Neurology, 48,* 151–157.

Sillanpaa, M. (1992). Epilepsy in children: Prevalence, disability, and handicap. *Epilepsia, 33,* 444–449.

Sipal, R., Schuengel, C., Voorman, J., Van Eck, M., & Becher, J. (2009). Course of behaviour problems of children with cerebral palsy: The role of parental stress and support. *Child Care, Health and Development, 36,* 74–84.

Spencer, N. J., Blackburn, C. M., & Read, J. M. (2009). Prevalence and social patterning of limiting long-term illness/disability in children and young people under the age of 20 years in 2001: UK census-based cross-sectional study. *Child: Care, Health, and Development, 36*, 566–573.

Spevack, T. V. (2007). A developmental approach to neuropsychological intervention. In S. J. Hunter & J. Donders (Eds.), *Pediatric neuropsychological intervention* (pp. 6–29). Cambridge, NY: Cambridge University Press.

Stiles, J., Nass, R. D., Levine, S. C., Moses, P., & Reilly, J. S. (2010). Perinatal stroke. In K. O. Yeates, M. D. Ris, H. G. Taylor, & B. F. Pennington (Eds.), *Pediatric neuropsychology: Research, theory, and practice* (2nd ed., pp. 181–210). New York: Guilford.

Straub, K., & Obrzut, J. E. (2009). Effects of cerebral palsy on neuropsychological function. *Journal of Developmental and Physical Disabilities, 21*, 153–167.

Stores, G. (1978). School-children with epilepsy at risk for learning and behavior problems. *Developmental Medicine and Child Neurology, 20,* 502–508.

Thompson, P. J., & Trimble, M. R. (1996). Neuropsychological aspects of epilepsy. In I. Grant & K. M. Adams (Eds.), *Neuropsychological assessment of neuropsychiatric disorders* (pp. 263–287). New York: Oxford University Press.

U.S. Department of Education, Office of Special Education and Rehabilitative Services, Office of Special Education Programs. (2009). *28th Annual Report to Congress on the implementation of the Individuals with Disabilities Education Act, 2006, vol. 1,* Washington, DC: U. S. Department of Education.

U.S. Department of Health and Human Services, Health Resources and Services Administration, Maternal and Child Health Bureau. (2008). *The National Survey of Children with Special Health Care Needs Chartbook 2005–2006.* Rockville, MD: U.S. Department of Health and Human Services.

U.S. Department of Health and Human Services, Health Resources and Services Administration, Maternal and Child Health Bureau. (2009). *The National Survey of Children's Health 2007.* Rockville, MD: U.S. Department of Health and Human Services.

Van Cleave, J., Gortmaker, S. L., & Perrin, J. (2010). Chronic health conditions and obesity among children and youth-Reply. *JAMA, 303*, 1915–1916.

Van der Burg, J. J. W., Didden, R., Jongerius, P. H., & Rotteveel, J. J. (2007). Behavioral treatment of drooling: A methodological critique of the literature with clinical guidelines and suggestions for future research. *Behavior Modification, 31*, 573–594.

Van der Lee, J. H., Mokkink, L. B., Grootenhuis, M. A., Heymans, H. S., & Offringa, M. (2007). Definitions and measurement of chronic health conditions in childhood: A systematic review. *JAMA, 297*, 2741–2751.

Wade, S. L., & Walz, N. C. (2010). Family, school, and community: Their role in the rehabilitation of children. In R. G. Frank, M. Rosenthal, & B. Caplan (Eds.), *Handbook of rehabilitation psychology* (2nd ed., pp. 345–354). Washington, DC: American Psychological Association.

Wagner, J. L., & Smith, G. (2007). Pediatric epilepsy: The role of the pediatric psychologist. *Epilepsy and Behavior, 11*, 253–256.

Wallander, J. L., Thompson, R. J., & Alriksson-Schmidt, A. (2003). Psychosocial adjustment of children with chronic physical conditions. In M. C. Roberts & R. G. Steele (Eds.) *Handbook of pediatric psychology* (pp. 141–158). New York: Guilford.

Warschausky, S. (2006). Physical impairments and disability. In J. E. Farmer, J. Donders, & S. Warschausky (Eds.), *Treating neurodevelopmental disabilities: Clinical research and practice* (pp. 81–97). New York: Guilford.

Warschausky, S., Argento, A. G., Hurvitz, E., & Berg, M. (2003). Neuropsychological status and social problem solving in children with congenital or acquired brain dysfunction. *Rehabilitation Psychology, 48,* 250–254.

Warschausky, S., & Kaufman, J. (2010). Neurodevelopmental conditions in children. In R. G. Frank, M. Rosenthal, & B. Caplan (Eds.), *Handbook of rehabilitation psychology* (2nd ed., pp. 329–335). Washington, DC: American Psychological Association.

Westerveld, M. (2010). Childhood epilepsy. In K. O. Yeates, M. D. Ris, H. G. Taylor, & B. R. Pennington (Eds.), *Pediatric neuropsychology: Research, theory, and practice* (2nd ed., pp. 71–91). New York: Guilford.

White, D. A., & Christ, S. E. (2005). Executive control of learning and memory in children with bilateral spastic cerebral palsy. *Journal of the International Neuropsychological Society, 11*, 920–924.

Whittingham, K., Wee, D, & Boyd, R. (2011). Systematic review of the efficacy of parenting interventions for children with cerebral palsy. *Child: Care, Health and Development, 37,* 475–483.

Williams, J. (2004). Seizure disorders. In R. T. Brown (Ed.), *Handbook of pediatric psychology in school settings* (pp. 221–239). New York: Guilford.

Williams, J., & Sharp, G. (1996). Academic achievement and behavioral ratings in children with absence and complex partial epilepsy. *Education and Treatment of Children, 19,* 143–152.

Williams, J., & Sharp, G. B. (2000). Epilepsy. In K. O. Yeates, M. D. Ris, & H. G. Taylor (Eds.), *Pediatric neuropsychology: Research, theory, and practice* (pp. 47–73). New York: Guilford.

Williams, P. D., Williams, A. R., Graff, J. C., Hanson, S., Stanton, A. et al. (2002). Interrelationships among variables affecting well siblings and mothers in families of children with a chronic illness or disability. *Journal of Behavioral Medicine, 25*, 411–424.

Witt, W. P., Riley, A. W., Coiro, M. J., Witt, W. P., Riley, A. W., & Coiro, M. J. (2003). Childhood functional status, family stressors, and psychosocial adjustment among school-aged children with disabilities in the United States. *Archives of Pediatrics and Adolescent Medicine, 157,* 687–695.

World Health Organization. (2001). *International classification of functioning, disability, and health.* Geneva, Switzerland: World Health Organization.

World Health Organization. (2007). *International classification of functioning, disability, and health-Children and youth version.* Geneva, Switzerland: World Health Organization.

Aging, Rehabilitation, and Psychology

Adam T. Gerstenecker *and* Benjamin T. Mast

Abstract

This chapter examines the role of psychologists in the rehabilitation of older adults. The chapter begins with a review of the changes expected to take place in the population demographics of the United States and its impact on geriatric rehabilitation. The next section highlights core concepts in geriatric rehabilitation, as well as predictors of successful outcome. In the final sections of the chapter, psychologists' roles within geriatric rehabilitation will be examined, with particular emphasis placed upon assessing cognitive impairment and depression, and specific interventions for treating depression in geriatric rehabilitation patients.

Key Words: Geriatric rehabilitation, geropsychology, medical rehabilitation, assessment, intervention, physical performance, disability, executive functioning, chronic pain, sleep disorders.

A Changing Population

There were 1.7 million more adults over the age of 65 living in the United Kingdom in 2009 than in 1984 (Office for National Statistics, 2009). This represents an increase from 15% to 16% of the total population, and this increase is expected to grow to 23% by 2034. Older adults over the age of 85 represent the fastest growing segment of this population and their numbers are expected to more than double in number to 3.5 million by 2034 (Office for National Statistics, 2009). In 2006, 37.3 million adults over the age of 65 lived in the United States, and this number is projected to more than double to 86.7 million by 2050 (Federal Interagency Forum on Aging-Related Statistics, 2008). Of the 37.3 million adults over the age of 65, 14% (5.3 million) are 85 years or older, but by 2050 the percent of older adults 85 years and older is expected to grow to 24% (20.9 million). This trend is expected to continue worldwide as life expectancy steadily increases in industrialized countries. As can be seen, the demographics of the population are quickly changing and adjustments to the current rehabilitation system will be needed in order to keep pace.

Older adults over the age of 65 are at an increased need for rehabilitation services in comparison to the general population, so a corresponding increase in the number of rehabilitation psychologists trained in working with older adults will be needed in the near future. Moreover, advances in medicine have led to an increased number of older adults living longer despite chronic disease. Lichtenberg and Schneider (2010) note that because people are living longer with chronic disease (i.e., heart disease), it is becoming much more common for rehabilitation psychologists to work with elders who have a wide range of comorbid medical conditions.

Geriatric Rehabilitation Concepts: Disability, Comorbidity, and Frailty

Numerous organizations and authors have outlined varying definitions of what constitutes rehabilitation. The World Health Organization (WHO) defines rehabilitation as all activities aimed at reducing the effects of functional limitation and handicapping conditions, enhancing the social integration of the individual and their ability to be active and fulfill vital goals with respect to family life, work, and leisure time (Wressle, Oberg, & Henriksson, 1999). Other definitions appear in the rehabilitation literature, but all are unified by the central theme of working toward the goal of overcoming disability to increase function. Applied to geriatric rehabilitation, this goal can be viewed as helping a person overcome functional or cognitive limitations due to aging, illness, or disability in order to achieve the highest possible independence and quality of life (QOL).

Several outcomes measures are most common in geriatric rehabilitation. Rehabilitation efficiency has been defined as the ratio of functional gains divided by the patient's length of stay (Patrick, Knoefel, Gaskowski, & Rexroth, 2001). Rehospitalization after discharge from a geriatric rehabilitation program has also been used to track long-term outcome. Finally, post-discharge placements to either the patient's home, or to an independent living, skilled nursing, or other long-term care facility have been used as common outcomes related to the effectiveness of geriatric rehabilitation.

In geriatric rehabilitation, it is important to differentiate disability from related terms like *frailty* and *comorbidity*. Once used to refer to the same concept, disability, frailty, and comorbidity are currently conceptualized as distinct despite possessing overlapping characteristics (Fried, Ferrucci, Darer, Williamson, & Anderson, 2004). These terms are important in geriatric rehabilitation because the amelioration of disability is often the primary goal, and comorbidity and frailty often affect the outcome of this goal.

Disability refers to the inability of a person to initiate, engage in, and carry out activities essential to daily living. Inherent in this definition is the notion that disability interferes on a direct level with activities of daily living (ADLs; i.e., eating, bathing, dressing, toileting, etc.) and with instrumental activities of daily living (IADLs; i.e., doing housework, driving a car, balancing a checkbook, etc.).

A person can experience disability through impairments in both physical and cognitive processes, and the risk for and acquisition of disability increases directly with age (Lichtenberg, 1998) and is associated with increased mortality (Gill, Richardson, & Tinetti, 1995; Landi et al., 2010) and hospitalization (Gill, Allore, Holford, & Guo, 2004; Ostir, Volpato, Kasper, Ferrucci, &

Guralnik, 2001). A central aim of geriatric rehabilitation is to increase performance in ADLs, mobility, IADLs, and subsequent independence. Therefore, the rehabilitation process is best conceptualized as a multifaceted intervention designed to reduce disability and its effects on the patient and family (Wressle et al., 1999).

Comorbidity is defined as the presence of multiple diagnoses and is distinct from both disability and frailty. Often besieged with multiple secondary illnesses (Stineman, 1997), older adults in rehabilitation frequently have to overcome obstacles other than the primary diagnoses that may have prompted admission to rehabilitation (e.g., stroke or lower extremity fracture), and medical comorbidity has been found to be one of the best predictors of rehabilitation efficiency (Patrick et al., 2001). Aside from medical comorbidity, psychiatric comorbidity has been observed in up to 73% of older adults in the rehabilitation setting (Patrick et al., 2001) and can affect the ability of older adults to perform optimally in a rehabilitation program.

Comorbidity has been found to be inversely (Patrick et al., 2001) or not significantly associated with the age of patients in geriatric rehabilitation (Lichtenberg, 1998), and this inverse association may be due to increased mortality among older adults with multiple medical diagnoses. This notion is bolstered by Arfken et al. (1999), who observed that comorbidity and not age was related to mortality in a follow-up study of 667 consecutive admissions to a rehabilitation hospital. In a geriatric rehabilitation patient population, Patrick et al. (2001) found musculoskeletal, vascular, cardiac, and psychiatric impairment dominant in the illness profiles of patients. In the overall older adult population, estimates place the percent living with heart disease at 30.9%, hypertension at 53.3%, diabetes at 18%, arthritis at 49.5%, cancer at 21.1%, stroke at 9.3%, and moderate to severe memory impairment at 12.7% (Federal Interagency Forum on Aging-Related Statistics, 2008).

Although not an inherent focus of the conceptualized aims of rehabilitation, *frailty* nevertheless plays a substantial role in the geriatric rehabilitation process. Experiencing impairment of function in multiple areas, frail older adults are at an increased risk for minor stressors causing a disproportionate amount of functional loss due to a decrease in physiological reserve (Young, Brown, Forster, & Clare, 1999). Frail older adults often experience wasting, loss of endurance, decreased balance and mobility, depressed performance, psychomotor retardation, and decreased cognitive capabilities that may hinder recovery and functional progress obtained in a rehabilitation program (Fried et al., 2004). Frailty increases with a person's age, and the more frail the person the greater the risk for mortality, disability (Gallucci, Ongaro, Amici, & Regini, 2009), and placement in a nursing home after discharge from an inpatient rehabilitation setting (Puts, Lips, Ribbe, & Deeg, 2005).

In addition to frailty and comorbidity, older adults in rehabilitation may have depression and/or cognitive impairment that can negatively impact rehabilitation outcomes.

Depression and Cognitive Impairment in Geriatric Rehabilitation

Depression

Depression has a strong influence on an older adult's ability to function optimally in the rehabilitation process. Up to 30–40% of older adults in inpatient medical rehabilitation demonstrate clinically significant elevations of depressive symptoms (Caplan & Moelter, 2000) compared to 14.4% of community-dwelling older adults (Federal Interagency Forum on Aging-Related Statistics, 2008). Depression has been identified as a significant predictor of physical recovery (Mossey, Mutran, Knott, & Craig, 1989) and hospital readmission following inpatient rehabilitation of older adults (Mast, Azar, MacNeill, & Lichtenberg, 2004). Therefore, all older adults in rehabilitation should be screened for symptoms of depression early in the process, regardless of the primary admitting diagnosis. High rates of depression in patients with stroke have long been emphasized in the literature (Andersen, Vestergaard, Riis, & Lauritzen, 1994; Gainotti & Marra, 2002; Robinson, Starr, Lipsey, Rao, & Price, 1984), but depression has been reported to be nearly as common in patients with lower extremity fracture as it was in patients with stroke (Mast, MacNeill, & Lichtenberg, 1999).

One reason for the high rates of depression in older adults in rehabilitation is that most present with significant comorbidity and functional dependence, both of which increase risk for depression both in the rehabilitation stay and after discharge. Older adults with greater vascular risk factors (i.e., hypertension, heart disease, diabetes, etc.) are at an increased risk of depression due to corresponding microvascular changes in the frontal and subcortical regions of the brain (Alexopoulos et al., 1997). These microvascular changes become more profound as the number of vascular risk factors increases, and rates of depression are also elevated in older adults with more vascular burden. For example, in a sample of 670 geriatric rehabilitation patients, clinically significant symptoms of depression were observed in 30.7% of patients presenting with one vascular risk factor, but that percent rose to 46.4 in patients presenting with two or more vascular risk factors (Mast, MacNeill, & Lichtenberg, 2004). Furthermore, geriatric rehabilitation patients with greater vascular burden demonstrated greater depression during their rehabilitation stay and were several times more likely to be depressed 6 and 18 months after discharge (Mast, MacNeill, & Lichtenberg, 2004; Mast, Neufeld, MacNeill, & Lichtenberg, 2004).

High rates of functional dependence are also strongly predictive of depression (Singh et al., 2000), and the functional limitations that prompt rehabilitation among older adults serve to increase rates of depression in this setting. Depression has been shown to be a significant predictor of disability even after controlling for medical illness (Koenig, Shelp, Goli, Cohen, & Blazer, 1989), so depressive symptoms may not be only a by-product of impairments in functioning but also a catalyst leading to their acquisition. No matter the direction of influence, rates of depression in older adults in the rehabilitative setting are high and have a neglected impact on rehabilitation outcomes.

Dementia and Cognitive Decline

Even though cognitive impairment can be classified as a comorbid medical disorder and can add to the frailty of an older adult, its impact upon the rehabilitation process is in need of special attention. Beginning at age 60, the probability of acquiring dementia doubles every 5 years and affects up to 45% of older adults over the age of 85 (Turner, 2003). In the rehabilitative setting, estimated rates of cognitive impairment and dementia in older adults vary by the assessment tools and samples utilized in a study, but a consensus in the literature concurs with the finding that the frequency of dementia is significantly greater in medical rehabilitation patients than in community-dwelling peers under age 80. In this cohort, dementia is twice as common in medical rehabilitation (Lichtenberg, 1998), and similar to depression, the rates of dementia in older adult medical patients are high regardless of principal medical diagnosis (Mast, MacNeill, & Lichtenberg, 1999).

The odds of succeeding in a medical rehabilitation program are up to 20 times less in older adults with dementia (Lieberman et al., 1996), but Huusko et al. (2000) found patients with mild dementia to achieve similar results in comparison to patients with normal cognition following intensive geriatric rehabilitation. Diminished cognition has been linked to an increased incidence of falls (Rösler, Krause, Niehuus, & von Renteln-Kruse, 2008) and hip fracture (Buchner & Larson, 1987) in the rehabilitation setting. Furthermore, rates of discharge to a more supervised setting for older adults who were living alone prior to rehabilitation (MacNeill, Lechtenberg, & LaBuda, 2000), rehospitalization within 3 months of discharge (Sullivan, 1992), and discharge from inpatient rehabilitation to a nursing home unit (Rösler et al., 2008) are all high in elders with cognitive impairment. Moreover, cognition was found to be a significant predictor accounting for up to 34% of unique variance in IADL performance (LaBuda & Lichtenberg, 1999), and poor performance on IADLs can also serve as a catalyst to loss of independence, rehospitalization, and nursing home placement (Wolinsky, Callahan, Fitzgerald, & Johnson, 1992).

Executive Dysfunction

Although the role of general cognitive functioning is well understood and identified as a point of focus, often executive functioning is not adequately tested by measures commonly used to screen for cognitive decline in older adults (see Mast & Gerstenecker, 2010, for a review). Executive functioning is highly involved in the ability to engage in goal-directed behavior, planning, and modifying actions and plans in response to feedback from the environment. Importantly, declines in executive functioning are predictive of functional capacity (Royall, Palmer, Chiodo, & Polk, 2004). Executive functioning has been demonstrated to be associated with physical performance after controlling for overall cognitive functioning and demographic characteristics and was implicated in increased disability risk in a sample comprised of predominantly older African American adults (Schneider & Lichtenberg, 2008).

Older adults with executive dysfunction have been found to experience difficulty managing complex tasks of the lower extremities (Ble et al., 2005). For example, walking at a normal pace is an overlearned activity requiring a minimal amount of attention. Walking at a brisk pace combined with managing simple obstacles, however, requires more attention and manipulation of the environment, and older adults with normal gait but executive dysfunction are more impaired at this task in relation

to their peers without executive dysfunction. Given its influence on mobility, functional capacity, and disability, executive functioning control should be given strong consideration when evaluating an older adult's ability to function independently (Lewis & Miller, 2007).

Assessment: A Critical Role of Psychologists Working in the Geriatric Rehabilitation Setting

Comprehensive assessment of a patient's needs requires input from the entire rehabilitation team (Young et al., 1999), and a lack of communication among team members can lead to underidentification patient needs (Cunningham et al., 1996). To effectively function as a contributing member of a rehabilitation team, psychologists require an understanding of relevant assessment tools and their psychometric properties. For the evaluation of cognitive impairment, time constraints limit the number of patients that can be assessed by a psychologist working in a rehabilitation unit. A full battery consisting of multiple measures designed to assess multiple cognitive domains is not needed or appropriate for every older adult beginning a rehabilitation program. However, every patient should be screened for cognitive impairment and recommendations for treatment and further testing made from the results. Screening should also take place at regular intervals throughout the rehabilitation process. By performing regular screens, the psychologist is better able to gauge a patient's ability to engage in interventions and also help to determine if interventions are increasing a patient's overall cognitive capabilities.

Although all cognitive screening instruments and brief batteries require evidence of clinical utility and validity, differing psychometric aspects of assessment measures may be emphasized depending upon the purpose of the assessment (Mast & Gerstenecker, 2010). Because instruments used for the early detection of dementia syndromes require high levels of sensitivity (percentage of people with cognitive impairment correctly identified), instruments used for the purpose of predicting functioning have greater need of predictive validity. As patients are identified as experiencing cognitive decline, the purpose of ongoing assessment shifts toward evaluating the impact of cognitive impairment on daily functioning and the potential need for enhanced environmental support within the rehabilitation stay and after discharge to ensure safety. Similarly, when recommendations for post-discharge living arrangements are being formulated, a psychologist should take the patient's environment into consideration in relation to cognitive capability. For those affected by more severe cognitive impairment, discharge to independent living may undermine safety and increase the potential for rehospitalization.

Short Screens

Depending upon time constraints and initial cognitive presentation, both short dementia screening measures and/or brief batteries can be employed to evaluate cognitive impairment. Unfortunately, the cognitive screening of older adults in a medical setting is often accomplished solely with the Mini Mental State Examination (MMSE; Folstein, Folstein, & McHugh, 1975), and this may lead to a large number of older adults with cognitive impairments not being correctly identified (Mast & Gerstenecker, 2010). The MMSE has a number of limitations, including a ceiling effect that renders it less sensitive to mild impairment, has limited focus on memory (3 points out of 30), and lacks an executive functioning component (Brodaty, Fay, Gibson, & Burns, 2006; Kahokehr, Siegert, & Weatherall, 2004; Lorentz, Scanlan, & Borson, 2002; Tombaugh & Mcintyre, 1992). Age and education effects can also significantly influence scores, but corrected norms designed to mitigate this limitation are available (Tombaugh, McDowell, Kristjansson, & Hubley, 1996). However, other measures exist that take less time to administer and exhibit psychometric properties superior to those of the MMSE.

Three separate reviews (Brodaty et al., 2006; Lorentz et al., 2002; Milne et al., 2008) have identified the Mini-Cog (Borson, Scanlan, Chen, & Ganguli, 2003), the Memory Impairment Screen (MIS; Buschke et al., 1999), and the General Practitioners Assessment of Cognition (GPCOG; Brodaty et al., 2002) as possessing promise for the rapid screening of older adults for cognitive impairments in a primary care setting. Although the previously mentioned reviews did not specifically evaluate the ability of the MIS, Mini-Cog, and GPCOG to detect cognitive impairment in older adults in inpatient rehabilitation, the psychometric properties of the measures may generalize because of the similarities in the samples (medically ill older adults recruited within a medical setting). And although the base rate of cognitive impairment and dementia in older adults evaluated in inpatient rehabilitation is higher than that seen in primary care, this difference is not expected to limit the generalization of the measures due to samples with varying base rates of cognitive impairment being utilized in validation studies. In the following section, the guidelines of administration and psychometric properties of the MIS, Mini-Cog, and GPCOG will be reviewed, along with a measure similar to the MMSE but with better operating characteristics (the Montreal Cognitive Assessment [MoCA]) and a measure useful when assessing older adults with sensory impairments (the Fuld Object Memory Evaluation [FOME]).

MINI-COG

Taking approximately 3 minutes to administer, the Mini-Cog employs a combination of clock drawing and the delayed recall of three words (Borson et al., 2003). The first step involves the patient listening to and repeating a list of three semantically unrelated words. The patient is then asked to draw the face of a clock and set the hands to "ten minutes after eleven." After completing the clock drawing, the patient is instructed to verbally retrieve the three semantically unrelated words, but this portion of the test is skipped if the patient cannot remember the words on the initial learning trial. Developed to improve the operating characteristics of traditional clock drawing while at the same time mitigating for bias effects from race, culture, education, and language (Borson, Scanlan, Brush, Vitaliano, & Dokmak, 2000), the Mini-Cog has been shown to be equally effective when administered by expert or naïve raters (Scanlan & Borson, 2001).

A sample of 249 ethnically diverse older adults with a dementia base rate of 50% was used when originally validating the measure. In the study, the Mini-Cog significantly exceeded the operating characteristics of the MMSE and demonstrated a sensitivity of 99% and a specificity (percentage of people correctly identified as not having cognitive impairment) of 93% (Borson et al., 2000). In a follow-up study utilizing 1,179 older adults from the MoVIES project, the Mini-Cog demonstrated a sensitivity of 76% and a specificity of 89%. However, the lower sensitivity and specificity observed in the follow-up study were not unexpected due to the differing base rates in the samples (50% vs. 6.4%) but were still superior to those of the MMSE (Borson et al., 2003).

MEMORY IMPAIRMENT SCREEN

Developed to be a simple yet accurate screening instrument for cognitive impairment, the MIS is a four-word test of delayed recall that can be administered in approximately 4 minutes (Kuslansky, Buschke, Katz, Sliwinski, & Lipton, 2002). To start the screen, four words belonging to unrelated semantic categories are presented to the patient on four flashcards. The word on the flashcard (e.g., New York) is then read and the patient is instructed to associate the word to the semantic category to which it belongs (e.g., city). After the process is completed for all four words, a 2–3 minute distracter task is initiated (counting from 1 to 20 forward and backward). After completion of the distracter task, the patient is asked to remember and recall as many words as he or she is able to recollect. If a word is not recalled in the free-recall trial, the associated semantic cue is verbally presented and the patient given a second opportunity to recall the word. Scores on the MIS range from 0 to 8 with 2 points given for each word recalled in the free-recall condition and 1 point given for each word recalled after the associated semantic category is presented. A screen is considered positive if scores fall below 4 (Buschke et al., 1999).

In the original validation study, the operating characteristics of the MIS were examined after being administered to 483 community volunteers with a 10% base rate of dementia. The area under the curve (AUC) was 0.94, and no bias effects due to education were observed. The MIS achieved a sensitivity of 80%, specificity of 96%, positive predictive value (PPV; number of people with positive results correctly identified) of 69%, and negative predictive value (NPV; number of people with negative results correctly identified) of 98% when evaluating for general cognitive impairment, and a sensitivity of 87% when evaluating only for dementia of the Alzheimer's type (AD) (Buschke et al., 1999) when using the recommended cutscore of 4. In a follow-up study, the MIS was administered to a sample of 240 community-dwelling older adults (12% dementia prevalence) (Kuslansky et al., 2002). No bias effects due to education were detected, and the MIS was found to outperform a conventional three-word memory screen in its ability to differentiate between older adults with cognitive impairment and older adults without cognitive impairment.

Even though its ease of administration and short duration make the MIS an attractive screen for use in a medical setting (Holsinger, Deveau, Boustani, & Williams, 2007), the lack of an executive functioning component may limit the overall effectiveness of the MIS. However, the potential for mitigation of this limitation may be possible by including measures with an executive functioning component, such as the Trail Making Test (TMT; Reitan, 1955) Parts A & B, or verbal fluency tasks to the distraction portion of the MIS. For example, the operating characteristics of the MIS were shown to be improved when used with the Isaacs Set Test (IST; Isaacs & Kennie, 1973) and animal naming in place of counting as the distracter task (Grober et al., 2008).

GENERAL PRACTITIONERS ASSESSMENT OF COGNITION

Administered in approximately 4–5 minutes, the GPCOG combines cognitive and informant data into a two-stage dementia screening instrument. Nine total points are possible on the cognitive portion with 1 point given for orientation to time, 1 point for awareness of a high-profile news story, 1 point for appropriate numbering and spacing, 1 point for placing the time as "ten minutes past eleven" on a clock drawing task, and 1 point for each unit when recalling "John, Brown, 42, West Street, Kensington." An optional informant section is included for patients scoring between 5 (positive screen) and 9 (negative screen). When an informant is utilized, comparisons of the patient's present functioning to that observed "a few years ago" are made. If the informant indicates the patient has more current difficulty with three or more of the six tasks in question (memory of recent conversations, misplacing items, word finding difficulties, money management, medication management, and need for travel assistance), then further evaluation is needed to rule out the presence of cognitive impairment (Brodaty, Kemp, & Low, 2004).

In the original validation study, a sample of 283 community-dwelling older adults with a dementia, a prevalence of 29% was examined. The GPCOG was found to be as effective or better than the MMSE by demonstrating a sensitivity of 85%, specificity of 86%, PPV of 71%, and an overall misclassification rate of 14%. However, in a follow-up study, sensitivity was found to be higher but sensitivity lower than that of the MMSE, so these results call into question the ability of the GPCOG to better differentiate older adults with cognitive impairment from those without cognitive impairment in comparison to the MMSE. The GPCOG has been found to be free of bias effects due to education, gender, and depression, but not to age (Brodaty et al., 2004).

MONTREAL COGNITIVE ASSESSMENT

The MoCA (Nasreddine et al., 2005) was designed to contain properties similar to those of the

MMSE while better detecting the presence of mild cognitive impairment in older adults scoring in the normal range on the MMSE. With administration time and scoring similar to the MMSE, the MoCA contains items assessing short-term memory, visuospatial abilities, executive functioning, attention, concentration, working memory, language, and orientation to time and place (Nasreddine et al., 2005). Thirty points are possible, and the recommended cutscore is 26 (Nasreddine et al., 2005). The MoCA is available in 27 languages, with administration instructions and normative data located at http://www.mocatest.org/.

The MoCA was administered to 93 older adults with Alzheimer's dementia, 94 older adults with mild cognitive impairment (MCI), and 90 older adults with no cognitive impairment (normal controls) (Nasreddine et al., 2005). With a sensitivity of 0.90 and 1.00 in the MCI and AD groups, respectively, the MoCA demonstrated utility superior to the MMSE. However, the specificity of the MoCA (0.87) was found to be slightly lower than that of the MMSE. For both cognitively impaired groups, the MoCA's PPV was observed to be 0.89 and its NPV was observed to be 0.91 for the MCI patients and 1.00 for the AD patients. Furthermore, changing the cutscore to 27 for older adults with over 12 years of education was recommended because of bias effects due to education being observed. At a cutscore of 26, subsequent studies have demonstrated a trend characterized by high sensitivity and low specificity (Luis, Keegan, & Mullan, 2009; Smith, Gildeh, & Holmes, 2007), but when a cutscore of 23 was used, both sensitivity (0.96) and specificity (0.95) were found to be excellent (Luis et al., 2009). The MoCA has also received empirical attention for its ability to detect cognitive impairment in people with Parkinson disease (PD) (Nazem et al., 2009; Zadikoff et al., 2008). The MoCA's range of specificity is wide across the few studies that have examined its clinical utility, and it has not been compared to screens other than the MMSE.

TESTING PATIENTS WITH SENSORY IMPAIRMENT: THE FOME

As a psychologist working in the rehabilitation setting, the probability of working with patients with poor hearing and/or vision is relatively high. The FOME (Fuld, 1981) is a useful measure to help in these instances (Chung & Ho, 2009). Developed to assess episodic memory function in an elderly population (Fuld, 1981), the FOME stands apart from other cognitive screening measures because it

allows patients to use tactile, auditory, and visual processes when encoding information. The tactile processing of information is utilized by patients during the first step of administering the measure, when the patient is asked to touch and identify an object in a bag without looking. The person then pulls the object out of the bag (visual encoding) and then the examiner repeats the name of the object (auditory encoding). The bag contains ten common objects (e.g., bottle, button, scissors), and the process is repeated until all ten objects are removed from the bag, with mistakes being corrected by the test administrator. The objects are then placed back into the bag by the test administrator so they are out of sight for recall trials. After completing a 60-second verbal fluency distracter task, the patient is asked to name as many objects as possible that he or she can remember removing from the bag. After the free-recall trial, the test administrator reminds the patient of the objects not recalled. There are five trials on the FOME, with 1 point being given for each correctly recalled object. A clinical cutoff of 30 is recommended (Wall, Deshpande, MacNeill, & Lichtenberg, 1998).

Numerous studies have demonstrated the FOME is a measure relatively unaffected by bias effects and has excellent operating characteristics across samples with differing rates of cognitive impairment (Chung, 2009; La Rue, 1989; Loewenstein, Duara, Arguelles, & Arguelles, 1995; Marcopulos et al., 1999; Mast, Fitzgerald, Steinberg, MacNeill, & Lichtenberg, 2001; Wall et al., 1998). The FOME may also be a more natural measure of memory than other memory tests because the learning and encoding of words occur at a slower pace, placing fewer demands on processing speed and reducing the partial confound that may exist between processing speed and memory in older adults (Salthouse, 1993, 1994). Furthermore, normative data is available for using only three of the five trials, and the decreased administration time when using the three-trial version may enhance its ability to be used as a cognitive screening instrument (Loewenstein et al., 2001).

Brief Batteries

If more time is available or a patient performs poorly on a short dementia screen, brief batteries can be administered that give a clearer picture of a patient's cognitive functioning. Two such measures are the Repeatable Battery for the Assessment of Neuropsychological Status (RBANS; Randolph, Tierney, Mohr, & Chase, 1998) and the Dementia

Rating Scale-2 (DRS-2; Jurica, Leitten, & Mattis, 2001).

REPEATABLE BATTERY FOR THE ASSESSMENT OF NEUROPSYCHOLOGICAL STATUS

The RBANS is designed to assess changes in cognitive functioning and can be administered in less than 30 minutes, and alternate forms that allow for the retesting of older adults are available (Randolph et al., 1998). Twelve subtests comprise the measure and span immediate memory, delayed memory, visual-spatial/constructional ability, attention, and language. Normative data is available for patients aged 20–89.

The ability of the RBANS to detect differences in the performance of 20 patients with AD and 20 patients with Huntington disease (HD) from 40 age- and education-matched normal controls was analyzed as part of the original validation study of the measure. Only one index score was found not to differ significantly (visual-spatial/constructional). Performance on the delayed memory and language indices was observed to be lower in the AD group, whereas attention and visual-spatial/constructional were lower in the HD group. Furthermore, the measure exhibited 90% sensitivity and 90% specificity when detecting for the presence or absence of cognitive impairment. The RBANS total score has been shown to be similar to estimates of premorbid intelligence in a community sample of older adults but significantly different in nursing home residents and older adults presenting to a neuropsychological clinic (Duff et al., 2008), and norms for a two-factor version of the RBANS have been developed from older adult medical patients (Duff et al., 2009).

The RBANS has also been examined in the OKLAHOMA (Oklahoma Longitudinal Assessment of Health Outcomes in Mature Adults) sample of 824 community-dwelling older adults. In the OKLAHOMA studies, age and education were found to significantly impact RBANS scores (Beatty, Mold, & Gontkovsky, 2003; Gontkovsky, Mold, & Beatty, 2002), and age and education correction norms have subsequently been made available (Duff et al., 2003). Furthermore, three of the five RBANS index scores and 10 of the 12 subtests were found to suffer from bias effects in a study evaluating the performance of 50 older adult African Americans to age-matched European Americans (Patton et al., 2003). Normative data for use with an older adult African American population were presented with the aforementioned study but suffer from low sample size ($n = 61$) thus limiting utility.

DEMENTIA RATING SCALE-2

Designed to be free of floor effects when assessing dementia severity over time, The Dementia Rating Scale-2 takes approximately 15–30 minutes to administer and is comprised of 32 stimulus cards and 36 tasks measuring cognitive functioning across six subscales: attention (8 items), initiation/perseveration (11 items), construction (6 items), conceptualization (6 items), and memory (5 items). The sample utilized when obtaining normative data for the DRS-2 was derived from the Mayo Older Adult Normative Study (MOANS; Lucas et al., 1998) and included 623 predominately well-educated, Caucasian elders aged 56–105. Because the demographic makeup of the original normative group lacked sufficient representation of ethnic minorities and people with less than 8 years of education, caution should be used when interpreting the scores of these groups (Mattis, Jurica, & Leitten, 2002). However, African American norms have been developed from older adults participating in the Mayo Older African American Normative Studies (MOAANS) (Rilling et al., 2005). The original version of the Dementia Rating Scale (DRS; Mattis, 1988) has been shown to be useful when testing older adults for cognitive impairment in medical rehabilitation (Bank, Yochim, MacNeill, & Lichtenberg, 2000; Yochim, Bank, Mast, MacNeill, & Lichtenberg, 2003) and in predicting ADL and IADL performance (Nadler et al., 1993), thus further demonstrating its potential for benefit in the rehabilitative setting. Normative data for use in medical rehabilitation with diverse samples have also been developed using the original DRS (Bank et al., 2000; Yochim et al., 2003). These abilities of the original DRS are expected to generalize to the DRS-2 because of the similarities between the two measures. An alternate form of the DRS-2 is also available that can be used when evaluating cognitive changes over time (DRS-2AF; Schmidt, 2004) and has operating characteristics similar to those of the DRS-2 (Schmidt, Mattis, Adams, & Nestor, 2005).

Another noteworthy aspect of the DRS-2 is its ability to identify different types of dementia based upon a patient's score presentation. For example, in a study comparing patients with AD to patients with frontotemporal dementia (FTD) by Rascovsky et al. (2008), correct identification of dementia type was achieved in 89% of the AD group and 82% of the FTD group. Furthermore, Aarsland et al. (2003) also demonstrated the ability of DRS-2 score presentation to correctly differentiate among patients with Parkinson disease dementia (PDD), dementia with Lewy bodies (DLB), progressive supranuclear palsy (PSP), and AD.

Evaluating for Depression in Older Adults in a Rehabilitative Setting

Assessing an older adult for depression is not as straightforward as assessing an older adult for cognitive impairment. Sophisticated measures with extensive normative data do not exist, thus rendering self- and informant-reports, clinical interviews, observation, and clinical judgment a more significant part of the process. Often, difficulty in the evaluation of depressive symptoms in older adults is experienced because of older adults presenting with anhedonia and somatic complaints instead of feelings of melancholy and dysphoria (Gallo, Anthony, & Muthén, 1994). Difficulty also arises because of the similarities that vegetative/somatic symptoms of depression share with certain organic diseases (House, 1988). However, self-report measures such as the Geriatric Depression Scale (GDS; Yesavage, 1982) are available that can aid a psychologist in assessing an older adult for symptoms of depression, and this measure in particular was designed to avoid the somatic symptoms that often confound depression assessment in medically ill older adults, thus making it appropriate for use in medical rehabilitation. As with any self-report measure, its main function is for screening rather than for diagnostic classification because of the possibility that the person may exaggerate symptom presentation or, more importantly, deny symptoms that are actually present.

The Geriatric Depression Scale

The GDS is a 30-item forced-choice self-report measure designed to detect the presence of depression in older adults. While being administered the GDS, the older adult is instructed to answer questions in relation to how he or she has "felt over the past week." A cutscore of 10 is recommended by the test developers, but Spreen and Strauss (1998) argue that using the following score ranges yield more accuracy: 0–9 "normal," 10–19 "mild," and 20–30 "severe." The GDS can be read to the patient or completed by the patient in written form. The GDS is also available in a 15-item short form (GDS-SF; Sheikh & Yesavage, 1986) to address potential issues of fatigue and concentration that may transpire during administration of the 30-item version.

Questions have been raised regarding the face validity of the GDS in medical patients due to the original scales being developed primarily with healthy community-dwelling older adults (Young et al., 1999). Also, debate exists in the literature, with some researchers arguing that older adults with cognitive impairment may experience difficulty remembering their emotional symptoms from the prior week (Burke, Houson, Boust, & Roccoforte, 1989; Kafonek et al., 1989); other studies have seemingly refuted this notion (Burke, Nitcher, Roccaforte, & Wengel, 1992; Feher, Larrabee, & Crook, 1992; Jackson & Baldwin, 1993; Lichtenberg, Marcopulos, Steiner, & Tabscott, 1992; Lichtenberg, Ross, Millis, & Manning, 1995; Lopez, Quan, & Carvajal, 2010; Maixner, Burke, Roccaforte, Wengel, & Potter, 1995; McGivney, Mulvihill, & Taylor, 1994; Shah, Phongsathorn, Bielawska, & Katona, 1996; Stiles & McGarrahan, 1998; Ward, Wadsworth, & Peterson, 1994).

Geriatric Depression Scale scores have been found to be predictive of rehospitalization within 6 months of discharge (Mast et al., 2004). Geriatric Depression Scale scores are also significantly associated with ADL performance at admission to geriatric rehabilitation and ADL performance (Nanna, Lichtenberg, Buda-Abela, & Barth, 1997) and loss of independence upon discharge from geriatric rehabilitation (MacNeill & Lichtenberg, 1998). It is imperative, however, to remain cognizant of the fact that the GDS is designed to be a screening instrument used in conjunction with multiple other tools when determining if a diagnosis of depression is warranted.

Treatment of Depression for Older Adults in the Rehabilitation Setting

When treating an older adult for depression in a rehabilitative setting, a psychologist faces unique challenges. Older adults in medical rehabilitation may be adjusting to new life roles, changes in function, changes in living arrangements, and the loss of family and friends. When these stressors are combined with factors such as multiple medical diagnoses, physical disabilities, chronic illnesses, and cognitive impairment, it becomes increasingly necessary for treatments to be flexible and tailored to the uniqueness of the rehabilitation setting and clients. Unlike treatment utilized in an outpatient setting, a psychologist working in rehabilitation often cannot simply rely upon weekly sessions using a single theoretical orientation but must instead use a multimodal framework, with focus given to a patient's behavior, mood, interpersonal functioning, activity level, and adherence to rehabilitation components (e.g., occupational therapy, physical therapy) and pharmacological regimens. The following descriptions highlight the need to utilize multimodal interventions when working with this population.

Behavioral Activation

Many older adults with depression in a rehabilitation program also have limited mobility and a decrease in the number of daily events experienced as positive and rewarding. Combined with the tendency for depressed people to find less enjoyment in activities once found pleasurable, reinforcing events can be greatly reduced for older adults in inpatient rehabilitation. Behavioral activation is an intervention designed to address both of these maintaining factors of depression.

Based upon Lewinsohn's theory of depression (Lewinsohn & Graf, 1973), behavioral activation interventions target a patient's day-to-day activities within his or her current environment. A patient is taught to monitor his or her mood so associations can be formed between activity engagement and fluctuations in mood (Lewinsohn, Sullivan, & Grosscap, 1980). As the process of associating behaviors with mood state is accomplished, patients schedule engagement in behaviors designed to make them more active and increase the probability of positive reinforcements being gradually introduced into daily life. The steps of behavioral activation are determined on a patient-by-patient basis and may begin as simple steps (i.e., not lying in bed between appointments with team members) or requiring more effort and movement (i.e., exercising for a half an hour a day) depending upon the functional capacity, level of current activity, and extent of depressive symptoms in the older adult. However, as treatment progresses, the older adult's rehabilitation program can be modified to maximize the total number of reinforcing events, thus keeping the patient active.

In a meta-analysis conducted by Mazzucchelli, Kane, and Rees (2009), behavioral activation therapy was found to have an overall effect size of 0.74 in patients meeting criteria for major depressive disorder. More specifically to older adults, behavioral activation therapy has been shown to be effective (Gallagher & Thompson, 1982; Rokke, Tomhave, & Jocic, 1999; Scogin, Jamison, & Gochneaur, 1989) and may be a particularly attractive alternative for older adults with cognitive impairment (Teri, Logsdon, Uomoto, & McCurry, 1997) who may not be viable candidates for treatments with a more cognitive- or insight-oriented focus. Furthermore, Lichtenberg et al. (1995) devised a highly structured program based upon behavior activation principles that can be utilized by occupational therapists in sessions with older adults in rehabilitation.

Cognitive-Behavioral Therapy

Cognitive-behavioral therapy (CBT) is based upon the theory by Aaron Beck that a depressed person's thinking is biased in a negative way. These negative biases are characterized by negative thoughts related to the self, the world, and the future, and comprise what is known as the "negative triad." Interventions based upon a CBT framework, therefore, are designed to identify the person's individual style of negative thinking and subsequently change his or her perceptions and thinking to counteract the negative cognitive schema currently held by the depressed person.

In a meta-analysis examining studies of CBT in older adults, Wilson, Mottram, and Vassilas (2008) found CBT to have the potential to benefit older adults with symptoms of depression. Studies giving support to the use of CBT in depressed older adults in a primary care setting have been conducted (Laidlaw et al., 2008; Serfaty et al., 2009; Wilson, Scott, Abou-Saleh, Burns, & Copeland, 1995). However, studies examining the effectiveness of CBT in inpatient rehabilitation are lacking, and initiating a treatment program with a cognitive orientation may not always be feasible in a rehabilitative setting (Lichtenberg & Schneider, 2010). Questions also remain as to the applicability of CBT as a treatment for depression in older adults with varying levels of cognitive impairment, and studies examining the use of CBT in the cognitively impaired (Kipling, Bailey, & Charlesworth, 1999; Walker, 2004) lack sufficient sample size and examinations across severity level for generalizations to be made. As Snow, Powers, and Liles (2006) note, no clinical trials examining CBT in older adults with dementia exist, but CBT may prove an effective intervention with the population due to it being shown to benefit people with mental retardation and traumatic brain injuries.

Interpersonal Therapy

Interpersonal therapy (IPT) as a treatment modality was originally developed with the sole purpose of treating symptoms of depression in adults (Klerman, Rounsaville, Chevron, Neu, & Weissman, 1979). Under the IPT framework, the core features of depression occur within a psychosocial and interpersonal context, and alleviating these symptoms is accomplished not only by directly treating the symptoms of depression but also by learning strategies to better function within the psychosocial and interpersonal environment. Interpersonal therapy may be an especially attractive option when treating older adults with depression who are engaged in a rehabilitation program because some of the identified targets of IPT interventions (i.e., grief, interpersonal role disputes, role transitions, and interpersonal deficits) are common issues faced by many older adults (Sholomskas, Chevron, Prusoff, & Berry, 1983).

The goal of IPT is to reduce social isolation by enhancing interactions with others and expanding the social support network of an older adult. Increased and more productive contact with others leads to an increase in positive reinforcement, which then becomes part of an older adult's daily life. Furthermore, the skills needed to enhance social relationships can potentially be learned and practiced in the rehabilitative setting and taken with the patient into the home environment upon discharge. Interpersonal therapy has been found to be an effective treatment for older adults with depression (Hinrichsen, 2006; Sholomskas et al., 1983), and modifications to standard IPT treatments are available for the treatment of older adults with cognitive impairment and to those in long-term care (Hinrichsen, 2008).

Other Points of Focus for Psychologists Working with Older Adults in a Rehabilitative Setting

Beyond the assessment of cognitive impairment and the assessment and treatment of depression, a rehabilitation psychologist will encounter other aspects of an older adult's mental and physical health that can be improved through psychological and behavioral interventions. In the following section, the impact of pain and sleep on an older adult's progress in a rehabilitation setting will be discussed. Also included in the discussion will be the assessment of and treatment for older adults experiencing high levels of pain and/or disturbances in sleep, and the patient's satisfaction with the rehabilitation process, with an emphasis on its impact on goal setting, progress, and motivation.

Pain

Chronic medical conditions such as arthritis, back problems, and bone and joint disorders increase sharply with age (American Geriatrics Society, 2002) and lead to increased instances of debilitating pain. Chronic pain affects up to 25–50% of

all community-dwelling older adults (Blyth et al., 2001; Helme & Gibson, 1999) and 80% of older adults in long-term care facilities (Charlton, 2005), and leads to decreased progress in a rehabilitation program (Yonan & Wegener, 2003). The pain experience has intrigued researchers for years, and theories on the cause of pain have changed sharply in light of the gate control theory (Melzack and Wall, 1965). No longer is the pain experience viewed as a phenomenon driven solely by physiological means; rather, it is now considered an interaction among physical, psychological, cultural, and social factors (Asmundson & Wright, 2004). Given this interaction, the pain experience varies between patients with the same medical condition and is amenable to psychological intervention.

The American Geriatrics Society (2002) recommends that all patients entering a rehabilitation program be evaluated for persistent pain as part of treatment planning. In rehabilitation, assessment begins with interviews and chart reviews, with particular emphasis given to the location and severity of pain; its impact on functioning mood and sleep; the patient's coping strategies, spirituality, and social support; comorbid disorders; environmental factors; beliefs and attitudes about pain; and overall life goals and expectations (Yonan & Wegener, 2003). Although patients are the most accurate indicator of their subjective pain experience (American Geriatrics Society, 1998), a number of instruments (i.e., pain scales, pain interviews, visual analog scales, and pain diaries) are designed to assist in the assessment of the presence and severity of pain and are available for use in and applicable to the rehabilitative setting (Tait, 1999).

After a patient has been evaluated for pain, and chronic pain has been indicated, a pain treatment plan can be developed that is tailored to the patient's needs. Patient education about pain mechanisms and pain treatments plays an important part in treating pain in older adults and should be ongoing throughout the rehabilitation process. Several treatment modalities have been demonstrated to be effective treatments for chronic pain in older adults and can be successfully used in the rehabilitative setting.

Two of the most common interventions for treating pain in older adults rely upon operant conditioning or cognitive behavioral principles (Yonan & Wegener, 2003). Using CBT principles, a psychologist may attempt to modify the feelings of helplessness, catastrophizing, and low self-efficacy often accompanying pain in an older adult.

For psychologists using operant conditioning, observable behaviors are modified through contingency management. Furthermore, these treatment modalities are not mutually exclusive and can be used in conjunction. Other treatments for pain in older adults include behavioral activation, mindfulness training, biofeedback, and relaxation training (Hadjistavropoulos, Hunter, & Dever Fitzgerald, 2009). A dearth of research exists, however, regarding the treatment of pain in older adults in the rehabilitative setting, and future studies should examine differing modalities of nonpharmacological treatments in the setting.

Sleep Disorders

Disorders of sleep affect up to 52% of older adults (Foley, Monjan, Brown, & Simonsick, 1995) and are primarily characterized by insomnia (difficulty falling or staying asleep at night) and excessive daytime sleepiness (difficulty staying awake and alert during the day) (Stepanski, Rybczyk, Lopez, & Stevens, 2003). Sleep disorders are associated with a decrease in QOL (Leger, Scheuermaier, Philip, Paillard, & Guilleminault, 2001) and an increase in nursing home placement when left untreated in older adults (Pollak, Perlick, & Linsner, 1990). Diminished cognition and motor function are also associated with poor sleep (Bonnet, 1986; Dinges et al., 1997) and can impair an older adult during daytime activities (Foley et al., 1995), rendering him or her less able to fully engage in a rehabilitation program. Disturbances affecting the quality and quantity of sleep in an older adult can be caused by myriad factors including irregular breathing during sleep, restless leg syndrome, periodic limb movement disorder, disruptions of circadian rhythm, parasomnias, age-related medical conditions, anxiety, and depression (Stepanski et al., 2003). In the following section, treatments for sleep disorders that can be implemented in rehabilitation are briefly reviewed. By treating sleep disturbances in older adults as they engage in a rehabilitation program, psychologists can increase energy and reduce fatigue in these patients. Furthermore, as a patient engages in more out of bed daytime activities, increases in motivation and energy can be gained that lead to the inclusion of more positive reinforcement into daily life and the possibility for more overall gains being made during the rehabilitative process.

Frequently, sleep disorders are treated solely with prescription medication while behavioral factors that maintain the disorder go unchecked and untreated. Good sleep hygiene (daily habits that can promote sleep quality and quantity) and relaxation techniques can be taught and used alone or in combination with interventions based upon behavioral/psychological paradigms and have been demonstrated to be effective treatments for most sleep disorders regardless of contributing factors (Rybarczyk et al., 2002). For example, due to a repeating cycle of sleep loss, an older adult often adopts negative cognitions about sleep that are amenable to modification using techniques adopted from CBT in combination with behavioral interventions.

Stimulus control is one example of a behavioral technique used to treat sleep problems (Bootzin, 1972). In stimulus control, a patient's bedroom activities are greatly limited with watching television, reading, eating, and all other activities not related to sleep or sex being contraindicated. Furthermore, if a patient is not able to fall asleep after lying in bed for 15–20 minutes, he or she is instructed to leave the bed and engage in a relaxing activity until sleepiness returns. This process is repeated until the patient is able to sleep. Another intervention based upon a behavioral paradigm is sleep restriction therapy. Using this technique, a patient's sleep schedule is manipulated to reflect the amount of time a patient indicates he or she is actually sleeping each night (Spielman, Saskin, & Thorpy, 1987). Morning wakeup remains at the same time but the time a patient goes to bed is pushed back. So, if a patient indicates sleep is only being maintained for 3 hours a night and wakeup time is at 6 am, the bedtime will be set to 3 am. Napping is not allowed during sleep restriction therapy, and bedtimes are moved ahead each week as the amount of time spent in bed sleeping increases.

Goal Setting and Its Impact on Patient Satisfaction

The subjective experience of the older adult as he or she engages in a rehabilitation program is a crucial aspect of the rehabilitation process (Ueda & Okawa, 2003) and understanding the patients perspective may help professionals gain a deeper insight into the needs of the patient (Aberg, 2008). Older adults who are more satisfied with their rehabilitation program will be more apt to engage in tasks and treatments to the fullest of their capacity, thus increasing the chances of successful rehabilitation. Although general satisfaction will undoubtedly be related to progress made during rehabilitation, not viewing the patient as an active member of the rehabilitation team can be a detriment to both patient satisfaction and the amount of progress achieved.

Goal setting is one aspect of rehabilitation that can increase an older adult's satisfaction with the process. Patients in rehabilitation programs are more aware of their functional limitations than is commonly believed and may modify goals to adapt to their functional capabilities (Aberg, 2008). Sometimes, these goals may appear to be minor aspects of the rehabilitative process (i.e., being able to use the toilet independently) but are in fact integral to the esteem of the person as he or she transitions into a post-rehabilitation environment. Unfortunately, patients are often not included in the goal-setting process, and goals are often not concrete enough for patients to conceptualize the progress that their rehabilitation team expects of them (Wressle et al., 1999). However, by discussing goals with the patient while being cognizant of functional capacity, and by serving as a negotiator between the patient and the rehabilitation team, a rehabilitation psychologist can make the older adult a part of the goal-setting process and thus generate more involvement for the patient in decision-making about his or her own individual program. Often, patients in inpatient rehabilitation exhibit a tendency to become more passive than necessary (Wressle et al., 1999) and therefore the rehabilitation psychologist can decrease this passivity while simultaneously improving a patient's satisfaction and increasing QOL through goal setting.

Working with Families

Although the patient works with professionals from multiple disciplines, family members also impact the level of success a patient will have during and after a rehabilitative stay. Families are not only associated with level of patient motivation exhibited while engaged in a rehabilitation program (Routasalo, Seija, & Sirkka, 2004) but also will ultimately act as caregivers and dictate the patient's environment after discharge. However, this is a stressful time for family members as they witness changes in the health status of a loved one. An adjustment in family roles and uncertainty about the future accompanies this change and is associated with an increased risk of depression in spouses and other family members (Tucker, 1993). To fully maximize the benefit families can have on outcome, therefore, families should be involved in the rehabilitation and decision-making process from the beginning (Routasalo et al., 2004). By collaborating with family members from the onset, treatment team members can enhance a sense of self-efficacy and hope.

However, interactions with family members should not be limited to collaboration and information gathering. Behavior-based programs designed to educate families and improve overall outcome should be included, with components including coping skills training, communication skills training, problem-solving skills training, and developing strategies to enhance social support (Karlson et al., 2004; Keefe et al., 2004). Finally, if a rehabilitation psychologist suspects a spouse or family member is experiencing clinically significant symptoms of depression, that family member should be approached with these concerns, treatment options given, and appropriate referrals made.

Managing Confusion

People over the age of 65 are at increased risk of experiencing confusion. This incidence is inflated in medical patients (Foreman, 1989), people with AD, and people with depression (Espino, Jules-Bradley, Johnston, & Mouton, 1998). Given the rates of older adults with medical issues, cognitive deficits, and depression in geriatric rehabilitation, it is almost certain that psychologists working in this setting will encounter patients suffering from both acute and chronic confusion. In these instances, the possible sources of confusion should be fully evaluated and strategies should be implemented that are designed to mitigate the impact of confusion on the rehabilitation process. Because of the increased incidence of morbidity and mortality associated with delirium (Gleason, 2003), all patients observed to experience a change in mental status during a rehabilitative stay need to be evaluated for delirium. If delirium is determined to be the cause of confusion, the underlying medical condition needs to be addressed before any further action is taken.

However, not all cases of confusion are due to delirium. If delirium is ruled out, steps can be taken to help the confused patient engage in the rehabilitation program to the best of his or her ability. Managing confusion means not only limiting situations that may bring about confusion but also managing accompanying features of confusion (i.e., anxiety, fatigue, agitation, etc). For a patient with confusion, the rehabilitation program needs to be designed so that the environment is as structured, predictable, and nonthreatening as possible (Williamson, Scott, & Adams, 1996). Strategies to accomplish this goal include limiting the patient to familiar surroundings, avoiding ambiguity by limiting unnecessary choices or decisions, limiting engagement in mental tasks exceeding the patient's cognitive ability, utilizing a highly structured daily routine, scheduling periods of sleep, limiting stimulant use (i.e., caffeine), providing adequate lighting, limiting television use, and limiting wandering behaviors (Williamson et al., 1996). Not all strategies are recommended for every patient, and an individualized program should be tailored to each patient in light of cognitive and functional capacities. Furthermore, once an individualized program is designed, the components of the program can be tailored for the home environment. Families can then be educated about the program so it can be implemented at home after discharge.

Environmental and Cognitive Stimulation

In geriatric rehabilitation, the simplest and arguably most effective method of adding enrichment to a patient's environment is through enhanced engagement in social activities. This can be accomplished by scheduling social and group events but also through participation in group treatment sessions. To increase participation in social activities, selective reinforcement may be used, as well as interventions adhering to behavioral activation principles.

Cognitive intervention techniques have also recently become a more commonly used way to enrich an older adult's environment. These techniques usually take on one of three forms: general cognitive stimulation, cognitive training, and cognitive rehabilitation. Although these techniques differ in theory, they are often difficult to distinguish in practice, and most cognitive intervention programs combine aspects of all three (Jean, Bergeron, Thivierge, & Simard, 2010). However, these techniques are not equally effective for all patient groups and may be more effective at increasing memory and QOL in patients with mild cognitive impairment than in patients with AD (Kurz, Pohl, Ramsenthaler, & Sorg, 2009). Furthermore, debate exists about the mechanisms underlying improvement and the role of increased social interaction (Clare & Woods, 2004) as these techniques are often applied in group format.

Conclusion

As the population continues to age, rehabilitation psychologists will increasingly work with older adults in the rehabilitation setting. For psychologists choosing to work in the setting, accurate and reliable assessment for cognitive impairment, and specifically for executive dysfunction, in older adults will be increasingly important. Moreover,

the rate of depression is substantially elevated for older adults engaged in a rehabilitation program, and psychologists will need to possess knowledge of how to effectively assess and treatment this condition in older patients. Rehabilitation psychologists working with older adults should also become familiar with nonpharmacologically based treatments for chronic pain and sleep problems as these conditions are quite common and can hinder the progress of rehabilitation participant. Finally, the older adult should be conceptualized as a unique individual who can make a valuable contribution to his or her own treatment plans and goals. By treating patients as contributing members of the team and by giving them a voice in the rehabilitation process, psychologists can increase their working alliance with older adults and motivate them to engage in the rehabilitation program to the best of their abilities.

Future Directions

• Given the changes expected in population demographics in the United States (i.e., increased number of older adults and increased number of ethnic minorities), rehabilitation programs will need to adapt and expand in order to accommodate older adults in need of rehabilitative services. Research will need to address normative data specific to different ethnic groups and develop reliable assessment instruments and effective treatment options for diverse elders in the rehabilitative setting.

• Alcohol abuse and its effects upon the rehabilitation process are not well understood, and treatments for alcohol abuse and dependence have not been sufficiently studied within the rehabilitative setting.

• Although cognitive impairment can negatively impact rehabilitation gains, some literature suggests that people with dementia nonetheless demonstrate some recovery over their rehabilitation stay. The mechanisms for these changes (e.g., reliance upon implicit memory, compensatory techniques) and methods to enhance functioning deserve further study.

References

Aarsland, D., Litvan, I., Salmon, D., Galasko, D., Wentzel-Larsen, T., & Larsen, J. P. (2003). Performance on the dementia rating scale in Parkinson's disease with dementia and dementia with Lewy bodies: Comparison with progressive supranuclear palsy and Alzheimer's disease. *Journal of Neurology, Neurosurgery and Psychiatry, 74*(9), 1215–1220.

Aberg, A. C. (2008). Care recipients' perceptions of activity-related life space and life satisfaction during and after geriatric rehabilitation. *Quality of Life Research, 17*(4), 509–520.

Alexopoulos, G. S., Meyers, B. S., Young, R. C., Kakuma, T., Silbersweig, D., & Charlson, M. (1997). Clinically defined vascular depression. *American Journal of Psychiatry, 154*(4), 562–565.

American Geriatrics Society. (2002). Panel on Chronic Pain in Older Persons. The management of persistent pain in older persons. *Journal of the American Geriatrics Society, 50*, 205–224.

American Geriatrics Society. (1998). Panel on Chronic Pain in Older Persons. The management of chronic pain in older persons. *Journal of the American Geriatrics Society, 46*, 635–651.

Andersen, G., Vestergaard, K., Riis, J., & Lauritzen, L. (1994). Incidence of post-stroke depression during the first year in a large unselected stroke population determined using a valid standardized rating scale. *Acta Psychiatria Scandinavia, 90*, 190–195.

Arfken, C. L., Lichtenberg, P. A., & Tancer, M. E. (1999). Cognitive impairment and depression predict mortality in medically ill older adults. *Journals of Gerontology: Series A: Biological Sciences and Medical Sciences, 54*(A), 152–156.

Asmundson, G. J. G., & Wright, K. (2004). Biopsychosocial approaches to pain. In T. Hadjistavropoulos & K. D. Craig (Eds.), *Pain: Psychological perspectives* (pp. 35–87). Mahwah, NJ: Erlbaum.

Bank, A. L., Yochim, B. P., MacNeill, S. E., & Lichtenberg, P. A. (2000). Expanded normative data for the Mattis Dementia Rating Scale for use with urban, elderly medical patients. *Clinical Neuropsychologist, 14*(2), 149–156.

Beatty, W. W., Mold, J. W., & Gontkovsky, S. T. (2003). RBANS performance: Influences of sex and education. *Journal of Clinical and Experimental Neuropsychology, 25*, 1065–1069.

Ble, A., Volpato, S., Zuliani, G., Guralnik, J. M., Bandinelli, S., Lauretani, F., et al. (2005). Executive function correlates with walking speed in older persons: The InCHIANTI study. *Journal of the American Geriatrics Society, 53*(3), 410–415.

Blyth, F. M., March, L. M., Brnabic, A. J., Jorm, L. R., Williamson, M., & Cousins, M. J. (2001). Chronic pain in Australia: A prevalence study. *Pain, 89*, 127–134.

Bonnet, M. H. (1986). Performance and sleepiness as a function of frequency and placement of sleep disruption. *Psychophysiology, 23*, 263–271.

Borson, S., Scanlan, J. M., Chen, P., & Ganguli, M. (2003). The Mini-Cog as a screen for dementia: Validation in a population-based sample. *Journal of the American Geriatric Society, 51*, 1452–1454.

Borson, S., Scanlan, J., Brush, M., Vitaliano, P., & Dokmak, A. (2000). The mini-cog: A cognitive "vital signs" measure for dementia screening in multi-lingual elderly. *International Journal of Geriatric Psychiatry, 15*, 1021–1027.

Brodaty, H., Fay, L. L., Gibson, L., & Burns, K. (2006). What is the best dementia screening instrument for general practitioners to use? *American Journal of Geriatric Psychiatry, 14*, 391–400.

Brodaty, H., Kemp, N. M., & Low, L. F. (2004). Characteristics of the GPCOG, a screening tool for cognitive impairment. *International Journal of Geriatric Psychiatry, 19*, 870–874.

Brodaty, H., Pond, D., Kemp, N. M., Luscombe, G., Berman, K., Harding, L., & Huppert, F. (2002). The GPCOG: A new screening test for dementia designed for general practice. Journal of the *American Geriatric Society, 50*, 530–534.

Buchner, D. M., & Larson, E. B. (1987). Falls and fractures in patients with the Alzheimer's type dementia. *Journal of the American Medical Association, 257*, 1492–1495.

Burke, W. J., Houston, M. J., Boust, S. J., & Roccoforte W. H. (1989). Use of the Geriatric Depression Scale in dementia of the Alzheimer's type. *Journal of the American Geriatrics Society, 37*, 856–860.

Burke, W. J., Nitcher, R. L., Roccaforte, W. H., & Wengel, S. P. (1992). A prospective evaluation of the Geriatric Depression Scale in an outpatient geriatric assessment center. *Journal of the American Geriatrics Society, 40*, 1227–1230.

Buschke, H., Kuslansky, G., Katz, M., Stewart, W. F., Sliwinski, M. J., Eckholdt, H. M., & Lipton, R. B. (1999). Screening for dementia with the Memory Impairment Screen (MIS). *Neurology, 52*, 231–237.

Caplan, B., & Moelter, S. (2000). Stroke. In R. Frank & T. Elliott (Eds.), *Handbook of rehabilitation psychology* (pp. 75–108). Washington, DC: American Psychological Association.

Charlton, J. E. (2005). *Core curriculum for professional education in pain* (3rd ed.). Seattle, WA: IASP Press.

Chung, J. C. C. (2009). Clinical validity of Fuld Object Memory Evaluation to screen for dementia in a Chinese society. *International Journal of Geriatric Psychiatry, 24*, 156–162.

Chung, J. C. C., & Ho, W. S. K. (2009). Validation of Fuld Object Memory Evaluation for the detection of dementia in nursing home residents. *Aging and Mental Health, 13*, 274–279.

Clare, L., & Woods, R. T. (2004). Cognitive training and cognitive rehabilitation for people with early-stage Alzheimer's disease: A review. *Neuropsychological Rehabilitation, 14*(4), 385–401.

Cunningham, C., Horgan, F., Keane, N., Connolly, P., Mannion, A., & O'Neill, D. (1996). Detection of disability by different members of an interdisciplinary team. *Clinical Rehabilitation, 10*, 247–254.

Dinges, D. F., Pack, F., Williams, K., Gillen, K. A., Powell, J. W., Ott, G. E., et al. (1997). Cumulative sleepiness, mood disturbance, and psychomotor vigilance performance decrements during a week of sleep restricted to 4–5 hours per night. *Sleep, 20*, 267–277.

Duff, K., Humphreys Clark, J. D., O'Bryant, S. E., Mold, J. W., Schiffer, R. B., & Sutker, P. B. (2008). Utility of the RBANS in detecting cognitive impairment associated with Alzheimer's disease: Sensitivity, specificity, and positive and negative predictive powers. *Archives of Clinical Neuropsychology, 23*, 603–612.

Duff, K., Langbehn, D. R., Schoenberg, M. R., Moser, D. J., Baade, L. E., Mold, J. W., et al. (2009). Normative data on and psychometric properties of Verbal and Visual Indexes of the RBANS in older adults. *Clinical Neuropsychologist, 23*(1), 39–50.

Duff, K., Pattern, D., Schoenberg, M. R., Mold, J., Scott, J. G., & Adams, R. L. (2003). Age- and education-corrected independent normative data for the RBANS in a community dwelling elderly sample. *Clinical Neuropsychologist, 17*, 351–366.

Espino, D. V., Jules-Bradley, A. C., Johnston, C. L., & Mouton, C. P. (1998). Diagnostic approach to the confused elderly patient. *American Family Physician, 57*(6), 1358–1366.

Federal Interagency Forum on Aging-Related Statistics. (2008). Older Americans 2008: Key Indicators of Well-Being. *Federal Interagency Forum on Aging-Related Statistics.* Washington, DC: U.S. Government Printing Office.

Feher, E. P., Larrabee, G. J., & Crook, T. H. (1992). Factors attenuating the validity of the Geriatric Depression Scale in a dementia population. *Journal of the American Geriatrics Society, 40,* 906–909.

Folstein, M. F., Folstein, S. E., & McHugh, P. R. (1975). Mini Mental State: A practical method for grading the cognitive state of patients for the clinician. *Journals of Gerontology: Series B: Psychological Sciences and Social Sciences, 12,* 189–198.

Foley, D. J., Monjan, A. A., Brown, S. L., & Simonsick, E. M. (1995). Sleep complaints among elderly persons: An epidemiologic study of three communities. *Sleep, 18,* 425–432.

Foreman, M. D. (1989). Confusion in the hospitalized elderly: Incidence, onset, and associated factors. *Research in Nursing and Health, 12,* 21–29.

Fried, L. P., Ferrucci, L., Darer, J., Williamson, J. D., & Anderson, G. (2004). Untangling the concepts of disability, frailty, and comorbidity: Implications for improved targeting and care. *Journals Of Gerontology. Series A, Biological Sciences And Medical Sciences, 59*(3), 255–263.

Fuld, P. A. (1981). *Fuld Object Memory Evaluation Instruction Manual.* WoodDale, IL: Stoelting.

Gainotti, G., & Marra, C. (2002). Determinants and consequences of post-stroke depression. *Current Opinion in Neurology, 15,* 85–89.

Gallagher, D. E., & Thompson, L. W. (1982). Treatment of major depressive disorder in older adult outpatients with brief psychotherapies. *Psychotherapy: Theory, Research, Practice, Training, 19,* 482–490.

Gallo, J. J., Anthony, J. C., & Muthén, B. O. (1994). Age differences in the symptoms of depression: A latent trait analysis. *Journal of Gerontology: Psychological Sciences, 49,* 251–264.

Gallucci, M, Ongaro, F, Amici, G. P., & Regini, C. (2009). Frailty, disability and survival in the elderly over the age of seventy: Evidence from "The Treviso Longeva (TRELONG) Study." *Archives of Gerontology and Geriatrics, 48*(3), 281–283.

Gill, T. M., Allore, H. G., Holford, T. R., & Guo, Z. (2004). Hospitalization, restricted activity, and the development of disability among older persons. *Journal of the American Medical Association, 292*(17), 2115–2124.

Gill, T. M., Richardson, E. D., & Tinetti, M. E. (1995). Evaluating the risk of dependence in activities of daily living among community-living older adults with mild to moderate cognitive impairment. *Journals of Gerontology. Series A, Biological Sciences and Medical Sciences, 50*(5), 235–241.

Gleason, O. C. (2003). Delirium. *American Family Physician, 67*(5), 1027–1034.

Gontkovsky, S. T., Mold, J. W., & Beatty, W. W. (2002). Age and educational influences on RBANS index scores in a non-demented geriatric sample. *Clinical Neuropsychologist, 16,* 258–263.

Grober, E., Hall, C., McGinn, M., Nicholls, T., Stanford, S., Ehrlich, A., et al. (2008). Neuropsychological strategies for detecting early dementia. *Journal of the International Neuropsychological Society, 14,* 130–142.

Hadjistavropoulos, T., Hunter, P., & Dever Fitzgerald, T. (2009). pain assessment and management in older adults: Conceptual issues and clinical challenges. *Canadian Psychology, 50*(4), 241–254.

Helme, R. D., & Gibson, S. J. (1999). Pain in older people. In I. K. Crombie, P. R. Croft, & S. J. Linton (Eds.), *Epidemiology of pain* (pp. 103–112). Seattle: IASP Press.

Hinrichsen, G. A. (2006). Interpersonal Factors and Late-Life Depression. *Clinical Psychology: Science and Practice, 12*(3), 264–275.

Hinrichsen, G. A. (2008). Interpersonal psychotherapy for late life depression: Current status and new applications. *Journal of Rational-Emotive and Cognitive Behavior Therapy, 26*(4), 263–275

Holsinger, T., Deveau, J., Boustani, M., & Williams, J. W. (2007). Does this patient have dementia? *Journal of the American Medical Association, 297,* 2391–2404.

House, A. (1988). Mood disorders in the physically ill: Problems of definition and measurement. *Journal of Psychosomatic Research, 32,* 345–353.

Huusko, T. M., Karppi, P., Avikainen, V., Kautiainen, H., & Sulkava, R. (2000). Randomised, clinically controlled trial of intensive geriatric rehabilitation in patients with hip fracture: Subgroup analysis of patients with dementia. *British Medical Journal, 321*(7269), 1107–1111.

Isaacs, B., & Kennie, A. T. (1973). The Set Test as an aid to the detection of dementia in old people. *British Journal of Psychiatry, 123,* 467–470.

Jackson, R., & Baldwin, B. (1993). Detecting depression in elderly medically ill patients: The use of the Geriatric Depression Scale compared with medical and nursing observations. *Age Aging, 22,* 349–353.

Jean, L., Bergeron, M., Thivierge, S., & Simard, M. (2010). Cognitive intervention programs for individuals with mild cognitive impairment: Systematic review of the literature. *American Journal of Geriatric Psychiatry, 18*(4), 281–296.

Jurica, P. J., Leitten, C. L., & Mattis, S. (2001). *Dementia Rating Scale-2: Professional manual.* Lutz, FL: Psychological Assessment Resources.

Kahokehr, A., Siegert, R. J., & Weatherall, M. (2004). The frequency of executive cognitive impairment in elderly rehabilitation inpatients. *Journal of Geriatric Psychiatry and Neurology, 17*(2), 68–72.

Kafonek, S., Ettinger, W. H., Roco, R., Kittner, S., Taylor, N., & German, P.S. (1989). Instruments for screening for depression and dementia in a long-term care facility. *Journal of the American Geriatrics Society, 37,* 29–34.

Karlson, E. W., Liang, M. H., Eaton, H., Huang, J., Fitzgerald, L., Rogers, M. P., Daltroy, L. H (2004). A randomized clinical trial of a psychoeducational intervention to improve outcomes in systemic lupus erythematosus. *Arthritis and Rheumatism, 50,* 1832–1841.

Keefe, F. J., Blumenthal, J., Baucom, D., Affleck, G., Waugh, R., Caldwell, D. S., et al. (2004). Effects of spouse-assisted coping skills training and exercise training in patients with osteoarthritic knee pain: A randomized controlled study. *Pain, 110,* 539–549.

Kipling, T., Bailey, M., & Charlesworth, G. (1999). The feasibility of a cognitive behavioral therapy group for men with mild/moderate cognitive impairment. *Behavioural and Cognitive Psychotherapy, 27*(2), 189–193.

Klerman, G., Rounsaville, B., Chevron, E., Neu, C., & Weissman, M. (1979). *Manual for short-term interpersonal therapy (IPT) of depression.* New Haven, CT: New Haven-Boston Collaborative Depression Project.

Koenig, H. G., Shelp, F., Goli, V., Cohen, H. J., & Blazer, D. G. (1989). Survival and health care utilization in elderly medical inpatients with major depression. *Journal of the American Geriatrics Society, 37*(7), 599–606.

Kurz, A., Pohl, C., Ramsenthaler, M., & Sorg, C. (2009). Cognitive rehabilitation in patients with mild cognitive impairment. *International Journal of Geriatric Psychiatry, 24*, 163–168.

Kuslansky, G., Buschke, H., Katz, M., Sliwinski, M., & Lipton, R. B. (2002). Screening for Alzheimer's disease: The Memory Impairment Screen versus the conventional three-word memory test. *Journal of the American Geriatric Society, 50*, 1086–1091.

LaBuda, J., & Lichtenberg, P. (1999). The role of cognition, depression, and awareness of deficit in predicting geriatric rehabilitation patients' IADL performance. *Clinical Neuropsychologist, 13*(3), 258–267.

Laidlaw, K., Davidson, K., Toner, H., Jackson, G., Clark, S., Law, J., et al. (2008). A randomized controlled trial of cognitive behaviour therapy vs treatment as usual in the treatment of mild to moderate late life depression. *International Journal of Geriatric Psychiatry, 23*, 843–850.

Landi, F., Liperoti, R., Russo, A., Capoluongo, E., Barillaro, C., Pahor, M., et al. (2010). Disability, more than multimorbidity, was predictive of mortality among older persons aged 80 years and older. *Journal of Clinical Epidemiology, 63*(7), 752–759.

La Rue, A. (1989). Patterns of performance on the Fuld Object Memory Evaluation in elderly inpatients with depression or dementia. *Journal of Clinical and Experimental Neuropsychology, 11*, 409–422.

Leger, D., Scheuermaier, K., Philip, K., Paillard, M., & Guilleminault, C. (2001). SF-36: Evaluation of quality of life in severe and mild insomniacs compared with good sleepers. *Psychosomatic Medicine, 63,* 49–55.

Lewinsohn, P. M., & Graf, M. (1973). Pleasant activities and depression. *Journal of Consulting and Clinical Psychology, 41,* 261–268.

Lewinsohn, P. M., Sullivan, J. M., & Grosscap, S. J. (1980). Changing reinforcing events: An approach to the treatment of depression. *Psychotherapy: Theory, Research and Practice, 17,* 322–334.

Lewis, M. S., & Miller, L. S. (2007). Executive control functioning and functional ability in older adults. *Clinical Neuropsychologist, 21*(2), 274–285.

Lichtenberg, P. A. (1998). *Mental health practice in geriatric healthcare settings.* New York: Hawthorn.

Lichtenberg, P. A., Kimbarow, M. L., MacKinnon, D., Morris, P. A., & Bush, J. V. (1995). An interdisciplinary behavioral treatment program for depressed geriatric rehabilitation inpatients. *Gerontologist, 35*(5), 688.

Lichtenberg, P. A., Marcopulos, B. A., Steiner, D. A., & Tabscott, J. A. (1992). Comparison of the Hamilton Depression Rating Scale and the Geriatric Depression Scale: Detection of depression in dementia patients. *Psychological Reports, 70,* 515–521.

Lichtenberg, P. A., Ross, T., Millis, S. R., & Manning, C. A. (1995). The relationship between depression and cognition in older adults: A cross-validation study. *Journal of Gerontology, 50,* 25–32.

Lichtenberg, P. A., & Schneider, B. (2010). Psychology and geriatric rehabilitation. In J. C. Cavanaugh, C. K. Cavanaugh, S. Qualls, & L. McGuire (Eds.), *Aging in America, Volume 2: Physical and mental health* (pp. 188–210). Santa Barbara, CA: Praeger/ABC-CLIO.

Lichtenberg, P. A., Schneider, B. C. (2010). Psychological assessment and practice in geriatric rehabilitation. In R. G. Frank, M. Rosenthal, & B. Caplan (Eds.), *Handbook of rehabilitation psychology* (2nd ed., pp. 95–106). Washington, DC: American Psychological Association.

Lieberman, D., Fried, V., Castel, H., Weitzmann, S., Lowenthal, M. N., & Galinsky, D. (1996). Factors related to successful rehabilitation after hip fracture: A case-control study. *Disability and Rehabilitation, 18*(5), 224–230.

Loewenstein, D. A., Argüelles, T., Acevedo, A., Freeman, R. Q., Mendelssohn, E., Ownby, R. L., et al. (2001). The utility of a modified object memory test in distinguishing between different age groups of Alzheimer's disease patients and normal controls. *Journal of Mental Health and Aging, 7*(3), 317–324.

Loewenstein, D. A., Duara, R., Arguelles, T., & Arguelles, S. (1995). Use of the Fuld Object Memory Evaluation in the detection of mild dementia among Spanish- and English-speaking groups. *American Journal of Geriatric Psychiatry, 3,* 300–307.

Lopez, M. N., Quan, N. M., & Carvajal, P. M. (2010). A psychometric study of the Geriatric Depression Scale. *European Journal of Psychological Assessment, 26*(1), 55–60.

Lorentz, W. J., Scanlan, J. M., & Borson, S. (2002). Brief screening tests for dementia. *Canadian Journal of Psychiatry, 47,* 723–733.

Lucas, J. A., Ivnik, R. J., Smith, G. E., Bohac, D. L., Tangalos, E. G., Kokmen, E., et al. (1998). Normative data for the Mattis Dementia Rating Scale. *Journal of Clinical and Experimental Neuropsychology, 20*(4), 536–547.

Luis, C. A., Keegan, A. P., & Mullan, M. (2009). Cross validation of the Montreal Cognitive Assessment in community dwelling older adults residing in the southeastern US. *International Journal of Geriatric Psychiatry, 24,* 197–201.

MacNeill, S. E., & Lichtenberg, P. A. (1998). Predictors for functional outcome in older rehabilitation patients. *Rehabilitation Psychology, 43*(3), 246–257.

MacNeill, S. E., Lichtenberg, P. A., & LaBuda, J. (2000). Factors affecting return to living alone following medical rehabilitation: A cross-validation study. *Rehabilitation Psychology, 45,* 356–364.

Maixner, S. M., Burke, W. J., Roccaforte, W. H., Wengel, S. P., & Potter, J. G. (1995). A comparison of two depression scales in a geriatric assessment clinic. *American Journal of Geriatric Psychiatry, 3,* 60–67.

Marcopulos, B. A., Gripshover, D. L., Broshek, D. K., McLain, C. A., & Brashear, H. R. (1999). Neuropsychological assessment of psychogeriatric patients with limited education. *Clinical Neuropsychologist, 13*(2), 147–156.

Mast, B. T., Azar, A. R., MacNeill, S. E., & Lichtenberg, P. A. (2004). Depression and activities of daily living predict rehospitalization within 6 months of discharge. *Geriatric Rehabilitation Rehabilitation Psychology, 49*(3), 219–223.

Mast, B., & Gerstenecker, A. (2010). Screening instruments and brief batteries for dementia. In P. Lichtenburg (Ed.), *Handbook of assessment in clinical gerontology.* New York: John Wiley & Sons.

Mast, B. T., Fitzgerald, J., Steinberg, J., MacNeill, S. E., & Lichtenberg, P. A. (2001). Effective screening for Alzheimer's disease among older African Americans. *Clinical Neuropsychologist, 15,* 196–202.

Mast, B. T., MacNeill, S. E., & Lichtenberg, P. A. (2004). Post-stroke and clinically-defined vascular depression in geriatric rehabilitation patients. *American Journal of Geriatric Psychiatry, 12*(1), 84–92.

Mast, B. T., MacNeill, S. E., & Lichtenberg, P. A. (1999). Geropsychological problems in medical rehabilitation: Dementia and depression among stroke and lower extremity fracture patients. *Journal of Gerontology, 54*(12), 607–612.

Mast, B., Neufeld, S., MacNeill, S., & Lichtenberg, P. (2004). Longitudinal support for the relationship between vascular risk and late life depressive symptoms. *American Journal of Geriatric Psychiatry, 12*(1), 93–101.

Mattis, S. (1988). *Dementia Rating Scale: Professional manual.* Odessa, FL: Psychological Assessment Resources.

Mattis, S., Jurica, P., & Leitten, C. (2002). *Dementia Rating Scale-2 Professional Manual.* Odessa, FL: Psychological Assessment Resources.

Mazzucchelli, T., Kane, R., & Rees, C. (2009). Behavioral activation treatments for depression in adults: A meta-analysis and review. *Clinical Psychology: Science and Practice, 16*(4), 383–411.

McGivney, S.A., Mulvihill, M., & Taylor, B. (1994). Validating the GDS depression screen in the nursing home. *Journal of the American Geriatrics Society, 42,* 490–492.

Melzack, R., & Wall, P. D. (1965). Pain mechanisms: A new theory. *Science, 150,* 971–979.

Milne, A., Culverwell, A., Guss, R., Tuppen, J., & Whelton, R. (2008). Screening for dementia in primary care: A review of the use, efficacy and quality of measures. *International Psychogeriatrics, 20*(5), 911–926.

Mossey, J. M., Mutran, E., Knott, K., & Craig, R. (1989). Determinants of recovery 12 months after hip fracture: The importance of psychosocial factors. *American Journal of Public Health, 79,* 279–285.

Nadler, J. D., Richardson, E. D., Malloy, P. F., Marran, M. E., & Hosteller Brinson, M. E. (1993). The ability of the Dementia Rating Scale to predict everyday functioning. *Archives of Clinical Neuropsychology, 8*(5), 449–460.

Nanna, M. J., Lichtenberg, P. A., Buda-Abela, M., & Barth, J. T. (1997). The role of cognition and depression in predicting functional outcome in geriatric medical rehabilitation patients. *Journal of Applied Gerontology, 16*(1), 120–132.

Nasreddine, Z. S., Phillips, N. A., Bedirian, V., Charbonneau, S., Whitehead, V., Collin, I., et al. (2005). The Montreal Cognitive Assessment, MoCA: A brief screening tool for mild cognitive impairment. *Journal of the American Geriatric Society, 53,* 695–699.

Nazem, S., Siderowf, A. D., Duda, J. E., Have, T. T., Colcher, A., Horn, S. S., et al. (2009). Montreal cognitive assessment performance in patients with Parkinson's disease with "normal" global cognition according to mini-mental state examination score. *Journal of the American Geriatrics Society, 57*(2), 304–308.

Office for National Statistics. (2009). Mid-year population estimates. Retrieved December 1, 2010, from http://www.statistics.gov.uk/cci/nugget.asp?id=949

Ostir, G. V., Volpato, S., Kasper, J. D., Ferrucci, L., & Guralnik, J. M. (2001). Summarizing amount of difficulty in ADLs: A refined characterization of disability. Results from the women's health and aging study. *Aging, 13*(6), 465–472.

Patrick, L., Knoefel, F., Gaskowski, P., & Rexroth, D. (2001). Medical comorbidity and rehabilitation efficiency in geriatric inpatients. *Journal of the American Geriatrics Society, 49*(11), 1471–1477.

Patton, D. E., Duff, K., Schoenberg, M. R., Mold, J., Scott, J. G., & Adams, R. L. (2003). Performance of cognitively normal African Americans on the RBANS in community dwelling older adults. *Clinical Neuropsychologist, 17*(4), 515–530.

Pollak, C. P., Perlick, D., & Linsner, J. P. (1990). Sleep problems in the community elderly as predictors of death and nursing home placement. *Journal of Community Health, 15,* 123–135.

Puts, M. T. E., Lips, P., Ribbe, M. W., & Deeg, D. J. H. (2005). The effect of frailty on residential/nursing home admission in the Netherlands independent of chronic diseases and functional limitations. *European Journal of Ageing, 2*(4), 264–274.

Randolph, C., Tierney, M. C., Mohr, E., & Chase, T. N. (1998). The Repeatable Battery for the Assessment of Neuropsychological Status (RBANS): Preliminary clinical validity. *Journal of Clinical and Experimental Neuropsychology, 20,* 310–319.

Rascovsky, K., Salmon, D. P., Hansen, L. A., & Galasko, D. (2008). Distinct cognitive profiles and rates of decline on the Mattis Dementia Rating Scale in autopsy-confirmed frontotemporal dementia and Alzheimer's disease. *Journal of the International Neuropsychological Society, 14*(3), 373–383.

Reitan, R. M. (1955). The relation of the trail making test to organic brain damage. *Journal of Consulting Psychology, 19*(5), 393–394.

Rilling, L. M., Lucas, J. A., Ivnik, R. J., Smith, G. E., Willis, F. B., Ferman, T. J., et al. (2005). Mayo's older African American normative studies: Norms for the Mattis Dementia Rating Scale. *Clinical Neuropsychologist, 19*(2), 229–242.

Robinson, R. G., Starr, L. B., Lipsey, J. R., Rao, K., & Price, T. R. (1984). A two-year longitudinal study of post-stroke mood disorders: Dynamic changes in associated variables over the first six months of follow-up. *Stroke, 15,* 510–517.

Rokke, P. D., Tomhave, J. A., & Jocic, Z. (1999). The role of client choice and target selection in self-management therapy for depression in older adults. *Psychology and Aging, 14,* 155–169.

Rösler, A., Krause, T., Niehuus, C., & von Renteln-Kruse, W. (2008). Dementia as a cofactor for geriatric rehabilitation-outcome in patients with osteosynthesis of the proximal femur: A retrospective, matched-pair analysis of 250 patients. *Archives of Gerontology and Geriatrics, 49*(1), 36–39.

Routasalo, P., Seija, A., & Sirkka, L. (2004). Geriatric rehabilitation nursing: Developing a model. *International Journal of Nursing Practice, 10,* 207–215.

Royall, D. R., Palmer, R., Chiodo, L. K., & Polk, M. J. (2004). Declining executive control in normal aging predicts change in functional status: The Freedom House Study. *Journal of the American Geriatrics Society, 52*(3), 346–352.

Rybarczyk, B., Lopez, M., Benson, R., Alsten, C., & Stepanski, E. (2002). The efficacy of two behavioral treatment programs for comorbid geriatric insomnia. *Psychology and Aging, 17,* 288–298.

Salthouse, T. A. (1993). Speed mediation of adult age-differences in cognition. *Developmental Psychology, 29,* 722–738.

Salthouse, T. A. (1994). The nature of the influence of speed on adult age-differences in cognition. *Developmental Psychology, 30,* 240–259.

Scanlan, J., & Borson, S. (2001). The mini-cog: Receiver operating characteristics with expert and naive raters. *International Journal Geriatric Psychiatry, 16,* 216–222.

Schmidt, K. S. (2004). *Dementia Rating Scale-2 Alternate Form: Manual supplement*. Lutz, FL: Psychological Assessment Resources.

Schmidt, K.S., Mattis, P., Adams, J., & Nestor, P. (2005). Alternate-form reliability of the Dementia Rating Scale-2. *Archives of Clinical Neuropsychology, 20*(4), 436–441.

Schneider, B. C., & Lichtenberg, P. A. (2008). Executive ability and physical performance in urban Black older adults. *Archives of Clinical Neuropsychology, 23*(5), 593–601.

Sholomskas, A. J., Chevron, E. S., Prusoff, B. A., & Berry, C. (1983). Short-term interpersonal therapy (IPT) with the depressed elderly: Case reports and discussion. *American Journal of Psychotherapy, 37*(4), 552–566.

Scogin, F., Jamison, C., & Gochneaur, K. (1989). Comparative efficacy of cognitive and behavioral bibliotherapy for mildly and moderately depressed older adults. *Journal of Consulting and Clinical Psychology, 57*, 403–407.

Serfaty, M. A., Haworth, D., Blanchard, M., Buszewicz, M., Murad, S., & King, M. (2009). Clinical effectiveness of individual cognitive behavioral therapy for depressed older people in primary care: A randomized controlled trial. *Archives of General Psychiatry, 66*(12), 1332–1340.

Shah, A., Phongsathorn, V., Bielawska, C., & Katona, C. (1996). Screening for depression among geriatric inpatients with short versions of the Geriatric Depression Scale. *International Journal of Geriatric Psychiatry, 11*, 915–918.

Sheikh, J. I., & Yesavage, J. A. (1986). Geriatric Depression Scale (GDS): Recent evidence and development of a shorter version. In T. L. Brink (Ed.), *Clinical gerontology: A guide to assessment and intervention* (pp. 165–173). New York: Haworth.

Singh, A., Black, S. E., Herrmann, N., Leibovitch, F. S., Ebert, P. L., Lawrence, J., & Szalai, J. P. (2000). Functional and neuroanatomic correlations in poststroke depression: The Sunnybrook Stroke Study. *Stroke, 31*(3), 637–644.

Smith, T., Gildeh, N., & Holmes, C. (2007). The Montreal Cognitive Assessment: Validity and utility in a memory clinic setting. *Canadian Journal of Psychiatry, 52*(5), 329–332.

Snow, A.L., Powers D., & Liles D., (2006). Cognitive-Behavioral Therapy for Long-Term Care Patients with Dementia. In: L. Hyer, & R. Intrieri (Eds.), Clinical Applied Gerontological Interventions In Long-term Care. (pp. 265–293). New York: Springer Publishing Company.

Spielman, A. J., Saskin, P., & Thorpy, M. J. (1987). Treatment of chronic insomnia by restriction of time in bed. *Sleep, 10*, 45–56.

Spreen, O., & Strauss, E. (1998). *A compendium of neuropsychological tests* (2nd ed.). New York: Oxford University Press.

Stepanski, E., Rybarczyk, B., Lopez, M., & Stevens, S. (2003). Assessment and treatment of sleep disorders in older adults: A review for rehabilitation psychologists. *Rehabilitation Psychology, 48*, 23–36.

Stiles, P.G., &McGarrahan, J.F. (1998). The Geriatric Depression Scale: A comprehensive review. *Journal of Clinical Geropsychology, 4*, 89–110.

Stineman, M. G. (1997). Measuring casemix, severity, and complexity in geriatric patients undergoing rehabilitation. *Medical Care, 36*, 106–112.

Sullivan, D. H. (1992). Risk factors for early hospital readmission in a select population of geriatric rehabilitation patients: The significance of nutritional status. *Journal of the American Geriatric Society, 40*, 792–798.

Tait, R. (1999). Assessment of pain and response to treatment in older adults. In P. A. Lichtenberg (Ed.), *Handbook of assessment in clinical gerontology* (pp. 555–584). New York: Wiley.

Teri, L., Logsdon, R. G., Uomoto, J., & McCurry, S. M. (1997). Behavioral treatment of depression in dementia patients: A controlled clinical trial. *Journal of Gerontology. Series B, Psychological Sciences Social Sciences, 52*, 159–166.

Tombaugh, T. N., & Mcintyre, N. J. (1992). The Mini-Mental-State-Examination: A comprehensive review. *Journal of the American Geriatrics Society, 40*, 922–935.

Tombaugh, T. N., McDowell, I., Kristjansson, B., & Hubley, A. M. (1996). Mini-Mental State Examination (MMSE) and the modified MMSE (3MS): A psychometric comparison and normative data. *Psychological Assessment, 8*, 48–59.

Tucker, N. J. (1993). Geriatric rehabilitation: Nursing challenge of the'90s. *Rehabilitation Nursing, 18*, 114–116.

Turner, R. S. (2003). Neurologic aspects of Alzheimer's disease. In P. A. Lichtenberg, D. L. Murman, & A. M. Mellow (Eds.), *Handbook of dementia: Psychological, neurological, and psychiatric perspectives* (pp. 1–25). Hoboken, NJ: Wiley.

Ueda, S., & Okawa, Y. (2003). The subjective dimension of functioning and disability: what is it and what is it for? *Disability and Rehabilitation, 25*(11–12), 596–601.

Walker, D. A. (2004). Cognitive behavioural therapy for depression in a person with Alzheimer's dementia. *Behavioural and Cognitive Psychotherapy, 32*(4), 495–500.

Wall, J. R., Deshpande, S. A., MacNeill, S. E., & Lichtenberg, P. A. (1998). The Fuld Object Memory Evaluation, a useful tool in the assessment of urban geriatric patients. *Clinical Gerontologist, 19*, 39–49.

Ward, L. C., Wadsworth, A. P., & Peterson, L. P. (1994). Concurrent validity of measures of anxiety, depression, and somatization in elderly, demented, male patients. *Clinical Gerontologist, 15*, 3–13.

Williamson, D., Scott, J., & Adams, R. (1996). Traumatic brain injury. In R. L. Adams, O. A. Parsons, & J. L. Culbertson (Eds.), *Neuropsychology for clinical practice: Etiology, assessment, and treatment*. Washington, DC: American Psychological Association

Wilson, K. C. M., Mottram, P. G., & Vassilas, C. A. (2008). Psychotherapeutic treatments for older depressed people. *Cochrane Database Systematic Review, 1*, CD004853.

Wilson, K. C. M., Scott, M., Abou-Saleh, M., Burns, R., & Copeland, D. (1995). Long term effects of cognitive behavioural therapy and lithium therapy on depression in the elderly. *British Journal of Psychiatry, 167*(5), 653–658.

Wolinsky, F. D., Callahan, C. M., Fitzgerald, J. F., & Johnson, R. J. (1992). The risk of nursing home placement and subsequent death among older adults. *Journals of Gerontology, 47*(4), 173–182.

Wressle, E., Oberg, B., & Henriksson, C. (1999). The rehabilitation process for the geriatric stroke patient—an exploratory study of goal setting and interventions. *Disability and Rehabilitation, 21*(2), 80–87.

Yesavage, J. A. (1982). Development and validation of a geriatric depression screening scale: A preliminary report. *Journal of Psychiatric Research, 22*, 37–49.

Yochim, B. P., Bank, A. L., Mast, B. T., MacNeill, S. E., & Lichtenberg, P. A. (2003). Clinical Utility of the Mattis Dementia Rating Scale in Older, Urban Medical Patients: An Expanded Study. *Aging, Neuropsychology, and Cognition, 10*(3), 230–237.

Yonan, C. A., & Wegener, S. T. (2003). Assessment and management of pain in the older adult. *Rehabilitation Psychology, 48*(1), 4–13.

Young, J., Brown, A., Forster, A., & Clare, J. (1999). An overview of rehabilitation for older people. *Reviews in Clinical Gerontology, 9*, 183–196.

Zadikoff, C., Fox, S. H., Tang-Wai, D. F., Thomsen, T., de Bie, R. M., Wadia, P., et al. (2008). A comparison of the mini mental state exam to the Montreal cognitive assessment in identifying cognitive deficits in Parkinson's disease. *Movement Disorders, 23*(2), 297–299.

PART 2

Clinical Contexts and Applications

Multiple Sclerosis

Kenneth I. Pakenham

Abstract

This chapter presents information on multiple sclerosis (MS) relevant to the psychologist's role in the care of persons with MS. Background information on the nature of MS, including prevalence, etiology, course, symptoms, and treatment is provided first. This is followed by a discussion of key issues related to cognitive impairment, mental health, and stress. Coping with MS is then discussed within a stress and coping framework, followed by a discussion of caregiving, and then a review of psychosocial interventions. Finally, future directions regarding psychological research and practice in MS are delineated.

Key Words: Multiple sclerosis, quality of life, rehabilitation, stress and coping, caregiving, cognitive impairment, depression, anxiety.

Multiple sclerosis (MS) is an inflammatory, demyelinating, neurodegenerative, autoimmune disease. The disease produces demyelination of the central nervous system (CNS) nerve fibers. The proposed pathogenetic mechanism is the activation of certain T cells that target proteins of the myelin sheath surrounding the axons of nerve cells. These cells enter the CNS through the blood–brain barrier, mount an "offensive" on the myelin sheath, and initiate a chronic inflammatory cascade that results in demyelination of axons. The damaged or scarred areas are called *lesions* or *plaques*. The particular symptoms that are experienced depend on the sites affected by plaques. Although diagnosis of MS can be difficult, the development of magnetic resonance imaging (MRI) techniques has greatly improved the accuracy and diagnosis of MS. Magnetic resonance imaging has become the gold standard technology for assessing brain lesions in MS.

Prevalence

Multiple sclerosis is the most common neurological disorder among young people; it is usually diagnosed between the ages of 20 and 40 and affects 2.5 million persons worldwide (World Health Organization, 2004). The prevalence is about twice as high in women as in men; however, MS tends to be less severe in women than in men (Matthews & Rice Oxley, 2001). In about 5% of cases, MS occurs in children or adolescents (Banwell, Ghezzi, Bar-Or, Mikaeloff, & Tardieu, 2007). A recent review of epidemiological data suggests that an increase in the prevalence of MS has occurred over the past few decades, largely due to longer survival and an overall increase in the incidence of MS in women (Koch-Henriksen & Sörensen, 2010).

Course

The disease course is variable and unpredictable, and acute exacerbations can occur unpredictably. Four disease courses have been identified (Lublin & Reingold, 1996). The most common course of illness is *relapsing-remitting*, which is characterized by disease exacerbations (or relapses) involving a sudden increase in symptoms that remit partially or fully in weeks or months. In about 85% of cases,

MS begins with a relapsing-remitting course characterized by exacerbations with baseline levels of functioning between relapses. In later stages, most patients develop a *secondary-progressive* course marked by decreasing numbers or cessation of relapses and increased progression. Of those who start with relapsing-remitting disease more than half will develop secondary-progressive MS within 10 years. About 10% of patients have a *primary-progressive* course from the onset, in which there is a steady increase in symptoms in the absence of relapses. The *progressive-relapsing* course is the least common, affecting approximately 5% of patients. It involves progressive disability from onset, but with relapses with or without full recovery. With respect to the two key clinical manifestations of the disease, relapses are usually associated with acute inflammatory lesions, whereas progression is thought to be triggered by permanent neuronal damage (Gold et al., 2005). Approximately 10–15% of patients begin with a *benign course* of MS, showing minimal disease activity; however, some of these patients go on to develop one of the more common disease presentations just described.

Prognostics

The prognosis in MS is variable and the rate of progression depends on type, severity, and location of MS. A high rate of severe relapses in the beginning is regarded as a predictor of worse outcome (Gold et al., 2005); however, the prognosis is difficult to predict early in the disease course (for further discussion of prognostic factors see Dahl, Stordal, Hydersen, & Midgard, 2009). D'hooghe, Nagels, Bissay, and De Keyser (2010) reviewed research that had investigated the association between modifiable factors and relapse and/or disability. They found strong evidence for an association between greater likelihood of relapse and infections, the postpartum period, and stressful life events, and a link between reduced relapse rate and pregnancy, exclusive breast-feeding, sunlight exposure, and higher vitamin D levels. Factors associated with increasing disability were stressful life events, radiotherapy to the head, low levels of physical activity, smoking, and low vitamin D levels. However, the authors acknowledged that some of these lifestyle factors may be linked to each other. In addition, the associations cannot be confidently interpreted with respect to causality.

Cause

The etiology of MS remains largely unknown and appears to include a complex relationship between individual genetic susceptibility and environmental factors. An increased risk of MS exists in close biological relatives of patients with MS, and the concordance rate in identical twins is about 25%, far higher than in dizygotic twins (see review in Koch-Henriksen & Sörensen, 2010). It appears that many genes affect the risk of MS. Regarding environmental causes of MS, a long held view is that MS is prevalent in regions where whites of Nordic origin live in temperate regions away from the equator, and in high-income countries. In contrast, MS is less common where non-whites live in low-income countries, and in tropical regions. However, a quantitative review of epidemiological data has challenged the theory of a latitudinal gradient of incidence of MS in Europe and North America, although the data supported this gradient for Australia and New Zealand (Koch-Henriksen & Sörensen, 2010). One physical effect of latitude is the exposure to solar ultraviolet radiation, the level of which has been found to be inversely associated with the prevalence of MS in some parts of the world (Sloka, Pryse-Phillips, & Stefanelli, 2008; van der Mei, Ponsonby, Blizzard, & Dwyer, 2001). Drawing on this data it has been proposed that greater exposure to solar ultraviolet radiation increases vitamin D_3, which is produced in the skin in response to sunlight which, in turn, has beneficial immunomodulatory effects in MS (Smolders, Damoiseaux, Menheere, & Hupperts, 2008). In summary, MS is likely to emerge as a result of multiple complex causal pathways and factors involving genetics, environmental factors, socioeconomic structure (e.g., access to medical facilities), and various biological mechanisms.

Symptoms

Clinical symptoms vary widely and include, but are not limited to, cognitive impairment, loss of balance, pain, sexual dysfunction, fatigue, loss of bowel or bladder control, mobility, visual and speech impairments, and emotional changes. Fatigue is the most common symptom affecting 50–75% of patients (Hadjimichael, Vollmer, & Oleen-Burkey 2008; Lerdal, Celius, Krupp, & Dalh 2007; Putzki, Katsarava, Vago, Diener, & Limmroth, 2008), and of these 14% regard it as their most disabling symptom (Fisk et al., 1994). Another relatively common symptom that has only recently begun to attract research attention is pain; the prevalence of pain ranges from 29% to 82% (Grasso et al., 2008). The Kurtzke Expanded Disability Status Scale (Kurtzke, 1983) is the primary instrument used by clinicians to assess neurological status, level of disability, and response to therapies. However, this scale is heavily weighted toward mobility and does not assess all the health-related quality of life (QOL) domains impacted by the disease (e.g., physical, mental, and emotional domains).

Psychosocial Impacts

Multiple sclerosis has profound social and psychological consequences, including disruptions in employment, sexual and family functioning, and activities of daily living (Simmons, 2010). Onset is most often in young adulthood, a developmental stage when chronic illness and disability are especially traumatic because they are likely to interfere with unrealized life plans. The psychosocial effects of MS are evident in data indicating that people with MS have a higher prevalence of emotional disorders relative to other patient groups with comparable degrees of physical disability (Rao, Huber, & Bornstein, 1992) and report lower QOL than community comparison groups (McCabe & McKern, 2002).

Treatment

Currently, there is no cure and often only minimal symptomatic relief (Rao et al., 1992). Clinical management of MS patients focuses on early acute treatment to reduce inflammatory processes in the CNS and ongoing treatment to reduce relapses and the progression of disability, symptoms, and disease activity as evident on MRI. Corticosteroid therapy is typically used for treating relapses, although evidence for the effectiveness of this treatment is sparse (see review Köpke, Kasper, Mühlhauser, Nübling, & Heesen, 2009). Licensed disease-modifying drug treatments (e.g., interferon [IFN] β-1a, IFN β-1b, glatiramer acetate) have been shown to offer improvements on clinical outcomes (e.g., relapses and disability progression) and MRI measures, and are now a first-line therapy for relapse-remitting MS (Freedman, 2006). Disease-modifying treatments suppress the inflammatory response evident on MRI and reduce exacerbation rates. However, given the limitations of these treatments, multidisciplinary rehabilitation programs are the mainstay of treatment. A recent Cochrane review of multidisciplinary rehabilitation programs in MS provided support for these programs using outcomes based on the International Classification of Functioning, Disability, and Health (Khan, Turner-Stokes, Ng, & Kilpatrick, 2008). There was strong evidence indicating that inpatient multidisciplinary rehabilitation programs can yield short-term gains in terms of activity (disability) and in overall ability to participate in society. Regarding high-intensity outpatient and home-based rehabilitation programs, there was limited evidence for short-term gains in symptoms, disability, QOL, and in participation in society. Low-intensity programs conducted over a longer period of time were associated with longer term improvements in QOL and benefits for caregivers.

Cognitive Impairment

Recent reviews of cognitive impairment in MS highlight cognitive deficits as a prominent issue requiring attention in the rehabilitation and clinical management of people with MS (Amato, Zipoli, & Portaccio, 2006; Patti, 2009). A general consensus exists that the frequency of cognitive impairment in MS ranges from 40% to 60% and that it is more common in the context of secondary-progressive disease and brain atrophy (Benedict, 2009). Cognitive impairment can occur in the early stage of MS and is sometimes the first manifestation of the disease (Amato et al., 1995, Haase, Tinnefield, Lienemann, Ganz, & Faustmann, 2003). For example, the prevalence of cognitive impairment in patients with a clinically isolated syndrome suggestive of MS is between 27% and 57%, and cognitive impairment has been shown to be a strong predictor of conversion to MS in these patients (Zipoli et al., 2010). Cognitive impairment has also been identified in those with low levels of disability. In a study using a large sample of mildly disabled relapsing-remitting MS patients, 20% of participants were identified as having cognitive impairment (Patti et al., 2009). Unfortunately remission of cognitive impairment is uncommon (Amato et al., 2006a).

Children may be especially vulnerable to cognitive impairment since the disease processes occur along with the myelination processes in the developing CNS, and illness-related difficulties are likely to interfere with timely movement through major developmental milestones (Amato et al., 2008). Although few studies have examined cognitive impairment in childhood and juvenile MS, those that have highlight the importance of cognitive impairment (Amato et al., 2008; Portaccio et al., 2009).

Cognitive impairment has profound adverse impacts on many areas of the patient's daily functioning (e.g., employment, interpersonal interactions, and driving) and consequently reduces QOL (e.g., Amato et al., 2006a; Wynia, Middel, van

Dijk, De Keyser, & Reijneveld, 2008). Cognitive impairment also adversely impacts on the caregiver. Figved et al. (2007) found that higher levels of cognitive impairment (and psychiatric symptoms) in people with MS were associated with poorer QOL and greater distress in caregivers over and above the effects of mobility problems.

Although a clear profile of cognitive impairment in MS is yet to be delineated, the cognitive functions most frequently affected are learning, memory (especially mnestic function), attention, processing speed, visuospatial abilities, and executive functions; however, the symptoms and severity of cognitive impairment vary widely (Patti, 2009; Rogers & Panegyres, 2007). Impairment of the retrieval of information from long-term memory is the most frequently reported cognitive impairment (Rogers & Panegyres, 2007). Language ability (e.g., repetition, fluency, and comprehension) and immediate, implicit, and recognition memory are usually unaffected in MS (Rogers & Panegyres, 2007).

There are mixed findings regarding the associations between cognitive impairment and neurological deficits or level of disability (Patti, 2009; Rogers & Panegyres, 2007). In fact, increasing cognitive impairment may indicate progressive disease in the presence of stable physical symptoms (Amato et al., 2001). However, moderate correlations between cognitive impairment and MRI disease measures have been reported (Patti, 2009), which suggest that cognitive impairment could reflect the disease processes within the brain. In addition, a range of factors have been identified that may influence the degree of cognitive impairment in MS, including location and extent of pathological lesions, progressive versus relapsing disease course, disease duration, CNS-active medication (e.g., antiepileptics, selective serotonin reuptake inhibitors, and baclofen), fatigue, and mood disturbance (Rogers & Panegyres, 2007). However, the causal directions of these associations have not been established. Risk factors for cognitive decline include advanced age, low intelligence or educational level (Randolph, Arnett, & Higginson, 2001), and depression (Haase et al., 2003), and cognitive decline early in the disease process is a risk for ongoing decline (Amato et al., 2006a). Patient-reported cognitive decline is not a sensitive marker for actual decline (Julian, Merluzzi, & Mohr, 2007). Nevertheless, Green, Pakenham, and Gardiner (2005) presented a model of subjective and objective indicators of cognitive impairment that proposes subjective perceptions of cognitive impairment as an important component

of QOL, and suggests that subjective measures of cognitive function correlate more strongly with psychosocial variables such as appraisal, coping, and emotions, than with objective cognitive function.

Assessment of Cognitive Impairment

Despite the high frequency of cognitive impairment in MS, cognitive function is not assessed routinely in clinical practice (Patti, 2009). Barriers to incorporating cognitive assessments as a routine part of clinical practice are perceptions of cognitive assessment as costly, time-consuming, complicated, burdensome for clients, and challenging to administer and interpret (Patti, 2009; Rogers & Panegyres, 2007). In addition, cognitive impairment in patients with mild physical handicap is often overlooked because of the low correlation between cognitive and physical deficits (Sartori & Edan, 2006). However, routine assessment of cognitive function in MS is essential because of: (a) the marked adverse effects of cognitive impairment on QOL, (b) the high prevalence of cognitive impairment, (c) cognitive impairment as a representative marker for disease progression (as evident by correlations with MRI indicators of brain lesion burden and atrophy), (d) the tendency of cognitive impairment to reduce a patient's ability to understand and adhere to treatment, and finally, (e) the adverse impact of a patient's cognitive impairment on his or her caregiver. Given that cognitive impairment can occur at all stages of MS, regular monitoring of cognitive functioning should be conducted and should commence as early as possible (Rogers & Panegyres, 2007). Sartori and Edan (2006) suggest that cognitive assessment should be performed at least 8 weeks after a relapse. The early detection of cognitive deficits is essential to enable intervention to alleviate symptoms and prevent further decline.

Comprehensive guidelines for cognitive assessment in MS are lacking and few cognitive tests have been validated on MS populations (Patti, 2009). However, Patti (2009) lists the neuropsychological test batteries (e.g., Rao's Brief Repeatable Battery) and individual cognitive tests (e.g., Paced Auditory Serial Addition Test) that have been shown to be suitable for the assessment of cognitive function in people with MS. Sartori and Edan (2006) have published recommendations for the optimal assessment of cognitive impairment in MS and also include a list of recommended tests for assessing cognitive functioning. Briefly, they suggest that neuropsychological tests should not rely on motor coordination or visuospatial ability, but should be sensitive to subtle cognitive changes, attention, speed, and working memory and the effects of fatigue. Rogers and Panegyres (2007) provide recommendations on instruments for screening for early cognitive impairment. Given the degree of specialization in the area of neuropsychology, it is likely that, in most settings, the assessment and management of cognitive impairment within psychology is best managed by neuropsychologists.

A critical aspect of the assessment process is the feedback to patients and their caregivers of results and the use of findings to inform and develop interventions. Regarding the latter, the process of giving feedback on the results of cognitive assessments that indicate cognitive decline must be managed with sensitivity and care, given the burdensome implications of such information for patient and caregiver. The discussion of cognitive deficits should be couched in the context of how the patient can maximize functioning and valued living despite such impairments. However, all too often practitioners invest considerable time and energy in assessment and invest few resources into the feedback and intervention phases.

Cognitive Rehabilitation

Although there are no clear guidelines for the optimal management of cognitive impairment in MS (Amato, Portaccio, & Zipoli, 2006b; Patti, 2009), cognitive rehabilitation should be multifaceted and include cognitive strategies, pharmacologic treatments, assistance with psychiatric problems, fatigue, psychosocial difficulties, and the inclusion of the primary caregiver and family members (Amato, Portaccio, & Zipoli, 2006a).

Regarding pharmacologic treatments, disease-modifying drug treatments for MS reduce brain lesion development or progressive brain atrophy and may therefore offer cognitive benefits for people with MS. Consistent with this view is emerging evidence for the cognitive benefits of these drug treatments for MS (see reviews by Amato, Portaccio, & Zipoli, 2006b; Patti, 2009). However, few disease-modifying drug trials include cognitive assessment; hence, the effects of these treatments on cognition are not well understood and the benefits remain unconfirmed (Amato, Portaccio, & Zipoli, 2006b; Patti, 2009).

Cognitive rehabilitation includes both remedial (direct retraining and targeting of specific skills) and compensatory (methods for working around deficits) approaches (Bagert, Camplair, & Bourdette, 2002). Environmental modification,

such as developing a quiet working space, may also be helpful. Education and counseling of patients and their families are important initial steps (Bagert et al., 2002) that can alleviate concerns and misperceptions associated with cognitive impairment. A variety of rehabilitation practitioners are likely to be involved in cognitive rehabilitation, including occupational therapists, speech therapists, and psychologists.

A dearth of research exists on cognitive rehabilitation strategies for people with MS, and the few studies that have been conducted have been criticized for a range of methodological weaknesses, including the neglect of experimental design parameters (Amato & Zipoli, 2003). A Cochrane review of psychological interventions in MS included a review of cognitive rehabilitation studies (Thomas, Thomas, Hillier, Galvin, & Baker, 2006). Three cognitive rehabilitation studies were reviewed and there was some evidence of gains on cognitive outcomes, although results were difficult to interpret because of the large number of outcome measures employed. Several subsequent controlled cognitive rehabilitation trials have yielded findings consistent with this review. A recent double-blind, controlled study of relapse-remitting MS patients with low levels of disability evaluated the efficacy of an individual, computer-based intensive cognitive rehabilitation program of 3 months' duration that targeted information processing, attention, and executive function, all of which were impaired in the 20 study participants (Flavia, Stampatori, Zanotti, Parrinello, & Capra, 2010). Relative to a comparison group, the cognitive rehabilitation participants after the intervention evidenced significantly greater improvement on tests of information processing, attention, and executive functions, as well as on a measure of depression. These findings were consistent with those of Hildebrandt, Lanz, Hahn, Hoffmann, and Schwarze (2007), who also used a computer-based cognitive rehabilitation intervention. In their controlled study, they found that intervention participants showed significant improvement in verbal and working memory performance, although they did not find an effect on depression or fatigue.

Mental Health

The two most common mental health issues that arise in MS are depression and anxiety, and these are discussed in more detail below. However, a range of other mental health problems can also arise in MS relatively frequently. Pathological laughing and crying occurs in about 5–15% of MS patients (Feinstein, Feinstein, Gray, & O'Connor, 1977; Surridge, 1969). Pathological laughing-crying involves periods of uncontrollable laughing, crying, or both in response to nonspecific stimuli in the absence of a corresponding mood state (Poeck, 1969). Pathological laughing-crying appears to be associated with cognitive impairment. For example, in a controlled study, Sartori, Belliard, Chevrier, Chaperon, and Edan (2006) found 36% of patients with cognitive impairment had pathological laughing-crying versus 8% of patients without cognitive deficit. A related and also relatively common problem is euphoria, which involves elevated mood. Another mental health issue is substance misuse. Quesnel and Feinstein (2004) found that 15% of MS patients abuse alcohol, and Korostil and Feinstein (2007) found alcohol abuse was associated with anxiety symptoms. In addition to clinical psychiatric diagnoses, subthreshold psychiatric symptoms and psychological distress are also frequently present (Feinstein & Feinstein, 2001), and MS patients have reported higher symptom load across a wide range of dimensions of psychological distress compared with healthy controls (Kern et al., 2009).

Depression

Depression is the most common psychiatric disorder in MS (Feinstein, 2004). A review of depression in MS by Siegert and Abernethy (2005) found an annual prevalence rate of around 20% and a lifetime prevalence rate of 50%. Clinically significant levels of depression occur more frequently in MS patients than in the general population (Dahl et al., 2009). A meta-analytic review of studies compared people with MS to healthy individuals and to people with other chronic conditions. This review found that mildly or moderately disabled people with MS have more depressive symptoms than healthy people (Dalton & Heinrichs, 2005). In comparison to people with other chronic conditions the differences were more variable, with people with MS reporting higher (spinal and neuromuscular), lower (chronic fatigue syndrome), and equivalent (mixed non-neurological conditions) levels of depressive symptoms (Dalton & Heinrichs, 2005).

Whether depression in MS is due to the disease itself or is a consequence of living with an unpredictable chronic disorder is not resolved. There has been speculation that depression may be related to specific disease processes (Mohr & Cox, 2001), such as autoimmune problems and the neurological

damage caused by these processes in the form of brain lesions. However, Siegert and Abernethy (2005) in their review concluded that the association between lesion sites in the CNS and the occurrence of depressive symptoms is weak. Depression may also be the result of the iatrogenic effects of some medications used to treat MS. Although earlier research found increases in depression following the initiation of IFN drugs, subsequent studies have found no increased risk of depression associated with these drugs. Multiple sclerosis exacerbations are treated with steroids, which can produce changes in mood and cognition. Dalton and Heinrichs (2005), in their review of depression in MS, concluded that the link between MS and depression is multifaceted and nonspecific.

Coping processes may also play a role in depression. The pattern of findings indicating associations between lower levels of disability and higher depressive symptoms (Dalton & Heinrichs, 2005), and between longer illness duration and lower depression (e.g., Chwastiak et al., 2002; Pakenham, 1999) suggests that patients adapt to the illness over time via coping processes, despite increasing disability (Dalton & Heinrichs, 2005). Several cross-sectional (Pakenham, 2001a; Pakenham, Stewart, & Rogers, 1997) and longitudinal (Pakenham, 1999, 2006) studies show that coping processes account for considerably more variance in measures of depressive symptoms than illness variables. The interpersonal context of the person with MS may also have a bearing on the patient's depression. This is consistent with interpersonal theories of depression and data showing that depressive symptoms in the person with MS are related to depression in their caregiver (Figved et al., 2007).

Depressive disorders are often overlooked and undertreated (Feinstein, 2007). For example, one study found that two-thirds of MS patients who met criteria for a depressive disorder were not treated for their psychiatric condition (Mohr, Hart, Fionareva, & Tasch, 2006). Making a diagnosis of depression is difficult because depressive symptoms are confounded with symptoms of MS. Clinicians and researchers have suggested particular standardized measures or modifications of such measures for assisting with the assessment of depression (e.g., Honarmand & Feinstein, 2009).

The Goldman Consensus statement on depression in MS reported that an integrated approach involving psychotherapy and medication was the gold standard for treatment, particularly for severe depression (Goldman Consensus Group, 2005).

Psychological treatments in MS are further elaborated below.

Anxiety

Far fewer studies have examined anxiety in MS compared with depression. Using a standardized clinical interview to diagnose *Diagnostic and Statistical Manual of Mental Disorders* (DSM-IV) anxiety disorders, two studies found a 36% lifetime prevalence rate for anxiety disorders (Galeazzi et al., 2005; Korostil & Feinstein, 2007). This finding is consistent with a recent, large, population-based study that used self-report of anxiety symptoms and found clinically significant levels of anxiety were reported by 30% of participants, which was higher than the frequency of elevated anxiety in the general population (Dahl et al., 2009). The lifetime prevalence rates for anxiety disorders in MS are higher than estimates for other medical conditions (Korostil & Feinstein, 2007). The most common anxiety disorders are panic disorder, obsessive-compulsive disorder, generalized anxiety disorder (Korostil & Feinstein 2007), and social anxiety (Poder et al., 2009). Although not widely researched, post-traumatic stress disorder (PTSD) also appears to be relatively common among people with MS. In a pilot study of 58 people with MS with an average illness duration of 8 years, Chalfant, Bryant, and Fulcher (2004) found that 16% met the DSM-IV criteria for PTSD assessed by a diagnostic interview. Regarding those who satisfied the re-experiencing criterion, 75% of participants reported intrusion related to future-oriented concerns about their prognosis (e.g., being restricted to a wheelchair or their future appearance). The presence or absence of PTSD and the severity of PTSD were unrelated to illness duration or severity. Risk factors for anxiety disorders in people with MS include being female, a comorbid diagnosis of depression, and limited social support (Korostil & Feinstein 2007).

Potential biomedical sources of anxiety are the effects of the disease process and some of the treatments. Regarding the latter, some of the common medications used to treat MS (e.g., glatiramer acetate and corticosteroids) can produce anxiety symptoms (Johnson et al., 1995), and anxiety has been found to be associated with self-injection (Mohr, Boudewyn, Likosky, Levine, & Goodkin, 2001). However, Korostil and Feinstein (2007) found that neurological variables, including treatment with disease-modifying drugs, were unrelated to anxiety in MS patients. Pakenham (2006) also found that illness-related variables (duration, disease course, and symptoms) were unrelated to anxiety, and Zorzon et al. (2001) found no cerebral correlates of anxiety using brain MRI. Another possible source of anxiety is the uncertainty and perceptions of potential threats that are characteristic of MS. In this regard, anxiety is likely to stem from the adjustment process. In support of this proposal, Korostil and Feinstein (2007) found that perceptions of increased stressors and decreased social supports were significantly related to the development of anxiety disorders. In addition, in longitudinal research, Pakenham showed that stress and coping variables (Pakenham, 2006) and meaning-making variables (Pakenham, 2007a; Pakenham & Cox, 2008) were stronger predictors of anxiety than were illness factors.

As with depressive disorders, anxiety disorders are often not recognized and treated (Korostil & Feinstein, 2007). In one study, about half of the MS patients diagnosed with an anxiety disorder were not receiving standard treatment for their anxiety (Korostil & Feinstein, 2007). A particular concern with the lack of formal diagnosis and treatment of anxiety and depressive disorders is the association between these two disorders and suicide in people with MS (Korostil & Feinstein 2007). Multiple sclerosis is one of the neurological disorders with the highest rates of suicidal intent and completed suicide (Feinstein, 2002), and MS has been shown to be associated with a twofold risk of suicide (Harris & Barraclough, 1997).

Positive Mental Health Outcomes

The growth of positive psychology (Seligman & Csikszentmihalyi, 2000) and its application to rehabilitation psychology (Dunn & Dougherty, 2005) has resulted in a broadened perspective on the outcomes of coping with illness that includes not only the adverse impacts, but also the positive outcomes and the strengths and virtues of humans. With respect to MS, several studies have documented the benefits and personal growth that people with MS have reported as a consequence of their having MS (e.g., Mohr et al., 1999; Pakenham, 2005a, 2007b). In recent years, researchers have conceptualized adjustment to MS as encompassing not only distress, but also positive outcomes such as positive affect, satisfaction with life, and positive states of mind (e.g., Pakenham, 2007a, 2005a). Preliminary data suggest that positive and negative adjustment outcomes have both common and unique coping antecedents (Pakenham, 2006). Increasing research attention has also been placed on factors that enhance well-being and growth in people with MS. Some of these "resilience" factors are described in more detail below but include optimism, acceptance, and benefit-finding. A similar application of positive psychology has also been extended to caregivers of persons with MS (e.g., Pakenham & Cox, 2008).

Stress

Multiple sclerosis is a complex disease that affects most areas of a person's life. Persons with MS therefore, face multiple physical and psychosocial stressors related to their illness that change over the course of the illness (e.g., Mohr et al., 1999; Pakenham et al., 1997). Despite MS being a physical illness, psychosocial problems are reported as frequently as physical health problems (Pakenham et al., 1997). Common physical health stressors include illness symptoms (e.g., symptom fluctuations, pain, fatigue, heat sensitivity, and disability) and treatment difficulties (e.g., negative side effects, self-administering of injections, and complex medical regimens). Multiple sclerosis-related problems occur in the following life domains:

- Employment and career (e.g., changing to less hours of employment, managing symptoms in the workplace, and changing career or jobs because of illness)
- Finances (e.g., decreased income and increased expenditure on medical treatments or home modifications)
- Education (e.g., learning impeded by fatigue and/or cognitive impairment)
- Social and interpersonal (e.g., dwindling support network, symptoms that interfere with sexual relations, stigma, and conflict with family members)
- Existential (e.g., coming to terms with one's mortality and physical limitation, and revisions to self-definition, life goals, and values)
- Psychological

Two related and common psychological issues faced by people with MS are fear of losing control and uncertainty. Multiple sclerosis is characterized by an uncertain course and unpredictable relapses and remissions. Loss of control over one's destiny and a sense of uncertainty about one's future can lead to fear, panic, and/or anxiety. Not being able to predict one's future makes forward planning difficult. Even during periods of stability, an underlying fear can persist about when the next deterioration will occur. Another common stressor is the conflict between the dependency imposed by increasing disability and the person's struggle to retain his or her independence. The frustration and anger resulting from not being independent in basic activities of daily living can lead to self-harm or pushing oneself beyond endurance levels. Multiple losses are faced by the person with MS including loss of employment, career, income, mobility, engagement in valued activities, energy, physical strength, and contact with some friends.

These stressors can produce lifestyle disruptions and functional deficits that have been referred to as *illness intrusiveness*, and these compromise QOL (Devins et al., 1993). Many of these stressors are directly related to MS; however, people with MS will also experience stressors and major life events that are independent of their disease (e.g., death of a loved one). Interestingly, Brown and colleagues (2006a) found that the disease-related stressors that people with MS reported were more likely to be chronic (i.e., >6 months duration), whereas disease-independent stressors were more often acute events (i.e., <6 months duration).

The Stress–Relapse Link

A common observation of many clinicians is that patients with MS will often report that stress triggered their first identified symptoms and/or that stress led to subsequent exacerbations of their disease. The proposal that psychological stress (e.g., grief or social disruptions) may trigger the onset of MS was first put forward by Charcot (1877). Since that time, considerable research has been undertaken to examine the potential association between stress and clinical exacerbations in MS.

A systematic meta-analysis of 14 prospective studies found a significant relationship between the occurrence of stressful life event and a greater risk for relapses (Mohr, Hart, Julian, Cox, & Pelletier, 2004), and the magnitude of this effect size ($d = 0.53$), although moderately large, has been considered clinically significant (Gold et al., 2005; Mohr et al., 2004). A more recent review of research on the potential link between stress and MS disease status also concluded that there is evidence to support the association between stressful life events and relapses in MS (Heesen et al., 2007). Research subsequent to these reviews has confirmed the association between stress and relapse in MS (e.g., Brown et al., 2006a,b; Golan, Somer, Dishon, Cuzin-Disegni, & Miller, 2008; Yamout, Itani, Hourany, Sibaii, & Yaghi, 2010). In addition, a recent review of modifiable factors influencing relapse and disability in MS found strong evidence for the association between stressful life events and relapse and disability (D'hooghe et al., 2010). However, it should be noted that the evidence supporting an association between stress and relapse is not conclusive and does not allow for firm causal inferences (Heesen et al., 2007).

The ways in which stress may affect MS and stress response systems in MS are not known, although several models of potential mechanisms have recently emerged. For example, Gold et al. (2005) presented a model to explain the role of stress in MS disease exacerbation. Consistent with their model, they proposed that disruptions in the communication between the immune system and the major stress response systems (the hypothalamic-pituitary-adrenal axis and the autonomic nervous system) are implicated in the pathogenesis and progression of MS. Gold et al. (2005) and Heesen et al. (2007) reviewed studies showing evidence of alterations in the major stress response systems in MS patients that are correlated with markers of disease activity and severity. However, it is not clear if and how these mechanisms may mediate the stress–relapse association, and this and other similar models lack evidence that unequivocally confirms or disconfirms associated predictions.

The link between stress and relapses in MS is likely to be complex, with a diverse range of psychological and biological factors influencing the association, including demographics (e.g., being male; Brown et al., 2006a), stressor characteristics, characteristics of the person, and viral infections. Regarding the latter, viral infections may be important precipitants of the disease, and stress can increase an individual's susceptibility to viral infections (Brown, Tennant, Dunn, & Pollard, 2005). With respect to stressor characteristics, certain types of stressors have been found to be associated with relapse (e.g., social conflicts and disruption in routine; Mohr et al., 2000). The severity of the stressor also seems to be important, with several studies showing that stressors of a moderate severity are more likely to be associated with relapse (see review Brown et al., 2005), although some studies have found that severity is unrelated to relapse (e.g., Brown et al., 2006a). The acute versus chronic dimension is another characteristic of the stressor that may impact on relapse. For example, in both cross-sectional and longitudinal analyses, Brown and colleagues (Brown et al., 2006a; 2006b) found that relapse was predicted by the frequency of acute stressors (i.e., <6 months duration), but not chronic stressors. However, other studies have found that protracted stressors are related to relapse (see review in Brown et al., 2005).

Regarding the characteristics of the person, as discussed below, stress and coping theory proposes numerous potential moderators and mediators of stress including the individual's coping strategies, coping resources, and appraisals. Numerous studies provide evidence that implicate these coping processes in the stress–relapse link (see review in Brown et al., 2005). For example coping strategies have been shown to moderate the effects of stress on disease outcomes (Mohr, Goodkin, Nelson, Cox, & Weiner, 2002) and have direct effects on relapse (Brown et al., 2006b). Consistent with stress and coping theory, Brown et al. (2006a) found that subjective appraisal of a stressor (ratings of emotional threat) was a stronger predictor of relapse than was objective measures of the stressor. Evidence that modifiable factors such as coping processes influence the stress–relapse association suggests a role for stress management interventions to enhance coping with MS. Randomised controlled trials of stress management interventions would also help to shed light on the stress–relapse link. Psychological interventions such as stress management and coping skills training programs are discussed below.

Coping with Multiple Sclerosis

Despite the difficulties associated with MS, there are considerable variations in adjustment among people with MS, and illness factors are typically not strong predictors of such variability (e.g., Dahl et al., 2009; Pakenham, 1999). How the individual copes with his or her illness appears to be a more potent determinant of a person's adjustment to MS, including some of the mental health problems mentioned above. Lazarus and Folkman's (1984) stress and coping theory has been used to guide much of the research into coping with MS. According to this theory, stress manifests when the relationship between the person and the environment is appraised as exceeding his or her resources and as threatening well-being. Beyond the effects of the person's biographical, illness, and treatment characteristics, adjustment to MS is determined by three coping processes: cognitive appraisal, coping strategies, and coping resources. Stress and coping theory proposes that when a person is confronted with a stressor, he or she appraises its potential for harm, threat, loss, controllability, and challenge and considers coping options. The person then employs various coping strategies and draws on resources to deal with the stressor. The person may alter his appraisals, modify his coping strategies, and/or use different resources according to how well he is adjusting to the event, and in this way coping becomes a dynamic, transactional process responsive to feedback loops. Given the evidence (reviewed above) suggesting an association between stress and relapses in MS, stress and coping theory has particular relevance because, according to this theory, appraisals, coping strategies, and coping resources have the potential to mitigate or exacerbate the negative physiological effects of stressful events.

The utility of stress and coping frameworks in explaining adjustment to MS has been supported in cross-sectional (e.g., McCartney Chalk, 2007; McCabe, McKern, & McDonald, 2004; Pakenham, 2001a; Pakenham et al., 1997) and longitudinal (e.g., Aikens, Fischer, Namey, & Rudick, 1997; McCabe, 2006; Pakenham, 1999, 2006) studies. Such frameworks have also been applied to caregiving in MS (Pakenham, 2001b, 2002, 2005b). Dennison, Moss-Morris, and Chalder (2009) reviewed research on the psychological correlates of adjustment in people with MS. They found varying degrees of support for many of the variables proposed by stress and coping theory to shape adjustment.

A diagrammatic summary of a stress and coping framework applied to the process of adapting to MS and caregiving is presented in Figure 12.1. The framework includes both patient and caregiver because, as mentioned above, variations of stress and coping theory have been applied to both. Although the framework is consistent with stress and coping theory, the diagrammatic summary presented in Figure 12.1 is not depicted as a tight theoretical model but as a working "map" of coping with MS and MS-related caregiving. The framework provides a conceptual map for practitioners that can be used to inform assessment, case formulations, and intervention. Each of the coping processes in Figure 12.1 subsumes a potentially wide range of factors, some of which are discussed below.

Cognitive Appraisal

Cognitive appraisal is an evaluative process that reflects the person's subjective interpretation of an event (Lazarus & Folkman, 1984). Events are generally appraised in terms of threat, challenge, and controllability (Lazarus & Folkman, 1984). The appraisal of an illness-related event as threatening to one's well-being, limiting opportunities for personal growth (i.e., not challenging), and/or uncontrollable is likely to negatively influence adjustment

to MS, given that these appraisals generate stress that may overwhelm the person's available coping skills and resources (Lazarus & Folkman, 1984). In the main, higher appraised stress has been shown to be related to poorer adjustment across a range of domains regardless of disease severity level (see review Dennison et al., 2009).

Two other cognitive processes associated with adjustment to MS include illness uncertainty (Mishel, 1981) and self-efficacy (Bandura, 1977). Higher illness uncertainty has been consistently linked with worse adjustment to MS (Dennison et al., 2009). Higher self-efficacy specific to managing MS-related challenges seems to be related to better adjustment, whereas generalized self-efficacy is not consistently related to adjustment (Dennison et al., 2009).

Coping Strategies

Coping strategies may be categorized as: *problem-focused* strategies that actively attempt to directly impact the stressor (e.g., problem solving, seeking information), *emotion-focused* strategies that deal with the distress associated with the stressor by avoidance (e.g., wishful thinking, escape, and use of alcohol or drugs) or approach (e.g., humor, identifying and expressing feelings, accepting the situation), and *meaning-focused* strategies that create, reinstate, or foster meaning (e.g., positive reframing, prayer, rearranging life priorities) (Lazarus & Folkman, 1984; Park & Folkman, 1997).

Cross-sectional (Mohr, Goodkin, Gatto & Van Der Wende, 1997; O'Brien, 1993; Pakenham, 2001a) and longitudinal (Aikens et al., 1997; Pakenham, 1999) MS studies have shown poorer adjustment to be related to reliance on avoidance-oriented emotion-focused coping strategies. Positive reappraisal coping and acceptance coping (which include elements of emotional approach coping and meaning-focused coping) and seeking social support (often assessed as a problem-focused strategy) have been found to be related to better adjustment, although this is a weaker pattern of findings (McCartney Chalk, 2007; Pakenham, 2001a, 2006). As mentioned above, there is also evidence that coping strategies may buffer the negative effects of stress on the MS disease process (e.g., Mohr et al., 2002).

Coping Resources

Coping resources are relatively stable characteristics of an individual's disposition and environment, and they refer to what is available when an individual evaluates a situation and develops his

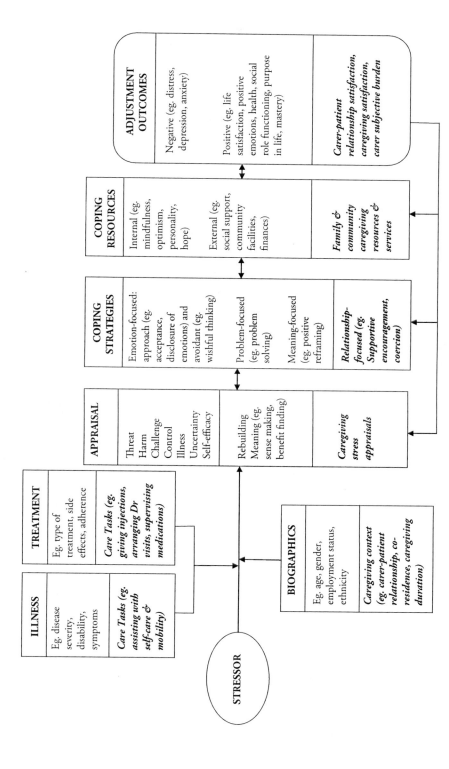

Figure 12.1 A modified version of Pakenham's (In press) working diagrammatic summary of a stress and coping framework for assessing and intervening in the coping processes that shape adjustment to MS and the caregiving role. Key generic variables applicable to both the person with MS and caregiver are depicted by regular font and caregiving specific variables are denoted by the bolded and shaded italics.

or her coping strategies (Moos & Billings, 1982). Of the potentially wide range of coping resources, optimism (a dispositional resource) and the availability of social support (an external resource) have received the most attention in the MS literature. Dennison et al.'s (2009) review showed that optimism (Scheier & Carver, 1985) and social support are associated with better adjustment across many domains. However, regarding social support, there is some evidence suggesting harmful impacts of support that is perceived as unsupportive (Wineman, 1990), overprotective (Schwartz & Frohner, 2005), and conflict (Stuifbergen, 1995).

Meaning-Making

Adverse events, such as the diagnosis of MS or a sudden deterioration in health, have the potential to disrupt fundamental assumptions regarding the benevolence and meaningfulness of the world and the worthiness of self. To the extent that an event undermines these assumptions, a sense of meaninglessness ensues that can cause existential distress which, in turn, is likely to trigger a rebuilding of meaning (Janoff-Bulman & Yopyk, 2004). Two ways to restore meaning are by finding reasons or an explanation for what has happened and by looking for the positive aspects of the event, referred to as *sense-making* and *benefit-finding*, respectively (Janoff Bulman & Yopyk, 2004). Although it is not clear whether meaning-making is better conceptualized as appraisal or coping processes within stress and coping theory, for the purposes of presenting a workable framework for understanding coping with MS, both are depicted as appraisal processes in Figure 12.1.

SENSE-MAKING

Making sense of adversity is achieved through developing new worldviews or via modifying existing assumptive worldviews that rebuild a sense of purpose, order, and self-worth. Pakenham (2008a) collected qualitative data from people with MS on how they made sense of their illness and found 16 sense-making themes (e.g., causal explanations, acceptance, experienced growth, spiritual/religious explanations). Based on this qualitative data, a multi-item Sense-making Scale was developed (Pakenham, 2007a). Over a third of those people with MS who could not make sense of their situation were able to anticipate comprehending it, and the strength of this anticipation was related to greater life satisfaction (Pakenham, 2008a). Sense-making has been shown to predict adjustment to MS concurrently

(Pakenham, 2008a) and over 12 months (Pakenham, 2007a). Sense-making dimensions characterized by perceptions of self-worth, controllability, and predictability were related to better adjustment, whereas those that involved perceptions that magnified the negatives of MS were related to poorer adjustment (Pakenham, 2007a).

BENEFIT-FINDING

Regarding benefit-finding, Pakenham (2007b) collected qualitative data from people with MS about the benefits related to their illness and identified seven themes (e.g., personal growth, strengthening of relationships, appreciation of life, new opportunities, health gains, and spiritual growth). Drawing on this data, Pakenham and Cox (2009) developed a multi-item benefit-finding scale (Benefit-finding in Multiple Sclerosis [BFiMS]) with seven subscales. Benefit-finding was found to be related to better adjustment to MS concurrently (Pakenham, 2005a) and over 12 months (Pakenham & Cox, 2009).

Many of the benefit-finding and sense-making themes reported by patients are qualitatively similar to those reported by their caregivers. There is also preliminary evidence showing that the sense-making and benefit-finding of the person with MS is correlated with the respective sense-making and benefit-finding of their caregiver (Pakenham, 2005c, 2008b). Furthermore, the sense-making and benefit-finding of one partner has been found to be associated with better adjustment of the other partner (Pakenham, 2005c, 2008b). Together, these findings suggest that people with MS and their caregivers engage in a process of shared meaning-making.

Practice Implications

It is difficult to draw robust practice guidelines from the above-mentioned research on coping with MS because of the numerous methodological weaknesses that characterize this body of research. A wide range of measures have been employed to assess each of the coping processes, and most researchers have used generic scales that do not tap aspects of the coping processes specific to managing MS that have emerged in recently developed measures that are more sensitive to the MS context (e.g., Pakenham, 2001a). A further limitation is that most studies have not examined coping processes in relation to specific MS-related stressors. As mentioned above, MS is associated with a range of stressors, and the types of coping strategies or coping resources that are likely to be effective in dealing with one type of stressor (e.g., fatigue) may not be effective in managing a different type of stressor (e.g., stigma). Indeed, in relation to coping strategies there is evidence suggesting that the effects of some strategies depend on the type of problem the person with MS is dealing with (Pakenham et al.,1997) and that the type of coping strategies a person relies on varies according to illness phase (Warren, Warren & Cockerill, 1991). A final limitation is the reliance on cross-sectional designs. Many of the concurrent associations between coping processes and adjustment do not hold when predicting change in adjustment over time.

Despite these limitations, several broad conclusions can be offered. One robust finding regarding coping strategies that does seem to hold in longitudinal designs and that is consistent with findings in other chronic illness research is that reliance on avoidance coping is associated with worse adjustment (Dennison et al., 2009). Hence, it would seem that avoidance in the context of dealing with a chronic illness is not adaptive, although when faced with an acute health problem, avoidance does appear to be effective (Clutton, Pakenham, & Buckley, 1999). Other coping processes that appear to hinder adjustment include those that are characterized by a focus on the negative aspects (e.g., threat) of stressors. Coping processes that appear to foster adjustment are those that are characterized by self-confidence in dealing with specific stressors (self-efficacy), a realistic optimistic outlook, seeking and utilizing social support, positive reappraisals of stressors, finding meaning in the illness, and acceptance of things that cannot be changed and actively dealing with things that can be modified.

The framework depicted in Figure 12.1 identifies variables that need to be assessed in order to identify coping deficits and strengths that will, in turn, inform the design of individualized interventions to build on assets and target weaknesses. Specific assessment instruments that may be used to assess the coping processes are described in detail elsewhere (Pakenham, in press). Interventions for fostering adaptive coping processes will be discussed below.

Caregivers

Informal caregivers are essential throughout the MS rehabilitation process since the disease affects both the caregiver and care recipient, and they appear to respond as a social unit (Pakenham, 1998). Caregivers can be a vital source of information about the functioning of the person living with MS and can be a resource in implementing rehabilitation plans.

Caregiving Activities

Caregivers perform a wide range of time-consuming and physically and emotionally demanding tasks (Finlayson & Cho, 2008; McKeown, Porter-Armstrong, & Baxter, 2003; Pakenham, 2007c), and some of these are depicted in Figure 12.1. Caregivers of persons with MS spend considerable time on these tasks, all of which are of immense economic value and make an essential contribution to the rehabilitation of persons living with MS (Aronson, Cleghorn, & Goldenberg, 1996; Carton, Loos, Pacolet, Versieck, & Vlietinck, 2000). Pakenham (2007c) developed the Caregiving Tasks in MS Scale (CTiMSS) from qualitative data obtained from MS caregivers and identified four dimensions of caregiving tasks: Instrumental Care (e.g., transportation, shopping), Activities of Daily Living Care (particularly intimate care such as toileting, bathing, and dressing), Psychological-Emotional Care (e.g., managing the care recipient's emotional and personality changes), and Social-Practical Care (e.g., providing emotional support and companionship). As MS disability increases, the number of hours spent caregiving increases and the nature of the caregiving tasks usually becomes more intimate.

Adjustment to Caregiving
NEGATIVE CAREGIVER ADJUSTMENT OUTCOMES

Reviews of the impacts of MS caregiving on caregivers (McKeown et al., 2003; Corry & While, 2009) suggest that caregivers experience adverse impacts on their QOL, physical health, psychological well-being, employment and career, social life, and financial situation. These negative caregiving impacts are often collectively referred to as *caregiver burden* (Pearlin, Mullan, Semple, & Skaff, 1990). Recent reviews of MS caregiving found that higher caregiver burden was consistently related to poorer psychological health in MS caregivers (Corry & While, 2009; McKeown et al., 2003). These negative impacts can emerge soon after diagnosis, before the emergence of marked physical disability and the related physical caregiving demands are apparent (Bogosian, Moss-Morris, Yardley, & Dennison, 2009; Janssens et al., 2003). Qualitative studies suggest that MS caregivers are confronted with a wide range of psychological issues including grief, confrontations with their own mortality, uncertainty about the future, lifestyle disruptions, challenges to their definition of self, and changes to their life goals. The emotional impact of caregiving in MS has been described as "chronic sorrow" (Hainsworth, 1996).

Compared to the general population, MS caregivers report higher levels of psychological distress (Sherman et al., 2007) and lower life satisfaction (Aronson, 1997). Between 24% (Janssens et al., 2003) and 28% (Pakenham, 2001b) of MS caregivers report clinically significant levels of global distress. Dewis and Niskala (1992) found that MS caregivers reported four times as many stress symptoms as the general population and one-third more than a heterogeneous group of caregivers. Regarding depressive symptoms, Pakenham (2001b) found that 9% and 17% of caregivers fell in the moderate–severe and mild ranges on the Beck Depression Inventory, respectively. Solari, Ferrari, and Radice (2006) found that 19% of caregivers reported depressed mood, which was twice as high as healthy controls. Janssens et al. (2003) found that 40% of spouse caregivers reported clinically significant levels of anxiety and, on average, they reported higher levels of anxiety than a comparison group. There is some evidence suggesting that spouse caregivers continue to report elevated anxiety and distress levels for 2–3 years after the diagnosis (Janssens et al., 2006). In view of data that suggest distress levels of caregivers and care recipients are correlated (e.g., Pakenham, 1998), a critical element of the rehabilitation process is attending to psychological and emotional distress in the patient's social system.

POSITIVE CAREGIVER ADJUSTMENT OUTCOMES

In addition to these negative impacts of MS caregiving are the rewards or benefits. Perrone, Gordon, and Tschopp (2006) compared MS caregivers with normative data and found that they reported greater love for their spouses than the normative sample. Hakim et al. (2000) found that 11% of spouses reported that their marital relationship had improved since the diagnosis of MS. Multiple sclerosis caregivers have reported a wide range of benefits associated with their caregiving, including greater insights into illness and hardship, caregiving gains, personal growth, the strengthening of relationships, increased appreciation of life, health gains, and a change in life priorities and personal goals (Pakenham, 2005c; Pakenham & Cox, 2008).

Multiple Sclerosis and the Family

Multiple sclerosis has direct and indirect effects on all family members. Findings from several studies provide support for the disruptive impact of MS on family functioning, including parenting tasks and roles (Deatrick, Brennan, & Cameron, 1998; Peters & Esses, 1985). Multiple sclerosis often occurs during young adulthood, a time when people typically consider marriage and starting a family. Hence, many people with MS confront the demands of parenting along with MS symptoms, such as fatigue and cognitive impairment, that can interfere with parenting roles and functions. Unfortunately, parental coping with MS has attracted little research attention, although several studies show that many parents with MS report concerns about the effects of their illness on their children (Braham, Houser, Cline, & Posner, 1975; De Judicibus & McCabe, 2004). There is very little data on the effects of parental MS on the partner and children, although the latter has been the focus of increasing research recently.

Young people who have a parent with MS often assume some responsibility for their care and for this reason some researchers have referred to them as "young caregivers." These young people take on many of the caregiving tasks that adults assume (described above). Some of these caregiving responsibilities necessitate the child assuming an adult caregiving role, and the provision of personal intimate care is particularly challenging for children. One study showed that compared to children of healthy parents, children of a parent with MS undertook significantly higher levels of family responsibilities (Pakenham & Bursnall, 2006). There is evidence to indicate that caring for a parent with MS can have a range of negative impacts on the child. Compared to children who have healthy parents, children of a parent with MS have been shown to have higher levels of distress and interpersonal difficulties, and lower life satisfaction and positive affect (Arnaud, 1959; Pakenham & Bursnall, 2006; Yahav, Vosburgh, & Miller, 2005). Other studies that have not employed comparison groups have also found somatic complaints (Friedemann & Tubergen, 1987) and emotional distress (Kikuchi, 1987) to be prominent in children of parents with MS. For a more detailed discussion of issues relevant to children caring for an ill or disabled family member, refer to Pakenham (2009).

Predictors of Caregiver Adjustment

The variations in the adjustment of MS caregivers can in part be explained by a range of patient and caregiver characteristics and stress and coping variables, as depicted in Figure 12.1. Patient illness characteristics that have been found to be related to lower caregiver well-being or QOL include psychiatric symptoms (particularly depression) and cognitive impairment (e.g., Chipchase & Lincoln, 2001; Figved, Myhr, Larsen, & Aarsland, 2007; Khan, McPhail, Brand, Turner-Stokes, & Kilpatrick, 2006), and greater functional disability and more severe disease progression (Chipchase & Lincoln 2001; Corry & While, 2009; Pakenham, 2001b; Pakenham & Bursnall, 2006). Caregiver-related factors associated with poorer caregiver adjustment include being female (Knight, Devereux, & Godfrey, 1997; Pakenham, 2001a), being the spouse of the person with MS (Aronson, 1997; Figved et al., 2007), longer caregiving duration (Aronson, 1997), and high levels of caregiving tasks (Pakenham, 2007c).

As mentioned above, Lazarus and Folkman's (1984) stress and coping theory has also been used to guide research into adaptation to MS caregiving, as summarized in Figure 12.1. In general, findings suggest that MS caregiver well-being is associated with lower stress appraisals, higher social support, less reliance on avoidant coping and relationship-focused coercion and criticism, and greater reliance on meaning-focused coping and relationship-focused supportive engagement (e.g., Knight et al., 1997; O'Brien, Wineman & Nealon, 1995; Pakenham, 2001b, 2002, 2005b). Pakenham and Bursnall (2006) found a similar pattern of findings in a study of young MS caregivers. With respect to coping strategies, evidence from one study suggests that whether caregivers and their care recipient rely on similar coping strategies may influence the adjustment of both partners (Pakenham, 1998).

The meaning-making processes of sense-making and benefit-finding that have been found to predict adjustment in the person with MS have also been found to predict adjustment in caregivers. Sense-making has been shown to predict caregiver adjustment concurrently (Pakenham, 2008b) and over 12 months (Pakenham, 2008c). Similarly, MS caregiver benefit-finding has been shown to be related to better caregiver adjustment concurrently (Pakenham, 2005c) and over 12 months (Pakenham & Cox, 2008).

Psychosocial Interventions

The most frequently used psychological intervention framework for fostering adjustment to MS is cognitive-behavioral therapy (CBT). A recent Cochrane review (Thomas et al., 2006) of the effectiveness of psychological interventions for people with MS concluded that there is reasonable evidence that CBT interventions help to improve depression, coping, and adjustment to MS. The majority of CBT interventions reviewed were delivered by psychologists. Cognitive-behavioral therapy interventions have been administered individually (Foley, Bedell, LaRocca, Scheinberg, & Reznikoff, 1987), in groups (Larcombe & Wilson, 1984), and by telephone (Mohr, Hart, et al., 2005), and recently electronic delivery has been examined (Hind et al., 2010). Regarding the latter, a recent qualitative study of generic computerized CBT interventions for people with MS found that these programs needed to be adapted for people with chronic physical conditions (Hind et al., 2010). The CBT intervention techniques used have varied widely and include relaxation training, self-monitoring, rehearsal of coping strategies, behavioral activation, cognitive restructuring strategies, problem-solving skills training, goal-setting, and coping skills training for dealing with specific symptoms and problems.

Many of these interventions have targeted the coping processes mentioned above. For example, one study showed that, relative to a control group, people with MS who received a CBT group stress management intervention demonstrated greater use of problem-focused coping strategies (Foley et al., 1987). Benedict et al. (2000) used CBT strategies to enhance self-control and behavior regulation to reduce socially aggressive behavior in people with MS with marked cognitive impairment. Cognitive-behavioral therapy has also been successfully used to help promote skills in managing fatigue in MS (van Kessel et al., 2008). Several interventions have focused on enhancing social skills (e.g., Benedict et al., 2000; Gordon, Lam, & Winter, 1977).

Other interventions that are not primarily CBT-based but have been used to promote adjustment to MS include exercise training, eclectic coping skills training programs, and lay-led self-management programs. A meta-analysis of the effects of exercise training on QOL in MS concluded that exercise training is associated with a small improvement in QOL (Motl & Gosney, 2008). A structured eclectic coping skills training program designed to teach coping flexibility for people with chronic illness was developed by Schwartz and Rogers (1994) and evaluated in a randomised trial using a sample of people with MS (Schwartz, 1999). Compared to participants in a peer telephone support program, the coping skills intervention participants reported increased functioning in psychosocial roles, less reliance on avoidant coping strategies, greater reliance on more active and approach-oriented coping strategies, and enhanced well-being. However, the peer telephone support intervention seemed most effective for those people with affective problems.

A generic lay-led community-based educational and self-management intervention called the Chronic Disease Self-Management Course has been developed for people with long-term health conditions, including MS (Lorig et al., 1999). The program has been delivered in numerous countries including the United Kingdom, the United States, Canada, and Australia. Generic topics are covered including self-management principles, exercise, pain management, depression, nutrition, communication, and goal setting. Reviews of the effectiveness of the Chronic Disease Self-Management Course showed that the intervention was, in the main, consistently associated with improvements in self-management, physical and mental health status, and self-efficacy (Griffiths, Foster, Ramsay, Eldridge, & Taylor, 2007; Lorig et al., 1999). A qualitative study of the experience of people with MS who participated in a Chronic Disease Self-Management Course showed that some participants learned new self-management techniques and found the goal-setting and mutual support from fellow participants particularly helpful (Barlow, Edwards, & Turner, 2009). However, some noted that the lack of MS-specific self-management techniques and information was a shortcoming of the program.

Considerable research on interventions designed to increase patient autonomy in treatment decision-making has been conducted in many chronic illnesses. One of the few studies to examine such an intervention in MS was conducted by Köpke and colleagues (2009). They evaluated an evidence-based decision aid that was delivered via a patient education program. Patients and their significant other attended a structured 4-hour education program on relapse management in MS. In comparison to the control group, intervention participants reported a reduction in physician-controlled therapies for managing relapses and reported greater decision autonomy.

There are no published studies of the application of a more recent variant of CBT (also referred to as a *third-wave behavior therapy*) called *Acceptance and Commitment Therapy* (ACT; Hayes, Strosahl, & Wilson, 1999) to people with MS. A key element of ACT is acceptance, which is defined as "the active and aware embracing of private events...without unnecessary attempts to change their frequency or form" (Hayes, Luoma, Bond, Masuda, & Lillis, 2006, p. 7). Acceptance and Commitment Therapy is likely to be applicable to people with MS in view of evidence indicating the beneficial effects of acceptance coping and acceptance sense-making in people with MS (e.g., McCartney Chalk, 2007; Pakenham, 2001a, 2006, 2007a). In addition, Pakenham and Fleming (2011) found that, after controlling for the effects of initial adjustment and relevant demographic and illness variables, greater ACT operationalized acceptance was related to better adjustment to MS over a 12-month interval. Furthermore, mindfulness (which is also used in ACT and encompasses acceptance) has been successfully applied to helping people with MS manage mobility difficulties (Mills & Allen, 2000) and improve QOL (Grossman, Kappos, Gensicke, D'Souza, Mohr, Penner, & Steiner, 2010). Acceptance and Commitment Therapy has been effectively applied to a range of chronic illnesses (e.g., see review Hayes et al., 2006).

The involvement of caregivers or family members in psychosocial interventions for people with MS has not been well investigated, although some of the above-mentioned interventions have included caregivers. The inclusion of family or caregivers is likely to be particularly important when the person with MS presents with interpersonal stressors, particularly given the evidence that suggests the coping strategies of both the person with MS and their caregiver influences dyadic adjustment (Pakenham, 1998).

Caregiver Interventions

Despite a great need for MS caregiver interventions, few have been published in the peer-reviewed literature. Finlayson, Garcia, and Preissner (2008) developed a group five-session program called Meeting the Challenges of MS, which focuses on building knowledge, skills, and self-efficacy in order to support caregivers in their caregiving role. The program is based on the self-management (Lorig & Holman, 2003) and person-environment-occupation (Law et al., 1996) frameworks. Single group pre- post-treatment pilot data showed that, after completing the program, participants reported being better prepared for their caregiving role and greater reliance on positive reframing and seeking practical assistance coping strategies (Finlayson, Preissner, & Garcia, 2009). Although CBT interventions have been found to be helpful to caregivers in other areas (e.g., caregivers of the frail elderly; Coon & Evans, 2009), published research on similar interventions with MS caregivers is absent. A range of practical services are designed to reduce caregiver burden by giving caregivers a break from their responsibilities, including respite care, day programs, and in-home health care aides. Several studies suggest that MS caregivers access these services at very low rates (e.g., Aronson et al., 1996). The extent to which utilization of these services reduces burden or enhances caregiver QOL has not been established.

In comparison to other disability groups, families with MS have been identified as having prominent psychosocial support needs (Olkin, Abrams, Preston, & Kirshbaum, 2006). Coles, Pakenham, and Leech (2007) conducted the only published evaluation of the efficacy of a psychosocial intervention for children of a parent with MS, in which both parents and children were included in the evaluation phases and received intervention resources. The 6-day camp intervention, called the Fun in the Sun Camp, involved both recreational activities and eight group sessions providing education about MS, opportunities to share experiences within a supportive environment, and training in various coping strategies and life skills. Single group pre- and post-treatment and 3-month follow-up pilot data showed that, after the intervention, children reported significant decreases in distress, stress appraisals, caregiving compulsion, and activity restrictions, and increases in social support and knowledge of MS (Coles et al., 2007). Parental data confirmed the significant increase in the children's knowledge of MS and, overall, the qualitative data supported the quantitative findings. Qualitative data showed that the intervention had indirect effects on some parents and families.

Conclusion

The complexity of MS is challenging for those who live with the illness, their caregivers and significant others, and health professionals involved in the care of these individuals. A wide range of symptoms are associated with MS, many of which are "invisible" to the observer. The course of MS is marked by unpredictability and fluctuations; MS has an onset typically in young adulthood, a developmental phase when a person is least prepared for physical limitation and disability. Disability can increase rapidly or gradually and can touch many, if not all, areas of a person's life and functioning. The extensive array of psychosocial issues associated with MS reflects the complexity of the illness. There is no cure for MS; hence, rehabilitation efforts are an important mainstay of treatment. Rehabilitation

interventions should reflect the multifaceted nature of the illness and its effects. Consequently, a range of health professionals need to collaborate in implementing well-coordinated rehabilitation interventions that target the many areas affected by MS. A potentially important member of this team is the caregiver, and, at times, the caregiver may in fact be the target of intervention. Psychologists are likely to play prominent roles in helping the person with MS and his or her caregiver manage cognitive impairment and mental health problems, and in promoting adaptive coping processes in dealing with the many and varied MS-related stressors. A flexible approach is required that may incorporate a range of intervention formats (e.g., individual, dyadic, family, and group), modalities (e.g., face-to-face, telephone, and self-help), and strategies (e.g., psychoeducation, coping skills training, psychotherapy, and marital therapy). Intervention starts with the individual human being; a person who is much more than his or her MS. Engagement and assessment are the early steps that inform intervention. The psychologist should have a workable framework for understanding how the person with MS adapts to his or her illness (like the one presented in this chapter), although not be blinkered by it. Such a framework should help the practitioner adopt a systematic and responsive approach to assessment and intervention.

This chapter has provided perspectives on MS from researchers, academics, and health professionals. Given that the person with MS has "expertise" and a perspective that differs from these individuals, it is important that the experience and views of people living with MS are also considered. To this purpose, the following is a brief self-narrated story of the experience of living with MS. It highlights many of the issues raised earlier in this chapter and infuses them with the lived experience of MS.

> I am a person living with MS, formally diagnosed in 1992.... For many years the impacts of symptoms of MS were minimal.... The past 5 years, however, have seen a more profound impact with the inability to work followed by a loss of function in my left hand and arm.
>
> I am now 46 years old and no longer work. I feel fatigued by the constant cycle of mourning and acceptance, never actually getting through the seven stages of grief before the next "loss" impacts. Over the last 3 years, I have been retrenched from my dream job, attempted to find work again with disastrous results and enormous impact on my

sense of self, which has always been linked with my profession as an architect. Then followed the drawn-out battle of making a claim on my salary continuation insurance, and then a "total and permanent disability" claim. This took over a year and had an enormous stress impact, contributing no doubt to worsening of symptoms. It was during this time that regular sessions with a psychologist with a particular interest in and understanding of life with MS was invaluable.

I have now lost function in my left hand and arm, cannot fulfil typical architectural drawing functions, type with one hand only. I've had to modify my bathroom, no longer drive a car. My world has continued to shrink to the range of my scooter. The other huge loss is that of not being able to visit my old friends. Most houses have steps at the entry. Usually, even if I can access the house, the toilet is inaccessible to me. I hardly ever see these people anymore; another source of grief and loss.

Now, with the physical symptoms so obvious, it is difficult to separate symptoms from the whole me. One is always aware of the impact of my mobility aid, a small scooter rather than a wheelchair, being the first thing people notice. Being waist high in a crowded function is difficult and no way to relate to people. It also sets up barriers to being taken seriously as a professional until I found my new niche of utilizing the synergy of my professional experience as an architect with my personal experience of a life with limited mobility. I have reinvented myself as an access consultant and now, all of a sudden, my "disability" has turned to something of an advantage. I feel buoyed and energized by the idea that I can contribute to change, however small, to the physical environment experienced by myself and others through the development of advocacy skills.

Future Directions

What follows is a summary of important future directions for psychological research and practice in MS that need to be addressed if we are to advance rehabilitation outcomes for people with MS. At a broad level, future research into the psychosocial aspects of MS should include subsamples representative of those people with extreme disabilities, which have been largely neglected in prior research. Future research into coping processes in MS should address the following methodological issues: use measures that are sensitive to the MS context, employ longitudinal designs, examine coping processes in relation to specific MS stressors, and consider a wider range of potential dispositional (e.g., hope and hardiness)

and external (e.g., financial and community assets) resources. Interdisciplinary research is required that continues to unravel the interplay between mental health problems (especially anxiety and depression) in MS and a wide range of factors, including biological and disease processes, biographical characteristics of the person with MS, and stress and coping processes.

With respect to intervention research, studies that investigate psychological treatment programs should assess their impact on objective measures of disease and illness, and examine the effects of stage of MS and other characteristics of the illness (e.g., cognitive impairment) to clarify how interventions need to be modified to match patient illness needs. The efficacy of the "third-wave" CBT interventions, such as ACT, also needs to be examined. Well-designed randomised controlled trials of stress management interventions that include objective measures of disease activity, illness symptoms and progression, and disability are required to further unravel the complex link between stress and relapse. Although multidisciplinary rehabilitations programs show promise in improving the QOL of people with MS, dismantling rehabilitation intervention research is required to clarify which components and structural aspects of these often complex programs best maximize outcomes. Future cognitive rehabilitation intervention research should clarify techniques that are most effective for specific cognitive impairment profiles. Further research is also needed to validate sensitive, cost-effective, and reliable cognitive screening instruments that can readily be used in clinical settings.

Regarding caregivers, given the dearth of MS caregiver intervention research, there is a pressing need for studies that examine the efficacy of caregiver-focused, patient- and caregiver-focused, and family-focused interventions and services. Studies are also needed that investigate and evaluate strategies used to engage caregivers in the rehabilitation process. Although MS often occurs during the child-rearing years, the children and partners of parents with MS have been neglected. Research is required that clarifies the needs and psychosocial issues of parents with MS and their children and partners.

Regarding future directions of the practice of psychology in MS, given the complexity of MS, practitioners should take a holistic approach to the care of persons with MS, one that takes into account the wide range of factors (summarized in Figure 12.1) that shape adaptation over the long haul of living with MS. Recent trends in psychology call for a widening of our approach to caring for people in the midst of hardship. For example, the positive psychology movement encourages us to go beyond pathology and harness human strengths and virtues even in the midst of adversity. The third-wave CBT therapies are more integrative of a wide range of therapy techniques and call for a more holistic treatment approach. Calls for a greater focus on existential issues in the management of people with chronic illness (e.g., Lee & McCormick, 2002) have long been ignored by practitioners involved in the care of people with MS. Only recently has there been a marked increase in research that addresses existential issues in MS. Given the prominence and the adverse prognostic implications of depression, anxiety, and cognitive impairment in MS, routine assessment of these should be incorporated into clinical protocols.

Illness is experienced and managed in an interpersonal context, hence, clinical management protocols need to clearly articulate the engagement and involvement of caregivers and the family. Supportive interventions to assist parents with MS, their partners, and children need to be developed and evaluated. The strategies, services, and interventions used to support people with MS need to reflect the complexity of the disease, the individual human being, and the social and cultural contexts.

References

Aikens, J. E., Fischer, J. S., Namey, M., & Rudick, R. A. (1997). A replicated prospective investigation of life stress, coping, and depressive symptoms in multiple sclerosis. *Journal of Behavioral Medicine, 20*(5), 433–445.

Amato, M. P., Goretti, B., Ghezzi, A., Lori, S., Zipoli, V., Portaccio, E., et al. (2008). Cognitive and psychosocial features of childhood and juvenile MS. *Neurology, 70*, 1891–1897.

Amato, M. P., Ponziani, G., Pracucci, G., Bracco, L., Siracusa, G., & Amaducci, L. (1995). Cognitive impairment in early-onset multiple sclerosis. Pattern, predictors, and impact on everyday life in a 4-year follow-up. *Archives of Neurology, 52*, 168–172.

Amato, M. P., Zipoli, V., & Portaccio, E. (2006a). Multiple sclerosis-related cognitive changes: A review of cross-sectional and longitudinal studies. *Journal of Neurological Sciences, 245*, 41–46.

Amato, M. P., Portaccio, E., & Zipoli, V. (2006b). Are there protective treatments for cognitive decline in MS? *Journal of Neurological Sciences, 245*, 183–186.

Amato, M. P., & Zipoli, V. (2003). Clinical management of cognitive impairment in multiple sclerosis: A review of current evidence. *International MS Journal, 10*(3), 72–83.

Amato, M.P., Ponziani, G., Siracusa, G., Sorbi, S. (2001). Cognitive dysfunction in early-onset multiple sclerosis: a reappraisal after 10 years, *Archives of Neurology, 58*, 1602–1606.

Arnaud, S. H. (1959). Some psychological characteristics of children of multiple sclerosis. *Psychosomatic Medicine, 21*, 8–22.

Aronson, K. J. (1997). Quality of life among persons with multiple sclerosis and their caregivers. *Neurology, 48*(1), 74–80.

Aronson, K. J., Cleghorn, G., & Goldenberg, E. (1996). Assistance arrangements and use of services among persons with multiple sclerosis and their caregivers. *Disability and Rehabilitation, 18*(7), 354–361.

Bagert, B., Camplair, P., & Bourdette, D. (2002). Cognitive dysfunction in multiple sclerosis: Natural history, pathophysiology and management. *CNS Drugs, 16*, 445–455.

Bandura, A. (1977). *Social learning theory*. Englewood Cliffs, NJ: Prentice Hall.

Banwell, B., Ghezzi, A., Bar-Or, A., Mikaeloff, Y., & Tardieu, M. (2007). Multiple sclerosis in children: Clinical diagnosis, therapeutic strategies, and future directions. *Lancet Neurology, 6*, 887–902.

Barlow, J., Edwards, R., & Turner, A. (2009). The experience of attending a lay-led, chronic disease self-management programme from the perspective of participants with multiple sclerosis. *Psychology and Health, 24*(10), 1167–1180.

Benedict, R. H. B. (2009). Standards for sample composition and impairment classification in neuropsychological studies of multiple sclerosis. *Multiple Sclerosis, 15*, 777–778.

Benedict, R. H. B., Shapiro, A., Priore, R., Miller, C., Munschauer, F., & Jacobs, L. (2000). Neuropsychological counseling improves social behavior in cognitively impaired multiple sclerosis patients. *Multiple Sclerosis, 6*, 391–396.

Bogosian, A., Moss-Morris, R., Yardley, L., & Dennison, L. (2009). Experiences of partners of people in the early stages of multiple sclerosis. *Multiple Sclerosis, 15*, 876–884.

Braham, S., Houser, H. B., Cline, A., & Posner, M. (1975). Evaluation of the social needs of non-hospitalized chronically ill persons: 1. Study of 47 patients with multiple sclerosis. *Journal of Chronic Diseases, 28*, 401–419.

Brown, R. F., Tennant, C. C., Dunn, S. M., & Pollard, J. D. (2005). A review of stress-relapse interactions in multiple sclerosis: Important features and stress-mediating and -moderating variables. *Multiple Sclerosis, 11*, 477–484.

Brown, R. F., Tennant, C. C., Sharrock, M., Hodgkinson, S., Dunn, S. M., & Pollard, J. D. (2006a). Relationship between stress and relapse in multiple sclerosis: Part I. Important features. *Multiple Sclerosis, 12*, 453–464.

Brown, R. F., Tennant, C. C., Sharrock, M., Hodgkinson, S., Dunn, S. M., & Pollard, J. D. (2006b). Relationship between stress and relapse in multiple sclerosis: Part II. Direct and indirect relationships. *Multiple Sclerosis, 12*, 465–475.

Carton, H., Loos, R., Pacolet, J., Versieck, K., & Vlietinck, R. (2000). A quantitative study of unpaid caregiving in multiple sclerosis. *Multiple Sclerosis, 6*, 274–279.

Chalfant, A. M., Bryant, R. A., & Fulcher, G. (2004). Posttraumatic stress disorder following diagnosis of multiple sclerosis. *Journal of Traumatic Stress, 17*(5), 423–428.

Charcot, J. M. (1877). *Lectures on diseases of the nervous system (G. Sigerson, Trans.)*. London: New Sydenham Society.

Chipchase, S. Y., & Lincoln, N. B. (2001). Factors associated with carer strain in carers of people with multiple sclerosis. *Disability and Rehabilitation, 23*, 768–776.

Chwastiak, L., Ehde, D. M., Gibbons, L. E., Sullivan, M., Bowen, J. D., & Kraft, G. H. (2002). Depressive symptoms and severity of illness in multiple sclerosis: Epidemiologic study of a large community sample. *American Journal of Psychiatry, 159*, 1862–1868.

Clutton, S., Pakenham, K. I., & Buckley, B. (1999). Predictors of emotional well-being following a 'false-positive' breast cancer screening result. *Psychology and Health, 14*(2), 263–275.

Coles, A. R., Pakenham, K. I., & Leech, C. (2007). Evaluation of an intensive psychosocial intervention for children of parents with multiple sclerosis. *Rehabilitation Psychology, 52*(2), 133–142.

Coon, D. W., & Evans, B. (2009). Empirically based treatments for family caregiver distress: What works and where do we go from here? *Geriatric Nursing, 30,* 426–436.

Corry, M., & While, A. (2009). The needs of carers of people with multiple sclerosis: A literature review. *Scandanavian Journal of Caring Sciences, 23*(3), 569–588.

D'hooghe, M. B., Nagels, G., Bissay, V., & De Keyser, J. (2010). Modifiable factors influencing relapses and disability in multiple sclerosis. *Multiple Sclerosis, 16,* 773–785.

Dahl, O., Stordal, E., Lydersen, S., & Midgard, R. (2009). Anxiety and depression in multiple sclerosis. A comparative population-based study in Nord-Trøndelag County, Norway. *Multiple Sclerosis, 15,* 1495–1501.

Dalton, E. J., & Heinrichs, R. W. (2005). Depression in multiple sclerosis: A quantitative review of the evidence. *Neuropsychology, 19,* 152–158.

De Judicibus, M. A., & McCabe, M. P. (2004). The impact of parental multiple sclerosis on the adjustment of children and adolescents. *Adolescence, 39*(155), 551–569.

Deatrick, J. A., Brennan, D., & Cameron, M. E. (1998). Mothers with multiple sclerosis and their children: Effects of fatigue and exacerbations on maternal support. *Nursing Research, 47*(4), 205–210.

Dennison, L., Moss-Morris, R., & Chalder, T. (2009). A review of psychological correlates of adjustment in patients with multiple sclerosis. *Clinical Psychology Review, 29,* 141–153.

Devins, G. M., Seland, T. P., Klein, G., Edworthy, S. M., et al. (1993). Stability and determinants of psychosocial well-being in multiple sclerosis. *Rehabilitation Psychology, 38*(1), 11–26.

Dewis, M. M. E., & Niskala, H. (1992). Nurturing a valuable resource: Family caregivers in multiple sclerosis. *Axon, 13,* 87–94.

Dunn, D. S., & Dougherty, S. B. (2005). Prospects for a positive psychology of rehabilitation. *Rehabilitation Psychology, 50*(3), 305–311.

Feinstein, A. (2002). An examination of suicidal intent in patients with multiple sclerosis. *Neurology, 59,* 674–678.

Feinstein, A. (2004). The neuropsychiatry of multiple sclerosis. *Canadian Journal of Psychiatry, 49,* 157–163.

Feinstein, A. (2007). Neuropsychiatric syndromes associated with multiple sclerosis. *Journal of Neurology, 25*(Suppl 2), 73–76.

Feinstein, A., & Feinstein, K. (2001). Depression associated with multiple sclerosis. Looking beyond diagnosis to symptom expression. *Journal of Affective Disorders, 66,* 193–198.

Feinstein, A., Feinstein, K., Gray, T., & O'Connor, P. (1977). Prevalence of neurobehavioral correlates of pathological laughing and crying in multiple sclerosis. *Archives of Neurology, 54,* 1116–1121.

Figved, N., Myhr, K. M., Larsen, J. P., & Aarsland, D. (2007). Caregiver burden in multiple sclerosis: The impact of neuropsychiatric symptoms. *Journal of Neurology, Neurosurgery, and Psychiatry, 78,* 1097–1102.

Finlayson, M., & Cho, C. (2008). A descriptive profile of caregivers of older adults with MS and the assistance they provide. *Disability and Rehabilitation, 30*(24), 1848–1857.

Finlayson, M., Garcia, J., & Preissner, K. (2008). Development of an education program for caregivers of people aging with multiple sclerosis. *Occupational Therapy International, 15*(1), 4–17.

Finlayson, M., Preissner, K., & Garcia, J. (2009). Pilot study of an educational programme for caregivers of people ageing with multiple sclerosis. *British Journal of Occupational Therapy, 72*(1), 11–19.

Fisk, J. D., Ritvo, P. G., Ross, L., Haase, D. A., Marrie, T. J., & Schlech, W. F. (1994). Measuring the functional impact of fatigue—initial validation of the Fatigue Impact Scale. *Clinical Infectious Diseases, 18,* S79–S83.

Flavia, M., Stampatori, C., Zanotti, D., Parrinello, G., & Capra, R. (2010). Efficacy and specificity of intensive cognitive rehabilitation of attention and executive functions in multiple sclerosis. *Journal of the Neurological Sciences, 288,* 101–105.

Foley, F. W., Bedell, J. R., LaRocca, N. G., Scheinberg, L. C., & Reznikoff, M. (1987). Efficacy of stress-inoculation training in coping with multiple sclerosis. *Journal of Consulting and Clinical Psychology, 55*(6), 919–922.

Freedman, M. S. (2006). Disease-modifying drugs for multiple sclerosis: Current and future aspects. *Expert Opinion on Pharmacotherapy, 7*(Suppl. 1), S1–S9.

Friedemann, M. L., & Tubergen, P. (1987). Multiple sclerosis and the family. *Archives of Psychiatric Nursing, 1*(1), 47–54.

Galeazzi, G. M., Ferrari, S., Giaroli, G., Mackinnon, A., Merelli, E., Motti, L., et al. (2005). Psychiatric disorders and depression in multiple sclerosis outpatients: Impact of disability and interferon beta therapy. *Neurological Sciences, 26,* 255–262.

Golan, D., Somer, E., Dishon, S., Cuzin-Disegni, L., & Miller, A. (2008). Impact of exposure to war stress on exacerbations of multiple sclerosis. *Annals of Neurology, 64,* 143–148.

Gold, S. M., Mohr, D. C., Huitinga, I., Flachenecker, P., Sternberg, E. M., & Heesen, C. (2005). The role of stress-response systems for the pathogenesis and progression of MS. *TRENDS in Immunology, 26,* 644–652.

Goldman Consensus Group. (2005). The Goldman Consensus statement on depression in multiple sclerosis. *Multiple Sclerosis, 11,* 328–337.

Gordon, P. A., Lam, C. S., & Winter, R. (1977). Interaction strain and persons with multiple sclerosis: Effectiveness of a social skills program. *Journal of Applied Rehabilitation Counselling, 28,* 5–11.

Grasso, M. G., Clemenzi, A., Tonini, A., Pace, L., Casillo, P., Cuccaro, A., et al. (2008). Pain in multiple sclerosis: A clinical and instrumental approach. *Multiple Sclerosis, 14,* 506–513.

Green, H. J., Pakenham, K. I., & Gardiner, R. A. (2005). Cognitive deficits associated with cancer: A model of subjective and objective outcomes. *Psychology, Health and Medicine, 10*(2), 145–160.

Griffiths, C., Foster, G., Ramsay, J., Eldridge, S., & Taylor, S. (2007). How effective are expert patient (lay-led) education programmes for disease? *BMJ, 334,* 1254–1256.

Grossman, P., Kappos, L., Gensicke, H., D'Souza, M., Mohr, D. C., Penner, I. K., & Steiner, C. (2010). MS quality of life, depression, and fatigue improve after mindfulness training. *Neurology, 75,* 1141–1149.

Haase, C. G., Tinnefeld, M., Lienemann, J., Ganz, R. E., & Faustmann, P. M. (2003). Depression and cognitive impairment in disability-free early multiple sclerosis. *Behavioural Neurology, 14,* 39–45.

Hadjimichael, O., Vollmer, T., & Oleen-Burkey, M. (2008). Fatigue characteristics in multiple sclerosis: The North American Research Committee on Multiple Sclerosis (NARCOMS) Survey. *Health and Quality of Life Outcomes, 6,* 100–111.

Hainsworth, M. A. (1996). Helping spouses with chronic sorrow related to multiple sclerosis. *Journal of Psychosocial Nursing, 34,* 36–40.

Hakim, E. A., Bakheit, A., Bryant, T., Roberts, M. W. H., McIntosh-Michaellis, S. A., Spackman, A. J., et al. (2000). The social impact of multiple sclerosis—a study of 305 patients and their relatives. *Disability and Rehabilitation, 22*(6), 288–293.

Harris, E. C., & Barraclough, B. (1997). Suicide as an outcome for mental disorders. A meta-analysis. *British Journal of Psychiatry, 170,* 205–228.

Hayes, S. C., Luoma, J. B., Bond, F. W., Masuda, A., & Lillis, J. (2006). Acceptance and commitment therapy: Model, processes and outcomes. *Behaviour Research and Therapy, 44,* 1–25.

Hayes, S. C., Strosahl, K., & Wilson, K. G. (1999). *Acceptance and commitment therapy: An experiential approach to behavior change.* New York: Guilford Press.

Heesen, C., Mohr, D. C., Huitinga, I., Then Bergh, F., Gaab, J., Otte, C., et al. (2007). Stress regulation in multiple sclerosis—current issues and concepts. *Multiple Sclerosis, 13,* 143–148.

Hildebrandt, H., Lanz, M., Hahn, H. K., Hoffmann, E., & Schwarze, B. (2007). Cognitive training in MS: Effects and relation to brain atrophy. *Restorative Neurology and Neuroscience, 25,* 33–43.

Hind, D., O'Cathain, A., Cooper, C. L., Parry, G. D., Isaac, C. L., Rose, A., et al. (2010). The acceptability of computerised cognitive behavioural therapy for the treatment of depression in people with chronic physical disease: A qualitative study of people with multiple sclerosis. *Psychology and Health, 25,* 699–712.

Honarmand, K., & Feinstein, A. (2009). Validation of the Hospital Anxiety and Depression Scale for use with multiple sclerosis patients. *Multiple Sclerosis, 15*(12), 1518–1524.

Janoff Bulman, R., & Yopyk, D. J. (2004). Random outcomes and valued commitments: Existential dilemmas and the paradox of meaning. In J. Greenberg, S. L. Koole & T. Pyszczynski (Eds.), *Handbook of experimental existential psychology* (pp. 122–138). New York: Guilford.

Janssens, A. C. J. W., Buljevac, D., Van Doorn, P. A., Van de Meche, F. G. A., Polman, C. H., Passchier, J., et al. (2006). Predictors of anxiety and distress following diagnosis of multiple sclerosis: A two year longitudinal study. *Multiple Sclerosis, 12,* 794–801.

Janssens, A. C. J. W., van Doorn, P. A., de Boer, J. B., van de Meche, F. G. A., Passchier, J., & Hintzen, R. Q. (2003). Impact of recently diagnosed multiple sclerosis on quality of life, anxiety, depression and distress of patients and partners. *Acta Neurologica Scandinavica, 108,* 389–395.

Julian, L., Merluzzi, N. M., & Mohr, D. C. (2007). The relationship among depression, subjective cognitive impairment, and neuropsychological performance in multiple sclerosis. *Multiple Sclerosis, 13,* 81–86.

Kern, S., Schrempf, W., Schneider, H., Schultheiß, T., Reichmann, H., & Ziemssen, T. (2009). Neurological disability, psychological distress, and health-related quality of life in MS patients within the first three years after diagnosis. *Multiple Sclerosis, 15,* 752–758.

Khan, F., McPhail, T., Brand, C., Turner-Stokes, L., & Kilpatrick, T. (2006). Multiple sclerosis: Disability profile and quality of life in Australian community report. *International Journal of Rehabilitation Research, 29,* 87–96.

Khan, F., Turner-Stokes, L., Ng, L., & Kilpatrick, T. (2008). Multidisciplinary rehabilitation for adults with multiple sclerosis. *Cochrane Database of Systematic Reviews 2007, 2,* CD006036.

Kikuchi, J. F. (1987). The reported quality of life of children and adolescents of parents with multiple sclerosis. *Recent Advances in Nursing, 16,* 163–191.

Knight, R. G., Devereux, R. C., & Godfrey, H. P. D. (1997). Psychosocial consequences of caring for a spouse with multiple sclerosis. *Journal of Clinical and Experimental Neuropsychology, 19*(1), 7–19.

Koch-Henriksen, N., & Sörensen, P. S. (2010). The changing demographic pattern of multiple sclerosis epidemiology. *Lancet Neurology, 9,* 520–532.

Köpke, S., Kasper, J., Mühlhauser, I., Nübling, M., & Heesen, C. (2009). Patient education program to enhance decision autonomy in multiple sclerosis relapse management: A randomised-controlled trial. *Multiple Sclerosis, 15,* 96–104.

Korostil, M., & Feinstein, A. (2007). Anxiety disorders and their clinical correlates in multiple sclerosis patients. *Multiple Sclerosis, 13,* 67–72.

Kurtzke, J. F. (1983). Rating neurological impairment in multiple sclerosis: An expanded disability status scale (EDSS). *Neurology, 33,* 1444–1452.

Larcombe, N. A., & Wilson, P. H. (1984). An evaluation of cognitive-behaviour therapy for depression in patients with multiple sclerosis. *British Journal of Psychiatry, 145,* 366–371.

Law, M., Cooper, B. A., Strong, S., Stewart, D., Rigby, P., & Letts, L. (1996). The Person-Environment-Occupational Model: A transactive approach to occupational performance. *Canadian Journal of Occupational Therapy, 63*(1), 9–23.

Lazarus, R. S., & Folkman, S. (1984). *Stress, appraisal, and coping.* NY: Springer.

Lee, Y., & McCormick, B. P. (2002). Sense making process in defining health for people with chronic illnesses and disabilities. *Therapeutic Recreation Journal, 36*(3), 235–246.

Lerdal, A., Celius, E. G., Krupp, L., & Dahl, A. A. (2007). A prospective study of patterns of fatigue in multiple sclerosis. *European Journal of Neurology, 14,* 1338–1343.

Lorig, K. R., & Holman, H. (2003). Self-management education: History, definition, outcomes, and mechanisms. *Annals of Behavioural Medicine, 26*(1), 1–7.

Lorig, K. R., Sobel, D. S., Stewart, A. L., Brown, B. W., Bandura, A., Ritter, P., et al. (1999). Evidence suggesting that a chronic disease self-management program can improve health status while reducing hospitalization: A randomized trial. *Medical Care, 37*(1), 5–14.

Lublin, F. D., & Reingold, S. C. (1996). Defining the clinical course of multiple sclerosis: Results of an international survey. *Neurology, 46,* 907–911.

Matthews, B., & Rice-Oxley, M. (2001). *Multiple sclerosis: The facts.* New York: Oxford University Press Inc.

McCabe, M. P. (2006). A longitudinal study of coping strategies and quality of life among people with multiple sclerosis. *Journal of Clinical Psychology in Medical Settings, 13,* 369–379.

McCabe, M. P., & McKern, S. (2002). Quality of life and multiple sclerosis: Comparison between people with multiple sclerosis and people from the general community. *Journal of Clinical Psychology in Medical Settings, 9*(4), 287–295.

McCabe, M. P., McKern, S., & McDonald, E. (2004). Coping and psychological adjustment among people with multiple sclerosis. *Journal of Psychosomatic Research, 56*, 355–361.

McCartney Chalk, H. (2007). Mind over matter: Cognitive-behavioral determinants of emotional distress in multiple sclerosis patients. *Psychology Health and Medicine, 12*(5), 556–566.

McKeown, L. P., Porter-Armstrong, A. P., & Baxter, G. D. (2003). The needs and experiences of caregivers of individuals with multiple sclerosis: A systematic review. *Clinical Rehabilitation, 17*, 234–248.

Mills, N., & Allen, J. (2000). Mindfulness of movement as a coping strategy in multiple sclerosis: A pilot study. *General Hospital Psychiatry, 22*, 425–431.

Mishel, M. H. (1981). The measurement of uncertainty of illness. *Nursing Research, 30*, 258–263.

Mohr, D. C., Boudewyn, A. C., Likosky, W., Levine, E., & Goodkin, D. E. (2001). Injectable medication for the treatment of multiple sclerosis: The influence of expectations and injection anxiety on adherence and ability to self-inject. *Annals of Behavioral Medicine, 23*, 125–132.

Mohr, D. C., & Cox, D. (2001). Multiple sclerosis: Empirical literature for the clinical health psychologist. *Journal of Clinical Psychology, 57*, 479–499.

Mohr, D. C., Dick, L. P., Russo, D., Pinn, J., Boudewyn, A. C., Likosky, W., et al. (1999). The psychosocial impact of multiple sclerosis: Exploring the patient's perspective. *Health Psychology, 18*(4), 376–382.

Mohr, D. C., Goodkin, D. E., Bacchetti, B., Boudewyn, A. C., Huang, L., Marietta, P., Cheuk, W., & Dee, B. (2000). Psychological stress and the subsequent appearance of new brain MRI lesion in MS. *Neurology, 55*, 55–61.

Mohr, D. C., Goodkin, D. E., Gatto, N., & Van der Wende, J. (1997). Depression, coping and level of neurological impairment in multiple sclerosis. *Multiple Sclerosis, 3*, 254–258.

Mohr, D. C., Goodkin, D. E., Nelson, S., Cox, D., & Weiner, M. (2002). Moderating effects of coping on the relationship between stress and the development of new brain lesions in multiple sclerosis. *Psychosomatic Medicine, 64*, 803–809.

Mohr, D. C., Hart, S. L., Fionareva, I., & Tasch, E. S. (2006). Treatment of depression for patients with multiple sclerosis in neurology clinics. *Multiple Sclerosis, 12*, 204–208.

Mohr, D. C., Hart, S. L., Julian, L., Catledge, C., Honos-Webb, L., Vella, L., et al. (2005). Telephone-administered psychotherapy for depression. *Archives of General Psychiatry, 62*, 1007–1014.

Mohr, D. C., Hart, S. L., Julian, L., Cox, D., & Pelletier, D. (2004). Association between stressful life events and exacerbation in multiple sclerosis: A meta-analysis. *BMJ, 328*, 731–735.

Moos, R. H., & Billings, A. G. (1982). Conceptualising and measuring coping resources and processes. In L. Goldberger & S. Breznitz (Eds.), *Handbook of stress: Theoretical and clinical aspects* (pp. 212–230). New York: Free Press.

Motl, R. W., & Gosney, J. L. (2008). Effect of exercise training on quality of life in multiple sclerosis: A meta-analysis. *Multiple Sclerosis, 14*, 129–135.

O'Brien, M. T. (1993). Multiple Sclerosis: The relationship among self-esteem, social support, and coping behaviour. *Applied Nursing Research, 6*, 54–63.

O'Brien, M. T., Wineman, N. M., & Nealon, N. R. (1995). Correlates of the caregiving process in multiple sclerosis.

Scholarly Inquiry for the Nursing Practice: An International Journal, 9, 323–338.

Olkin, R., Abrams, K., Preston, P., & Kirshbaum, M. (2006). Comparison of parents with and without disabilities raising teens: Information from the NHIS and two national surveys. *Rehabilitation Psychology, 51*(1), 43–49.

Pakenham, K. I. (1998). Couple coping and adjustment to multiple sclerosis in care receiver-carer dyads. *Family Relations: Interdisciplinary Journal of Applied Family Studies, 47*(3), 269–277.

Pakenham, K. I. (1999). Adjustment to multiple sclerosis: Application of a stress and coping model. *Health Psychology, 18*(4), 383–392.

Pakenham, K. I. (2001a). Coping with multiple sclerosis: Development of a measure. *Psychology, Health and Medicine, 6*(4), 411–428.

Pakenham, K. I. (2001b). Application of a stress and coping model to caregiving in multiple sclerosis. *Psychology, Health and Medicine, 6*(1), 13–27.

Pakenham, K. I. (2002). Development of a measure of coping with multiple sclerosis caregiving. *Psychology and Health, 17*(1), 97–118.

Pakenham, K. I. (2005a). Benefit finding in multiple sclerosis and associations with positive and negative outcomes. *Health Psychology, 24*(2), 123–132.

Pakenham, K. I. (2005b). Relations between coping and positive and negative outcomes in carers of persons with Multiple Sclerosis. *Journal of Clinical Psychology in Medical Settings, 12*(1), 25–38.

Pakenham, K. I. (2005c). The positive impact of multiple sclerosis on carers: Associations between carer benefit finding and positive and negative adjustment domains. *Disability and Rehabilitation, 27*(17), 985–997.

Pakenham, K. I. (2006). Investigation of the coping antecedents to positive outcomes and distress in Multiple Sclerosis (MS). *Psychology and Health, 21*(3), 633–649.

Pakenham, K. I. (2007a). Making sense of multiple sclerosis. *Rehabilitation Psychology, 52*, 380–389.

Pakenham, K. I. (2007b). The nature of benefit finding in multiple sclerosis. *Psychology, Health and Medicine, 12*(2), 190–196.

Pakenham, K. I. (2007c). The nature of caregiving in multiple sclerosis: Development of the Caregiving Tasks in Multiple Sclerosis Scale. *Multiple Sclerosis, 13*, 929–938.

Pakenham, K. I. (2008a). Making sense of illness or disability: The nature of sense making in multiple sclerosis (MS). *Journal of Health Psychology, 13*(1), 93–105.

Pakenham, K. I. (2008b). The nature of sense making in caregiving for persons with multiple sclerosis (MS). *Disability and Rehabilitation, 30*(17), 1263–1273.

Pakenham, K. I. (2008c). Making sense of caregiving for persons with multiple sclerosis (MS): The dimensional structure of sense making and relations with positive and negative adjustment. *International Journal of Behavioral Medicine, 15*, 241–252.

Pakenham, K. I. (2009). Children who care for their parents: The impact of disability on young lives. In Marshall, C. A., Kendall, E., Banks, M., & Gover, R.M.S. (Eds.), *Disability: Insights from across fields and around the world* (Vol. II, pp. 39–60). Westport, CT: Praeger Press.

Pakenham, K. I. (In press). Coping with MS. In Finlayson, M. (Ed.), *Multiple sclerosis rehabilitation: From impairment to participation*. New York: Taylor & Francis.

Pakenham, K. I., & Bursnall, S. (2006). Relations between social support, appraisal and coping and both positive and negative outcomes for children of a parent with MS and comparisons with children of healthy parents. *Clinical Rehabilitation, 20*, 709–723.

Pakenham, K. I., & Cox, S. (2008). Development of the Benefit Finding in Multiple Sclerosis (MS) Caregiving Scale: A longitudinal study of relations between benefit finding and adjustment. *British Journal of Health Psychology, 13*, 583–602.

Pakenham, K. I., & Cox, S. (2009). The dimensional structure of benefit finding in multiple sclerosis and relations with positive and negative adjustment: A longitudinal study. *Psychology and Health, 24*(4), 373–393.

Pakenham, K. I., & Fleming, M. (2011). Relations between acceptance of multiple sclerosis and positive and negative adjustment. *Psychology and Health, 26*, 1292–1309.

Pakenham, K. I., Stewart, C. A., & Rogers, A. (1997). The role of coping in adjustment to multiple sclerosis-related adaptive demands. *Psychology, Health and Medicine, 2*(3), 197–211.

Park, C. L., & Folkman, S. (1997). Meaning in the context of stress and coping. *Review of General Psychology, 1*(2), 115–144.

Patti, F. (2009). Cognitive impairment in multiple sclerosis. *Multiple Sclerosis, 15*, 2–8.

Patti, F., Amato, M. P., Trojano, M., Bastianello, S., Tola, M. R., Goretti, B., et al. (2009). Cognitive impairment and its relation with disease measures in mildly disabled patients with relapsing-remitting multiple sclerosis: Baseline results from the Cognitive Impairment in Multiple Sclerosis (COGIMUS) Study. *Multiple Sclerosis, 15*, 779–788.

Pearlin, L. I., Mullan, J. T., Semple, S. J., & Skaff, M. M. (1990). Caregiving and the stress process: An overview of concepts and their measures. *The Gerontologist, 30*, 583–594.

Perrone, K. M., Gordon, P. A., & Tschopp, M. K. (2006). Caregiver marital satisfaction when a spouse has multiple sclerosis. *Journal of Applied Rehabilitation Counselling, 37*, 26–32.

Peters, L. C., & Esses, L. M. (1985). Family environment as perceived by children with a chronically ill parent. *Journal of Chronic Diseases, 38*(4), 301–308.

Poder, K., Ghatavi, K., Fisk, J. D., Campbell, T. L., Kisely, S., Sarty, I., et al. (2009). Social anxiety in a multiple sclerosis clinic population. *Multiple Sclerosis, 15*, 393–398.

Poeck, K. (1969). Pathophysiology of emotional disorders associated with brain damage. In P. J. Vinken & G. W. Bruyn (Eds.), *Handbook of clinical neurology* (pp. 343–367). Amsterdam: North Holland Publishing.

Portaccio, E., Goretti, B., Lori, S., Zipoli, V., Centorrino, S., Ghezzi, A., et al. (2009). The brief neuropsychological battery for children: A screening tool for cognitive impairment in childhood and juvenile multiple sclerosis. *Multiple Sclerosis, 15*, 620–626.

Putzki, N., Katsarava, Z., Vago, S., Diener, H. C., & Limmroth, V. (2008). Prevalence and severity of multiple sclerosis-associated fatigue in treated and untreated patients. *European Neurology, 59*, 136–142.

Quesnel, S., & Feinstein, A. (2004). Multiple sclerosis and alcohol: A study of problem drinking. *Multiple Sclerosis, 10*, 197–201.

Randolph, J. J., Arnett, P. A., & Higginson, C. I. (2001). Metamemory and tested cognitive functioning in multiple sclerosis. *Clinical Neuropsychologist, 15*, 357–368.

Rao, S. M., Huber, S. J., & Bornstein, R. A. (1992). Emotional changes with multiple sclerosis and Parkinson's disease. *Journal of Consulting and Clinical Psychology, 60*(3), 369–378.

Rogers, J. M., & Panegyres, P. K. (2007). Cognitive impairment in multiple sclerosis: Evidence-based analysis and recommendations. *Journal of Clinical Neuroscience, 14*, 919–927.

Sartori, E., Belliard, S., Chevrier, C. P., Chaperon, J., & Edan, G. (2006). From psychometry to neuropsychological disability in multiple sclerosis: A new brief French cognitive screening battery and cognitive risk factors. *Review Neurology, 162*(5), 603–615.

Sartori, E., & Edan, G. (2006). Assessment of cognitive dysfunction in multiple sclerosis. *Journal of Neurological Sciences, 245*, 169–175.

Scheier, M. F., & Carver, C. S. (1985). Optimism, coping, and health: Assessment and implications of generalized outcome expectancies. *Health Psychology, 4*, 219–247.

Schwartz, C., & Frohner, R. (2005). Contribution of demographic, medical and social support variables in predicting the mental health dimension of quality of life among people with multiple sclerosis. *Health and Social Work, 30*, 203–212.

Schwartz, C. E. (1999). Teaching coping skills enhances quality of life more than peer support: Results of a randomized trial with multiple sclerosis patients. *Health Psychology, 18*(3), 211–220.

Schwartz, C. E., & Rogers, M. (1994). Designing a psychosocial intervention to teach coping flexibility. *Rehabilitation Psychology, 39*(1), 57–72.

Seligman, M. E. P., & Csikszentmihalyi, M. (2000). Positive psychology. *American Psychologist, 55*(1), 5–14.

Sherman, T. E., Rapport, L. J., Hanks, R. A., Ryan, K. A., Keenan, P. A., Khan, O., et al. (2007). Predictors of well-being among significant others of persons with multiple sclerosis. *Multiple Sclerosis, 13*, 238–249.

Siegert, R. J., & Abernethy, D. A. (2005). Depression in multiple sclerosis: A review *Journal of Neurology, Neurosurgery and Psychiatry, 76*, 469–475.

Simmons, R. D. (2010). Life issues in multiple sclerosis. *Nature Reviews Neurology, 6*, 603–610.

Sloka, J. S., Pryse-Phillips, W. E., & Stefanelli, M. (2008). The relation of ultraviolet radiation and multiple sclerosis in Newfoundland. *Canadian Journal of Neurological Science, 35*, 69–74.

Smolders, J., Damoiseaux, J., Menheere, P., & Hupperts, R. (2008). Vitamin D as an immune modulator in multiple sclerosis, a review. *Journal of Neuroimmunology, 194*, 7–17.

Solari, A., Ferrari, G., & Radice, D. (2006). A longitudinal survey of self-assessed health trends in a community cohort of people with multiple sclerosis and their significant others. *Journal of Neurological Sciences, 243*, 13–20.

Stuifbergen, A. (1995). Health-promoting behaviors and quality of life among individuals with multiple sclerosis. *Scholarly Inquiry for the Nursing Practice: An International Journal, 9*, 31–55.

Surridge, D. (1969). An investigation into some psychiatric aspects of multiple sclerosis. *British Journal of Psychiatry, 115*, 749–764.

Thomas, P. W., Thomas, S., Hillier, C., Galvin, K., & Baker, R. (2006). Psychological interventions for multiple sclerosis (Review). *Cochrane Database of Systematic Reviews, 1*, CD004431 van der Mei, I., Ponsonby, A. L., Blizzard, L., & Dwyer, T. (2001). Regional variation in multiple sclerosis prevalence in Australia and its association with ambient ultraviolet radiation. *Neuroepidemiology, 20*, 168–174.

van Kessel, K., Moss-Morris, R., Willoughby, E., Chalder, T., Johnson, M., & Robinson, E. (2008). A randomized controlled trial of cognitive behavior therapy for multiple sclerosis fatigue. *Psychosomatic Medicine, 70*, 205–213.

Warren, S., Warren, K. G., & Cockerill, R. (1991). Emotional stress and coping in multiple sclerosis (MS) exacerbations. *Journal of Psychosomatic Research, 35*(1), 37–47.

Wineman, N. M. (1990). Adaptation to multiple sclerosis: The role of social support, functional disability, and perceived uncertainty. *Nursing Research, 39*(5), 294–299.

World Health Organization. (2004). *Atlas: Country Resources for Neurological Disorders. Results of a collaborative study of World Health Organization and World Federation of Neurology. Programme for Neurological Diseases and Neurosciences Department of Mental Health and Substance Abuse.* Geneva: World Health Organization.

Wynia, K., Middel, B., van Dijk, J. P., De Keyser, J. H. A., & Reijneveld, S. A. (2008). The impact of disabilities on quality of life in people with multiple sclerosis. *Multiple Sclerosis, 14*, 972–980.

Yahav, R., Vosburgh, J., & Miller, A. (2005). Emotional responses of children and adolescents to parents with multiple sclerosis. *Multiple Sclerosis, 11*, 464–468.

Yamout, B., Itani, S., Hourany, R., Sibaii, A. M., & Yaghi, S. (2010). The effect of war stress on multiple sclerosis exacerbations and radiological disease activity. *Journal of the Neurological Sciences, 288*, 42–44.

Zipoli, V., Benedetta, G., Hakiki, B., Siracusa, G., Sorbi, S., Portaccio, E., et al. (2010). Cognitive impairment predicts conversion to multiple sclerosis in clinically isolated syndromes. *Multiple Sclerosis, 16*, 62–67.

Zorzon, M., de Masi, R., Nasuelli, D., Ukmar, M., Mucelli, R. P., Cazzato, G., et al. (2001). Depression and anxiety in multiple sclerosis. A clinical and MRI study in 95 subjects. *Journal of Neurology, 248*, 416–421.

Stroke and Rehabilitation: Psychological Perspectives

Jane Barton

Abstract

It is important to recognize the traumatic experience of stroke and the psychological factors that are important in rehabilitation and recovery. A range of psychological experiences often occur following stroke, including grief and bereavement reactions, depression, and anxiety, as well as more problematic symptoms of post-traumatic stress. How people deal with and respond to these experiences will differ, and these responses, to some extent, will be influenced by other psychological factors, including patient beliefs and attitudes. Treatment programs should take account of psychological factors in recovery, with interventions being targeted at the level of the organization and health care system, as well as at the level of the individual.

Key Words: Psychological adjustment, trauma, disability, depression, cognitive impairment, emotional adjustment, care environments, psychological therapy.

Perhaps the starting point for this chapter is to acknowledge the complex relationship that exists between physical, emotional, and mental health (Prince et al., 2007). Taking the World Health Organization (WHO) definition of health as, "a state of complete physical, mental and social well-being, and not merely the absence of disease or infirmity," it is fundamentally important to see why, when we are talking about the experience, recovery, and rehabilitation of people with medical conditions such as stroke, it is essential that we do not overlook the importance of psychological factors in this relationship. The experience of stroke and the variations that exist in terms of how people respond to and recover from stroke, fits very well within the biopsychosocial model of illness proposed by Engel in 1977. In this view, he proposed that any model of illness should take into account the complex inter-actions among biological, psychological, and social factors in patient illness experience; that is, the person him- or herself, the social context in which he

or she lives, and the role of health care workers and systems. This model of thinking is in direct contrast to the more established biomedical model of illness, in which there is believed to be a direct relationship between the degree and severity of physical illness and the degree and extent of the recovery made.

Before exploring in detail the psychological aspects of stroke experience and recovery, it is help-ful to have some understanding of the nature, prev-alence, and physical implications of stroke. A stroke is caused when there is a disruption of blood flow to the brain, which results in the brain being deprived of oxygen. There are two ways in which this can occur, either through a blockage in an artery that feeds blood to the brain (an *ischemic stroke*), or through a burst blood vessel that results in bleeding in and around the brain (a *haemorrhagica stroke*). The incidence of stroke is high, with approximately 800,000 people in the United States (American Heart Association, 2009) and 130,000 people in England and Wales (Stroke Association, 2009) suffering a stroke each year. Stroke does not only affect older people. Approximately 10% of people affected will be under the age of 55, with approximately 1,000 people under the age of 20.

Although many stroke patients make a good physical recovery, a significant proportion are left with some permanent disability, and one-third of all stroke patients will die within the first 3 months of having had the stroke. Stroke is estimated to be the single largest cause of disability in the United Kingdom. No two strokes are the same, and the severity of the stroke, as well as the location of the stroke in the brain, will determine what physical effects occur. Some of the more common physical effects include weakness or paralysis on one side of the body (hemiparesis); communication difficulties, which might include difficulties with word fining, reading, writing, and understanding what is said (aphasia), slurring of speech (dysarthria), and difficulties with swallowing (dysphagia); disturbed vision; urinary and incontinence problems; and an overwhelming fatigue (Stroke Association, 2009). It is estimated that approximately one-third of stroke patients will end up with a permanent disability, and that a significant proportion will end up moving into long-term nursing or residential care. In view of these devastating and long-lasting physical effects of stroke, it is hardly surprising that there is also likely to be a huge emotional response to the event.

The Traumatic Impact of Stroke

Having a stroke is often seen as a traumatic and devastating experience for stroke patients and their families (Field, Norman, & Barton, 2008; Merriman, Norman, & Barton, 2007). In many cases, the stroke will come completely "out of the blue," and, as such, will totally disrupt the person's life in mid flow. Patients frequently report that it feels as if their lives have been completely turned upside down (Lanza, 2006), and this is also very often the experience of families and partners as well (Carek, Norman, & Barton 2010). In view of this, it can be helpful to think about the experience of stroke within the context of psychological trauma. In recent years, the Department of Health has reclassified stroke as a medical emergency, and this inevitably highlights the traumatic nature of stroke, rather than stroke being seen as a health condition specific to older age. Understanding stroke within this context of trauma is important in helping to understand what the emotional experience of patients might be, and what we as professionals might be able to do to

help. It is important to recognize that the degree of emotional distress that can occur following a stroke can be huge, in some cases being associated with the more common symptoms of post-traumatic stress, such as intrusion and avoidance (Eccles, House, & Knapp, 1999), although this does not always manifest as an actual clinical disorder. It is nonetheless crucial that this emotional distress is acknowledged and dealt with effectively, by the whole of the multidisciplinary team, as failing to do so will inevitably lead to greater psychological distress in patients. This will, in turn, have a detrimental effect on the process of rehabilitation and recovery (Remer-Osborn, 1998) and, in some cases, may even increase the risk of a further stroke (Surtees et al., 2008).

Psychological Consequences of Stroke

There is no uniform way in which people react to events, and this is certainly the case with stroke. The ways in which people experience illness in general, and stroke specifically, will vary enormously. Despite this, a number of common themes emerge when we look at how a stroke is experienced emotionally, and great commonality also exists in the psychological consequences that often occur (Clark & Smith, 1999). This can be seen on a number of levels, from the fact that the process of being ill and hospitalized can often be a huge emotional burden for patients, to the more specific clinical emotional disorders that some patients develop following the stroke.

The Hospital Experience

Being unwell and hospitalized, irrespective of whether this is due to having had a stroke or some other medical condition, can be extremely stressful; as such, it can often result in impoverished psychological well-being (Bowman, 2001). Many accounts in the literature highlight the psychological experiences of hospitalized patients. A number of common themes tend to emerge from these patients, specifically stroke patients (e.g. Lanza, 2006). First, the trauma of being hospitalized. Regaining consciousness in hospital can be a terrifying experience as the person realizes that he or she may be unable to either speak, move, or both, and may have no understanding of why this might be so. Patients often have no understanding of what stage of recovery they are at, or indeed how long the recovery process is likely to take. Even the process of transferring patients to an alternative ward can be terrifying, particularly as patients often expect the worst, and often fear that this move may mean that they are going to die. Second, patients often experience a range of emotions while hospitalized, and these tend to fluctuate over time. Some may feel quite depressed, and others may feel quite anxious. Most are often fearful about the future, wondering what effect their stroke will have on their lives and the lives of their families and loved ones. Perhaps one of the most difficult feelings to cope with at this stage is the feeling of no longer being in control and in losing independence. Third, although most patients are very keen to leave a hospital and return home, they are nonetheless often faced with mixed feelings. In particular, patients often fear missing the safety of the hospital, where they have nurses on hand 24 hours a day to respond to their needs and concerns. This perceived safety net will not be present when they return home. In addition, hospitalized patients often do not realize the full implications of their disability and presume that, when they return to their own home environment, they will automatically be able to function as well, or nearly as well, as they did prior to the stroke. Returning home can therefore be the point of realization for patients regarding the extent of their disability, and it is at this point that mood can often take a significant dip.

Emotional Distress and Adjustment

Although many stroke patients will not develop specific emotional disorders in the aftermath of their stroke, the majority will show signs of emotional distress, and a significant proportion may report negative cognitions about how they see themselves and how they now view the world (Field et al., 2008; Hackett, Yang, Anderson, Horrocks, & House, 2010; Thomas & Lincoln, 2008). Ellis-Hill and Horn (2000) showed that some stroke patients may report a negative change in their perceived self-identity, seeing themselves as being less interested, less independent, and less capable than they were prior to the stroke. Although there is debate in the literature, many stroke patients and their families will experience a range of emotions following the stroke, and this has been likened by some to the process of grieving following a bereavement (Carek et al., 2010). However, there remains dispute as to whether the pattern and course of emotional reactions following a bereavement actually follow a stage theory of grieving (e.g., Maciejewski, Zhang, Block, & Prigerson, 2007; Silver & Wortman, 2007), and as such, it is not expected that stroke patients will necessarily progress through an orderly sequence of grief stages. Some authors highlight the interaction between appraisal of the stroke event

and the coping behavior of the stroke patient and stress the importance of education and support in helping the patient adapt to the aftermath of stroke (Rochette, Bravo, Desrosiers, St-Cyr/Tribble, & Bourget, 2007).

Nonetheless, a significant proportion of stroke patients and their families will experience a range of quite intense emotional reactions following the stroke, many which are considered to be entirely normal, and these should not necessarily be seen as being of clinical significance. In fact, it is often believed that for a patient not to experience such intense negative feelings after a stroke this might be problematic in itself, particularly when one reflects upon the extent to which the person's life has been disrupted. For some, however, this "normal" emotional experience can become problematic, and patients may find themselves stuck in cycles of despair or hopelessness. In such cases, distinct clinical disorders can emerge.

Clinical Conditions

Depression is perhaps the most common emotional clinical problem that occurs following a stroke. Estimates vary, but probably between 30% and 50% of stroke patients will suffer depression at some point following their stroke (De Wit et al., 2008; Gordon & Hibbard, 1997). The course of depression is not uniform, with some people developing depression in the early stages following their stroke and others developing depression much later (De Wit et al., 2008). Depression is often associated with the experience of loss, and for many stroke patients, there will be great feelings of loss in relation to many aspects of their former life and health. The presence of mood disorders can have far-reaching effects on patient recovery and rehabilitation (Goodwin, Devanand & Devangere, 2008). In cases in which mood disorders persist, patients have been shown to make fewer gains in recovery and, in extreme cases, this may be associated with increased risk of mortality (Ellis, Zhao, & Egede, 2010; House, Knapp, Bamford, & Vail, 2001; Naess, Lunde, Brogger, & Waje-Andreassen, 2010; Pohjasvaara, Vataja, Leppavuori, Kaste, & Erkihjuntti, 2001). The exact mechanism at work here is unknown; however, given what we know about the effects of depression on ways of thinking and behavior, it is reasonable to assume that stroke patients who are suffering from depression will be less likely to take a proactive role in their rehabilitation and recovery, will be less likely to engage with their physiotherapy and speech therapy sessions, will be less likely to eat and sleep properly, and will be less likely to take their medication regularly. All these effects will have a cumulative negative impact on overall recovery.

Although it is understood that an organic basis exists for some depression after stroke, it is generally believed that a number of psychological and psychosocial variables are relevant, such as perceptions of social support, being younger, experiencing problems with activities of daily living (Gainotti, 2000; Kneebone & Dunmore, 2000; van de Port, Kwakkel, Bruin, & Lindeman, 2007), having an external locus of control (Thomas & Lincoln, 2006), and having a past history of mental health problems (Storor and Byrne, 2006). Within this context, depression appears to be related to the losses that people perceive to result from the stroke, and a discrepancy between the real self and the ideal self. In some more extreme cases, patients may develop a pervading sense of hopelessness regarding the future, and feelings of depression can become so severe that they no longer want to continue living. It is estimated that stroke patients are at twice the risk of the general population for committing suicide, and that this risk is greater in younger people if they have already had a previous stroke, and related to length of stay in a hospital (Stenager, Madsen, Stenager, & Boldsen, 1998). In the majority of cases, suicidal ideation is strongly associated with having a diagnosis of severe depression.

Anxiety following a stroke is also common, with approximately 20–40% of people being affected at any one time (Burvill et al., 1995; De Wit et al., 2008). In some cases, these levels remaining high at 3 years post stroke (Morrison, Pollard, Johnston, & MacWalter, 2005). The experience of anxiety is often associated with feelings of threat. Given the enormous threat that a stroke presents to a person's life, it is perhaps not surprising then that many stroke patients suffer anxiety. Anxiety tends to be characterized in terms of its physical experience (bodily sensations), how patients think about their situation (cognitive), and what they actually do to cope with their worries and concerns (behavior). Generalized feelings of anxiety are the most common. Patients and their families often express concerns about how they are going to cope in the future; how the stroke will change their lives; the impact of their stroke on their relationships, families, and friends; and whether they are likely to have another, potentially life-threatening stroke in the future. A certain degree of anxiety is expected, and be considered normal under the circumstances

(as discussed earlier) as patients and families face the challenge of coping with the crisis of the stroke. In some cases, though, these feelings of anxiety can become so intense that they impact negatively on the rehabilitation process and prevent patients from engaging fully with their therapy, thus reducing the degree of functional improvement made (Schultz, Castillo, Kosier, & Robinson, 1997; Shimoda & Robinson, 1998).

Panic is a specific type of anxiety sometimes experienced by stroke patients. It tends to be characterized by very rapid or deep breathing. The effect is that the amount of oxygen in the bloodstream will be reduced, and this can in turn lead to a range of unpleasant body sensations, such as faintness, dizziness, tingling, headaches, racing heart, flushes, nausea, chest pain, and shakiness. These sensations can be extremely worrying for the patient and are often misinterpreted as something medically wrong, such as having another stroke. Fears and concerns then intensify, which results in further overbreathing, and hence a vicious circle of panic can develop. Vignette 1 describes the case of a man with problematic levels of anxiety.

Vignette 1

Bob was a 62-year-old man who had made a fairly good physical recovery following his stroke. However, Bob had a family history of stroke, with his father dying at age 66 after a series of severe strokes, and as such believed that he, too, would follow the same course that his father had done. Bob started to become aware of different body sensations, for example, a slight twinge in his leg, a small sensation of breathlessness, a pain down the side of his body, becoming fixated to the point where he believed that these were signs that he was about to have another stroke. This misperception and misattribution of the cause of these sensations led Bob to worry to the extent that his breathing was affected, and he would start to hyperventilate. Thus, a vicious circle developed whereby the initial misattribution of bodily sensations led to panic symptoms that affected his breathing, which in turn reinforced Bob's view that he was about to have another stroke. His strong belief that these were signs that he was about to have another stroke led to extreme actions, with Bob telephoning the emergency ambulance on a number of occasions.

Phobias are another form of anxiety that can develop after a stroke; they are characterized by a sometimes unrealistic fear of a particular object, person, or situation, which results in avoidant behavior. Specific phobias that sometimes develop during rehabilitation include fear of transferring, sometimes from the bed to a chair, or from the chair to the toilet; fear of tackling the stairs; and fear of mixing with people and of being in social situations. This latter fear, often known as *social phobia*, is very common after a stroke. Many patients experience intensely negative feelings about reintegrating into their previous social networks. Patients often report that they feel very different, believe that they look very different (even if they do not), and worry about their ability to communicate with people. Patients often report experiencing feelings of shame, and the last thing they want is for people to feel sorry for them. Hence, they tend to avoid situations that will bring them into contact with acquaintances.

An emerging body of literature highlights the traumatic nature of physical illness and the role that this can have in the development of post-traumatic stress disorder (PTSD). For example, PTSD symptoms have been shown to exist following myocardial infarction (Kutz, Shabtai, Solomon, Neumann, & David, 1994) and following subarachnoid haemorrhage (Berry, 1998). Stroke is one of these conditions, with estimates of the number of people suffering from post-traumatic stress symptoms following a stroke ranging from 9% to 25% (Bruggimann et al., 2006; Merriman et al., 2007; Sembi, Tarrier, O'Neill, Burns, & Farragher, 1998). It is not uncommon to observe signs of psychological trauma in people who have experienced a stroke, either in relation to psychologically re-experiencing the events of the stroke and possibly having flashbacks, or alternatively, developing avoidant behavior regarding anything to do with the stroke or that reminds them of having the stroke. The following vignette describes a woman who developed post-traumatic stress symptoms following her stroke.

Vignette 2
Alice was a 69-year-old woman who had experienced her stroke while gardening at home. Alice did not lose consciousness during her stroke, so had a very clear memory of the stroke happening and of her being carried away in an ambulance to the hospital. For many months following her stroke, Alice had flashbacks of what had happened when she had the stroke. She remembered being in the garden and suddenly starting to feel paralysed down one side of her body. She also remembered trying to call out for her husband, but that no words actually came out of her mouth. This was a terrifying experience for Alice. Although Alice did not actually want to remember the events of her stroke, she found that images and memories of the event kept flashing into her mind and that she felt helpless to

prevent these. This was very distressing. Alice also found that she could not face returning to the spot where she had had her stroke because of the distressing memories associated with it. This meant that Alice avoided going out into the garden. It is likely that Alice was suffering from PTSD.

Cognitive Problems

In the early days following a stroke, the majority of patients will experience some cognitive problems. These typically include:

- *Confusion and disorientation.* Patients are often unaware of the time, where they are, or what has happened to them.
- *Memory problems.* These might include remembering important information about themselves and their families, remembering new information, or remembering recent events.
- *Concentration.* Problems often manifest during therapy sessions, or when patients are attempting to read a book or watch a television program.
- *Perceptual problems.* These might include problems with the detection of shapes in space, or indeed of themselves in space.
- *Executive functioning.* Problems are often associated with reasoning and planning, and with the initiation and regulation of behavior.
- *Attention.* Problems tend to be characterized in terms of dividing, switching, selecting, or sustaining attention.

Many of these cognitive problems resolve over time, but approximately 38% of those people who survive a stroke will be left with some longer term cognitive impairment (Tatemichi et al., 1994). Cognitive problems are often seen as a hidden disability, as in many cases these will not necessarily be obvious to others. Cognitive problems can sometimes be misinterpreted. For example, someone who does not follow through with the exercises that a physiotherapist has prescribed might be thought to be apathetic about their recovery, whereas this might be a problem of poor initiation of behavior that can occur following damage to the brain's executive system. Many cognitive problems can have a significant detrimental impact on physical rehabilitation and recovery (Galski, Bruno, Zorowitz, & Walker, 1993; Robertson, Ridgeway, Greenfield, & Parr, 1997). This is often seen when patients have problems with their memory, particularly in relation to assimilating new information. Progress in rehabilitation can become extremely difficult when patients are not able to remember what it is the physiotherapist or the occupational therapist has told them to do (e.g., which foot to step forward with first), and, indeed, cognitive impairment has been shown to be associated with reduced social and functional independence in the longer term (Shimoda & Robinson, 1998).

Psychological Factors Affecting Recovery

When thinking about the factors that are important in influencing recovery and rehabilitation following a stroke, understanding the relationship between impairment and disability is vital. *Impairment* refers to "any loss or abnormality of psychological, physiological or anatomical structure or function," whereas *disability* refers to "any restriction or lack (resulting from an impairment) of an ability to perform an activity in the manner or within the range considered normal for a human being" (Wood, 1980). The former therefore refers to disturbances at the level of the organ, whereas the latter refers to disturbances at the level of the individual person. Thinking in this way, then, it is important to acknowledge that no direct relationship exists between impairment and disability, and that people can react very differently to the same event. This is seen, for example, in the case of depression. The experience and severity of depression is not directly related to the severity of the physical impairment. For example, a stroke patient who ends up with very little physical impairment following his or her stroke might actually become more depressed than a stroke patient with quite a severe physical impairment. Thus, it is fundamentally important to recognize and understand that psychological factors will play a crucially important role in a patient's recovery.

Twining (1988) offers some insight into the complex understanding of the relationship between impairment and disability. He argues that how a person responds and adjusts to the impact of illness and subsequent disability can be seen as an interaction between the person and the handicap. He describes a range of individual factors, including personality, attitudes, social relationships, interests, and activities, and outlines how these will interact with aspects of the illness impairment (e.g., the severity, extent, prognosis, history, and cause of the illness) to affect a person's emotional adjustment. An example of this might be that a keen reader will be more devastated by a stroke that affects language but leaves his or her limbs unaffected, whereas a keen gardener may cope better with a communication impairment, but not so well if his or her limbs were affected. What is important is how aspects of both the individual and the handicap interact with each other.

An important variable is the way that people respond to their illness in terms of the beliefs that they hold about it. According to Leventhal, Diefenbach, and Leventhal (1992), the beliefs that a person holds about the identity, cause, consequences, potential cure, or control of the illness will significantly influence how they manage their illness. He refers to this a *self-regulatory model of illness behavior*. For example, a stroke patient who believes that engaging in any form of physical exertion following their stroke will lead to a further catastrophic stroke, is less likely to fully engage in physiotherapy rehabilitation. Similarly, someone who believes that his unhealthy eating habits prior to the stroke made no contribution to his subsequent stroke is unlikely to change any of these habits in the future.

Most individuals believe that people hold a degree of personal control over events; this may influence how a person thinks about his stroke or his individual contribution to recovery. It has been shown that the degree to which a person thinks that he or she can influence his or her own recovery varies between people, and that those people who believe that they have more personal control over their recovery actually do better in rehabilitation (Bonetti & Johnston, 2008; Johnston, Gilbert, Partridge & Collins, 1992; Johnson, Pollard, Morrison, & MacWalter, 2004; Johnston, Morrison. It has also been shown that it is in fact possible for health professionals to influence a patient's perceived level of personal control in the direction of internality; that is, increasing the person's belief that he or she has personal control over his or her recovery (Johnston, Gilbert, Partridge, & Collins, 1992). This concept is known as *recovery locus of control*.

Psychologically Informed Interventions

Not only have psychologically informed interventions been shown to be effective in treating emotional disorders following stroke (Hackett, Anderson, & House, 2008), but they have also been shown to be effective in preventing the development of depression post stroke (Buchanan, 2009). Some useful models help us to think about how and when it might be best to intervene with patients on a psychological level. This is, of course, not an exact science; rather, the models provide guidance about we know is important to patients at different stages of their recovery.

Moos and Schaefer (1984) describes the time phases of a physical illness and differentiates between the early days and weeks following the event (the crisis phase), the longer term phase of living with the condition (chronic phase), and the end phase (terminal phase). He describes the psychological (and physical) tasks that patients and families need to undertake to cope with the situation that they face. For many stroke patients, the early months following the stroke are very often experienced as a crisis phase. According to Moos, the psychologically adaptive tasks that a person and his or her family need to undertake within this crisis phase include: (a) creating a meaning for the illness event that maximizes a preservation of a sense of mastery and competency; (b) grieving for the loss of the preillness identity; (c) moving toward a position of acceptance of permanent change while maintaining a sense of continuity between past and future; (d) pulling together to undergo short-term crisis reorganization; and (e) in the face of uncertainty, developing flexibility toward future goals.

Building on this model, Barton, Goudie, and Scott (2003), recognizing the huge impact of the stroke on the wider family system, highlight the importance of tailoring interventions to both stroke patients and their families in the time following the stroke. They describe how the emotional needs of patients and their families will differ in the different time phases of recovery following the stroke, and that psychosocial interventions need to take these varying needs into account.

Interventions at the Level of the Organization

It is important to consider the context in which care is delivered. Although many health service settings would argue that they provide good psychological care, the general consensus is that what care is offered is often patchy and inconsistent (Nichols, 1994). Nichols (2003) has written extensively about this, and argues that a scheme of delivering psychological care is required that can match the level of physical care given. He argues that good psychological care needs to consist of more than purely being a caring professional who helps a patient with his problems as and when they arise, and that environments that are psychologically sophisticated deliver emotional care in a systematic and routine way. The question that he asks is: Can the service be confident that the psychological care that it delivers is both timely and meaningful? And, can it be confident that this will be available for all patients? He thus argues that a system of psychological care must be in place that is structured, routine, and timely for

all patents, and that this is fundamentally crucial for addressing the emotional well-being of patients.

Drawing on the work and ideas of Nichols, discussed above, if the multidisciplinary team (MDT) is to become successful in ensuring that good psychological care is delivered to all hospitalized patients, then a structure needs to be put into place to make this happen. One way that this can be achieved is through the introduction of care plans for each patient; these plans are specifically devoted to the emotional and psychological care of a particular patient. The use of care plans is well established within physical health (and particularly nursing) settings and primarily tend to focus on monitoring aspects of physical care. Introducing care plans that focus on the psychological needs of patients helps to ensure that patient mood is systematically and routinely assessed and monitored while the patient is hospitalized, and that timely and appropriate interventions are offered. At the same time, the plan also clearly highlights that this is the responsibility of the whole MDT, not just the task of the clinical psychologist or the mental health practitioner. Some of the key principles to consider when trying to develop both routine and systematic psychological care are presented in Table 13.1. In addition, it is important to address the training needs of the MDT, and in particular those of the nursing staff, to develop skills in basic counseling techniques and in providing basic psychological care (Bennett, 1996; Ross, Barton, & Read, 2009).

Building on this concept, it is also important to consider the impact that the behavior of professionals caring for the stroke patient can have on his or her general psychological well-being and motivation to engage in therapy. Staff who are more responsive to the psychological needs of patients, who address the information and education needs of patients, and who encourage realistic expectations of recovery appear to impact positively on a patient's motivation to engage in rehabilitation. Thus, factors beyond the individual patient's control can affect his or her motivation to engage (Maclean, Pound, Wolfe, & Rudd, 2008; Wiles, Ashburn, Payne, & Murphy, 2002) and have an influence on their overall quality of life (Western, 2007).

Interventions at the Level of the Individual

When thinking about interventions aimed at individuals, it is important to consider what type of intervention might be most appropriate, and who the best person might be to deliver it. Some of the work of the National Institute for Clinical Excellence (NICE) (2009) has been extremely significant in

Table 13.1 Key principles in developing emotional care

1. Insert emotional care plans routinely into all patients' notes at the start of treatment.

2. Insert emotional care plans into notes regardless of whether or not the person appears to be suffering with mood. This is partly to take account of the fact that problems with mood following a stroke can fluctuate. Some patients may not show any signs or symptoms of low mood at one point in time, but this can change very quickly and thus needs to be continually monitored.

3. Introduce a system of key workers whereby one person is responsible for ensuring that the emotional care plans are completed appropriately, and any necessary action is taken. However, it is important to remember that it is not the total responsibility of the key worker to provide all the emotional care for the patient, but rather the responsibility of the whole MDT to deliver this care by incorporating this into the routine aspects of their work.

4. To ensure that routine emotional care is provided, a step-by-step approach should be detailed on the care plan, in order that the key worker can follow a prescribed set of steps. This helps to standardize the process and ensure that all patients are receiving the same standard of care and monitoring.

5. Provide options on the care plan as to the most appropriate screening tools to use, depending on whether or not the patient has any communication difficulties, and if so, the extent of these difficulties. These options should be based on the best available evidence from within the literature.

6. Any action to be taken, based on the results of the assessment measures, should be clearly identified on the care plan, and some guidance given as to who is responsible for doing this. For example, a comprehensive diagnostic assessment interview might be requested by one of the medical staff if the patient scores above the cutoff point on any of the screening measures.

7. A range of possible interventions to address emotional distress should be listed that are primarily evidence based, as detailed, for example, in the NICE guidelines for the management of depression. These can then be tailored to what the service can actually offer, largely in terms of what skills and resources are available to the team.

8. Perhaps most importantly, the process of developing emotional care plan should be the work of the whole multidisciplinary team and the different professional groups. This helps to ensure that all members of staff feel some ownership of the process, and as a result will be more likely to engage with the process.

helping staff make these decisions. For example, the guidelines that NICE have produced on managing depression are extremely helpful in guiding health care staff on what level of assessment and intervention should be delivered by different staff members. NICE (2009) proposes a stepped model of care in which the basic recognition, assessment, and treatment of depression ought to be undertaken by the generic MDT. Only when these attempts do not prove successful in alleviating the depression should more intensive and specialist treatments be offered by members of the staff who have specialist training in mental health conditions and management. Thus, it is recognized and expected that all members of the MDT can play a part in the assessment and treatment of mood disorders, depending on the severity of the presentation (e.g. Brumfitt & Barton, 2006).

EMOTIONAL ADJUSTMENT AND COUNSELLING

One of the lower intensity interventions for depression and anxiety is supportive counseling, and this can be undertaken by a range of health professionals within the MDT. Talking through the events of the stroke can be crucial in helping both patients and families to emotionally process the trauma of the event and to start to adapt to this life-changing experience (Barton & Scott, 2003; Bennett, 1996; Murray & Harrison, 2004). In addition, applying motivational interviewing approaches in the early stages following stroke has also been shown to have a beneficial impact on patient mood (Watkins et al., 2007). Key aspects of counseling include adopting an empathic approach, listening to what the client is saying, summarizing what has been said, and reflecting this back to check understanding and to let the patient know that he has been heard. Perhaps most importantly, patients need to be listened to, and even if they are emotionally upset, the last thing they want is for this distress to be minimized and brushed aside. Table 13.2 summarizes some of the basic factors to consider when responding to emotional distress.

In some cases, bringing patients together in a safe and supportive group that gives them the

Table 13.2 Tips on how to respond to emotional distress

1. Listening to the patient is perhaps the most crucial skill. This is not always easy, but using a combination of verbal and nonverbal methods of communication can help.

2. Let the patient know that you have heard what he is saying' and that you understand. If you do not understand what the patient is trying to communicate, it is important to acknowledge this with the patient and suggest that you will need to do some more exploration of what the problem is.

3. Try to concentrate on what the patient is trying to communicate to you. Focus on how the patient is behaving, as well as what he is saying.

4. Remember that if a patient is distressed or is crying, it is important to acknowledge this distress with the patient, not avoid it or shy away from it. The last thing that patients want to hear when they are upset is that "everything will be all right." Of course, patients do want reassurance, but they also want to have their distress acknowledged and validated.

5. Remember to make eye contact with the patient, and try to keep an open body posture, so that the patient knows that you are interested in what he is trying to communicate to you.

opportunity to reflect on and share their own individual experiences of loss and their worries and concerns with others can be extremely helpful in the adjustment process (Barton & Scott, 2003; Bennett & Barnston, 2007; Gurr, 2009). The sharing of experiences and the mutual support that develops within the group can have added benefit.

ANXIETY MANAGEMENT

Anxiety management includes regulating breathing, physical and mental relaxation, identifying alternative thoughts, and distraction. These approaches can be helpful in tackling most aspects of anxiety, particularly when anxiety is generalized and largely related to the person's general rehabilitation and recovery and his or her plans for the future. Frequently, with older people and those who have had a stroke, pain is an issue in considering what relaxation methods to utilize. Hypnotic or imagery techniques are less likely to produce or exacerbate pain than are those that rely on tensing and relaxing muscles. The psychologist or occupational therapist can teach the patient basic anxiety management skills, and these can be reinforced by the rest of the therapy team. Phobic anxiety is tackled through the process of systematic desensitization. In this approach, the psychologist, working in conjunction with the therapy team, helps the patient to gradually make contact with the feared object or situation through a series of graded steps. The principle here is of approach rather than avoidance of the feared object or situation. In the case of post-traumatic stress symptoms, cognitive-behavioral therapy (CBT) approaches have been shown to be helpful. A referral to the psychologist should be made in such cases.

PSYCHOLOGICAL THERAPY

Psychological therapy is recommended for those patients suffering either with depression or anxiety symptoms that have not responded to lower intensity interventions. Despite the fact that depressed stroke patients have been shown to have disproportionately more negative than positive cognitions (Thomas & Lincoln, 2008), there are mixed results regarding the effectiveness of CBT with stroke patients (Hackett, Anderson, House, & Xia, 2008; Lincoln, Flannaghan, Sutcliffe, & Rother,1997; Rasquin, van de Sande, Praamstra, & van Heugten 2009). Cognitive-behavioral therapy approaches with depressed older people in general are known to be effective (Laidlaw, Thompson, Dick-Siskin & Gallagher-Thompson 2003; Laidlaw and Knight 2008). Cognitive-behavioral therapy approaches tend to focus on helping clients to challenge and evaluate their negative styles of thinking and to replace these with more adaptive and realistic thinking patterns. This approach can be helpful with stroke patients who may catastrophize the negative outcome of their stroke, believing, for example, that because they are no longer able to walk independently, they will never be able to leave the house again. This type of psychological therapy is usually undertaken by trained clinical psychologists, in one-to-one or group sessions with the client. Behavior therapy is another type of psychological approach that is known to be helpful with depressed older people. The theory underpinning this construct is that mood is linked to behavior and that increasing the positive experiences that people have will lead to an improvement in mood. With stroke patients, building previously enjoyed interests and activities into the day can be extremely helpful. Most patients who are depressed find it difficult to motivate themselves to engage in activities, and this is where professional involvement is helpful. All members of the MDT can participate in encouraging patients to participate in activity.

EDUCATION AND INFORMATION

Patients and families need to gain some understanding of the stroke experience, and they need for information and education to achieve this. Indeed, providing information to stroke patients (and their caregivers) has been shown to improve depression (Smith et al., 2008). According to Moos and Schaefer (1984), the psychological tasks that patients need to undertake in the early part of their recovery include trying to make sense of what has happened to them and learning to understand their medical condition. They also need to start to get to know the staff and the hospital system, and understand what rehabilitation means. Information needs differ, however, among patients and their families, and are known to change over time. How information is given and in what quantity are also important factors. Care needs to be taken not to overload patients with information, taking account the impact of primacy and recency effects in what people remember. For example, when faced with a number of things to remember, it is not uncommon for people to remember the first and last few items. Thus, keeping the number of items to remember short may be beneficial. It is also suggested that people remember pieces of information best if they are delivered in multiples of three. For information to be remembered, it is important that it is thought to be meaningful. Thus, it is important to consider what information is presented to people at different stages in their recovery. For example, discussing access to financial benefits might be less relevant to stroke patients in the first weeks of their recovery than are the principles behind bladder retraining and catheterization. It is also important to remember that many pieces of information will need to be given on more than one occasion, as many patients and families will not necessarily remember what they have been told. The Stroke Association has produced a series of fact sheets of different aspects of stroke that can be downloaded and given to patients and families as required. Formal education programs have been shown to be helpful in reducing emotional distress (e.g., Johnson & Pearson, 2000; Smith, Forster & Young, 2004), while Barton (2002), in describing the benefits of a group approach to stroke education, highlights the importance of timing in the delivery of information.

COGNITIVE REHABILITATION

The purpose of cognitive rehabilitation is not to retrain impaired cognitive functions through drill and exercise, but rather to help reduce the negative impact of cognitive problems on a person's everyday life and functioning. Although there is limited evidence supporting the usefulness of memory rehabilitation on improving functional outcomes in stroke patients (das Nair, & Lincoln, 2007), cognitive rehabilitation still remains a promising approach. Wilson (1997) provides an overview of the different approaches to cognitive rehabilitation. In clinical rehabilitation settings, the usual practice is for the results of the cognitive assessment to inform the rehabilitation program. This is usually developed jointly by the psychologist, occupational therapist, physiotherapist, and other members of the MDT. Compensatory strategies are extremely helpful in relation to memory functioning and executive functioning. *Errorless learning* is an approach that works well with memory-impaired people (Evans et al., 2000). In this approach, when learning new information, the person is prevented from making a mistake, so that only correct information is actually encoded. This is different from the trial-and-error approach to learning most commonly used. Different strategies and techniques can also be used to help people to remember, and these can be built into the rehabilitation program (for a comprehensive review of working with memory problems,

Table 13.3 Strategies for working with memory and executive functioning problems

Problems with executive functioning:
- General principle is to provide structure
- Plan and talk through a task prior to activity
- Continually prompt and guide through a task
- Encourage self-reflection and monitoring of behaviour

Memory problems:
- Encourage patients to use external memory aids (e.g., diaries, electronic organizers, Dictaphones)
- Simplify information and provide written instructions
- Divide information into small chunks
- Use errorless learning techniques

Attention and concentration problems:
- Minimize unnecessary distractions
- Focus on one thing at a time
- Provide warning and preparation when the patient needs to switch his attention to a new task

see Clare & Wilson, 1997). Table 13.3 lists of some strategies that are helpful when working with memory problems and problems with executive functioning.

Conclusion

It is important to recognize the traumatic impact that a stroke can have on an individual, as well as on their families and friends. There is a huge diversity in the ways that individuals respond to trauma, and, as such, it is essential that psychological factors involved in the experience of this event, as well as in the rehabilitation, recovery, and adjustment, are fully recognized and taken into account when planning treatment programs. Psychological factors are known to interact in a complex way with physical and medically related factors, and as such ought to be given the same degree of consideration when treating patients since failure to do so will inevitably result in impoverished recovery. Understanding the psychological factors that are important in illness is essential for all staff working in health care environments, and ways to address these factors ought to be considered at the level of the organization, as well as at the level of the individual.

References

American Heart Association. (2009). Heart disease and stroke statistics 2009 update: A report from the American Heart Association Statistics Committee and Stroke Statistics Subcommittee. *Circulation, 119*, e21–e181.

Barton, J. (2002). Stroke: A group learning approach. *Nursing Times, 98*(7), 34–35.

Barton, J., Goudie, F., & Scott, S. (2003). Emotional adjustment following stroke: A family affair. *PSIGE Newsletter, 84*, 18–21.

Barton, J., & Scott, S. (2003). Emotional adjustment to stroke: A group therapeutic approach. *PSIGE Newsletter, 84*, 13–15.

Bennett, B. (1996). How nurses in a stroke rehabilitation unit attempt to meet the psychological needs of patients who become depressed following a stroke. *Journal of Advanced Nursing, 23*, 314–321.

Bennett, B., & Barnston, S. (2007). Emotional support after stroke, part 1: Two models from hospital practice. *British Journal of Neuroscience Nursing, 3*, 2–6.

Berry, E. (1998). Post traumatic stress disorder after subarachnoid haemorrhage. *British Journal of Clinical Psychology, 37*, 365–367.

Bonetti, D., & Johnston, M. (2008). Perceived control predicting the recovery of individual-specific walking behaviours following stroke: Testing psychological models and constructs. *British Journal of Health Psychology, 13*, 463–478.

Bowman, G. (2001). Emotion and illness. *Journal of Advanced Nursing, 34*(2), 256–263.

Bruggimann, L., Annoni, J.M., Staub, F., von Steinbuchel, N., van der Linden, M., & Bogousslavsky, J. (2006). Chronic posttraumatic stress symptoms after nonsevere stroke. *Neurology, 66*, 513–516

Brumfitt, S., & Barton, J. (2006). Evaluating well-being in people with aphasia using speech therapy and clinical psychology. *International Journal of Therapy and Rehabilitation, 13*, 305–310.

Buchanan, D. (2009). Review: Psychological interventions prevent depression after stroke. *Evidence-Based Nursing, 12*, 23.

Burvill, P., Johnson, G., Jamrozik, K., Anderson, C., Stewart-Wynne, E., & Chakera, T. (1995). Anxiety disorders after stroke: Results from the Perth Community Stroke Study. *British Journal of Psychiatry, 166*, 328–332.

Carek, V., Norman, P., & Barton, J. (2010). Cognitive appraisals and post traumatic stress disorder symptoms in informal carers of stroke survivors. *Rehabilitation Psychology, 55*(1), 91–96.

Clare, L., & Wilson, B. A. (1997). *Coping with memory problems.* Bury St Edmunds: Thames Valley Test Company.

Clark, M., & Smith, D. (1999). Psychological correlates of outcome following rehabilitation from stroke. *Clinical Rehabilitation, 13/2*(129–140), 0269–2155;1477–0873.

das Nair R., & Lincoln N. (2007). Cognitive rehabilitation for memory deficits following stroke. *Cochrane Database of Systematic Reviews, 3*, CD002293. doi: 10.1002/14651858. CD002293.pub2.

De Wit, L., Putman, K., Baert, I., Lincoln, N., Angst, F., Beyens, H., et al. (2008). Anxiety and depression in the first six months after stroke: A longitudinal multicentre study. *Disability and Rehabilitation, 30*, 1858–1866.

Eccles, S., House, A., & Knapp, P. (1999). Psychological adjustment and self reported coping in stroke survivors with and without emotionalism. *Journal of Neurology, Neurosurgery and Psychiatry, 67/1*, 125–126, 0022–3050.

Ellis, C, Zhao, Y, Egede, L. (2010). Depression and increased risk of death in adults with stroke. *Journal of Psychosomatic Research, 68*, 545–551.

Ellis-Hill, C., & Horn, S. (2000). Change in identity and self-concept: A new theoretical approach to recovery following a stroke. *Clinical Rehabilitation, 14*, 279–287.

Engel, G.L. (1977). The need for a new medical model: A challenge for biomedicine. *Science, 196*, 129–136.

Evans, J., Wilson, B., Schuri, U., Andrade, J., Baddley, A., Brua, O., et al. (2000). A comparison or errorless and trial-and-error learning methods for treating individuals with acquired memory deficits. *Neuropsychological Rehabilitation, 10*, 67–101.

Field, E.L., Norman, P., & Barton, J. (2008). Cross-sectional and prospective associations between cognitive appraisals and posttraumatic stress disorder symptoms following stroke. *Behaviour Research and Therapy, 46*, 62–70.

Gainotti, G. (2000). Psychological model of post-stroke major depression.: Reply. *British Journal of Psychiatry, 176*, 295–296.

Galski, T., Bruno, R., Zorowitz, R., & Walker, J. (1993). Predicting length of stay, functional outcome and aftercare in the rehabilitation of stroke patients: The dominant role of higher-order cognition. *Stroke, 24*, 1794–1800.

Goodwin, R, Devanand, R., & Devangere P. (2008). Stroke, depression, and functional health outcomes among adults in the community. *Journal of Geriatric Psychiatry and Neurology, 21*, 41–46.

Gordon, W.A., & Hibbard, M.R. (1997). Post-stroke depression: An examination of the literature. *Archives of Physical Medicine and Rehabilitation, 78*, 658–663.

Gurr, B. (2009). A psychological well-being group for stroke patients. *Clinical Psychology Forum, 202*, 12–17.

Hackett, M. L., Anderson, C. S., House, A., & Xia, J. (2008). Interventions for treating depression after stroke. *Cochrane Database of Systematic Reviews, 4*, 1469493X: CD003437. doi: 10.1002/14651858.CD003437.pub3

Hackett, M. L., Yang, M., Anderson, C. S., Horrocks, J. A., & House A. (2010). Pharmaceutical interventions for emotionalism after stroke. *Cochrane Database of Systematic Reviews, 2*, CD003690. doi: 10.1002/14651858.CD003690.pub3

House, A., Knapp, P., Bamford, J., & Vail, A. (2001). Mortality at 12 and 24 months after stroke may be associated with depressive symptoms at 1 month. *Stroke, 32*, 696–701.

Johnson, J., & Pearson, V. (2000). The effects of a structured education course on stroke survivors living in the community. *Rehabilitation Nursing, 25*, 59–65.

Johnston, M., Gilbert, P., Partridge, C., & Collins, J. (1992). Changing perceived control in patients with physical disabilities: An intervention study with patients receiving rehabilitation. *British Journal of Clinical Psychology, 31*, 89–94.

Johnston, M., Pollard, B., Morrison, V., & MacWalter, R. (2004). Functional limitations and survival following stroke: psychological and clinical predictors of 3-year outcome. *International Journal of Behavioral Medicine, 11*, 187–196.

Kneebone, I., & Dunmore, E. (2000). Psychological management of post stroke depression. *British Journal of Clinical Psychology, 39*, 53–65.

Kutz, I., Shabtai, H., Solomon, Z., Neumann, M., & David, D. (1994). Posttraumatic stress disorder in myocardial infarction patients—prevalence study. *Israel Journal of Psychiatry, and Related Sciences, 31*, 48–56.

Laidlaw, K, Thompson, L, Dick-Siskin, L, Gallagher-Thompson, D. (2003). *Cognitive Behaviour Therapy with Older People.* Chichester: Wiley

Laidlaw, K & Knight, B (2008). *Handbook of emotional disorders in later life.* Oxford: Oxford University Press.

Lanza, M. (2006). Psychological impact of stroke: A recovering nurse's story. *Issues in Mental Health Nursing, 27*, 765–774.

Leventhal, H., Diefenbach, M., & Leventhal, E.A. (1992). Illness cognition: Using common sense to understand treatment adherence and affect cognition interactions. *Cognitive Therapy and Research, 16*, 143–163.

Lincoln, N., Flannaghan, T., Sutcliffe, L., & Rother, L. (1997). Evaluation of cognitive behavioural treatment for depression after stroke: A pilot study, *Clinical Rehabilitation, 11*, 114–122.

Maciejewski, P., Zhang, B., Block, S., & Prigerson, H. (2007). The stage theory of grief—reply. *Journal of the American Medical Association, 297*, 2693–2694.

Maclean, N., Pound, P., Wolfe, C., & Rudd, A. (2008). Qualitative analysis of stroke patients' motivation for rehabilitation. *British Medical Journal, 321*, 1051–1054.

Merriman, C., Norman, P., & Barton, J. (2007). Psychological correlates of PTSD symptoms following stroke. *Psychology, Health and Medicine, 12*(5), 592–602.

Moos, R. H., & Schaefer, J, A. (1984). The crisis of physical illness. In R. H. Moos (Ed), *Coping with physical illness*, 3–25, New York: Plenum.

Morrison, V., Pollard, B., Johnston, M. & MacWalter, R. (2005). Anxiety and depression 3 years following stroke: Demographic, clinical, and psychological predictors. *Journal of Psychosomatic Research, 59*, 209–213.

Murray, C.D., & Harrison, B. (2004). The meaning and experience of being a stroke survivor: An interpretative phenomenological analysis. *Disability and Rehabilitation, 26*(13), 808–816.

Naess, H., Lunde, L., Brogger, J., & Waje-Andreassen, U. (2010). Depression predicts unfavourable functional outcome and higher mortality in stroke patients: The Bergen Stroke Study. *Acta Neurologica Scandinavica, 122*(190), 34–38.

National Institute for Health and Clinical Excellence (NICE). (2009). *Depression in adults with a chronic physical health problem.* Clinical Guideline 91. London: NICE.

Nichols, K. (1994). Preventive psychological care for the physically ill. *Journal of Mental Health, 3*, 443–446.

Nichols, K. (2003). *Psychological care for ill and injured people: A clinical guide.* Maidenhead: Open University Press.

Pohjasvaara, T., Vataja, R., Leppavuori, A., Kaste, M., & Erkihjuntti, T. (2001). Depression is an independent predictor of long-term functional outcome post-stroke. *European Journal of Neurology, 8*(4), 315–319.

Prince, M., Patel, V., Saxena, S., Maj, M., Maselko, J., Phillips, M., & Rahman, A. (2007). No health without mental health. *The Lancet, 370*, 859–877.

Rasquin, S. M. C., van de Sande, P., Praamstra, A. J., & van Heugten, C. M. (2009). Cognitive-behavioural intervention for depression after stroke: Five single case studies on effects and feasibility. *Neuropsychological Rehabilitation, 19*, 208–222.

Remer-Osborn, J. (1998). Psychological, behavioral, and environmental influences on post-stroke recovery. *Topics in Stroke Rehabilitation, 5/2*, 45–53.

Robertson, I., Ridgeway, V., Greenfield, E., & Parr, A. (1997). Motor recovery after stroke depends on intact sustained attention: A two year follow-up study. *Neuropsychology, 11*, 290–295.

Rochette, A., Bravo, G., Desrosiers, J., St-Cyr/Tribble, D., & Bourget, A. (2007). Adaptation process, participation and depression over six months in first-stroke individuals and spouses. *Clinical Rehabilitation, 21*, 554–562.

Ross, S., Barton, J., & Read, J. (2009). Staff in-service training on post stroke psychological and communication issues. *International Journal of Therapy and Rehabilitation, 16*, 342–348.

Schultz, S., Castillo, C., Kosier, T., & Robinson, R. (1997). Generalized anxiety and depression: Assessment over 2 years after stroke. *American Journal of Geriatric Psychiatry, 5*, 229–237.

Sembi, S., Tarrier, N., O'Neill, P., Burns, A., & Farragher, B. (1998). Does post traumatic stress disorder occur after stroke: A preliminary study. *International Journal of Geriatric Psychiatry, 13*, 315–322.

Shimoda, K., & Robinson, R. (1998). Effect of anxiety disorder on impairment and recovery from stroke. *Journal of Neuropsychiatry and Clinical Neurosciences, 10*, 34–40.

Silver, R., & Wortman, C. (2007). The stage theory of grief. *Journal of the American Medical Association, 297*, 2692.

Shimoda, K., & Robinson, R. (1998). The relationship between social impairment and recovery from stroke. *Psychiatry, 61*, 101–111.

Smith, J., Forster, A., House, A., Knapp, P., Wright, J. J., & Young, J. (2008). Information provision for stroke patients and their caregivers. *Cochrane Database of Systematic Reviews, 2*, CD001919. doi: 10.1002/14651858.CD001919.pub2

Smith, J., Forster, A. & Young, J. (2004). A randomised trial to evaluate an education programme for patients and carers after stroke. *Clinical Rehabilitation, 18*, 726–736.

Stenager, E. N., Madsen, C., Stenager, E., & Boldsen, J. (1998). Suicide in patients with stroke: Epidemiological study. *British Medical Journal, 316,* 1206.

Storor, D., & Byrne, G. (2006). Pre-morbid personality and depression following stroke. *International Psychogeriatrics, 18,* 457–469.

Stroke Association. (2009). Facts and figures about stroke. Retrieved from www.stroke.org.uk/media_centre/facts_and_figures/index.html

Surtees, P. G., Wainwright, N. W. J., Luben, R. N., Wareham, N. J., Bingham, S. A., & Khaw, K. T. (2008). Psychological distress, major depressive disorder, and risk of stroke. *Neurology, 70*(10), 788–794.

Tatemichi, T. K., Desmond, D. W., Stern, Y., Palik, M., Sano, M., & Bagella, E. (1994). Cognitive impairments after stroke: Frequency, patterns, and relationship to functional abilities. *Journal of Neurology, Neurosurgery and Psychiatry, 57,* 202–207.

Thomas, S., & Lincoln, N. (2006). Factors relating to depression after stroke. *British Journal of Clinical Psychology, 45,* 49–61.

Thomas, S. A., & Lincoln, N. B. (2008). Depression and cognitions after stroke: Validation of the Stroke Cognitions Questionnaire Revised (SCQR). *Disability and Rehabilitation: An International, Multidisciplinary Journal, 30,* 1779–1785.

Twining, C. (1988). *Helping older people: A psychological approach.* New York: John Wiley.

van de Port, I., Kwakkel, G., Bruin, M., & Lindeman, E. (2007). Factors relating to depression after stroke. *Disability and Rehabilitation, 29,* 353–358.

Watkins, C., Auton, M., Deans, C., Dickinson, H., Jack, C., Lightbody, C., et al. (2007), Motivational interviewing early after acute stroke: A randomised controlled trial. *Stroke, 38,* 1004–1009.

Western, H. (2007). Altered living: Coping, hope and quality of life after stroke. *British Journal of Nursing, 16,* 1266–1270.

Wiles, R., Ashburn, A., Payne, S., & Murphy, C. (2002). Patients' expectations of recovery following stroke: A qualitative study. *Disability and Rehabilitation, 24,* 841–850.

Wilson, B. A. (1997). Cognitive rehabilitation: How it is and how it might be. *Journal of the International Neuropsychological Society, 3,* 487–496.

Wood, P. (1980). *International Classification of impairments, disabilities and handicaps.* Geneva: World Health Organization.

Traumatic Brain Injury

Robyn L. Tate

Abstract

This chapter provides an overview of the current clinical and research literature on traumatic brain injury (TBI), as it pertains to rehabilitation psychology. The background context is provided first, describing the epidemiology of TBI, mechanisms of the injury, recovery process, and outcome. The section concludes with the role of assessment in rehabilitation, drawing on the International Classification of Functioning, Disability, and Health. The next section focuses on the psychological rehabilitation of TBI, initially by describing principles of evidence-based clinical practice and resources such as PsycBITE (http://www.psycbite.com) to facilitate rapid identification of relevant research and critical appraisal. Inpatient and community models of rehabilitation are described, and the final section of the chapter reports results of systematic reviews on the types and effectiveness of interventions for cognitive, behavioral, and emotional disorders commonly encountered after TBI.

Key Words: Brain injuries, neuropsychology, cognition disorders, disability, rehabilitation, evidence-based clinical practice, systematic reviews, PsycBITE, International Classification of Functioning, Disability, and Health (ICF).

Background and Context

Traumatic brain injury (TBI) is an important health condition, if for no other reason than it mainly involves previously healthy, young people in their prime of life; moreover, it is caused by an external mechanical force and hence is potentially preventable. Indeed, TBI is the most common cause of acquired disability in healthy, young people (Thurman, Alverson, Dunn, Guerrero, & Sniezek, 1999), and it is often referred to as the "silent epidemic" (Goldstein, 1990). Severe degrees of TBI can cause life-long disability, effectively precluding the person from participating in the workforce, living independently, and enjoying life and love.

There are numerous personal accounts of the tragedy caused by TBI and the struggles to rebuild shattered lives—usually both for the person with brain injury, as well as for the family who shares the journey (e.g., Dann, 1984; Graham, 1985; Koenig, 2008; Osborn, 1998). To date, the research literature on the consequences of TBI for the person and family members has focused on negative consequences and losses, but, increasingly, a more balanced perspective recognizes post-traumatic growth (e.g., Ownsworth & Fleming, 2011) seen in the courage, resilience, and resourcefulness displayed by patients and their families as they adjust to the consequences of the injury, often working toward different life goals and, in the process, developing personal strengths and qualities. Rehabilitation is integral to this process.

The World Health Organization (WHO) website (http://www.who.int/topics/rehabilitation/en/) defines rehabilitation as a process that enables people "to reach and maintain their optimal physical, sensory, intellectual, psychological, and social functional levels. Rehabilitation provides disabled people with the tools they need to attain independence and self-determination." Rehabilitation psychology has a broad brief in TBI, including assessment and provision of specific therapies targeting those cognitive and behavioral deficits that are a direct consequence of the injury, as well as other therapies addressing secondary effects, including emotional adjustment. Commonly, the recipient is the person with brain injury, but rehabilitation may also include the adjustment process for family members (see Anderson et al., 2009; Blais & Boisvert, 2005; Boschen, Gargaro, Gan, Gerber, & Brandys, 2007; Kreutzer, Marwitz, Godwin, & Arango-Lasprilla, 2010; Oddy & Herbert, 2003; Perlesz, Kinsella, & Crowe, 1999; Sinnakaruppan & Williams, 2001). A large literature on psychological rehabilitation after brain injury is available, and commonly used reference works include Christensen and Uzzell (2000), Eslinger (2002), Ponsford (2004), Ponsford, Sloan, and Snow (2012), Prigatano (1999), Sohlberg and Mateer (2001), and Wilson (2003a).

This chapter presents an overview of TBI, with special reference to rehabilitation psychology. An introductory section provides the background and context of TBI, followed by brief description of the International Classification of Functioning, Disability, and Health (ICF; World Health Organization [WHO], 2001) as a useful way to conceptualize the consequences of TBI and their measurement. The main focus of the chapter is on interventions relevant to rehabilitation psychology. Many specific rehabilitation techniques are available, and the clinician/researcher needs to select the best intervention for the individual patient. Given the sheer volume of the available intervention literature, this can be a daunting task. The chapter thus includes a description of resources to facilitate quick and effective searching of the evidence-based literature. Descriptions of rehabilitation interventions are provided at both the systems and individual levels. The focus of the individual interventions in this chapter is on the results of systematic reviews of therapies for cognitive, behavioral, and emotional consequences of TBI.

Epidemiology, Mechanisms of Injury, Course of Recovery and Outcome

Traumatic brain injury is defined as "craniocerebral trauma, specifically, an occurrence of injury to the head (arising from blunt or penetrating trauma or from acceleration–deceleration forces) that is associated with any of these occurrences attributable to the injury: decreased level of consciousness, amnesia, other neurologic or neuropsychological abnormalities, skull fracture, diagnosed intracranial lesions, or death" (Thurman et al., 1999, p. 603). Traumatic brain injury refers equally to the fleeting loss of consciousness seen in a child who falls off a swing as it does to the months of prolonged impaired consciousness accompanied by lifelong, profound disability in a person injured in a road traffic crash. Both examples are simply polar ends of a spectrum of injury.

EPIDEMIOLOGY

For a variety of methodological reasons (Corrigan, Selassie, & Orman, 2010; Kraus & McArthur, 1996; Tate, McDonald, & Lulham, 1998), it is difficult to ascertain the precise incidence of TBI. Incidence figures are generally confounded by the inclusion of large numbers of people who are head injured but not brain injured (see Tate et al., 1998, for discussion). Although the terms "head injury" and "brain injury" are often used synonymously, arguably, the health condition of interest is injury to the brain, which is encased within the head (skull)—specifically, *traumatic* brain injury (as opposed to brain injury of other etiology, such as stroke). Estimates of the annual occurrence of hospital-treated TBI ranging between 175 and 200/100,000 are regarded as reliable (Kraus & McArthur, 1996; Thurman et al., 1999). In the United States alone, it is estimated that each year one-quarter of a million people are hospitalized with nonfatal TBI, with just under half of those having long-term disability (Corrigan et al., 2010). In warfare, however, the incidence of TBI is orders of magnitude higher: 14% of survivors and 19% of casualties from U.S. armed forces sustained head injury in the Vietnam war (Salazar, Schwab, & Grafman, 1995), with similar figures for the Iraq and Afghanistan conflicts (French & Parkinson, 2008).

Traumatic brain injury is more common in males (ratio of males to females is at least 2:1 and for severe injury 3:1). In civilians, TBI most commonly occurs in young adults—for example, in the series of Tate et al. (1998), the peak incidence escalated from 100/100,000 overall to almost 400/100,000 in 15- to 24-year-old males. Cause of injury differs by age: falls are the most common in very young and older persons, sports injuries in school aged children, and road traffic crashes in young adults (Kraus & McArthur, 1996; Tate et al., 1998). The occurrence of gunshot wounds and assaults is more variable and largely related to specific settings; blast injuries are considered the signature type of TBI in modern warfare.

In civilian hospital admissions for TBI, mild degree of injury (73% in the series of Kraus et al., 1984) far outstrips moderate and severe injury (8% each, with the remainder being dead on arrival to hospital). For mild TBI, the evidence from the systematic review by Holm, Cassidy, Carroll, and Borg (2005) indicates that, although cognitive symptoms are common in the acute stages after mild injury, full recovery occurs for the majority within the first 12 months. At the other end of the injury spectrum, because of advances in emergency retrieval, early treatment, and newly developed interventions, many people who previously would have died now survive (Eker et al., 2000). Consequently, increasing numbers of people with minimally conscious states are admitted to rehabilitation wards, and their outcomes are extremely variable (see Giacino & Kalmar, 1997; Lammi, Smith, Tate, & Taylor, 2005).

MECHANISMS OF INJURY

Injury to the brain in civilian TBI is largely due to acceleration–deceleration forces. These forces occur because the brain, in motion within the skull (acceleration), comes into abrupt contact with an immobile surface (deceleration; such as the dashboard of a car in a road traffic crash, or the ground in a fall or assault). The sudden halt causes the jelly-like cerebral tissue of the brain to collide against the bony ridges of the interior surface of the skull, causing a variety of damage (see below). In addition to these contact phenomena are the inertial effects, in which the continued movement of the brain causes rotation of the brain tissue with consequent shearing and tearing of nerve fibres (Adams, Gennarelli, & Graham, 1982; Katz, 1992). This type of acceleration–deceleration injury (also referred to as blunt injury) is classified as a *closed injury* when the dura mater (the tough protective lining between the brain and skull) is not pierced, and an *open injury* if the dura mater is ruptured. Reasons that the dura mater may be pierced include skull fracture and neurosurgery.

The characteristic (but not the only) neuropathologies arising from acceleration–deceleration forces are contusions and diffuse axonal injury, which in turn have predictable locations, mapping directly to the types of impairments observed after TBI:

• *Contusions* are streaks of punctuate haemorrhage or bruising and are commonly found on the crests of the gyri of the brain. Irrespective of the site of impact, they occur most frequently in those areas of the brain situated in the anterior and middle cranial fossa of the skull—the frontal poles, orbital gyri, peri-Sylvan area, inferior and lateral surfaces of the temporal lobes, and inferolateral angle of the occipital lobes. The frontal lobes also feature as the site of the most severe contusions, closely followed in severity by the temporal lobes. In lacerations, where brain substance is torn, commonly on the bony protuberances of the skull such as the sphenoidal ridges, the damage is worse.

• *Diffuse axonal injury* (or nerve fiber damage) is largely restricted to the subcortical white matter of the cerebral hemispheres, cerebellum, and brain stem. Additionally, consistent sites of focal lesions (which may be observed macroscopically) are the corpus callosum and rostral brain stem proximal to the superior cerebellar peduncles.

The functional consequences of damage to the frontal and temporal lobes from contusions, along with damage to subcortical white matter from diffuse axonal injury, are largely responsible for compromised executive/behavior regulation processes, memory/learning functions, and processing speed, respectively. Additionally, the aforementioned mechanical events set in train a series of biochemical reactions that have the potential to cause further damage to the brain. The biochemical and neurological sequelae (e.g., intracerebral haemorrhage, ischaemia, infections, etc.) are varied and complex, and further information is available from sources such as Gordon et al. (2006); Jennett and Teasdale (1981); Whyte, Hart, Laborde, and Rosenthal (2005); and Zasler, Katz, and Zafonte (2006).

COURSE OF RECOVERY

Immediately following acceleration–deceleration injury, there is a predictable set of three phases in the course of recovery: the acute period, post-acute recovery phase, and long-term outcome. The duration of each phase is extremely variable among patients, this being a direct reflection of the severity of the injury.

The *initial acute phase* is life-threatening and treated in medical emergency and intensive care units. A characteristic feature is a coma or loss of consciousness in which the patient is not responsive to external stimuli and cannot be roused. Coma, as operationalized on the Glasgow Coma Scale (GCS; Teasdale & Jennett, 1974), is a state of unconsciousness characterized by three features: absence of eye opening, no comprehensible verbalization, and no motor response to commands. The GCS has been adapted for children to take account of developmental stages in babies to 5 years of age (Simpson, Cockington, Hanieh, Raftos, & Reilly, 1991; British Paediatric Neurological Association, 2001; http://www.bpna.org.uk/audit/GCS.PDF)

Coma, and more specifically, the GCS score, is also one of the two most commonly used indexes to determine injury severity. The GCS scores range from 3 to 15, with injury severity (ideally, GCS score taken at 6 hours post-trauma) classified as follows:

- Score of 3–8: severe injury
- Score of 9–12: moderate injury
- Score of 13–15: mild injury

Emergence from coma is signaled by eye opening and return of autonomic functions (e.g., sleep–wake cycles). In extremely severe injuries, the patient may emerge from coma to higher levels of impaired consciousness, including the vegetative and minimally conscious states (see Giacino et al., 2002, for description). For the majority of patients, however, emergence from coma heralds the post-acute phase of recovery.

In the *early post-acute phase*, patients are in post-traumatic amnesia (PTA), a state of impaired consciousness sharing similar behavioral features to delirium or acute confusion. Post-traumatic amnesia is a temporary state of altered consciousness following coma "during which the patient is confused, amnesic for ongoing events, and likely to evidence behavioral disturbance" (Levin, O'Donnell, & Grossman, 1979, p. 675). It can be measured prospectively with instruments such as the Galveston Orientation and Amnesia Test (Levin et al., 1979), Westmead PTA Scale (Shores, Marosszeky, Sandanam, & Batchelor, 1986), and other similar scales. Adapted versions of these respective scales for children are also available (Ewing-Cobbs, Levin, Fletcher, Miner, & Ensenberg, 1990; Rocca, Wallen, & Batchelor, 2008). Additionally, procedures are available to estimate duration of PTA retrospectively (King et al., 1997; McMillan, Jongen, & Greenwood, 1996), and these are useful when PTA has not been measured prospectively while the patient is hospitalized, or if results of such testing are not available.

Along with coma depth, PTA duration is the other commonly used index of injury severity. The original classification was initially described by

Russell and Smith (1961), and later expanded by Jennett and Teasdale (1981) as follows:

- <5 minutes: very mild injury
- 5–60 minutes: mild injury
- 1–24 hours: moderate injury
- 1–7 days: severe injury
- 1–4 weeks: very severe injury
- >1 month: extremely severe injury

In the recent research literature, this traditional classification of injury severity in relation to PTA duration has been questioned (e.g., Nakase-Richardson et al., 2011). The WHO Collaborating Task Force on Mild Traumatic Brain Injury (Carroll, Cassidy, Holm, Kraus, & Coronado, 2004) has revised the definition of mild injury to include PTA durations up to 24 hours, thereby subsuming the moderate injury classification. In cases in which the GCS score suggests one injury severity classification and PTA duration indicates a different classification, the rule of thumb takes the more severe category (Von Holst & Cassidy, 2004).

The post-acute recovery phase is also a period of active improvement in functional abilities in physical, cognitive, and behavioral domains. There is general consensus (but limited empirical evidence) that this middle period lasts up to 6 or 12 months post-trauma (Stuss & Buckle, 1992). Rehabilitation efforts are maximized during this period, as well as during the final long-term phase, and interventions used are described in detail in subsequent sections of this chapter.

In the *final phase*, spontaneous recovery will have reached a plateau, with the patient attaining a variable level of outcome. It must be stressed that outcome is not necessarily fixed and immutable; a range of internal as well as external environmental factors can result in subsequent functional adaptations and hence influence outcome. Thus, although level of outcome is largely determined by injury severity, it is not the case that a severe injury invariably results in a severe outcome. Predictors of outcome are as yet incompletely understood. A widely used classification of outcome is the Glasgow Outcome Scale (Jennett & Bond, 1975), which takes into account the sum total of physical and mental disability, along with their effects on social functioning. The Glasgow Outcome Scale has five main categories: death, persistent vegetative state, severe disability, moderate disability, and good recovery, with the last three categories being divided into upper and lower levels of outcome (Jennett, Snoek, Bond, &

Brooks, 1981). An extended version of the Glasgow Outcome Scale, using an interview format, has been published (Teasdale, Pettigrew, Wilson, Murray, & Jennett, 1998).

OUTCOME

A large literature exists documenting psychosocial outcomes after TBI, ranging from those studies that focus on the early stage within a few months of injury to those examining the very long-term, decades post-trauma. A seminal cohort study is that of Dikmen, Ross, Machamer, and Temkin (1995), who examined TBI at 12 months post-trauma. This study has a number of features that makes it important: the source of participants was consecutive admissions to a Level 1 trauma hospital and thus the range of severity levels was represented, the sample size was large ($n = 466$), and two control groups were included ($n = 88$ friends and $n = 124$ (non-TBI) trauma patients). Not surprisingly, in the TBI sample, severity of the initial injury was related to global outcome on the Glasgow Outcome Scale: more than 80% of those with mild injury were classified as having good recovery and, at the other extreme, just under 50% of those with severe injury were classified at the severe levels (approximately 35% were classified as having severe disability, and the remaining were in the persistent vegetative state or had died). Yet, it needs to be said that, in this series, a significant proportion of those with severe injury (approximately 25%) were classified as good recovery, thus reinforcing the observation that a severe injury does not necessarily result in severe disability.

Compared with the control groups, the TBI group had more problems. Whereas 93–94% of the control groups lived independently, this was the case for 76% of the TBI group as a whole, ranging from 89% for the least severely injured subgroup to 23% for the most severely injured. Similarly 82% and 63% of the control groups (friend and trauma controls respectively) had returned to work by 12 months post-trauma, compared with 49% of the TBI group (injury severity subgroup range: 6–64%). On the Sickness Impact Profile, 0% and 6% of the respective control groups were classified as having dysfunction, compared with 9% for the TBI groups as a whole (injury severity subgroup range: 7–17%). For this latter most severely injured TBI group, the rank order of dysfunction in the 12 Sickness Impact Profile dimensions was as follows: work (47%), recreation and pastimes (28%), home management (20%), alertness behavior (20%), sleep

and rest (19%), communication (18%), ambulation (16%), emotional behavior (14%), social interaction (14%), mobility (14%), body care and movement (12%), and eating (4%).

The functional outcomes at 2 years post-trauma were reported by Ponsford, Olver, and Curren (1995) for a rehabilitation sample ($n = 175$). Although most participants were independent in areas such as feeding, personal hygiene, and dressing (93%, 88%, and 87%, respectively), only about two-thirds of the group were independent in more demanding activities, such as mobility for walking, running, and jumping (60%); home activities (68%); and independence in use of public transport/driving a car (65%). Reported problems in areas of cognition (74%), behavior (44%), and mood (58–59%) were very common. Olver, Ponsford, and Curren (1996) compared a subset ($n = 103$) of the above sample at both 2 and 5 years post-trauma. Although there were overall slight improvements in some community activities (e.g., number able to drive increased from 40% to 48%), key areas such as employment decreased from 41% to 34%, and the reported problems in cognitive, behavioral, and emotional domains remained relatively high (e.g., forgetfulness in 71%, irritability in 66%, depression in 56%). The longer term outcome from 10 years up to 25 years post-trauma has been studied (e.g., Draper, Ponsford, & Schönberger, 2007; Hoofien, Gilboa, Vakil, & Donovick, 2001; Tate, Broe, Cameron, Hodgkinson, & Soo, 2005; Wood & Rutterford, 2006). Although there is variability among findings of the studies, which is largely a function of sample composition and measuring instruments, relatively high rates of neuropsychological and emotional morbidity remain, which exert an adverse effect on everyday functioning.

The Role of Assessment in Traumatic Brain Injury Rehabilitation

Good assessment is fundamental to effective rehabilitation; the black-box approach to rehabilitation, in which therapy commences in the absence of detailed knowledge of the person's strengths and limitations, is to be eschewed. Moreover, pre-intervention assessment is necessary to provide the essential baseline against which the effect of an intervention can be measured, whether this is therapy for skill acquisition or psychological adjustment. In people with TBI (and other health conditions), two types of assessment are required to provide the crucial context in which an intervention is applied. These assessments can be conceptualized along a dimension of increasing specificity, as depicted in Figure 14.1. The first type of assessment pertains to the overall level of functioning using health status measures and standardized tests (cf. Levels 1 and 2 of Figure 14.1), and the second type of assessment relates to the specific behaviors that are the target of therapy (cf. Level 3 of Figure 14.1).

ASSESSMENT OF OVERALL LEVEL OF FUNCTION

Increasingly, the ICF (WHO, 2001) is being applied in the field of rehabilitation. Its singular advantage is that it provides a comprehensive overview of functioning from all perspectives: at the body function (impairment) level, functional (activities) level, and social (participation) level, together with consideration of contextual factors that influence outcome, both environmental and personal (see Bruyère, van Looy, & Peterson, 2005; Üstün, Chatterji, Bickenbach, Kostanjsek, & Schneider, 2003). It is worth noting, however, that a number of concepts are pertinent to rehabilitation psychology in TBI that are not covered by the ICF. These include concepts such as quality of life (QOL) and psychological adjustment; additionally the personal factors component of the ICF, highly relevant to rehabilitation psychology, is yet to be delineated. The ICF is essentially a taxonomy, comprising a list of approximately 1,500 alphanumeric codes representing various aspects of functioning. The codes are grouped in a hierarchical, nested structure of parts, components, domains, and categories, described as a stem-branch-leaf arrangement; Tate and Perdices (2008) have graphically depicted this structure as an "ICF tree" to fit to a single page. The basic ICF tree of parts, components, and domains (along with codes) is shown in Figure 14.2; ICF trees for the categories are also presented in the above reference.

Because the ICF is intended to be applicable to all health conditions, the codes take on varying relevance in different health conditions. Consequently,

ICF "core sets" have been identified for specific health conditions. They constitute the minimum number of codes that are necessary yet sufficient to describe a health condition, and hence provide a guide for comprehensive and targeted outcome measurement. Core sets have been developed for selected neurological (and other) conditions, including stroke (Geyh et al., 2004), as well as in different settings, such as early post-acute rehabilitation (Stier-Jarmer et al., 2005). Development of a core set for TBI is currently in progress (Bernabeu et al., 2009) and, when validated, the items will provide guidance as to the areas of functioning that should be assessed after TBI.

The ICF is not an assessment tool itself, but a checklist is available for this purpose, being a summary form of the ICF classification. The ICF Checklist (http://www.who.int/classifications/icf/training/icfchecklist.pdf) uses 29 items for the domains and 123 items for the categories. Ratings are made on a 5-point scale from 0 (not present) to 4 (complete impairment/difficulty; 96–100%). When the TBI core set is validated, the identified categories will be able to be selected from the ICF Checklist, thereby providing a tailor-made assessment of TBI-relevant factors within the ICF model. Until that time, however, Koskinen, Hokkinen, Sarajuuri, and Alaranta (2007) identified 15 ICF domains and 30 categories as the most relevant problem areas for people with TBI (see Table 14.1). In turn, these categories provide the context, basis, and direction for general assessment and for measuring the effect of rehabilitation interventions.

A wide variety of standardized instruments is necessary to assess all the foregoing domains of function. Many of these will be objective neuropsychological tests, and texts such as Lezak, Howieson, and Loring (2004) are a good resource; Sohlberg and Mateer (2001) also provide a helpful listing of various instruments targeting specific functions

Level 1	Level 2	Level 3
Health status measures (assessing Activities/Participation; Environmental Factors)	Standardized impairment-based measures	Target behavior to be treated
e.g., WHODAS II, CHIEF	e.g., RBMT; D-KEFS	e.g., memory failures, aggressive behavior

Increasing specificity →

Figure 14.1 Levels of measurement in rehabilitation.
Note: WHODAS II, World Health Organization Disability Assessment Schedule II; CHIEF, Craig Hospital Inventory of Environmental Factors; RBMT, Rivermead Behavioural Memory Test; D-KEFS, Delis-Kaplan Executive Function Scale.

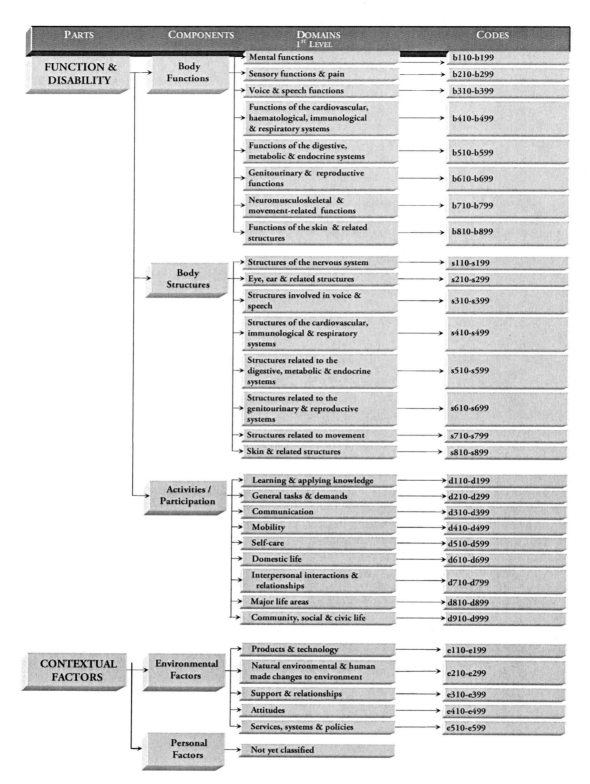

Figure 14.2 Structure of the International Classification of Functioning, Disability, and Health
Acknowledgement: Adapted from Tate and Perdices (2008), with permission.

Table 14.1 International Classification of Functioning, Disability, and Health (ICF) domains and categories pertinent to TBI (after Koskinen et al., 2007)

Component	Domain	Category
Body Functions	b1: Mental functions	• Memory: 100% • Higher level cognitive (Executive) functions: 100% • Attention: 96% • Emotional functions: 96% • Energy and drive functions: 86% • Language functions: 76% • Sleep: 73% • Perceptual functions: 36%
	b2: Sensory functions and pain	• Pain: 69% • Vestibular: 67% • Seeing: 46%
	b7: Neuromusculoskeletal and movement related functions	• Muscle power: 47%
Body Structures	s1: Nervous system	• Brain (% not specified in report, but >30%)
Activities/Participation	d1: Learning and applying knowledge	• Solving problems: 60%
	d2: General tasks and demands	• Undertaking multiple tasks: 58%
	d3: Communication	• Conversation: 89% • Speaking: 82% • Communication—receiving spoken messages: 40%
	d4: Mobility	• Fine hand use: 46% • Driving: 35%
	d6: Domestic life	• Acquisition of goods and services: 58% • Doing housework: 38%
	d7: Interpersonal interactions and relationships	• Complex interpersonal interactions: 69%
	d8: Major life areas	• Remunerative employment: 100%

(see Chapter 4, Table 4.2 of their volume), although more recently published tests will not be included. Rating scales covering the Activities/Participation and Environmental Factors components (as well as Mental Functions) are also available in compendia, such as Tate (2010).

A pre-intervention evaluation using a selection of pertinent instruments (Levels 1 and 2 in Figure 14.1) will provide the necessary context for application of a therapy program, which nonetheless may need to be tailored to take account of (different) compromised areas of functioning. For example, in a patient with challenging behavior, knowing that he or she experiences pain, fatigue, or major memory problems is important information in terms of the structure of a program to manage the challenging behaviors. Indeed, addressing the pain, fatigue, or memory problems in their own right may in fact ameliorate the challenging behaviors.

In terms of specific instruments selected to measure effect of interventions, one of the first systematic reviews of cognitive rehabilitation (Carney et al.,1999) was critical of the tendency of many researchers to restrict examination of (cognitive) therapy outcomes at the intermediate level (i.e., standard neuropsychological tests and impairment-based measures; cf. Level 2 measures in Figure 14.1) and not include health status measures (cf. Level 1) to document whether treatments had any practical effects on everyday functioning. The importance of this is highlighted in a systematic review of treatments for meta-cognitive (executive) impairments.

Kennedy et al. (2008) showed that changes after executive treatments were more likely to be observed at the level of Activities/Participation in daily life rather than on standardized tests. Wilson (2003b) also agreed that neuropsychological tests are not the appropriate measure of treatment effectiveness, and she gave the example of Jay, a 20-year-old man, who became densely amnesic after a subarachnoid haemorrhage. Notwithstanding the major restrictions imposed by his memory disorder, Jay learned to live alone and independently, and was also a successfully self-employed craftsman. In spite of his undeniable rehabilitation success, Jay continued to score zero on any test of delayed memory. Thus, if the neuropsychological test score were used as a measure of therapy outcome, then the result would be an undeniable rehabilitation failure. There is no contradiction here; the rehabilitation strategy used for Jay (and many other people with brain injury) was training in use of compensatory techniques, rather than restoring the underlying impairment. It stands to reason that, in this situation, the appropriate measures should be effective use of compensatory techniques and their effect on everyday behaviors (cf. Levels 1 and 3 in Figure 14.1), not evaluation of the underlying impairment (viz., integrity of the memory system as assessed by standard memory tests; cf. Level 2), given that this was not the aim of treatment. In other words, as noted by Kennedy and Turkstra (2006), the outcome measure(s) selected should be those that best represent the treatment results.

ASSESSMENT OF SPECIFIC BEHAVIORS TARGETED IN THERAPY

Jay's example also demonstrates that assessment using generic instruments is too nonspecific to capture the target behavior that is to be the subject of an intervention in an individual patient, particularly those interventions that involve skill acquisition. To implement a memory therapy program, for example, it is necessary to know and measure not only the nature and severity of the client's memory disorder in general terms (available from a standardized memory test), but also much more specific information, such as the frequency of memory failures, the types of failures, the situations in which the failures occur, and so forth (which require measures at Level 3 of Figure 14.1). Similarly, rehabilitation of challenging behaviors requires specification of the precise behavior (e.g., throwing objects, hitting people) and detailed knowledge of the frequency and intensity of the behavior, as well as the antecedents to

and settings in which the behavior occurs. With some exceptions, this information will only be furnished by a specific measure tailor-made to evaluate the specific behavior exhibited by the specific individual. It follows that such measures may need to be developed by the clinician/researcher for the individual patient/client. In this endeavor, the principles of applied behavior analysis are relevant.

Applied behavior analysis is a method by which to identify and specify the behavior to be targeted for treatment, then break down a behavior into its component parts. There is a large literature in this area and the interested reader is referred to chapters on assessment in texts such as those by Barlow, Nock, and Herson (2009) and Kazdin (2011). The crucial features of target behavior(s) are that they must be defined operationally in specific and measurable terms and have the capacity for repeated measurement. An example of the precision with which the target behavior is specified is given by Treadwell and Page (1996), who treated, inter alia, spitting behavior in a patient with TBI. Spitting was defined as "spittle landing within 1 foot of another person" (p. 65). Often, a task analysis of the target behavior is conducted; as Kazdin notes, if one is treating "bed-making" or "table-setting,", then one will identify the 20 or 30 specific behaviors that are involved in bed-making or table-setting. Single-case experimental designs are advocated as a rigorous way by which to implement evidence-based rehabilitation interventions, and the above texts provide methodological guidance in this area. The methodological rating scale for single-case experimental designs (Tate et al., 2008; 2011) can also be used as a checklist for designing and critically appraising such therapy programs. A wide variety of statistical procedures is available, some of which are simple to execute and suitable for examining treatment effect in the individual patient (see Kazdin, 2011; Perdices & Tate, 2009).

Closely related to the selection of target behaviors for treatment are patient goals. There is, however, some controversy about the procedures used in goal setting. McMillan and Sparkes (1999), for instance, make the distinction between client-centered patient goals and staff action plans, in which "a 'fog' of energetic staff activity...masks the absence of any real progress or improvement" (p. 244). Moreover, Malec (1999) cites the work of Ottenbacher and Cusick (1990), who "criticized traditional clinical goal setting as vague, global, and without definite timelines for achievement, often resulting in goals that are 'irrelevant, unmeasurable, or unattainable'"

(p. 254). Nonetheless, the potential benefits of goal setting are reflected in the systematic review of Cullen et al. (2007), who concluded that there was moderate evidence to support the direct involvement of patients in goal setting. The cited study was that of Webb and Glueckauf (1994), who demonstrated greater gains in goal attainment in community rehabilitation programs when patients were directly involved in the process of goal setting than when they had low involvement.

When goals are highly individualized, goal attainment scaling is advocated as providing a standardized, quantitative method by which to measure treatment effect, and it has been used in TBI rehabilitation (Malec, Smigielski, & DePompolo, 1991; Malec, 1999). Malec (1999) describes goal attainment scaling as a six-step process:

1. Select goal(s).
2. Weight goals in terms of their importance (weighting, however, is commonly regarded as an optional procedure).
3. Define the time frame within which goal(s) will be assessed.
4. Operationally define the expected outcome of the goal(s) when achieved, in precise and measurable terms; this level is usually assigned score zero.
5. Operationally define other (less/more than expected) outcomes. Usually, goal attainment is measured on a 5-point scale, from -2 (much less than expected) to +2 (much more than expected).
6. Take pre- and post-treatment measures of the patient's status with respect to the goal(s). The effect of the treatment on goal attainment can be determined statistically. (See Malec, 1999, for details)

Psychological Rehabilitation in Traumatic Brain Injury
Evidence-Based Clinical Practice
GENERAL CONSIDERATIONS

Clinical practice in the contemporary context is charged with the goal of being evidence-based. Evidence-based clinical practice in medicine is defined as "the integration of best research evidence with clinical expertise and patient values.... When these three elements are integrated, clinicians and patients form a diagnostic and therapeutic alliance which optimizes clinical outcomes and quality of life" (Sackett, Straus, Richardson, Rosenberg, & Haynes, 2000, p. 1). *Best research evidence* refers to the methodology used to evaluate interventions.

Many different research designs are used for this purpose, but some methodologies are better than others in that they minimize the risk of bias and produce more reliable results. Group designs for intervention research have an established hierarchy of levels or classes of evidence (see Oxford Centre for Evidence-based Medicine, CEBM; http://www.cebm.net). Systematic reviews of randomized controlled trials (RCT) provide the best (Level 1) evidence, with case series and expert opinion providing much lower levels of evidence (Levels 4 and 5, respectively).[1] The new guidelines of the Oxford CEBM (Levels2) place the *n-of-1 trial* as Level 1 evidence, on an equal footing to systematic reviews of multiple RCTs (Howick et al., 2011). It stands to reason that more store should be placed on the results of studies using methodologies that provides a high level of evidence.

Single-participant designs (including n-of-1 trials) provide an alternative methodology to group designs for the evaluation of treatment effect and, they are also well-suited to implementing evidence-based practice in the clinical setting (see Guyatt et al., 1986; Guyatt, Jaeschke & McGinn, 2002; Perdices & Tate, 2009). Like group designs, variability also exists in the methodological rigor of single-participant designs. High-level evidence can be obtained from those single-participant designs that provide experimental control and manipulation of variables, such as withdrawal/reversal (A-B-A) and multiple-baseline designs (Barlow et al., 2009; Kazdin, 2011; Perdices & Tate, 2009). Indeed, Guyatt and colleagues (2002) consider the randomized n-of-1 trial to provide the best level of evidence for clinical decision-making in individual patients, above both systematic reviews and RCTs, as now reflected in the Oxford CEBM Levels2. Other single-participant designs, such as studies in which measures are not taken during treatment (essentially a pre-/post-design more suitable to group methodology) or B-phase training studies, provide low levels of evidence of treatment effect.

Systematic reviews and meta-analyses of the literature are valuable in that they provide exhaustive searches of the literature, use explicit methodology and selection criteria for inclusion of individual studies, and synthesize and critically appraise the research findings from included studies. Systematic reviews archived in the Cochrane Database of Systematic Reviews (http://www.cochrane.org) are widely regarded as providing high-quality reviews. Those systematic reviews that also translate their findings to make recommendations for clinical practice based on the strength of the evidence are particularly helpful. Cicerone and colleagues (2000, 2005; 2011), among others, used a three-tiered system of practice standards, practice guidelines, and practice options; Kennedy et al. (2008) have further incorporated terminology recommended by the Quality Standards Subcommittee of the American Academy of Neurology (AAN; http://www.aan.com) to describe four levels:

• *Practice standards* relate to interventions with positive results used in studies with a high level of evidence (at least one well-designed Class I RCT, as well as very strong evidence from Class II or III studies); comparable to Level A of the AAN—such interventions "should be used."

• *Practice guidelines* relate to interventions with a moderate degree of certainty, furnished from well-designed Class II studies; comparable to Level B of the AAN—such interventions "should be considered."

• *Practice options* relate to interventions from Class II and III studies; comparable to Level C of the AAN—such interventions "may be considered."

• *Level D* of the AAN—the intervention has insufficient data to make a recommendation for clinical practice.

Sackett and colleagues (2000) identify five steps in the practice of evidence-based medicine: (1) formulating an answerable question, (2) tracking down the evidence, (3) critically appraising the evidence, (4) integrating critical appraisal with clinical expertise and patient factors, and (5) self-evaluation of the effectiveness of this process and ways it could have been improved. It is particularly for steps 2 (identifying the evidence) and 3 (critical appraisal) that the busy clinician encounters barriers in implementing an evidence-based approach to clinical practice. The processes involved in locating the research evidence about interventions and critically appraising that evidence are time-consuming. Critical appraisal of methodology is important because the more rigorous methodological designs (e.g., controlled studies with randomization vs. case series without control groups) reduce the risk of bias and thus produce more reliable results. Yet, even within controlled studies, marked variability in method quality exists, as demonstrated in a number of surveys of RCTs (e.g., Moseley, Sherrington, Herbert, & Maher, 2000; Perdices et al., 2006). Similar variability of methodological quality has been found for single-participant designs (Tate et al., 2011). Systematic reviews also vary in quality, and the PRISMA statement (Moher et al., 2009) provides a checklist of important characteristics of a systematic review that should be reported, such as describing methods used for assessing risk of bias; providing summary data for each intervention from each study, along with effect sizes and confidence intervals; and so forth. A method quality rating scale for systematic reviews, AMSTAR, was described by Shea et al. (2007). [2] Moreover, unlike in previous decades, part of the difficulty in identifying and appraising the literature is not because of the dearth of available evidence; rather, the volume of published literature on health conditions (including TBI) is overwhelming. Fortunately, resources are available to facilitate the steps of identifying and critically appraising the literature.

RESOURCES TO FACILITATE EVIDENCE-BASED CLINICAL PRACTICE, FEATURING PSYCBITE

A number of websites compile evidence-based resources lists (see, e.g., http://www.ecu.edu.au/library/faculty/pdf/chs/facEvidencebasedhealth.htm; http://www.otcats.com/links/databases.html). Among the facilities listed on these websites is an Australian suite of evidence-based databases that are available free of charge (see http://www.pedro.org.au; http://www.psycbite.com; http://www.otseeker.com; http://www.speechbite.com); these use a single model, PEDro, developed by the Centre for Evidence-based Physiotherapy (Herbert, Moseley & Sherrington, 1998/1999), as a structure. The majority of these databases are discipline-specific, although recognizing the overlap in roles among rehabilitation allied health professionals. The database of most relevance to the present chapter is PsycBITE, the Psychological Database for Brain Impairment Treatment Efficacy (http://www.psycbite.com).

PsycBITE, whose development and procedures are described in detail elsewhere (Tate et al., 2004), contains all of the published literature on nonpharmacological interventions for the psychological consequences of acquired brain impairment, and currently archives more than 3,000 records. Seven electronic databases are searched simultaneously (Allied and Alternative Medicine Database, AMED; Cumulated Index to Nursing and Allied Health Literature, CINAHL; Cochrane Library; Excerpta Medica Database (EMBASE); Educational Resource Information Centre database (ERIC); Medline; and PsycINFO). All references generated from the searches are processed online to identify those meeting five eligibility criteria: The report is

(1) a full-length publication in a peer-reviewed, scientific journal that (2) addresses humans with brain impairment of acquired etiology, (3) specifically in people older than 5 years of age, and (4) it provides empirical, quantitative data on interventions, with (5) such interventions comprising at least one intervention that is psychologically based and/or targets at least one psychological consequence of acquired brain impairment.

All levels of evidence are included on PsycBITE, providing that the report contains empirical (quantitative) data on treatment effectiveness: this includes systematic reviews (10% of the current records), RCTs (22%), controlled clinical trials that are not randomized (non-RCTs; 12%), case series (21%), and single-participant designs (35%). Studies using qualitative methodology are not currently included on PsycBITE. Eligible articles are indexed against 126 terms in six domains: problem or target area (58 areas), intervention type (37 types), service delivery mode (10 modes), neurological group (13 groups), age group (3 groups), and study design (5 designs).

Studies using RCT/non-RCT designs and some single-participant designs (those using single-case experimental designs [SCED], i.e., withdrawal/reversal designs, multiple-baseline designs) are critically appraised and rated for methodological quality, using a slightly adapted version of the PEDro Scale (Maher, Sherrington, Herbert, Moseley, & Elkins, 2003) for RCT/non-RCT designs and the SCED Scale (Tate et al., 2008, 2011) for single-participant designs. The PEDro and SCED scales are brief and reliable; both have a similar structure, but differ in content as appropriate to the specific methodological designs.

Reports are ranked on PsycBITE according to levels of evidence and method quality: systematic reviews are ordered first because they represent the strongest level of evidence, followed by RCTs, non-RCTs, and case series. Single-participant designs are ranked last, not because they use an inherently inferior methodology to the other research designs, but rather because the methodology (i.e., not group-based studies) represents a unique research design. Within single-participant designs, the methodologically stronger designs with control conditions (e.g., withdrawal/reversal [A-B-A], multiple-baseline) are ranked above single-participant designs without control conditions (e.g., A-B, "pre-/post" designs, B-phase training studies).

Using the PsycBITE website to search for evidence is very easy. Searches can be conducted by using drop-down menus that tap into the 126 indexing terms, or alternatively, key words can be used. Figure 14.3 provides a screen shot of the search page of PsycBITE using the drop-down menus for neurological group (TBI) and method (systematic review). The results of this search are described in the final section of the chapter.

Rehabilitation at the Systems Level

This section describes the macrosystem of rehabilitation for TBI within which specific evidence-based interventions, such as those described in the next section, are implemented. It is argued that the most effective rehabilitation is offered through an integrated system of specialized and multidisciplinary services, as has been demonstrated in a Cochrane systematic review for stroke (Stroke Unit Trialists' Collaboration, 2007).

A range of TBI-specific rehabilitation services has been developed in different countries. Some of these services offer a hospital-based inpatient program, often commencing in the post-acute stage as soon as the patient is medically stable. Generally, the goals at the inpatient stage involve functional rehabilitation, focusing on basic self-care skills, mobility, communication, and instrumental activities of daily living. The TBI Model Systems in the United States (see Dijkers, Harrison-Felix, & Marwitz, 2010), the Rivermead Rehabilitation Centre—Oxford Centre for Enablement in the United Kingdom, and the Brain Injury Rehabilitation Program for New South Wales (NSW) in Australia are some examples. Some of these services continue rehabilitation in the community—it is recognized that many people with severe injury experience continuing disabilities that necessitate clinical service provision after hospital discharge. In the community rehabilitation model, the focus generally changes from physical and functional goals to psychosocial ones, thereby going beyond the medical model.

A different type of rehabilitation service for TBI specializes in neuropsychological rehabilitation, often using a holistic model. Such services may be nonresidential and occur at a later stage in the recovery time frame, months or even years post-trauma. Examples include the Barrow Neurological Institute, in Phoenix, Arizona; the Brain Injury Day Treatment Program in New York City, New York; the Center for Rehabilitation in Brain Injury in Copenhagen, Denmark; and the Oliver Zangwill Centre (OZC) in Ely, United Kingdom. These and similar neuropsychological programs are described by contributors to Christensen and Uzzell (2000).

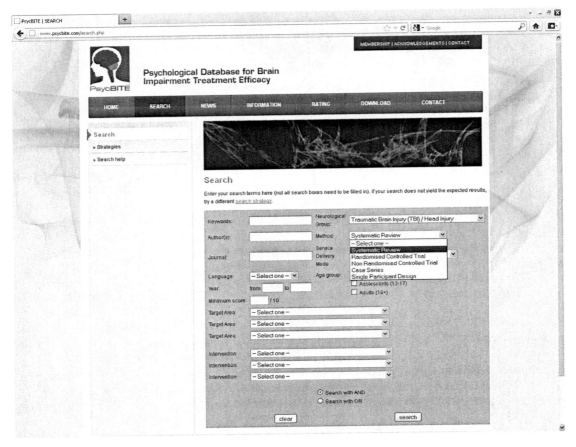

Figure 14.3 PsycBITE search page.
Acknowledgement: Reproduced with permission from Dr. Tate.

Two examples of TBI rehabilitation services representing a comprehensive, health-based service commencing at the early post-acute stage, and a nonresidential program providing specialist neuropsychological rehabilitation within a holistic framework, are described below.

A COMPREHENSIVE, POST-ACUTE REHABILITATION SERVICE

In the acute and post-acute stages after TBI, the nature and extent of impairments and disabilities of people with more severe degrees of injury are such that hospitalization is a necessity. The Australian NSW Brain Injury Rehabilitation Program is distinctive in that it is a government-funded, regionally based, specialist TBI rehabilitation service that was planned using epidemiological data to determine the number of beds and location of the units required to service the occurrence of TBI. It incorporates both hospital- and community-based

models of rehabilitation. Specifically, the program comprises a networked system of 14 centers located throughout the state of NSW, which has a population of approximately 7 million people and covers a geographical region of some 800,600 square kilometers (see Figure 14.4). Three of the 14 centers are dedicated to pediatric TBI and 11 to adult TBI. Five centers (three adult and two pediatric) are located in the state capital of Sydney; the remaining nine centers (including the third pediatric center) are located in regional centers that outreach to rural and remote areas of the state. Each of the three urban centers has 12 to 16 beds, with transitional living units and community outreach/outpatient teams. In total, the 14 centers receive approximately 1200 new admissions per annum (2009 data).

The networked NSW Brain Injury Rehabilitation Program commenced in 1989. Admission criteria are few and liberal: the patient's age at injury is generally less than 65 years (age 16 years being

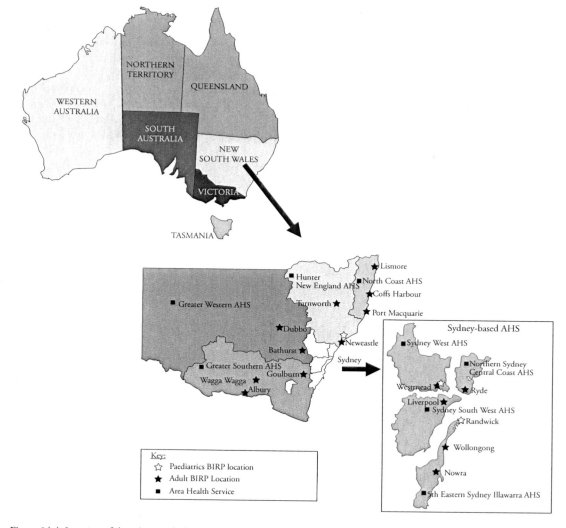

Figure 14.4 Location of the 14 networked service units of the Brain Injury Rehabilitation Program for New South Wales (Australia).

the threshold for admission to an adult or pediatric unit), the patient is a resident in the geographical catchment area served by the center, and the patient has sustained a TBI. The program operates on the principle of universal access and no-one is excluded on the grounds of health insurance credentials, psychosocial or economic backgrounds, or the nature, severity, and combination of impairments arising from the TBI. Virtually all inpatient admissions are for severe injury, with less than 5% of admissions having mild injury. Early referral to the program is encouraged, and patients are admitted to the inpatient units as soon as they are medically stable, although referral to any stage of the service at any time post-trauma is possible. The urban centers take on responsibility to provide inpatient services to all

residents of the state, and transfer to transitional living and community outreach services occur as appropriate. The services are multidisciplinary and the program has a strong commitment to longer term service provision in the community, as long as either the patient or the family has needs that are related to the TBI. The majority of people requiring rehabilitation after TBI in NSW are referred to the networked rehabilitation program.

One of the urban services for adults is located at Liverpool Hospital in the south-western region of Sydney. It contains five service components: (1) a 16-bed, post-acute inpatient unit, (2) a four-bed transitional living unit (described in Simpson et al., 2004), and (3) a community service (described in Tate, Strettles, & Osoteo, 2003) which includes case management and clinical service provision, as well as (4) a four-bed community living unit providing respite and therapy services and (5) the *Head-2-Work* program. In 2010, approximately 75 full-time equivalent (FTE) positions covered the five service components. Staffing is multidisciplinary including medical (3.8 FTE); nursing staff (20.0 FTE) and residential care workers (7.25 FTE); physiotherapy (3.6 FTE); occupational therapy (9.0 FTE); speech pathology (3.0 FTE); diversional therapy (1.0 FTE); rehabilitation assistants (1.5 FTE); clinical, neuro-, and rehabilitation psychology (5.1 FTE); social work (4.2 FTE); case managers (5.0 FTE); vocational instructor (1.0 FTE); rehabilitation counselor (1.0 FTE); and service coordinators and liaison (4.25 FTE). Consultant services of medical specialists (e.g., neurology, orthopaedics, psychiatry), dieticians, and so forth are available as required. The staffing configuration differs in the five service components, as a function of the variety of patient needs at different stages of recovery.

The inpatient unit of the Liverpool service necessarily operates within a medical model, as is appropriate for the early post-acute stage of recovery after TBI. Our survey of consecutive inpatient admissions during the calendar year 2000 documented that, on admission, 8% of patients (5/61) were in a minimally conscious state, 69% (42/61) were in post-traumatic amnesia (PTA), and 23% (14/61) had emerged from PTA (Tate, Perdices, Pfaff, & Jurjevic, 2001). The main roles of the psychologist at the inpatient level include monitoring patients during post-traumatic amnesia, neuropsychological assessment that occurs when the patient stabilizes after emergence from PTA, liaison with rehabilitation staff and family members regarding the cognitive and behavioral impairments, management of patients who exhibit agitated and challenging behaviors, and cognitive rehabilitation as appropriate. Following discharge from the inpatient service, patients are referred to the community team—some, but not all, will require a transitional living program before discharge to the community.

Given the fixed number of inpatient beds, services at the inpatient level are finite, but the community team grapples with a large and cumulative caseload. A survey of the work profile of the community team for the calendar year 2000 documented staffing levels of 16.7 FTE, with services provided to 467 individual clients and families, totaling 8,046 occasions of service (Tate, Strettles, & Osoteo, 2004). Moreover, because of the nonrestrictive admission criteria, the service has a large proportion of people with major functional disability: in the above series, 18% were classified as having severe disability on the Glasgow Outcome Scale, 28% as having moderate disability, and 54% as having good recovery (all at the lower level). Level of functional ability obviously impacts on goal setting and attainment.

The work of the community team has a psychosocial focus. The staffing configuration is distinctive in that case managers (5.0 FTE) work alongside therapists (FTE 5.6), psychologists (FTE 3.1), and social workers (FTE 2.2) in providing a range of clinical services to clients and their families. Services are both center-based, as well as provided in the home or community. The work of the community team thus goes beyond the coordination and service liaison roles of case management. People referred to the community service may be new clients or previous clients of the service who were discharged but have been re-referred, usually because of new issues requiring assistance.

Upon referral to the community service, the client attends a clinic where a rehabilitation physician identifies pertinent issues via a psychosocial interview, as well as providing medical review. The weekly case conference, attended by representative members of the community team, is the central mechanism by which a management plan is formulated, and subsequently monitored, reviewed, and adjusted as necessary. The rehabilitation plan is tailored to each client's unique configuration of impairments, functional disabilities, environmental circumstances, and personal factors, thereby providing a needs-driven, goal-based, community-focused rehabilitation program. The roles of the psychologist are to provide neuropsychological assessment (including capacity assessment when indicated), along with individual or group-based therapies for cognitive, emotional, interpersonal, and behavioral sequelae, often in collaboration with other therapy staff (see next section for specific therapeutic interventions).

A HOLISTIC, NEUROPSYCHOLOGICAL REHABILITATION SERVICE

Increasingly, the medical model that largely characterizes post-acute, inpatient rehabilitation programs is recognized as representing but one stage of the rehabilitation process after TBI. In the longer term, it is neuropsychological sequelae, by and large, that are responsible for restricting a person's resumption of previous roles and lifestyle. The OZC (Wilson et al., 2000; Wilson, Gracey, Malley, Bateman, & Evans, 2009) is an example of a nonresidential unit with a focus on addressing cognitive, emotional, and social sequelae of acquired brain injury (including, but not restricted to TBI).

The OZC was established in 1996, at the Princess of Wales Hospital, Ely, near Cambridge, United Kingdom. It was modeled on the holistic neuropsychological rehabilitation programs pioneered in the United States by Ben-Yishay in New York and Prigatano in Phoenix. Wilson et al. (2009) describe the holistic approach as recognizing "that it does not make sense to separate the cognitive, emotional, and social consequences of brain injury as how we feel and think affects how we behave. Ben-Yishay's (1978) model follows a hierarchy of stages through which the patient or client should work in rehabilitation. These stages are engagement, awareness, mastery, control, acceptance, and identity" (p. 47). The components of the OZC program, and the model and principles on which it is based, are described in detail in Wilson, Gracey, Evans, and Bateman (2009). The book also contains helpful worksheets for specific program modules.[3]

Referrals to the OZC are accepted if the person has a nonprogressive acquired brain injury, is aged between 16 and 60 years, and is medically stable. Funding is generally met by the local health authority or personal injury lawyers. Staffing comprises a multidisciplinary team with the clinical manager having an allied health (not medical) background. The team includes clinical psychologists (3.0 FTE), occupational therapists (2.5 FTE), speech and language therapists (1.5 FTE), and physiotherapists (1.0 FTE). The rehabilitation team is supported by psychology assistants (2.0 FTE), a rehabilitation assistant (1.0 FTE), and administrative support. A consultant neuropsychiatrist and a neurologist are available when required. The program caters to a maximum of eight clients at any one time, affording a staff-to-client ratio of approximately 1:1.

Upon referral to the OZC, the client and (usually) a family member participate in a 1-day assessment to determine whether the team is able to help the client and whether the client is willing to participate in the program. This is followed by a 2-week formal evaluation that includes administration of tests, interviews, questionnaires, and functional assessments. During this phase, the client also attends selected therapy groups, and the formal goal planning process commences. Each client is appointed an individual program coordinator, who meets regularly with the client to review goals and ensure the program is coordinated and meets the client's needs. The rehabilitation program itself is divided into two phases. The first intensive phase involves attendance for 4 or 5 days per week, followed by the reintegration phase, in which the client attends OZC for 2 or 3 days per week with the focus on establishing work experience, further education, and independent living skills as appropriate. The program, which runs from 10 AM to 4 PM, contains a mix of individual and group sessions. Group sessions are structured around the following themes: understanding brain injury, attention and goal management, memory, mood management, psychological support, communication and social skills, working with families, strategy application, and various other project-based and functional groups. Individual therapy sessions for specific cognitive, emotional, and social issues are driven by client need (see next section for specific therapeutic interventions).

Systematic Reviews of the Effectiveness of Psychological Rehabilitation at the Individual Level

The systems of rehabilitation described in the foregoing section use a range of specific interventions to treat the impairments and disabilities of the patients/clients. How are the best interventions to be identified in a world defined by a knowledge explosion? Sackett and colleagues (2000) advise that, for the busy clinician, a useful way to identify evidence-based interventions is to focus on systematic reviews in which the literature is already summarized. A search was conducted of PsycBITE (http://www.psycbite.com) and other electronic databases to identify systematic reviews of interventions for people with TBI (Tate & Rosenkoetter, submitted). More than 50 systematic reviews and meta-analyses involving people with TBI were identified, with approximately 30 being relevant to the present chapter in that they evaluated interventions for specific cognitive, behavioral, or emotional disorders for people with TBI in the post-acute stage (after emergence from PTA) or later; provided a critical appraisal of the included studies; and were published relatively recently (since 2000). These systematic reviews provide a lot of information regarding evidence-based interventions pertinent to rehabilitation psychology in TBI.

Results of the reviews are classified into interventions targeting cognitive impairments (viz., visuospatial, praxis, language/communication, attention, memory, and executive), behavioral deficits (both challenging behaviors and mood disturbances), and comprehensive-holistic interventions. Two of the 30 reviews specifically examined pediatric TBI (Laatsch et al., 2007; Limond & Leeke, 2005) and two addressed mild TBI (Holm et al., 2005; Snell, Surgenor, Hay-Smith, & Siegert, 2009). A number of reviews focused on rehabilitation service configuration (e.g., optimal timing of rehabilitation, length of stay, intensity of rehabilitation; Cullen et al., 2007; Turner-Stokes, Disler, Nair, & Wade, 2005). Reviews of neurorehabilitation strategies frequently focus on specific domains, and an important systematic review is that of Erlhardt et al. (2008), who examined the evidence for the best instructional procedures for people with acquired brain impairment. The value of this review lies in its applicability to all areas of neurorehabilitation, not just cognition or memory function. They reported on 51 studies that met selection criteria and recommended seven key instructional practices, as follows:

• Delineate target behaviors and/or use task analysis when training in multistep procedures.
• Limit errors (e.g., using errorless learning procedures) when acquiring new (or relearning) information/skills.
• Provide sufficient practice.
• Distribute practice.
• Vary stimuli (e.g., use multiple exemplars).
• Use strategies to promote effortful processing.
• Select and train for ecologically valid tasks.

COGNITIVE IMPAIRMENTS

Reviews of multiple cognitive domains identified a number of interventions with empirical evidence for their effectiveness. The earliest systematic reviews of cognitive rehabilitation interventions for TBI were those of Carney et al. (1999) and Chestnut et al. (1999), but these reviews are now dated. Cicerone and colleagues systematically reviewed the literature on cognitive interventions for TBI and stroke published up to 2008 (Cicerone et al., 2000, 2005; 2011), and their reviews are considered the most exhaustive search of the literature to date (Rohling, Faust, Beverly, & Demakis, 2009). Together, the three systematic reviews yielded 370 empirical intervention studies, of which 65 studies (18%) were Class I prospective RCTs and 54 (15%) were Class II studies with controls (including multiple-baseline across participants designs). The remaining two-thirds of the studies ($n = 251$, 68%), however, were uncontrolled Class III studies providing low levels of evidence. In making recommendations for clinical practice, Cicerone et al. took into account the strength of evidence afforded by the research designs of the studies they included. The individual studies in the Cicerone et al. (2000, 2005; 2011) reviews were categorized into the following cognitive domains: attention, visuospatial, apraxia, language/communication, memory, executive functioning/problem solving/awareness, and comprehensive-holistic cognitive rehabilitation. The systematic review of Rees et al. (2007), which identified 64 studies meeting selection criteria, focused on four domains of intervention (attention, memory, executive, and "general cognitive approaches") and additionally considered pharmacological treatments for these cognitive disorders.

In their 2011 report, Cicerone et al. concluded that "there is now sufficient information to support evidence-based clinical protocols, and to design and implement a comprehensive program of empirically supported treatments for cognitive disability after TBI and stroke" (p. 527).

Interventions for visuospatial, praxis, and language impairments are most commonly studied in stroke populations, in which such deficits occur more frequently than in the TBI population. The studies provide good evidence for their effectiveness, each being recommended as a practice standard. Although there are few RCTs of their application in TBI, when a patient has one of these problems, such an intervention may be helpful. Examples of RCTs providing Class I evidence in these areas include the classic study by Weinberg et al. (1977), who used a scanning machine to deliver graded visual stimuli to promote left-sided scanning; the work by Donkervoort, Dekker, Stehmann-Saris, and Deelman (2001), who treated apraxia with strategy training using internal and external compensations (e.g., self-verbalizations, pictorial sequences); and in treating aphasia, Pulvermüller et al.'s (2001) applied principles of constraint-induced practice for the massed practice of speech acts with which the patients experienced difficulty. Cognitive-communication disorders after TBI are common and are a new area of investigation. Cicerone et al. (2011) recommends such interventions as a practice standard. For example, Dahlberg et al. (2007) and McDonald et al. (2008) separately developed social skills training to improve interpersonal communication.

A targeted systematic review of communication interventions was conducted by Rispoli, Machalicek, and Lang (2010), searching the literature from 1980 to 2009. They identified 21 studies that met their criteria and which addressed seven communication skill areas (social conversation, labeling items, requests, receptive language, sentence construction, decreasing verbosity, and multiple skill areas). The authors applied rigorous criteria, finding that outcomes were conclusive in only four studies and were unable to be determined in the remaining 17 due to poor methodology (no experimental control), treatment effect not demonstrated, absence of sufficient data to replicate the study, or reliability of outcome assessment not established. Consequently, although 12 studies reported positive outcomes, only three of these were classified as providing a reliable result: (1) in patients with severe aphasia, augmented and alternative communication devises were effective in increasing sentence production (Koul, Corwin, & Hayes, 2004); (2) written scripts (graphic support) were effective in increasing conversation duration and number of exchanges in a patient with Broca's aphasia (Garrett & Huth, 2002); and (3) use of prompts increased correct verbal responding (labeling objects, food, etc.; Wesolowski, Zencius, McCarthy-Lydon, & Lydon, 2005). The authors concluded that "identification of a specific 'research-based best practice' is not possible" (p. 149), although at a more general level behavioral interventions were "potentially effective."

Attention interventions have been the subject of systematic reviews from a number of research groups (Cicerone et al., 2000, 2005; 2011; Park & Ingles, 2001; Rees et al., 2007; Riccio & French, 2004). All reviews are consistent in concluding that there is no evidence for the effectiveness of direct training methods (e.g., drill and practice often using computer programs to restore/strengthen the underlying impaired attention function). The Park and Ingles meta-analysis, which identified 30 eligible studies from their searches, found a small, statistically nonsignificant effect size (ES = 0.15). By contrast, strategy training for attention was more effective and classified as a practice standard by Cicerone and colleagues. The Park and Ingles review described the study of Kewman, Seigerman, Kinter, Chu, Henson, and Reeder (1985), who used a specific-skill approach to improve driving ability that specifically targeted attentional components relevant to driving and found a large effect size (ES = 1.15).

Memory treatments commonly involve use of compensatory techniques, either internal strategies or external aids. The Cicerone et al. (2000, 2005; 2011) reviews recommend strategy training as a practice standard for people with mild memory impairment. Other internal strategies, such as visual imagery, are also effective. Ownsworth and McFarland (1999), for example, used a combination

of internal strategies (self-instruction) and external compensations (diary use) that was found to be more effective than diary use alone in reducing (self-reported) memory problems. More specific guidance regarding internal strategies is provided from the meta-analysis of Kessels and de Haan (2003), who searched the literature to 2002 to compare the efficacy of two types training approaches: errorless learning and vanishing cues. Of 27 studies identified, 13 did not include control conditions, and, in the remaining studies, the effect size for the errorless learning method was large (ES = 0.87), whereas that for the vanishing cues method was small (ES = 0.27). The critical review of Clare and Jones (2008), however, identified variability in the findings of errorless learning studies and concluded that the evidence was strongest for people with severe memory impairment.

For moderate to severe impairments, memory interventions using external assistive devices are classified as a practice guideline by Cicerone et al. (2011). Wilson, Emslie, Quirk, and Evans (2001), for example, conducted a randomized cross-over trial using an externally directed portable pager and demonstrated that it was effective in improving completion of everyday activities in people with memory disorders, many of whom had failed to improve in previous memory rehabilitation programs. The recommendation of a practice guideline is supported by the systematic review of Sohlberg et al. (2007), who examined the literature to 2003 regarding the efficacy of external memory aids. They identified 21 eligible studies and made the same practice recommendation. Rees et al. (2007) also reported strong evidence for the use of internal strategies and external aids. Rees et al. additionally considered studies examining the traditional "memory group" as an intervention and concluded that the available evidence was *not* supportive of their efficacy in terms of improving memory function.

Interventions for *executive impairments* using problem-solving strategy training were previously recommended as a practice guideline (Cicerone et al., 2005), and Rees et al. (2007) also concluded that there was moderate evidence for goal management training. The more recent review by Kennedy et al. (2008), who reviewed 15 eligible studies, suggested that meta-cognitive training, which focuses exclusively on aspects of executive functioning involved in organization, planning, problem-solving, and multitasking, should be considered a practice standard for young to middle-aged adults with TBI when the goal is improvement in everyday, functional tasks, and this practice standard has been confirmed in the 2011 updated review of Cicerone et al. Von Cramon, Mathes-von Cramon, and Mai (1991), for example, developed a meta-cognitive strategy training program, with specific modules in which patients were trained to analyze tasks by breaking down problems into small steps. Participants receiving the strategy training showed greater improvements than did those participating in a control (memory) treatment. The Kennedy et al. (2008) review also conducted meta-analyses. Similar effect sizes were found for both the strategy (mean ES = 0.41) and control (mean ES = 0.37) conditions for outcomes measured at the impairment level; however, for outcomes measured at the activity/participation level, the strategy condition had a significantly larger effect size than did the control condition (mean ES = 0.57 and 0.38, respectively).

The intervention literature on self-awareness was reviewed by Fleming and Ownsworth (2006), but they found that very few interventions specifically designed to address self-awareness had been rigorously tested for their treatment effectiveness of self-awareness per se. Cicerone et al. (2011) updated the available evidence regarding the effectiveness of meta-cognitive strategy training to increase awareness and recommended this as a practice standard. As noted in the section describing interventions for language impairments, Cicerone et al. (2011) recommended social communication skills interventions as a practice standard for treating interpersonal and pragmatic communication impairments.

IMPAIRMENTS IN BEHAVIOR AND EMOTION

Interventions for problems with *behavior regulation* were addressed in the reviews of Ylvisaker et al. (2007) and Cattelani, Zettin and Zoccolotti (2010), and the latter review additionally addressed the broader domain of psychosocial functioning. The types of treatments were classified by Cattelani et al. as follows:

- Interventions using the clinical application of learning theory (applied behavior analysis), including (i) contingency management using operant procedures to addresses consequences of behavior, such as verbal praise, token economies, time out, response cost; and (ii) positive behavioral supports targeting antecedents of behaviors using techniques resulting in skill acquisition, such as fading, shaping, feedback, stress inoculation, redirection, planned assurance

- Cognitive-behavioural therapy (CBT) using techniques such as education, cognitive restructuring, self-monitoring, self-talk training
- Comprehensive holistic interventions (for emotional and psychosocial functioning rather than challenging behaviors per se—the components of the Cattelani review addressing this area are considered in the section below on comprehensive, holistic rehabilitation).

Cattelani et al. (2010) identified 63 studies meeting selection criteria. The more focused review of Ylvisaker et al. (2007) addressed interventions using applied behavior analysis. Both contingency management procedures and positive behavioral supports were examined, yielding 65 studies with 172 participants. Only two class I RCTs were identified. An example of contingency management procedures was given in the study of Alderman, Fry, and Youngson (1995), who implemented a reversal (A-B-A-B) design using response-cost and successfully treated repetitive verbal utterances in a patient with encephalitis. In terms of addressing antecedents, Medd and Tate (2000), for example, successfully treated anger management problems in an RCT by using positive behavior supports and CBT strategies, including education, self-awareness training, stress inoculation training, and anger management strategies.

Both reviews noted that, in spite of the large number of studies reviewed, "serious methodological concerns weaken this body of evidence" (Ylvisaker et al., 2007, p. 780) and consequently recommended contingency management and positive behavior supports as practice options, although Ylvisaker et al. concluded that "behavioral interventions (not otherwise specified)" met criteria for a practice guideline.

The Ylvisaker et al. (2007) review commented on the poverty of studies of "internalizing disorders" (such as apathy, poor motivation, withdrawal, lack of initiative). Two systematic reviews by Lane-Brown and Tate (2009a, 2009b) have examined the evidence for apathy treatments. In a Cochrane systematic review of RCTs for apathy (Lane-Brown & Tate, 2009a), a single RCT was identified, but no evidence was provided to support use of the intervention (cranial electrotherapy stimulation). A second review (Lane-Brown & Tate, 2009b) examined a broader range of neurological conditions and research designs, including single-participant designs, and identified 28 studies, four of which addressed apathy in patients with TBI. For example, Burke, Zencius, Wesolowski, and Doubleday

(1991) successfully used self-initiation checklists in patients with TBI who exhibited multiple neuropsychological impairments, including poor initiation, a component of apathy.

Treatments for *emotional disorders* are, given their frequent occurrence, surprisingly sparse, with only two systematic reviews being identified from PsycBITE, albeit they addressed the most common emotional consequences, depression (Fann, Hart, & Schomer, 2009) and anxiety (Soo & Tate, 2007). Fann et al. considered both pharmacological and psychological treatments. They identified 27 studies meeting criteria, 19 using pharmacological or other biological interventions and eight using behavioral treatments. They found evidence to support use of selective serotonin reuptake inhibitors as antidepressant medication (specifically Sertraline, 25–150 mg/day). The eight nonpharmacological treatment studies were limited in that none was designed specifically to treat depression (although depression was one of the outcome areas in each study). The review thus concluded that there was insufficient evidence to support general psychotherapeutic/rehabilitation programs as a treatment for depression after TBI. In their Cochrane systematic review, Soo and Tate (2007) focused on nonpharmacological treatments for anxiety and identified three RCTs. They concluded that there was some evidence for the efficacy of CBT and neurorehabilitation for treating anxiety symptomatology after TBI. For example, Byrant, Moulds, Guthrie, and Nixon (2003) treated acute anxiety disorder in patients with mild TBI using CBT techniques.

COMPREHENSIVE–HOLISTIC INTERVENTIONS

For people with moderate to severe TBI, comprehensive–holistic interventions were classified as a practice guideline by Cicerone et al. (2005): in two class II controlled studies, the U.S.-based programs of the New York Brain Injury Day Treatment Program (Rattock et al., 1992) and Barrow Neurological Institute (Prigatano et al., 1984) were shown to be effective compared with standard treatment or no treatment, respectively. The review of Cattelani et al. (2010) upgraded the evidence to a practice standard, as did Cicerone et al. (2011). Included in their reviews was the RCT of Cicerone et al. (2008), who examined the efficacy of a 240-hour program conducted over 4 months to provide intensive and integrated interventions targeting cognitive, interpersonal, and functional deficits within a therapeutic environment. The program

resulted in greater gains in community integration (ES = 0.59) and QOL (ES = 0.30) than did standard neurorehabilitation, and gains were maintained at 6 months. Yet, the recommendation of Cattelani et al. and Cicerone et al. (2011) is at variation with that drawn by Geurtsen, van Heugten, Martina, and Geurts (2010), who examined 13 studies meeting criteria for their systematic review of comprehensive rehabilitation programs for severe brain injury. Notwithstanding the positive results of the Cicerone et al. (2008) RCT, taking all studies into account, Geurtsen and colleagues concluded that the evidence in this area remained insufficient to make a definitive practice recommendation.

The integrated approach to rehabilitation characterizing the comprehensive–holistic program is in stark contrast to isolated "cognitive retaining" exercises, which are generally delivered via computer programs. Rees et al. (2007) concluded that there was some limited evidence indicating that such interventions were *not* effective; Cicerone et al. (2011) made a more definitive statement concluding that "sole reliance on repeated use of computer-based tasks without some involvement and intervention by a therapist is not recommended". (p. 522).

Conclusion

It is well recognized that the neuropsychological consequences of TBI, in large part, restrict social participation and community integration. A comprehensive armamentarium of appropriate instruments is currently available to measure such consequences. Additionally, a large number of clinical trials have been conducted over the past three decades, the results of which are synthesized in systematic reviews described in this chapter. Although the literature suggests that further work still lies ahead, the major gaps have certainly been identified. Moreover, therapies are available that systematic reviews have recommended at the level of practice guidelines and standards and these interventions have the potential to improve the functioning and outcomes of people with TBI and their families. This is an exciting time for rehabilitation psychology in the field of TBI. The clinician has sound information about the effectiveness of a range of evidence-based interventions and researchers have their work cut out for them to improve that evidence base.

Notes

1. There is some variation in the literature regarding the description of levels of evidence. Many systematic reviews in the neurorehabilitation literature (including reviews cited in this

chapter) simply refer to three classes of evidence: Class I, RCTs; class II, controlled clinical trials that are not randomized or RCTs with flaws; and class III, case series. Some systematic reviews also include single-participant designs with control conditions (e.g., multiple baseline designs) as class II evidence.

2. A useful resource for accessing reporting guidelines for various research designs is the EQUATOR Network (http://www.equator-network.org/); see also Tate and Douglas (2011).

3. Another resource that also contains practical worksheets and strategy lists for the rehabilitation of cognitive, behavioral, and emotional sequelae of acquired brain injury is Sohlberg and Mateer (2001).

References

Adams, J. H., Gennarelli, T. A., & Graham, D. I. (1982). Brain damage in non-missile head injury: Observations in man and subhuman primates. In W. T. Smith & J. B. Cavanagh (Eds.), *Recent advances in neuropathology* (vol. 2, pp. 165–190). Edinburgh: Churchill-Livingstone.

Alderman, N., Fry, R. K., & Youngson, H. A. (1995). Improvement of self-monitoring skills, reduction of behaviour disturbance and the dysexecutive syndrome: Comparison of response cost and a new programme of self-monitoring training. *Neuropsychological Rehabilitation, 5*(3), 193–221.

Anderson, M. I., Simpson, G. K., Morey, P. J., Mok, M. M., Gosling, T. J., & Gillett, L. E. (2009). Differential pathways of psychological distress in spouses vs parents of people with severe traumatic brain injury (TBI): Multi-group analysis. *Brain Injury, 23*(12), 931–943.

Barlow, D. H., Nock, M. K., & Hersen, M. (2009). *Single case experimental designs: Strategies for studying behavior change* (3rd ed.). Boston: Pearson Education, Inc.

Ben-Yishay, Y. (Ed.). (1978). *Working approaches to remediation of cognitive deficits in brain damaged persons*. Rehabilitation Monograph No.59, New York: New York University Medical Centre.

Bernabeu, M., Laxe, S., Lopez, R., Stucki, G., Ward, A., Barnes, M., et al. (2009). Developing core sets for persons with traumatic brain injury based on the International Classification of Functioning, Disability and Health. *Neurorehabilitation and Neural Repair, 23*(5), 464–467.

Blais, M. C., & Boisvert, J-M. (2005). Psychological and marital adjustment in couples following a traumatic brain injury (TBI): A critical review. *Brain Injury, 19*(14), 1223–1235.

Boschen, K., Gargaro, J., Gan, C., Gerber, G., & Brandys, C. (2007). Family interventions after acquired brain injury and other chronic conditions: A critical appraisal of the quality of evidence. *NeuroRehabilitation, 22*, 19–41.

British Paediatric Neurological Association (2001). *Child's Glasgow Coma Scale*. Retrieved 15 February, 2012, from http://www.bpna.org.uk/audit/GCS.PDF

Bruyère, S. M., Van Looy, S. A., & Peterson, D. B. (2005). The International Classification of Functioning, Disability and Health: Contemporary literature overview. *Rehabilitation Psychology, 50*(2), 113–121.

Burke, W. H., Zencius, A. H., Wesolowski, M. D., & Doubleday, F. (1991). Improving executive function disorders in brain-injured clients. *Brain Injury, 5*(3), 241–252.

Byrant, R. A., Moulds, M., Guthrie, R., & Nixon, R. D. V. (2003). Treating acute distress disorder following mild traumatic brain injury. *The American Journal of Psychiatry, 160*(3), 585–587.

Carney, N., Chestnut, R. M., Maynard, H., Mann, N. C., Patterson, P., & Helfand, M. (1999). Effect of cognitive rehabilitation on outcomes for persons with traumatic brain injury: A systematic review. *Journal of Head Trauma Rehabilitation, 14*(3), 277–307.

Carroll, L. J., Cassidy, J. D., Holm, L., Kraus, J., & Coronado, V. G. (2004). Methodological issues and research recommendations for mild traumatic brain injury: The WHO Collaborating Centre Task Force on mild traumatic brain injury. *Journal of Rehabilitation Medicine, 43*(Suppl.), 113–125.

Cattelani, R., Zettin, M., & Zoccolotti, P. (2010). Rehabilitation treatments for adults with behavioral and psychosocial disorders following acquired brain injury: A systematic review. *Neuropsychology Review, 20*(1), 52–85.

Chestnut, R. M., Carney, N., Maynard, H., Mann, N. C., Patterson, P., & Helfand, M. (1999). Summary report: Evidence for the effectiveness of rehabilitation for persons with traumatic brain injury. *Journal of Head Trauma Rehabilitation, 14*(2), 176–188.

Christensen, A-L., & Uzzell, B. P. (Eds.). (2000). *International handbook of neuropsychological rehabilitation*. New York: Klewer Academic.

Cicerone, K. D., Dahlberg, C., Kalmar, K., Langenbahn, D. M., Malec, J. F., Berquist, T. F., et al. (2000). Evidence-based cognitive rehabilitation: Recommendations for clinical practice. *Archives of Physical Medicine and Rehabilitation, 81*, 1596–1615.

Cicerone, K. D., Dahlberg, C., Malec, J. F., Langenbahn, D. M., Felicetti, T., Kneipp, S., et al. (2005). Evidence-based cognitive rehabilitation: Updated review of the literature from 1998 through 2002. *Archives of Physical Medicine and Rehabilitation, 86*, 1681–1692.

Cicerone, K. D., Langenbahn, D. M., Braden, C., Malec, J. F., Kalmar, K., Fraas, M., et al. (2011). Evidence-based cognitive rehabilitation: Updated review of the literature from 2003 through 2008. *Archives of Physical Medicine and Rehabilitation, 92*, 519–530.

Cicerone, K. D., Mott, T., Azulay, J., Sharlow-Galella, M. A., Ellmo, W. J., Paradise, S, & Friel, J. C. (2008). A randomized controlled trial of holistic neuropsychologic rehabilitation after traumatic brain injury. *Archives of Physical Medicine and Rehabilitation, 89*, 2239–2249.

Clare, L., & Jones, R. S. P. (2008). Errorless learning in the rehabilitation of memory impairment: A critical review. *Neuropsychology Review, 18*, 1–23.

Corrigan, J. D., Selassie, A. W., & Orman, J. A. (2010). The epidemiology of traumatic brain injury. *Journal of Head Trauma Rehabilitation, 25*(2), 72–80.

Cullen, N., Chundamala, J., Bayley, M., & Jutai, J. (2007). The efficacy of acquired brain injury rehabilitation. *Brain Injury, 21*(2), 113–132.

Dahlberg, C., Cusick, C. P., Hawley, L., Newman, J. K., Morey, C. E., Harrison-Felix, C. L., & Whiteneck, G. G. (2007). Treatment efficacy of social communication skills training after traumatic brain injury: A randomized treatment and deferred treatment controlled trial. *Archives of Physical Medicine and Rehabilitation, 88*, 1561–1573.

Dann, M. D. (1984). Loss of self. *Journal of Cognitive Rehabilitation, 2*, 11–12.

Dijkers, M. P., Harrison-Felix, C., & Marwitz, J. H. (2010). The Traumatic Brain Injury Model Systems: History and contributions to clinical service and research. *Journal of Head Trauma Rehabilitation, 25*(2), 81–91.

Dikmen, S. S., Ross, B. L., Machamer, J. E., & Temkin, N. R. (1995). One year psychosocial outcome in head injury. *Journal of the International Neuropsychological Society, 1,* 67–77.

Donkervoort, M., Dekker, J., Stehmann-Saris, F. C., & Deelman, B. G. (2001). Efficacy of strategy training in left hemisphere stroke patients with apraxia: A randomized clinical trial. *Neuropsychological Rehabilitation, 11,* 549–566.

Draper, K., Ponsford, J., & Schönberger, M. (2007). Psychosocial and emotional outcomes 10 years following traumatic brain injury. *Journal of Head Trauma Rehabilitation, 22*(5), 278–287.

Eker, C., Schalén, W., Asgeirsson, B., Grände, P.-O., Ranstam, J., & Nordström, C.-H. (2000). Reduced mortality after severe head injury will increase the demands for rehabilitation services. *Brain Injury, 14*(7), 605–619.

Erlhardt, L. A., Sohlberg, M. M., Kennedy, M., Coelho, C., Ylvisaker, M., Turkstra, L., & Yorkston, K. (2008). Evidence-based practice guidelines for instructing individuals with neurogenic memory impairments: What have we learned in the past 20 years? *Neuropsychological Rehabilitation, 18*(3), 300–342.

Eslinger, P. (Ed.). (2002). *Neuropsychological interventions. Clinical research and practice.* New York: Guildford.

Ewing-Cobbs, L., Levin, H. S., Fletcher, J. M., Miner, M. E., & Eisenberg, H. M. (1990). The Children's Orientation and Amnesia Test: Relationship to severity of acute head injury and to recovery of memory. *Neurosurgery, 27*(5), 683–691.

Fann, J. R., Hart, T., & Schomer, K. G. (2009). Treatment for depression after traumatic brain injury: A systematic review. *Journal of Neurotrauma, 26*(12), 2383–2402.

Fleming, J. M., & Ownsworth, T. (2006). A review of awareness interventions in brain injury rehabilitation. *Neuropsychological Rehabilitation, 16*(4), 474–500.

French, L. M., & Parkinson, G. W. (2008). Assessing and treating veterans with traumatic brain injury. *Journal of Clinical Psychology, 64,* 1004–1013.

Garrett, K. L., & Huth, C. (2002). The impact of graphic contextual information and instruction on the conversational behaviours of a person with severe aphasia. *Aphasiology, 16*(4/5/6), 523–536.

Geurtsen, G. J., van Heugten, C. M., Martina, J. D., & Geurts, A. C. H. (2010). Comprehensive rehabilitation programmes in the chronic phase after severe brain injury: A systematic review. *Journal of Rehabilitation Medicine, 42*(2), 97–110.

Geyh, S., Cieza, A., Schouten, J., Dickson, H., Frommelt, P., Zaliha, O., Kostanjsek, N., Ring, H., & Stucki, G. (2004). ICF core sets for stroke. *Journal of Rehabilitation Medicine, 44*(Suppl), 135–141.

Giacino, J. T., Ashwal, S., Childs, N., Cranford, R., Jennett, B., Katz, D. I., et al. (2002). The minimally conscious state: Definition and diagnostic criteria. *Neurology, 58*(3), 349–353.

Giacino, J. T., & Kalmar, K. (1997). The vegetative and minimally conscious states: A comparison of clinical features and functional outcome. *Journal of Head Trauma Rehabilitation, 12*(4), 36–51.

Goldstein, M. (1990). Editorial. Traumatic brain injury: A silent epidemic. *Annals of Neurology, 27*(3), 327.

Gordon, W. A., Zafonte, R., Cicerone, K., Cantor, J., Brown, M., Lombard, L., Goldsmith, R., & Chandna, T. (2006). Traumatic brain injury rehabilitation: State of the science. *American Journal of Physical Medicine and Rehabilitation, 85,* 343–382.

Graham, S. (1985). Something more valuable than life. *Journal of Cognitive Rehabilitation, 3,* 4–6.

Guyatt, G., Jaeschke, R., & McGinn, T. (2002). *N-of-1 randomized controlled trials.* In G Guyatt, D Rennie, MO Meade, & DJ Cook (Eds). *Users' guide to the medical literature: A manual for evidence-based clinical practice* (2nd ed., pp.179–192). New York: McGrawHill Medical and American Medical Association.

Guyatt, G., Sackett, D., Taylor, D. W., Chong, J., Roberts, R., & Pugsley, S. (1986). Determining optimal therapy—randomised trials in individual patients. *The New England Journal of Medicine, 314*(14), 889–892.

Herbert, R., Moseley, A., & Sherrington, C. (1998/99). PEDro: A database of RCTs in physiotherapy. *Health Information Management, 28,* 186–188.

Holm, L., Cassidy, J. D., Carroll, L. J., & Borg, J. (2005). Summary of the WHO collaborating centre for neurotrauma task force on mild traumatic brain injury. *Journal of Rehabilitation Medicine, 37,* 137–141.

Hoofien, D., Gilboa, A., Vakil, E., & Donovick, P. J. (2001). Traumatic brain injury (TBI) 10–20 years later: A comprehensive outcome study of psychiatric symptomatology, cognitive abilities and psychosocial functioning. *Brain Injury, 15*(3), 189–209.

Howick, J., Chalmers, I., Glasziou, P., Greenhalgh, T., Heneghan, C., Liberati, A., & Thornton, H. (2011). The 2011 Oxford CEBM evidence table (introductory document). *Oxford Centre for Evidence-Based Medicine.* Retrieved from http://www.cebm.net/index.aspx?o = 5653

Jennett, B., Bond, M. (1975). Assessment of outcome after severe brain damage. A practical scale. *Lancet, i*(1), 480–484.

Jennett, B., Snoek, J., Bond, M. R., & Brooks, N. (1981). Disability after severe head injury: Observations on the use of the Glasgow Outcome Scale. *Journal of Neurology, Neurosurgery, and Psychiatry, 44,* 285–293.

Jennett, B., & Teasdale, G. (1981). *Management of head injuries.* Philadelphia: F. A. Davis Company.

Kazdin, A. E. (2011). *Single-case research designs: Methods for clinical and applied settings* (2nd ed.). New York: Oxford University Press.

Katz, D. I. (1992). Neuropathology and neurobehavioral recovery from closed head injury. *Journal of Head Trauma Rehabilitation, 7*(2), 1–15.

Kennedy, M. R., Turkstra, L. (2006). Group intervention studies in the cognitive rehabilitation of individuals with traumatic brain injury: Challenges faced by researchers. *Neuropsychology Review, 16,* 151–159.

Kennedy, M. R. T., Coelho, C., Turkstra, L., Ylvisaker, M., Sohlberg, M. M., Yorkston, K., et al. (2008). Intervention for executive functions after traumatic brain injury: A systematic review, meta-analysis and clinical recommendations. *Neuropsychological Rehabilitation, 18*(3), 257–299.

Kessels, R. P. C., & de Haan, E. H. F. (2003). Implicit learning in memory rehabilitation: A meta-analysis on errorless learning and vanishing cues methods. *Journal of Clinical and Experimental Neuropsychology, 25*(6), 805–814.

Kewman, D. G., Seigerman, C., Kintner, H., Chu, S., Henson, D., & Reeder, C. (1985). Simulation training of psychomotor skills: Teaching the brain-injured to drive. *Rehabilitation Psychology, 30*(1), 11–27.

King, N. S., Crawford, S., Wenden, F. J., Moss, N. E. G., Wade, D. T., & Caldwell, F. E. (1997). Measurement of posttraumatic amnesia: How reliable is it? *Journal of Neurology, Neurosurgery and Psychiatry, 62,* 38–42.

Koenig, C. (2008). *Paper cranes. A mother's story of hope, courage and determination*. Auckland: Exile Publishing Ltd.

Koskinen, S., Hokkinen, E-M., Sarajuuri, J., & Alaranta, H. (2007). Applicability of the ICF Checklist to traumatically brain-injured patients in post-acute rehabilitation settings. *Journal of Rehabilitation Medicine, 39,* 467–472.

Koul, R., Corwin, M., & Hayes, S. (2004). Production of graphic symbol sentences by individuals with aphasia: Efficacy of a computer-based augmentative and alternative communication intervention. *Brain and Language, 92,* 58–77.

Kraus, J. F., Black, M. A., Hessol, N., Ley, P., Rokaw, W., Sullivan, C., et al. (1984). The incidence of acute brain injury and serious impairment in a defined population. *American Journal of Epidemiology, 119*(2), 186–201.

Kraus, J. F., & McArthur, D. L. (1996). Epidemiologic aspects of brain injury. *Neurologic Clinics, 14*(2), 435–450.

Kreutzer, J. S., Marwitz, J. H., Godwin, E. E., & Arango-Lasprilla, J. C. (2010). Practical approaches to effective family intervention after brain injury. *Journal of Head Trauma Rehabilitation, 25*(2), 113–120.

Laatsch, L., Harrington, D., Hotz, G., Marcantuono, J., Mozzoni, M. P., Walsh, V., & Hersey, K. P. (2007). An evidence-based review of cognitive and behavioral rehabilitation treatment studies in children with acquired brain injury. *Journal of Head Trauma Rehabilitation, 22*(4), 248–256.

Lammi, M. H., Smith, V. H., Tate, R. L., & Taylor, C. M. (2005). The minimally conscious state and recovery potential: A follow-up study 2–5 years after traumatic brain injury. *Archives of Physical Medicine and Rehabilitation. 86,* 746–754.

Lane-Brown, A., & Tate, R. (2009a). Interventions for apathy after traumatic brain injury. *Cochrane Database of Systematic Reviews, 2,* CD006341.

Lane-Brown, A. T., & Tate, R. L. (2009b). Apathy after acquired brain impairment: A systematic review of non-pharmacological interventions. *Neuropsychological Rehabilitation, 19*(4), 481–516.

Levin, H. S., O'Donnell, V. M., & Grossman, R. G. (1979). The Galveston Orientation and Amnesia Test. A practical scale to assess cognition after head injury. *Journal of Nervous and Mental Disease, 167*(11), 675–684.

Lezak, M. D., Howieson, D. B., & Loring, D. W. (2004). *Neuropsychological assessment* (4th ed.). Oxford: Oxford University Press.

Limond, J., & Leeke, R. (2005). Practitioner review: Cognitive rehabilitation for children with acquired brain injury. *Journal of Child Psychology and Psychiatry, 46,* 339–352.

Maher, C. G., Sherrington, C., Herbert, R. D., Moseley, A. M., & Elkins, M. (2003). Reliability of the PEDro scale for rating quality of RCTs. *Physical Therapy, 83,* 713–721.

Malec, J. F. (1999). Goal attainment scaling in rehabilitation. *Neuropsychological Rehabilitation, 9*(3/4), 253–275.

Malec, J. F., Smigielski, J. S., & DePompolo, R. W. (1991). Goal attainment scaling and outcome measurement in postacute brain injury rehabilitation. *Archives of Physical Medicine and Rehabilitation, 72,* 138–143.

McDonald, S., Tate, R., Togher, L., Bornhofen, C., Long, E., Gertler, P., & Bowen, R. (2008). Social skills treatment for people with severe, chronic acquired brain injuries: A multicentre trial. *Archives of Physical Medicine and Rehabilitation, 89,* 1648–1659.

McMillan, T. M., & Sparkes, C. (1999). Goal planning and neurorehabilitation: The Wolfson Neurorehabilitation Centre approach. *Neuropsychological Rehabilitation, 9*(3/4), 241–251.

McMillan, T. M., Jongen, E. L. M. M., & Greenwood, R. J. (1996). Assessment of post-traumatic amnesia after severe closed head injury: Retrospective or prospective? *Journal of Neurology, Neurosurgery and Psychiatry, 60,* 422–427.

Medd, J., & Tate, R. L. (2000). Evaluation of an anger management therapy programme following acquired brain injury: A preliminary study. *Neuropsychological Rehabilitation. 10,* 185–201.

Moher, D., Liberati, A., Tetzlaff, J., Altman, D. G., & the PRISMA group. (2009). Preferred reporting items for systematic reviews and meta-analyses: The PRISMA statement. *PLoS Medicine, 6*(7), e1000097.

Moseley, A., Sherrington, C., Herbert. R., & Maher, C. (2000). The extent and quality of evidence in neurological physiotherapy: An analysis of the Physiotherapy Evidence Database (PEDro). *Brain Impairment, 1*(2), 130–140.

Nakase-Richardson, R., Sherer, M., Seel, R. T. Hart, T., Hanks, R., Arango-Lasprilla, J. C., et al. (2011). Utility of post-traumatic amnesia in predicting 1-year productivity following traumatic brain injury: Comparison of the Russell and Mississippi PTA classification levels. *Journal of Neurology, Neurosurgery and Psychiatry.* [E-published ahead of print, January 17, 2011.] doi 10.1136/jnnp.2010. 222489.

Oddy, M., & Herbert, C. (2003). Intervention with families following brain injury: Evidence-based practice. *Neuropsychological Rehabilitation, 13*(1/2), 259–273.

Olver, J. H., Ponsford, J. L., & Curran, C. A. (1996). Outcome following traumatic brain injury. A comparison between 2 and 5 years after injury. *Brain Injury, 10*(11), 841–848.

Osborn, C. L. (1998). *Over my head. A doctor's own story of head injury from the inside looking out.* Kansas City, MO: Andrews McMeel Publishing.

Ottenbacher, K. J., & Cusick, A. (1990). Goal attainment scaling as a method of clinical service evaluation. *The American Journal of Occupational Therapy. 44*(6), 519–525.

Ownsworth, T. L., & Fleming, J. (Eds.) (2011). Adopting a growth perspective in brain injury research: theoretical perspectives and empirical findings. *Special issue of Brain Impairment. 12*(2).

Ownsworth, T. L., & McFarland, K. (1999). Memory remediation in long-term acquired brain injury: Two approaches to diary training. *Brain Injury, 13*(8), 605–626.

Park, N. W., & Ingles, J. L. (2001). Effectiveness of attention rehabilitation after an acquired brain injury: A meta-analysis. *Neuropsychology, 15*(2), 199–210.

Perdices, M., Schultz, R., Tate, R., McDonald, S., Togher, L., Savage, S., Winders, K., & Smith, K. (2006). The evidence base of neuropsychological rehabilitation in acquired brain impairment (ABI): How good is the research? *Brain Impairment, 7*(2), 119–132.

Perdices, M., & Tate, R. L. (2009). Single-subject designs as a tool for evidence-based clinical practice: Are they unrecognised and undervalued? *Neuropsychological Rehabilitation. 19*(6), 904–927.

Perlesz, A., Kinsella, G., & Crowe, S. (1999). Impact of traumatic brain injury on the family: A critical review. *Rehabilitation Psychology, 44*(1), 6–35.

Ponsford, J. (Ed.). (2004). *Cognitive and behavioral rehabilitation: From neurobiology to clinical practice.* New York: Guildford.

Ponsford, J. L., Olver, J. H., & Curran, C. (2012). A profile of outcome 2 years after traumatic brain injury. *Brain Injury, 9*(1), 1–10.

Ponsford, J., Sloan, S., & Snow, P. (2012). *Traumatic brain injury: Rehabilitation for everyday adaptive living* (2nd ed.). Hove, UK: Psychology Press.

Prigatano, G. P., Fordyce, D. J., Zeiner, H. K., Rouche, J. R., Pepping, M., & Wood, B. C. (1984). Neuropsychologial rehabilitation after closed head injury in young adults. *Journal of Neurology, Neurosurgery and Psychiatry, 47*, 505–513.

Prigatano, G. P. (1999). *Principles of neuropsychological rehabilitation.* New York: Oxford University Press.

Pulvermüller, F., Neininger, B., Elbert, T., Mohr, B., Rockstroh, B., Koebbel, P., & Taub, E. (2001). Constraint-induced therapy of chronic aphasia after stroke. *Stroke, 32*, 1621–1626.

Rattock, J., Ben-Yishay, Y., Ezrachi, O., Lakin, P., Piastetsky, E., Ross, B., et al. (1992). Outcome of different treatment mixes in a multidimensional rehabilitation program. *Neuropsychology, 6*, 395–415.

Rees, L., Marshall, S., Hartridge, C., Mackie, D., Weiser, M., for the ERABI Group. (2007). Cognitive interventions post acquired brain injury. *Brain Injury, 21*(2), 161–200.

Riccio, C. A., & French, C. L. (2004). The status of empirical support for treatments of attention deficits. *The Clinical Neuropsychologist, 18*, 528–558.

Rispoli, M. J., Machalicek, W., & Lang, R. (2010). Communication interventions for individuals with acquired brain injury. *Developmental Neurorehabilitation, 13*(2), 141–151.

Rocca, A., Wallen, M., & Batchelor, J. (2008). The Westmead Post-traumatic Amnesia Scale for Children (WPTAS-C) aged 4 and 5 years old. *Brain Impairment, 9*(1), 14–21.

Rohling, M. L., Faust, M. E., Beverly, B., & Demakis, G. (2009). Effectiveness of cognitive rehabilitation following acquired brain injury: A meta-analytic re-examination of Cicerone et al.'s (2000, 2005) systematic reviews. *Neuropsychology, 23*(1), 20–39.

Russell, W. R., & Smith, A. (1961). Post-traumatic amnesia in closed head injury. *Archives of Neurology, 5*, 16–29.

Sackett, D. L., Straus, S. E., Richardson, W. S., Rosenberg, W., & Haynes, R. B. (2000). *Evidence-based medicine. How to practice and teach EBM* (2nd ed.). Edinburgh: Churchill-Livingstone.

Salazar, A. M., Schwab, K., & Grafman, J. H. (1995). Penetrating injuries in the Vietnam war. Traumatic unconsciousness, epilepsy, and psychosocial outcome. *Neurosurgery Clinics of North America, 6*, 715–726.

Simpson, D. A., Cockington, R. A., Hanieh, A., Raftos, J., & Reilly, P. L. (1991). Head injuries in infants and young children: The value of the Pediatric Coma Scale. *Child's Nervous System, 7*, 183–190.

Simpson, G., Secheny, T., Lane-Brown, A., Strettles, B., Ferry K., & Phillips, J. (2004). Post-acute rehabilitation for people with traumatic brain injury: A model description and evaluation of the Liverpool Hospital Transitional Living Program. *Brain Impairment, 5*(1), 67–80.

Sinnakaruppan, I., & Williams, D. M. (2001). Family carers and the adult head-injured: A critical review of carers' needs. *Brain Injury, 15*(8), 653–672.

Shea, B. J., Grimshaw, J. M., Wells, G. A., Boers, M., Andersson, N., Hamel, C., et al. (2007). Development of AMSTAR: A measurement tool to assess the methodological quality of systematic reviews. *BioMed Central Medical Research Methodology, 7*, 10.

Shores, E., A., Marosszeky, J. E., Sandanam, J., & Batchelor, J. (1986). Preliminary validation of a clinical scale for measuring the duration of post-traumatic amnesia. *Medical Journal of Australia, 144*(11), 569–572.

Sohlberg, M. M., Kennedy, M., Avery, J., Coelho, C., Turkstra, L., Ylvisaker, M., & Yorkston, K. (2007). Evidence-based practice for the use of external aids as memory compensation technique. *Journal of Medical Speech-Language Pathology, 15*(1), xv–li.

Sohlberg, M. M., & Mateer, C. A. (2001). *Cognitive rehabilitation. An integrative neuropsychological approach.* New York: Guildford.

Soo, C., & Tate, R. (2007). Psychological treatment for anxiety in people with traumatic brain injury. *Cochrane Database of Systematic Reviews, 3*, CD005239.

Snell, D. L., Surgenor, L. J., Hay-Smith, E. J. C., & Siegert, R. J. (2009). A systematic review of psychological treatments for mild traumatic brain injury: An update on the evidence. *Journal of Clinical and Experimental Neuropsychology, 31*(1), 20–38.

Stier-Jarmer, M., Grill, E., Ewert, T., Bartholomeyczik, S., Finger, M., Mokrusch, T., Kostanjsek, N., & Stucki, G. (2005). ICF Core Set for patients with neurological conditions in early post-acute rehabilitation facilities. *Disability and Rehabilitation, 27*(7/8), 389–395.

Stroke Unit Trialists' Collaboration. (2007). Organised inpatient (stroke unit) care for stroke. *Cochrane Database of Systematic Reviews, 4*, CD000197.

Stuss, D. T., & Buckle, L. (1992). Traumatic brain injury: Neuropsychological deficits and evaluation at different stages of recovery and in different pathologic subtypes. *The Journal of Head Trauma Rehabilitation, 7(2)*, 40–49.

Tate, R. L. (2010). *A compendium of tests, scales and questionnaires: The practitioner's guide to measuring outcomes after acquired brain impairment.* Hove, UK: Psychology Press.

Tate, R. L., & Rosenkoetter U. (submitted). Interventions for treating consequences of traumatic brain injury: What systematic reviews tell us.

Tate, R. L., Broe, G. A., Cameron, I. D., Hodgkinson, A. E., & Soo, C. A. (2005). Pre-injury, injury and early post-injury predictors of long-term functional and psychosocial recovery after severe traumatic brain injury. *Brain Impairment, 6*(2), 75–89.

Tate, R. L., & Douglas, J. (2011). Special editorial. Use of reporting guidelines in scientific writing: PRISMA, CONSORT, STROBE, STARD and other resources. *Brain Impairment, 12*(1), 1–21.

Tate, R. L., McDonald, S., & Lulham, J. M. (1998). Incidence of hospital-treated traumatic brain injury in an Australian community. *Australian and New Zealand Journal of Public Health, 22*, 419–423.

Tate, R. L., McDonald, S., Perdices, M., Togher, L., Schultz, R., & Savage, S. (2008). Rating the methodological quality of single-subject designs and n-of-1 trials: Introducing the Single-case Experimental Design (SCED) Scale. *Neuropsychological Rehabilitation, 18*(4), 385–401.

Tate, R. L., & Perdices, M. (2008). Applying the International Classification of Functioning Disability and Health (ICF) to clinical practice and research in acquired brain impairment. *Brain Impairment, 9*(3), 282–292.

Tate, R. L., Perdices, M., McDonald, S., Togher, L., Moseley, A., Winders, K., et al. (2004). Development of a database of rehabilitation therapies for the psychological consequences of acquired brain impairment. *Neuropsychological Rehabilitation, 15*(5), 517–534.

Tate, R. L., Perdices, M., Pfaff, A., & Jurjevic, L. (2001). Predicting duration of posttraumatic amnesia (PTA) from early PTA measurements. *Journal of Head Trauma Rehabilitation, 16,* 525–542.

Tate, R. L., Strettles, B., & Osoteo, T. (2003). Enhancing outcomes after traumatic brain injury: A social rehabilitation approach. In BA Wilson (Ed.), *Neuropsychological rehabilitation: Theory and practice* (pp. 137–169). Lisse, the Netherlands: Swets & Zeitlinger.

Tate, R. L., Strettles, B., & Osoteo, T. (2004). The clinical practice of a community rehabilitation team for people with acquired brain injury. *Brain Impairment, 5*(1), 81–92.

Tate, R. L., Togher, L., Perdices, M., McDonald, S., Rosenkoetter, U., Godbee, K., et al. (2011). (Abstract). Rehabilitating neuropsychological impairments using single-participant research designs: A survey of methodological quality of withdrawal/reversal (A-B-A), multiple-baseline, A-B, and other designs. *Brain Impairment, 12*(Suppl), 70–71.

Teasdale, G., & Jennett, B. (1974). Assessment of coma and impaired consciousness: A practical scale. *The Lancet, 2*(7873), 81–84.

Teasdale, G. M., Pettigrew, L. E. L., Wilson, J. T., Murray, G., & Jennett, B. (1998). Analyzing outcome of treatment of severe head injury: A review and update on advancing the use of the Glasgow Outcome Scale. *Journal of Neurotrauma, 15*(8), 587–597.

Thurman, D. J., Alverson, C., Dunn, K. A., Guerrero, J., & Sniezek, J. E. (1999). Traumatic brain injury in the United States: A public health perspective. *Journal of Head Trauma Rehabilitation, 14*(6), 602–615.

Treadwell, K., & Page, T. J. (1996). Functional analysis: Identifying the environmental determinants of severe behavior disorders. *Journal of Head Trauma Rehabilitation, 11*(1), 62–74.

Turner-Stokes, L., Disler, P. B., Nair, A., & Wade, D. T. (2005). Multi-disciplinary rehabilitation for acquired brain injury in adults of working age. *Cochrane Database of Systematic Reviews, 3,* CD004170.

Üstün, T. B., Chatterji, S., Bickenbach, J., Kostanjsek, N., & Schneider, M. (2003). The International Classification of Functioning, Disability and Health: A new tool for understanding disability and health. *Disability and Rehabilitation, 25*(11–12), 565–571.

Von Cramon, D. Y., Mathes-von Cramon, G., & Mai, N. (1991). Problem-solving deficits in brain-injured patients: A therapeutic approach. *Neuropsychological Rehabilitation, 1,* 45–64.

Von Holst, H., Cassidy, J. D. (2004). Mandate of the WHO Collaborating Centre Task Force on Mild Traumatic Brain Injury. *Journal of Rehabilitation Medicine, 43*(Suppl), 8–10.

Webb, P. M., & Glueckauf, R. L. (1994). The effects of direct involvement in goal setting on rehabilitation outcome for persons with traumatic brain injuries. *Rehabilitation Psychology, 39*(3), 179–188.

Weinberg, J., Diller, L., Gordon, W. A., Gerstman, L. J., Lieberman, A., Lakin, P., Hodges, G., & Ezrachi, O. (1977). Visual scanning training effect on reading-related tasks in acquired right brain damage. *Archives of Physical Medicine and Rehabilitation, 58,* 479–486.

Wesolowski, M. D., Zenicius, A. H., McCarthy-Lydon, D., & Lydon, S. (2005). Using behavioral interventions to treat speech disorders in persons with head trauma. *Behavioral Interventions, 20,* 67–75.

Whyte, J., Hart, T., Laborde, A., & Rosenthal, M. (2005). Rehabilitation issues in traumatic brain injury. In DeLisa, J. A., Gans, B. M., Walsh, N. E., et al. (Eds.), *Physical medicine and rehabilitation: Principles and practice* (4th ed., vol. 2, p. 1677–1713). Philadelphia: Lippincott Williams & Wilkins.

Wilson, B. A. (Ed.). (2003a). *Neuropsychological rehabilitation: Theory and practice.* Lisse, the Netherlands: Swets & Zeitlinger.

Wilson, B. (2003b). Goal planning rather than neuropsychological tests should be used to structure and evaluate cognitive rehabilitation. *Brain Impairment, 4*(1), 25–30.

Wilson, B. A., Evans, J. J., Brentnall, S., Bremner, S., Keohane, C., & Williams, H. (2000). The Oliver Zangwill Center for Neuropsychological Rehabilitation: A partnership between health care and rehabilitation research. In Christensen, A-L., & Uzzell, B. P. (Eds.). (2000). *International handbook of neuropsychological rehabilitation* (pp. 231–246). New York: Klewer Academic.

Wilson, B. A., Emslie, H. C., Quirk, K., & Evans, J. J. (2001). Reducing everyday memory and planning problems by means of a paging system: A randomized control crossover study. *Journal of Neurology, Neurosurgery and Psychiatry, 70,* 477–482.

Wilson, B. A., Gracey, F., Evans, J. J., & Bateman, A. (2009). *Neuropsychological Rehabilitation. Theory, models, therapy and outcome.* Cambridge: Cambridge University Press.

Wilson, B. A., Gracey, F., Malley, D., Bateman, A., & Evans, J. J. (2009). The Oliver Zangwill Centre approach to neuropsychological rehabilitation. In B. A. Wilson, F. Gracey, J. J. Evans, & A. Bateman (Eds.), *Neuropsychological rehabilitation. theory, models, therapy and outcome* (pp. 47–67). Cambridge: Cambridge University Press.

Wood, R. L., & Rutterford, N. A. (2006). Psychosocial adjustment 17 years after severe brain injury. *Journal of Neurology, Neurosurgery, and Psychiatry, 77,* 71–73.

World Health Organization. (2001). *International classification of functioning, disability and health.* Geneva: World Health Organization.

Ylvisaker, M., Turkstra, L., Coehlo, C., Yorkston, K., Kennedy, M., Sohlberg, M. M., & Avery, J. (2007). Behavioural interventions for children and adults with behaviour disorders after TBI: A systematic review of the evidence. *Brain Injury, 21*(8), 769–805.

Zasler, N., Katz, D., & Zafonte, R. (Eds.). (2006). *Brain injury medicine: Principles and practice.* New York: Demos Medical Publishing.

Post-Acute Rehabilitation

Jeri Morris

Abstract

Post-acute brain injury rehabilitation was initially developed in the early 20th century by some of the most brilliant thinkers in medicine and psychology. Remarkably, the pioneers in post-acute rehabilitation had such insights and vision that their work remains the bases for brain injury treatment a century later. Stimulated by the effects of wars and impeded at times by social and political forces, the field draws intensely caring professionals, and techniques continue to be refined and innovations put into practice.

Key Words: Brain injury, traumatic brain injury, post-traumatic brain injury treatment, neurorehabilitation, cognitive rehabilitation.

Unlike may other areas of science and medical practice wherein striking new discoveries cause great changes and even paradigm shifts in how key ideas are conceptualized, to a large extent neurorehabilitation of brain injured individuals has involved building on the work of the earliest contributors to the field. Emphases have differed at times, and the practice of neurorehabilitation has undergone change, but the fundamental principles have been understood for nearly the entirety of the history of post-acute treatment. Treatment has been refined through the years, new techniques have been and continue to be developed, and post-acute treatment has continued to evolve, although its history, both with regard to refinement of theories and to practice, has been punctuated by setbacks caused by social and political pressures. To appreciate the underlying principles involved in post-acute treatment and to understand how these principles have been put into practice, it is helpful to have a historical perspective, beginning with the inception of the field following World War I and continuing to this day.

The Aftermath of World War I

Rehabilitation of brain injured individuals has a history dating from World War I. The field owes its origins to some of the greatest minds and most innovative thinkers of the 20th century Western world.

Generally considered the father of brain injury treatment, Kurt Goldstein (1878–1965) pioneered the development of a holistic theory that inspired the most influential therapists and scientists in the field of brain injury treatment (Votsmeier, 1996). Originally a medical student at the University of Breslau, Goldstein studied under Carl Wernike, the German physician and neuropathologist whose contributions in the area of aphasia were critical to our current understanding of functional neuroanatomy. Differing sharply from the localizationist theories (Landreth & Richardson, 2004), Goldstein based his work on what he termed the *organismic approach,* in which the activities of the organism as a whole, rather than individual aspects of the person (e.g. eyes, legs, and brain) were conceptualized to work in synchrony to achieve the adaptive capacities that account for human behavior (Goldstein, 1942). His work led him away from simple classification of patients into syndromes toward attention to the individual involved in various cognitive tasks and over many situations. With this emphasis on the individual, in his research he pioneered the use of single-case study methodology to investigate language and nonlinguistic disturbances. In 1914, Goldstein established the Institute for Research on the After-Effects of Brain Injury at the Frankfurt Neurological Institute (Goldstein, 1942). At that facility, he treated the many injured soldiers sent to him from the warfront in a cooperative effort with neurosurgeons, neurologists, and psychologists, thus setting the stage for the team approach that is the core of modern treatment of the effects of brain injury and, in fact, of much of the field of physical and neurorehabilitation.

Investigations of individual veterans led Goldstein to relate cognitive capacities to personality, and even in his early investigations, personality-related issues were addressed. For example, Goldstein's work with color and object sorting tests led him to make a distinction between two modes of behavior, the concrete and the abstract. He observed, "The abstract and concrete behaviors are dependent upon two corresponding attitudes which are psychologically so basic that one may speak of them almost as levels. The normal person is capable of assuming both, whereas the abnormal individual is confined to but one type of behavior—the concrete" (Goldstein & Scheerer, 1941, p. 1).

Thus, his work with assessment of cognitive processes led Goldstein to postulate a number of concepts that are still considered relevant. The first is the relationship between head injury and specific changes in the individual's capacities and the effect of those changes on the individual's ability to function in the more holistic sense of general adaptive behaviors (Goldstein, 1942). The second is the implication, later elaborated on by others (Morris, 1986; Prigatano, 1999) that there is a *qualitative* and not simply a quantitative change that occurs in many after brain injury that alters the brain injured individual's personality. As explained by Goldstein and Scheerer (1941):

> In some ways, the use of the term "attitude" may disturb the psychologist who would prefer the more legitimate terminology of "*mental set*" or "*approach*" as being the more common designations. Both expressions, however, are either too "partitive" and "temporal" in meaning or bear certain behavioristic

connotations; and the latter leave little room for an explanatory concept not adhering to the monopolizing claims of "past experience" or "acquired traits." The meaning the authors try to convey by the term *attitude* is rather unique in one respect. Our concept of attitude implies a *capacity level* of the total personality in a specific plane of activity. (p. 2)

That abstract or concrete attitude referred to either outer-world situations or inner experiences, and in his various writings, Goldstein (1942) described that individual with a concrete attitude as one who is limited to the immediate understanding and grasp of one's situation rather than one mediated by reasoning beyond the specific instance, and he speaks of the brain injured individual as having to "surrender to experiences of an unreflective character" (Goldstein & Scheerer, p. 2).

Remarkably, Goldstein also identified another critical component to understanding and treating those with brain injuries, what he termed the "catastrophic reaction" (Goldstein, 1939). To Goldstein, "Anxiety is the subjective experience of the organism in a catastrophic condition" (Teuber, 1966). In effect, a patient might encounter a task that once was very easy but that now, since his brain injury, he no longer can perform. Those working with brain injured patients have all seen the panic this can engender in the individual under those circumstances. In fact, it is frequently referred to by patients themselves as "brain freeze" or other similarly expressive terms that describe the paralyzing fear they experience when they cannot respond adequately to the demands of a situation they realize would have presented no challenge to them prior to their injury.

Thus, from horrific injuries incurred by soldiers in World War I came the fundamentals of the next phase of brain injury treatment wherein a team approach became the norm for rehabilitative treatment of the "whole person," who was seen to have cognitive deficits affecting adaptive abilities and personality functions.

The Aftermath of World War II

Born in Kazan near Moscow, Alexander Romanovich Luria (1902–1977), now considered the father of neuropsychology, originally studied and practiced medicine before beginning his clinical work with mentally retarded and brain-impaired individuals. Interestingly, while still a student, he formed the Kazan Psychoanalytic Association. A student of Lev Vygotsky, Luria became interested in Vygotsky's "cultural-historical psychology," which was an attempt to counter what Vygotsky saw as the narrow view of behaviorism (Homskaya & Tupper, 2001). Luria's work focused on an emphasis on the effects of culture on higher mental functions, such as perception and problem-solving.

Luria's influence on the modern understanding of brain–behavior relationships is extraordinary. Utilizing an approach similar to that of a physician, Luria administered what now might be thought of as an extended mental status examination, working with each individual in a nonstandardized manner, covering various domains of functioning (e.g. speech, visuospatial abilities), but exploring areas in depth as he saw fit, given what was suggested to him. Through these methods and after extensively evaluating thousands of brain-impaired patients, Luria developed an elaborate and comprehensive theory of brain functioning founded on the concept that the brain is a functional system wherein its various parts work in concert, ultimately to produce complex activities requiring input from areas of the brain that may be quite distant from each other. He described this system as hierarchical, with the most basic functions present in a manner we might now call "hardwired." These involve functions such as those governing the autonomic nervous system, as well as those controlling the reticular activating system responsible for arousal and awakening. Other portions of the brain that are hardwired into the system are the primary areas for receiving sensory information (hearing, vision, audition, somatosensory information). Secondary areas received information from primary areas but were affected to a large degree by experience. For example, while the primary auditory area takes in sounds, the secondary area interprets the sounds depending on the experience of the individual, learning to interpret the language to which the individual is exposed. Tertiary areas, largely found only in humans, permit the integration of information from the unisensory-modal primary and secondary areas, thus allowing for the performance of complex tasks such as reading, which requires input from auditory and visual areas. In the United States, research has been largely based on a systematic empirical approach in which subjects are given standardized tests that provide for comparisons between subjects, between patient groups and controls, and between the individual subject across multiple time periods. Further, we now have enormous amounts of information from neurologic laboratory tests (e.g., magnetic resonance imaging [MRI], computed tomography [CT], positron emission tomography [PET] scans,

electroencephalograms [EEGs]) and from neurosurgical records, Wada tests, and medication trials. We have been awed to learn that the brain of each individual contains approximately 10 billion neurons that have connections with as many as 10,000 other cells. Remarkably, these discoveries have largely (of course, not perfectly) confirmed Luria's theory of brain functioning (Homskaya & Tupper, 2001).

During and after World War II, Luria worked with brain injured patients at an army hospital. Engaging in rehabilitation with those individuals, Luria focused on teaching compensatory techniques and remediation strategies to address deficits relating to functions such as motor planning, visuospatial deficits, language dysfunction, and problem-solving deficits (Luria, 1964, 1979). Luria promoted an individualized approach in treatment planning, as he had with regard to assessment, and Luria's treatment involved increasing a patient's awareness of his deficits through feedback during the rehabilitation process as a means of gaining the patient's motivation for treatment. His ideas were promulgated in part because he wrote so expressively, in a manner akin to other scientist-poetic writers such as Lewis Thomas, the physician/poet who authored *Lives of a Cell* (1978) and *Medusa and the Snail* (1995), books that allowed us to envision what was being described. For example, Luria, with the assistance of his colleagues, wrote *The Mind of a Mnemonist: A Little Book About a Vast Memory* (Luria, Solotaroff, & Bruner, 1987), in which they described an individual whose memory was so outstanding that he could recall a table of numbers he learned years earlier but who was handicapped in his functioning because he could not think abstractly or make normal logical connections when reasoning in everyday life situations. Along with his students Lynn Solotaroff and Oliver Sacks, Luria also wrote *The Man with a Shattered World: The History of a Brain Wound* (1987), using such descriptive language that the reader is able to imagine the patient and the problems the brain injury caused to this specific individual. Thus, Luria's work encompassed theoretical foundations for understanding the brain as a functional system, and he provided vividly written examples of how his theories are expressed, the latter in a manner that can be appreciated even by laymen.

In this same period following World War II, Oliver Zangwill (1913–1987), professor of experimental psychology at the University of Cambridge, made other valuable contributions, particularly adding to our understanding of lateralization of functions, amnesia, and memory problems in brain injured individuals, and visuospatial deficits in right hemisphere injured individuals. Whereas Luria had focused a great deal on compensation and the remediation of various deficits and utilized the patient's intact functions, Zangwill emphasized the importance of understanding the positive attributes the patient might have, encouraging his patients to make good use of the abilities in which they retained strengths despite their injuries (Zangwill, 1947). The Oliver Zangwill Centre for Neuropsychological Rehabilitation, part of the National Health Services (NHS) Primary Care Trust, continues to carry out his important legacy.

The Aftermath of the Yom Kippur War

The Yom Kippur War in Israel was brief, lasting only from October 6 to October 25, 1973, but it produced numerous casualties, including head injuries. The Israeli government sought out the assistance of two neuropsychologists, Yehuda Ben-Yishay and Leonard Diller, at the Rusk Institute of Rehabilitation at the New York University School of Medicine. Ben-Yishay and Diller (1983) have written extensively about the program of post-acute rehabilitation they developed, which they based upon key concepts of Kurt Goldstein's holistic theory. In their program at the Rusk Institute, Ben-Yishay and Diller built their brain injury treatment program on a therapeutic milieu approach. The outcome of their initial work produced data from a pilot study that assessed the efficacy of this holistic neuropsychological rehabilitation program, conducted during 1974–1976 with a group of Israeli war veterans who had sustained head injuries (Ben-Yishay, 1981, 1996) in the Rusk Institute Brain Injury Day Treatment Program. The program underwent a large-scale study in 1978, and as a part of a 5 -year U.S. federally funded grant, the program was formally implemented in 1983. This program, described by Ben-Yishay and Gold (1990), involved interventions delivered in three phases, with expressly designed exercises within a structured program but delivered in a milieu setting that provided treatment within what a was referred to as a "therapeutic community." The community provided a unique opportunity in that it allowed for support from peers, the persuasive influence of peers to encourage participation, and transition from a rehabilitation setting to home and work. Phase One involved intensive interventions designed to both prepare the "trainee"—the preferred term rather than "patient" or "client"—for the program and to initiate remediations. A major

focus of this phase was helping the individual to gain an understanding of the consequences of his or her injury and to gain realistic self-acceptance while fostering optimism about what might be improved through the program of interventions. Ben-Yishay and Diller (1983) formulated treatment based upon the proposition that brain injured individuals profit most from treatment when they understand in explicit terms their specific problems and how those problems are to be addressed. Remediations were presented in the form of "training modules," as well as in individualized exercises in a 4-day-per week, 5-hour per day plan lasting 20 consecutive weeks. This structured program was delivered in a group, consisting of 10–12 trainees who remained together for the entire 20 weeks of Phase One. As many as half the trainees were "veterans" who had been through one cycle and were returning for additional intensive treatment. The inclusion of the "veterans" facilitated the adjustment of the new trainees. In addition to working on remediation modules, the program included personal counseling sessions, family/significant other counseling, and weekly sessions in which the families of all trainees met together so that staff could keep them informed of the features of the program and help them understand the nature of the program, as well as of the effects of brain injury and how they might best help their injured family member. Further, family members were given guidelines for coaching the trainee at home. This is important for increasing the generalizability of the results. At the completion of Phase One, the trainee was assessed in five primary areas of training, and, if ready, advanced to Phase Two. Phase Two generally lasted for 3 months or longer and concentrated on individualized pre-work or work experiences in conjunction with a vocational counselor. Ideally, the work was done through in vivo work experiences and was given on-site work supervision with assistance from the vocational counselor. Individual and group vocational counseling also are incorporated into the program. Phase Three, the follow-up/maintenance portion of the program, provided individualized therapeutic support either from the program staff, if they lived near New York City, or from treatment providers in the areas in which the trainees resided. Thus, the Brain Injury Day Treatment Program, in its current form, functions as the outgrowth of the principles articulated by Kurt Goldstein, with treatment delivered within a milieu setting that addresses cognitive, interpersonal, and vocational issues in a systematic manner. It utilizes remediation methods and compensatory techniques to directly treat specific, acquired cognitive deficits and train compensatory techniques, and it also addresses adjustment to and acceptance of the long-term sequelae of brain injury.

The "Golden Age" of Brain Injury Rehabilitation

Following the development of this program, other facilities instituted post-acute milieu day treatment programs based on the Ben-Yishay/Diller milieu day treatment model. Some, like that led by George Prigatano in Oklahoma City, were primarily developed from that model but expanded upon it by further emphasizing psychotherapeutic treatment (Prigatano, 1999).

In addition, in the 1980s, free-standing rehabilitation hospitals, as well as departments in primary care hospitals, provided acute and post-acute programs. The nature of third-party (private insurance, Medicare, Medicaid) payment at the time was such that individuals who had sustained head injuries were allowed to remain in acute care rehabilitation treatment for long periods, often 6 months to a year for those with serious sequelae. At that time, there was little oversight by third-party payers, and treatment generally was provided for as long as therapists felt the patient was benefitting from it. This acute care treatment was aimed at remediation of cognitive deficits and restoration of function, to the extent possible. Even after many months of treatment, acute care rehabilitation professionals remained hopeful for their patients' further recovery, and referrals to post-acute programs were commonplace. Those post-acute programs thrived, and outcome studies showed the value of those programs to quality of life and return to home and work for many injured individuals.

Principles of Treatment

This "Golden Age," in which financial resources were plentiful, allowed treatment team members the time to work with patients to produce new and effective treatment techniques. In doing so, various neurocognitive rehabilitationists, often working separately, developed theories of what brings about change in brain injured individuals. Although those theories differ to various degrees in form and content, many (Morris, 2007; Luria, 1964; Prigatano, 1999) came to focus on the importance of awareness in the process of cognitive rehabilitation. Thus, many who treated individuals who had sustained head injuries came to believe that, after such an injury, cognitive functions that once were automatic now must be performed on a conscious or intentional basis or they

would not take place. However, the injured individuals often have no realization of having any acquired cognitive deficits and have little understanding of the specifics of their problem. Consequently, they are unable to make productive attempts to compensate for or remediate their deficits. Further, without awareness, it is difficult for the patient to understand the purpose of strategies being offered by the treatment team, making generalization to real-life situations unlikely. Understanding the importance of awareness in bringing about meaningful change led treatment members to address awareness directly. When awareness is seen as the cornerstone of treatment, it becomes obvious that a clear delineation of specific deficits by the treatment team is a primary requisite for developing a treatment plan. Helping the injured individual to become aware of these specific deficits and how they can be addressed through remediations or compensations can then help that individual to become an active participant in the process, increasing motivation in treatment settings and generalization of the results to situations outside the treatment settings. Thus, in many rehabilitation facilities, theory of what brings about change in the brain injured individual drove the treatment process.

The Influence of the Commission on Accreditation of Rehabilitation Facilities

The Commission on Accreditation of Rehabilitation Facilities (CARF) also contributed to the promulgation of post-acute rehabilitation and, in significant ways, altered the focus of treatment. Founded in 1966 as the Commission on Accreditation of Rehabilitation Facilities, now functioning as CARF International, the organization is an independent, nonprofit accreditor of various areas of health and human services. In January 1988, the Standards Manual for Organizations Serving People with Disabilities added new standards in the area of post-acute brain injury programs. In addition to setting forth the minimal standards required in such programs, a primary goal of those standards was to promote program evaluation systems that emphasize quality. Further, CARF formally introduced the concept of "functional goals." To that point, many post-acute programs, as well as most acute rehabilitation programs, focused on remediations and compensations for specific cognitive deficits, as described in the Ben Yishea/Diller program discussed above. Particularly until the last phase of those post-acute programs, functional considerations remained in the background. Rather than teaching a patient how to get to their place of employment, they were taught the underlying cognitive skills (e.g., divided attention; visuospatial abilities) needed to solve a novel problem when they encountered one. Thus, with restored or compensated-for cognitive functions, the individual could solve novel problems (e.g., of how one might find a way by train, bus, or the like, to get from one place to another). CARF began requiring a treatment plan that included a statement of functional goals with a time frame for accomplishing them. Functional goals include tasks such as keeping a checkbook, shopping, cooking, and ambulating various distances. The CARF standards undoubtedly improved the quality of rehabilitation by defining and requiring appropriate and standardized record-keeping, the eligibility and constitution of the rehabilitation team, and a format for defined treatment plans. The standards also encouraged inclusion of the patient and his or her family members into the rehabilitation team, encouraging those individuals to be full participants in the process, including goal setting. However, nowhere in the CARF treatment plan was there a requirement to record the process of how the team would move the patient "from here to there." In other words, the team was required to state the functional goal and time frame to accomplish the functional goal, but there was no requirement for the team to state what treatment would be utilized to accomplish the functional goal. Consequently, the focus of the practice of rehabilitation was shifted dramatically toward achieving functional goals and away from remediating and developing compensatory strategies for underlying impaired cognitive abilities. This effect of the introduction of the CARF standards had the positive result of steering the treatment team toward practical, real-world solutions for the brain injured individual and, in addition, also promoted more cost- and time-efficient treatment, foreshadowing the modern constraints now facing treatment teams. However, although likely unintentional and, in fact, unnoticed by many rehabilitation professionals, the regulations created a sea change in post-acute rehabilitation because they took the focus away from two key aspects of the rehabilitation process: articulating the treatment and directly treating impaired cognitive processes. With no emphasis on articulation of treatment, methods were no longer the focus of team meetings, and, importantly, the methods used by one team member were not communicated to another, thus lessening the coordinated use of the same methods across disciplines. The focus toward achieving functional goals and away from treating underlying cognitive processes limited the scope of treatment.

Health Care Financial Crisis

Beginning in the mid to late 1980s, intensifying greatly in the 1990s, and continuing to this time, the financial crisis that has enveloped U.S. health care in general has had devastating effects on post-acute rehabilitation. In the "Golden Age" of the 1980s, with virtually no financial constraints, brain injury rehabilitation had undergone a burst of innovative treatments. In effect, since patients could be maintained in acute and post-acute programs almost indefinitely, treatment providers were able to try new methods and fine-tune their work. This led to wide-sweeping improvements in care but also to considerable costs. Therapists attempted to remediate or compensate for cognitive impairments, and little was spared by the treatment team in the trying. Often, particularly before the CARF post-acute care standards were implemented, functional goals were considered almost as an afterthought, a capitulation to the failure of their treatments to restore the person to their pre-trauma levels of cognitive functioning.

The refinements made to rehabilitative treatment of brain injured individuals in the "Golden Age" led to an exponential growth of new brain injury rehabilitation programs for both acute and post-acute treatment. Length of stay was considerable (often months, sometimes years), permitted by what often seemed to be nearly inexhaustible resources from private payment sources (e.g., insurance companies) and by state and federal government programs (e.g., Medicaid; Medicare). With regard to post-acute programs, specialized treatment also began to be offered for those diagnosed with mild traumatic brain injuries. Although most who experience "mild" injuries substantially recover, some are left with devastating, life-long problems. This was a problem that had largely gone unnoticed and untreated prior to the "Golden Age," and treatment programs were developed to address the needs of those individuals through cognitive rehabilitation. Funding has never been strong for those with less severe and less obvious injuries, thus spurring rehabilitation professions—and especially those working with patients classified as having "mild" injuries—to document the evidence for the efficacy of their treatments, as discussed below.

By the mid to late 1980s and continuing to the present, health care costs in the United States have been spiraling alarmingly. During the Clinton presidency, national attention was brought to this issue, and various solutions were implemented. For example, there was wide promotion of Health Care Maintenance programs, initially provided for by the Health Maintenance Organization (HMO) Act, approved by President Nixon in 1973. Unlike traditional insurance policies, an HMO covers care only by providers (e.g., hospitals, rehabilitation settings, doctors) who have agreed to participate in the HMO's restrictions and within the HMO-dictated fee schedules. With extensive enrollment in HMO group plans by employers wishing to contain costs, doctors and hospitals felt a pressure to join or face losing much of their patient population. As the popularity of those plans has grown, more claims were denied, less money was paid to doctors and hospitals for the same services, and pre-approval through primary care "gate-keepers" was required. Post-acute rehabilitative treatment often was denied. At least as great an influence on health care as the HMO is the diagnosis-related group (DRG) prospective payment system developed for Medicare. This system classifies hospital-related illnesses into one of more than 700 groups, based on International Classification of Function, Disability, and Health (ICD) diagnoses. With the goal of limiting the amount of the national budget spent on health care, DRGs have been utilized since 1983 to determine how much Medicare will pay a hospital for each illness category, since patients within each category theoretically are expected to require the same amount of hospital resources.

> The change was nothing short of revolutionary. For the first time, the federal government gained the upper hand in its financial relationship with the hospital industry. Medicare's new prospective payment system with DRGs triggered a shift in the balance of political and economic power between the providers of medical care (hospitals and physicians) and those who paid for it—power that providers had successfully accumulated for more than half a century. (*Mayes*, 2007, p. 22)

As the DRG system was applied to acute (non-rehabilitation) hospital treatment, funding for patient care was reduced in virtually every category. Consequently, patients were transferred to rehabilitation facilities after much shorter stays in the acute hospital, resulting in the introduction to acute rehabilitation facilities of patients who were less recovered and who often required considerable nursing care. Initially, rehabilitation facilities were able to make accommodations for these more medically involved individuals because they were not regulated by DRGs. There was hope that these regulations would not be extended to rehabilitation settings, which accounted for less than 1% of medical costs. However, by 2003, a prospective payment system was instituted that led to extreme cuts in payment by Medicare, and private insurance payers followed suit (Evashwick, 2005). Cutbacks continued to a point where, now, although patients arrive in acute rehabilitation settings much more medically involved and, therefore, considerably less able to benefit from treatments, the length of stay in acute care rehabilitation has been reduced from many months (as during the "Golden Age") to only 2–3 weeks, and in some cases even less. Often, this means patients are returning home while still in post-traumatic amnesia. Further, post-acute rehabilitation is rarely covered, and those programs have been drastically reduced in number. A few programs (e.g., the Ben-Yishay/Diller program; the Cicerone program) exist, especially in very large metropolitan areas, but the number of patients serviced is small and often services are very limited.

Complicating the introduction of the prospective payment system into rehabilitation was the inclusion into that system of the Functional Independence Measure (FIM). This is an 18-item outcome measure, initially introduced as a way of assessing progress during inpatient rehabilitation, ostensibly for the purpose of providing evidence for the utility of treatment that would garner greater acceptance and, therefore, greater funding for rehabilitation by third-party payers (Wright, 2000). The FIM has been subject to controversy since its inception (Merbitz, Morris, & Grip, 1989; Morris, 1994) because it uses statistical procedures involving ordinal scales, whereby individual, disparate items are totaled (e.g., adding independence ratings for bowel control and ambulation) and then averaged. Further, interrater reliability, questioned by Merbitz, Morris, and Grip in their 1989 article, has again come into question, as a recent article examining this issue showed poor agreement between raters from two rehabilitation units (Kohler, Redmond, Dickson, & Connolly, 2010). Beyond the questionable meaning of FIM results, when the instrument was incorporated into the reimbursement process, including the current use of the prospective payment system, comparison between rehabilitation programs was encouraged, thus engendering competition rather than cooperation between facilities. As a consequence, rather than providing evidence for the utility of treatment and thereby bringing about greater, more appropriate funding for rehabilitation by third-party payers, the use of the instrument pitted programs against one another, with each program attempting to show it could bring about the same benefit or greater for lower costs. Thus, as rehabilitation funding continued to shrink dramatically, with terrible consequences to patient care, treatment programs provided outcome data that contributed to the problem. No one could seriously believe that what was once accomplished in several months could now be done at bare-bones expense in 2–3 weeks, but programs were induced by the FIM, which had been incorporated into the prospective payor system, to fight against each other to prove they could do the job for less rather than joining together to plead the case to third-party payers for sufficient funding to provide adequate rehabilitative services. Perhaps a compromise in length of stay and provision of services was prudent and wise, and it can certainly be argued that some efforts of the "Golden Age" were excessive, but certainly the pendulum has swung, and it is not an exaggeration to conclude that both acute and post-acute rehabilitation programs for brain injured individuals, which account for only a very small fraction of medical expenditures and which have been proved over the last century to be of such benefit to these patients, have been largely decimated.

In August 2007, the Center for Medicare Services (CMS) finalized this proposal, and CMS Acting Deputy Administrator Herb Kuhn stated that Medicare payments for inpatient services "will be more accurate and better reflect the severity of the patient's condition." The CMS says it adopted severity-based DRGs to prevent abuses under the prevalent system.

The replacement of the old DRG (CMS-DRG) system, which was relatively stable since its 1983 inception, meant that hospitals and, in particular, physicians and HMO, coding, and quality improvement departments must carefully work within the new system to ensure accurate reimbursement.

The new severity-based DRG System applied for all discharges after October 1, 2007. The rule creates 745 new severity-adjusted DRGs to replace the current 538 DRGs. The 745 Medicare severity-based DRGs (MS-DRGs) are divided into three severity levels: MCC, CC, and Non-CC. The familiar complication and comorbidity (CC) classification has been expanded to include CCs and major CCs (MCCs), which are conditions that require double the additional resources of a normal CC.

Additionally, the list of complications and comorbidities has changed. Some complications and comorbidities have been deleted, and several have been added. Examples of secondary diagnoses that were previously considered complications and comorbidities but have been removed from the list include unspecified congestive heart failure or other heart failure, unspecified chronic airway obstruction (COPD), and renal dialysis status.

The Iraq and Afghanistan Wars

Unfortunately, once again we are confronted with an upsurge in the numbers of brain injured patients as a consequence of war. In fact, the Iraq and Afghanistan conflicts have provided a new cause of brain injuries: the introduction of improvised explosive devices (IEDs) has brought about a shift in the source of injuries sustained by U.S. military personnel and the allied multinational forces. These popular homemade explosive devices have been used extensively against coalition forces. By the end of 2007, they were responsible for approximately 60% of coalition deaths in Iraq (Taber, Warden, & Hurley, 2006) and over 70% of coalition casualties in Afghanistan. The use of IEDs accounts for the deaths of thousands of soldiers, but, in addition to inflicting mortal wounds, IEDs are responsible for extremely high numbers of head injuries because they cause concussive injuries to those not directly hit by objects. These *blast injuries* bring about head injuries with affects similar to those seen in acceleration–deceleration injuries (e.g., car crashes Sayer et al., 2008). Blast injuries have occurred with such frequency in the Iraq and Afghanistan conflicts (they are estimated to account for at least 10% of U.S. troop injuries (Warden, 2006) that they have come to be called the "signature wound" of these wars.

Army field studies have shown that more than 10% of troops in Iraq and Afghanistan have suffered at least one concussion or brain injury, the vast majority of those from exposure to a homemade bomb or IED. Five percent to 15% of mild TBI patients develop lasting problems with concentration, short-term memory, fatigue, and chronic headaches.

In response to a growing awareness of these devastating injuries, the Veterans Administration (VA) and the Department of Defense (DoD) have initiated numerous programs designed to identify soldiers who have sustained head injuries and to treat them through programs of acute and post-acute rehabilitation. In the attempt to identify those injured and the sequelae of these injuries, soldiers are given abbreviated neuropsychological evaluations before deployment and at discharge. In addition, various tests have been implemented to assess soldiers on the battlefield to determine if, after experiencing a blast injury, they are fit to return to duty (Brener et al., 2010). In addition, implementation of post-acute treatment in specialized VA and military hospital settings is growing. The military is also particularly concerned by the fact that an increasing number of head injured soldiers and veterans have committed suicide. Given the enormity of these problems, an intensive effort is being made through various projects funded by the VA and by DoD to address key issues. Some funding is being directed to very innovative programs. For example, I am a team leader on a project by the Defense Advanced Research Projects Agency (DARPA), an agency of the U.S. DoD. The project involves delivery of services and information to brain injured individuals and their spouses via an online chat room format led by a rehabilitation professional (Department of Defense Advance Research Projects Agency (DARPA), 2011). Yet again, the tragedy of war is the stimulating factor for the increase in post-acute brain injury programs and is the impetus for advancements in brain injury treatment techniques.

Evidenced-Based Cognitive Rehabilitation

For at least the past two decades, serious efforts have been made to find evidence for the positive outcomes of cognitive rehabilitation. Such research on the effects of brain injury treatment is methodologically complex as it is difficulty to design studies that account for the differences in subjects prior to their injuries, the differences between the effects of brain injury to different individuals, and the differences in treatment methods. Consequently, amassing sufficient rigorously conducted studies has been a slow process. In recent years, this effort has been driven in part by the need to prove to third-party payers that cognitive rehabilitation, as delivered (however infrequently) primarily in post-acute settings, is effective and brings about meaningful change and, therefore, should be reimbursed. The reality is that the delivery of post-acute brain injury treatment cannot be done for free, and most third-party payers, public and private, have refused to sufficiently recognize its significance to the quality of life of brain injured individuals.

The importance of acquiring evidence of the efficacy of treatment cannot be understated. First and foremost, evidence informs our clinical judgment. Those working with brain injured patients often have experience with treatment that leads them to have strong opinions about what is helpful and what is not, but those opinions can only be bolstered or disproved

with actual data. Further, evidence of the effectiveness of treatment protects patients and treatment providers from squandering resources. Treatments that appear logical are not necessarily effective. For example, reading paragraphs and practicing retaining the details may intuitively seem like a helpful exercise in improving memory processes when it is actually ineffective and, therefore, a waste of time and money.

Additionally, publishing well-designed studies on treatment allows for experience and outcomes to be shared between therapists and rehabilitation programs. Without these efforts, proven techniques, exercises, and approaches are not easily disseminated, and therapists can find themselves rediscovering ideas that should be discarded or have already been proved effective. Evidenced-based cognitive rehabilitation allows for an escape from subjectivity and brings brain injury treatment from art to science.

One of the most important sources for understanding evidenced-based treatment of brain-impaired individuals stems from the work conducted over more than the past decade by the Cognitive Rehabilitation Task Force of the Brain Injury Special Interest Group (BI-ISIG) of the American Congress of Rehabilitation Medicine (ACRM). The Task Force, led by Keith Cicerone, has published a series of articles reviewing the evidence for and against specific cognitive treatments and making recommendations for clinical practice based on that evidence (Cicerone et al., 2000, 2005).

These review articles define cognitive rehabilitation as "A systematic, functionally oriented service of therapeutic activities that is based on assessment and understanding of the patient's brain-behavioral deficits" (Cicerone, et al., 2000, p. 1596). As in other areas of medicine that consider evidenced-based treatments (Ezzo, Bausell, Moerman, Berman, & Hadhazy, 2001), the ACRM Task Force recognized that the most reliable evidence comes from randomized controlled trials (RCTs) in which studies are considered to fall into one of four classes. Class I studies are well-designed, prospective, RCTs. Class Ia studies are prospective studies with "quasi-randomized" assignment to treatment conditions. Class II studies are prospective, but are nonrandomized cohort studies, retrospective nonrandomized case–control studies, or multiple base–baseline studies that allow for a direct comparison between treatment conditions. Class III studies have no concurrent control subjects or are single-subject studies that include adequate quantification and analysis. In their review articles, Cicerone and his colleagues considered cognitive rehabilitation techniques used in patients who either sustained a TBI or suffered a cerebral vascular accident (CVA). Both produce similar cognitive deficits and are commonly treated in groups, with both diagnoses found in post-acute brain injury treatment programs.

In the second of the reviews of evidenced-based findings in studies of cognitive rehabilitation, the Task Force evaluated the literature reporting all class I studies from 1998 to 2002 (Cicerone et al., 2005) and compared the differential treatment effects of cognitive rehabilitation with alternative treatment or control conditions.

They reported that in ten studies that compared cognitive rehabilitation with other treatments (e.g., psychosocial treatment; traditional therapy), involving a total of 290 patients, 60% of the comparison showed benefit in favor of cognitive rehabilitation. Those receiving actually cognitive rehabilitation showed 66.7% greater improvement in comparison to those receiving pseudotreatment. In eight studies that compared cognitive rehabilitation with no treatment whatever, involving a total of 342 patients, 100% of the comparison showed benefit in favor of those receiving the cognitive rehabilitation. In all, the article reviewed a total of 47 class I studies involving 1,891 patients, and 78.7% of comparisons showed benefit in favor of cognitive rehabilitation.

The ACRM Task Force found sufficient evidence in these rigorously conducted class I studies to recommend 19 practice standards for the neurorehabilitation of individuals with TBIs and with CVAs. Some of the 19 involve recommendations for specific therapies, while others indicate treatments that are not supported by research studies. These findings are summarized as follows:

• With regard to visuospatial rehabilitation, studies showed that treatment for visual neglect, particularly after right hemisphere strokes, is recommended. However, they found that existing class I studies did not support optokinetic stimulation for visual neglect.

• Treatments involving cognitive-linguistic therapies were recommended during both the acute and post-acute rehabilitation processes for persons with language deficit secondary to left hemisphere dysfunction, particularly following CVAs.

• Treatments involving specific interventions for deficits to functional communication were recommended for individuals who have sustained TBIs. These included training for pragmatic conversational skills, so often impaired following head trauma.

• Research addressing specific training for apraxias was found to be efficacious, particularly for persons who have sustained left hemisphere damage secondary to CVAs.

• Memory training involving the use of internal strategies (e.g., visual imagery), as well as that involving external strategies (e.g., memory notebooks) was recommended, particularly for individuals with mild memory deficits resulting from TBI.

• Recommendations were made involving treatment of attentional problems, particularly during the post-acute rehabilitation of individuals who have sustained TBIs. This post-acute treatment was differentiated from acute-rehabilitations efforts, in which there was little support for the effects of treatment. The lack of support for the treatment during the acute phase of rehabilitation may be due to spontaneous recovery or more general cognitive treatments provided within the acute-rehabilitation process.

• Scanning training was highly recommended, considered even a critical facet of rehabilitation for persons with severe visuoperceptual impairment following CVAs.

• Treatments for specific language deficits, such as impairments to reading comprehension or language formulation, were recommended after either TBI or CVAs.

• The use of external compensations (e.g., calculators, hand-held computer devices, memory notebooks) was recommended, particularly when they have direct application to specific functional activities and goals. These compensatory techniques were recommended for individuals after TBI or CVA.

• Training in formal problem-solving strategies was recommended for those in post-acute rehabilitation programs, particularly when the application of the training was geared toward everyday situations and functional activities.

• Evidence was found for comprehensive-holistic neuropsychological rehabilitation during post-acute rehabilitation and was recommended for reducing cognitive and functional disabilities, particularly in individuals with moderate to severe TBIs or CVAs.

• The results of the class I studies did not provide support for isolated computer exercises geared toward treating unilateral left-side neglect, and such treatment was not recommended due to the fact that it did not appear effective.

• Systematic training of organizational skills was recommended for consideration for individuals with visual perceptual deficits without visual neglect, particularly soon after injury or CVA.

• Evidence was found for inclusion of limb activation or electronic technologies for visual scanning, and these treatments were recommended, particularly soon after injury or CVA.

• Computer-based interventions specifically intended to produce extension of damaged visual fields was recommended for consideration after TBI or stroke.

• Computer-based interventions also are recommended for consideration for cognitive and linguistic deficits if used in conjunction with clinician-guided treatments.

• The Task Force found that the class I studies showed no improvement in individuals when treatment consisted of sole reliance on repeated exposure and practice with computer programs, with no intervention by a therapist. Consequently, they recommended against such a program of treatment.

• The evidence demonstrated that treatments that promote internalization of self-regulation strategies (e.g., through self-instruction) are recommended for consideration following TBIs, particularly alongside treatment for deficits in attention, neglect, and memory.

• In general, the class I studies reviewed showed evidence for improvement in functioning for individuals with TBIs through individualized cognitive rehabilitation therapies that are provided within the context of a comprehensive neuropsychological rehabilitation program.

Some have seen the power of class I RTC designs to be so great as to allow for the revelation of the ultimate scientific bases for all of treatment. As an example, Hollon (2006, p. 105) stated,

> I find the power of RCTs both humbling and reassuring. I do not have to be free of prejudices to come to know the truth; all I have to do is apply the kinds of controls that protect me from my biases. Doing science is a delightful way of groping toward enlightenment and doing experiments is the most powerful way of determining causal efficacy. For any therapist who wants to have an effect, attending to the results of well-constructed RCTs is one of the best ways to make sure that what he or she does will truly make a difference.

Conclusion

To whatever degree one finds the scientific process a "delightful way of groping toward enlightenment," it is important to take a dispassionate and realistic view of the challenges we face in further substantiating the effectiveness of post-acute rehabilitation. Rehabilitation of brain injured individuals is complex and cannot easily be compared to medical treatments, such as prescribing medications. Our patients differ from one another both prior to and after their injuries, and treatment that is useful for one may not be productive for another. Although specific treatments may have been found to be effective, philosophies of treatment differ from one program to another. These include assumptions about what brings about change or the importance of the order in which treatment is delivered, assumptions that are difficult to address through research. Further, it is important to acknowledge that treatment providers differ. We are offering help to actual individuals, and how we connect with them is also a factor in the effectiveness of treatment. As an example, we are required to deliver information to our patients that can be terribly difficult to receive. No one wants to learn that they have a specific cognitive deficit they need to become aware of and acknowledge. No one wants to be less intelligent or capable than they once were. Therapists will differ in their capacity to relate to patients, especially in these sensitive areas, and the therapist's ability to earn the trust and respect of the individual patient may remain more art than science, at least for the foreseeable future.

Nevertheless, the work of Cicerone and his colleagues in summarizing rigorously conducted class I studies provides strong support for the effectiveness of treatment of individuals with TBIs. This evidence is necessary, given the fact that limited financial resources and the current "politics" of health care in general, and post-acute treatment programs in particular, work against delivery of services to many who might benefit. The challenge is to find a path that will allow us to advance our understanding of which of our methods are genuinely valuable in post-acute rehabilitation and to convince others to let us do it. Taking a lesson from Dr. Esther Duflo (2010), whose work has made great and meaningful contributions toward curing illnesses in impoverished children around the world, "We recognize that the problem is huge, and we do not always know if we are doing the right thing, but evidence is powerful and can prompt action."

To appreciate the development of theory and practice of post-acute rehabilitation requires an historical view. The one constant throughout the century of treatment is the intense desire of rehabilitation treatment team professionals to provide the utmost help to those who have sustained brain injuries. Sometimes the goals may be set too high and the practical social and political realities difficult to accept, but the dedication of those working with brain injured individuals remains strong, and progress continues to be made.

References

Ben-Yishay, Y. (1981). Cognitive remediation: Toward a definition of its objectives, tasks, and conditions. In Ben-Yishay, Y. (Ed.), *New York University Medical Center, Rehabilitation Monograph*, No. 62, pp. 14–42.

Ben-Yishay, Y. (1996). Reflections on the evolution of the therapeutic milieu concept. *Neuropsychological Rehabilitation, 6*, 327–343.

Ben-Yishay, Y., & Diller, L. (1983). Cognitive remediation. In M. Rosenthal, E. R. Griffith, M. R. Bond, & J. D. Miller (Eds.), *Rehabilitation of the head injured adult* (pp. 367–380). Philadelphia: F. A. Davis.

Ben-Yishay, Y., & Gold, J. (1990). Therapeutic milieu approach to neuropsychological rehabilitation. In R. L. Wood (Ed.), *Neurobehavioral sequelae of traumatic brain injury* (pp. 194–215). London: Taylor and Francis.

Brenner, L. A., Terrio, H., Homaifar, B.Y., Gutierrez, P.M., Staves, P.J., Harwood, J.E.F., Reeves, D, Adler, L. E., Ivins, B.J., Helmick, K., & Warden, D. (2010). Neuropsychological test performance in soldiers with blast-related mild TBI. *Neuropsychology, 24*(2), 160–167.

Cicerone, K. D., Dahlberg, C., Kalmer, K., Langenbahn, D. M., Malec, J. F., Berquist, T. F., et al. (2000). Evidence-based cognitive rehabilitation for clinical practice. *Archives of Physical Medicine and Rehabilitation, 81*, 1596–1615.

Cicerone, K. D., Dahlberg, C., Malec, J. F., Langenbahn, D. M., Felicetti, T., Kneipp, S., et al. (2005). Evidenced-based cognitive rehabilitation: Updated review of the literature from 1998–2002. *Archives of Physical Medicine and Rehabilitation, 86*, 1681–1692.

Department of Defense Advance Research Projects Agency (DARPA, 2011). Healing Hero's Project: Detection and Computational Analysis of Psychological Signals, Grant Contract Number N66001-11-C-4007.

Duflo, E. (2010). *Social experiments to fight poverty.* Retrieved October 2, 2010, from http://www.ted.com/talks/esther_duflo_social_experiments_to_fight_poverty.html

Evashwick, C. (2005). *The continuum of long term care, 3rd edition.* Clifton, New York: Thompson Delmore Learning.

Ezzo, J., Bausell, B., Moerman, D. E., Berman, B., & Hadhazy, V. (2001). Reviewing the reviews. How strong is the evidence? How clear are the conclusions? *International Journal of Technology Assess Health Care, 17*(4), 457–466.

Goldstein, K. (1939). Theoretical reflections on the function of the nervous system as foundation for a theory of the organism. *The organism: A holistic approach to biology derived from pathological data in man.* Salt Lake City, Utah: American Book Publishing.

Goldstein, K. (1942). *After effects of brain injuries in war.* New York: Grune & Stratton.

Goldstein, K., & Scheerer, M. (1941). Abstract and concrete behavior: An experimental study with special tests. *Psychological Monographs, 53*(2), 1–151.

Hollon, S. D. (2006). Randomized clinical trials. In J. C. Norcross, L. E. Beutler, & R. F. Levant (Eds.), *Evidenced-based practices in mental health: Debate and dialogue on the fundamental questions* (pp. 96–105). Washington, DC: American Psychological Association.

Homskaya, E. D., & Tupper, D. E. (Eds.). (2001). *Alexander Romanovich Luria: A scientific biography.* New York: Springer.

Kohler, F., Redmond, H., Dickson, H., & Connolly, C. (2010). Interrater reliability of functional status scores for patients transferred from one rehabilitation center to another. *Archives of Physical Medicine and Rehabilitation, 91*(7), 1031–1037.

Landreth, A., & Richardson, R. (2004). Localization and the new phrenology. [Review of the book *The new phrenology*]. *Philosophical Psychology, 17*, 107–123.

Luria, A., Cole, M. & Cole, S. (1979). The making of mind: A personal account of Soviet psychology. Cambridge, Mass: Harvard University Press.

Luria, A. R., Solotaroff, L., & Bruner, J. (1987). *The mind of a mnemonist: A little book about a vast memory.* Cambridge, MA: Harvard University Press.

Luria, A. R., Solotaroff, L., & Sacks, O. (1987). *The man with a shattered world: The history of a brain wound.* Cambridge, MA: Harvard University Press.

Mayes, R. (2007). The origins, development, and passage of Medicare's revolutionary prospective payment system. *Journal of the History of Allied Sciences, 62*(1), 21–55.

Merbitz, C., Morris, J., & Grip, J. C. (1989). Ordinal scales and foundations of misinference. *Archives of Physical Medicine and Rehabilitation, 70*, 308–312.

Morris, J. (1994). Some cautions when using functional assessment scales. *Geriatric Rehabilitation, 9* (3), 2–7.

Morris, J. (2007). Cognitive rehabilitation. In J. Young (Ed.), *Physical medicine and rehabilitation clinics of North America: Traumatic brain injury: New directions and treatment approaches* (pp. 27–42). Philadelphia, PA: W. B. Saunders Company.

Morris, J., & Bleiberg, J. (1986). Neuropsychological rehabilitation and traditional psychotherapy. *International Journal of Clinical Neuropsychology, 8*, 133–135.

Prigatano, G. P. (1999). *Principles of neuropsychological rehabilitation.* New York: Oxford University Press.

Sayer, N.A., Chiros, C.E., Sigford, B., Scott, S., Clothier, B., Pickett, T., & Lew, H.L. (2008). Characteristics and rehabilitation outcomes among patients with blast and other injuries sustained during the global war on terror. *Archives of Physical Medicine and Rehabilitation, 89*(1), 163–170.

Taber, K. H., Warden, D. L., & Hurley, R. A. (2006). Blast-related traumatic brain injury: What is known? *Journal of Neuropsychiatry and Clinical Neurology, 18*(2), 141–145.

Thomas, L. (1978). *Lives of a cell: Notes of a biology watcher.* New York: Penguin.

Thomas, L. (1995). *Medusa and the snail: More notes of a biology watcher.* New York: Penguin.

Teuber, H. (1966). Kurt Goldstein's role in the development of neuropsychology. *Neuropsychologia, 4*(4), 299–310.

Votsmeier, A. (1996). *Kurt Goldstein and holism.* Retrieved November 2, 2010, from www.gestaltpsychotherapie.de/LAgo1_ho.pdf

Warden, D. (2006). Military TBI during the Iraq and Afghanistan wars. *Journal of Head Trauma Rehabiliation, 21*(5), 398–402.

Wright, J. (2000). The FIM(TM). *The center for outcome measurement in brain injury.* Retrieved December 2, 2010, from http://www.tbims.org/combi/FIM

Zangwill, O. L. (1947). Psychological aspects of rehabilitation in cases of brain injury. *British Journal of Psychology, 37*, 60–69.

Spinal Cord Injuries

Paul Kennedy *and* Emilie F. Smithson

Abstract

The neurological injury and resulting losses in sensation and movement is only one of the numerous consequences of damage to the spinal cord. Sustaining a spinal cord injury (SCI) not only leads to major changes in an individual's physical ability, but also to changes in his or her occupational status, in the leisure activities with which he or she engages, in social participation and in intimate relationships. In recent years, there has been increasing interest in the psychological and social repercussions of SCI; research has looked into how these factors in turn affect adjustment to injury, self-care, quality of life, and morbidity, and professionals working in SCI rehabilitation have begun to consider how to promote positive adjustment in hospital settings. This chapter discusses psychological, social, and physical issues relating to SCI rehabilitation and covers the psychological interventions utilized in rehabilitation settings.

Key Words: Depression, Adjustment, Coping, Pain, Appraisals, Coping Effectiveness Training

Factors Affecting Acute Spinal Cord Injury Rehabilitation

To anyone unfamiliar with spinal cord injury (SCI), the process of rehabilitation may be misunderstood as consisting of the initial medical and surgical treatment, of being taught adaptive techniques for getting around and performing day-to-day tasks, and physiotherapy. However, SCI is frequently complicated by a number of additional factors that must be considered to ensure the provision of appropriate support for the patient's needs. This section discusses research findings and psychological approaches for managing complications during SCI rehabilitation.

A vast majority of individuals sustain SCIs through traumatic circumstances, such as falls, road traffic, and sports accidents (Spinal Cord Injury Information Network, 2009). As a consequence of these circumstances, it is not unusual for patients admitted to specialist SCI centers to present with comorbid traumatic brain injury (TBI). Although the cognitive and behavioral effects of TBI can vary between individuals, cognitive deficits in arousal, attention, concentration, memory, information processing, and capacity for learning new information are frequently reported in this population group, while behavioral changes in motivation, initiation, disinhibition, aggression, and depression can also be observed (see Morris & Tate, this volume, for more information).

Cognitive impairments to attentional processes, memory, and problem-solving in people with SCI have been estimated in up to 50% of individuals (Davidoff, Morris, Roth, & Bleiberg, 1985; Davidoff, Roth, & Richards, 1992), whereas estimates of TBI in the spinal cord injured population range from 16% to 59%. However, it has been argued that identification and classification of TBI is varied and at times unreliable. In a prospective study of 198 admissions to a traumatic SCI rehabilitation center, Macciocchi and colleagues (Macciocchi, Seel, Thompson, Byams, & Bowman, 2008) used stringent diagnostic measures and found that 60% of patients admitted to a center following an SCI had also sustained a TBI.

For patients with both SCI and TBI, the dual diagnosis can pose challenges to clinical rehabilitation over and above those elicited by either diagnosis on its own (Bradbury et al., 2008). Rehabilitation following SCI requires the relearning of skills or the introduction of new compensatory techniques to manage the changes resulting from injury. The neuropsychological changes resulting from sustaining a TBI would understandably impede the patient's ability to process large amounts of information and acquire the new knowledge necessary for increasing independence. A review of the complications arising from brain injury demonstrated how cognitive deficits can interfere with the SCI patient's capacity to learn new skills and achieve optimum independence (Arzaga, Shaw, & Vasile, 2003). Bradbury and colleagues (2008) conducted a study looking at the impact of comorbid TBI on SCI rehabilitation, finding the TBI-SCI group to show more behavioral and critical incidents (defined as aggressive or emotional outbursts to others, verbal or physical violence, and injuries arising from risk-taking behaviors); increased scores on measures of paranoia/schizophrenia, attention, and speed of information processing; and memory impairments than the group with SCI alone. Clinically, not only can these sequelae have a deleterious effect on the patient's progress in rehabilitation, but if the TBI is left undiagnosed, they could lead to frustrations within the treating team and other patients, who might consequently label the patient as being "difficult." In those cases in which the presence of TBI is established, the type of emotional, psychological, and clinical support offered to the patient will need to be modified according to his or her need.

In addition to the complications arising from traumatic injury, cognitive functions and subsequent rehabilitation outcomes are also found to be affected by pre-injury substance or alcohol misuse. Intoxication at time of injury is implicated in 39–50% of SCI cases (Burke, Linden, Zhang, Maiste, & Shields, 2001; Heinemann, Keen, Donohue, & Schnoll, 1988) and has been documented as both a pre- and post-injury problem for those with SCI. With pre-injury alcohol use patterns found to be strongly related to consumption following injury, continued misuse can lead to longer hospitalization and increased likelihood of depression, pressure ulcers, and urinary tract infections (Tate, Forchheimer, Krause, Meade, & Bombardier). One study (Kolakowsky-Haynor et al., 2002) found that 96% of consecutive newly injured admissions reported pre-injury alcohol use, with 57% assessed as being heavy drinkers, whereas a second study (Elliot, Kurylo, Chen, & Hicken, 2002) found 23% of inpatients had significant alcohol problems. Elliot and colleagues also found those individuals with alcohol misuse problems scored higher on measures of depressive behavior, and were also over two and a half times more likely to develop a pressure sore in the 3 years following injury.

Research has found substance misuse to be linked to greater use of avoidance coping strategies and less acceptance of injury (Kennedy, Duff, Evans, & Beedie, 2003) compared to those who do not abuse alcohol. These avoidant coping strategies have also been associated with poorer adjustment and increased likelihood of psychological difficulties. Furthermore, pre-injury alcoholism has also been found to account for a significant proportion of variance in functional improvement (as measured using the Functional Independence Measure [FIM]; Bombardier, Stroud, Esselman, & Rimmele, 2004; Hamilton & Granger, 1990) and can therefore act as a barrier to rehabilitation progress.

In addition to the negative impact on rehabilitation and psychological adjustment, people with alcohol problems have been found to report greater interference and intensity of pain following injury. Tate and colleagues (2004) conducted a retrospective analysis of 3,041 people with SCI, finding that the 14% of participants classified as having alcohol abuse problems were more likely to develop a pressure ulcer and reported significantly worse pain outcomes and lower life satisfaction scores than those without substance misuse problems.

Chronic pain is a commonly reported problem following SCI, with prevalence estimates ranging from 25% to 45% (Richards, 1992) and up to 96% (Dijkers, Bryce, & Zanca, 2009). It results from disruption to the signaling of nerve fibers (meaning that the pain signal is sent in the absence of any noxious stimulus) and has been associated with poor adjustment, depression, and with lower scores on ratings of life satisfaction and quality of life (QOL) measures. Chronic pain can not only lead to difficulties in mobility, but also impacts on social participation, life satisfaction (Norrbrink Budh & Österåker, 2007), and QOL (Putzke, Richards, Hicken, & DeVivo, 2002). Neuropathic pain has been related to lower scores on measures of physical health status (Noonan, Kopec, Zhang, & Dvorak, 2008) and has been found to have a negative effect on occupational status after injury (Meade, Barrett, Ellenbogen, & Jackson, 2006), with those reporting higher pain intensity and interference less likely to be in full time employment.

A variety of demographic and injury-related variables such as age, sex, completeness of lesion, and duration of injury have been investigated in relation to risk factors for developing chronic pain; however, results have been inconsistent and inconclusive. One major difficulty in ascertaining reliable risk factors for the development of chronic pain after SCI is the lack of consensus on classification of pain subtypes (see Sipski & Richards, 2006, for a review). Higher ratings of pain have been linked to affectivity and psychopathology such as expressed anger and negative cognitions (Summers, Rapoff, Varghese, Porter, & Palmer, 1991), and higher pain severity has been linked to lower scores on measures of acceptance of injury (Wade, Price, Hamer, Schwartz, & Hart, 1990) and greater catastrophizing (Turner, Jensen, Warms, & Cardenas, 2002). A study of 190 individuals with SCI by Widerström-Noga and colleagues (2007) found a small group of individuals to report low psychosocial impact of pain despite experiencing moderately high pain severity. When the characteristics of these individuals were explored, analysis revealed significantly higher levels of positive interpersonal support from significant others compared to people with moderately high pain severity and high psychosocial impact. These findings reinforce the importance of social support to many aspects of rehabilitation and adjustment for people with SCI.

Pressure ulcers are the most commonly occurring complication of SCI, with estimations of 85% of people with SCI developing complications of this sort during their lifespans. Pressure ulcers are localized areas of tissue necrosis that are caused when soft tissue is exposed to prolonged periods of unrelieved pressure. By nature, the individual with SCI is at high risk of pressure ulcer development if appropriate preventative measures are not in place.

A range of factors have been associated with an increased risk for pressure ulcer development. Impairments directly resulting from the injury such as the individual's American Spinal Injury Association (ASIA) classification of functioning, autonomic dysreflexia, faecal or urinary incontinence, and muscle tone abnormality; medical conditions such as diabetes, malnutrition, urinary tract infections, and pulmonary disease; the immediate

management after injury such as the duration of time left immobile; demographic factors such as age, education, gender, and duration of injury; behavioral factors such as substance misuse, smoking, and noncompliance with skin care routine; and psychological factors such as impaired cognition, lack of social support, and poor problem-solving abilities have all been associated with risk for pressure ulcer development.

Not only does the occurrence of pressure ulcers lead to prolonged periods of bed rest, time away from family, and disruption to work and social life, but, due to complications and septicemia, the development of a pressure ulcer can even increase the risk of death (Devivo et al., 1989; Lidal et al., 2007).

What is interesting about the high incidence rate of pressure ulcer development following SCI is the degree to which it is avoidable if a regular skin care routine is followed. During rehabilitation, the prevention of pressure ulcers remains a focus of education through instruction and practice of pressure relief techniques, regular skin checks, increasing the patients' awareness of factors that can increase the risk of damage to skin, and encouraging a healthy and balanced diet to prevent malnutrition. Although education of the patient and regular checks are important factors in reducing the likelihood of secondary complications, the level of educational information that families or caregivers receive has also been found to be important to the maintenance of a healthy skin care regime.

In an evaluation of the knowledge families and caregivers of bedridden patients had on pressure sore prevention, Kwiczala-Szydlowska and colleagues (2005) found that only 11% of questioned person knew what the pressure ulcer was, 42% of caregivers were not aware of possible pressure ulcer causes, and 54.8% were not able to name any pressure ulcer risk factor. The researchers suggested a need to implement educational program for caregivers in order to prevent complications after discharge. However, the support that interpersonal relationships provide may alone be an important factor in the development of secondary conditions such as pressure sores.

Although the provision of education and instruction on how to prevent pressure ulcer development undoubtedly lowers the incidence in this population, research has found that the level of knowledge about pressure ulcer prevention is not related to subsequent skin care behavior (King, Porter, & Vertiz, 2008). Despite participants expressing beliefs of their own susceptibility to pressure ulcer development and an awareness of the importance of preventative care, contradictory statements about beliefs and behavior were frequent. The researchers hypothesized that this may be due to the individuals' beliefs about their "personal efficacy" or ability to carry out the required behaviors, or that the consequences of not caring for their skin were too far in the future and outweighed by favorable priorities.

Coping with the challenges that SCI brings requires daily ongoing self-care. Health programs seeking to reduce post-discharge complications have focused on increasing levels of exercise (Martine-Ginis, 2003), active coping skills (Sable, Craig, & Lee, 2000), and an emphasis on self-management and increased knowledge (Hughes, Nosek, Howland, Groff, & Mullen, 2003). The development of pressure ulcers has been found to be significantly related to ineffective problem-solving in cross-sectional (Herrick, Elliot, & Crew, 1994) and prospective (Elliott & Bush, 2003) studies of people living with SCI, and other programs have built on cognitive behavioral strategies to build self-efficacy (Smarr et al., 1997) and effective problem-solving abilities.

The incidence and prevalence of pressure sores continues to be problematic for the spinal cord injured population and a vast amount of the literature and research has focused on physiological variables and medical risk factors. However, despite evidence to suggest that psychological variables may be more reliable predictors of mortality than demographic or medical status (Krause & Crewe, 1987), the majority of research continues to focus on biomechanical issues. Given that the occurrence of pressure ulcers can be devastating to an individual's QOL, and in some cases to his or her psychological well-being, more research into the potentially modifiable variables should be conducted. Additionally, if such secondary complications are to be successfully reduced in people with SCI living in the community, proactive measures are required. The past four decades have shown strong implication that pressure ulcer risk assessment should not only include physiological and medical markers but also those psychosocial factors that continue to appear in research.

Psychosocial Factors in Spinal Cord Injury Rehabilitation

Although suggestions were initially made that individuals would have to go through a period of depression (Siller, 1969) or through a set path of psychological phases similar to bereavement in order to adjust to life after SCI, research has found that people can respond and adjust to injury in very different ways. Although it is common and understandable that individuals will experience a certain amount of negative emotion toward the injury, the percentage for which these emotions develop into clinically significant psychological problems is relatively low (around 25–30%), and the majority of people sustaining a SCI go on to lead satisfying and rewarding lives. This section will introduce research findings on the psychosocial factors involved in SCI rehabilitation.

The 19th-century psychologist William James postulated that emotional experiences arise from the subjective interpretation of autonomic changes in bodily states such as heart rate, perspiration, and blood pressure (James, 1884), which are influenced by changes in regional cerebral activity and communicated through the spinal cord. In light of James' theory of emotion, there has been much debate as to whether the emotional experiences of individuals who sustain injuries to the spinal cord are subsequently affected. Driven by personal experience, an early paper by George Hohmann, in 1966, used structured interviews to obtain patient perspectives of their own emotional experiences before and after SCI. The main findings of the study were of a perceived overall change in the way that emotions were experienced by the participants, and that this degree of change was in some way related to the severity of the injury. However, the early investigation was hampered by a number of methodological limitations, and as psychological research developed, this early evidence has not been confirmed. A recent paper by Deady and colleagues (Deady, North, Allan, Smith, & O'Carroll, 2010) investigated emotionality and memory for emotional material in a sample of participants with SCI in comparison to participants without injury and orthopaedic surgery controls, finding no significant decrease in either measure.

Simultaneously, as some researchers focus on whether people with SCI show significant emotional impairment, a considerable amount of literature has accumulated to investigate the emotional and psychological sequelae of SCI and the prevalence of emotional disturbance post injury. A study by Quale and colleagues (Quale, Schanke, Frøslie, & Røise, 2009) found that 6% of a sample of severely injured patients met diagnostic criteria for posttraumatic stress disorder (PTSD) and 9% were classified as subthreshold. On looking at the risk factors related to PTSD, the research team found that females, those with symptoms of anxiety, and those with negative attitudes to emotional expression were more likely to develop PTSD, whereas injury-related data or severity of injury did not impact on subsequent psychological distress. A review by Craig and colleagues (2009) found estimates of depression during rehabilitation to be approximately 30%, while 37% of a community sample investigated in a study by Migliorini and colleagues (2008) experienced problems of depression; 30%, anxiety; 25%, stress; and 8.4% met diagnostic criteria for PTSD. An investigation of PTSD symptoms in a large sample of people with long-standing SCI (defined by a minimum of 7 years post injury) found the prevalence of PTSD to be similar to that of the general population (Krause, Saunders, & Newman, 2010). Furthermore, the study acknowledged that the item on which participants with SCI scored highly on was the difficulty of remembering important aspects of the event. The authors point out that for many individuals sustaining an SCI the circumstances are commonly traumatic and frequently associated with a loss of consciousness or TBI; therefore, endorsement of this item may be due to organic rather than psychological reasons.

Recently, Kennedy and colleagues (2010) investigated depression and anxiety in 281 participants with SCI across six European countries. The study found that at 6 weeks post injury, 40% were above clinical threshold for anxiety and 44% for depression. At 12 weeks post injury, these figures had dropped to 38% and 39%, respectively. Using a longitudinal design, Quale and Schanke (2010) identified the trajectories, characterized by resilience, recovery, or distress, of psychological adjustment to acquired physical disability. Classification into a particular trajectory was based on symptoms of psychological distress such as depression, anxiety, and PTSD; the most common trajectory in the sample was found to be one of resilience, with 54% of patients falling into this trajectory of adjustment. Twenty-five percent of the sample fell into the recovery category, meaning that 21% were classified into the distress trajectory.

Pollard and Kennedy (2007) reported longitudinal results from a study of emotional impact in people with SCI. Questionnaires completed at 12 weeks post-injury and again at a 10-year follow-up found rates of depression to remain relatively stable after 10 years; 38% of the sample reached clinical cutoff scores on the Becks Depression Inventory at 12 weeks and 35% at 10 years post injury. One prospective study (Dryden et al., 2004) followed people

sustaining a SCI for 6 years to gather information on the incidence of clinical depression when compared to demographically matched controls. Analysis found that 27.5% of those with SCI received treatment for depression during the follow-up interval compared with 10.8% of the control group.

In rehabilitation settings, clinical guidelines developed to identify risk of, assessment of, and treatment for depression (Paralyzed Veterans of America, 1998) recommend that routine screening should take place at the initial assessment and should continue to take place at annual reviews thereafter. The guidelines also suggest that thorough risk assessments, including previous or family history of depressive disorder, social support, chronic pain, coping style, substance abuse, and cognitive factors, should take place for people receiving rehabilitation following SCI.

Suicide rates in SCI populations have been estimated as up to six times more prevalent than in the general population. However, the reliability of these estimations has been questioned by researchers due to the inclusion of people sustaining spinal injury following a suicide attempt (Kennedy, Rogers, Speer, & Frankel, 1999). They suggested that the exaggerated estimations may be due to pre-injury psychological difficulties and not representative of the SCI population as a whole. The research group conducted a retrospective review of mortality in individuals sustaining an injury following deliberate self-harm and found that 24% of deaths were as a result of suicide. However, over 60% of deaths could be attributed to medical complications, such as bladder infections. In the SCI population, indirect forms of self-harm, such as self-neglect or alcohol and substance abuse, are more prevalent than actual suicide attempts, which themselves can lead to potentially fatal medical complications, such as bladder infections and pressure ulcers.

Scores obtained on QOL measures from SCI populations are generally found to be lower than those of the general population (Martz, Livneh, Priebe, Wuersmer, & Ottomanelli, 2005). However, further investigation has found that such ratings are linked more to secondary complications, activity limitations, and barriers to participation (Barker et al., 2009; Lund, Nordlund, Bernspång, & Lexell, 2007) rather than to factors relating to the injury itself or degrees of physical ability (Manns & Chad, 1999; Westgren & Levi, 1998). Indeed, the majority of people with SCI report that they are happy and satisfied with life (Carpenter, Forwell, Jongbloed, & Backman, 2007).

Contrary to what most people would expect, research has found that it is not the severity of injury or loss of function that determines how well an individual copes with and adjusts to the changes arising from spinal injury. This may explain why it is that two people with similar injuries can respond in psychologically polarized fashion following their injury.

In relation to risk or protective factors to the development of psychological distress, research has found that the presence of psychosocial issues or difficulties adjusting to injury is related more to the emotional responses and coping strategies used in response to the injury than to injury or impairment variables (Martz et al., 2005). A recent paper examined the influence of injury severity, global meaning-making, and perceived loss of functioning on psychological adjustment after SCI. The study found that, although medically determined injury severity was not related to psychological functioning and well-being, participants' *perceived* loss of functioning did have an impact on their psychological adjustment. Furthermore, the study found that global meaning-making partially mediated this relationship and suggested that these psychological factors are important variables that influence adaptation after SCI (deRoon-Cassini, de St Aubin, Valvano, Hastings, & Horn, 2009).

A review by Galvin and Godfrey (2001) highlighted the role of psychological variables in predicting the variance in adjustment to injury, particularly the way people think about or "appraise" their injury and the coping strategies they use in response to these appraisals. Negative coping strategies, such as disengagement or avoidance, have been linked to increased levels of depression and emotional distress in persons with SCI (Kennedy, Marsh, Lowe, Grey, Short, & Rogers, 2000) and decreased levels of life satisfaction and participation (Hansen & Tate, 1994), whereas positive adjustment to injury is found to be associated with active coping and positive reinterpretation (Pollard & Kennedy, 2007). A study investigating the relationship between appraisals, coping, and adjustment found that those people who initially interpret the injury as a challenge are more likely to use adaptive coping strategies, such as acceptance. At a 1-year follow-up, these individuals scored considerably better than those who initially interpreted their injury as a loss or a threat on measures of QOL, anxiety, and depression (Kennedy et al., 2010). In the previously discussed paper by Quale and Schanke (2010), the results found a relationship between resilience and trait positive and

negative affect, suggesting these variables to be an important factor in the long-term adjustment to acquired physical disability.

The vast amount of literature and research into the relationship of appraisals, coping, and adjustment has led to the development of appraisal and coping measures specific to people with SCI—the Appraisals of Disability: Primary and Secondary Scale (ADAPSS; Dean & Kennedy, 2009) and the Spinal Cord Lesion-Related Coping Strategies Questionnaire (Elfström, Rydén, Kreuter, Persson, & Sullivan, 2002). Not only can these measures be used in furthering our understanding of the adjustment process in people with SCI, but they can assist in tailoring cognitive behavioral therapies to suit the specific appraisal and coping patterns of the individual. Pollard and Kennedy (2007) completed a 10-year investigation of coping and adjustment, concluding that the stability of coping strategies suggest them to be a dispositional factor and therefore requiring of more in-depth interventions. Such interventions are discussed in more detail later in this chapter.

A further research development has revealed a significant relationship between psychological appraisals and coping strategies and the patient's *functional* outcomes following SCI (Kennedy, Lude, Elfström, & Smithson, (2010). In a longitudinal study using a large sample from four European spinal injury rehabilitation centers, appraisals and coping variables at 12 weeks post injury explained 25% of the variance in FIM scores at 1 year post injury. Most significantly, a strong contribution to this variance was found to be made by the coping strategy of social reliance. The type of statements that would be endorsed by people using this method of coping would be phrases such as "I feel helpless without support" and "my injury has taught me that I am dependent on others." Clearly, the results from these analyses suggest that the use of social reliance as a method of coping with spinal injury has a negative longitudinal effect.

Similarly, the salient appraisal process *negative perceptions of disability* (from the ADAPSS) has been found to be related to functional independence in a community sample of spinal cord injured patients (Kennedy et al., 2010). From these two studies, it may be interpreted that negative appraisals of injury may increase the degree to which the individual perceives his or her situation as unmanageable and that he or she doesn't have the resources to cope. This may in turn lead the individual to contribute minimal effort to the rehabilitation process or to show an increased dependency or "social reliance" on other people. Research findings such as these underscore the impact of psychological factors not only on adjustment to injury but to functional rehabilitation outcomes and independence.

Studies looking into the variations of scores between people with SCI on measures of life satisfaction have found scores to be directly related to involvement in productive activities such as employment and leisure pursuits (Buck & Hohmann, 1981), while qualitative research highlights the importance of meaningful relationships, responsibility, sense of personal control, and engagement in meaningful activity on QOL ratings (Alexander, Hwang, & Sipski, 2002). Kortte and colleagues (2010) examined the relationships between psychological variables and ratings on life satisfaction measures during acute rehabilitation and again at 3 months after discharge. Their findings suggested that positive "facilitators," such as hope and positive affect, were related to higher ratings of life satisfaction at both time points. A second study (White, Driver, & Warren, 2010) investigated the relationships between resilience, life satisfaction, depression, spirituality, and independence during hospital rehabilitation and found significant correlations between these factors. These hypothesized links may therefore provide valuable frameworks around which to structure interventions to facilitate positive outcomes.

Social support is also found to be related to psychological outcomes and adjustment after SCI (North, 1999), has been identified as a predictor of early mortality (Krause & Carter, 2009) and associated with low hopelessness and depression scores (Beedie & Kennedy, 2002). Qualitative findings have underscored the benefit in services providing informal support and advice to people with SCI throughout rehabilitation since family and peer support have been reported as facilitating the adjustment process.

Following discharge from the hospital, partners or family members often adopt the role of primary caregiver. At times, families can assume this role with little or no education and support, which may lead to problems with overload, financial strain, impaired QOL, and health and emotional problems (Post, Bloemen, & de Witte, 2005; Vitaliano, Zhang, & Scanlan, 2003). Chan (2000) looked at the coping strategies used by partners of people with SCI and found that those who used distancing and escape-avoidance strategies reported higher levels of depression and caregiving burden.

In terms of the adjustment of children of people with SCI, research has found children of fathers with SCI to be well adjusted, emotionally stable, and not affected in terms of body image, recreation interests, and personal relationships (Buck & Hohmann, 1981), whereas Alexander and colleagues (2002) found no differences in the personalities of children of mothers with SCI and children of mothers without injury. Ghidini and colleagues (2009) investigated the impact of pregnancy and childbearing in women with SCI, finding that 96% reported motherhood to have increased their QOL and that they would consider having more children in the future.

With respect to marriage and divorce in the spinal cord injured population, researchers have generally found a marginally higher rate of divorce in the spinal injured population compared to national norms, and that the greatest risk of divorce occurs in the first year following injury, before declining to rates similar to that of the general population. In contrast, marriages that take place following the acquired injury have been found to be more stable (see Kreuter, 2000, for a review). Furthermore, studies have found that people with SCI who are married report significantly higher levels of QOL, life satisfaction, and participation than do their single counterparts.

Problems with sexual dysfunction are commonly experienced following SCI due to the neurological changes incurred as a result of the injury. Such difficulties can lead to emotional distress for the individual with SCI and have a negative impact on his or her QOL and social relationships. Furthermore, patient concerns about bowel and bladder accidents, altered body image, autonomic dysreflexia, pain interference, and spasm have been reported as factors that discourage the pursuit of physical relationships (Anderson, Borisoff, Johnson, Steines, & Elliot, 2007). Anderson and colleagues (2007) found that the majority of respondents on an internet survey reported that their injury had affected their sexual sense of self and that improvements in sexual function would improve their QOL. Phelps and colleagues (2001) found that 42% of a sample of married men with SCI were dissatisfied with their sex lives and 50% had experienced feelings of sexual inadequacy. Decreased sexual activity was reported as one of the areas with which people were most dissatisfied in the first 18 months following discharge from hospital. In a study to describe women's experience of sexual activity and functioning after spinal injury, Kreuter and colleagues (2010) completed a cross-sectional survey of 392 women who had engaged in sexual activity following spinal injury. Many of the women included in the study reported that their injury had a negative impact on their sexuality and resulted in major changes to their sex lives. As previously discussed, some of these changes were physical in nature (e.g., changes in sensation, movement, and positioning, and bladder or bowel problems); however, some women reported more psychological changes with regards to their sexuality, such as feeling unattractive, reduced self-confidence, and difficulties in meeting a partner.

Clearly, this is an area in which rehabilitation services may be improved with the provision of further support and information for patients following the occurrence of SCI (Kennedy et al., 2009). Continued sexual health is important for all people, including those with acquired disability, and it is therefore important for any holistic service to include and support the sexual health and well-being of their service users. The *recognition model* (Couldrick, Sadlo, & Cross, 2010) is a team-based approach to support and provide advice on the sexual health of service users in disability rehabilitation services. It recognizes the importance of the sexual needs of the service user and the importance of affirming the relevance and priority of questions posed regarding sexual expression. The model was based on a research study developed in consultation with disabled people and is targeted at health and social care professionals working in multiprofessional disability teams, thus highlighting how shared skills can be used to "protect, support, or restore the sexual health of disabled people."

Psychological Interventions Following Spinal Cord Injury

During the acute period following SCI, the purpose of rehabilitation is to maximize the patient's independence, autonomy, and participation. During this period, it is important for the clinical team to recognize that, although the patient will undoubtedly require a high intensity of support and be dependent on the assistance of others, ultimately, the goal of rehabilitation is to maximize independence in the community. In practice, facilitating an assertive and independent way of communicating is not as straightforward as it may seem. In the early stages, the patient's high level of dependence and need for assistance from others may communicate the message that he or she is incapable of self-direction; decisions are made for them, schedules are set according to nursing practices, and an overly assertive manner may be misinterpreted as "difficult" or

"challenging." As previously discussed, perceived control and manageability have been associated with positive adjustment. This section will discuss those psychological interventions that have been found to promote positive appraisals of injury and increase patients' beliefs that they can manage the challenges arising from SCI.

The association between appraisals and coping strategies and scores on measures of anxiety and depression (Kennedy et al., 2000, 2010) has led to the development of psychoeducational intervention programs specifically tailored for use in the SCI population. *Coping effectiveness training* (CET; Kennedy et al., 2003) aims to equip patients with the knowledge and confidence to apply adaptive coping strategies to manage the changes arising from a spinal injury. It is based on the premise that coping serves two functions—to alter the problem causing distress and to regulate the emotional response to the problem. For those aspects of the problem that can be changed, the individual is trained to use problem-focused coping strategies, while for unchangeable aspects of the problem, the individual is encouraged to use emotion-focused strategies. The content of CET includes a range of standardized cognitive-behavioral strategies, such as activity scheduling and challenging negative thoughts, in addition to training in relaxation techniques and problem-solving skills. In the first session, the concept of stress is introduced and stress reactions are normalized. During sessions, patients are encouraged to think about how stressful situations are interpreted or "appraised," and what behaviors are selected to manage or "cope" with the stressful situation. The second and third sessions discuss in more detail critical appraisal skills and effective problem-solving, while the fourth session adopts a cognitive-behavioral framework in examining the relationship among thoughts, feelings, and behaviors. The fifth session looks at recognizing negative appraisals and how to overcome them, while the final two sessions integrate patients' knowledge on how to select the appropriate coping response for a particular situation.

A study by Kennedy and colleagues (2003) compared patients completing the CET program against matched controls. The study found significantly reduced anxiety and depression scores in the active treatment group compared to controls both immediately post intervention and at a 6-week follow-up. In addition to the psychological benefits, qualitative data obtained from patients participating in CET highlighted the importance of group discussion to the newly injured person and the benefit felt through information sharing with peers, thus reiterating the need for services to provide patients with the opportunity for informal peer support during rehabilitation. A later evaluation was carried out by Duchnick and colleagues (2009); it compared the effectiveness of CET against an alternative therapy condition. Although no differences were found between treatment groups on measures of anxiety, depression, and adjustment, symptom reductions were achieved with fewer sessions of CET than in the comparison group.

The overarching aim of SCI rehabilitation is to equip the individual with the necessary skills and confidence to manage the changes and challenges arising from injury and to encourage a sense of personal responsibility. The rehabilitation team can encourage this through involving the patient in problem-solving activities and allowing him or her to make informed choices about his or her care and rehabilitation. One way in which this has been implemented in clinical care is with the Needs Assessment and Goal Planning Programme (NAC; Kennedy & Hamilton, 1999), which is integrated into patient care at the National Spinal Injuries Centre (NSIC) at Stoke Mandeville Hospital, England (see Kennedy and Smithson, Chapter 7 for more information). Goal setting theory has endorsed the individual's involvement in the process as essential to its success and to the maintenance of change. In SCI, the patient may have to relearn basic skills and also acquire new techniques to maintain health, in addition to receiving large amounts of information and advice on various aspects of his injury. The NAC functions to identify areas of need through standardized assessment of knowledge and ability across rehabilitation domains. What differentiates this measure from most outcome measures, and highlights its suitability to the spinal cord injured population, is the acknowledgment of both physical and verbal independence. From the NAC, key areas of need are identified, and the multidisciplinary team works with the patient in a goal planning meeting to set clearly identifiable and achievable goals to work toward during rehabilitation. Following the introduction of the program at the NSIC, patients were found to spend more time participating in therapy and involved in rehabilitation activities when on the ward, showing that goal planning was an effective way of reducing the disengagement of patients and increasing their activity levels and involvement in therapy.

A significant development to the goal planning approach has seen the integration of "action plans

and coping plans." Coping planning for anticipated difficult or challenging situations allows an individual to prepare strategies that will prioritize a planned behavior in favor of an instinctive reaction. Strategies can consist of self-regulatory techniques, such as self-motivational statements, cognitive restructuring, and emotional regulation. Coping planning differs from typical action or goal planning in that it takes into consideration situational and environmental cues that may lead to an undesired behavioral response, and it elicits behaviors that may not be linked directly to an intended goal. Action planning and coping planning are therefore hypothesized to work in synchrony toward goal attainment through specifying details of the actions required to achieve the goals and those strategies to implement it in the face of challenges. The effectiveness of action planning with coping planning on participant's leisure time physical activity was evaluated in a sample of people with SCI living in the community (Arbour-Nicitopoulos, Ginis, & Latimer, 2009). These researchers found that those allocated to a combined treatment condition reported significantly greater activity levels and improved scheduling and self-efficacy in comparison to those completing action plans only. This study highlights how encouraging problem-solving and self-efficacy can be beneficial in overall scheduling and activity planning in the community.

Cognitive-behavioral approaches have been frequently applied as a therapeutic intervention in the spinal cord injured population due to the strong evidence base for positive outcomes. Cognitive-behavioral techniques can be applied to challenge negative cognitions about disability, thus decatastrophizing and supporting patients during the acute phase of injury or continuing with ongoing care for those with a preexisting history of psychological problems. Craig and colleagues (Craig, Hancock & Dickson, 1999) found that patients receiving cognitive-behavioral therapy (CBT) during hospital admission were less likely to be readmitted 2 years after injury, less likely to use prescription or illegal drugs, and were more likely to report themselves as having adjusted to living with SCI compared to a control group receiving care as usual. One recent study (Dorstyn, Mathias, & Denson, 2009) investigated the effectiveness of individualized CBT on psychological adjustment of patients with SCI undergoing acute rehabilitation when compared to standard clinical care. Patients in the treatment condition were found to show significant improvements in depression, anxiety, and stress throughout treatment; however, following the discontinuation of therapy, depression symptoms were found to worsen. The study highlighted the benefit of individualized care but also suggested the need for patients to have access to specialized psychological services post discharge.

Norrbrink Budh, Kowalski, and Lundeberg (2006) developed a comprehensive cognitive, behavioral, and educational program for neuropathic pain, designed specifically for people with SCI. Although no significant changes in pain intensity were found following the intervention, results from a 12-month follow-up found levels of anxiety and depression to be decreased when compared to baseline measures, suggesting that the intervention enabled the patients to cope effectively with the pain they experienced and minimize the psychological impact. A second study by Perry and colleagues (2010) evaluated the effectiveness of a group-based cognitive-behavioral pain management intervention for people with SCI-related chronic pain. The study found that at the end of the program, those who had received the cognitive-behavioral intervention reported significantly less anxiety, pain catastrophizing, and interference from pain and more improvements in mood compared to the group receiving usual care. However, the study also found that the initial improvements observed in this group were not maintained at a 9-month follow-up, suggesting the potential need for pain management interventions specifically tailored for the SCI population, while taking into consideration further psychological variables that may be specific to SCI and therefore impact on patients' ability to benefit from generic pain management programs.

What these studies highlight, and as discussed in a review by Gault and colleagues (2009), is that the psychological management of neuropathic pain has beneficial effects on the associated symptoms of chronic pain such as anxiety, depression, fatigue, and sleep disorder, rather than on the intensity of pain itself. However, in affording patients with chronic pain those skills with which to manage and cope with their pain effectively, clinicians can nevertheless improve their QOL and psychological well-being.

Families play an important role in providing the social support found to facilitate healthy adjustment in the spinal cord injured patient. However, the nature of injury means that the patient's social network often experience a high level of distress during both the acute and rehabilitation stages of injury, and psychological interventions have also been found to be beneficial in improving caregiver social and physical functioning. Elliot and Berry (2009) completed a randomised controlled trial to evaluate the effectiveness of a brief individualized problem-solving intervention for family and friends close to people with SCI. Although the intervention group did not show observable decreases in depression compared to controls, the group did report a significant decrease in dysfunctional problem-solving styles and an increase in beneficial effects on social and physical functioning. A second study compared the efficacy of two psychosocial interventions for caregivers of older persons with SCI (Schulz et al., 2009). They compared the outcomes on measures of depressive symptoms, burden, social support and integration, self-care problems, and physical health symptoms after a caregiver-only treatment or caregiver plus care recipient intervention. They found that the dual-target condition had significantly greater increases in QOL and improvements in depressive symptoms and burden compared to the control group, and significantly fewer physical health problems than both the caregiver-only condition and the controls. This study highlighted not only that caregivers can likewise benefit from psychological support, but that these benefits are most effective when intervention strategies target both the caregiver and care recipient. Future work should focus on the added benefit of increased support for families and caregivers on patient rehabilitation and adjustment.

Conclusion

Spinal cord injury is an event that may lead to profound changes, not only to an individual's physical and neurological functioning, but to his or her everyday life, psychological health, and social relationships. This chapter has highlighted that, for most people with SCI, their lives continue to be satisfying and fulfilling. The majority of people with SCI go on to enjoy strong and rewarding relationships with family and friends and participate fully in a variety of vocational and leisure activities. However, the impact of SCI for some people is such that they experience enduring adjustment difficulties that can lead to significant psychological problems. Previous research has revealed a link between secondary complications and QOL, and a recent commentary (Hammell, 2010) reported how people with SCI identify issues such as pain, fatigue, and pressure sores as areas in which they consider more research would be beneficial in improving the lives of people with SCI. Hammell also argues that further research is necessary to elucidate the link between secondary complications and QOL and the impact of environmental barriers on community and vocational participation. In order to obtain valuable insights into the complexity of factors facing those people with SCI, innovative research partnerships and patient consultation should take place in the development of new research initiatives.

The issues discussed here have highlighted the need for comprehensive, person-centered rehabilitation services incorporating theoretical models of appraisals, coping, and adjustment into therapeutic care.

Future Directions

• Work should continue to investigate the ways in which psychological interventions during rehabilitation can encourage reappraisal strategies and encourage adaptive coping strategies.

• Research partnerships should be fostered through consultation with patient representatives and SCI charities in order to ensure that the concerns and needs of the spinal cord injured population are being addressed.

• There remains relatively little work on the impact of SCI on children and siblings. Research should focus on the way in which family members adjust and cope with the changes arising from a family member sustaining a life-changing injury, and whether links exist between the way in which family and patient cope with injury. Such work may lead to beneficial long-term outcomes if family members receive similar support during the early stages of rehabilitation.

References

Alexander, C. J., Hwang, K., & Sipski, M. L. (2002). Mothers with spinal cord injuries: Impact on marital, family and children's adjustment. *Archives of Physical Medicine and Rehabilitation, 83*, 24–30.

Anderson, K. D., Borisoff, J. F., Johnson, R. D., Stiens, S. A., & Elliot, S. L. (2007). The impact of spinal cord injury on sexual function: Concerns of the general population. *Spinal Cord, 45*, 328–337.

Arbour-Nicitopoulos, K. P., Ginis, K. A., & Latimer, A. E. (2009). Planning, leisure time physical activity, and coping self-efficacy in persons with spinal cord injury: A randomized controlled trial. *Archives of Physical Medicine and Rehabilitation, 90*(12), 2003–2011.

Arzaga, D., Shaw, V., & Vasile, A. T. (2003). Dual diagnosis: The person with spinal cord injury and a concomitant brain injury. *SCI Nursing, 20*(2), 86–92.

Barker, R. N., Kendall, M. D., Amsters, D. I, Pershouse, K. J., Haines, T. P., & Kuipers, P. (2009). The relationship between quality of life and disability across the lifespan for people with spinal cord injury. *Spinal Cord, 47*(2), 149–155.

Beedie, A., & Kennedy, P. (2002). Quality of social support predicts hopelessness and depression post spinal cord injury. *Journal of Clinical Psychology in Medical Settings, 9*, 227–234.

Bombardier, C. H., Stroud, M. W., Esselman, P. C., & Rimmele, C. T. (2004). Do preinjury alcohol problems predict poorer rehabilitation progress in persons with spinal cord injury? *Archives of Physical Medicine and Rehabilitation, 85*(9), 1488–1492.

Bradbury, C. L., Wodchis, W. P., Mikulis, D. J., Pano, E. G., Hitzig, S. L., McGillivray, C. F., et al. (2008). Traumatic brain injury in patients with traumatic spinal cord injury: Clinical and economic consequences. *Archives of Physical Medicine and Rehabilitation, 89*(12 Suppl 2), S77–S84.

Buck, F. M., & Hohmann, G. (1981). Personality, behavior, values and family relations of children of fathers with spinal cord injury. *Archives of Physical Medicine and Rehabilitation, 62*, 432–438.

Burke, D. A., Linden, R. D., Zhang, Y. P., Maiste, A. C., & Shields, C. B. (2001). Incidence rates and populations at risk for spinal cord injury: A regional study. *Spinal Cord, 39*, 274–278.

Carpenter, C., Forwell, S. J., Jongbloed, L. E., & Backman, C. L. (2007). Community participation after spinal cord injury. *Archives of Physical Medicine and Rehabilitation, 88*, 427–433.

Chan, R. C., (2000). Stress and Coping in Spouses following Spinal Cord Injuries. *Clinical Rehabilitation, 14*(2), 137–144.

Couldrick, L., Sadlo, G., & Cross, V. (2010). Proposing a new sexual health model of practice for disability teams: The recognition model. *International Journal of Therapy and Rehabilitation, 17*(6), 290–293.

Craig, A., Hancock, K., & Dickson, H. (1999). Improving the long-term adjustment of spinal cord injured persons. *Spinal Cord, 37*(5), 345–350.

Craig, A., Tran, Y., & Middleton, J. (2009). Psychological morbidity and spinal cord injury: A systematic review. *Spinal Cord, 47*(2), 108–114.

Davidoff, G., Morris, J., Roth, E., & Bleiberg, J. (1985). Cognitive dysfunction and mild closed head injury in traumatic spinal cord injury. *Archives of Physical Medicine and Rehabilitation, 66*, 489–491.

Davidoff, G. N., Roth, E. J., & Richards, J. S. (1992). Cognitive deficits in spinal cord injury: Epidemiology and outcome. *Archives of Physical Medicine and Rehabilitation, 73*, 275–284.

Deady, D. K., North, N. T., Allan, D., Smith, M. J., & O'Carroll, R. E. (2010). Examining the effect of spinal cord injury on emotional awareness, expressivity and memory for emotional material. *Psychology, Health and Medicine, 15*(4), 406–419.

Dean, R., & Kennedy, P. (2009). Measuring appraisals following spinal cord injury: A preliminary psychometric analysis of the appraisals of disability. *Rehabilitation Psychology, 54*, 222–231.

DeVivo, M. J., Kartus, P. L., Stover, S. L., Rutt, R. D., & Fine, P. R. (1989). Cause of death for patients with spinal cord injuries. *Archives of Internal Medicine, 149*(8), 1761–1766.

Dijkers, M., Bryce, T., & Zanca, J. (2009). Prevalence of chronic pain after traumatic spinal cord injury: A systematic review. *Journal of Rehabilitation Research and Development, 46*, 13–29.

Dorstyn, D. S., Mathias, J. L., & Denson, L. A. (2010). Psychological intervention during spinal rehabilitation: A preliminary study. *Spinal Cord, 48*, 756–761.

Dryden, D., Saunders, L., Rowe, B., May, L. A., Yiannakoulias, N., Svenson, L. W., et al. (2004). Utilization of health services following spinal cord injury: A 6-year follow up study. *Spinal Cord, 42,* 513–525.

Duchnick, J. J., Letsch, E. A., & Curtiss, G. (2009). Coping effectiveness training during acute rehabilitation of spinal cord injury/dysfunction: A randomized clinical trial. *Rehabilitation Psychology, 54*(2), 123–132.

Elfström, M. L., Rydén, A., Kreuter, M., Persson, L. O., & Sullivan, M. (2002). Linkages between coping and psychological outcome in the spinal cord lesioned: Development of SCL-related measures. *Spinal Cord, 40,* 23–29.

Elliott, T. R., & Berry, J. (2009). W. Brief problem-solving training for family caregivers of persons with recent-onset spinal cord injuries: A randomized controlled trial. *Journal of Clinical Psychology, 65*(4), 406–422.

Elliott, T., & Bush, B. (2003). *Social problem solving abilities and pressure sore occurrence among persons with spinal cord injury.* Paper presented at the mid-winter conference of the Division of Rehabilitation Psychology/APA and the American Board of Rehabilitation Psychology, Tucson, AZ.

Elliott, T. R., Kurylo, M., Chen, Y., & Hicken, B. (2002). Alcohol abuse history and adjustment following spinal cord injury. *Rehabilitation Psychology, 47,* 278–290.

Galvin, L. R., & Godfrey, H. P. D. (2001). The impact of coping on emotional adjustment to spinal cord injury (SCI): Review of the literature and application of a stress appraisal and coping formulation. *Spinal Cord, 39,* 615–627.

Gault, D., Morel-Fatio, M., Albert, T., & Fattal, C. (2009). Chronic neuropathic pain of spinal cord injury: What is the effectiveness of psychocompartmental management? *Annals of Physical and Rehabilitation Medicine, 52*(2), 167–172.

Ghidini, A., Healey, A., Andreani, M., & Simonson, M. R. (2009). Pregnancy and women with spinal cord injuries. *Obstetrical and Gynaecological Survey, 64,* 141–142.

Hamilton, B. B., & Granger, C. V. (1990). *Guide for the use of the uniform data set for medical rehabilitation.* Buffalo, New York: Research Foundation of State University of New York.

Hammell, K. R. (2010). Spinal cord injury rehabilitation research: Patient priorities, current deficiencies and potential directions. *Disability and Rehabilitation, 32*(14), 1209–1218.

Hansen, N., & Tate, D. (1994). Avoidance coping, perceived handicap, and coping strategies of persons with spinal cord injury. *SCI Psychosocial Processes, 7,* 195.

Heinemann, A. W., Keen, M., Donohue, R., & Schnoll, S. (1988). Alcohol use in persons with recent spinal cord injuries. *Archives of Physical Medicine and Rehabilitation, 69,* 619–624.

Herrick, S., Elliott, T. R., & Crew, F. (1994). Self-appraised problem solving skills and the prediction of secondary complications among persons with spinal cord injuries. *Journal of Clinical Psychology in Medical Settings, 1*(3), 269–283.

Hohmann, G. W. (1966). Some effects of spinal cord lesions on experienced emotional feelings. *Psychophysiology, 3*(2), 143–156.

Hughes, R. B., Nosek, M. A., Howland, C. A., Groff, J. Y., & Mullen, P. D. (2003). Health promotion for women with physical disabilities: A pilot study. *Rehabilitation Psychology, 48,* 182–188.

James, W. (1884). What is an emotion? *Mind, 9,* 188–205.

Kennedy, P., & Hamilton, L.R. (1999). The Needs Assessment Checklist: A clinical approach to measuring outcome. *Spinal Cord, 37* (2), 136–9

Kennedy, P., Duff, J., Evans, M., & Beedie, A. (2003). Coping effectiveness training reduces depression and anxiety following traumatic spinal cord injuries. *British Journal of Clinical Psychology, 41,* 41–52.

Kennedy, P., Lude, P., Elfström, M., & Smithson, E. (2010). Cognitive appraisals, coping and psychological outcomes: A multi-centre study of spinal cord injury rehabilitation. *Spinal Cord.* Advance online publication. doi: 10.1038/sc.2010.20

Kennedy P, Lude P, Elfström ML & Smithson E.F. (2010). Psychological contributions to functional independence: a longitudinal investigation of spinal cord injury rehabilitation. *Archives of Physical Medicine and Rehabilitation, 92,* 597–602.

Kennedy, P., Marsh, N., Lowe, R., Grey, N., Short, E., & Rogers, B. (2000). A longitudinal analysis of psychological impact and coping strategies following spinal cord injury. *British Journal of Health Psychology, 5,* 157–172.

Kennedy, P., Rogers, B., Speer, S., & Frankel, H. (1999). Spinal cord injuries and attempted suicide: A retrospective review. *Spinal Cord, 37*(12), 847–852.

Kennedy, P., Sherlock, O., McClelland, M., Short, D., Royle, J., & Wilson, C. (2009). A multi-centre study of the community needs of people with spinal cord injuries: The first eighteen months. *Spinal Cord, 48,* 15–20.

Kennedy, P., Smithson, E., McClelland, M., Short, D., Royle, J., & Wilson, C. (2010). Life satisfaction, appraisals and functional outcomes in spinal cord injured people living in the community. *Spinal Cord, 48*(2), 144–148.

King, R. B., Porter, S. L., & Vertiz, K.B. (2008). Preventative skin care beliefs of people with spinal cord injury. *Rehabilitation Nursing, 33*(4), 154–162.

Kolakowsky-Haynor, S., Gourley, E., Kreutzer, J., Marwitz, J. H., Meade, M., & Cifu, D. X. (2002). Post injury substance abuse among persons with brain injury and persons with spinal cord injury. *Brain Injury, 16,* 583–592.

Kortte, K. B., Gilbert, M., Gorman, P., & Wegener, S. T. (2010). Positive psychological variables in the prediction of life satisfaction after spinal cord injury. *Rehabilitation Psychology, 55*(1), 40–47.

Krause, J. S., & Carter, R. E. (2009). Risk of mortality after spinal cord injury: Relationship with social support, education, and income. *Spinal Cord, 47,* 592–596.

Krause, J. S., & Crewe, N. (1987). Prediction of long term survival of persons with spinal cord injury: An 11-year prospective study. *Rehabilitation Psychology, 32,* 205–213.

Krause, J. S., Saunders, L. L., & Newman, S. (2010). Posttraumatic stress disorder and spinal cord injury. *Archives of Physical Medicine and Rehabilitation, 91,* 1182–1187.

Kreuter, M. (2000). Spinal cord injury and partner relationships. *Spinal Cord, 38,* 2–6.

Kreuter, M., Taft, C., Siösteen, A., & Biering-Sørensen, F. (2011). Women's sexual functioning and sex life after spinal cord injury. *Spinal Cord, 49,* 154–160.

Kwiczala-Szydłowska, S., Skalska, A., & Grodzicki, T. (2005). Pressure ulcer prevention-evaluation of awareness in families of patients at risk. *Przegadl Lekarski, 62*(12), 1393–1397.

Lidal, I. B., Snekkevik, H., Aamodt, G., Hjeltnes, N., Stanghelle, J. K., & Biering-Sørenson, F. (2007). Mortality after spinal cord injury in Norway. *Journal of Rehabilitation Medicine, 39,* 145–151.

Lund, M. L., Nordlund, A., Bernspång, B., & Lexell, J. (2007). Perceived participation and problems in participation are determinants of life satisfaction in people with spinal cord injury. *Disability Rehabilitation, 29*(18), 1417–1422.

Macciocchi, S., Seel, R. T., Thompson, N., Byams, R., & Bowman, B. (2008). Spinal cord injury and co-occurring traumatic brain injury: Assessment and incidence. *Archives of Physical Medicine and Rehabilitation, 89*(7), 1350–1357.

Manns, P., & Chad, K. (1999). Determining the relation between quality of life, handicap, fitness and physical activity for persons with spinal cord injury. *Archives of Physical Medicine and Rehabilitation, 80*, 1566–1571.

Martin-Ginis, K. A., Latimer, A. E., McKechinie, K., Ditor, D. S., McCartney, N., Hicks, A. L., et al. (2003). Using exercise to enhance subjective well being among people with spinal cord injury: The mediating influences of stress and pain. *Rehabilitation Psychology, 48*(3), 157–164.

Martz, E., Livneh, H., Priebe, M., Wuermser, L. A., & Ottomanelli, L. (2005). Predictors of psychosocial adaptation among people with spinal cord injury or disorder. *Archives of Physical Medicine and Rehabilitation, 86*, 1182–1192.

Meade, M. A., Barrett, K., Ellenbogen, P. S., & Jackson, M. N. (2006). Work intensity and variations in health and personal characteristics of individuals with Spinal Cord Injury (SCI). *Journal of Vocational Rehabilitation, 25*, 13–19.

Migliorini, C., Tonge, B., & Taleporos, G. (2008). Spinal cord injury and mental health. *Australian and New Zealand Journal of Psychiatry, 42*(4), 309–314.

Noonan, V., Kopec, J., Zhang, H., & Dvorak M. (2008). Impact of associated conditions resulting from spinal cord injury on health status and quality of life in people with traumatic central cord syndrome. *Archives of Physical Medicine and Rehabilitation, 89*, 1074–1082.

Norrbrink Budh, C., & Österåker, A. L. (2007). Life satisfaction in individuals with a spinal cord injury and pain. *Clinical Rehabilitation, 21*, 89–96.

Norrbrink Budh, C., Kowalski, J., & Lundeberg, T. (2006). A comprehensive pain management programme comprising educational, cognitive and behavioural interventions for neuropathic pain following spinal cord injury. *Journal of Rehabilitation Medicine, 38*(3), 172–180.

North, N. T. (1999). The psychological effects of spinal cord injury: A review. *Spinal Cord, 37*, 671–679.

Paralyzed Veterans of America (1998). *Depression following spinal cord injury: A clinical practice guideline for primary care physicians.* Washington, DC: PVA.

Perry, K. N., Nicholas, M. K., & Middleton, J. W. (2010). Comparison of a pain management program with usual care in a pain management center for people with spinal cord injury related chronic pain. *Clinical Journal of Pain, 26*(3), 206–216.

Phelps, J., Albo, M., Dunn, K., & Joseph, A. (2001). Spinal cord injury and sexuality in married or partnered men: Activities, function, needs and predictors of sexual adjustment. *Archives of Sexual Behaviour, 30*, 591–602.

Pollard, C., & Kennedy, P. (2007). A longitudinal analysis of emotional impact, coping strategies and post-traumatic psychological growth following spinal cord injury: A 10-year review. *British Journal of Health Psychology, 12*, 347–362.

Post, M. W. M., Bloemen, J., & de Witte, L. P. (2005). Burden of support for partners of persons with spinal cord injuries. *Spinal Cord, 43*, 311–319.

Putzke, J. D., Richards, J. S., Hicken, B. L., & DeVivo, M. J. (2002). Interference due to pain following spinal cord injury: Important predictors and impact on quality of life. *Pain, 100*(3), 231–242.

Quale, A. J., & Schanke, A. K. (2010). Resilience in the face of coping with a severe physical injury: A study of trajectories of adjustment in a rehabilitation setting. *Rehabilitation Psychology, 55*(1), 12–22.

Quale, A. J., Schanke, A. K., Frøslie, K. F., & Røise, O. (2009). Severity of injury does not have any impact on posttraumatic stress symptoms in severely injured patients. *Injury, 40*(5), 498–505.

Richards, J. S. (1992). Chronic pain and spinal cord injury: Review and comment. *Clinical Journal of Pain, 8*(2), 119–122.

deRoon-Cassini, T. A., de St Aubin, E., Valvano, A., Hastings, J., & Horn, P. (2009). Psychological well-being after spinal cord injury: Perception of loss and meaning making. *Rehabilitation Psychology, 54*(3), 306–314.

Sable, J., Craig, P., & Lee, D. (2000). Promoting health and wellness: A research based case report. *Therapeutic Recreational Journal, 34*, 348–361.

Schulz, R., Czaja, S. J., Lustig, A., Zdaniuk, B., Martire, L. M., & Perdomo, D. (2009). Improving the quality of life of caregivers of persons with spinal cord injury: A randomized controlled trial. *Rehabilitation Psychology, 54*(1), 1–15.

Siller, J. (1969). Psychological situation of the disabled with spinal cord injuries. *Rehabilitation Literature, 30*, 290–296.

Sipski, M. L., & Richards, J. S. (2006). Spinal cord injury rehabilitation: State of the science. *American Journal of Physical Medicine and Rehabilitation, 85*(4), 310–342.

Smarr, K. L., Parker, J. D., Wright, G. E., Stucky-Ropp, R. C., Buckelew, S. P., Hoffman, R. W., et al. (1997). The importance of enhancing self-efficacy in rheumatoid arthritis. *Arthritis Care and Research, 10*, 18–26.

Spinal Cord Injury Information Network. (2009). *Spinal cord injury facts and statistics at a glance.* Retrieved from http://images.main.aub.edu/spinalcord/pdffiles/factsApr09.pdf

Summers, J. D., Rapoff, M. A., Varghese, G., Porter, K., & Palmer, R. E. (1991). Psychosocial factors in spinal cord injury pain. *Pain, 47*, 183–189.

Tate, D. G., Forchheimer, M. B., Krause, J. S., Meade, M. A., & Bombardier, C. H. (2004). Patterns of alcohol and substance use and abuse in persons with spinal cord injury: Risk factors and correlates. *Archives of Physical Medicine and Rehabilitation, 85*, 1837–1847.

Turner, J. A., Jensen, M. P., Warms, C. A., & Cardenas, D. D. (2002). Catastrophizing is associated with pain intensity, psychological distress, and pain-related disability among individuals with chronic pain after spinal cord injury. *Pain, 98*, 127–134.

Vitaliano, P. P., Zhang, J., & Scanlan, J. (2003). Is caregiving hazardous to one's health? A meta-analysis. *Psychological Bulletin, 129*, 946–972.

Wade, J. B., Price, D. D., Hamer, R. M., Schwartz, S. M., & Hart, R. P. (1990). An emotional component analysis of chronic pain. *Pain, 40*, 303–310.

Westgren, N., & Levi, R. (1998). Quality of life and traumatic spinal cord injury. *Archives of Physical Medicine and Rehabilitation, 79*, 1433–1439.

White, B., Driver, S., & Warren, A. M. (2010). Resilience and indicators of adjustment during rehabilitation from a spinal cord injury. *Rehabilitation Psychology, 55*(1), 23–32.

Widerström-Noga, E. G., Felix, E. R., Cruz-Almeida, Y., & Turk, D. C. (2007). Psychosocial subgroups in persons with spinal cord injuries and chronic pain. *Archives of Physical Medicine and Rehabilitation, 88*(12), 1628–1635.

Persistent and Chronic Pain

Elizabeth J. Richardson *and* J. Scott Richards

Abstract

Chronic pain impacts a significant portion of the general population and often poses barriers to optimal functioning in a variety of activities of daily living. Our understanding of chronic pain has progressed considerably from a unidirectional pain processing model of afferent sensation to one involving a complex interplay of multiple factors including biological, psychological, and sociological components. This chapter discusses the complex interface of cognition, behavior, and pathophysiology on persistent pain, and its psychological and behavioral comorbidities. Current and emerging treatment paradigms and interventional contexts reflecting the multidimensionality of the chronic pain syndrome are also presented. Finally, future directions of study to advance the field of chronic pain psychology are proposed.

Key Words: Chronic pain, depression, anxiety, pain behavior, assessment, outcomes, multidisciplinary treatment.

Pain is a necessary, protective mechanism that promotes survival in our environment. Pain functions as a warning to protect an organism from sustaining damage or to facilitate healing when significant damage has occurred. The International Association for the Study of Pain defines pain as "an unpleasant sensory and emotional experience associated with actual or potential tissue damage, or described in terms of such damage" (Merskey & Bogduk, 1994, p. 210). An important aspect of this definition is that pain is understood as a subjective experience and not necessarily the sole consequence of an external stimulus. Defining pain in this way can account for the many pain syndromes seen in clinical situations.

Pain can be categorized as acute or chronic. *Acute pain* is of short duration, typically lasting no more than 3 months (Merskey, 1986), although a marker of 6 months is more typically applied (Doleys, 2000; Russo & Brose, 1998). It is often associated with apparent tissue damage which, when healed, leads to the elimination of pain (Walsh, Dumitru, Schoenfeld, & Ramamurthy, 1998). *Chronic pain,* on the other hand, continues despite apparent healing of the tissues involved, or it may be secondary to long-standing disease or other pathology (Walsh et al., 1998). However, the experience of pain is more than just afferent sensation. It is a complex interplay of multiple factors including biological, psychological/affective, and sociological components. It is for this reason that alterations or changes in any one or more of these factors can result in a maladaptive pain state with its attendant negative physiological changes, increased emotional distress, strained interpersonal relationships, and substantial economic burden from lost work days and incurred treatment costs.

A recent U.S. national survey indicated that 26% of Americans over the age of 20 reported experiencing a problem with pain, with 42% of those experiencing pain for more than 1 year (National Centers for Health Statistics, 2006). Others (Elliott, Smith, Penny, Smith, & Chambers, 1999) have found that up to 46.5% of the general U.S. population suffers from some form of chronic pain. Pain is the primary reason for most physician or medical consultations (Abbott & Fraser, 1998), and in 2000, it was reported that more than 312 million analgesic medications were prescribed (Turk, 2002a). Many, however, continue to experience pain despite provision of pharmacologic or surgical interventions. Cousins (1995) posited that the health care cost of treating chronic pain possibly exceeds that of heart disease, cancer, and AIDS combined. Indirect costs through lost work productivity secondary to common chronic pain conditions among workers were estimated to be $61.2 billion per year (Stewart, Ricci, Chee, Morganstein, & Lipton, 2003).

Chronic pain estimates across European populations have ranged from 12% to 30%, with lower rates in Spain, Ireland, and the United Kingdom (12%, 13%, and 13%, respectively) and highest rates in Italy, Poland, and Norway (26%, 27%, and 30%, respectively; Breivik, Collett, Ventafridda, Cohen, & Gallacher, 2006). Rates of chronic pain have been found to be lower in Asian countries, such as Singapore, where approximately 8.7% of the population reported experiencing pain for at least 3 months (Yeo & Tay, 2009). In the United Kingdom, production losses, absenteeism, and informal care costs from back pain conditions alone were approximated at £10.7 billion in 1998 UK £s (Maniadakis & Gray, 2000). The need persists to clarify current estimates of economic burden from chronic pain conditions in non-U.S. countries (Juniper, Le, & Mladsi, 2009).

Chronic Pain Subtypes and Pathophysiology

Pain can be further categorized into two broad types: nociceptive or neuropathic. *Nociceptive pain* is the most common form and occurs when pain nerve fiber endings, called *nociceptors*, are stimulated by tissue damage resulting from trauma or disease. Acute nociceptive pain conditions include postsurgical pain, trauma, obstetric pain, and pain from acute medical diseases, whereas more chronic nociceptive pain syndromes include headache, low back pain, and other musculoskeletal forms of pain (Raj, 1996). Neuropathic pain is understood as the product of damage to the peripheral or central nervous system (CNS) that alters the normal functioning of the nociceptive system (Bennett, 1994).

Neuropathic pain is a common physical sequela of deafferentation conditions such as amputation and spinal cord injury, or other conditions associated with nerve damage (e.g., diabetic neuropathy). This form of pain often presents a paradox, as neuropathic pain is often experienced in insensate, paralyzed, or in the case of amputation, even missing areas of the body. Neuropathic pain descriptively differs from nociceptive pain, as it is often reported as burning, electric, pricking, or tingling (Boureau, Doubrere, & Luu, 1990).

Until Melzack and Wall's (1965) seminal paper on the gate control mechanisms of pain processing, the predominant view was that pain resulted from a unidirectional relationship between peripheral stimulation from tissue damage and perception in the brain, and that the severity of pain perceived was essentially proportional to the degree of damage sustained. The *gate control theory* posited that incoming pain sensations did not pass to the cortex unaltered; rather, at specialized synapses in the dorsal horn of the spinal cord, a "gate" could be closed that reduced the amount of pain perceived (Melzack & Wall, 1965). In the periphery, pain is transmitted by two types of fibers: small, myelinated, and therefore fast, A-delta (Aδ) fibers and small, unmyelinated and slower C-fibers. Larger, non–pain transmitting A-beta (Aβ) fibers that relay pressure, touch, and vibration also synapse in the dorsal horn, and when stimulated, can override transmission of the Aδ and C pain fibers and thus attenuate pain sensation. This is believed to underlie the phenomenon of pain alleviation from rubbing or massaging an injured area. The gating mechanism is also thought to be the reason for the effectiveness of alternative treatments such as acupuncture (Man & Chen, 1972) and transcutaneous electrical nerve stimulation for pain (Sluka & Walsh, 2003).

The work of Melzack and Wall (1965) was seminal in fomenting a new, dynamic era in pain research, shifting the trajectory of investigative focus to additional biological, behavioral, and psychological factors that may modify the pain experience. The gate theory was later expanded by Melzack and Casey (1968) into a broader theoretical model of pain processing in higher CNS centers to explain how descending modulation of pain could occur. According to Melzack and Casey (1968), ascending pathways from the gating system in the dorsal horn of the spinal cord activate, in parallel, separate neural substrates associated with sensory discrimination (location and severity) and affective-motivational (fear, distress, and a desire to terminate or escape) components of pain. Higher CNS processes then evaluate these simultaneous inputs in light of past experiences, memories, and context, and exert a descending modulatory influence. However, the affective dimension of pain does not always coincide with pain severity. In clinical pain states, for instance, the affective components of pain may be greater than the sensory levels of that clinical pain, whereas the converse is seen in induced experimental pain (Price, Harkins, & Baker, 1987). Evidence for separate, but simultaneously operating pain dimensions led Price (1988) to conceptualize the pain experience as a sequential process in which the affective response to pain is mediated by cognitive appraisal of that pain and the situation in which it occurs. Further, how one appraises incoming pain sensations is affected by a host of other psychological factors, including memories, prior experiences, attitudes, and beliefs. Price's (1988) model indicated that affective distress in response to nociceptive stimulation could be differentially reduced by restructuring cognitive appraisals.

Evidence also implicates a high degree of plasticity in the neurochemical and cellular processes of nociception that may underlie the development and maintenance of chronic pain. The phenomenon of central sensitization is premised on a dynamically operating system and is believed to underlie pain hypersensitivity even after an injury has healed (Woolf, 1983). Central sensitization can occur following repeated afferent nociceptive input which increases the excitability of dorsal horn nociceptive neurons by alterations in neurochemistry and synaptic contacts (Woolf & Salter, 2006). As a result, dorsal horn nociceptors are "sensitized" via an increase in synaptic strength, and the threshold for afferent excitation is reduced (Ji, Kohno, Moore, & Woolf, 2003). Stimulation of non-pain sensory fibers may easily evoke potentials from hypersensitive nociceptors in the dorsal horn, producing a sensation of pain in the periphery. Allodynia, or a sensation of pain evoked by non-noxious stimulation, and hyperalgesia, or the increased sensitivity to noxious stimulation, are forms of chronic neuropathic pain believed to be caused by central sensitization mechanisms (Bolay & Moskowitz, 2002; Woolf & Mannion, 1999).

Plasticity in pain processing has also been identified in supraspinal pain circuitry. Long-term potentiation (LTP)—or the strengthening of synaptic contacts—is most associated with biological underpinnings of learning and memory. However, this mechanism has recently been implicated in chronic pain. Long-term potentiation has been shown to occur in the anterior cingulate cortex (ACC), a cortical region involved in processing pain unpleasantness and severity (Zhou, 2007). Johansen and Fields (2004) found that the ACC serves an important role in acquisition of memory for aversion in the presence of noxious stimulation. Changes in synaptic transmission following continued exposure to pain have also been observed in other cortical areas including the amygdala, medial prefrontal cortex, and thalamus (for a review, see Apkarian, Baliki, & Geha, 2009). The overlap in synaptic plasticity with pain and memory likely has adaptive benefit, as following exposure to a harmful stimulus, an organism has an increased chance for survival if thresholds for sensing similar stimuli are reduced in the future (Ji et al., 2003). Assimilating what is known about both the broader neural network connections and synaptic mechanisms of pain and memory, Apkarian and colleagues (2009) proposed viewing chronic pain as an old memory trace of previous injury in the prefrontal cortex—a region implicated in emotion and learning. This conceptualization of pain draws from basic Pavlovian learning but is recast in modern understanding of neurobiology. In essence, new pain experiences can trigger synaptic changes which, in turn, affect how one experiences a pain experience in the future. Chronic pain, or the continued exposure to pain, results in the memory of pain from an initial injury persisting, with a consequent inability to extinguish that pain memory (Apkarian et al., 2009).

Psychological and Behavioral Correlates of Chronic Pain
Depression

Psychological and affective comorbidities commonly exist with chronic pain; however, the most investigated is depression. Approximately half of chronic pain patients exhibit a substantial level of depressive symptomatology (Fishbain, Goldberg, Meagher, Steele, & Rosomoff, 1986; Romano & Turner, 1985; Turk, Okifuji, & Scharff, 1995). Among the various chronic pain populations, chronic low back pain is associated with the highest prevalence of depressive symptoms, with rates falling between 70% and 73% (Richardson et al., 2009; Gallagher, Moore, & Chernoff, 1995; Krishnan, France, Pelton, & McCann, 1985). When depression and chronic pain are comorbid, poor outcomes can occur in a variety of domains. People who experience depression in the context of a chronic pain condition are more likely to experience pain-related disability (Arnow et al., 2006; Ericsson et al., 2002) and incur greater health care costs (Greenberg, Leong, Birnbaum, & Robinson, 2003). Moreover, the presence of pain contributes to the risk of suicide in persons who are depressed (Gensichen, Teising, König, Gerlach, & Petersen, 2010).

The frequency with which depression coexists with chronic pain has fostered considerable debate about causality. Since limited longitudinal data exist, there remain mostly theories in the literature to describe the pain–depression relationship. Theories posited include depression as an antecedent, depression as a consequence, or that pain and depression are dynamic, concurrent states due to similar biological mechanisms (Brown, 1990; Fishbain, Cutler, Rosomoff, & Rosomoff, 1997). Views of depression as a consequence typically incorporate behavioral or cognitive factors as moderating and/or mediating variables. Continued efforts by the patient to pursue a pain "cure" may potentially become all-consuming, inadvertently drawing from psychological resources and energy that could otherwise be devoted to important aspects of living (McCracken, Carson, Eccleston, & Keefe, 2004). A sense of helplessness, an aspect of a depressive state, may ensue as the pain becomes increasingly perceived as outside one's locus of control (Crisson & Keefe, 1988). Deprivation of positively reinforcing activities as the result of pain may also contribute to negative affect (Fordyce, 1976). The chronic pain–depression relationship within the context of Beck's cognitive model (Beck, Rush, Shaw, & Emery, 1979) can be understood as erroneous thought patterns, such as catastrophizing about pain, that adversely affect emotional states (Sullivan et al., 2001). Distortions in thinking stem from maladaptive schemas that form from and are perpetuated by multiple pain experiences over time, as occurs in chronic pain (Sullivan et al., 2001). In this manner, pain catastrophizing—or the distorted thought process surrounding pain-related information—may not only be associated with depressive symptoms but also may precipitate a generalized depressive schema. Indeed, evidence indicates that greater catastrophizing at earlier time points has been found to significantly predict depression at subsequent time points (Keefe, Brown, Wallston, & Caldwell, 1989; Keefe et al., 1991).

Banks and Kerns (1996) applied a diathesis–stress model to explain depression in chronic pain. This model is consistent with the idea that depression stems from chronic pain, but it further describes the dynamic interaction between premorbid characteristics that may increase vulnerability to the development of psychopathology following the onset of a chronic pain condition. Banks and Kerns (1996) conceptualized diatheses to be preexisting traits or tendencies, such as attributional styles or maladaptive schemas that, when combined with the negative psychosocial stress from chronic pain, produce a depressive state.

Conversely, there is evidence to also suggest that negative affective states may precede chronic pain syndromes. Theories that view depression as a possible antecedent factor primarily stem from knowledge of shared biological pathways between nociceptive and affective processes. Limbic structures are implicated in the efferent pathways that aid in modulating pain (Fields, Basbaum, & Heinricher, 2006). This relay system includes serotonergic and noradrenergic neurons that can attenuate afferent pain sensations (Hirakawa, Tershrer, & Fields, 1999). Thus, a potential consequence of dysregulation of these neurotransmitters would be painful sensation from otherwise innocuous peripheral stimulation (Bair, Robinson, Katon, & Kroenke, 2003). Tricyclic antidepressants, such as amitriptyline, have a long history of showing positive results in reducing some forms of neuropathic pain (Watson, Chipman, & Monks, 2006), but more recently, serotonin and norepinephrine reuptake inhibitors (SNRIs) have been found to be of benefit in alleviating diabetic neuropathy pain and other chronic pain syndromes (Jann & Slade, 2007). Arnold and colleagues (2004), in a double-blind, placebo-controlled study, similarly found that an SNRI reduced pain among fibromyalgia patients with and without comorbid major depressive disorder.

Unraveling both causal and reciprocal relationships between pain and depression remains somewhat elusive. A single theoretical model may not always apply to the clinical situation, as the chronic pain–depression symptom constellation may depend on the pathology of the chronic pain itself and the unique individual factors that may predispose (or protect) from developing depression.

Anxiety and Pain-Related Fear

Comorbid anxiety has received less attention relative to depression in the chronic pain literature, although this trend appears to be changing (Asmundson & Katz, 2009). McWilliams, Cox, and Enns (2003) found that community-dwelling persons with chronic pain were almost three times as likely to have an anxiety disorder. Specifically, the associations between chronic pain and both panic disorder and post-traumatic stress disorder (PTSD) were found to be higher than that of depression. Demyttenaere and colleagues (2007) analyzed data cross-nationally and found that persons with chronic back or neck pain were 2.7 and 2.6 times as likely to have co-occurring generalized anxiety disorder and PTSD, respectively. However, it is important to note that an individual with chronic pain may not have an anxiety disorder exclusive of other forms of psychological or emotional distress. Means-Christensen et al. (2008) found that the relationship between anxiety disorders and pain was explained by the presence of depression. Individuals with chronic pain therefore may not experience a fixed affective state; rather, there is likely vacillation between depressed and anxious states depending on fluctuations of pain levels and changes in the context in which pain is experienced.

An area of pain-related anxiety that has received considerable attention has been that of *fear-avoidance* (Leeuw et al., 2007; Vlaeyen, Kole-Snijders, Boeren, & van Eek, 1995; Vlaeyen & Linton, 2000). Fordyce (1976) originally explained maladaptive behaviors from chronic pain using an operant learning model. From this perspective, a reduction in pain from the avoidance of activity serves as reinforcement to continue the avoidance behavior. In fact, the decrease in anxiety that results from avoiding experiences that are merely suspected to increase pain can serve as reinforcement, as well as the reduction social anxiety from avoiding social or performance situations in which one's pain or physical condition is thought to potentially interfere (Asmundson, Norton, & Jacobson, 1996). With continued avoidance behavior, increased physical deconditioning and disability, in addition to greater attentional focus on bodily symptoms can occur (Asmundson, Norton, & Norton, 1999). Eventually, reinforcement of avoidance behaviors shifts from a direct reduction in pain to more indirect means, such as social responsiveness and medication use (Fordyce, 1976).

The role of maladaptive cognitions, such as negative appraisals, low self-efficacy, and reduced perceived control, has also been implicated in pain anxiety (Turk, Meichenbaum, & Genest, 1983; Turk & Rudy; 1989). Vlaeyen and Linton (2000) incorporated cognitive postulates into instrumental theory to explain negative outcomes associated with chronic musculoskeletal pain. In their fear-avoidance model, if an individual who is injured catastrophizes about the pain (e.g., perceives the pain as a significant threat), this leads to pain-related fear, hypervigilance to somatic symptoms, avoidance, and, ultimately, disuse and disability. Here, an individual's interpretation or appraisal of the pain initially is a key cognitive precursor to a subsequent negative cycle of fear of pain and avoidance, or a more positive route of adaptation and recovery (Vlaeyen & Linton, 2000).

Catastrophizing about pain can be a powerful influence on various pain outcomes (Jensen, Turner, Romano, & Karoly, 1991; Sullivan et al., 2001). Catastrophizing has broadly been conceptualized as a construct comprised of both cognitive appraisal and affective elements (Jensen et al., 1991; Jones, Rollman, White, Hill, & Brooke, 2003) and is a process that involves an exaggeration or magnification of the perceived threat of incoming pain sensations (Sullivan et al., 2001; Turner & Aaron, 2001). Consistent with the fear-avoidance model, persons with chronic pain who catastrophize report greater pain-related disability (Keefe et al., 1989; Severeijns, Vlaeyen, van den Hout, & Weber, 2001), more negative affective ratings of pain (Geisser, Robinson, Keefe, & Weiner, 1994; Sullivan, Lynch, & Clark, 2005), and also more severe pain ratings in general (Richardson et al., 2009; Sullivan, Bishop, & Pivik., 1995).

Post-Traumatic Stress Disorder

Post-traumatic stress disorder (PTSD) is precipitated by an extreme stressor perceived as providing the potential for death or serious harm, and involves intense fear or helplessness as a response to the stressor. Post-traumatic stress disorder has been shown to have a high prevalence rate in chronic pain populations. In a longitudinal study of persons who sustained various forms of traumatic injuries, Jenewein, Wittmann, Moergeli, Creutzig, and Schnyder (2009) found that at 6 and 12 months post injury, greater PTSD symptoms were associated with increased pain severity from injury. Others (Norman, Stein, Dimsdale, & Hoyt, 2008) have found that increased pain severity at the time of a traumatic injury, but not persistent pain, is a risk factor for later development of PTSD. A symptom cluster observed frequently with PTSD (e.g., hypervigilance, increased somatic awareness, and avoidance behaviors) is not uncommon in chronic pain (Asmundson, Coons, Taylor, & Katz, 2002; Vlaeyen & Linton, 2000). To this end, a mutual maintenance model has been proposed to explain the association, whereby symptoms of chronic pain perpetuate PTSD and vice versa (Sharp &

Harvey, 2001). Chronic pain elicits continual reminders of the trauma which cancause increased arousal and subsequent avoidance behavior.

In addition to the shared external factors associated with onset (e.g., traumatic event), others have noted a dispositional style that may increase vulnerability for the development of chronic pain and/or PTSD. Termed *anxiety sensitivity*, this predisposition is the tendency to respond with increased fear to anxiety-related cognitions and bodily sensations (Taylor, 1999), often accompanied by a belief that such symptoms will have harmful consequences (Reiss, 1991; Reiss & McNally, 1985; Taylor, 1999). Anxiety sensitivity is considered a significant susceptibility factor for PTSD (Elwood, Hahn, Olatunji, & Williams, 2009), and when measured acutely following trauma, high anxiety sensitivity has been found to be predictive of subsequent PTSD symptom development (Feldner, Zvolensky, Schmidt, & Smith 2008; Marshall, Miles, & Stewart, 2010). In a study of persons with work-related injury and chronic pain, anxiety sensitivity was found to be significantly and positively related to comorbid PTSD symptom severity (Asmundson, Norton, Allerdings, Norton, & Larsen, 1998).

Similar to a diathesis stress model, anxiety sensitivity may explain preexisting vulnerability to developing and maintaining a chronic pain syndrome. This trait is associated with greater pain-related fear, negative affect, pain-related anxiety, and higher use of pain medications (Asmundson & Norton, 1995). Using structural equation modeling to clarify the role of anxiety sensitivity in chronic pain outcomes, Asmundson and Taylor (1996) found that anxiety sensitivity amplified fear of pain and led to pain-related escape and avoidance behaviors. In a recent meta-analysis of the association between anxiety sensitivity and pain, Ocañez, McHugh, and Otto (2010) found a strong, positive association between anxiety sensitivity and fear of pain, a key factor in the fear-avoidance model of the perpetuation of pain and disability.

Treatment Approaches in Chronic Pain

First-line treatment of chronic pain has often involved pharmacologic regimens; however, medication use has been moderately effective at best (Curatolo & Bogduk, 2001; Turk, 2002a). Moreover, many of the pharmacological treatments, such as opioids, show minimal long-term efficacy and increase the risk for addiction or aberrant medication use (Martell et al., 2007). Other treatments for chronic pain include invasive techniques such as surgery, intrathecal pumps and anesthetic procedures (e.g., nerve blocks). Although these modalities may be effective for many suffering chronic pain, the goal is usually not a cure per se; rather, the inherent objective is management of chronic pain.

Behavioral Paradigms

Fordyce (1976) was an early influence in alternative routes to targeting experienced pain intensity and associated sequelae. Fordyce and others (1976) diverged from the long-standing disease model of pain treatment with a proposed behavioral modification approach to treatment. Fordyce, Fowler, Lehman, and De Lateur (1968) developed an operant pain treatment program that systematically controlled environmental contingencies with the goal of increasing well behaviors, such as participating in activities, while reducing pain behaviors, such as activity avoidance and overuse of medications. A central feature of behavioral pain therapy is addressing the interpersonal dynamics maintaining pain behaviors. Solicitous responses from others to pain behaviors exhibited by the patient are conceptualized as reinforcing, and as such, should be discouraged. In Fordyce's (1976) program, rehabilitation staff members were to be socially nonresponsive and neutral to displayed pain behaviors. Spouses and key family members can also serve as discriminative stimuli eliciting maladaptive pain behaviors. Solicitous responses from spouses have been associated with more severe pain and less engagement in activities among individuals with chronic pain (Flor, Kerns, & Turk, 1987; Turk, Kerns, & Rosenberg, 1992), thus, modification of social interactions is crucial in promoting well behavior and optimizing functioning.

Another important tenet of behavioral pain management was shifting the contingency of medication use from displayed pain behaviors to fixed intervals of time. In this way, pain no longer served as a cue to take medications, thus reducing the potential for habituation and dependence. In addition to adherence to a structured daily medication schedule, medications were delivered via a "pain cocktail," whereby a patient's medications were delivered via a taste- and color-masked liquid vehicle. Using this method, medications were reduced over time, with patients themselves blinded to the exact tapering schedule (Fordyce, 1976). It has been found that, when incorporated in a comprehensive pain management program, time-contingent administration of analgesic medications with gradual reduction in dosages across time has been associated with either no change or an actual decrease in self-reported pain (Cairns, Thomas, Mooney, & Pace, 1976; Roberts & Reinhardt, 1980). Ralphs and colleagues (1994) subsequently examined the efficacy of staff-controlled delivery of the "pain cocktail" versus a patient-controlled opiate reduction schedule among 108 persons admitted to an inpatient pain program. At discharge, 89% of those who underwent staff-controlled "cocktail" reduction were off of all opiates, compared to 68% of those whose reduction schedules were self-controlled. However, follow-up assessments revealed no difference and even a significant increase in opiate use among those receiving the pain cocktail at 6 months post-discharge (Ralphs, Williams, Richardson, Pither, & Nicholas, 1994). However, subjects in this study were allowed to opt for which method of reduction they preferred, and therefore group selection was not randomized. Moreover, the patients who opted for the staff-controlled pain cocktail reported less confidence in their own ability to cope without their pain medications, suggesting that cognitive factors such as self-efficacy may contribute to lasting abstinence and well behaviors.

Since overt behavior and functioning, rather than the pain itself, is the primary criterion for behavioral pain management outcomes, level of activity engagement is often a primary focus. Exercise is seen as a form of physical activity engagement that is incompatible with pain behaviors. Fordyce (1976) implemented a quota system, in which exercises were reduced to quantifiable amounts, such as repetitions of specific movements. Baseline level of performance and tolerance were determined, and exercise increments gradually increased over time at an individualized pace. An important aspect in determining exercise quotas was developing an exercise program that maximized the probability of success. Persons with chronic pain show steady and gradual increases in activity levels when exercise quotas are established (Cairns & Pasino, 1977; Doleys, Crocker, & Patton, 1982). Dolce and colleagues (1986) found that, in addition to increasing exercise, the use of quota systems promoted self-efficacy and lessened anxiety and pain-related fear. These researchers concluded that the success of exercise quota systems was due to exposure to activity rather than mere reinforcement for achieving a certain level of that activity (Dolce, Crocker, Moletteire, & Doleys, 1986). More recently, Kernan and Rainville (2007) similarly found that persons with chronic low back pain undergoing quota-based physical therapy experienced less fear of reinjury, pain, and

disability, and these positive outcomes were maintained when reassessed at 1 year post-discharge. However, persons with acute pain do not show real benefit from exercise therapy (Hayden, van Tulder, Malmivaara, & Koes, 2005). As fear-avoidance is a cycle that is believed to develop with chronicity of pain, a lessening of fear via exposure may indeed be the mediating factor in successful outcomes of exercise therapy. Regardless of the mechanism by which the positive outcomes are produced, exercise therapy is typically seen as an important component of pain management. In a systematic review of 37 randomized controlled trials (RCTs) in chronic low back pain populations, van Middelkoop and colleagues (2010) concluded that exercise therapy improved pain intensity, disability, and long-term functioning.

Cognitive-Behavioral Paradigms

Coinciding with the general paradigm shift of the time, Turk, Meichenbaum, and Genest (1983) developed a model of pain based on Beck's (1964) cognitive-behavioral theory. The cognitive-behavioral treatment (CBT) model, when used to conceptualize chronic pain outcomes, views the patient with chronic pain as more than a reactive agent in his or her environment who is bound by the contingencies of reinforcement or conditioning. In this model, the patient is understood to actively predict, appraise, and interpret pain cues via cognitive schema that lead to selected behavior. There are a variety of techniques and components under the umbrella of CBT, and a given CBT protocol used may often be a conglomerate of behavioral strategies and other techniques discussed later in this section. What is common among virtually all CBT approaches, however, is that it is often time-limited, sessions are structured, and there is a focus on targeting present issues or problems. Cognitive-behavioral therapy approaches also encourage the patient to be an active participant in the process, to continuously question his or her thinking, and reappraise interpretations to gain a sense of control over his or her plight (Turk & Flor, 2006; Turk, Swanson, & Tunks, 2008).

Turk and others (2008) note that education, skill learning, and generalization of these new skills are important components for promoting efficacy of CBT in chronic pain. Patients are taught the links among thinking, emotion, and behavior, and how restructuring common errors in thought processes can bring about positive change. Distortions in thought, such as overgeneralization, catastrophizing, and all-or-nothing thinking are similar to cognitive errors identified in generic CBT (Beck, 1995). Applying CBT in chronic pain often targets these same errors in thinking but in pain-related contexts (Thorn, 2004). The goal of skill learning is to provide the patient with the means to ultimately self-manage responses to pain and problematic situations and thinking that may exacerbate pain. Negative thought stopping, positive self-talk, problem-solving, assertiveness training, and more behavioral tactics, such as breathing and activity pacing, are common components of chronic pain CBT programs (Turk & Flor, 2006). Homework and assignments are often given to the patient with the aim of consolidating and generalizing these skills in various settings in order to maintain positive outcomes.

Presently, psychological treatments based on cognitive-behavioral principles are widely used in chronic pain populations (Eimer & Freeman, 1998; Thorn, 2004; Turk, 2002b; Turk & Flor, 2006). In an early quantitative review of heterogeneous groups of nonmedical treatments (Malone & Strube, 1988), treatments incorporating cognitive-behavioral components were found to be effective in improving outcomes generally. However, as efficacy was examined by an aggregate of affective and physical outcomes, specific domains in which CBT may provide particular benefit were unclear. Turner (1996) later conducted a meta-analysis of a small set of RCTs of cognitive-behavioral treatments in chronic low back pain. Results from this study revealed significant improvement on measures of pain report, self-reported pain behaviors, and disability. Observed pain behaviors or depression did not improve significantly, but lack of effect in these domains may have been from a floor effect, as participants in this study were recruited from the community and not necessarily to specialized pain programs in which overt pain behaviors and depression may be more salient in a patient's presenting symptom cluster (Turner, 1996). Morley and others (1999) conducted a systematic review of 25 RCTs that utilized CBT for chronic pain. In this analysis, CBT was compared with both wait-list control groups and also standard active treatments that included physiotherapy and regular pain clinic visits. From results based on all 1,672 persons with chronic pain, CBT significantly improved mood symptoms, positive coping and appraisals, pain behaviors, activity engagement, and social functioning. When CBT was compared to the standard treatments, the effects of increased positive coping and reduced pain behaviors remained, albeit to a smaller degree; CBT was not, however,

better at improving mood or social role functioning (Morley et al., 1999). Eccleston, Williams, and Morley (2009) have conducted the largest review to date with a meta-analysis of 40 studies for a total of 4,781 persons with chronic pain. Results from this investigation indicated that CBT approaches were effective at improving mood but only produced small effects in terms of pain severity and disability (Eccleston et al., 2009). Although these reviews do suggest benefit, CBT has not been shown to affect specific outcome domains consistently.

However, analysis of the aggregate often precludes understanding of how individual treatment process variables may mediate successful outcome from CBT for chronic pain. Consideration of initial presentation of the patient, baseline psychological functioning, nature of chronic pain, and available instrumental support can aid in determining for whom CBT may be most effective (for a review, see McCracken & Turk, 2002).

Biofeedback

In some cases, pain is believed to be maintained by dysregulation of autonomic system activity. Biofeedback is any psycho-physiological technique designed to increase one's self-control over certain physiological functions (Arena & Blanchard, 1996; Olton & Noonberg, 1980). This procedure is often employed using equipment that records one or more types of physiological responses from the patient, such as muscle tension, skin conductance, heart rate, skin temperature, and respiration. The biofeedback equipment then conveys this information back to the patient via fluctuations in auditory tones or computerized display of this information graphed in real-time. The main objective of biofeedback is to teach the patient to control these signals by way of regulating his or her own physiological processes.

The type of biofeedback equipment utilized and the placement of sensors depends on the form of chronic pain. Arena, Bruno, Hannah, and Meador (1995) used electromyographic (EMG) biofeedback to treat individuals suffering from chronic tension headache, placing the EMG feeds at the trapezius muscle or forehead. Results from this study indicated that, following 12 sessions, all participants in the trapezius group, as compared to 50% of the forehead EMG group, showed sustained decreases in headache 3 months following treatment. Thermal biofeedback aids individuals in gaining volitional control over peripheral vasodilation, and as such, has been found effective at reducing pain associated with migraine and vascular headache (Arena & Blanchard, 1996). Given evidence implicating autonomic dysfunction in fibromyalgia (Clauw, Radulovic, Heshmat, & Barbey, 1996), Hassett and others (2007) gathered pilot data on the effectiveness of heart rate variability biofeedback on pain associated with this condition. These researchers found no difference in pain levels immediately following treatment, but, reported fibromyalgia pain was significantly reduced 3 months later.

Self-regulatory techniques have recently advanced with the developing field of real-time functional magnetic resonance imaging (rtfMRI). Utilizing this method as a source of feedback, De Charms and colleagues (2005) trained a group of healthy individuals exposed to experimental pain to control activity in the neural cortex associated with pain perception, the rostral anterior cingulate cortex (rACC), a region that has been implicated in both opioid and placebo analgesia (Petrovic, Kalso, Petersson, & Ingvar, 2002). Following training, self-induced changes in rACC activation were found to positively correlate with the intensity of the experimental pain. These researchers also had eight chronic pain patients follow a similar feedback training protocol and examined effects on the severity of their chronic pain rather than an externally applied pain. Interestingly, the chronic patients reported significant reductions in their chronic pain, with the rtfMRI training protocol showing superior results compared to standard autonomic biofeedback training (de Charms et al., 2005). Although promising, the small sample size of this study and paucity of other data in rtfMRI feedback warrants further investigation to determine its potential viability in chronic pain treatment.

Relaxation and Imagery

Relaxation is a technique designed to reduce psychological and physiological tension while simultaneously promoting greater awareness of bodily sensations and responses. Benson (1975) first described the physiological benefits of relaxation, including reduced heart rate, lowered blood pressure, slower breathing, and less muscle tension, which he collectively termed the *relaxation response*. However, it was in the first half of the 20th century that Johannes Schultz developed autogenic training involving repetition of suggestive phrases (e.g., "my right arm is heavy and warm"), which is often conducted in a sequential manner across various parts of the body (Schultz & Luthe, 1959). Jacobson also (1929) developed a technique in which muscle groups were tensed and relaxed, similarly in sequence. Known as *progressive muscle relaxation* (PMR), it is considered to be one of the most commonly used methods, especially in easing tension-related chronic pains (Arena & Blanchard, 1996).

In a review of RCTs of various forms of behavioral therapy, two studies were identified showing PMR as more effective than wait-list control groups at reducing chronic low back pain, at least acutely following treatment (Ostelo et al., 2005). However, an earlier review (Carroll & Seers, 1998) of a larger number of studies revealed only a third of the RCTs reporting significant benefit of relaxation therapy for chronic pain. The inconsistency in findings may be, in part, due to the heterogeneity in relaxation methods used or that relaxation strategies better target psychological sequelae of chronic pain rather than pain perception per se. Gustavsson and von Koch (2006) conducted a pilot study examining the benefit of applied relaxation for chronic neck pain and found that those undergoing relaxation, as compared to standard physical therapy, reported no change in severity of pain but did report increased adaptive coping for that pain. Similar results have been reported among individuals with chronic rheumatoid arthritis pain, in that relaxation decreased anxiety and depressive symptoms but failed to decrease joint pain severity (Bagheri-Nesami, Mohseni-Bandpei, & Shayesteh-Azar, 2006).

Guided imagery or visualization is often coupled with relaxation techniques. Guided imagery is the use of mental images, often facilitated by the therapist, to aid in diverting attention from the experience of pain (visualizing pleasant scenes) or to mentally modify the severity of the pain. In the latter, an individual may be guided to objectify his or her pain, such as visualizing a block with sharp edges that get "sanded smooth." In an RCT examining the efficacy of guided imagery on chronic fibromyalgia pain, Menzies, Taylor, and Bourguignon (2006) found that those individuals supplemented with guided imagery in their usual care across 6 weeks had improved functional status and sense of self-efficacy for managing symptoms of fibromyalgia. However, there were no differences in pain ratings between the usual care group and those receiving additional guided imagery. In a subsequent pilot study in the use of guided imagery among Hispanics with fibromyalgia pain, Menzies and Kim (2008) similarly noted improved functional status and self-efficacy, but found reductions only in pain intensity ratings and not the sensory or affective ratings of their chronic pain. Among individuals with osteoarthritis, use of guided imagery and PMR led to reductions in pain and improved mobility (Baird & Sands, 2004).

A promising new form of visual imagery treatment is based on a growing understanding regarding the modulating role of the motor cortex in the experience of pain. It has been posited that the CNS is a dynamically operating feedback mechanism, with motor cortical activity continuously modulated by afferent, intersensory processes including proprioception and visual feedback (Harris, 1999). A disruption in this motor cortical–sensory feedback system, as occurs in such states as amputation, may result in a chronic sensation of pain (Harris, 1999). Clinical evidence to support this notion comes from studies that aim to artificially reinstate one of the sensory mechanisms, visual feedback, by use of a technique called "mirror box," "mirror visual feedback," or "mirror therapy." In such studies, individuals with post-amputation "phantom" pain experience significant relief from that pain when given the illusion that the missing limb appears to exist and move (Chan et al., 2007; Ramachandran & Altschuler, 2009). This illusion is accomplished with the use of a mirror, often positioned in an individual's mid-sagittal plane, so that the individual observes a reflection of his or her remaining limb. Ramachandran, Brang, and McGeoch (2009) have also found that when the mirror image of the missing limb is given the appearance of decreasing in size, persons with amputations will similarly report a decrease in phantom pain. Mirror visual feedback has also shown utility in reducing pain associated with complex regional pain syndrome (CRPS; Karmarkar & Lieberman, 2006; McCabe et al., 2003; Selles, Schreuders, & Stam, 2008). Cacchio, De Blasis, Necozione, di Orio, and Santilli (2009) found that in addition to reducing CRPS-related pain, edema and motor functioning in the affected limb also improved. Murray and colleagues (2007) expanded the limited spatial dimensions of the mirror box paradigm in an immersive virtual reality environment with an avatar of the intact limb to produce phantom limb pain relief. However, as Moseley, Gallace, and Spence (2008) appropriately note, data indicating positive analgesic effects reported in mirror visual feedback and immersive virtual reality were mainly from case studies or anecdotal reports, and larger RCTs are needed to determine whether mirror therapy may indeed serve as a viable treatment approach to treat nerve injury-related chronic pain.

Hypnosis

Among many in the public realm, the term "hypnosis" often conjures images of the proverbial swinging pendulum, inducing an enigmatic trance that results in one person being under the behavioral control of another. However, among clinicians using this technique, it is typically considered a state of focused attention in which one's peripheral awareness and perceptions are altered. A hypnotic procedure often makes use of an individual's imagination in guiding and encouraging responses "to suggestions for changes in subjective experience, alterations in perception, sensation, emotion, thought, or behavior" (Green, Barabasz, Barrett, & Montgomery, 2005, p. 262). Although hypnosis comprises a heterogeneous group of technical components (e.g., visual imagery and/or relaxation), it typically involves an induction phase when suggestions are presented to aid in shifting focus away from bodily sensation to an internal experience. Once the induction phase is complete, the clinician may then pose suggestions for pain control. Syrjala and Abrams (2002) used suggestion consistent with an individual's pain quality. For example, an effective analgesic suggestion may be utilizing snow or ice for pain that is hot or burning in nature. Other suggestions can include imaginal escape to a pleasant place or the use of metaphors, such as traveling away from the physical discomfort (Syrjala & Abrams, 2002). Post-hypnotic suggestions can be incorporated and can include a suggestion that whenever pain increases, one may retrieve the state of relaxation and analgesia. In fact, the ultimate goal is for the chronic pain patient to learn self-hypnosis and acquire the skills needed to generalize alterations in pain outside of sessions (Jensen & Patterson, 2006). Thus, a common practice is to provide the individual with a CD or audio recording of sessions to practice at home. Overall, systematic reviews of the literature to date indicate hypnosis for the treatment of chronic pain is more efficacious than standard care, such as physical and pharmacological therapy, but similar to other psychological treatments that include similar components to hypnosis (e.g., relaxation techniques) and some forms of CBT (Jensen & Patterson, 2006; Stoelb, Molton, Jensen, & Patterson, 2009).

Individual factors contributing to the analgesic effects of hypnosis have also been studied. One characteristic is hypnotic suggestibility, or the degree to which an individual is likely to respond to hypnotic suggestions. A number of data indicate that those scoring high on hypnotic susceptibility questionnaires respond more favorably to analgesic suggestions provided during hypnosis (Montgomery, DuHamel, & Redd, 2000) and report even greater analgesic effects when asked to recall the pain and distress during the hypnotic treatment (De Pascalis, Cacace, & Massicolle, 2008). Thus, hypnotic techniques may be of greatest benefit among a subset of individuals. Electroencephalogram neurofeedback training has been shown to enhance hypnotic susceptibility, but not in those with low levels of susceptibility prior to that training (Batty, Bonnington, Tang, Hawken, & Gruzelier, 2006). Jensen (2009) discusses the potential future role for immersive virtual reality environments to guide attention and facilitate induction among chronic pain patients who do not respond to traditional hypnotic techniques. Patterson, Jensen, Wiechman, and Sharar (2010) found hypnosis, delivered via virtual reality, was associated with greater reductions in pain intensity and unpleasantness among patients recovering from traumatic injuries when compared to virtual reality without hypnosis or standard analgesic care. To explore the potential effects on chronic, refractory forms of pain, Oneal and others (2009) conducted a case study of an individual who suffered chronic spinal cord injury-related neuropathic pain. Of note, was that this individual also scored low on a hypnotizability measure. Following treatments with immersive virtual reality hypnosis, there was a 36% decrease in pain intensity, but analgesic benefits did not persist at 1-month follow-up.

Advances in neuroimaging technology have enabled greater neurophysiological insight into the mechanism of action in hypnosis. Rainville, Duncan, Price, Carrier, and Bushnell (1997) applied experimental pain to healthy individuals and found that hypnotic suggestions for decreasing pain unpleasantness differentially altered regional cerebral blood flow in the anterior cingulate cortex but not primary somatosensory cortex, suggesting that hypnosis readily modulates the affective and distressing component of pain. Using a different hypnotic technique among healthy individuals in an experimental pain paradigm, Faymonville and others (2000) found reductions in both affective and sensory ratings of pain, and these decreases in pain were modulated by the anterior cingulate cortex. Fewer data are available regarding hypnosis and the associated neurobiological substrates among persons with chronic pain. However, there have been recent attempts to dissect components of hypnosis to determine if it is the hypnotic state itself or the suggestions posed during hypnosis that are effective. Derbyshire, Whalley, and Oakley (2009) provided suggestions for pain reduction during hypnosis or wakefulness among persons with chronic fibromyalgia pain. Regardless of the condition, decreases in reported pain occurred when suggestions were provided; however, the greatest benefit was found when suggestions were delivered during hypnosis. Moreover, functional MRI (fMRI) activation in pain-related cortices correlated with changes in reported pain, with greatest activation in some regions, including the anterior mid-cingulate cortex, when suggestions were provided during a hypnotic state (Derbyshire et al., 2009).

Mindfulness and Acceptance-Based Approaches

Historically, an effort has been made to identify barriers to optimal outcomes, and rightly so, given the preponderance of data suggesting significant negative effects of emotional distress on outcomes in chronic pain. Pain acceptance has been the focus of more recent interest in elucidating positive factors that promote psychological well-being and optimal day-to-day functioning despite the presence of chronic pain. Acceptance has been found to be positively associated with work activity and physical functioning in heterogeneous chronic pain samples (McCracken & Eccleston, 2005). Viane, Crombez, Eccleston, Devulder, and De Corte (2004) found that individuals who showed greater acceptance of their pain reported that they devoted less attention to that pain and engaged in more daily activities. In a group of chronic low back pain patients, Vowles and colleagues (2007) found that patients taught to emphasize acceptance rather than pain control showed the greatest improvements in physical functioning.

Acceptance has been conceptualized as an adaptive factor facilitating the pursuit of important goals and activities notwithstanding feelings, thoughts, or beliefs—whatever their valence may be (Hayes, Luoma, Bond, Masuda, & Lillis, 2006). *Acceptance and commitment therapy* (ACT; Hayes, 2004) is a treatment paradigm that aims to increase acceptance in order to buffer the negative influence of negative thinking on functioning. The ACT approach has been utilized in chronic pain populations with success in terms of physical functioning outcomes (McCracken, Vowles, & Eccleston, 2005; Vowles & McCracken, 2008). A principle of acceptance-based therapies in chronic pain is promoting the view that reducing negative thoughts or emotions is not required to engage in an activity or pursue valued goals. By developing a sense of acceptance, the potential negative influence of certain thoughts, emotions, or sensations (e.g., catastrophizing about pain) on adaptive functioning can be buffered. Whereas traditional cognitive approaches aim to reduce the frequency and change the content of distorted negative thoughts, ACT focuses more on neutralizing the influence of those thoughts (Hayes & Wilson, 1995). Individuals may use their emotions or thoughts to guide selected behaviors or action (i.e., a negative cognition or appraisal of an event may be interpreted as true and one may act in a manner so as to reduce the assumed negative outcome). In the context of chronic pain, one may be faced with the possibility of engaging in a task, have the thought that the pain will become excruciating, and thus avoid that task in order to reduce the fear or anxiety that the thought produced. This "experiential avoidance" (Blackledge & Hayes, 2001 p. 244) becomes maladaptive when it begins to obstruct the pursuit of valued goals and life activities.

Levels of acceptance among those with chronic pain have been found to be inversely related to depression and anxiety (McCracken & Eccleston, 2005), and even negative appraisals such as catastrophizing (Nicholas & Asghari, 2006; Richardson et al., 2009; Viane et al., 2003). However, evidence exists to suggest that negative psychological processes and positive ones, such as acceptance, are more than two sides of the same coin. Acceptance has been found to be a better predictor of functional outcomes, whereas catastrophizing and negative coping were better predictors of emotional functioning (Esteve, Ramírez-Maestre, & López-Martínez, 2007; Richardson et al., 2010). In a study of chronic low back pain patients, a component of acceptance was found to buffer the negative effect of catastrophizing on objective task performance during an experimental pain procedure (Richardson et al., 2010).

In ACT generally (Hayes et al., 2006) and in acceptance based treatments for chronic pain (McCracken, 2005; McCracken, MacKichan, & Eccleston, 2007; McCracken, Vowles, & Eccleston, 2005; Vowles & McCracken, 2008), mindfulness is considered an additional key mechanism by which adaptive functioning is achieved and techniques aimed at increasing mindfulness are often included in the acceptance-based treatment package as a whole. Mindfulness has been described as viewing oneself as the "self as process," whereby one's thoughts are simply described for what they are as they enter and exit awareness, without judgment or

using them to evaluate present or future circumstances or outcomes (Hayes, 2004; Hayes et al., 2006). The converse of mindfulness, or the restriction of awareness in a given context—can result in negative thoughts and emotions dictating behavior, ultimately leading to disability in chronic pain (Gauntlett-Gilbert & Vowles, 2007; McCracken, 2005). Being mindful of the natural fluctuation of thoughts and emotions allows for increased behavioral and psychological flexibility in a situation, rather than using internal experiences as automatic rules by which behavior and action are guided. Thus, the thought, "My pain will be unbearable," and corresponding apprehension and fear can be seen as fleeting and transient rather than something inevitably governing behavior in a given context.

Mindfulness training has its roots in Eastern religious philosophy and meditation practices; however, approximately 30 years ago, Kabat-Zinn (1982) described use of mindfulness-based stress reduction (MBSR) in medical populations including individuals with chronic pain. In addition to group sessions teaching body scanning and breathing techniques, individuals were encouraged to practice mindfulness in everyday activities by giving momentary notice to their thoughts and emotions but returning attention to the present context (Kabat-Zinn, 1982). Kabat-Zinn and colleagues (1985) found that chronic pain patients who participated in MBSR reported less pain, reduced use of pain medications, improved mood, increased involvement in activity, increased self-esteem, and better body image. Mindfulness interventions have been found beneficial in improving physical functioning and acceptance in older persons with chronic low back pain (Morone, Greco, & Weiner, 2008) and in decreasing emotional distress in persons with chronic rheumatoid arthritis pain (Pradhan et al., 2007). Rosenzweig and others (2010) found that MBSR resulted in less pain intensity and physical limitations, and that home practice of the mindfulness meditation techniques that were taught during the intervention was associated with improved emotional well-being and self-rated health.

Similarly, McCracken, Gauntlett-Gilbert, and Vowles (2007) found that when individuals with chronic pain were more mindful in day-to-day activities, they reported less physical disability, pain-related anxiety, and depression. These researchers also found that when considered in a statistical model examining functional outcomes, both acceptance of one's pain and mindfulness contributed significantly. From these results, McCracken and his colleagues (2007) posited that both acceptance of one's pain, in conjunction with a present-focused, behaviorally neutral, and nonreactive mindful state maximize engagement in valued goals while minimizing suffering.

Both constructs of acceptance and mindfulness are included as subprocesses in the larger, theoretically driven model of what is termed *psychological flexibility*, a broader mechanism that is fundamental to ACT intervention (Hayes et al., 2006). Results from two investigations indicated that patients with greater psychological flexibility, conceptualized as higher levels of mindfulness, acceptance, and values-based action, exhibited better functioning across a variety of domains above and beyond traditional pain management strategies such as pacing and use of positive self-talk (McCracken & Vowles, 2007; Vowles & McCracken, 2010). Among chronic pain patients in a primary care setting, McCracken and Velleman (2010) similarly found psychological flexibility associated with less visits to their general practitioner for pain and better self-reported social, emotional, and physical functioning. Jointly, these results suggest that psychological flexibility is important in adaptive functioning in chronic pain. Less clear, however, is the differential importance of the processes comprising what is deemed psychological flexibility, and how inclusion of all six subprocesses originally outlined (Hayes, 2004; Hayes et al., 2006) would apply to the clinical situation in chronic pain. Although McCracken and his colleagues (McCracken, 2005; McCracken, MacKichan, & Eccleston, 2007; McCracken et al., 2005; Vowles & McCracken, 2008) incorporate mindfulness in their acceptance-based treatment for chronic pain with significant positive outcomes, more research is needed to clarify the efficacy of individual components of acceptance-based therapies and differentiate the specific outcomes of interest to which these benefits apply.

In sum, acceptance-based approaches focus on contextual factors, with the goal of defusing the thought–behavior connection within a context, so that the individual can engage in meaningful activities. This is thought to occur by promoting both mindfulness and acceptance of thoughts and emotions that may arise in various situations. Thus, in the context of engaging in positive activities counter to negative pain behaviors, one would acknowledge but not give credence to the thought telling one that he cannot or should not complete the task at hand because his pain is too great or further damage would ensue. The acceptance-based approach is in contrast to traditional cognitive-behavioral theory in that it removes the focus from thoughts or other negative internal experiences, whereas CBT targets such thoughts so as to change any errors in thinking. Where CBT would aim to restructure catastrophizing about pain in a given context, acceptance-based models teach the individual that the presence of catastrophic thinking does not matter; life activities and goals can be pursued regardless.

Assessment of Pain

Pain measurement is necessary to determine progress of an individual seen in the clinical setting and for determining efficacy of new chronic pain treatments in research trials. Variations of the Numeric Rating Scales (NRS), the Verbal Rating Scale (VRS), and the Visual Analog Scale (VAS) are most commonly used to quantify levels of or changes in pain severity (Jensen & Karoly, 2001). An NRS is often verbally given and consists of sequential numbers, usually a 0–10 scale, with the lowest and highest number anchored with "no pain" and "worst imaginable pain" respectively. The VRS consists of numerically ranked verbal descriptors (e.g., no pain, mild, moderate, or severe) that reflect the degree of pain severity. The VAS is visually presented, and consists of a straight line, often 10 cm in length, on which individuals are asked to make a mark on the line to denote severity of their the level of pain (Jensen & Karoly, 2001). Use of unidimensional pain scales may be problematic among those with cognitive impairments (Closs, Barr, Briggs, Cash, & Seers, 2004; Ferrell, Ferrell, & Rivera, 1995) and higher opioid usage has been associated with less accurate VAS scores (Kremer, Atkinson & Ignelzi, 1981; Paice & Cohen, 1997). Nonetheless, brevity and simple administration are practical advantages in administering these scales in various clinical settings.

Chronic pain is comprised of empirically distinct sensory and emotional components (Price et al., 1987; Price, 1988); therefore, a single pain intensity rating may be insufficient, particularly when these dimensions of pain may respond differently to treatment (Kupers, Konings, Adriaensen, & Gybels, 1991). The NRS, VRS, and VAS scaled format is commonly used to also measure the degree of pain unpleasantness along with pain intensity. The Short Form McGill Pain Questionnaire (SF-MPQ; Melzack, 1987) is a psychometrically sound measure designed specifically to assess the multiple dimensions of pain. This measure consists of 15 verbal descriptors that are associated with both sensory and affective aspects of pain. The degree to which each descriptor is experienced (e.g., severe burning versus mild burning) is also quantified using a Likert scale ranging from 0 (none) to 3 (severe). Both sensory and affective pain scores are derived from the sum of the intensity rank values of the words chosen for the associated descriptors. In addition to providing assessment of different dimensions of pain, instruments such as the SF-MPQ can also provide qualitative information of the nature of the pain itself. For example, an individual with chronic low back pain may reveal a different endorsement pattern of descriptors than someone with spinal cord injury-related neuropathic pain.

It is well accepted that subjective pain rating scales are crucial in the assessment of treatment outcomes. In chronic pain, however, pain levels per se are not exclusive of a broader symptom constellation comprised of functioning across various life domains. Thus, indicators of functioning across multiple domains are important when evaluating overall treatment effects. Over the past decade, a consortium of experts from academia, the pharmaceutical industry, and regulatory agencies convened for the Initiative on Methods, Measurement, and Pain Assessment in Clinical Trials (IMMPACT) to develop a consensus for a core set of the chronic pain outcome domains (Turk et al., 2003) to be assessed when conducting clinical trials. From this effort, six domains were identified: physical functioning, emotional functioning, patient/participant ratings of improvement and satisfaction with treatment, symptoms and adverse events, and participant disposition, in addition to the sensory, affective, and evaluative components of pain itself.

Using a priori criteria including good reliability, validity, low participant burden, responsiveness, and content, the IMMPACT group subsequently recommended instruments for measuring outcomes of the aforementioned core domains (Dworkin et al., 2005). In addition to assessing subjective pain intensity with the NRS, the IMMPACT forum suggested measuring pain interference in activities of daily living with the interference scale of the Brief Pain Inventory (BPI; Cleeland & Ryan, 1994) or the Multidimensional Pain Inventory Interference Scale (MPI; Kerns, Turk, & Rudy, 1985). These measures of pain interference are general and therefore should be complemented by disease-specific measures of pain interference when possible (Dworkin et al., 2005), such as use of the Roland Morris Back Pain Disability Scale (Roland & Morris, 1983), when analyzing treatment outcomes among persons

with chronic low back pain. For affective functioning in chronic pain, recommendations were made for use of the Beck Depression Inventory (BDI; Beck, Ward, Mendelson, Mock, & Erbaugh, 1961) and the Profile of Mood States (POMS; McNair, Lorr, & Droppleman, 1971). A driving factor for organizing a forum to identify a set of measures was to reduce variability and provide a basis for comparison across clinical trials (Dworkin et al., 2005; Turk et al., 2003). A higher degree of standardization would also solidify an empirical reference for determining significant improvement in the clinical situation. However, a criticism has been that the IMMPACT endeavor was heavily North American, and taking a proscriptive stance to assessment may exclude important input from international chronic pain researchers (McQuay, 2005). Moreover, the IMMPACT group has cautioned that these core measures should not be mechanistically applied; scientific or clinical rationale take precedence when ultimately selecting measures to be used (Dworkin et al., 2005). For example, assessing chronic pain-related outcomes in a cognitively impaired group may require caregiver instruments, whereas pencil-and-paper questionnaires may need to be modified or substituted among persons with physical disabilities.

Another issue to consider when assessing chronic pain is the temporal quality of the experienced pain. Chronic pain can be continuous or paroxysmal. Breakthrough pain can denote an episode of severe pain in the context of the background chronic pain. Emotional and physical functioning may also parallel an individual's fluctuations in pain. Thus, capturing the frequency with which these episodes occur, along with the temporal patterning of pain severity, may provide richer understanding of the nature of the chronic pain syndrome. An average NRS score from asking the chronic pain patient to provide ratings across a previous time frame is often used; however, there can be discrepancy between an individual's present pain versus retrospective descriptions of his or her pain experience, usually in the form of overestimation (Broderick et al., 2008; Jamison, Sbrocco, & Parris, 1989). Respondent error aside, evidence suggests that mean fluctuations in chronic pain do not remain stable across time, and nonlinear methods for assessing temporal aspects of chronic pain may provide a more accurate reflection of the temporal qualities of that pain (Foss, Apkarian, & Chialvo, 2006). Foss and colleagues (2006) utilized fractal analysis to characterize potentially unique temporal dynamics and fluctuations of spontaneous pain in chronic low back pain and postherpetic neuropathy patients. These researchers found that the fractal properties were distinctly different for the pain reported by individuals with chronic pain when compared to nonchronic, induced pain experienced by healthy individuals. Although IMMPACT has recommended including temporal aspects of pain as a secondary outcome measure (Dworkin et al., 2005), it is clear that when the variable of time is introduced, pain assessment can become quite complicated. Further research is needed to develop valid methods of assessing the frequency and intensity of chronic pain intervals.

Conclusion

Chronic pain is developed and maintained by a multitude of biopsychosocial factors. Moreover, the various components of chronic pain do not simply co-occur but are dynamically interacting; for example, chronic pain may produce negative psychosocial sequelae which, in turn, may magnify the experience of that pain. Ideally, treatment of persistent and chronic pain should reflect the multidimensionality of the chronic pain syndrome via coordinated, integrated care from relevant fields in health care (Loeser, 1991). Meta-analytic and systematic reviews across various chronic pain populations have found multidisciplinary treatment paradigms to potentiate positive outcomes not only in terms of reducing pain severity, but in decreasing functional interference from pain, improving mood, and increasing the number of patients returning to work (Flor, Fydrich, & Turk, 1992; Scascighini, Toma, Dober-Spielmann, & Sprott, 2008; Turk, 2002a). Collectively, however, a common limitation mentioned by many reviewers is the lack of methodological soundness in individual study design, which may obviate detection of true effects. To some degree this issue has been addressed by the efforts of the IMMPACT forum to standardize RCT methodology in chronic pain treatment and their call to researchers in the field to meet higher standards in this arena (Dworkin et al., 2005; Turk et al., 2003). Yet, another confounding issue is the heterogeneity of techniques, both inter- and intradisciplinary, falling under the umbrella of "multidisciplinary." It remains unclear as to which components are truly effective and which, if any, may be less so or even perhaps not effective at all. Interventional pain medicine in general and pain psychology in particular would benefit from future work aimed at disassembling current multimodal treatment packages to determine efficacy of individual techniques. Those methods found to be clinically beneficial could be retained in a more streamlined approach.

Future Directions

The value of evidence-based medicine has afforded our field with exponential growth in technology and new treatments for chronic pain. Some (Boswell & Giordano, 2009) have noted that the ardent quest for novelty and efficacy at the bench may have diverted attention from fulfilling our ultimate purpose at bedside. As our repertoire of effective treatments increases, effectiveness, practicality, and feasibility in patients' day-to-day functioning may be lost. In some regions, managed care and third-party payers have begun to apply their own "Occam's razor" by selecting the individual techniques approved for coverage, with a potential negative impact on patients (Robbins et al., 2003). It is therefore important that health care professionals in their respective fields promote efficacious, as well as pragmatic and effective, approaches for chronic pain. This will ensure quality treatment for patients that is likewise amenable to criteria applied by third-party providers, who are relied upon by many individual patients for access to care. Efforts to improve multidisciplinary programs would be amiss, however, if different chronic pain diagnoses are not taken into consideration. Mechanistically applying a treatment approach "standardized" across chronic pain generally would ignore the needs and unique issues associated with a particular condition. An attempt has been made to tease apart the effects of multidisciplinary programs according to chronic pain diagnosis, with more favorable results for fibromyalgia and chronic back pain patients than for patients with chronic pain of mixed etiology (Scascighini et al., 2008). Here again, however, what constituted multidisciplinary treatments provided, even within a given chronic pain subtype, was not held constant in order to determine any true main effects. What may also aid in developing a tailored constellation of effective techniques is gaining a better understanding of symptom profiles and prognostic indicators characteristic of a particular diagnosis. Porter-Moffitt and others (2006) investigated the biopsychosocial profiles of seven chronic pain diagnostic groups and found that the levels of psychosocial and physical functioning can vary according to diagnosis. This would suggest that emphasis on a particular technique within a structured multidisciplinary program should vary according to what chronic pain diagnosis has been applied. In sum, the field of chronic pain psychology would greatly benefit from adopting an orientation that values both efficacy and effectiveness to optimize not only quality, but efficiency and access to care for those depending upon third-party coverage. Identifying the truly effective components of a multidisciplinary program will allow for customizing, through a degree of emphasis on specific psychotherapeutic techniques, according to the chronic pain diagnosis.

On average, individuals have experienced chronic pain for approximately 7 years before presenting at a multidisciplinary pain treatment facility (Flor et al., 1992). This emphasizes the need to identify those individuals at risk for developing and maintaining a negative chronic pain course. Musculoskeletal pain is a common presenting problem in the acute care setting (Abbott & Frasier, 1998), and many are likely to find relief from single-modality treatments. However, there are those whose pain remains rather refractory to each successive treatment option tried, and a pain clinic is considered the last resort. A key area for further study is possible prevention to reduce the functional interference and cost incurred during the time the patient and clinician are searching for the appropriate treatment. Based on identified risk factors, Gatchel, Polatin, Noe, Gardea, Pulliam, and Thompson (2003) developed a statistical algorithm to classify patients at greater risk for going on to develop chronic low back pain. These researchers then implemented a multidisciplinary early intervention treatment protocol that included biofeedback and pain management for those considered at high risk for the development of chronic pain. Results indicated that, 1 year later, those at risk but who received the early intervention protocol reported less functional and occupational disability, pain, and medication use compared to those considered at risk but who did not receive early intervention (Gatchel et al., 2003). More data are needed to determine both the clinical and cost utility of identifying those at risk and the benefits to applying secondary prevention protocols. Although the results from Gatchel et al. (2003) are promising for low back pain, it remains unclear as to how such an algorithm may work in other pain conditions with different prognostic indicators of chronicity.

There are those too, however, who continue to live with refractory chronic pain but are not ultimately treated at multidisciplinary clinics. The lack of access to chronic pain health care and treatment may be due to a number of reasons, but racial and demographic disparities have unfortunately been identified (Green et al., 2003; Richardson et al., 2009). Developing approaches to deliver treatment without the proviso of clinic visits may lessen barriers for many. Wegener and colleagues (2009) found that among those with limb amputations, self-management programs delivered in the community by trained volunteers who also had limb loss, resulted in increased self-efficacy and improved physical functioning compared to those involved with a community support group only. Recently, the use of technology via web-based platforms and telephone have emerged as approaches to reduce barriers and increase access to care in many chronic illness populations (Rosser, Vowles, Keogh, Eccleston, & Mountain, 2009). Both rural and urban dwelling individuals receiving a telephone-based intervention had significant improvements with depressive symptoms and severity of cancer pain (Kroenke et al., 2010). Chiauzzi and others (2010) found that when persons with chronic low back pain were provided with an interactive web program, as compared to those with printed material, improved coping with pain was the result. However, only those recruited online, versus those recruited in clinics, experienced improved coping and reduced pain, suggesting possible inherent differences in the characteristics of those living in the community and those presenting at clinics (Chiauzzi et al., 2010).

In a similar vein, it is important to consider that those treated for chronic pain at multidisciplinary clinics likely represent only a subset of those living with chronic pain. Since clinician-researchers often work within this setting and have convenient access to this population, investigational hypotheses are often foundationally narrow and limited to one side of the chronic pain "distribution." Studying individuals in the community who are able to live fully despite having chronic pain may offer insights into factors facilitating successful self-management and adaptation to secondary limitations (May, 2010). Recent interest in positive psychology has developed in the field generally, and the subfield of chronic pain psychology would profit from following suit. In the literature of psychosocial outcomes following adverse events such as loss or trauma, the construct of resilience, or the ability of an individual to maintain stability and adapt amidst adversity, has expanded our understanding of positive biopsychosocial trajectories that can ensue (Bonanno, 2004). As noted by Sturgeon and Zautra (2010), expanding focus to the behaviors, personal traits, and skills of resilient individuals with chronic pain will be of heuristic benefit, in both a broader understanding of a continuum of possibilities in the human response to chronic pain and new directions for treatment.

References

Abbott, F. V., & Fraser, M. I. (1998). Use and abuse of over-the-counter analgesic agents. *Journal of Psychiatry and Neuroscience, 23*, 13–34.

Apkarian, A. V., Baliki, M. N., & Geha, P. Y. (2009). Towards a theory of chronic pain. *Progress in Neurobiology, 87*, 81–97.

Arena, J. G., & Blanchard, E. B. (1996). Biofeedback and relaxation therapy for chronic pain disorders. In R. J. Gatchel, & D. C. Turk (Eds.), *Psychological approaches to pain management: A practitioner's handbook* (pp. 179–230). New York: Guilford.

Arena, J. G., Bruno, G. M., Hannah, S. L., & Meador, K. J. (1995). A comparison of frontal electromyographic biofeedback training, trapezius electromyographic biofeedback training, and progressive muscle relaxation therapy in the treatment of tension headache. *Headache, 35*, 411–419.

Arnold, L. M., Lu, Y., Crofford, L. J., Wohlreich, M., Detke, M. J., Iyengar, S., et al. (2004). A double-blind, multicenter trial comparing duloxetine with placebo in the treatment of fibromyalgia patients with or without major depressive disorder. *Arthritis and Rheumatism, 50*, 2974–2984.

Arnow, B. A., Hunkeler, E. M., Blasey, C. M., Lee, J., Constantino, M. J., Fireman, B., et al. (2006). Comorbid depression, chronic pain, and disability in primary care. *Psychosomatic Medicine, 68*, 262–268.

Asmundson, G. J., Coons, M. J., Taylor, S., & Katz, J. (2002). PTSD and the experience of pain: Research and clinical implications of shared vulnerability and mutual maintenance models. *Canadian Journal of Psychiatry, 47*, 930–937.

Asmundson, G. J. G., & Katz, J. (2009). Understanding the co-occurrence of anxiety disorders and chronic pain: State-of-the-art. *Depression and Anxiety, 26*, 888–901.

Asmundson, G. J., & Norton, G. R. (1995). Anxiety sensitivity in patients with physically unexplained chronic back pain: A preliminary report. *Behaviour Research and Therapy, 33*, 771–777.

Asmundson, G. J. G., Norton, G. R., Allerdings, M. D., Norton, P. J., & Larsen, D. K. (1998). Posttraumatic stress disorder and work-related injury. *Journal of Anxiety Disorders, 12*, 57–69.

Asmundson, G. J., Norton, G. R., & Jacobson, S. J. (1996). Social, blood/injury, and agoraphobic fears in patients with physically unexplained chronic pain: Are they clinically significant? *Anxiety, 2*, 28–33.

Asmundson, G. J., Norton, P. J., & Norton, G. R. (1999). Beyond pain: The role of fear and avoidance in chronicity. *Clinical Psychology Review, 19*, 97–119.

Asmundson, G. J. G., & Taylor, S. (1996). Role of anxiety sensitivity in pain-related fear and avoidance. *Journal of Behavioral Medicine, 19*, 577–586.

Bagheri-Nesami, M., Mohseni-Bandpei, M. A., & Shayesteh-Azar, M. (2006). The effect of Benson relaxation technique on rheumatoid arthritis patients: Extended report. *International Journal of Nursing Practice, 12*, 214–219.

Bair, M. J., Robinson, R. L., Katon, W., & Kroenke, K. (2003). Depression and pain comorbidity: A literature review. *Archives of Internal Medicine, 163*, 2433–2445.

Baird, C. L., & Sands, L. (2004). A pilot study of the effectiveness of guided imagery with progressive muscle relaxation to reduce chronic pain and mobility difficulties of osteoarthritis. *Pain Management Nursing, 5*(3), 97–104.

Banks, S. M., & Kerns, R. D. (1996). Explaining high rates of depression in chronic pain: A diathesis-stress framework. *Psychological Bulletin, 119*, 95–110.

Batty, M. J., Bonnington, S., Tang, B. K., Hawken, M. B., & Gruzelier, J. H. (2006). Relaxation strategies and enhancement of hypnotic susceptibility: EEG neurofeedback, progressive muscle relaxation, and self-hypnosis. *Brain Research Bulletin, 71*, 83–90.

Beck, A. T. (1964). Thinking and depression: II. Theory and therapy. *Archives of General Psychiatry, 10*, 561–571.

Beck, J. S. (1995). *Cognitive therapy: Basics and beyond.* New York: Guilford.

Beck, A. T., Rush, A. J., Shaw, B. F., & Emery, B. F. (1979). *Cognitive therapy of depression.* New York: Guilford.

Beck, A. T., Ward, C. H., Mendelson, M., Mock, J., & Erbaugh, J. (1961). An inventory for measuring depression. *Archives of General Psychiatry, 4*, 561–571.

Bennett, G. J. (1994). Neuropathic pain. In P. D. Wall, & R. Melzack (Eds.), *Textbook of pain* (pp. 201–224). London: Churchill Livingstone.

Benson, H. (1975). *The relaxation response.* New York: Morrow.

Blackledge, J. T., & Hayes, S. C. (2001). Emotion regulation in Acceptance And Commitment Therapy. *Journal of Clinical Psychology, 57*, 243–255.

Bolay, H., & Moskowitz, M. A. (2002). Mechanisms of pain modulation in chronic syndromes. *Neurology, 59*(Suppl 2), S2–S7.

Bonanno, G. A. (2004). Loss, trauma, and human resilience: Have we underestimated the human capacity to thrive after extremely aversive events? *American Psychologist, 59*, 20–28.

Boswell, M. V., & Giordano, J. (2009). Reflection, analysis and change: The decade of pain control and research and its lessons for the future of pain management. *Pain Physician, 12*, 923–928.

Boureau, F., Doubrere, J. F., & Luu, M. (1990). Study of verbal description in neuropathic pain. *Pain, 42*, 145–152.

Breivik, H., Collett, B., Ventafridda, V., Cohen, R., & Gallacher, D. (2006). Survey of chronic pain in Europe: Prevalence, impact on daily life, and treatment. *European Journal of Pain, 10*, 287–333.

Broderick, J. E., Schwartz, J. E., Vikingstad, G., Pribbernow, M., Grossman, S., & Stone, A. A. (2008). The accuracy of pain and fatigue items across reporting periods. *Pain, 139*, 146–157.

Brown, G. K. (1990). A causal analysis of chronic pain and depression. *Journal of Abnormal Psychology, 99*, 127–137.

Cacchio, A., De Blasis, E., Necozione, S., di Orio, F., & Santilli, V. (2009). Mirror therapy for chronic complex regional pain syndrome type 1 and stroke. *The New England Journal of Medicine, 361*, 634–636.

Cairns, D., & Pasino, J. (1977). Comparison of verbal reinforcement and feedback in the operant treatment of disability of chronic low back pain. *Behavior Therapy, 8*, 621–630.

Cairns, D., Thomas, L., Mooney, V., & Pace, J. B. (1976). A comprehensive treatment approach to chronic low back pain. *Pain, 2*, 301–308.

Carroll, D., & Seers, K. (1998). Relaxation for the relief of chronic pain: A systematic review. *Journal of Advanced Nursing, 27*, 476–487.

Chan, B. L., Witt, R., Charrow, A. P., Magee, A., Howard, R., Pasquina, P. F., et al. (2007). Mirror therapy for phantom limb pain. *The New England Journal of Medicine, 357*, 2206–2207.

Chiauzzi, E., Pujol, L. A., Wood, M., Bond, K., Black, R., Yiu, E., et al. (2010). painACTION-back pain: A self-management website for people with chronic back pain. *Pain Medicine, 11*, 1044–1058.

Clauw, D. J., Radulovic, D., Heshmat, Y., & Barbey, J. T. (1996). Heart rate variability as a measure of autonomic dysfunction in patients with fibromyalgia. *Arthritis and Rheumatism, 39*, S276.

Cleeland, C. S., & Ryan, K. M. (1994). Pain assessment: Global use of the brief pain inventory. *Annals of the Academy of Medicine, Singapore, 23*, 129–138.

Closs, S. J., Barr, B., Briggs, M., Cash, K., & Seers, K. (2004). A comparison of five pain assessment scales for nursing home residents with varying degrees of cognitive impairment. *Journal of Pain and Symptom Management, 27*, 196–205.

Cousins, M. J. (1995). Foreword. In W. E. Fordyce (Ed.), *Back pain in the workplace: Management of disability in nonspecific conditions. Task force report* (p. ix). Seattle: IASP Press.

Crisson, J. E., & Keefe, F. J. (1988). The relationship of locus of control to pain coping strategies and psychological distress in chronic pain patients. *Pain, 35*, 147–154.

Curatolo, M., & Bogduk, N. (2001). Pharmacologic pain treatment of musculoskeletal disorders: Current perspectives and future prospects. *The Clinical Journal of Pain, 17*, 25–32.

De Charms, R. C., Maeda, F., Glover, G. H., Ludlow, D., Pauly, J. M., Soneji, D., et al. (2005). Control over brain activation and pain learned by using real-time functional MRI. *Proceedings of the National Academy of Sciences of the United States of America, 102*, 18626–18631.

Demyttenaere, K., Bruffaerts, R., Lee, S., Posada-Villa, J., Kovess, V., Angermeyer, M. C., et al. (2007). Mental disorders among persons with chronic back or neck pain: Results from the world mental health surveys. *Pain, 129*, 332–342.

De Pascalis, V., Cacace, I., & Massicolle, F. (2008). Focused analgesia in waking and hypnosis: Effects on pain, memory, and somatosensory event-related potentials. *Pain, 134*, 197–208.

Derbyshire, S. W., Whalley, M. G., & Oakley, D. A. (2009). Fibromyalgia pain and its modulation by hypnotic and non-hypnotic suggestions: An fMRI analysis. *European Journal of Pain, 13*, 542–550.

Dolce, J. J., Crocker, M. F., Moletteire, C., & Doleys, D. M. (1986). Exercise quotas, anticipatory concern and self-efficacy expectancies in chronic pain: A preliminary report. *Pain, 24*, 365–372.

Doleys, D. M. (2000). Chronic pain. In R. G. Frank, & T. R. Elliott (Eds.), *Handbook of rehabilitation psychology* (pp. 185–203). Washington, DC: American Psychological Association.

Doleys, D. M., Crocker, M., & Patton, D. (1982). Response of patients with chronic pain to exercise quotas. *Physical Therapy, 62*, 1111–1114.

Dworkin, R. H., Turk, D. C., Farrar, J. T., Haythornthwaite, J. A., Jensen, M. P., Katz, N. P., et al. (2005). Core outcome measures for chronic pain clinical trials: IMMPACT recommendations. *Pain, 113*, 9–19.

Eccleston, C., Williams, A. C., & Morley, S. (2009). Psychological therapies for the management of chronic pain (excluding headache) in adults. *Cochrane Database of Systematic Reviews, 2*, CD007407.

Eimer, B. N., & Freeman, A. (1998). *Pain management psychotherapy.* New York: Wiley.

Elliott, A. M., Smith, B. H., Penny, K. I., Smith, W. C., & Chambers, W. A. (1999). The epidemiology of chronic pain in the community. *Lancet, 354*, 1248–1252.

Elwood, L. S., Hahn, K. S., Olatunji, B. O., & Williams, N. L. (2009). Cognitive vulnerabilities to the development of PTSD: A review of four vulnerabilities and the proposal of an integrative vulnerability model. *Clinical Psychology Review, 29*, 87–100.

Ericsson, M., Poston, W. S., Linder, J., Taylor, J. E., Haddock, C. K., & Foreyt, J. P. (2002). Depression predicts disability in long-term chronic pain patients. *Disability and Rehabilitation, 24*, 334–340.

Esteve, R., Ramírez-Maestre, C., & López-Martínez, A. E. (2007). Adjustment to chronic pain: The role of pain acceptance, coping strategies, and pain-related cognitions. *Annals of Behavioral Medicine, 33*, 179–188.

Faymonville, M. E., Laureys, S., Degueldre, C., Del Fiore, G., Luxen, A., Franck, G. et al. (2000). Neural mechanisms of antinociceptive effects of hypnosis. *Anesthesiology, 92*, 1257–1267.

Feldner, M. T., Zvolensky, M. J., Schmidt, N. B., & Smith, R. C. (2008). A prospective test of anxiety sensitivity as a moderator of the relation between gender and posttraumatic symptom maintenance among high anxiety sensitive young adults. *Depression and Anxiety, 25*, 190–199.

Ferrell, B. A., Ferrell, B. R., & Rivera, L. (1995). Pain in cognitively impaired nursing home patients. *Journal of Pain and Symptom Management, 10*, 591–598.

Fields, H. L., Basbaum, A. I., & Heinricher, M. M. (2006). Central nervous system mechanisms of pain modulation. In S. B. McMahon, & M. Koltzenburg (Eds.), *Wall and Melzack's textbook of pain* (5th ed., pp. 125–142). Philadelphia: Elsevier/Churchill Livingstone.

Fishbain, D. A., Cutler, R., Rosomoff, H. L., & Rosomoff, R. S. (1997). Chronic pain-associated depression: Antecedent or consequence of chronic pain? A review. *The Clinical Journal of Pain, 13*, 116–137.

Fishbain, D. A., Goldberg, M., Meagher, B. R., Steele, R., & Rosomoff, H. (1986). Male and female chronic pain patients categorized by DSM-III psychiatric criteria. *Pain, 26*, 181–197.

Flor, H., Fydrich, T., & Turk, D. C. (1992). Efficacy of multidisciplinary pain treatment centers: A meta-analytic review. *Pain, 49*, 221–230.

Flor, H., Kerns, R. D., & Turk, D. C. (1987). The role of spouse reinforcement, perceived pain, and activity levels of chronic pain patients. *Journal of Psychosomatic Research, 31*, 251–259.

Fordyce, W. E. (1976). *Behavioral methods for chronic pain and illness.* St Louis: Mosby.

Fordyce, W. E., Fowler, R., Lehmann, J., & De Lateur, B. (1968). Some implications of learning in problems of chronic pain. *Journal of Chronic Disabilities, 21*, 179–190.

Foss, J. M., Apkarian, A. V., & Chialvo, D. R. (2006). Dynamics of pain: Fractal dimension of temporal variability of spontaneous pain differentiates between pain states. *Journal of Neurophysiology, 95*, 730–736.

Gallagher, R. M., Moore, P., & Chernoff, I. (1995). The reliability of depression diagnosis in chronic low back pain. *General Hospital Psychiatry, 17*, 399–413.

Gatchel, R. J., Polatin, P. B., Noe, C., Gardea, M., Pulliam, C., & Thompson, J. (2003). Treatment- and cost-effectiveness of early intervention for acute low-back pain patients: A one-year prospective study. *Journal of Occupational Rehabilitation, 13*, 1–9.

Geisser, M. E., Robinson, M. E., Keefe, F. J., & Weiner, M. L. (1994). Catastrophizing, depression and the sensory, affective and evaluative aspects of chronic pain. *Pain, 59*, 79–83.

Gensichen, J., Teising, A., König, J., Gerlach, F. M., & Petersen, J. J. (2010). Predictors of suicidal ideation in depressive primary care patients. *Journal of Affective Disorders, 125*, 124–127.

Green, C. R., Anderson, K. O., Baker, T. A., Campbell, L. C., Decker, S., Fillingim, R. B., et al. (2003). The unequal burden of pain: Confronting racial and ethnic disparities in pain. *Pain Medicine, 4*, 277–294.

Green, J. P., Barabasz, A. F., Barrett, D., & Montgomery, G. H. (2005). Forging ahead: The 2003 APA division 30 definition of hypnosis. *Journal of Clinical and Experimental Hypnosis, 53*, 259–264.

Greenberg, P. E., Leong, S. A., Birnbaum, H. G., & Robinson, R. L. (2003). The economic burden of depression with painful symptoms. *Journal of Clinical Psychiatry, 64*, 17–23.

Gustavsson, C., & von Koch, L. (2006). Applied relaxation in the treatment of long-lasting neck pain: A randomized controlled pilot study. *Journal of Rehabilitation Medicine, 38*, 100–107.

Harris, A. J. (1999). Cortical origin of pathological pain. *Lancet, 354*, 1464–1466.

Hassett, A. L., Radvanski, D. C., Vaschillo, E. G., Vaschillo, B., Sigal, L. H., Karavidas, M. K., et al. (2007). A pilot study of the efficacy of heart rate variability (HRV) biofeedback in patients with fibromyalgia. *Applied Psychophysiology and Biofeedback, 32*, 1–10.

Hayden, J. A., van Tulder, M. W., Malmivaara, A. V., & Koes, B. W. (2005). Meta-analysis: Exercise therapy for nonspecific low back pain. *Annals of Internal Medicine, 142*, 765–775.

Hayes, S. C. (2004). Acceptance and Commitment Therapy, relational frame theory, and the third wave of behavioral and cognitive therapies. *Behavior Therapy, 35*, 639–665.

Hayes, S. C., Luoma, J. B., Bond, F. W., Masuda, A., & Lillis, J. (2006). Acceptance and Commitment Therapy: Model, processes and outcomes. *Behaviour Research and Therapy, 44*, 1–25.

Hayes, S. C., & Wilson, K. G. (1995). The role of cognition in complex human behavior: A contextualistic perspective. *Journal of Behavior Therapy and Experimental Psychiatry, 26*, 241–248.

Hirakawa, N., Tershrer, S. A., & Fields, H. L. (1999). Highly deltal selective antagonists in the RVM attenuate the antinociceptive effect of PAG DAMGO. *Neuroreport, 10*, 3125–3129.

Jacobson, E. (1929). *Progressive relaxation.* Chicago: University of Chicago Press.

Jamison, R. N., Sbrocco, T., & Parris, W. C. V. (1989). The influence of physical and psychosocial factors on accuracy of memory for pain in chronic pain patients. *Pain, 37*, 289–294.

Jann, M. W., & Slade, J. H. (2007). Antidepressant agents for the treatment of chronic pain and depression. *Pharmacotherapy, 27*, 1572–1587.

Jenewein, J., Wittmann, L., Moergeli, H., Creutzig, J., & Schnyder, U. (2009). Mutual influence of posttraumatic stress disorder symptoms and chronic pain among injured accident survivors: A longitudinal study. *Journal of Traumatic Stress, 22*, 540–548.

Jensen, M. P. (2009). Hypnosis for chronic pain management: A new hope. *Pain, 146*, 235–237.

Jensen, M. P., & Karoly, P. (2001). Self-report scales and procedures for assessing pain in adults. In D. C. Turk, & R.

Melzack (Eds.), *Handbook of pain assessment* (pp. 15–34). New York: Guilford.

Jensen, M., & Patterson, D. R. (2006). Hypnotic treatment of chronic pain. *Journal of Behavioral Medicine, 29*, 95–124.

Jensen, M. P., Turner, J. A., Romano, J. M., & Karoly, P. (1991). Coping with chronic pain: A critical review of the literature. *Pain, 47*, 249–283.

Ji, R. R., Kohno, T., Moore, K. A., & Woolf, C. J. (2003). Central sensitization and LTP: Do pain and memory share similar mechanisms? *Trends in Neurosciences, 26*, 696–705.

Johansen, J. P., & Fields, H. L. (2004). Glutamatergic activation of anterior cingulate cortex produces an aversive teaching signal. *Nature Neuroscience, 7*, 398–403.

Jones, D. A., Rollman, G. B., White, K. P., Hill, M. L., & Brooke, R. I. (2003). The relationship between cognitive appraisal, affect, and catastrophizing in patients with chronic pain. *The Journal of Pain, 4*, 267–277.

Juniper, M., Le, T. K., & Mladsi, D. (2009). The epidemiology, economic burden, and pharmacological treatment of chronic low back pain in France, Germany, Italy, Spain and the UK: a literature-based review. *Expert Opinion on Pharmacotherapy, 10*, 2581–2592.

Kabat-Zinn, J. (1982). An outpatient program in behavioral medicine for chronic pain patients based on the practice of mindfulness meditation: Theoretical considerations and preliminary results. *General Hospital Psychiatry, 4*, 33–47.

Kabat-Zinn, J., Lipworth, L., & Burney, R. (1985). The clinical use of mindfulness meditation for the self-regulation of chronic pain. *Journal of Behavioral Medicine, 8*, 163–190.

Karmarkar, A., & Lieberman, I. (2006). Mirror box therapy for complex regional pain syndrome. *Anaesthesia, 61*, 412–413.

Keefe, F. J., Brown, G. K., Wallston, K. A., & Caldwell, D. S. (1989). Coping with rheumatoid arthritis pain: Catastrophizing as a maladaptive strategy. *Pain, 37*, 51–56.

Keefe, F. J., Caldwell, D. S., Martinez, S., Nunley, J., Beckham, J., & Williams, D. A. (1991). Analyzing pain in rheumatoid arthritis patients. Pain coping strategies in patients who have had knee replacement surgery. *Pain, 46*, 153–160.

Kernan, T., & Rainville, J. (2007). Observed outcomes associated with a quota-based exercise approach on measures of kinesophobia in patients with chronic low back pain. *The Journal of Orthopaedic and Sports Physical Therapy, 37*, 679–687.

Kerns, R. D., Turk, D. C., & Rudy, T. E. (1985). The West Haven-Yale Multidimensional Pain Inventory (WHYMPI). *Pain, 23*, 345–356.

Kremer, E., Atkinson, J. H., & Ignelzi, R. J. (1981). Measurement of pain: Patient preference does not confound pain measurement. *Pain, 10*, 241–248.

Krishnan, K., France, R., Pelton, S., & McCann, S. (1985). Chronic pain and depression: 1. Classification of depression in chronic low back patients. *Pain, 22*, 279–287.

Kroenke, K., Theobald, D, Wu, J., Norton, K., Morrison, G., Carpenter, J., et al. (2010). Effect of telecare management on pain and depression in patients with cancer: A randomized trial. *Journal of the American Medical Association, 304*, 163–171.

Kupers, R. C., Konings, H., Adriaensen, H., & Gybels, J. M. (1991). Morphine differentially affects the sensory and affective pain ratings in neurogenic and idiopathic forms of pain. *Pain, 47*, 5–12.

Leeuw, M., Goossens, M. E., Linton, S. J., Crombez, G., Boersma, K., & Vlaeyen, J. W. (2007). The fear-avoidance model of musculoskeletal pain: current state of scientific evidence. *Journal of Behavioral Medicine, 30*, 77–94.

Loeser, J. D. (1991). Desirable characteristics for pain treatment facilities: Report of the IASP taskforce. In M. R. Bond, J. E. Charlton, & C. J. Woolf (Eds.), *Pain Research and Clinical Management, 4,* 411–415.

Malone, M. D., & Strube, M. J. (1988). Meta-analysis of non-medical treatments for chronic pain. *Pain, 34,* 231–244.

Man, P. L., & Chen, C. H. (1972). Mechanism of acupunctural anesthesia. The two-gate control theory. *Diseases of the Nervous System, 33,* 730–735.

Maniadakis, N., & Gray, A. (2000). The economic burden of back pain in the UK. *Pain 84,* 95–103.

Marshall, G. N., Miles, J. N., & Stewart, S. H. (2010). Anxiety sensitivity and PTSD symptom severity are reciprocally related: Evidence from a longitudinal study of physical trauma survivors. *Journal of Abnormal Psychology, 119,* 143–150.

Martell, B. A., O'Connor, P. G., Kerns, R. D., Becker, W. C., Morales, K. H., Kosten, T., et al. (2007). Systematic review: Opioid treatment for chronic back pain: Prevalence, efficacy, and association with addiction. *Annals of Internal Medicine, 146,* 116–127.

May, S. (2010). Self-management of chronic low back pain and osteoarthritis. *Nature Reviews. Rheumatology, 6,* 199–209.

McCabe, C. S., Haigh, R. C., Ring, E. F., Halligan, P. W., Wall, P. D., & Blake, D. R. (2003). A controlled pilot study of the utility of mirror visual feedback in the treatment of complex regional pain syndrome (type 1). *Rheumatology (Oxford), 42,* 97–101.

McCracken, L. M. (2005). *Contextual cognitive-behavioral therapy for chronic pain: Progress in pain research and management.* Seattle: IASP.

McCracken, L. M., Carson, J. W., Eccleston, C., & Keefe, F. J. (2004). Acceptance and change in the context of chronic pain. *Pain, 109,* 4–7.

McCracken, L. M., & Eccleston, C. (2005). A prospective study of acceptance of pain and patient functioning with chronic pain. *Pain, 118,* 164–169.

McCracken, L. M., Gauntlett-Gilbert, J., & Vowles, K. E. (2007). The role of mindfulness in a contextual cognitive-behavioral analysis of chronic pain-related suffering and disability. *Pain, 131,* 63–69.

McCracken, L. M., MacKichan, F., & Eccleston, C. (2007). Contextual cognitive-behavioral therapy for severely disabled chronic pain sufferers: Effectiveness and clinically significant change. *European Journal of Pain, 11,* 314–322.

McCracken, L. M., & Turk, D. C. (2002). Behavioral and cognitive-behavioral treatment for chronic pain: Outcome, predictors of outcome, and treatment process. *Spine, 27,* 2564–2573.

McCracken, L. M., & Velleman, S. C. (2010). Psychological flexibility in adults with chronic pain: A study of acceptance, mindfulness, and values-based action in primary care. *Pain, 148,* 141–147.

McCracken, L. M., & Vowles, K. E. (2007). Psychological flexibility and traditional pain management strategies in relation to patient functioning with chronic pain: An examination of a revised instrument. *The Journal of Pain, 8,* 700–707.

McCracken L. M., Vowles, K. E., & Eccleston, C. (2005). Acceptance-based treatment for persons with complex, long standing chronic pain: A preliminary analysis of treatment outcome in comparison to a waiting phase. *Behaviour Research and Therapy, 43,* 1335–1346.

McNair, D. M., Lorr, M., & Droppleman, L. F. (1971). *FITS manual for the profile of mood states.* San Diego: Educational & Industrial Testing Service.

McQuay, H. (2005). Consensus on outcome measures for chronic pain trials. *Pain, 113,* 1–2.

McWilliams, L. A., Cox, B. J., & Enns, M. W. (2003). Mood and anxiety disorders associated with chronic pain: An examination in a nationally representative sample. *Pain, 106,* 127–133.

Means-Christensen, A. J., Roy-Byrne, P. P., Sherbourne, C. D., Craske, M. G., & Stein, M. B. (2008). Relationships among pain, anxiety, and depression in primary care. *Depression and Anxiety, 25,* 593–600.

Melzack, R. (1987). The short-form McGill Pain Questionnaire. *Pain, 30,* 191–197.

Melzack, R., & Casey, K. L. (1968). Sensory, motivational, and central control determinants of pain: A new conceptual model. In D. Kenshalo (Ed.), *The skin senses* (pp. 423–443). Springfield, IL: Thomas.

Melzack, R., & Wall, P. (1965). Pain mechanisms: A new theory. *Science, 150,* 971–979.

Menzies, V., & Kim, S. (2008). Relaxation and guided imagery in Hispanic persons diagnosed with fibromyalgia: A pilot study. *Family and Community Health, 31,* 204–212.

Menzies, V., Taylor, A. G., & Bourguignon, C. (2006). Effects of guided imagery on outcomes of pain, functional status, and self-efficacy in persons diagnosed with fibromyalgia. *The Journal of Alternative and Complementary Medicine, 12,* 23–30.

Merskey, H. (1986). Classification of chronic pain: Description of chronic pain syndromes and definitions of pain terms. *Pain,* (Suppl. 3), S1-S225.

Merskey, H., & Bogduk, N. (1994). *Classification of chronic pain* (2nd ed.). Seattle: IASP.

Montgomery, G. H., DuHamel, K. N., & Redd, W. H. (2000). A meta-analysis of hypnotically induced analgesia: How effective is hypnosis? *International Journal of Clinical and Experimental Hypnosis, 48,* 138–153.

Morley, S., Eccleston, C., & Williams, A. (1999). Systematic review and meta-analysis of randomized controlled trials of cognitive behaviour therapy and behaviour therapy for chronic pain in adults, excluding headache. *Pain, 80,* 1–13.

Morone, N. E., Greco, C. M., & Weiner, D. K. (2008). Mindfulness meditation for the treatment of chronic low back pain in older adults: A randomized controlled pilot study. *Pain, 134,* 310–319.

Moseley, G. L., Gallace, A., & Spence, C. (2008). Is mirror therapy all it is cracked up to be? Current evidence and future directions. *Pain, 138,* 7–10.

Murray, C. D., Pettifer, S., Howard, T., Patchick, E. L., Caillette, F., Kulkarni, J., et al. (2007). The treatment of phantom limb pain using immersive virtual reality: Three case studies. *Disability and Rehabilitation, 29,* 1465–1469.

National Centers for Health Statistics. (2006). *Health, United States, 2006 with chartbook trends in the health of Americans. Special feature: Pain* (pp. 68–87). Hyattsville, MD: Author.

Nicholas, M. K., & Asghari, A. (2006). Investigating acceptance in adjustment to chronic pain: Is acceptance broader than we thought? *Pain, 124,* 269–279.

Norman, S. B., Stein, M. B., Dimsdale, J. E., & Hoyt, D. B. (2008). Pain in the aftermath of trauma is a risk factor for post-traumatic stress disorder. *Psychological Medicine, 38,* 533–542.

Ocañez, K. L., McHugh, K. R, & Otto, M. W. (2010). A meta-analytic review of the association between anxiety sensitivity and pain. *Depression and Anxiety, 27,* 760–767.

Olton, D. S., & Noonberg, A. R. (1980). *Biofeedback: Clinical applications in behavioral medicine*. Englewood Cliffs, NJ: Prentice Hall.

Oneal, B. J., Patterson, D. R., Soltani, M, Teeley, A., & Jensen, M. P. (2009). Virtual reality hypnosis in the treatment of chronic neuropathic pain: A case report. *The International Journal of Clinical and Experimental Hypnosis, 56*, 451–462.

Ostelo, R. W. J. G., van Tulder, M. W., Vlaeyen, J. W. S., Linton, S. J., Morley, S., & Assendelft, W. J. J. (2005). Behavioural treatment for chronic low-back pain. *Cochrane Database of Systematic Reviews, 1*, CD002014.

Paice, J. A., & Cohen, F. L. (1997). Validity of a verbally administered numeric rating scale to measure cancer pain intensity. *Cancer Nursing, 20*, 88–93.

Patterson, D. R., Jensen, M. P., Wiechman, S. A., & Sharar, S. R. (2010). Virtual reality hypnosis for pain associated with recovery from physical trauma. *The International Journal of Clinical and Experimental Hypnosis, 58*, 288–300.

Petrovic, P., Kalso, E., Petersson, K. M., & Ingvar, M. (2002). Placebo and opioid analgesia: Imaging a shared neuronal network. *Science, 295*, 1737–1740.

Porter-Moffitt, S., Gatchel, R. J., Robinson, R. C., Deschner, M., Posamentier, M., Polatin, P., et al. (2006). Biopsychosocial profiles of different pain diagnostic groups. *The Journal of Pain, 7*, 308–318.

Pradhan, E. K., Baumgarten, M., Langenberg, P., Handwerger, B., Gilpin, A. K., Magyari, T., et al. (2007). Effect of mindfulness-based stress reduction in rheumatoid arthritis patients. *Arthritis and Rheumatism, 57*, 1134–1142.

Price, D. D. (1988). *Psychological and neural mechanisms of pain*. New York: Raven.

Price, D. D., Harkins, S. W., & Baker, C. (1987). Sensory-affective relationships among different types of clinical pain and experimental pain. *Pain, 28*, 297–307.

Rainville, P., Duncan, G. H., Price, D. D., Carrier, B., & Bushnell, M. C. (1997). Pain affect encoded in human anterior cingulate but not somatosensory cortex. *Science, 277*, 968–971.

Raj, P. P. (1996). *Pain medicine: A comprehensive review*. Mosby: St. Louis, MO.

Ralphs, J. A., Williams, A. C. de C., Richardson, P. H., Pither, C. E., & Nicholas, M. K. (1994). Opiate reduction in chronic pain patients: A comparison of patient-controlled reduction and staff controlled cocktail methods. *Pain, 56*, 279–288.

Ramachandran, V. S., & Altschuler, E. L. (2009). The use of visual feedback, in particular mirror visual feedback, in restoring brain function. *Brain, 132*, 1693–1710.

Ramachandran, V. S., Brang, D., & McGeoch, P. D. (2009). Size reduction using Mirror Visual Feedback (MVF) reduces phantom pain. *Neurocase, 15*, 357–360.

Reiss, S. (1991). Expectancy theory of fear, anxiety, and panic. *Clinical Psychology Review, 11*, 141–153.

Reiss, S., & McNally, R. J. (1985). The expectancy model of fear. In S. Reiss, & R. R. Bootzin (Eds.), *Theoretical issues in behavior therapy* (pp. 107–121). New York: Academic Press.

Richardson, E. J., Ness, T. J., Doleys, D. M., Baños, J. H., Cianfrini, L., & Richards, J. S. (2009). Depressive symptoms and pain evaluations among persons with chronic pain: Catastrophizing, but not pain acceptance, shows significant effects. *Pain, 147*, 147–152.

Richardson, E. J., Ness, T. J., Doleys, D. M., Baños, J. H., Cianfrini, L., & Richards, J. S. (2010). Catastrophizing, acceptance, and interference: Laboratory findings, subjective report, and pain willingness as a moderator. *Health Psychology, 29*, 299–306.

Robbins, H., Gatchel, R. J., Noe, C., Gajraj, N., Polatin, P., Deschner, M., et al. (2003). A prospective one-year outcome study of interdisciplinary chronic pain management: Compromising its efficacy by managed care policies. *Anesthesia and Analgesia, 97*, 156–162.

Roberts, A. H., & Reinhardt, L. (1980). The behavioral management of chronic pain: Long-term follow-up with comparison groups. *Pain, 8*, 151–162.

Roland, M., & Morris, R. (1983). A study of the natural history of back pain. Part I: Development of a reliable and sensitive measure of disability in low back pain. *Spine, 8*, 141–144.

Romano, J. M., & Turner, J. A. (1985). Chronic pain and depression: Does the evidence support a relationship? *Psychological Bulletin, 97*, 18–34.

Rosenzweig, S., Greeson, J. M., Reibel, D. K., Green J. S., Jasser, S. A., & Beasley, D. (2010). Mindfulness-based stress reduction for chronic pain conditions: Variation in treatment outcomes and role of meditation practice. *Journal of Psychosomatic Research, 68*, 29–36.

Rosser, B. A., Vowles, K. E., Keogh, E., Eccleston, C., & Mountain, G. A. (2009). Technologically-assisted behavior change: A systematic review of studies of novel technologies for the management of chronic illness. *Journal of Telemedicine and Telecare, 15*, 327–338.

Russo, C. M., & Brose, W. G. (1998). Chronic pain. *Annual Review of Medicine, 49*, 123–133.

Scascighini, L., Toma, V., Dober-Spielmann, S., & Sprott, H. (2008). Multidisciplinary treatment for chronic pain: A systematic review of interventions and outcomes. *Rheumatology, 47*, 670–678.

Schultz, J. H., & Luthe, W. (1959). *Autogenic training: A psychophysiologic approach in psychotherapy*. New York: Grune & Stratton.

Selles, R. W., Schreuders, T. A., & Stam, H. J. (2008). Mirror therapy in patients with causalgia (complex regional pain syndrome type II) following peripheral nerve injury: Two cases. *Journal of Rehabilitation Medicine, 40*, 312–314.

Severeijns, R., Vlaeyen, J. W. S., van den Hout, M. A., & Weber, W. E. J. (2001). Pain catastrophizing predicts pain intensity, disability, and psychological distress independent of the level of physical impairment. *The Clinical Journal of Pain, 17*, 165–172.

Sharp, T. J., & Harvey, A. G. (2001). Chronic pain and post-traumatic stress disorder: Mutual maintenance? *Clinical Psychology Review, 21*, 857–877.

Sluka, K. A., & Walsh, D. (2003). Transcutaneous electrical nerve stimulation: Basic science mechanisms and clinical effectiveness. *The Journal of Pain, 4*, 109–121.

Stewart, W. F., Ricci, J. A., Chee, E. Morganstein, D., & Lipton, R. (2003). Lost productive time and cost due to common pain conditions in the US workforce. *Journal of the American Medical Association, 290*, 2443–2454.

Stoelb, B. L., Molton, I. R., Jensen, M. P., & Patterson, D. R. (2009). The efficacy of hypnotic analgesia in adults: A review of the literature. *Contemporary Hypnosis, 26*, 24–39.

Sturgeon, J. A., & Zautra, A J. (2010). Resilience: A new paradigm for adaptation to chronic pain. *Current Pain and Headache Reports, 14*, 105–112.

Sullivan, M. J. L., Bishop, S. R., & Pivik, J. (1995). The Pain Catastrophizing Scale: Development and validation. *Psychological Assessment, 7*, 524–532.

Sullivan, M. J. L., Lynch, M. E., & Clark, A. J. (2005). Dimensions of catastrophic thinking associated with pain experience and disability with neuropathic pain conditions. *Pain, 113*, 310–315.

Sullivan, M. J. L., Thorn, B., Haythornthwaite, J. A., Keefe, F., Martin, M., Bradley, L. A., et al. (2001). Theoretical perspectives on the relation between catastrophizing and pain. *The Clinical Journal of Pain, 17*, 52–64.

Syrjala, K. L., & Abrams, J. R. (2002). Hypnosis and imagery in the treatment of pain. In D. C. Turk, & R. J. Gatchel (Eds.), *Psychological approaches to pain management: A practitioner's handbook* (pp. 187–209). New York: Guilford.

Taylor, S. (1999). Anxiety sensitivity: Theoretical perspectives and recent findings. *Behavior Research and Therapy, 33*, 243–258.

Thorn, B. E. (2004). *Cognitive therapy for chronic pain: A step by step guide*. New York: Guilford.

Turk, D. C. (2002a). Clinical effectiveness and cost-effectiveness of treatments for chronic pain patients. *The Clinical Journal of Pain, 18*, 355–365.

Turk, D. C. (2002b). A cognitive-behavioral perspective on treatment of chronic pain patients. In D. C. Turk, & R. J. Gatchel (Eds.), *Psychological approaches to pain Management* (2nd ed., pp. 138–158). New York: Guilford.

Turk, D. C., Dworkin, R. H., Allen, R. R., Bellamy, N., Brandenburg, N., Carr, D. B., et al. (2003). Core outcome domains for chronic pain clinical trials: IMMPACT recommendations. *Pain, 106*, 337–345.

Turk, D. C., & Flor, H. (2006). The cognitive-behavioural approach to pain management. In S. B. McMahon, & M. Koltzenburg (Eds.), *Wall and Melzack's textbook of pain*. (5th ed., pp. 339–348). Philadelphia: Elsevier/Churchill Livingstone.

Turk, D. C., Kerns, R. D., & Rosenberg, R. (1992). Effects of marital interaction on chronic pain and disability: Examining the down-side of social support. *Rehabilitation Psychology, 37*, 259–274.

Turk, D. C., Meichenbaum, D., & Genest, M. (1983). *Pain and behavioural medicine: A cognitive-behavioural perspective*. New York: Guilford.

Turk, D. C., Okifuji, A., & Scharff, L. (1995). Chronic pain and depression: Role of perceived impact and perceived control in different age cohorts. *Pain, 61*, 93–101.

Turk, D. C., & Rudy, T. E. (1989). Assessment of cognitive factors in chronic pain: A worthwhile enterprise? *Journal of Consulting and Clinical Psychology, 54*, 760–768.

Turk, D. C., Swanson, K. S., & Tunks, E. R. (2008). Psychological approaches in the treatment of chronic pain patients: When pills, scalpels, and needles are not enough. *The Canadian Journal of Psychiatry, 53*, 213–223.

Turner, J. A. (1996). Educational and behavioral interventions for back pain in primary care. *Spine, 21*, 2851–2859.

Turner, J. A., & Aaron, L. A. (2001). Pain-related catastrophizing: What is it? *The Clinical Journal of Pain, 17*, 65–71.

van Middelkoop, M., Rubinstein, S. M., Verhagen, A. P., Ostelo, R. W., Koes, B. W., & van Tulder, M. W. (2010). Exercise therapy for chronic non-specific low back pain. *Best Practice and Research Clinical Rheumatology, 24*, 193–204.

Viane, I., Crombez, G., Eccleston, C., Devulder, J., & De Corte, W. (2004). Acceptance of the unpleasant reality of chronic pain: Effects upon attention to pain and engagement with daily activities. *Pain, 112*, 282–288.

Viane, I., Crombez, G., Eccleston, C., Poppe, C., Devulder, J., Van Houdenhove, B., et al. (2003). Acceptance of pain is an independent predictor of mental well-being in patients with chronic pain: Empirical evidence and reappraisal. *Pain, 106*, 65–72.

Vlaeyen, J. W., Kole-Snijders, A. M., Boeren, R. G., & van Eek, H. (1995). Fear of movement/(re)injury in chronic low back pain and its relation to behavioral performance. *Pain, 62*, 363–372.

Vlaeyen, J. W. S., & Linton, S. J. (2000). Fear-avoidance and its consequences in chronic musculoskeletal pain: A state of the art. *Pain, 85*, 317–332.

Vowles, K. E., & McCracken, L. M. (2008). Acceptance and values-based action in chronic pain: A study of treatment effectiveness and process. *Journal of Consulting and Clinical Psychology, 76*, 397–407.

Vowles, K. E., & McCracken, L. M. (2010). Comparing the role of psychological flexibility and traditional pain management coping strategies in chronic pain treatment outcomes. *Behaviour Research and Therapy, 48*, 141–146.

Vowles, K. E., McNeil, D. W., Gross, R. T., McDaniel, M. L., Mouse, A., Bates, M., et al. (2007). Effects of pain acceptance and pain control strategies on physical impairment in individuals with chronic low back pain. *Behavior Therapy, 38*, 412–425.

Walsh, N. E., Dumitru, D., Schoenfeld, L. S., & Ramamurthy, S. (1998). Treatment of the patient with chronic pain. In J. A. DeLisa, & B. M. Gans (Eds.), *Rehabilitation medicine: Principles and practice* (3rd ed., pp. 1385–1421). Philadelphia: Lippincott-Raven.

Watson, C. P. N., Chipman, M. L., & Monks, R. C. (2006). Antidepressant analgesics: A systematic review and comparative study. In S. B. McMahon, & M. Koltzenburg (Eds.), *Wall and Melzack's textbook of pain* (5th ed., pp. 481–497). Philadelphia: Elsevier/Churchill Livingstone.

Wegener, S. T., Mackenzie, E. J., Ephraim, P., Ehde, D., & Williams, R. (2009). Self-management improves outcomes in persons with limb loss. *Archives of Physical Medicine and Rehabilitation, 90*, 373–380.

Woolf, C. J. (1983). Evidence for a central component of post-injury pain hypersensitivity. *Nature, 306*, 686–688.

Woolf, C. J., & Mannion, R. J. (1999). Neuropathic pain: Aetiology, symptoms, mechanisms, and management. *Lancet, 353*, 1959–1964.

Woolf, C. J., & Salter, M. W. (2006). Plasticity and pain: Role of the dorsal horn. In S. B. McMahon, & M. Koltzenburg (Eds.), *Wall and Melzack's textbook of pain* (5th ed., pp. 91–105). Philadelphia: Elsevier/Churchill Livingstone.

Yeo, S.N., & Tay, K.H. (2009). Pain prevalence in Singapore. *Annals of the Academy of Medicine, Singapore, 38*, 937–942.

Zhou, M. (2007). A synaptic model for pain: Long-term potentiation in the anterior cingulate cortex. *Molecules and Cells, 23*, 259–271.

Pulmonary Rehabilitation in Chronic Obstructive Pulmonary Disease

Margreet Scharloo, Maarten J. Fischer, Esther van den Ende, *and* Adrian A. Kaptein

Abstract

This chapter starts with a description of the main disease characteristics and psychosocial consequences of chronic obstructive pulmonary disease (COPD), a multisystem disease with significant comorbidities. Comprehensive pulmonary rehabilitation programs (PRPs) aim at tackling these systemic consequences of COPD by combining self-management education, exercise training, nutritional intervention, and psychosocial and support interventions. Research on the effects of psychosocial interventions within programs is scarce. Studies on cognitive-behavioral interventions for anxiety and depression provide proof that a combination of strategies can add extra results to the positive effects that pulmonary rehabilitation in itself has on COPD symptoms. The results from studies on relaxation techniques for stress management and relieving breathlessness do not suggest much specific benefit for progressive muscle relaxation or other strategies. Currently, the evidence is largely absent that should guide "who does what and how" in the psychosocial components of pulmonary rehabilitation.

Key Words: chronic obstructive pulmonary disease (COPD), pulmonary rehabilitation programs (PRPs), systemic consequences, psychosocial interventions, cognitive behavioral interventions, anxiety and depression.

At its first appearance in the 1950s, pulmonary rehabilitation (PR) was initially met with skepticism based upon the lack of improvement in biochemical markers of exercise adaptation (Carlin, 2009). In the 1990s, research trials showed benefits in other outcome measures, such as dyspnea and quality of life (QOL). These encouraging improvements have fueled the development of evidence-based PR guidelines since the late 1990s. Today, PR is embraced as a key component in the management of patients with chronic obstructive pulmonary disease (COPD), and it has outgrown its reputation of being a "last ditch" resort for patients with invariably poor prognosis (Carlin, 2009; Global Initiative for Chronic Obstructive Lung Disease [GOLD], 2010). Unfortunately, despite the recommendations by the majority of scientific societies to include PR as an important part of treatment for COPD, and

despite the good evidence concerning the benefits of PR, findings on the low availability of PR indicate that the implementation of PR still has a long way to go (Güell-Rous & Diez-Betoret, 2010).

Over the previous decade, there has been an increasing appreciation of the importance of the systemic manifestations of COPD. Clearly, progressive airflow limitation results in the most predominant symptom experienced by patients: the sensation of breathlessness. However, as the disease progresses, its extrapulmonary features include systemic inflammation, muscular weakness, and alterations in body mass index, thus putting patients at an increased risk of osteoporosis, chronic anemia, depression, and cardiovascular disease (Decramer et al., 2008; GOLD, 2010; Nici et al., 2006). Comprehensive PR programs aim at tackling these systemic consequences of COPD, in combining (at the least) self-management education, exercise training, and nutritional intervention (GOLD, 2010).

With regard to the position of psychosocial interventions in PR, the most recent guidelines state that "current practice and expert opinion support the inclusion of psychosocial interventions as a component of comprehensive pulmonary rehabilitation programs for patients with COPD" (Ries et al., 2007, p. 29S), and that "psychologic and social support provided within the pulmonary rehabilitation setting can facilitate the adjustment process by encouraging adaptive thoughts and behaviors, helping patients to diminish negative emotions, and providing a socially supportive environment" (Nici et al., 2006, p. 1399).

This chapter will focus on the available evidence to support this notion. It will start with a case study to illustrate why psychologists should be involved in PR programs (PRPs). Next, the main features of COPD and the definition and content of PRPs will be described. We will take a closer look at the involvement of psychologists in PRPs, and at guideline recommendations regarding psychosocial assessment and psychosocial interventions. Randomized controlled studies on the effects of psychosocial and behavioral interventions in COPD will be reviewed, and the chapter will end with suggestions for future research.

The Downward Spiral

Ms. B, a 62-year-old woman is enrolled in an inpatient PR program. A diagnosis of COPD was made 9 years ago, and Ms. B is on long-term oxygen therapy for the last year. Nursing staff reports that Ms. B's behavior is very unpredictable. She can be social, cheerful, and pleasant, but at times she reacts cynically, is expressing a demanding attitude and engages in splitting (a mental mechanism in which the self or others are reviewed as all good or all bad, with failure to integrate the positive and negative qualities of self and others into cohesive images). If Ms. B has a bad day, she often cancels her therapies (endurance training, strength training, and educational sessions). She frequently asks for consultations with the respiratory specialist, and the answers she gets are never satisfying to her.

From intake assessments (questionnaires, exercise tests, and interviews), it appears that Ms. B suffers from anxiety, depression, and a strong tendency to somatize. She expresses a need for social support, but tries to get this in an indirect manner. For a number of physical complaints that are less obviously related to COPD, she insists on seeing a physician.

Because of the frequency of her demands she gets varying reactions, and she has the feeling that she is not heard and not taken seriously. When searching for support and confirmation, she plays the nursing staff, therapists, and her caregivers against each other. In the meantime, her worsening dyspnea evokes a great deal of anxiety and panic, which raises her need for support and strengthens her demanding attitude, at the same time reducing her self-care activities and leading to growing passivity.

Chronic Obstructive Pulmonary Disease
Definition, Diagnosis, Symptoms, and Severity

The current working definition of COPD reflects the acknowledgment that COPD should be regarded as a pulmonary disease, but that significant comorbidities must be taken into account:

> Chronic obstructive pulmonary disease is a preventable and treatable disease with some significant extrapulmonary effects that may contribute to the severity in individual patients. Its pulmonary component is characterized by airflow limitation that is not fully reversible. The airflow limitation is usually progressive and associated with an abnormal inflammatory response of the lung to noxious particles or gases. (GOLD, 2010, p. 2)

The characteristic symptoms of COPD are chronic and progressive dyspnea, cough, and sputum production. The diagnosis is established by spirometric testing, which requires the patient to take a maximum inspiration and then blow out all of the air in his lungs into a spirometer as forcefully and as rapidly as possible. The volume of air exhaled within 1 second is referred to as forced expiratory volume in 1 second (FEV_1) and is expressed in liters. Predicted forced expiratory volumes are expressed in terms of a normal range for age, sex, and height. Airflow abnormality is usually demonstrated by a decreased FEV_1 and a decrease in the ratio of FEV_1 to forced vital capacity (FVC). Forced vital capacity values represent the maximum volume of air that can be forcibly expelled after inhaling as deeply as possible. The current spirometric classification of severity of COPD (GOLD, 2010) includes four stages. At the initial stage of COPD (stage 1: "mild"; FEV_1 ≥80% predicted, FEV_1/FVC <70%) patients may have symptoms such as chronic cough and sputum production. However, patients are usually unaware that their lung function is already abnormal, and they often accept their symptoms as normal "smoker's cough."

When the disease progresses (stage 2: "moderate"; FEV_1 ≥50% and <80% predicted, FEV_1/FVC <70%), symptoms of breathlessness are only present at exertion, such as running and uphill bicycling, and cough and sputum production are sometimes also present. This often is the first stage at which medical attention is sought due to symptoms or an exacerbation. Acute exacerbations are episodes of worsened dyspnea, increased sputum production, and increased sputum purulence resulting from lung infections or irritation.

With deteriorating lung function (stage 3: "severe"; FEV_1 ≥30% and <50% predicted, FEV_1/FVC <70%), shortness of breath is already present when patients perform less strenuous activities, such as climbing the stairs or (hurried) walking, and patients experience fatigue and repeated exacerbations.

With worsening airflow limitation and chronic respiratory failure (stage 4: "very severe"; FEV_1 <30% predicted, or FEV_1 <50% predicted plus chronic respiratory failure), the respiratory system fails in oxygenation and/or carbon dioxide elimination, sentencing patients to chronic oxygen therapy. In this stage, people are often short of breath even at rest and exacerbations may be life-threatening. Also respiratory failure may lead to effects on the heart, such as right-sided heart failure.

Systemic Consequences

Although the prevalence of systemic consequences increases with increasing severity of airflow obstruction, both systemic consequences and comorbidities are already present in moderate COPD. For example, the proportion of patients with weight loss and cachexia (excessive weight loss in the setting of ongoing disease, associated with disproportionate muscle wasting) is already 10–15% in mild to moderate COPD. Also, the risk of reduced bone mass increases by 30% in moderate COPD, and in patients with mild to moderate COPD cardiovascular diseases account for 40–50% of all hospital admissions (for an overview, see Decramer et al., 2008). The mechanisms by which systemic consequences develop are yet unclear, but two key factors have been suggested: systemic inflammation and inactivity/deconditioning. Both processes contribute to the vicious cycle in COPD, with airflow obstruction leading to air trapping (retention of air in the lungs after expiration) and hyperinflation (abnormally increased lung volume), resulting in exertional breathlessness, fatigue, and activity limitation. Dyspnea may then cause anxiety and

distress, which increases the breathing rate, thereby enhancing air trapping. Activity limitation leads to progressive muscle deconditioning, which increases the need for oxygen and can lead to further air trapping. Local and systemic inflammation during exacerbations contribute to the development of airflow obstruction and the progression of the disease (Decramer et al., 2008; Tkáč, Man, & Sin, 2007).

Psychosocial Impact of Chronic Obstructive Pulmonary Disease

As the downward physical spiral continues, the disease is accompanied by considerable psychosocial comorbidity. Impairments related to emotional functioning, energy levels, sleep and rest, mobility, social interaction, activities of daily living, recreation, work, finance, and satisfaction with life have been documented.

EMOTIONAL FUNCTIONING

The primary focus of much of the research into the psychological effects of COPD has been on anxiety and depression. The reported prevalence of anxiety among patients with COPD is considerable, with 33% of patients having moderate to severe anxiety and 41% having panic disorder (Brenes, 2003). Although precise data on depression rates in patients with COPD are lacking and prevalence estimates of depression vary widely, there also appears to be a high incidence of depression in COPD. In stable COPD, the prevalence of clinical depression ranges between 10% and 42%. In patients who have recently recovered from an acute exacerbation of COPD, the prevalence of depression ranges between 19.4% and 50%. In patients with severe disease, the prevalence of depression ranges from 37% to 71%, with the highest rates found in oxygen-dependent patients (Maurer et al., 2008). These figures are comparable to or higher than prevalence rates in other advanced diseases (van den Bemt et al., 2009).

ENERGY LEVELS

Fatigue is a highly prevalent symptom in patients with COPD and may manifest itself as physical or mental tiredness, or loss of attention, concentration, or motivation. Studies suggest worse scoring on all these dimensions for patients with COPD as compared to healthy elderly subjects (Lewko, Bidgood, & Garrod, 2009).

SLEEP

Sleep-related complaints are ranked third, after dyspnea and fatigue, in frequency of complaints of patients with COPD, with nearly twice as many COPD patients classified as poor sleepers (61%) as healthy elderly controls (31.9%) (Lewis, Fergusson, Eaton, Zeng, & Kolbe, 2009). Delayed sleep onset, reduced rapid eye movement (REM) sleep, decreased sleep time, and frequent changes in sleep stages have been described in patients with COPD (Nunes et al., 2009).

COGNITIVE FUNCTION

Cognitive dysfunction is also increasingly recognized in patients with COPD, especially in those with hypoxemia. Studies have shown that patients with COPD have significant cognitive impairment, either globally or in domains such as perception, memory, and motor functions (Dodd, Getov, & Jones, 2010; Hung, Wisnivesky, Siu, & Ross, 2009; Klein, Gauggel, Sachs, & Pohl, 2010). Also, during exacerbations, COPD patients were reported to have impaired information processing and a tendency to worse attention and memory (Kirkil et al., 2007).

SELF-EFFICACY

The gradual physical incapacitation necessitates increasing dependence (on medication, oxygen, support and help from spouses, family members, etc.), which often compromises a patient's sense of autonomy and self-efficacy. Several studies have demonstrated the erosion of patients' feelings of self-efficacy (Arnold et al., 2006b; Barnett, 2005; Kanervisto, Kaistila, & Paavilainen, 2007; Nicolson & Anderson, 2003).

SOCIAL AND ROLE FUNCTIONING

The pervasive influence of COPD on social and role functioning is demonstrated in studies comparing COPD with other illnesses and age-matched controls (Arne et al., 2009; Katz et al., 2010; Stavem, Lossius, Kvien, & Guldvog, 2000). Social isolation, loneliness, sexual dysfunction, and impairments in valued life activities are frequently reported (Barnett, 2005; Kaptein et al., 2008; Kara & Mirici, 2004; Rennard et al., 2002; Sturesson & Bränholm, 2000), with substantial impairment in physical and daily life activities and in family and economic factors already present in patients with moderate disease severity (Rodriguez Gonzalez-Moro et al., 2009).

Impact of Psychosocial Issues on Health-Related Behavior and Functioning

Unfortunately, and understandably, the wide-ranging psychosocial consequences of living with COPD affect treatment-related behavior and treatment outcome in these patients.

Generally, depression severely limits the effectiveness of smoking cessation programs (Cinciripini et al., 2003; Freedland, Carney, & Skala, 2005), predicts reductions in activities of daily living (Felker et al., 2001; Yohannes, Baldwin, & Connolly, 2003), increases the likelihood of disturbed sleep (Bellia et al., 2003), diminishes the likelihood of adherence to PR (Fan et al., 2008; Garrod, Marshall, Barley, & Jones, 2006), and inhibits self-management (Dowson, Town, Frampton, & Mulder, 2004). The important consequences of depression for health outcomes in COPD are demonstrated in studies showing effects on mortality, hospital (re)admission, symptom burden, functional status, exacerbations, and QOL (Dahlén & Janson, 2002; Fan et al., 2007; Ng, Niti, Fones, Yap, & Tan, 2009; de Voogd et al., 2009; Xu et al., 2008).

The few studies that examined the effect of anxiety on health behavior and treatment outcome in COPD found that anxiety, too, diminishes the likelihood of adherence to PR (Fan et al., 2008) and is associated with submaximal exercise performance (Cully et al., 2006; Eisner et al., 2010; Giardino et al., 2010). State anxiety is associated with worse health-related QOL, more functional limitations, and greater shortness of breath in patients with moderate to severe COPD, after accounting for the influence of age, gender, lung functioning, and depression (Eisner et al., 2010; Giardino et al., 2010). Also, the risk of exacerbations and (re)hospitalization is increased in anxious COPD patients (Benzo et al., 2010; Eisner et al., 2010; Gudmundsson et al., 2005). Some authors suggest that anxiety is a more salient condition for patients with COPD (relative to depression) because the symptom of dyspnea, which is a cardinal manifestation of COPD, can be a potent stimulus for anxiety. Anxiety, in turn, increases disability in COPD by increasing vigilance for and amplification of distressing respiratory sensations, leading anxious COPD patients to avoid any activity that might produce these sensations. (Cully et al., 2006; Dowson, Kuijer, & Mulder, 2004; Giardino et al., 2010).

Fatigue has a strong, direct, and negative effect on performance of day-to-day activities in patients with COPD and is closely related to levels of dyspnea, depressed mood, and sleep quality (Kapella, Larson, Patel, Covey, & Berry, 2006; Reishtein, 2005). Patients who experience severe fatigue report significantly more limitations in cognitive, physical, and psychosocial functioning, compared with those patients reporting moderate fatigue (Theander, Jakobsson, Torstensson, & Unosson, 2008). Quality of sleep in itself also has a major impact on health-related QOL in COPD. Most affected by impaired sleep are the areas of social and professional life and the psychological condition of the patient (Nunes et al., 2009).

Cognitive dysfunction in COPD has been associated with poor medication adherence and incorrect inhaler use. One study found that impaired frontal executive function, which affects planning and sequencing, is an important determinant of inadequate inhaler self-administration technique in subjects with or without overt cognitive impairment (Allen, Jain, Ragab, & Malik, 2003). Another study shows that verbal memory declines in patients with advanced COPD are due to the impairment of active recall and passive recognition, and that this decline is associated with poor medication adherence (Incalzi et al., 1997). Some studies have found that cognitive dysfunction in COPD may also be associated with mortality (Antonelli-Incalzi et al., 2006) and mobility-related functional impairment, such as walking up or down stairs, or walking for at least 400 m (Antonelli-Incalzi et al., 2005; Hung et al., 2009).

Expectations that COPD patients have for their own self-efficacy or perceived control over the disease have been found to predict exercise tolerance, self-management strategies, success in PR, and variance in functional ability (Dowson, Kuijer, & Mulder, 2004; Garrod, Marshall, & Jones, 2008; Gormley, Carrieri-Kohlman, Douglas, & Stulbarg, 1993; Kaplan, Ries, Prewitt, & Eakin, 1994; Siela, 2003). Greater exercise self-regulatory efficacy is associated with increased exercise behaviors (Davis, Figueredo, Fahy, & Rawiworrakul, 2007). Other psychosocial factors that have been reported to influence self-management and treatment-related behavior in patients with COPD are social support at home, increased self-confidence, and higher confidence in treatment (positive influence on continued adherence to PR; Arnold, Bruton, & Ellis-Hill, 2006; Fischer et al., 2009, 2012).

With so many systemic consequences of the disease in the physiological and psychological field and in terms of social consequences, it is increasingly recognized that the lifetime management of patients with symptomatic COPD requires incorporating multiple modalities, such as advice on smoking cessation, nutritional intervention, exercise training, and self-management education. The

strong evidence-based support for the effectiveness of comprehensive programs suggests PR as a state-of-the-art intervention in reversing or stabilizing the systemic consequences of COPD. However, one must bear in mind that "the last thing that a depressed, demoralized, cognitively compromised and physically weak patient wants to do is pursue a consistent exercise program, go to doctors and treatment centers, and reengineer social aspects of his/her life" (Alexopoulos, Raue, Sirey, & Arean, 2008, p. 449).

Pulmonary Rehabilitation
Definition and Principles

In the joint statement of the American Thoracic Society (ATS) and the European Respiratory Society (ERS) (Nici et al., 2006), PR is defined as:

[A]n evidence-based, multidisciplinary, and comprehensive intervention for patients with chronic respiratory diseases who are symptomatic and often have decreased daily life activities. Integrated into the individualized treatment of the patient, PR is designed to reduce symptoms, optimize functional status, increase participation, and reduce health care costs through stabilizing or reversing systemic manifestations of the disease. (p. 1391)

The Global Initiative for Chronic Obstructive Lung Disease (GOLD, 2010) states that, to accomplish the principal goals (reducing symptoms, improving QOL, and increasing physical and emotional participation in everyday activities), PR should cover a range of nonpulmonary problems, such as exercise deconditioning, relative social isolation, altered mood states, muscle wasting, and weight loss.

Exercise is the centerpiece of all PRPs. Although PR does not improve lung mechanisms or gas exchange, it optimizes the function of other body systems, thereby increasing exercise tolerance, reducing dyspnea, and improving QOL (see Figure 18.1).

Program Components

The essential components of PR, as stated in the ATS/ERS guidelines (Nici et al., 2006), are exercise training, treating body composition abnormalities, self-management education, psychosocial and social support interventions, and outcomes assessment.

EXERCISE TRAINING

Exercise training is indicated for patients who have decreased exercise tolerance, exertional dyspnea or fatigue, and/or impairments in activities

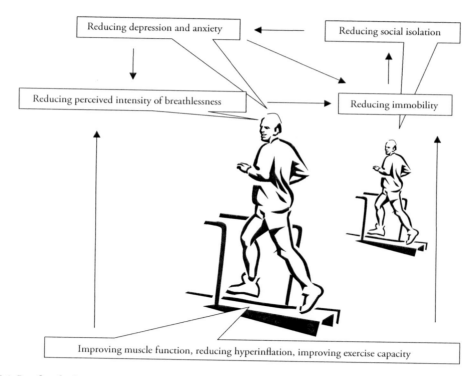

Figure 18.1 Benefits of pulmonary rehabilitation in chronic obstructive pulmonary disease (COPD): breaking the cycle.

of daily living. It is recommended that both lower (treadmill or stationary cycle ergometer) and upper (arm cycle ergometer, free weights, elastic bands) extremity exercises are incorporated into the training program. Endurance training (cycling and/or walking in >30 minutes exercise sessions at >60% of maximal work rate) and strength training should be combined. A minimum of 20 sessions is recommended, which should be given at least three times per week.

BODY COMPOSITION ABNORMALITIES

Interventions to treat body composition abnormalities are necessary because of the strong associations of muscle wasting and weight loss with morbidity and mortality, the extra caloric requirements from exercise training, and to enhance the benefits of exercise and strength training. Caloric supplementation (adaptation in the patient's dietary habits and energy-dense supplements) is indicated for underweight patients, patients with rapid involuntary weight loss, or with depletion in fat-free mass. Depletion in fat-free mass can also occur in weight-stable patients and can be countered by strength training. Obesity is associated with respiratory disturbances, obstructive sleep apnea, pulmonary hypertension, and heart problems. It should be

treated in patients with obesity-related respiratory disorders and when obesity contributes to functional limitations. Specific interventions include nutritional education, meal planning, encouragement, and psychological support.

SELF-MANAGEMENT EDUCATION

Self-management education is considered to be a core component of comprehensive PR. Ideally, the style of teaching should *not* be in the form of didactic lectures, but should teach self-management skills that emphasize illness control through health behavior modification, thus increasing self-efficacy. Strategies to enhance self-efficacy include the practice of self-management skills, feedback on and reinforcement of the patient's ability to use these skills, addressing prior negative experiences, and vicarious learning from successful peers. Education should include instructions in the prevention and early treatment of exacerbations, instructions in breathing strategies (such as pursed-lip breathing, active expiration, diaphragmatic breathing, adapting specific body positions, and coordinating paced breathing with activities), and bronchial hygiene techniques for clearing airway secretion (such as postural drainage, percussion, and forced expiration) in patients with mucus hypersecretion. Additionally, education could include topics such as proper use of medication; benefits of exercise; energy conservation; avoidance of irritants; indications for calling for help; leisure, travel, and sexuality; coping with COPD; end-of-life planning; anxiety and panic control; relaxation techniques; and stress management. Individualized patient self-management capabilities are considered essential in promoting long-term adherence to therapeutic interventions. It is increasingly recognized that the transference of educational training and exercise adherence to the home setting to produce long-lasting benefits involves assisting patients to adopt PR as a starting point of creating a balance that needs to be maintained with routine training and insightful daily management of one's condition.

PSYCHOLOGICAL AND SOCIAL INTERVENTIONS

Psychological and social interventions include the individual assessment of the concerns patients have about their psychosocial adjustment to their disease. According to the guidelines, questions should cover perception of QOL, ability to adjust to the disease, self-efficacy, motivation, adherence, and neuropsychological impairment. Also, patients should be screened for significant anxiety and depression, and psychological counseling should be considered when patients are depressed. Common concerns and feelings include guilt, anger, resentment, abandonment, fears, anxieties, helplessness, isolation, grief, pity, sadness, poor sleep, poor marital relations, poor sexual functioning, and failing health of the spouse caregiver. Supportive counseling to address concerns could be offered, either individually, in a couples format, or in (small) group sessions. Developing an adequate patient support system is considered important and, if possible, significant caregivers or spouses should be involved to explore issues related to dependency, interpersonal conflict, and intimacy. To tackle dyspnea and controlling panic, patients should be trained in stress-management techniques.

OUTCOMES ASSESSMENT

According to the guidelines, assessment of patient-centered outcomes should be an integral component of PR. Most commonly, assessments focus on symptom evaluation, performance evaluation, exercise capacity, and QOL measurements. With regard to symptoms, dyspnea or fatigue during exercise testing or training is most frequently measured (Borg scale or Visual Analogue Scale) and sometimes cough and sputum production

is also measured. Assessment of functional performance is important because improvements in exercise capacity do not necessarily translate into increases in activities of daily living. Most PRPs rely on patient self-reports to assess activity levels using both the patient's report on the intensity of dyspnea with activities and the degree to which a patient may perform real-life activities. Also, activity monitors or motion detectors (pedometers) are sometimes used to provide an objective measure of patients' daily activity. Exercise capacity is usually expressed in walking distance, measured with either the self-paced 6-minute walking distance (6MWD) or the externally paced shuttle walk test. For measuring QOL, both generic and respiratory-specific questionnaires are used in the PR setting. The two most widely used respiratory-specific questionnaires are the Chronic Respiratory Disease Questionnaire (CRQ) and the Saint George's Respiratory Questionnaire (SGRQ).

Psychosocial Interventions in Pulmonary Rehabilitation Programs: A Closer Look

Pulmonary rehabilitation guideline papers, clinical competency guidelines, and recent national representative surveys do not offer much (detailed) guidance on the contents of psychosocial interventions for COPD patients in PRPs, let alone guidance on who should deliver these components. According to a 2001 national representative survey in the United Kingdom, 43% of the hospitals offering PRPs reported having a social worker, and 21% had a psychologist as member of their team (Yohannes & Connolly, 2004). A 2005 national survey across Canada reported that 61% of the outpatient PRPs employed a social worker, and psychologists were not mentioned (Brooks et al., 2007). A 2007 Northern Ireland PR audit revealed that psychologists were involved in the deliverance of education in less than 2% of the hospitals offering PRPs and that the most common deficit reported was the lack of input or funding of health care professionals, such as psychologists (O'Neill & Bradley, 2007). No studies could be identified investigating in what kind of PR components psychologists (if they participated at all) are commonly involved. However, the American Association of Cardiovascular and Pulmonary Rehabilitation (AACVPR, Nici et al., 2007) have published guidelines for the clinical competency of rehabilitation professionals, and it provides some information on what personnel involved in psychosocial assessment and psychosocial intervention should be capable of. Also, in its most recent guideline, it provides some practical information on psychosocial assessment and psychosocial interventions (American Association of Cardiovascular and Pulmonary Rehabilitation [AACVPR], 2011).

Psychosocial Assessment in Pulmonary Rehabilitation Programs

According to the AACVPR guidelines, personnel involved in psychosocial assessment should

1) [U]tilize active listening and behavioral observation skills in assessing and evaluating impairments in interpersonal functioning, level of family and social support, psychosocial adaptation to illness, and screening for the presence of maladaptive behaviors and psychopathology; 2) demonstrate an understanding of the psychosocial issues affecting adherence to various intervention strategies and the development of an integrated plan; 3) assess individual patient needs for additional psychosocial services in addition to the PR intervention.
(*Nici* et al., 2007, p. 357)

Translated into practical aspects of assessing psychosocial morbidity, the most recent (and most detailed) guideline (AACVPR, 2011) advises screening for major depressive disorder, anxiety and panic disorder, cognitive impairment, motivation, coping, social support, and chemical dependency issues. The AACVPR guideline also provides some information on what instruments could be used. The guideline suggests the Primary Care Evaluation of Mental Disorders (PRIME-MD, Kunik et al., 2007) as an appropriate screening tool to identify patients who need further evaluation for depression and/or anxiety disorders. Other (more) established tools, such as the Geriatric Depression Scale (GDS), the Center for Epidemiological Studies Depression Scale (CES-D), the General Anxiety Disorder-7 (GAD-7), or the Penn State Worry Questionnaire (PSWQ-A), could be used for assessing outcome. The Mini-Mental State Examination (MMSE) is considered to be the gold standard for brief cognitive assessment, with those scoring 23 or lower being at risk for difficulty remembering the education or instructions provided in PR. Other topics that should be incorporated in initial assessments are issues that could interfere with potential improvements, such as (lack of) motivation (e.g. "On a scale of 1 to 10, how ready are you to commit to attending PR?," "Do you see barriers?" "Benefits?"), (inadequate) coping (e.g. "Are there issues you are dealing with that interfere with successfully completing PR?"),

(insufficient) social support, medication (non)adherence, addictions (smoking, drugs, alcohol), and (lack of) self-efficacy or concerns about exercising. Tools for determining nicotine dependence include the Fagerström Test for Nicotine Dependence (FTND), and questions should be asked about the patient's desire to quit and experiences with previous quit attempts.

Guidelines recommend screening for psychosocial issues in COPD patients entering PR, but only very few studies have been published on the prevalence of these issues. Studies have reported clinically relevant symptoms of anxiety in 29–38%, and depression in 20–42% of patients upon admission, using cutoff scores on the Hospital Anxiety and Depression Scale of ≥10 and/or Beck's Depression Inventory of ≥19 as a criterion (Janssen et al., 2010; Trappenburg et al., 2005; de Voogd et al., 2009; de Voogd, Sanderman, Postema, van Sonderen, & Wempe, 2010). One study also reported severe adjustment problems in the psychosocial domain in 59% of patients, using the Psychosocial Adjustment to Illness Scale–Self-Report (PAIS-SR) as a screening tool. The PAIS-SR measures health care orientation, vocational environment, domestic environment, sexual relationships, extended family relationships, social environment, and psychological distress. No problems in levels of social support were identified (Trappenburg et al., 2005). With regard to smoking, the available studies show that being diagnosed with COPD and even the referral to PR is not always a sufficient threat to motivate smokers to quit. Studies reporting percentages of patients who are smokers at the start of their PR show that current smoking ranges from 10% (de Godoy et al., 2005; Brazil), 14% (Garrod et al., 2006; UK), 17% (Wong, Goodridge, Marciniuk, & Rennie, 2010; Canada), 27% (Trappenburg et al., 2005; Belgium), 35% (Bentsen, Wentzel-Larsen, Henriksen, Rokne, & Wahl, 2010; Norway), to even 50% (Janssen et al., 2010; the Netherlands).

Psychosocial Intervention

The AACVPR clinical competency guidelines for professionals involved in psychosocial intervention, state that personnel should

1) [P]rovide supportive counsel to all participants, with special emphasis on mild to moderate psychological distress (i.e., depression, anxiety/panic, anger); 2) understand and utilize self-help techniques, materials, and resources offering additional referral when needed to mental healthcare

professionals, support groups, community, and home care services; 3) involve family members or significant others as appropriate in counseling to enhance social support; and 4) address long-term planning issues including advance directives and, as appropriate, end-of-life/hospice information. (*Nici* et al., 2007, p. 358)

Translated into practical aspects of psychosocial interventions, the AACVPR guideline (2011) focuses on suggestions for building support systems and for smoking cessation/treating nicotine dependency. Suggestions for enhancing social support include patient involvement in support groups offering educational presentations and encouragement in sharing disease-related information, successful coping skills, personal experiences, and emotions. A patient's spouse or support person should be encouraged to participate in these support groups, and if interpersonal or family conflicts surface, referral to a counselor is recommended. As for smoking cessation, tobacco use and dependence are considered to be chronic disorders and should be treated with a combination of pharmacological strategies (nicotine replacement, bupropion, and varenicline) and counseling. Within the PR setting, individual counseling is advised, employing strategies such as self-monitoring, solving barriers to quitting, setting a quit date, using social support, relapse prevention strategies, motivational interviewing, and cravings management. As a framework for health care providers to help patients stop smoking the 5-A's could be used (Ask, Advise, Assess, Assist, Arrange; for more information on this framework see, Glasgow, Emont, & Miller, 2006).

The available data from national representative surveys show that with regard to (education on) smoking cessation there is still much to gain. Smoking cessation care (or at least education) is offered in 30% of outpatient PRPs, and in 25% of inpatient PRPs (Canada, 2005), 49% (Australia, 2000), 26% (Northern Ireland, 2007), and 50% (UK, 2001). Although maybe anecdotal, data from a more recent regional PR service audit from the internet (Lothian Pulmonary Rehabilitation Service Audit; Mackenzie, McNarry, Leith, & Hewitt, 2009) provide a more positive outlook: all smoking patients (32%) were offered smoking cessation advice, and 52% of these were referred to smoking cessation services (with 43% of the patients accepting).

A few national surveys offer information on the provision of support groups as aftercare. In Canada (Brooks et al., 2007), support groups were offered in 20% of the centers after inpatient PR, and in 30% after outpatient PR. In the United Kingdom (Yohannes & Connolly, 2004), 17% of the centers ran a support group, and 28% combined periodic assessment and supervised maintenance sessions with a support group. According to the Northern Ireland report (O'Neill & Bradley, 2007), 78% of the PRPs had access to support groups for patients, and 87% provided patients with information about the existing networks for maintenance of social support. All programs encouraged patients to continue to engage with support and exercise activities after the programs and follow-up stopped. The function of these support groups was reported as social (85%), educational (85%), peer support (70%), service awareness (23%), and to fund-raise (8%). Most groups were charity or self-funded and were meeting on a monthly basis. Although all groups reported that partners/spouses/caregivers were invited to attend the meetings, these were primarily attended by patients and a small number of "others"(4:1). Involvement of partners/spouses/caregivers in the formal PRP also seems to be suboptimal. Although invited to participate, only 4% generally attended the exercise sessions, and only 17% attended any of the education sessions.

Randomized Controlled Studies on the Effects of Psychosocial and Behavioral Interventions in Chronic Obstructive Pulmonary Disease

In the first review of empirical papers on the effect of psychosocial support in PR, Kaptein and Dekker (2000) identified 10 studies with a randomized controlled design. The types of psychosocial support used in these studies included relaxation, coping skills training, stress-management, cognitive and/or behavior modification, panic control, supportive discussions, and symptom control. The review showed significant improvements in QOL, dyspnea, functional capacity, and self-efficacy. More recently, reviews have concentrated on the available randomized controlled trials (RCTs) to examine efficacy of psychosocial interventions for depression and anxiety in COPD patients (Coventry & Gellatly, 2008; Putman-Casdorph & McCrone, 2009; Rose et al., 2002). Other areas in which RCTs have been published include treatment for panic disorder, relaxation and dyspnea management strategies, smoking cessation, cognitive training, and the efficacy of support groups/maintenance interventions.

Cognitive-Behavioral Interventions for Anxiety and Depression

A small number of RCTs have assessed the efficacy of cognitive-behavior therapy (CBT) on depression and anxiety in COPD patients. Within a PR setting Emery, Schein, Hauck, and MacIntyre (1998) examined the effect of a CBT-based education intervention (with or without exercise) in comparison to a wait-list control group. Participants received four 1-hour educational lectures a week (lectures on anatomy and physiology of the lungs, medications, interpreting pulmonary function tests, etc.) and a weekly 1-hour group meeting for stress management and psychosocial support (progressive muscle relaxation, raising awareness of cognitive distortions, and discussing emotional consequences). As expected, patients in the CBT-plus-exercise condition achieved significant gains in cardiopulmonary endurance and experienced reduced depression and anxiety compared to the wait-list control group. However, patients in the CBT-only condition experienced more distress, suggesting that cognitive-behavioral education without exercise is counterproductive in alleviating anxiety. De Godoy and de Godoy (2003) examined the effectiveness of CBT added to exercise and education in comparison with an exercise and education only group. After the 12-week PR period, reductions in depression and anxiety were reported only among patients who participated in the therapy sessions (one group session per week). These sessions addressed the patient's psychosocial needs and included his or her social, marital, work, health, and interpersonal philosophy and habits. In another RCT (De Godoy et al., 2005), individual CBT sessions (one session per week) addressed difficulties in social and marital life, at work and with health, and offered maintenance of anxiety control. Patients with moderate or severe COPD were randomized into one of three groups: PR with exercise and CBT sessions, PR with CBT but without exercise, and PR with exercise but without CBT. Results showed that post PRP reduction in anxiety and depression was significantly greater in patients receiving CBT sessions than in those not receiving those sessions. These studies apparently suggest that neither exercise and/or education alone nor CBT and/or education alone can account for improvements in anxiety and depression in COPD patients enrolled in PRPs.

Randomized controlled trials outside the PR setting involving CBT have also shown improvements in anxiety and depression scores. In an elderly population of COPD outpatients, a single 2-hour group session of CBT was compared with education only (Kunik et al., 2001). A small effect size in favor of the CBT group was calculated.

In a larger RCT, Kunik et al. (2008) selected COPD patients with moderate anxiety and/or moderate depression and compared CBT group treatment with educational sessions (both eight 1-hour sessions). The CBT protocol included education and awareness training focused on anxiety, depression, and associated physiological, cognitive, and behavioral symptoms; relaxation training; increasing pleasurable activity and decreasing anxiety-related avoidance; cognitive therapy (alternative thoughts, encouraging self-statements, and thought-stopping); problem-solving techniques; sleep management skills; and skills review and planning for maintenance of gains (a more extensive review of the protocol can be found in Stanley, Veazey, Hopko, Diefenbach, & Kunik, 2005). The control intervention included COPD education (lectures and discussions). Topics included breathing strategies and airway management; pathophysiology of lung disease; medications; use of oxygen; avoidance of environmental irritants; nutrition; exercise; smoking cessation; and end-of-life planning. Both CBT group treatment for anxiety and depressive symptoms and COPD education significantly improved QOL, anxiety, depression, and 6MWD, with no significant differences between groups, and improvement was maintained during the following 44 weeks. In another RCT of CBT for anxiety and depression (Hynninen, Bjerke, Pallesen, Bakke, & Nordhus, 2010), COPD patients with clinically significant comorbid anxiety or depression attended seven weekly CBT group sessions. The CBT intervention was based on the same therapy manual as used in the study by Kunik et al. (2008), and was modified to include six components in seven longer (2-hour) sessions. Key components were psychoeducation/awareness, relaxation, cognitive therapy, behavioral activation, fear-based exposure, and sleep management skills. Participants in the control group (enhanced standard care) received 5–10 minutes of telephone contact (monitoring of psychological status) every 2 weeks in addition to standard care. Compared to the enhanced standard care, the CBT intervention resulted in improvements in symptoms of anxiety and depression that were sustained at 8-month follow-up, with no significant changes in the control group. Although the results from this study are promising, the authors report a large number of patients who did not wish to participate (58% of eligible patients). High refusal rates are not uncommon in studies involving COPD patients (Dowson, Kuijer, & Mulder, 2004) and underline the need for integration of self-management and mental health care into PRPs.

Panic and Panic Disorder

One recent RCT could be identified that specifically target panic in COPD. Livermore, Sharpe, and McKenzie (2010) selected 41 patients with moderate to severe COPD without panic disorder or depression who had already undergone PR to test an intervention designed to prevent panic attacks and panic disorder. The standardized CBT intervention comprised four, individually administered 1-hour sessions and included psychoeducation about CBT, the effects of the stress response on breathing, the cycle of panic anxiety in COPD, training in cognitive challenging of unhelpful cognitions, training in pursed-lip breathing, reinforcement of activity planning and pacing, the development of a coping plan, and problem-solving to address barriers to good coping. At 18-month follow-up, 60% of patients in the routine care control group had experienced at least one panic attack, whereas no CBT participant experienced any panic attacks, with a significant difference also in the number of hospital admissions between 6- and 12-month follow-ups. Although the sample size in this study was small, the fact that patients who were selected for *not* being anxious went on to develop panic attacks presents a strong case for including this kind of self-management routinely into the care for all COPD patients.

Relaxation Therapy and Dyspnea Management Strategies

Strategies to control the distressing experience of breathlessness have been taught to patients with COPD for a long time. As early as 1944, Ronald V. Christie, M.D. (1944) tried to convince his colleagues that respiratory exercises (instead of a forcefully created pneumothorax) could considerably increase tolerance to exercise: "More popular in this country, and less dangerous, are respiratory exercises designed to teach the patient to deflate the lung and to increase the use of the diaphragm" (p. 145).

A remarkable statement, especially when we look at his explanation of the causes of COPD in the same lecture: the wear and tear of forceful and repeated coughing—not a word about cigarettes.

And even more remarkable when taking into account the ideas of his colleagues:

> It is also a striking testimony to the conservatism of medical teaching that there is scarcely a textbook of medicine which does not quote glass-blowing and the blowing of wind instruments as probable or possible causes of emphysema; and this in spite of ample evidence in the literature that no such aetiological relationship exists (Christie, 1939). The original statement of Laennec, made in 1819, based on no actual cases, has been copied from textbook to textbook over a period of 120 years. (p. 144)

Much more recently, RCTs have been conducted on the effects of a whole range of interventions to reduce stress and breathlessness. In a recent Cochrane systematic review Bausewein, Booth, Gysels, and Higginson (2008) studied the available nonpharmacological and noninvasive interventions to relieve breathlessness. The authors concluded there was a low strength of evidence that acupuncture/acupressure is helpful, and not enough data to judge the evidence for distractive auditory stimuli (music), relaxation, fans, counseling and support, counseling and support with breathing-relaxation training, case management and psychotherapy. Since then, a few new RCTs have been published examining the effectiveness of these kind of interventions.

The effect of added progressive muscle relaxation (PMR) training on anxiety and depression in COPD patients receiving PR was studied by Lolak, Connors, Sheridan, and Wise (2008). Both the PMR group and the standard care PR group demonstrated statistically significant reductions in anxiety and depression over an 8-week period, but the differences between the groups were not statistically significant. These findings suggest that adding PMR to a well-established PRP does not confer additional benefit in the further reduction of anxiety and depression.

Researchers designing RCTs outside the PR setting are often quite imaginative. Results from an RCT designed to determine if listening to relaxing music was more effective than PMR showed that the music condition (offering a choice from a selection of non-lyric Indian classical instrumental music) successfully reduced anxiety, dyspnea, and systolic blood pressure (Singh, Rao, Prem, Sahoo, & Keshav Pai, 2009). A mindfulness-based breathing therapy trial (MBBT, Mularski et al., 2009) found no measurable improvements in patients with COPD receiving 8 weeks of MBBT compared to a support group (on dyspnea, 6MWT, QOL, symptoms or stress levels). This intervention is unlikely to be an important therapeutic option for those with moderate to severe COPD, not only because of the lack of results, but also because of the 50% withdrawal rate before or right after the first MBBT session. A small pilot in patients with moderate to severe COPD offered tai chi training consisting of twice weekly classes (gentle movement, relaxation, meditation, and breathing techniques). When compared to usual care (general exercise advise), the training showed some benefits in the emotion domain of the Chronic Respiratory Questionnaire but not on dyspnea or functional exercise capacity (Yeh et al., 2010). Weekly singings classes (for 24 weeks) were compared to handcraft work. Between-groups comparisons showed small and transitory reductions of pulmonary dynamic hyperinflation, but no differences in improvements in QOL or dyspnea (Bonilha, Onofre, Vieira, Prado, & Martinez, 2009). In another RCT, COPD patients were randomized into a group that received singing classes and a no-intervention control group. The singing program improved QOL and anxiety but did not improve the control of breathing measures or functional exercise capacity (Lord et al., 2010).

If anything, these studies seem to suggest that observed improvements in anxiety and QOL have been due to regular contact with a social group and that some of the activities (regardless of which one, as long as it is not mindfulness-based) could be a nice addition to the schedule of support groups for patients with COPD.

Smoking Cessation

Although smoking cessation plays a central role in the treatment of COPD, data regarding smoking cessation interventions among COPD patients are remarkably sparse. No studies could be identified on the effectiveness of smoking cessation interventions offered in PRPs, smoking cessation is not recorded as an outcome measure in PRPs, and few controlled trials have specifically addressed the effectiveness of smoking cessation interventions in patients with COPD. A recent review concluded that smoking cessation care (SCC) plus nicotine replacement therapy (NRT) had the greatest effect on prolonged abstinence rates in patients with COPD who smoke, followed by SCC in combination with an antidepressant. Smoking cessation care without additional drug treatment was only slightly superior over usual care. High-intensity SCC tended to be more effective than low-intensity SCC, but the trend was only statistically significant when combined with NRT (Strassmann et al., 2009).

Cognitive Training

One RCT could be identified directly targeting cognitive abilities of patients with hypoxemic COPD (Antonelli-Incalzi et al., 2008). After baseline assessment, patients were randomized to receive standardized multidimensional care (pharmacological therapy, health education, selection of inhalers according to patient's ability, respiratory rehabilitation, nutritional counseling, oxygen therapy, and control visits) with or without cognitive training aimed at stimulating attention, learning, and logical-deductive thinking. Both intervention and control groups showed no significant changes in cognitive performance except for a trend toward improvement in verbal fluency and verbal memory, but no differences between groups. Thus, specific cognitive training seems ineffective in COPD, but the fact that cognitive status did not change substantially over the 6-month period in both study and control patients shows that a multidimensional standardized therapeutic approach could help to slow or prevent cognitive decline.

Building Support Groups and Aftercare

Since the effects of a specific PRP package wane if exercise, education, and psychosocial support are not maintained, support groups (SGs) have the potential to promote continuation of activities and information and reduce social isolation. Moullec and Ninot (2010) examined the effects of a maintenance integrated health care program compared to a usual aftercare group in COPD patients with moderate disease severity. Only patients who had no previous involvement in PR were selected. The program started after all patients had first completed a 4-week inpatient PR. Patients allocated to the intervention group joined a regional health care network that included local self-help associations of patients who had also completed a PR. Coordinated sessions (96 spread over 1 year) included 72 sessions (3.5 hours/week) of supervised individualized exercise training, 12 sessions (2 hours/month) of health education by professionals, and 12 sessions (1 hour/ month) psychosocial support with discussion groups (supervised by a psychologist). Discretionary leisure activities, such as outings, could be added if desired by members. Patients in the usual aftercare group received a PR discharge letter outlining the recommended home-based exercise program. At 1 year, the maintenance intervention not only sustained the effects from the initial PR, but actually produced improvements in functional and emotional dimension scores of QOL and an increase in exercise tolerance. In patients in the control group, functional dimension scores stayed at PR discharge level, but emotional scores and exercise tolerance had deteriorated.

No studies have been done (yet) to examine the feasibility of involvement of the partners/significant others of COPD patients in PRPs. A large RCT is under way in which an approach to patient care will be studied in which caregivers are used to assist in the delivery of coping skills training to patients with COPD (albeit not in a PR setting). The authors of this study believe this approach has the potential to change the way in which COPD patients are routinely managed in order to reduce distress, enhance QOL, and potentially improve medical outcomes (Blumenthal et al., 2009).

Conclusion

Reflecting back to this chapter's section on disease characteristics and psychosocial consequences, it can be concluded that COPD is a multisystem disease with significant comorbidities that requires a multifaceted approach. The many lengthy guideline papers on treatments for COPD and PR support this notion and include sections on self-management education and psychological and social support. Pulmonary guideline papers suggest that: "current practice and expert opinion support the inclusion of psychosocial interventions.... " (Ries et al., 2007, p. 29S) and "psychologic and social support provided within the pulmonary rehabilitation setting can facilitate the adjustment process" (Nici et al., 2006, p. 1399). The available proof, the RCTs, and review studies to support "current practice," "expert opinion," and "can" are presented in this chapter. Unfortunately research on the effects of psychosocial interventions within PRPs is scarce. Cognitive-behavioral intervention for anxiety and depression is the relatively most well-researched area, and there is indeed some proof that a combination of strategies can add extra results to the positive effects that PR in itself has on symptoms of anxiety and depression. The other area in which some studies are available is relaxation techniques for stress management and relieving breathlessness. Since no detailed reports are available on the provision of psychosocial components in PRPs, it is not clear in how many rehabilitation centers the subject

is taught or how this is done. The results from the reviewed studies outside PRP settings, however, do not suggest much specific benefit of PMR or other strategies. The single RCTs on cognitive training and panic control provided some evidence that they could be useful in a PRP setting. No RCTs could be identified on SCC within a PRP and on interventions to strengthen social support. Overall, it can be concluded that much more research is needed to establish the role of psychosocial interventions in the management of COPD patients enrolled in PR. Currently, the evidence is largely absent that should guide "who does what and how" in the psychosocial components of PRPs.

Future Directions

This chapter mainly focused on psychosocial interventions in the traditional inpatient and outpatient programs offered in hospital settings or health care facilities. Although PRPs for patients with COPD are well-established, they are also expensive and not accessible by the majority of patients; many eligible patients decline or drop-out of participation; and the decline in exercise adherence following PR limits long-term benefits. Home-based PRPs without direct patient supervision have been shown to be of equivalent benefit to hospital-based programs (Vieira, Maltais, & Bourbeau, 2010) and have been proposed as an alternative (Bourbeau, 2010). A study is under way to directly compare the effectiveness of PR to a self-management approach (Chang et al., 2008). As in other chronic illnesses, the approach in COPD patients is moving toward collaborative care and the chronic care model (Kaptein et al., 2009). In shifting from management by health care providers to management by patients themselves, emphasis is shifted toward programs that produce durable changes in health behavior. These programs already incorporate and could greatly benefit from the (theoretical and practical) input of psychologists.

With regard to the more "traditional" PRPs, future research using randomized controlled designs with adequate sample sizes are needed. Studies with psychosocial support added as an extra experimental condition to PR are needed to enable the evaluation of the additional value of psychosocial support for COPD patients. In addition, in these trials, the content of psychosocial support should be precisely defined and theoretically based, and trials should provide directions for the qualifications of health care providers responsible for the psychosocial support. Areas in which any information would be most welcome are smoking cessation programs in PR, and the involvement of partners/significant others for enhancing social support. Also, it is striking how little information is available on the magnitude of the psychosocial problems of patients (apart from anxiety and depression) entering PRPs. The data are probably "out there" and need to be published.

References

Alexopoulos, G. S., Raue, P. J., Sirey, J. A., & Arean, P. A. (2008). Developing an intervention for depressed, chronically medically ill elders: A model from COPD. *International Journal of Geriatric Psychiatry, 23*, 447–453.

Allen, S. C., Jain, M., Ragab, S., & Malik, N. (2003). Acquisition and short-term retention of inhaler techniques require intact executive function in elderly subjects. *Age and Ageing, 32*, 299–302.

Antonelli-Incalzi, R., Corsonello, A., Pedone, C., Corica, F., Carbonin, P., Bernabei, R., & GIFA Investigators. (2005). Construct validity of activities of daily living scale: A clue to distinguish the disabling effects of COPD and congestive heart failure. *Chest, 127*, 830–838.

Antonelli-Incalzi, R., Corsonello, A., Pedone, C., Trojano, L., Acanfora, D., Spada, A., et al. (2006). Drawing impairment predicts mortality in severe COPD. *Chest, 130*, 1687–1694.

Antonelli-Incalzi, R. A., Corsonello, A., Trojano, L., Pedone, C., Acanfora, D., Spada, A., et al. (2008). Cognitive training is ineffective in hypoxemic COPD: A six-month randomized controlled trial. *Rejuvenation Research, 11*, 239–250.

Arne, M., Janson, C., Janson, S., Boman, G., Lindqvist, U., Berne, C., & Emtner, M. (2009). Physical activity and quality of life in subjects with chronic disease: Chronic obstructive pulmonary disease compared with rheumatoid arthritis and diabetes mellitus. *Scandinavian Journal of Primary Health Care, 27*, 141–147.

Arnold, E., Bruton, A., & Ellis-Hill, C. (2006a). Adherence to pulmonary rehabilitation: A qualitative study. *Respiratory Medicine, 100*, 1716–1723.

Arnold, R., Ranchor, A. V., Koëter, G. H., de Jongste, M. J., Wempe, J. B., ten Hacken, N. H., et al. (2006b). Changes in personal control as a predictor of quality of life after pulmonary rehabilitation. *Patient Education and Counseling, 61*, 99–108.

American Association of Cardiovascular and Pulmonary Rehabilitation (AACVPR). (2011). *Guidelines for pulmonary rehabilitation programs—4th edition*. Champaign, Ill: Human Kinetics publishers.

Barnett, M. (2005). Chronic obstructive pulmonary disease: A phenomenological study of patients' experiences. *Journal of Clinical Nursing, 14*, 805–812.

Bausewein, C., Booth, S., Gysels, M., & Higginson, I. J. (2008). Non-pharmacological interventions for breathlessness in advanced stages of malignant and non-malignant diseases. *Cochrane Database of Systematic Reviews, 2*, CD005623. DOI: 10.1002/14651858.CD005623.pub2

Bellia, V., Catalano, F., Scichilone, N., Incalzi, R. A., Spatafora, M., Vergani, C., & Rengo, F. (2003). Sleep disorders in the elderly with and without chronic airflow obstruction: The SARA study. *Sleep, 26*, 318–323.

Bentsen, S. B., Wentzel-Larsen, T., Henriksen, A. H., Rokne, B., & Wahl, A. K. (2010). Self-efficacy as a predictor of improvement in health status and overall quality of life in pulmonary rehabilitation-an exploratory study. *Patient Education and Counseling, 81*, 5–13.

Benzo, R. P., Chang, C. C., Farrell, M. H., Kaplan, R., Ries, A., Martinez, F. J., et al. (2010). Physical activity, health status and risk of hospitalization in patients with severe chronic obstructive pulmonary disease. *Respiration, 80*, 10–18.

Blumenthal, J. A., Keefe, F. J., Babyak, M. A., Fenwick, C. V., Johnson, J. M., Stott, K., et al. (2009). Caregiver-assisted coping skills training for patients with COPD: Background, design, and methodological issues for the INSPIRE-II study. *Clinical Trials, 6*, 172–184.

Bonilha, A. G., Onofre, F., Vieira, M. L., Prado, M. Y., & Martinez, J. A. (2009). Effects of singing classes on pulmonary function and quality of life of COPD patients. *International Journal of Chronic Obstructive Pulmonary Disease, 4*, 1–8.

Bourbeau, J. (2010). Making pulmonary rehabilitation a success in COPD. *Swiss Medical Weekly, 140*, w13067. doi:10.4414/smw.2010.13067

Brenes, G. A. (2003). Anxiety and chronic obstructive pulmonary disease: Prevalence, impact, and treatment. *Psychosomatic Medicine, 65*, 963–970.

Brooks, D., Sottana, R., Bell, B., Hanna, M., Laframboise, L., Selvanayagarajah, S., & Goldstein, R. (2007). Characterization of pulmonary rehabilitation programs in Canada in 2005. *Canadian Respiratory Journal, 14*, 87–92.

Carlin, B. W. (2009). Pulmonary rehabilitation: An historical perspective. *Seminars in Respiratory and Critical Care Medicine, 30*, 629–635.

Chang, A. T., Haines, T., Jackson, C., Yang, I., Nitz, J., Low Choy, N., & Vicenzino, B. (2008). Rationale and design of the PRSM study: Pulmonary rehabilitation or self management for chronic obstructive pulmonary disease (COPD), what is the best approach? *Contemporary Clinical Trials, 29*, 796–800.

Christie, R. V. (1939). Chronic Hypertrophic Emphysema: Aetiology and cause of some of its signs and symptoms. *Edinburgh Medical Journal, 46*, 463

Christie, R. V. (1944). Emphysema of the Lungs-II. *British Medical Journal, 1*(4334), 143–146.

Cinciripini, P. M., Wetter, D. W., Fouladi, R. T., Blalock, J. A., Carter, B. L., Cinciripini, L. G., & Baile, W. F. (2003). The effects of depressed mood on smoking cessation: Mediation by postcessation self-efficacy. *Journal of Consulting and Clinical Psychology, 71*, 292–301.

Coventry, P. A., & Gellatly, J. L. (2008). Improving outcomes for COPD patients with mild-to-moderate anxiety and depression: A systematic review of cognitive behavioural therapy. *British Journal of Health Psychology, 13*, 381–400.

Cully, J. A., Graham, D. P., Stanley, M. A., Ferguson, C. J., Sharafkhaneh, A., Souchek, J., & Kunik, M. E. (2006). Quality of life in patients with chronic obstructive pulmonary disease and comorbid anxiety or depression. *Psychosomatics, 47*, 312–319.

Dahlén, I., & Janson, C. (2002). Anxiety and depression are related to the outcome of emergency treatment in patients with obstructive pulmonary disease. *Chest, 122*, 1633–1637.

Davis, A. H., Figueredo, A. J., Fahy, B. F., & Rawiworrakul, T. (2007). Reliability and validity of the Exercise Self-Regulatory Efficacy Scale for individuals with chronic obstructive pulmonary disease. *Heart Lung, 36*, 205–216.

Decramer, M., Rennard, S., Troosters, T., Mapel, D. W., Giardino, N., Mannino, D., et al. (2008). COPD as a lung disease with systemic consequences—Clinical impact, mechanisms, and potential for early intervention. *COPD, 5*, 235–256.

de Godoy, D. V., & de Godoy, R. F. (2003). A randomized controlled trial of the effect of psychotherapy on anxiety and depression in chronic obstructive pulmonary disease. *Archives of Physical Medicine and Rehabilitation, 84*, 1154–1157.

de Godoy, D. V., Godoy de, R. F., Becker, B. Jr., Vaccari, P. F., Michelli, M., Teixeira, P. J., & Palombini, B. C. (2005). The effect of psychotherapy provided as part of a pulmonary rehabilitation program for the treatment of patients with chronic obstructive pulmonary disease. *Jornal Brasileiro de Pneumologia, 31*, 449–505.

de Voogd, J. N., Wempe, J. B., Koëter, G. H., Postema, K., van Sonderen, E., Ranchor, A. V., et al. (2009). Depressive symptoms as predictors of mortality in patients with COPD. *Chest, 135*, 619–625.

de Voogd, J. N., Sanderman, R., Postema, K., van Sonderen, E., & Wempe, J. B. (2011). Relationship between anxiety and dyspnea on exertion in patients with chronic obstructive pulmonary disease. *Anxiety, Stress, and Coping, 24*, 439–449.

Dodd, J. W., Getov, S. V., & Jones, P. W. (2010). Cognitive function in COPD. *European Respiratory Journal, 35*, 913–922.

Dowson, C. A., Kuijer, R. G., & Mulder, R. T. (2004). Anxiety and self-management behaviour in chronic obstructive pulmonary disease: What has been learned? *Chronic Respiratory Disease, 1*, 213–220.

Dowson, C. A., Town, G. I., Frampton, C., & Mulder, R. T. (2004). Psychopathology and illness beliefs influence COPD self-management. *Journal of Psychosomatic Research, 56*, 333–340.

Eisner, M. D., Blanc, P. D., Yelin, E. H., Katz, P. P., Sanchez, G., Iribarren, C., & Omachi, T. A. (2010). Influence of anxiety on health outcomes in COPD. *Thorax, 65*, 229–234.

Emery, C. F., Schein, R. L., Hauck, E. R., & MacIntyre, N. R. (1998). Psychological and cognitive outcomes of a randomized trial of exercise among patients with chronic obstructive pulmonary disease. *Health Psychology, 17*, 232–240.

Fan, V. S., Giardino, N. D., Blough, D. K., Kaplan, R. M., Ramsey, S. D., & Nett Research Group. (2008). Costs of pulmonary rehabilitation and predictors of adherence in the National Emphysema Treatment Trial. *COPD, 5*, 105–116.

Fan, V. S., Ramsey, S. D., Giardino, N. D., Make, B. J., Emery, C. F., Diaz, P. T., & National Emphysema Treatment Trial (NETT) Research Group. (2007). Sex, depression, and risk of hospitalization and mortality in chronic obstructive pulmonary disease. *Archives of Internal Medicine, 26*, 2345–2353.

Felker, B., Katon, W., Hedrick, S. C., Rasmussen, J., McKnight, K., McDonnell, M. B., & Fihn, S. D. (2001). The association between depressive symptoms and health status in patients with chronic pulmonary disease. *General Hospital Psychiatry, 23*, 56–61.

Fischer, M. J., Scharloo, M., Abbink, J. J., van 't Hul, A. J., van Ranst, D., Rudolphus, A., et al. (2009). Drop-out and attendance in pulmonary rehabilitation: The role of clinical and psychosocial variables. *Respiratory Medicine, 103*, 1564–1571.

Fischer, M. J., Scharloo, M., Abbink, J., van 't Hul, A., van Ranst, D., Rudolphus, A., et al. (2012). Concerns about exercise are related to walk test results in pulmonary rehabilitation for patients with COPD. *International Journal of Behavioral Medicine, 19*, 39–47.

Freedland, K. E., Carney, R. M., & Skala, J. A. (2005). Depression and smoking in coronary heart disease. *Psychosomatic Medicine, 67*, S42–S46.

Garrod, R., Marshall, J., Barley, E., & Jones, P. W. (2006). Predictors of success and failure in pulmonary rehabilitation. *European Respiratory Journal, 27*, 788–794.

Garrod, R., Marshall, J., & Jones, F. (2008). Self-efficacy measurement and goal attainment after pulmonary rehabilitation. *International Journal of Chronic Obstructive Pulmonary Disease, 3*, 791–706.

Giardino, N. D., Curtis, J. L., Andrei, A. C., Fan, V. S., Benditt, J. O., Lyubkin, M., et al. (2010). Anxiety is associated with diminished exercise performance and quality of life in severe emphysema: A cross-sectional study. *Respiratory Research, 9*, 29. doi:10.1186/14659921–1129–

Glasgow, R. E., Emont, S., & Miller, D. C. (2006). Assessing delivery of the five "As" for patient-centered counseling. *Health Promotion International, 21*, 245–255.

Global Initiative for Chronic Obstructive Lung Disease (GOLD). (2010). *Global strategy for diagnosis, management and prevention of COPD*. Retrieved from http://www.goldcopd.org

Gormley, J., Carrieri-Kohlman, V., Douglas, M., & Stulbarg, M. (1993). Treadmill self-efficacy and walking performance in patients with COPD. *Journal of Cardiopulmonary Rehabilitation, 13*, 424–431.

Gudmundsson, G., Gislason, T., Janson, C., Lindberg, E., Hallin, R., Ulrik, C. S., et al. (2005). Risk factors for rehospitalisation in COPD: Role of health status, anxiety and depression. *European Respiratory Journal, 26*, 414–419.

Güell-Rous, M. R., & Diez-Betoret, J. L. (2010). Is pulmonary rehabilitation really implemented today? *Clinical Pulmonary Medicine, 17*, 57–60.

Hung, W., Wisnivesky, J. P., Siu, A. L., & Ross, J. S. (2009). Cognitive decline among patients with chronic obstructive pulmonary disease. *American Journal of Respiratory and Critical Care Medicine, 180*, 134–137.

Hynninen, M. J., Bjerke, N., Pallesen, S., Bakke, P. S., & Nordhus, I. H. (2010). A randomized controlled trial of cognitive behavioral therapy for anxiety and depression in COPD. *Respiratory Medicine, 104*, 986–994.

Incalzi, R. A., Gemma, A., Marra, C., Capparella, O., Fuso, L., & Carbonin, P. (1997). Verbal memory impairment in COPD: Its mechanisms and clinical relevance. *Chest, 112*, 1506–1513.

Janssen, D. J., Spruit, M. A., Leue, C., Gijsen, C., Hameleers, H., Schols, J. M., et al. (2010). Symptoms of anxiety and depression in COPD patients entering pulmonary rehabilitation. *Chronic Respiratory Disease, 7*, 147–157.

Kanervisto, M., Kaistila, T., & Paavilainen, E. (2007). Severe chronic obstructive pulmonary disease in a family's everyday life in Finland: Perceptions of people with chronic obstructive pulmonary disease and their spouses. *Nursing and Health Sciences, 9*, 40–47.

Kapella, M. C., Larson, J. L., Patel, M. K., Covey, M. K., & Berry, J. K. (2006). Subjective fatigue, influencing variables, and consequences in chronic obstructive pulmonary disease. *Nursing Research, 55*, 10–17.

Kaplan, R. M., Ries, A. L., Prewitt, L. M., & Eakin, E. (1994). Self-efficacy expectations predict survival for patients with chronic obstructive pulmonary disease. *Health Psychology, 13*, 366–368.

Kaptein, A. A., & Dekker, F. W. (2000). Psychosocial support. *European Respiratory Monograph, 13*, 58–69.

Kaptein, A. A., van Klink, R. C., de Kok, F., Scharloo, M., Snoei, L., Broadbent, E., et al. (2008). Sexuality in patients with asthma and COPD. *Respiratory Medicine, 102,* 198–204.

Kaptein, A. A., Scharloo, M., Fischer, M. J., Snoei, L., Hughes, B. M., Weinman, J., et al. (2009). 50 years of psychological research on patients with COPD—road to ruin or highway to heaven? *Respiratory Medicine, 103,* 3–11.

Kara, M., & Mirici, A. (2004). Loneliness, depression, and social support of Turkish patients with chronic obstructive pulmonary disease and their spouses. *Journal of Nursing Scholarship, 36,* 331–336.

Katz, P. P., Gregorich, S., Eisner, M., Julian, L., Chen, H., Yelin, E., & Blanc, P. D. (2010). Disability in valued life activities among individuals with COPD and other respiratory conditions. *Journal of Cardiopulmonary Rehabilitation and Prevention, 30,* 126–136.

Kirkil, G., Tug, T., Ozel, E., Bulut, S., Tekatas, A., & Muz, M. H. (2007). The evaluation of cognitive functions with P300 test for chronic obstructive pulmonary disease patients in attack and stable period. *Clinical Neurology and Neurosurgery, 109,* 553–560.

Klein, M., Gauggel, S., Sachs, G., & Pohl, W. (2010). Impact of chronic obstructive pulmonary disease (COPD) on attention functions. *Respiratory Medicine, 104,* 52–60.

Kunik, M. E., Azzam, P. N., Souchek, J., Cully, J. A., Wray, N. P., Krishnan, L. L., et al. (2007). A practical screening tool for anxiety and depression in patients with chronic breathing disorders. *Psychosomatics, 48,* 16–21.

Kunik, M. E., Braun, U., Stanley, M. A., Wristers, K., Molinari, V., Stoebner, D., & Orengo, C. A. (2001). One session cognitive behavioural therapy for elderly patients with chronic obstructive pulmonary disease. *Psychological Medicine, 31,* 717–723.

Kunik, M. E., Veazey, C., Cully, J. A., Souchek, J., Graham, D. P., Hopko, D., et al. (2008). COPD education and cognitive behavioral therapy group treatment for clinically significant symptoms of depression and anxiety in COPD patients: A randomized controlled trial. *Psychological Medicine, 38,* 385–396.

Lewis, C. A., Fergusson, W., Eaton, T., Zeng, I., & Kolbe, J. (2009). Isolated nocturnal desaturation in COPD: Prevalence and impact on quality of life and sleep. *Thorax, 64,* 133–138.

Lewko, A., Bidgood, P. L., & Garrod, R. (2009). Evaluation of psychological and physiological predictors of fatigue in patients with COPD. *BMC Pulmonary Medicine, 21,* 47. Retrieved from http://www.biomedcentral.com/14712466–/9/47

Livermore, N., Sharpe, L., & McKenzie, D. (2010). Prevention of panic attacks and panic disorder in COPD. *European Respiratory Journal, 35,* 557–563.

Lolak, S., Connors, G. L., Sheridan, M. J., & Wise, T. N. (2008). Effects of progressive muscle relaxation training on anxiety and depression in patients enrolled in an outpatient pulmonary rehabilitation program. *Psychotherapy and Psychosomatics, 77,* 119–125.

Lord, V. M., Cave, P., Hume, V. J., Flude, E. J., Evans, A., Kelly, J. L., et al. (2010). Singing teaching as a therapy for chronic respiratory disease—a randomised controlled trial and qualitative evaluation. *BMC Pulmonary Medicine, 3,* 41. Retrieved from http://www.biomedcentral.com/14712466–/10/41

Mackenzie, A., McNarry, S., Leith, CTC, & Hewitt, N. (2009). *Lothian pulmonary rehabilitation service audit, 2009.* Retrieved from http://www.lothianrespiratorymcn.

scot.nhs.uk/wp-content/uploads/2010/08/Pulmonary-Rehabilitation-Service-Audit-2009-v1.0.pdf

Maurer, J., Rebbapragada, V., Borson, S., Goldstein, R., Kunik, M. E., Yohannes, A. M., et al. (2008). Anxiety and depression in COPD: Current understanding, unanswered questions, and research needs. *Chest, 134,* 43S–56S.

Moullec, G., & Ninot, G. (2010). An integrated programme after pulmonary rehabilitation in patients with chronic obstructive pulmonary disease: Effect on emotional and functional dimensions of quality of life. *Clinical Rehabilitation, 24,* 122–136.

Mularski, R. A., Munjas, B. A., Lorenz, K. A., Sun, S., Robertson, S. J., Schmelzer, W., et al. (2009). Randomized controlled trial of mindfulness-based therapy for dyspnea in chronic obstructive lung disease. *Journal of Alternative and Complementary Medicine, 15,* 1083–1090.

Ng, T. P., Niti, M., Fones, C., Yap, K. B., & Tan, W. C. (2009). Co-morbid association of depression and COPD: A population-based study. *Respiratory Medicine, 103,* 895–901.

Nici, L., Donner, C., Wouters, E., Zuwallack, R., Ambrosino, N., Bourbeau, J., et al. (2006). American Thoracic Society/European Respiratory Society statement on pulmonary rehabilitation. *American Journal of Respiratory and Critical Care Medicine, 15,* 1390–1413.

Nici, L., Limberg, T., Hilling, L., Garvey, C., Normandin, E. A., Reardon, J., et al. (2007). Clinical competency guidelines for pulmonary rehabilitation professionals: American Association of Cardiovascular and Pulmonary Rehabilitation position statement. *Journal of Cardiopulmonary Rehabilitation and Prevention, 27,* 355–358.

Nicolson, P., & Anderson, P. (2003). Quality of life, distress and self-esteem: A focus group study of people with chronic bronchitis. *British Journal of Health Psychology, 8,* 251–270.

Nunes, D. M., Mota, R. M., de Pontes Neto, O. L., Pereira, E. D., de Bruin, V. M., & de Bruin, P. F. (2009). Impaired sleep reduces quality of life in chronic obstructive pulmonary disease. *Lung, 187,* 159–163.

O'Neill, B., & Bradley, J. (2007). *Northern Ireland Pulmonary Rehabilitation Audit.* Retrieved from http://www.gain-ni.org/Library/Audit/RMAG_Book_insidecover.pdf

Putman-Casdorph, H., & McCrone, S. (2009). Chronic obstructive pulmonary disease, anxiety, and depression: State of the science. *Heart and Lung, 38,* 34–47.

Reishtein, J. L. (2005). Relationship between symptoms and functional performance in COPD. *Research in Nursing and Health, 28,* 39–47.

Rennard, S., Decramer, M., Calverley, P. M., Pride, N. B., Soriano, J. B., Vermeire, P. A., & Vestbo, J. (2002). Impact of COPD in North America and Europe in 2000: Subjects' perspective of Confronting COPD International Survey. *European Respiratory Journal, 20,* 799–805.

Ries, A. L., Bauldoff, G. S., Carlin, B. W., Casaburi, R., Emery, C. F., Mahler, D. A., et al. (2007). Pulmonary rehabilitation: Joint ACCP/AACVPR evidence-based clinical practice guidelines. *Chest, 131,* 4S–42S.

Rodriguez Gonzalez-Moro, J. M., de Lucas Ramos, P., Izquierdo Alonso, J. L., López-Muñiz Ballesteros, B., Antón Díaz, E., Ribera, X., & Martín, A. (2009). Impact of COPD severity on physical disability and daily living activities: EDIP-EPOC I and EDIP-EPOC II studies. *International Journal of Clinical Practice, 63,* 742–750.

Rose, C., Wallace, L., Dickson, R., Ayres, J., Lehman, R., Searle, Y., & Burge, P. S. (2002). The most effective psychologically-based treatments to reduce anxiety and panic in patients with chronic obstructive pulmonary disease (COPD): A systematic review. *Patient Education and Counseling, 47,* 311–318.

Siela, D. (2003). Use of self-efficacy and dyspnea perceptions to predict functional performance in people with COPD. *Rehabilitation Nursing, 28,* 197–204.

Singh, V. P., Rao, V., Prem, V., Sahoo, R. C., & Keshav Pai, K. (2009). Comparison of the effectiveness of music and progressive muscle relaxation for anxiety in COPD—A randomized controlled pilot study. *Chronic Respiratory Disease, 6,* 209–216.

Stavem, K., Lossius, M. I., Kvien, T. K., & Guldvog, B. (2000). The health-related quality of life of patients with epilepsy compared with angina pectoris, rheumatoid arthritis, asthma and chronic obstructive pulmonary disease. *Quality of Life Research, 9,* 865–871.

Stanley, M. A., Veazey, C., Hopko, D., Diefenbach, G., & Kunik, M. E. (2005). Anxiety and depression in chronic obstructive pulmonary disease: A new intervention and case report. *Cognitive and Behavioral Practice, 12,* 424–436.

Strassmann, R., Bausch, B., Spaar, A., Kleijnen, J., Braendli, O., & Puhan, M. A.(2009). Smoking cessation interventions in COPD: A network meta-analysis of randomised trials. *European Respiratory Journal, 34,* 634–640.

Sturesson, M., & Bränholm, I. B. (2000). Life satisfaction in subjects with chronic obstructive pulmonary disease. *Work, 14,* 77–82.

Theander, K., Jakobsson, P., Torstensson, O., & Unosson, M. (2008). Severity of fatigue is related to functional limitation and health in patients with chronic obstructive pulmonary disease. *International Journal of Nursing Practice, 14,* 455–462.

Tkáč, J., Man, S. F., & Sin, D. D. (2007). Systemic consequences of COPD. *Therapeutic Advances in Respiratory Disease, 1,* 47–59.

Trappenburg, J. C., Troosters, T., Spruit, M. A., Vandebrouck, N., Decramer, M., & Gosselink, R. (2005). Psychosocial conditions do not affect short-term outcome of multidisciplinary rehabilitation in chronic obstructive pulmonary disease. *Archives of Physical Medicine and Rehabilitation, 86,* 1788–1792.

van den Bemt, L., Schermer, T., Bor, H., Smink, R., van Weel-Baumgarten, E., Lucassen, P., & van Weel, C. (2009). The risk for depression comorbidity in patients with COPD. *Chest, 135,* 108–114.

Vieira, D. S. R., Maltais, F., & Bourbeau, J. (2010). Home-based pulmonary rehabilitation in chronic obstructive pulmonary disease patients. *Current Opinion in Pulmonary Medicine, 16,* 134–143.

Wong, C. J., Goodridge, D., Marciniuk, D. D., & Rennie, D. (2010). Fatigue in patients with COPD participating in a pulmonary rehabilitation program. *International Journal of Chronic Obstructive Pulmonary Disease, 5,* 319–326.

Xu, W., Collet, J. P., Shapiro, S., Lin, Y., Yang, T., Platt, R. W., et al. (2008). Independent effect of depression and anxiety on chronic obstructive pulmonary disease exacerbations and hospitalizations. *American Journal of Respiratory and Critical Care Medicine, 178,* 913–920.

Yeh, G. Y., Roberts, D. H, Wayne, P. M., Davis, R. B., Quilty, M. T., & Phillips, R. S. (2010). Tai chi exercise for patients with chronic obstructive pulmonary disease: A pilot study. *Respiratory Care, 55,* 1475–1482.

Yohannes, A. M., Baldwin, R. C., & Connolly, M. J. (2003). Prevalence of sub-threshold depression in elderly patients with chronic obstructive pulmonary disease. *International Journal of Geriatric Psychiatry, 18,* 412–416.

Yohannes, A. M., & Connolly, M. J. (2004). Pulmonary rehabilitation programmes in the UK: A national representative survey. *Clinical Rehabilitation, 18,* 444–449.

Cardiovascular Rehabilitation

Paul Bennett

Abstract

This chapter provides an overview of the psychological impact of the acute onset of coronary heart disease before addressing how cardiac rehabilitation may moderate any negative consequences of such an event. The chapter identifies three key goals for cardiac rehabilitation programs: helping people adjust physically and emotionally to their illness, symptom control, and changing behaviors that maintain or increase risk for cardiac disease. The chapter considers the comparative impact of educational and "behavioral interventions" based on Bandura's social cognitive theory, live versus distance approaches, interventions targeting those most in need, and more specific interventions on each of these goals. It concludes that "behavioral interventions" are central to maximizing the impact of rehabilitation; that distance interventions appear to be as effective as clinic-based interventions, but no more cost-effective; and that the next generation of research may best focus on who benefits most from each type of intervention.

Key Words: Cardiac rehabilitation, risk, emotion, behavior, disease progression.

Cardiac rehabilitation is now widely, but by no means universally (Leon et al., 2005; Thompson & Clark, 2009), available to patients who have experienced an acute cardiac event. The key goals of most rehabilitation programs involve:

- Changing behaviors, such as smoking and low levels of exercise, that maintain or increase risk for cardiac disease
- Helping people adjust physically and emotionally to their illness
- Symptom control

These goals may be achieved both directly and indirectly. Participation in an exercise program, for example, may both improve cardiovascular fitness and reduce depression or anxiety (Milani & Lavie, 2009) as the individual feels that he or she is gaining control over his or her illness and life. Changes in depression or anxiety may improve adherence

to medication or exercise regimens. They may also have direct implications for physical recovery following myocardial infarction (MI; Van Dixhoorn & White, 2005). Nevertheless, psychological interventions can be divided broadly into those that address behavioral change and those that address emotional issues. The chapter first considers any spontaneous behavioral and emotional reactions to the onset of coronary disease, before moving to address the impact of interventions designed to facilitate appropriate behavioral and emotional change.

The Consequences of Disease Onset
Behavioral Consequences of Disease

Studies of the behavioral impact of cardiac disease are surprisingly sparse. However, what evidence there is suggests that disease onset may trigger appropriate behavior change, although some changes may be relatively short-term. Hajek, Taylor, and Mills

(2002), for example, found that by 6 weeks following an MI, 60% of previous smokers who did not receive any form of intervention reported not smoking. One year after their MI, the figure had dropped to 37%. Similarly, Dornelas, Sampson, Gray, Waters, and Thompson (2000) found that 43% of previous smokers were not smoking at 6-month follow-up: by 12 months, this figure had fallen to 34%. Diet may also change in the short-term (Bennett, Mayfield, Norman, Lowe, & Morgan, 1999), although old habits may return. Leslie, Hankey, Matthews, Currall, and Lean (2004), for example, found that 65% of cardiac patients in their dietary counseling program achieved the target of five portions of fruit and vegetables per day. Thirty-one percent of their control group achieved this goal. The percentage of those eating healthily in the intervention group fell over a 1-year follow-up period and did not differ from the control group by this time. Similar levels of adherence were found by Luszczynska and Cieslak (2009), who found that less than 20% of cardiac patients met recommended guidelines for fruit and vegetable intake immediately following a cardiac rehabilitation program, and that this figure reduced to 12% at 1-year follow-up. Changes in exercise levels may also be modest and reduce over time. Bennett, Mayfield, Norman, Lowe, and Morgan (1999) found significant spontaneous changes in mild-moderate exercise levels in the 3 months following MI. By contrast, Lear et al. (2003) reported minimal changes from baseline on measures of leisure time exercise and treadmill performance 1-year following MI despite participants taking part in a general rehabilitation program.

Emotional Consequences of Disease

The emotional consequences of acute cardiac events may be profound and persistent. Wiklund, Sanne, Vedin, and Wilhelmsson (1984) interviewed a number of patients who had experienced an MI 1 year previously. Over a third thought about their heart disease frequently, and 74% worried about their cardiac state. Fifty-eight percent reported that they were protected from physical exertion by friends and family, frequently as a consequence of anxiety rather than symptom severity. Clinical interviews or psychometric measures confirm these high levels of distress. Dickens et al. (2004) reported a 20% depression rate based on clinical interviews in the period immediately following infarction. Twenty-one percent of those not depressed at this time became depressed over the following year. Again using clinical interviews, Strik, Lousberg,

Cheriex, and Honig (2004) found that 31% of a cohort of MI patients developed major or minor depression in the year following first MI. The highest incidence rate was in the first month following MI. Using psychometric measures, Lane, Carroll, Ring, Beevers, and Lip (2002) found a 31% prevalence rate of elevated depression scores during hospitalization. The 4- and 12-month prevalence rates were 38% and 37%, respectively. The same group reported the prevalence of elevated anxiety to be 26% in the hospital, 42% at 4-month follow-up, and 40% at the end of 1 year. They also reported high levels of comorbidity between anxiety and depression. Interest in the rates of post-traumatic stress disorder (PTSD) as a consequence of MI has recently increased, with prevalence rates typically being around 8–10% up to 1 year following infarction (e.g., Bennett, Owen, Koutsakis, & Bisson, 2002). Of note is that the onset of disease may not be the only cause for anxiety. Some treatments may themselves trigger such emotions. Jacq et al. (2009), for example, found an 8% prevalence of anxiety disorders among patients with an implantable cardioverter defibrillator (ICD) that had not fired: a prevalence rate of 37.5% was found among those that had experienced an ICD shock. Finally, despite consistent findings of negative emotional reactions to MI, the obverse may also be found. Petrie, Buick, Weinman, and Booth (1999) reported that nearly two-thirds of their sample of patients who had survived an MI reported some personal gains as a result of their illness some 3 months after its onset. The most highly endorsed positive outcome—by over 60% of respondents—was a change to a healthier lifestyle, although improvements in relationships, an appreciation of health and life, a change in life priorities, and gains in empathy were also reported.

The Consequences of Emotional Distress

One important outcome of high levels of anxiety and/or depression is their influence on health care usage. Depressed and anxious individuals are less likely to attend cardiac rehabilitation classes than are those with less distress (e.g., McGrady, McGinnis, Badenhop, Bentle, & Rajput, 2009). Paradoxically, they are more likely to contact doctors and make and attend outpatient appointments, as well as have more readmissions in the year following infarction (Strik, Lousberg, Cheriex, & Honig, 2004). Many of these visits will be due to worry and health concerns rather than validated cardiac problems. The impact of mood on health behaviors appears to be modest—although high-quality longitudinal data addressing this issue are surprisingly lacking. Nevertheless, there is evidence that depression is predictive of lower levels of smoking cessation following infarction. Both Perez, Nicolau, Romano, and Laranjeira (2008) and Huijbrechts, Duivenvoorden, and Deckers (1996) found that between 5 and 6 months following infarction, key predictors of smoking relapse were high levels of depression and anxiety. Similarly, Havik and Maeland (1988) reported that the MI patients least likely to quit smoking were those who had become increasingly depressed in the months immediately following their MI. Bennett et al. (1999) reported a modest association between low levels of exercise and depression, but no differences between depressed and nondepressed individuals on levels of smoking, alcohol consumption, or diet. Luyster, Hughes, and Gunstad (2009) found that depression was predictive of low levels of adherence to dietary recommendations in patients with heart failure. Finally, Shemesh et al. (2004) found that high levels of PTSD symptoms, but not depression or global distress scores, were significant predictors of nonadherence to aspirin.

Occupational factors mean that white collar, male, and young workers are most likely to retain their jobs. However, mood and expectations will also significantly influence return to work. Depression has been consistently associated with delayed or failure to return to previous work after rehabilitation and low ratings of work or social satisfaction. Söderman, Lisspers, and Sundin (2003), for example, found depression to predict low levels of resumption of full-time work and reduced working hours. Delay in returning to work was predicted by greater concerns about health and low social support. Resuming work at a lower activity level than before infarction was associated with older age, higher health concerns, and patients' expectations of lower working capacity (independently of actual capacity).

Emotional outcomes may also impact directly on disease and prognosis. Following seminal work by Frasure-Smith, Lespérance, and Talajic (1995) showing depression to be a significant and independent risk factor of reinfarction within the first 6 months following MI, with some notable exceptions (Lane, Carroll, Ring, Beevers, & Lip, 2002; Mayou et al., 2000) the majority of research has replicated this finding. In North America, Frasure-Smith has found depression to predict cardiac mortality in patients with atrial fibrillation and heart failure (Frasure-Smith et al., 2009), whereas in the United Kingdom, Dickens et al. (2004) reported that depression with onset following MI doubled the risk of cardiac mortality over a 1-year period, independently of other risk factors. No relationship was found between depression pre-MI and subsequent mortality. Other recent work has found a more complex association between depression, anxiety, and MI. Rutledge et al. (2009) found that depression scores were significant predictors of cardiac events only among women with low anxiety scores; not among those with higher levels of anxiety.

Cognitive Responses

The mechanisms through which depression and other negative emotions influence behavior have not been fully investigated in cardiac patients. However, the likelihood is that any impact on behavior is mediated by cognitive processes. One framework through which these have been investigated in cardiac patients involves the illness perceptions questionnaire. Using this, Petrie et al. (2002) found that attendance at cardiac rehabilitation was significantly related to a stronger belief during admission that the illness could be cured or controlled. Return to work within 6 weeks was significantly predicted by the perception that the illness would last a short time and have less serious consequences for the patient. Patients' belief that their heart disease would have serious consequences was significantly related to later disability in work around the house, recreational activities, and social interaction. A strong illness identity was significantly related to greater sexual dysfunction at both 3 and 6 months. Although they did not investigate it, these negative attributions and expectations are likely to be associated with depression and/or anxiety.

Impact and Interaction with Partners

Finally, it should be noted that the partners of patients also experience high levels of distress, often greater than those reported by the patient. Moser and Dracup (2004) also found that patients' adjustment to illness was worse when their partners were more anxious or depressed than themselves and was best when patients were more anxious or depressed than their partners. Stern and Pascale (1979) found that the women at greatest risk of depression or anxiety were those married to men who denied their infarction. In this situation, partners experienced high levels of anxiety when their partner engaged in what they considered unsafe behaviors, such as high levels of physical exertion or continued smoking, which they were unable to control. In addition, many wives appear to inhibit angry or sexual feelings and become overprotective of their husbands (Stewart, Davidson, Meade, Hirth, & Makrides, 2000). Bennett and Connell (1999) found two contrasting processes to influence anxiety and depression in patients' partners. The primary causes of partner anxiety were the physical health consequences of the MI, and in particular the perceived physical limitations imposed on their partner by their MI. In contrast, the strongest predictors of partner depression were the emotional state of their spouse, the quality of the marital relationship, and the wider social support available to them. Three disease factors were particularly associated with anxiety: the severity of the MI, and the patients' perceptions of their health and physical limitations as a consequence of disease. Two patient coping responses to the MI, mental withdrawal and seeking instrumental social support, were also associated with partner anxiety.

Summary

Although many people recover well from an MI and other cardiac disorders and make appropriate behavioral changes, many do not. In addition, a significant minority of individuals experience significant and long-term negative emotional consequences. These may impact on all areas of life, from the social, psychological, to the economic. Any of these changes may be mediated by cognitive processes.

Models of Cardiac Rehabilitation

As cardiac rehabilitation now forms a mainstream intervention, the form it takes is becoming increasingly standardized. In the United States, the American Heart Association/American Association of Cardiovascular and Pulmonary Rehabilitation's (2007) guidelines recommended that cardiovascular rehabilitation should involve: baseline patient assessment, nutritional counseling, risk factor management (lipids, blood pressure, weight, diabetes mellitus, and smoking), psychosocial interventions, physical activity counseling, and exercise training. In addition, they placed a strong emphasis on enhancing adherence to preventive medications, such as lipid-lowering drugs, and close collaboration between the cardiac rehabilitation team and patients' cardiologists and primary care physicians. Detailed procedures and treatment goals in relation to each of these outcomes are provided. In the United Kingdom, the British Association for Cardiac Rehabilitation (BACR, 2007) has established a similar set of guidelines. They also call for the involvement of patients, caregivers, and relatives in any program.

These inputs are usually provided in a program lasting between 6 and 8 weeks, usually conducted on an outpatient basis, and in a group format. The opportunity to see individual patients is typically limited. Indeed, most cardiac patients do not receive any form of intervention, even in countries with relatively well-funded health care systems such as the United Kingdom (Thompson & Clark, 2009) and United States (Leon et al., 2005). In addition, access to cardiac rehabilitation programs may be influenced by a number of nonclinical factors, including gender, race, and economic factors. Stewart Williams (2009) calculated that 18% of the gender differences in referral to cardiac rehabilitation programs (with men favoring women) were "discriminatory" and not explained by medical or other variables. In addition, despite carrying more risk factors for disease progression, white Americans are twice as likely to be referred to cardiac rehabilitation programs as their African American counterparts (Gregory, LaVeist, & Timpson, 2006). Income, race, and gender may also interact to influence referral to cardiac rehabilitation. Allen et al. (2004), for example, found that women were less likely to be referred to cardiac rehabilitation than men, African American women were less likely to be referred than white women, and people with incomes of less than $20,000 were less likely to be enrolled than those with higher incomes.

Education Versus Problem-Focused/Behavioral Approaches

The most frequently conducted cardiac rehabilitation programs involve a significant educational element. They may be of benefit, but the effects can be limited. Bellman, Hambraus, Lindbäck, and Lindahl (2009), for example, found benefits in smoking but no other outcome measure following a general cardiac educational program. Similarly, Jiang, Sit, and Wong (2007) found a nurse-led educational program resulted in improvements relative to a control group on measures of walking and medication adherence, although the impact of the program on smoking and cholesterol levels was limited. Zullo, Dolansky, and Jackson (2010) also reported long-term gains on consumption of fruit and vegetables, but not physical activity or body mass index (BMI) among attenders of cardiac rehabilitation programs following MI.

Most formal educational programs are relatively didactic in their content. However, evidence from a range of domains suggests that the type of program most likely to result in behavioral change is based on the social cognition model of Bandura (1986). This suggests that the optimum context for learning new skills occurs when participants are shown how to achieve any required behavioral change, plan how to achieve change in the context of their own lives, and gradually introduce any changes using clearly identified and progressive behavioral goals. The intrinsic reinforcement of achieving behavioral change may encourage continued change and progression toward longer term goals. Group processes may also provide extrinsic reinforcers of change. The work of Lorig in the self-management of chronic diseases such as arthritis (e.g., Lorig, Ritter, & Jacquez, 2005) provides excellent testimony to the effectiveness of this approach. In this chapter, this approach will be labeled as a "behavioral" approach or intervention.

One early comparison of didactic education versus the behavioral approach in the context of cardiac rehabilitation was conducted by Oldenburg, Allam, and Fastier (1989). They compared the effectiveness of a didactic educational group intervention, a behavioral program, and a "standard intervention" (which at that time comprised outpatient appointments with a cardiologist). At 1-year follow-up, there was a gradation of outcomes on a variety of measures including weight loss, smoking, resumption of previous leisure activities, depression, vigor, and adopting the "invalid role." The educational program proved more effective than the standard intervention but not as effective as the behavioral program. More recently, this type of work has been extended to examine risk behaviors and hard physical outcomes. Giannuzzi et al. (2008) compared a "long-term (3-year), reinforced, multifactorial educational and behavioral intervention" with standard (didactic education) cardiac rehabilitation, and achieved significant additional improvements on coronary risk behaviors including exercise, diet, psychosocial stress, and a number of coronary outcomes. Total reinfarction and nonfatal MI rates in the behavioral intervention group were half those in the standard rehabilitation group. Similarly, Lisspers et al. (2005) reported differences in cardiovascular mortality rates of 2.2% versus 14.6% in their intensive behavioral intervention and standard rehabilitation groups.

The mixed intervention approaches frequently adopted by rehabilitation programs, combining, for example, education with counseling, exercise, relaxation or stress management procedures (Barlow, Lehrer, Woolfolk, & Sime, 2008), makes it difficult to identify systematic differences in effect size attributable to educational or behavioral interventions. However, a number of reviews have begun to hint at the benefits of this extended approach. Edwardson (2007), for example, suggested that although educating patients with heart failure may be of benefit, supplementing this with "continuing reinforcement, symptom monitoring, and behavioral reinforcement" is likely to add to the benefits of a simple educational approach. Similarly, Welton, Caldwell, Adamopoulos, and Vedhara (2009) suggested that the most beneficial cardiac rehabilitation programs in terms of reducing disease burden were those that incorporated a behavioral component. There seems to be an emerging consensus that interventions with a strong behavioral component are likely to be most effective.

"Live" or Distant

One important cardiac rehabilitation program that has adopted a behavioral approach was developed by Lewin, Robertson, Irving, and Campbell (1992). Originally focused on patients with an MI, the approach has now been adapted for use with patients with angina (Lewin et al., 2002) or an implantable cardioverter defibrillator (ICD; Lewin, Coulton, Frizelle, Kaye, & Cox, 2009). In each, patients are provided with a workbook that provides a progressive behavioral change program utilizing various aspects of Bandura's social cognition model. In the MI program, a loose-leaf A4 size book (the *Heart Manual*) provides a 6-week graduated program of behavioral change, focusing on increasing exercise, use of stress management procedures including positive self-talk and relaxation, and dietary and smoking change. During each week, patients are encouraged to plan and monitor their progress. Patients are contacted on three occasions by telephone to discuss adherence to the program—but they are not encouraged to use the telephone call as a counseling contact. Similar programs are established for the angina and ICD patients. These programs have the clear advantage of ease of provision and cost. The phone calls are relatively brief, and patients do not have to attend a hospital. So, if the program works, both patients and providers may find the program time- and cost-effective. The first study of the *Heart Manual* reported equivocal results. Lewin et al. (1992) found that patients who received the intervention reported greater benefits on measures of distress at 6- and 12-month follow-up than did those who received placebo information plus nurse contact similar to that in the Heart Manual group. They also made an average of two to three fewer visits to their general practitioners in the year following their infarction, and had a significantly lower readmission rate to a hospital (8% vs. 24%) over the first 6 months following discharge. This benefit was no longer evident at 12-month follow-up. Unfortunately, no behavioral data were reported. Even more powerful evidence was reported over a decade later, when Jolly et al. (2009) reported the outcome of the Birmingham Rehabilitation Uptake Maximisation Study (BRUM). They compared the *Heart Manual* with a standard outpatient rehabilitation program that provided a "live" version of the manual in a culturally diverse group of patients who had sustained an MI. By 6-month follow-up, patients in both groups reported significant improvements in measures of total cholesterol, smoking prevalence, self-reported physical activity, and diet, as well as in anxiety scores. Equally importantly, they found no clinically or statistically significant differences on any outcome measure between the two groups. The angina (Lewin et al., 2002) and ICD Plans (Lewin et al., 2009) appear to be equally effective.

The Lewin model involves minimal contact with professional staff. Phone calls are designed to encourage adherence to the written program, rather than problem-solving or forming an intervention in themselves. However, a number of programs have used the telephone contact as a significant part of the intervention. In one relatively early study of this approach, Hartford, Wong, and Zakaria (2009) used a telephone contact program for patients who had had a coronary artery bypass graft (CABG) and their partners. The program provided information on a number of issues to aid recovery, including a graded activity and exercise plan, coping with pain, and dealing with psychosocial problems, diet, and medication use. The program began with a meeting between a specialist nurse and the patient and their partner on the day of discharge, when they were provided with information about medication for pain, distances to walk, rest stops on the way home, the nurse's 24-hour telephone number, and a time when they would phone again. This was followed by six telephone calls at increasing intervals over the next 7 weeks, during which problems were assessed and relevant information provided. Despite its emphasis on changing behavior, it proved effective in reducing both patient and partner levels of anxiety. Interestingly, adherence to home-based interventions may be higher than those based in hospitals

(Piotrowicz et al., 2009). In addition, patients who fail or who are unable to attend standard cardiac rehabilitation appear to benefit from a subsequently offered telephone intervention. Furber, Butler, Phongsavan Mark, and Bauman (2010) reported the outcomes of a telephone based exercise program involving self-monitoring of physical activity combined with behavioral counseling and goal setting. After the 6-week program, improvements in total physical activity time, total physical activity sessions, walking time, and walking sessions in the intervention group were significantly higher than in the control group after adjusting for baseline differences, and remained so for 6 months. Confirming these generally positive findings, a systematic review and meta-analysis by Jolly, Taylor, Lip, and Stevens (2006) and an update by Taylor, Dalal, Jolly, Moxham, and Zawada (2010) found no differences between hospital and distance learning approaches on measures of both behavioral change and cardiac outcome. The review did note, however, that the cost per patient of both approaches is similar: there are no financial gains from intervening in the home settings.

Targeting Interventions

The previously described interventions have targeted whole populations of patients. But there is the possibility that some individuals will not need any intervention. The Life Stress Monitoring Program (Frasure-Smith & Prince, 1985) followed a cohort of men following an MI who either received no intervention or a "low contact" counseling intervention. In this, they were contacted once a month via telephone by a nurse who completed the General Health Questionnaire (a measure of psychological morbidity). If they reached a score indicating some degree of distress, they were visited by a nurse and received "counseling" for any cardiac-related problems they may have been experiencing at the time. This counseling was not specified and was dependent on the problems being experienced, but included advice on symptoms and medication, and referral to cardiologists, as well as issues that could be more directly addressed by the patients. By the end of the year-long program, half the participants in the intervention condition had been visited by the nursing team, with an average of 6 hours contact per patient. At this time, the program seemed effective. The total death rate in the control group was 9%. That of the intervention group was 5%: a significant difference. Unfortunately, this apparent success was somewhat mitigated by problems caused by a complex recruitment process that resulted in the intervention group having a greater prevalence of white collar workers than did the control group, making the prognosis in this group likely to be better than that of the control group. The findings were therefore far from unequivocal. To determine whether this was a true effect, and to show whether any benefit generalized to women, the study was replicated with the addition of a sample of women. The Montreal Heart Attack Re-adjustment Trial (M-HART; Frasure-Smith et al., 1997) reported no benefits for men—reinfarction rates in the first year were 2.4% in the intervention group and 2.5% in the control group. Worse, women in the intervention group proved *more* at risk of reinfarction than those in the control group—with 1-year reinfarction rates of 10% and 5%, respectively—an effect maintained to 5-year follow-up. Frasure-Smith hypothesized that this result occurred because the nurses who provided the counseling were skilled in the highly complex environment of the coronary care unit, but were not skilled counselors. As a consequence, they may have provided poor counseling and even added to patients' distress rather than reducing it. As evidence to support this assertion, Cossette, Frasure-Smith, and Lespérance (2001) reported that those patients who did report a reduction in distress following the counseling were marginally less likely to die of all causes and significantly less likely to die of cardiac problems than were those who showed no such benefit. The equivocal nature of the two trials, however, has meant that this model of rehabilitation has not been adopted.

Summary

Two clear conclusions can be drawn from the evidence considered so far. First, programs that target and provide effective strategies to promote behavioral change—and perhaps also reward such changes—are likely to be more effective than standardized educational programs. Second, in many cases, this approach can be delivered at a distance as effectively as in hospital or clinic settings. Indeed, by encouraging change within the home setting, this may generalize and continue for sustained periods, perhaps more so than changes in clinic-based interventions. Whether this approach will work for all patients is not clear. From a psychosocial perspective, those who are depressed, lack confidence, or are socially isolated, for example, may benefit from group work within hospitals. In addition, some individuals may have poor cardiac function and require medical expertise on hand during

rehabilitation. Nevertheless, both the content and setting of cardiac rehabilitation programs may shift in the next decade as service providers adopt these new ways of working.

Outcomes of Cardiac Rehabilitation

Having concluded that behaviorally focused programs are likely to be the most effective means of delivering cardiac rehabilitation, this section considers in more detail some of the approaches and outcomes of interventions that may form components of any comprehensive rehabilitation program. We first consider whether these components can effectively change emotional sequelae to the onset of disease or behaviors that increase risk for disease progression. In the next section, we consider whether these and other approaches can reduce the risk of future cardiac events.

Reducing Distress

Given the substantial evidence that cognitive-behavioral interventions, including cognitive restructuring, positive self-talk, and hypothesis testing (e.g., Beck, 1993), can reduce both clinical levels of depression and anxiety in a wide variety of clinical settings, it would be surprising if these types of interventions did not have a similar effect in cardiac patients. And this is, indeed, the case. Most interventions have targeted levels of anxiety, usually with significant effect (Rees et al., 2005). Even relatively simple interventions that employ teaching relaxation techniques have proven effective in reducing distress and (when measured) proximal physiological markers of stress such as cortisol. Van Dixhoorn and White (2005) reported outcomes of a meta-analysis of studies using relaxation techniques either alone or as part of a more complex cognitive-behavioral intervention. They found similar and significant reductions in anxiety and depression in both sets of studies. Such reductions are typically greater than would be expected following a typical cardiac rehabilitation program (Neves, Alves, Ribeiro, Gomes, & Oliveira, 2009). A second potentially beneficial area for stress management interventions involves helping people cope with the stress associated with the use of implantable cardioverter defibrillators (ICDs). Research in this area is still limited. However, Sears et al. (2007) compared two active stress management programs following ICD implantation, one lasting a full day, the other involving six, weekly, sessions. Both interventions were associated with short-term reductions in anxiety and cortisol levels—although the lack of no treatment control group allows the possibility that these changes would have occurred naturally as patients adapted to having the ICD.

Programs targeting depression have been conducted less frequently than those targeting anxiety, but also appear effective. The largest of these studies, the ENRICHD study (Berkman et al., 2003) provided an intervention lasting up to 1 year for people identified as depressed immediately following their MI. All participants in the active intervention arm received two or three treatment components, each aimed at improving their emotional state: group cognitive-behavior therapy based on the work of Beck (1993), social support, and training in the social skills required to develop a social support network, and antidepressant medication for nonresponders to the psychosocial intervention. The intervention proved effective in reducing depression in the intervention group relative to a usual treatment control condition, although the scale of the intervention suggests it has limited applicability in health services where cost-effectiveness is a driving issue. In addition, its impact on cardiac prognosis was limited—an issue that is returned to later in the chapter.

Symptom Control

A second area in which stress management techniques may prove of benefit is helping to moderate day-to-day symptoms of angina. Episodes of angina may be triggered by emotional as well as by physical stresses. Accordingly, a number of studies have explored the potential benefits of stress management procedures in people with this condition. One of the first was reported by Bundy, Carroll, Wallace, and Nagle (1998), who found that patients who took part in a stress management program reported greater reductions in the frequency of angina symptoms, were less reliant on medication, and performed better on a treadmill test than a control group that did not receive the intervention. A much larger study, involving hundreds of participants, was reported by Gallacher, Hopkinson, Bennett, and Yarnell (1997), who compared a less intensive intervention, involving a stress management program delivered in booklet form and three group meetings, with a no-treatment control condition. At 6-month follow-up, patients in the intervention condition reported significantly fewer episodes of angina triggered by stress, but not exercise—a finding consistent with the intervention impacting directly on the stress mechanisms that led to the episodes of angina. Using a similar approach, Lewin, Furze, Robinson,

Griffith, Wiseman, Pye, and Boyle (2002) found a reduction of three episodes of angina per week in their active intervention group compared to a reduction of 0.4 episodes per week in a control condition.

Risk Behavior Change
SMOKING

Interventions that specifically target smoking cessation appear to be of benefit. In a Cochrane review of the evidence, Barth, Critchley, and Bengel (2008) reported that the 16 randomised controlled trials of smoking cessation programs so far conducted achieved significant benefit at both 6- and 12-month follow-up assessments, although these gains were no longer evident at 5-year follow-up. Outcomes varied with the intensity of the intervention, with more "intense" interventions achieving better quit rates. Among these, however, there was no evidence for the superiority of any one intervention, with behavioral, telephone support, and self-help achieving similar outcomes—around a 50% greater quit rate than that found in control conditions. Brief interventions were found to be no more effective than usual care. A more recent study (Smith & Burgess, 2009), compared a minimal intervention involving advice from physicians and nurses and two pamphlets with a complex program involving an hour bedside counseling, take-home materials, and seven nurse-initiated counseling telephone calls over the 2 months following discharge. The biologically confirmed 12-month cessation rates were 53% in the intensive therapy group and 35% in the minimal intervention. Of those who quit smoking immediately following their CABG, 57% of those in the intensive intervention group and 37% in the minimal intervention group remained abstinent at this time. Similar outcomes have been achieved by other nurse-led interventions (e.g., Quist-Paulsen & Gallefoss, 2003).

DIET

Modest gains in dietary intake may be achieved by goal setting. Leslie, Hankey, Matthews, Currall, and Lean (2004) randomly allocated MI patients who had already undergone a standard cardiac rehabilitation program to either a no-treatment group or additional dietary counseling. This involved setting quantifiable dietary targets focusing on eating more fruit (five portions a day), oily fish (two to three times per week), and a reduction in saturated fat intake. Participants also made a folder including information, recipes, and "tools to encourage and consolidate...dietary changes." Those in the counseling group reported higher fruit and vegetable intake 12 weeks following the counseling. However, these gains were no longer evident at 1-year follow-up. Planning behavioral change may be more effective. One extremely brief intervention that is currently being developed across a range of settings and health problems is based on theories that have identified two phases to behavioral change (Gollwitzer, 1999; Schwarzer, 2008). The first involves increasing motivation; the second involves enacting intentions based on this motivation. The latter is by no means certain. In fact, the widespread failure to translate intentions into actions has been given a name: the *intention–behavior gap*. One way of reducing this gap involves active planning of actions. This process, known as an *implementation intention* (Gollwitzer & Sheeran, 2006), has now been formalized into a program known as *implementation intention training* (e.g., Luszczynska, Scholz, & Sutton, 2007). This involves identifying specific desired behavioral changes and identifying when, where, and how they can be achieved. In a study with cardiac patients, they enrolled participants (who had experienced an MI) 2 weeks following a standard cardiac rehabilitation program into an implementation intentions training program designed to reduce their intake of saturated fat. Compared to participants who had cardiac rehabilitation alone, they found a reduction in saturated fat intake from 22.88 g at 2 months after MI to 19.71 g at 6-month follow-up.

EXERCISE

Exercise programs increase exercise, although adherence to exercise typically falls following cessation of programs. Interestingly, home-based interventions may have higher adherence levels than those based in hospitals. King, Haskell, Taylor, Kraemer, and DeBusk (1991) reported adherence to a long-term exercise program of around 75% for a home-based exercise program and 52% for a center-based program 1 year following the program. Similar adherence levels were reported by Jolly et al. (2009). Exercise programs also increase short-term markers of fitness and health. In a meta-analysis of functional gains following home-based exercise programs for people with chronic heart failure, Hwang and Marwick (2009) found gains relative to no intervention on measures of peak oxygen consumption, exercise duration, and distance on the 6-minute walk test. In a Cochrane review of all exercise programs, Rees, Taylor, Singh, Coats, and Ebrahim (2004) noted similar gains, as well as increases in maximal oxygen consumption (VO_2 max). Finally, Tabet et al. (2009) noted immunological benefits, reductions in vascular resistance, and improvements in ventilatory capacity. Given these benefits, the contribution of psychology in this domain may be to increase adherence to exercise programs. Petter et al. (2009) found that six variables, most of which are subsumed within the health action process model (Schwarzer, 2008), were consistently related to exercise (self-regulatory self-efficacy, health status, intention, perceived control, beliefs/benefits, and previous physical activity). Several variables were also related to exercise in three of four contexts (e.g., task self-efficacy, perceived barriers, attitude, action planning, gender, and employment status). Together, these studies suggest that teaching and instigating self-regulatory skills may prove an effective intervention in this context. Evidence that this, indeed, is the case can be found in the work of Sniehotta, Scholz, and Schwarzer (2006). They allocated patients who had already completed a standard rehabilitation program into one of three conditions: standard care; developing action plans (implementation intentions) concerning when, where, and how to exercise; or action planning plus developing coping plans on how to deal with anticipated barriers to exercise. Participants in the combined planning group engaged in significantly more physical exercise 2 months post-discharge than did those in the other groups. An alternative, and perhaps simpler, intervention reported by Arrigo et al. (2008) involved patients writing a diary of physical activities combined with quarterly group meetings to discuss issues around exercise. In comparison to a standard care group, significantly more patients reported engaging in regular physical activity (73% vs. 40%) at 1-year follow-up. They also showed better outcomes on measures of BMI and lipid values.

PREVENTING DISEASE PROGRESSION

Most cardiac rehabilitation programs are multicomponential, including both educational and exercise processes, and systematic reviews attempt to divide a somewhat complex range of intervention strategies into those that are primarily exercise-based and those that are psychosocial. The two descriptors are not mutually exclusive, as many programs may include both an exercise and relaxation component. In addition, "psychosocial" has frequently included educational, stress management, and counseling approaches under one umbrella. Accordingly, some caution is required in the interpretation of these general conclusions. Reflecting this proviso, in their meta-analysis of the effectiveness of cardiac exercise programs, Taylor et al. (2006) noted that although mortality rates following exercise training post MI, angina, or revascularization were 28% lower than in control conditions, only half of this was attributable to exercise per se. Half were attributable to other behavioral changes, in particular reductions in smoking. Although a number of meta-analyses examining the effectiveness of psychosocial therapies have been reported, these have generally suffered from evaluating the effects of a variety of types of program, alone or in combination with other cardiac rehabilitation interventions (e.g., Clark, Hartling, Vandermeer, & McAlister, 2005; Rees et al., 2005). Accordingly, although they have shown reductions in risk behaviors, improvements in mood, and reductions in cardiovascular morbidity, assigning these effects to particular components of the intervention is problematic. Linden, Phillips, and Leclerc (2007) specified their psychological interventions as those that involved multicomponent stress management, cognitive-behavioral, or behavioral interventions. Excluded were individual interventions they considered as biological/self-regulation- based, which included meditation, autogenic training, and deep muscle relaxation. Also excluded from the analysis were interventions that combined psychological and other interventions. Overall, cardiac patients who received a psychological intervention evidenced a reduction in mortality of 27% at follow-up of 2 years or less and reduced event recurrence at follow-up of 2 years or longer (43% reduction) in comparison to control conditions. In addition, they found that gains in mortality were only found following successful reductions in distress. Van Dixhoorn and White's (2005) meta-analysis of relaxation interventions also showed significant reductions in cardiac mortality in their pooled data. Two particular studies of cognitive-behavioral interventions are of particular interest. Historically, perhaps the strongest evaluation of the effectiveness of stress management in the context of cardiac disease was provided by Friedman et al. (1986), who reported on a trial known as the Recurrent Coronary Prevention Program. This targeted men high on a measure of type A behavior who had experienced an MI. Participants were allocated to one of three groups: cardiac rehabilitation, cardiac rehabilitation plus type A management, and a usual care control. The rehabilitation program involved small group meetings over a period of 4.5 years, in which participants received information on medication, exercise, and diet, as well as social support from the group. The type A management group received the same information in addition to engaging in a sustained program of behavioral change involving training in relaxation, cognitive techniques, and specific behavioral change plans in which they reduced the frequency of their type A behavior. Evidence of the effectiveness of this process was compelling. Over the 4.5 years of the intervention, those in the type A management program were at half the risk of further infarction than those in the traditional rehabilitation program, with total infarction rates over this time of 13% and 21% in each group, respectively. Rates of nonfatal MI were 8% and 14%, respectively. This remains one of the most convincing studies of the effectiveness of stress management on survival following an MI, although whether most health care services could provide such an expensive long-term intervention is debatable. A second intervention was more disappointing. The ENRICHD study (Berkman et al., 2003) targeted patients who were depressed following an MI. Using a comprehensive year-long approach to reducing depression, including group cognitive-behavioral therapy, social skills training, and (if necessary) pharmacological intervention, they were successful in reducing depression more than a usual care condition. However, there were no differences in survival between the two groups over the 2 years following infarction. These data have led some to claim that there are no benefits to treating depression in MI patients—and they certainly seem to indicate this to be the case. However, the sheer size of the study meant that the investigators had limited control over the interventions received by patients in both arms of the study. This meant that the usual care received by some people in the control condition was, in fact, very similar to that provided by the ENRICHD study. In addition, attendance at the ENRICHD intervention was less than optimal, with most patients attending about 11 sessions—an attendance not that different to many of the control group interventions. Perhaps because of these factors, the differences in levels of depression between the two groups, although statistically significant, were not that great. Accordingly, it remains possible that the reductions in depression in the ENRICHD condition relative to the control condition were not sufficiently large enough to bring about reductions in risk for further MI.

Conclusion

A number of conclusions can now be drawn from the cardiac rehabilitation literature. Important recent studies have shown that the most effective interventions (in terms of emotional, behavioral, and physical outcomes) involve an element of behavioral or planning interventions. These are likely to be superior to didactic educational programs. In addition, the context of the program need no longer be the hospital. Home-based programs appear to have similar outcomes to hospital-based programs. However, the nature of the differing programs means that neither type of program appears to be more cost-effective than the other. In addition, it is not clear whether some patients, such as those with low levels of cardiac damage, good social support, and high levels of self-efficacy, may benefit more from such programs than those with less benign physical or psychological profiles.

Future Directions

We now know which programs are likely to benefit most patients most of the time. The next phase of research needs to identify the optimal intervention (within the limits of practicability) for differing types of individual. Who benefits most from home-based interventions? Do some people benefit from the social or other benefits of group interventions? In addition, given the poor outcome of targeted interventions, yet the potential benefits of focusing resources on those most in need, are there models of this type of intervention that could be developed based on different decision criteria and perhaps adopting types of intervention different from those used by Frasure-Smith? Or, would perhaps the best strategy be to provide a menu of issues from which patients may self-select? At a more fundamental level, a number of simpler yet important questions can be addressed. When is the optimal time to start rehabilitation—in hospital, or some weeks after, when the initial shock has receded and the challenges to be faced are more apparent? How long and intensive do any interventions need to be? Some of the research reported involves programs lasting several years. This is impractical in the face of financial hurdles facing all health services within the next decade. We know much about the components of what to provide: now we need to address the optimal cost-effective means of providing them.

References

Allen, J. K., Scott, L. B., Stewart, K. J., & Young, D. R. (2004). Disparities in women's referral to and enrollment in outpatient cardiac rehabilitation. *Journal of General Internal Medicine, 19,* 747–753.

Arrigo, I., Brunner-LaRocca, H., Lefkovits, M., Pfisterer, M., & Hoffmann, A. (2008). Comparative outcome one year after formal cardiac rehabilitation: The effects of a randomized intervention to improve exercise adherence. *European Journal of Cardiovascular Prevention and Rehabilitation, 15,* 306–311.

Bandura, A. (1986). *Social foundations of thought and action: A social cognitive theory.* Englewood Cliffs, NJ: Prentice-Hall.

Barlow, D. H., Lehrer, P. M., Woolfolk, R. L., & Sime, W. E. (Eds.). (2008). *Principles and practice of stress management.* New York: Guilford Press.

Barth, J., Critchley, J., & Bengel, J. (2008). Psychosocial interventions for smoking cessation in patients with coronary heart disease. *Cochrane Database of Systematic Reviews, 1,* CD006886.

Bellman, C., Hambraeus, K., Lindbäck, J., & Lindahl, B. (2009). Achievement of secondary preventive goals after acute myocardial infarction: A comparison between participants and nonparticipants in a routine patient education program in Sweden. *Journal of Cardiovascular Nursing, 24,* 362–368.

Beck, A. (1993). *Cognitive therapy and the emotional disorders.* New York: Penguin.

Bennett, P., Mayfield, T., Norman, P., Lowe, R., & Morgan M. (1999). Affective and social cognitive predictors of behavioural change following myocardial infarction. *British Journal of Health Psychology, 4,* 247–256.

Bennett, P., Owen, R., Koutsakis, S., & Bisson, J. (2002). Personality, social context, and cognitive predictors of post-traumatic stress disorder in myocardial infarction patients. *Psychology and Health, 17,* 489–500.

Bennett, P., & Connell, H. (1999). Dyadic responses to myocardial infarction. *Psychology, Health and Medicine, 4,* 45–55.

Berkman, L. F., Blumenthal, J., Burg, M., Carney, R. M., Catellier, D., Cowan, M. J., et al. (2003). Effects of treating depression and low perceived social support on clinical events after myocardial infarction: The Enhancing Recovery in Coronary Heart Disease Patients (ENRICHD) randomized trial. *Journal of the American Medical Association, 289,* 3106–3116.

British Association for Cardiac Rehabilitation. (2007). *Standards and core components for cardiac rehabilitation (2007).* London: BACR.

Bundy, C., Carroll, D., Wallace, L., & Nagle, R. (1998). Stress management training in chronic stable angina pectoris. *Psychology and Health, 13,* 147–155.

Clark, A. M., Hartling, L., Vandermeer, B., & McAlister, F. A. (2005). Meta-analysis: Secondary prevention programs for patients with coronary artery disease. *Annals of Internal Medicine, 143,* 659–672.

Cossette, S., Frasure-Smith, N., & Lespérance, F. (2001). Clinical implications of a reduction in psychological distress on cardiac prognosis in patients participating in a psychosocial intervention program. *Psychosomatic Medicine, 63,* 257–266.

Dickens, C. M., Percival, C., McGowan, L., Douglas, J., Tomenson, B., Cotter, L., et al. (2004). The risk factors for depression in first myocardial infarction patients. *Psychological Medicine, 34,* 1083–1092.

Dornelas, E. A., Sampson, R. A., Gray, J. F., Waters, D., & Thompson, P. D. (2000). A randomized controlled trial of smoking cessation counseling after myocardial Infarction. *Preventive Medicine, 30,* 261–268.

Edwardson, S. R. (2007). Patient education in heart failure. *Heart and Lung, 36,* 244–252.

Frasure-Smith, N., Lespérance, F., & Talajic, M. (1995). Depression and 18-month prognosis after myocardial infarction. *Circulation, 91,* 999–1005.

Frasure-Smith, N., Lespérance, F., Habra, M., Talajic, M., Khairy, P., Dorian, P., et al. (2009). Elevated depression symptoms predict long-term cardiovascular mortality in patients with atrial fibrillation and heart failure. *Circulation, 120*, 134–140.

Frasure-Smith, N., Lespérance, F., Prince, R. H., Verrier, P., Garber, R. A., Juneau, M., et al. (1997). Randomised trial of home-based psychosocial nursing intervention for patients recovering from myocardial infarction. *Lancet, 350*, 473–479.

Frasure-Smith, N., & Prince, R. (1985). The ischemic heart disease life stress monitoring program: Impact on mortality. *Psychosomatic Medicine, 47*, 431–445.

Friedman, M., Thoresen, C. D., Gill, J. J., Ulmer, D., Powell, L. H., Price, V.A., et al. (1986). Alteration of Type A behaviour and its effect on cardiac recurrences in post myocardial infarction patients: Summary results of the recurrent coronary prevention project. *American Heart Journal, 112*, 653–665.

Furber, S., Butler, L., Phongsavan, P., Mark, A., & Bauman, A. (2010). Randomised controlled trial of a pedometer-based telephone intervention to increase physical activity among cardiac patients not attending cardiac rehabilitation. *Patient Education and Counseling, 80*, 212–218.

Gallacher J., Hopkinson J., Bennett P., & Yarnell, J. (1997). Stress management in the treatment of angina. *Psychology and Health, 12*, 523–532.

Giannuzzi, P., Temporelli, P. L., Marchioli, R., Maggioni, A. P., Balestroni, G., Ceci, V., et al. (2008). Global secondary prevention strategies to limit event recurrence after myocardial infarction: Results of the GOSPEL study, a multicenter, randomized controlled trial from the Italian Cardiac Rehabilitation Network. *Archives of Internal Medicine, 168*, 2194–2204.

Gollwitzer, P. M. (1999). Implementation intentions: Strong effects of simple plans. *American Psychologist, 54*, 493–503.

Gollwitzer, P. M., & Sheeran, P. (2006). Implementation intentions and goal achievement: A meta-analysis of effects and processes. *Advances in Experimental Social Psychology, 38*, 69ñ119.

Gregory, P. C., LaVeist, T. A., & Simpson, C. (2006). Racial disparities in access to cardiac rehabilitation. *American Journal of Physical Medicine and Rehabilitation, 85*, 705–710.

Hajek, P., Taylor, T. Z., & Mills, P. (2002). Brief intervention during hospital admission to help patients to give up smoking after myocardial infarction and bypass surgery: Randomised controlled trial. *British Medical Journal, 324*, 87–89.

Hartford, K., Wong, C., & Zakaria, D. (2009). Randomized controlled trial of a telephone intervention by nurses to provide information and support to patients and their partners after elective coronary artery bypass graft surgery: Effects of anxiety. *Heart and Lung, 31*, 199–206.

Havik, O. E., & Maeland, J. G. (1988). Verbal denial and outcome in myocardial infarction patients. *Journal of Psychosomatic Research, 32*, 145–157.

Huijbrechts, I. P., Duivenvoorden, H. J., & Deckers, J. W. (1996). Modification of smoking habits five months after myocardial infarction: Relationship with personality characteristics. *Journal of Psychosomatic Research, 40*, 369–378.

Hwang, R., & Marwick, T. (2009). Efficacy of home-based exercise programmes for people with chronic heart failure: A meta-analysis. *European Journal of Cardiovascular Prevention and Rehabilitation, 16*, 527–535.

Jacq, F., Foulldrin, G., Savouré, A., Anselme, F., Baguelin-Pinaud, A., Cribier, A., & Thibaut, F. (2009). A comparison of anxiety, depression and quality of life between device shock and nonshock groups in implantable cardioverter defibrillator recipients. *General Hospital Psychiatry, 31*, 266–273.

Jiang, X., Sit, J. W., & Wong, T. K. (2007). A nurse-led cardiac rehabilitation programme improves health behaviours and cardiac physiological risk parameters: Evidence from Chengdu, China. *Journal of Clinical Nursing, 16*(10), 1886–1897.

Jolly, K., Taylor, R. S., Lip, G. Y., & Stevens, A. (2006). Home-based cardiac rehabilitation compared with centre-based rehabilitation and usual care: A systematic review and meta-analysis. *International Journal of Cardiology, 111*, 343–351.

Jolly, K., Lip, G. Y., Taylor, R. S., Raftery, J., Mant, J., Lane, D., et al. (2009). The Birmingham Rehabilitation Uptake Maximisation study (BRUM): A randomised controlled trial comparing home-based with centre-based cardiac rehabilitation. *Heart, 95*, 36–42.

King, A. C., Haskell, W. L., Taylor, C. B., Kraemer, H. C., & DeBusk R. F. (1991). Group- vs home-based exercise training in healthy older men and women. *Journal of the American Medical Association, 266*, 1535–1542.

Lane, D., Carroll, D., Ring, C., Beevers, D. G., & Lip, G. Y. (2002). The prevalence and persistence of depression and anxiety following myocardial infarction. *British Journal Health Psychology, 7*, 11–21.

Lane, D., Carroll, D., Ring, C., Beevers, D. G., & Lip, G. Y. (2002). In-hospital symptoms of depression do not predict mortality 3 years after myocardial infarction. *International Journal of Epidemiology, 31*, 1179–1182.

Lear, S. A. Ignaszewski, A., Linden, W., Brozic, A., Kiess, M., Spinelli, J. J., et al. (2003). The Extensive Lifestyle Management Intervention (ELMI) following cardiac rehabilitation trial. *European Heart Journal, 24*, 1920–1927.

Leon, A. S., Franklin, B. A., Costa, F., Gary J., Balady, G. J., Berra, K. A., et al. (2005). AHA scientific statement. Cardiac rehabilitation and secondary prevention of coronary heart disease. *Circulation, 111*, 369–376.

Leslie, W. S., Hankey, C. R., Matthews, D., Currall, J. E., & Lean, M. E. (2004). A transferable programme of nutritional counselling for rehabilitation following myocardial infarction: A randomised controlled study. *European Journal of Clinical Nutrition, 58*, 778–786.

Lewin, R. J., Coulton, S., Frizelle, D. J., Kaye, G., & Cox, H. (2009). A brief cognitive behavioural preimplantation and rehabilitation programme for patients receiving an implantable cardioverter-defibrillator improves physical health and reduces psychological morbidity and unplanned readmissions. *Heart, 95*, 63–69.

Lewin, R. J. P., Furze, G., Robinson, J., Griffith, K., Wiseman, S., Pye, M., & Boyle R. (2002). A randomised controlled trial of a self-management plan for patients with newly diagnosed angina. *British Journal of General Practice, 52*, 194–201.

Lewin, B., Robertson, I. H., Irving, J. B., & Campbell, M. (1992). Effects of self-help post-myocardial-infarction rehabilitation on psychological adjustment and use of health services. *Lancet, 339*, 1036–1040.

Linden, W., Phillips, M. J., & Leclerc, J. (2007). Psychological treatment of cardiac patients: A meta-analysis. *European Heart Journal, 28*, 2972–2984.

Lisspers, J., Sundin, O., Ohman, A., Hofman-Bang, C., Rydén, L., & Nygren, A. (2005). Long-term effects of lifestyle behavior change in coronary artery disease: Effects on recurrent coronary events after percutaneous coronary intervention. *Health Psychology, 24*, 41–48.

Lorig, K.R., Ritter, P.L. & Jacquez, A. (2005). Outcomes of border health Spanish/English chronic disease self-management programs. *Diabetes Education, 31*, 401–409.

Luszczynska, A. & Cieslak, R. (2009). Mediated effects of social support for healthy nutrition: fruit and vegetable intake across 8 months after myocardial infarction. *Behavioral Medicine, 35*, 308.

Luszczynska, A., Scholz, U., & Sutton, S. (2007). Planning to change diet: A controlled trial of an implementation intentions training intervention to reduce saturated fat intake among patients after myocardial infarction. *Journal of Psychosomatic Research, 63*, 491–497.

Luyster, F. S., Hughes, J. W., & Gunstad, J. (2009). Depression and anxiety symptoms are associated with reduced dietary adherence in heart failure patients treated with an implantable cardioverter defibrillator. *Journal of Cardiovascular Nursing, 24*, 10–17.

Mayou, R. A., Gill, D., Thompson, D. R., Day, A., Hicks, N., Volmink, J., & Neil, A. (2000). Depression and anxiety as predictors of outcome after myocardial infarction. *Psychosomatic Medicine, 62*, 212–219.

McGrady, A., McGinnis, R., Badenhop, D., Bentle, M., & Rajput, M. (2009). Effects of depression and anxiety on adherence to cardiac rehabilitation. *Journal of Cardiopulmonary Rehabilitation and Prevention, 29*, 358–364.

Milani, R.V., & Lavie, C. J. (2009). Reducing psychosocial stress: A novel mechanism of improving survival from exercise training. *American Journal of Medicine, 122*, 931–938.

Moser, D. K., & Dracup, K. (2004). Role of spousal anxiety and depression in patients' psychosocial recovery after a cardiac event. *Psychosomatic Medicine, 66*, 527–532.

Neves, A., Alves, A. J., Ribeiro, F., Gomes, J. L., & Oliveira, J. (2009). The effect of cardiac rehabilitation with relaxation therapy on psychological, hemodynamic, and hospital admission outcome variables. *Journal of Cardiopulmonary Rehabilitation and Prevention, 29*, 304–309.

Oldenburg, B., Allam, R., & Fastier, G. (1989). The role of behavioral and educational interventions in the secondary prevention of heart disease. *Clinical and Abnormal Psychology, 27*, 429–438.

Perez, G. H., Nicolau, J. C., Romano, B. W., & Laranjeira, R. (2008). Depression: A predictor of smoking relapse in a 6-month follow-up after hospitalization for acute coronary syndrome. *European Journal of Cardiovascular Prevention and Rehabilitation, 15*, 89–94.

Petrie, K. J., Buick, D. L., Weinman, J., & Booth, R. J. (1999). Positive effects of illness reported by myocardial infarction and breast cancer patients. *Journal of Psychosomatic Research, 47*, 537–543.

Petrie, K. J., Cameron, L. D., Ellis, C. J., Buick, D., & Weinman, J. (2002). Changing illness perceptions after myocardial infarction: An early intervention randomized controlled trial. *Psychosomatic Medicine, 64*, 580–586.

Petrie, K. J., Weinman, J., Sharpe, N., & Buckley, J. (1996). Role of patients' view of their illness in predicting return to work and functioning after myocardial infarction: Longitudinal study. *British Medical Journal, 312*, 1191–1194.

Petter, M., Blanchard, C., Kemp, K.A., Mazoff, A.S. & Ferrier, S.N. (2009). Correlates of exercise among coronary heart disease patients: review, implications and future directions. *European Journal of Cardiovascular Prevention and Rehabilitation, 16*, 515–526.

Piotrowicz, E., Baranowski, R., Bilinska, M., Stepnowska, M., Piotrowska, M., Wójcik, A., et al. (2009). A new model of home-based telemonitored cardiac rehabilitation in patients with heart failure: Effectiveness, quality of life, and adherence. *European Journal of Heart Failure, 12*, 164–171.

Quist-Paulsen, P., & Gallefoss, F. (2003). Randomised controlled trial of smoking cessation intervention after admission for coronary heart disease. *British Medical Journal, 327*, 1254–1257.

Rees K., Bennett P., West, R., Davey Smith, S. G., & Ebrahim, S. (2005). Stress management for coronary heart disease. *Cochrane Database of Systematic Reviews, 2*: Chichester: John Wiley and Sons.

Rees, K., Taylor, R. S., Singh, S., Coats, A. J., & Ebrahim, S. (2004). Exercise based rehabilitation for heart failure. *Cochrane Database of Systematic Reviews, 3*: Chichester: John Wiley and Sons.

Rutledge, T., Linke, S. E., Krantz, D. S., Johnson, B. D., Bittner, V., Eastwood, J. A., et al. (2009). Comorbid depression and anxiety symptoms as predictors of cardiovascular events: Results from the NHLBI-sponsored Women's Ischemia Syndrome Evaluation (WISE) study. *Psychosomatic Medicine, 71*, 958–964.

Sears, S. F., Sowell, L. D., Kuhl, E. A., Kovacs, A. H., Serber, E. R., Handberg, E., et al. (2007). The ICD shock and stress management program: A randomized trial of psychosocial treatment to optimize quality of life in ICD patients. *Pacing and Clinical Electrophysiology, 30*, 858–864.

Schwarzer, R. (2008). Modeling health behavior change: How to predict and modify the adoption and maintenance of health behaviours. *Applied Psychology: An International Review, 57*, 1–29.

Shemesh, E., Yehuda, R., Milo, O., Dinur, I., Rudnick, A., Vered, Z., & Cotter, G. (2004). Posttraumatic stress, nonadherence, and adverse outcome in survivors of a myocardial infarction. *Psychosomatic Medicine, 66*, 521–526.

Smith, P. M., & Burgess, E. (2009). Smoking cessation initiated during hospital stay for patients with coronary artery disease: A randomized controlled trial. *Canadian Medical Association Journal, 180*, 1297–1303.

Sniehotta, F. F., Scholz, U., & Schwarzer, R. (2006). Action plans and coping plans for physical exercise: A longitudinal intervention study in cardiac rehabilitation. *British Journal of Health Psychology, 11*, 23–37.

Söderman, E., Lisspers, J., & Sundin, O. (2003). Depression as a predictor of return to work in patients with coronary artery disease. *Social Science and Medicine, 56*, 193–202.

Söderman, E., Lisspers, J., & Sundin, O. (2007). Impact of depressive mood on lifestyle changes in patients with coronary artery disease. *Journal of Rehabilitation Medicine, 39*(5), 412–417.

Stern, M. J., & Pascale, L. (1979). Psychosocial adaption post-myocardial infarction: The spouses' dilemma. *Journal of Psychosomatic Research, 23*, 83–87.

Stewart, M., Davidson, K., Meade, D., Hirth, A., & Makrides, L. (2000). Myocardial infarction: Survivors' and spouses' stress, coping, and support. *Journal of Advanced Nursing, 31*, 1351–1360.

Stewart Williams, J. A. (2009). Using non-linear decomposition to explain the discriminatory effects of male-female differentials in access to care: A cardiac rehabilitation case study. *Social Science and Medicine, 69,* 1072–1079.

Strik, J. J., Lousberg, R., Cheriex, E. C., & Honig, A. (2004). One year cumulative incidence of depression following myocardial infarction and impact on cardiac outcome. *Journal Psychosomatic Research, 56,* 59–66.

Tabet, J. Y., Meurin, P., Driss, A. B., Weber, H., Renaud, N., Grosdemouge, A., et al. (2009). Benefits of exercise training in chronic heart failure. *Archives of Cardiovascular Disease, 102,* 721–730.

Taylor, R. S., Dalal, H., Jolly, K., Moxham, T., & Zawada, A. (2010). Home-based versus centre-based cardiac rehabilitation. *Cochrane Database Systematic Review, 1,* CD007130.

Taylor, R. S., Unal, B., Critchley, J. A., & Capewell, S. (2006). Mortality reductions in patients receiving exercise-based cardiac rehabilitation: How much can be attributed to cardiovascular risk factor improvements? *European Journal of Cardiovascular Prevention and Rehabilitation, 13,* 369–374.

Thompson, D. R., & Clark, A. M. (2009). Cardiac rehabilitation: Into the future. *Heart, 95,* 1897–1900.

van Dixhoorn, J., & White, A. (2005). Relaxation therapy for rehabilitation and prevention in ischaemic heart disease: A systematic review and meta-analysis. *European Journal of Cardiovascular Prevention and Rehabilitation, 12,* 193–202.

Welton, N. J., Caldwell, D. M., Adamopoulos, E., & Vedhara, K. (2009). Mixed treatment comparison meta-analysis of complex interventions: Psychological interventions in coronary heart disease. *American Journal of Epidemiology, 169,* 1158–1165.

Wiklund, I., Sanne, H., Vedin, A., & Wilhelmsson, C. (1984). Psychosocial outcome one year after a first myocardial infarction. *Journal of Psychosomatic Research, 28,* 309–321.

Zullo, M. D., Dolansky, M. A., & Jackson, L. W. (2010). Cardiac rehabilitation, health behaviors, and body mass index post-myocardial infarction. *Journal of Cardiopulmonary Rehabilitation and Prevention, 30,* 28–34.

Limb Amputation

Deirdre M. Desmond, Laura Coffey, Pamela Gallagher, Malcolm MacLachlan, Stephen T. Wegener, *and* Fiadhnait O'Keeffe

Abstract

Limb amputation is both a life-saving procedure and a life-changing event. The aims of rehabilitation following amputation are to restore acceptable levels of functioning that allow individuals to achieve their goals, facilitate personal health, and improve participation in society and quality of life, either with or without a prosthesis. Individual responses to limb loss are varied and complex; some individuals experience functional, psychological, and social dysfunction; many others adjust and function well. This chapter highlights critical psychological and social issues in amputation, summarizes current knowledge in these domains, and provides a brief overview of psychological interventions designed to address these issues.

Key Words: Adjustment, amputation, limb, pain, participation, psychology, rehabilitation.

The multiple pathways that may lead to limb amputation include disease (e.g., diabetes, peripheral vascular disease, malignant tumors), traumatic injury (e.g., motor vehicle and industrial accidents), and congenital causes. In many cases, limb amputation is both a life-saving procedure and a life-changing event. Individual responses to limb loss are varied and complex, and are influenced by a range of personal, clinical, social, physical, and environmental factors. No single professional group can address all of the multifaceted care needs that patients and their families present; comprehensive, effective, patient-centered rehabilitation after amputation requires an interdisciplinary team approach in partnership with the patient. Psychologists play vital roles in assessment of cognitive and psychological functioning, in the formulation of the patient's presenting difficulties, and in the design and delivery of interventions to optimize mental health and adjustment outcomes. However, the totality of the rehabilitation experience and the entire rehabilitation team can impact on the patient's psychological and

social well-being. Working within the limits of their professional competencies, team members, including the patient and their family, share responsibility for attending to psychosocial health across the continuum of care (Wegener, Hofkamp, & Ehde, 2008). This chapter highlights critical psychological and social issues in amputation, summarizes current knowledge in these domains, and provides a brief overview of psychological interventions designed to address these issues.

Epidemiology of Amputation
Incidence and Prevalence of Amputation

The global incidence of amputation is unknown; available data evidence considerable variation both between and within countries (Ephraim, Dillingham, Sector, Pezzin, & MacKenzie, 2003; Renzi, Unwin, Jubelirer, & Haag, 2006; Unwin, 2000). Using a standard protocol for data collection, the Global Lower Extremity Amputation Study Group (Unwin, 2000) assessed the incidence of lower limb amputation in ten different locations worldwide and reported marked differences among test sites in their annual rates of lower limb amputation. Comparison of all-cause amputation rates during the 1995–1997 period revealed lowest age-adjusted rates of first major lower limb amputation in Madrid, Spain (0.5 per 100,000 women, 2.8 per 100,000 men), whereas highest rates were reported in the Navajo region of the United States (22.4 per 100,000 women, 43.9 per 100,000 men). In the United States, it is estimated that one out of every 190 persons has lost a limb; the number of persons living with amputation in the United States is projected to increase over twofold to 3.6 million by 2050 if current trends continue (Ziegler-Graham, MacKenzie, Ephraim, Travison, & Brookmeyer, 2008). Internationally, men are more likely than women to undergo amputation, and there is an age-related increase in lower limb amputation secondary to dysvascular disease (Ephraim et al., 2003; Heikkinen, Saarinen, Suominen, Virkkunen, & Salenius, 2007).

Cause and Level of Amputation

Amputation may involve a single limb (unilateral), both the upper or lower limbs (bilateral), or a combination of upper and lower limb amputations (multiple amputations). Amputation may be performed at various anatomical levels. Lower limb amputation may involve removal of one or more toes, part of the foot, ankle disarticulation (disarticulation is the amputation of a body part through a joint), transtibial (below the knee) amputation, knee disarticulation, transfemoral (above the knee) amputation, hip disarticulation, and hemipelvectomy (removal of half of the pelvis). Upper limb amputation may involve the removal of one or more fingers, wrist disarticulation, below-elbow amputation, elbow disarticulation, above-elbow amputation, shoulder disarticulation, and forequarter amputation (amputation of the arm, clavicle, and scapula).

In high-income countries, dysvascularity is the foremost cause of amputation; as a corollary, the majority of amputations involve the lower limbs (Ziegler-Graham et al., 2008). The typical dysvascular patient with an amputation is older than 60 years of age and commonly experiences comorbidities; postoperative morbidity and mortality rates are high (Dillingham & Pezzin, 2008; Dillingham, Pezzin, & Shore, 2005; Ploeg, Lardenoye, Vrancken Peeters, & Breslau, 2005; Schofield et al., 2006). Among individuals with dysvascular amputations, higher amputation levels are generally indicative of more advanced disease stage. Furthermore, older age is associated with higher levels of amputation, reflecting the progression of vascular disease with advancing age. The risk of losing the contralateral limb following unilateral amputation ranges from 15% to 20% in the first 2 years after the initial procedure, and rises to 40% by 4 years post amputation (Cutson & Bongiorni, 1996); patients with amputation secondary to diabetes have elevated morbidity (Schofield et al., 2006). The patient's overall health status complicates the challenge of amputation rehabilitation. Traumatic amputation (associated with mechanical, chemical, thermal, and/or electrical injuries), is more common among working-age adults who are otherwise in good health. Trauma is the most common cause of acquired upper limb amputation (National Amputee Statistical Database, 2009) and the most common cause of all-level amputations in nonindustrialized countries (Ephraim et al., 2003). Amputation as a result of military conflict or civilian violence continues to constitute a serious public health problem in some regions (Burger, Marincek, & Jaeger, 2004; Fergason, Keeling, & Bluman, 2010; Williams, Rajput-Ray, Lassalle, Crombie, & Lacoux, 2011). It is clear that the circumstances surrounding disease-related amputation differ substantially from those surrounding traumatic amputation, whether military or civilian (Dougherty, 2001). Nonetheless, much of the literature is based on mixed samples that include individuals with disease-related and traumatic amputations; with notable exceptions, relatively little research has addressed outcomes of amputation related to trauma as a specific focus (Desmond, 2007; Desmond & MacLachlan, 2004, 2006b; Dillingham, Pezzin, & MacKenzie, 1998; Dougherty, 2003; Pezzin, Dillingham, & MacKenzie, 2000).

Physical Adjustment to Amputation

The primary goals of rehabilitation following amputation are to restore acceptable levels of functioning that allow individuals to achieve their goals, to facilitate personal health, and to improve participation in society and quality of life (QOL; van Velzen et al., 2006), either with or without a prosthesis. Individuals with amputations have a complex range of rehabilitation needs and are faced with multiple and evolving physical, psychological, and social threats and challenges including impairments in physical functioning, pain, prosthesis use, alterations in body image and self-concept, changes in close personal relationships, employment status or occupation, and disruptions to valued activities and lifestyle (Desmond & Gallagher, 2008; Desmond & MacLachlan, 2006b; Horgan & MacLachlan, 2004; Rybarczyk, Edwards, & Behel, 2004). Comprehensive rehabilitation requires an interdisciplinary team approach in collaboration with the patient and their family.

The medical and physical consequences of amputation serve as the centerpiece in acute care and are commonly at the forefront of prosthetic rehabilitation. Prosthetic prescription aims to compensate for functional and/or cosmetic losses where possible (van Velzen et al., 2006). Prostheses may be considered "intimate extensions of the body" (Biddiss & Chau, 2007a, pp. 236) and consequently prosthesis users often have a wide range of personal requirements, expectations, and priorities that pose challenges for prosthetic prescription, fabrication, and delivery and are influential across the continuum of care (Biddiss & Chau, 2007a; Smit & Plettenburg, 2010). Attrition in the use of prescribed prostheses is high, particularly among individuals with upper limb amputations, and there is substantial variability in the extent of prosthesis usage (Biddiss & Chau, 2007b). (Note: the amputation literature lacks standardized comprehensive definitions of *successful prosthetic fit* or *use*; such definition is rendered difficult because of differences in expectations and priorities expressed by patients and clinicians, and because outcomes of importance differ from person to person [Bhangu, Devlin, & Pauley, 2009; Schaffalitzky, Gallagher, MacLachlan, & Ryall, 2010; Schaffalitzky et al., 2009]). Reasons for non-referral for prosthetic fitting, unsuccessful prosthetic restoration, and prosthesis abandonment include mortality, comorbidities, cognitive deficits, residual limb condition and length, pain, delayed prosthetic fitting, limited device functionality, patient preference, patient dissatisfaction, and pre-amputation ambulatory status (lower limb amputation) (e.g., Biddiss & Chau, 2007a, 2008; O'Neill, 2008). Individuals who are not candidates for prosthetic use or who do not use their prostheses may require alternative assistive devices (e.g., wheelchairs), and such assistive technologies may in themselves require significant self-image and lifestyle adaptations (MacLachlan & Gallagher, 2004).

The main phases of prosthetic rehabilitation are pre-prosthetic management; postoperative care; prosthetic training; and long-term follow-up care (including community reintegration and vocational rehabilitation) (Esquenazi, 2004). During prosthetic training, the patient must learn how to don and doff the prosthesis appropriately and must practice the skills necessary to perform activities of daily living in different environmental conditions. Basic training serves as a foundation for more complex skills that are learned with progressively less physical support and supervision over the course of rehabilitation. The complex behavioral tasks inherent in prosthetic rehabilitation require both an adequate level of physical fitness and the cognitive capacity to learn new skills and adapt them to different situations and environments. Persons with cognitive deficits may struggle to retain this new information or to initiate new behaviors necessary for optimal rehabilitation (Larner, Van Ross, & Hale, 2003; O'Neill, Moran, & Gillespie, 2010; O'Neill, 2008). Cognitive screening may be beneficial in identifying impairments and potential barriers to new learning, in informing, planning and setting of rehabilitation goals and, when appropriate, in identifying compensatory strategies to assist in achieving rehabilitation goals (O'Neill et al., 2010; O'Neill & Evans, 2009; O'Neill, 2008). For example, cognitive rehabilitation techniques and compensatory strategies, such as errorless learning and vanishing cues techniques, may be of benefit in the amputation rehabilitation process for those with cognitive impairments.

Pain secondary to limb amputation is a very common occurrence and may be manifest at multiple anatomical sites (Desmond & MacLachlan, 2006a, 2010; Ehde & Wegener, 2008). The spectrum of potential pain problems experienced after amputation includes phantom limb pain (PLP; painful sensation perceived in the amputated body part), residual limb/stump pain (pain emanating from the residual or remaining portion of the limb/stump), and pain in regions beyond the amputated limb, which may be associated with comorbidities, increased forces on the intact limb, alterations in the biomechanics of movement associated with prosthesis use, and secondary musculoskeletal pathologies (Gailey, Allen, Castles, Kucharik, & Roeder, 2008). Chronic back pain is a significant problem among individuals with lower limb amputations in particular; prevalence estimates are approximately double those documented in the general population (Ehde et al., 2000, 2001; Ehde & Wegener, 2008; Hagberg & Brånemark, 2001). Although estimates vary considerably (see Borsje, Bosmans, Van der Schans, Geertzen, & Dijkstra, 2004, for details), both PLP and residual limb pain (RLP) appear to be common and persistent in the long term (at least intermittently) for a substantial number of persons with limb loss (lower limb amputation:

PLP prevalence. ~60–80%; RLP prevalence, ~60–70%; upper limb amputation: PLP prevalence, ~40–83%; RLP prevalence, ~10–50%) (Desmond & MacLachlan, 2010; Dijkstra, Geertzen, Stewart, & van der Schans, 2002; Dudkiewicz, Gabrielov, Seiv-Ner, Zelig, & Heim, 2004; Ehde et al., 2000; Ephraim, Wegener, MacKenzie, Dillingham, & Pezzin, 2005). Among individuals with amputations, pain has been associated with a variety of negative outcomes, such as poor adjustment, affective distress, decrements in QOL, interference with prosthesis use, and activity and participation restriction (Desmond, Gallagher, Henderson-Slater, & Chatfield, 2008; van der Schans, Geertzen, Schoppen, & Dijkstra, 2002; Whyte & Carroll, 2004; Williamson & Schulz, 1995). Appropriate pain management is critical to ameliorate the potentially profound impact of pain on the individual. In keeping with other persistent pain conditions, the interplay of physiological and psychological factors (e.g., pain coping responses and pain-related cognitions) is central to pain experience post-amputation. Thus, multidisciplinary pain management, integrating physical, psychological, and social factors, has the greatest potential to achieve optimal outcomes. For a review of the management of pain after limb loss, refer to Ehde and Wegener (2008).

Psychological and Social Adjustment to Amputation

Amputation is a distressing experience that is likely to pose considerable challenges in terms of psychological and social adjustment. Not only does this procedure incur permanent physical loss, it may also lead to restrictions in many other important life domains. Limb amputation can lead to significant psychological and social dysfunction among some individuals, whereas many others adjust and function well (Desmond & MacLachlan, 2006a; Pezzin et al., 2000). Models delineating important factors in such variation (e.g., Livneh, 2001; Taylor, 1983) describe a complex interplay between *risk factors*, including disease/disability parameters, functional limitation, and psychosocial stressors, and *resistance factors* or *psychosocial assets* including stress processing factors, intrapersonal factors, and social-ecological factors such as social support and family environment (Desmond & Gallagher, 2008). According to Livneh and Antonak (1997), adaptation is a dynamic and evolving process through which the individual strives to approach an optimal state of congruence with his or her environment. Adjustment is the final phase in an evolving

process of adaptation distinguished by maintaining psychosocial equilibrium; achieving a state of reintegration; positively engaging in the pursuit of life goals; evidencing positive self-esteem, self-concept, and self-regard; and experiencing positive attitudes toward oneself, others, and one's disability. The multidimensional nature of psychosocial adjustment (Antonak & Livneh, 1995; Livneh & Antonak, 1997) has stimulated investigation of a range of outcomes, resulting in a snapshot of particular indicators of adjustment, typically at one time point. Negative impacts of amputation (e.g., depression, anxiety) have formed the central focus of most of the research (absence of psychological disorder is interpreted as an indicator of favorable adjustment) (Desmond & Gallagher, 2008). Despite this emphasis, there is little consensus regarding the prevalence of clinically significant psychological dysfunction following limb amputation, either in the short or longer terms (Desmond & MacLachlan, 2006a), and understanding of the processes through which favorable outcomes emerge is limited (Murray, 2010).

Affective Distress

Depressive symptomatology is the most commonly documented mood disturbance following amputation, and estimates suggest that between 13% and 32% of individuals with limb amputations might experience significant depressive symptoms at any one time (Atherton & Robertson, 2006; Cavanagh, Shin, Karamouz, & Rauch, 2006; Desmond & MacLachlan, 2006a; Phelps, Williams, Raichle, Turner, & Ehde, 2008; Rybarczyk et al., 1992). Disparities in such estimates are attributable to methodological differences in assessment of depression and heterogeneity in study samples in terms of demographic and amputation-related factors such as age, amputation etiology, preexisting psychological morbidity, and time since amputation (Cavanagh et al., 2006; Horgan & MacLachlan, 2004; MacLachlan, 2004; Singh et al., 2009). Converging evidence suggests that the initial 2 years following amputation may be a period of elevated risk (see Horgan & MacLachlan, 2004, for review), however, this does not preclude the possibility of depression much later on. The presence of depressive symptomatology has been linked with a wide variety of negative outcomes such as increased pain intensity, activity restriction, anxiety, public self-consciousness, vulnerability, body image anxiety, and reduced QOL (Asano, Rushton, Miller, & Deathe, 2008; Atherton & Robertson, 2006; Behel,

Rybarczyk, Elliott, Nicholas, & Nyenhuis, 2002; Donovan-Hall, Yardley, & Watts, 2002; Ephraim et al., 2005; Hanley et al., 2004; Jensen et al., 2002; Rybarczyk, Nyenhuis, Nicholas, Cash, & Kaiser, 1995; Williamson, Schulz, Bridges, & Behan, 1994).

Increased anxiety is common in the early postoperative period and among inpatients. However, similar findings also emerge in other patient groups and are considered an *"appropriate"* response in light of potentially life-threatening surgery or injury and prolonged hospitalization (e.g., Kennedy & Rogers, 2000). Anxiety does not appear to persist in the long term following limb amputation (Horgan & MacLachlan, 2004). Potential for post-traumatic stress disorder (PTSD) following limb amputation is widely recognized yet poorly researched, even among those with traumatic limb loss (Desmond & MacLachlan, 2004; Wegener et al., 2008). Available estimates suggest that between 15% and 26% of people with limb loss might experience PTSD (Desmond & MacLachlan, 2006a; Fukunishi, Sasaki, Chishima, Anze, & Saijo, 1996; Phelps et al., 2008). The relationship between PTSD and cause of amputation is unclear; two recent studies have examined PTSD symptoms in samples with mixed amputation etiologies. Cavanagh et al. (2006) interviewed 26 rehabilitation patients, an average of 6 weeks after amputation surgery, and found that only one of 23 patients with nontraumatic amputations in the sample met the criteria for PTSD (the patient had previously experienced combat-related PTSD); whereas two of the three persons with traumatic amputations in this sample met the criteria for PTSD, the third demonstrated elevated scores just under the threshold for diagnosis. Phelps and colleagues (2008) failed to observe a significant relationship between amputation etiology and PTSD symptomatology in their sample ($n = 83$), two-thirds of whom had lost their limb due to illness.

Body Image Disturbance

The image of one's body is a critical element of the individual's formulation of the "sense of self" (Klapheke, Marcell, Taliaferro, & Creamer, 2000). Experiences of one's own body are the basis for all other life experiences (Novotny, 1991), hence the disruption of body image engendered by amputation can have significant and long-lasting impact on the individual's sense of identity and agency (MacLachlan, 2004), as well as on personal relationships and interactions with others (Desmond &

MacLachlan, 2002; Rybarczyk et al., 1995). Gallagher, Horgan, Franchignoni, et al. (2007) propose that limb loss necessitates adjustment to changed images of the body: from the "complete" or familiar body before the limb loss, to the traumatized body, the healing body, and the extended body (i.e., a body supplemented with prosthetic devices and/ or mobility aids). Rybarczyk and Behel (2008) note that, for some, the transformative impact of amputation on body image and self-concept is tolerated with minimal distress, whereas for others it results in long-lasting negative self-appraisals. Anxiety may be experienced over the changes in one's body image that occur as a result of limb loss. In an evaluation of a counseling service for persons with amputations, Price and Fisher (2002) noted that 31% of clients sampled raised the issue of body image in their counseling sessions. Body image anxiety following amputation is associated with depression, anxiety, reduced QOL, lower self-esteem, greater public self-consciousness, and poorer psychosocial adjustment to amputation and participation in physical activity (Atherton & Robertson, 2006; Breakey, 1997; Coffey, Gallagher, Horgan, Desmond, & MacLachlan, 2009; Donovan-Hall et al., 2002; Murray & Fox, 2002; Rybarczyk et al., 1995).

Pereira, Kour, Leow, et al. (1996) argue that, in some circumstances, prostheses can act to substantially "repair" compromised body image, in addition to restoring relatively normal appearance and form, and improving physical capabilities. Examination of the role of prostheses in mediating body image distress by Fisher and Hanspal (1998) revealed an association between moderate satisfaction with one's prosthesis and low levels of body image disruption. Similarly, Murray and Fox (2002) reported an association between higher levels of prosthesis satisfaction and lower levels of body image disturbance. Findings from a qualitative study by Gallagher and MacLachlan (2001) suggest that prosthesis appearance is an integral component in establishing positive self-image. In their focus group discussions, concerns regarding public appearance and desires to appear *normal* emerged as dominant themes, and many participants indicated that taking delivery of their prostheses was an important element in restoring normality to their lives.

Social Impact

The social impact of amputation can be substantial. Recovery and rehabilitation encompasses reintegration into the family, community, and, for some, the workplace, and may require negotiation of evolving roles, relationships, and identities. Major lower limb amputation that significantly compromises mobility can necessitate significant adaptations to the patient's home or transition into residential care. Changes and restrictions in participation are commonly reported after limb amputation and may be related to personal (e.g., functional abilities, balance confidence, social discomfort, public self-consciousness, emotional impact of amputation, changes in goals and priorities) and/or external constraints (e.g., lack of accessibility, climate, transportation issues) (Couture, Caron, & Desrosiers, 2010; Donovan-Hall et al., 2002; Gallagher, Donovan, Doyle, & Desmond, 2011; Hamill, Carson, & Dorahy, 2010; Miller, Deathe, Speechley, & Koval, 2001; Rybarczyk et al., 1995; Sjödahl, Gard, & Jarnlo, 2004). Limb amputation also impacts on sexual functioning, relationships, and satisfaction (Geertzen, Van Es, & Dijkstra, 2009; Ide, 2004). Despite the importance of sexual expression in contributing to QOL, research on sexuality among individuals with amputations is very limited. A recent review of sexuality and amputation identified just 11 published studies addressing issues of sex and sexuality over the past 60 years (Geertzen et al., 2009). For individuals of working age, return to work and issues of employment are pertinent, and changes in occupation and alterations in work practices and patterns may be required (Burger & Marincek, 2007; Schoppen et al., 2001; van der Sluis, Hartman, Schoppen, & Dijkstra, 2009).

Positive Psychological and Social Consequences of Amputation

The majority of research on adjustment to amputation has tended to focus on negative outcomes and to interpret the absence of psychological disorder as an indicator of favorable adjustment (Desmond & Gallagher, 2008). This unidimensional conceptualization of adjustment is by no means unique to the study of persons with amputation and can be observed across the literature on adaptation to chronic illness and disability (Bishop, 2005). However, the emerging emphasis on resilience and adaptive psychological processes evident in the general psychological literature has led to growing consideration of positive indicators of adjustment in the amputation field. A number of qualitative studies have detailed positive adjustment and growth among individuals who have experienced the loss of a limb (Couture, Desrosiers, & Caron, 2011; Gallagher & MacLachlan, 2000b; Oaksford, Frude, & Cuddihy, 2005; Saradjian, Thompson, & Datta, 2007). For example, men with upper limb amputations reported having gained a high sense of self-worth from their success in overcoming the functional and psychosocial challenges posed by limb loss and being able to fulfill personally meaningful activities and roles (Saradjian et al., 2007). Oaksford and colleagues (2005) noted that 10 out of the 12 people with lower limb amputations interviewed for their study reported they had experienced psychological growth as a result of their limb loss. Benefits included gaining a new appreciation of what it is like to live with a disability, being more inclined to help others, having greater patience, and having more appreciation of one's own resilience, as well as of the kindness of others.

A small but growing body of quantitative research also addresses positive psychosocial adjustment to amputation (e.g., Oaksford et al., 2005; Phelps et al., 2008; Unwin, Kacperek, & Clarke, 2009). For example, Dunn (1996) examined the salutary effects of finding positive meaning in the experience of amputation among 138 members of a golfing association for persons with amputation. More than three-quarters of participants reported that something positive had happened since their limb loss. Of these, 60% found benefits such as becoming more outgoing or making positive life changes. Others found positive meaning in their experiences by engaging in downward social comparison or focusing on the positive aspects of their limb loss. Those who were able to see a positive side to their amputation experienced significantly fewer symptoms of depression than those who were unable to find a "silver lining." Benefit-finding among persons with amputations was also observed in a study by Gallagher and MacLachlan (2000b), in which 46% of participants reported that something good had happened as a result of their limb loss. The beneficial effects of amputation reported included gaining independence through the use of a prosthetic limb, developing a more positive outlook, leading a better life, viewing the experience as character-building, and experiencing less pain as a result of amputation. Finding positive meaning in amputation was associated with better self-reported health and physical capability, and greater adjustment to limitations.

Factors Associated with Adjustment to Amputation

Attempts to identify specific factors that may account for the diversity of responses to amputation have stimulated investigation of an array of medical/amputation-related factors (e.g., amputation etiology, level of amputation), demographic variables (e.g., age), and individual psychological variables (e.g., perceived social support, coping). In general, relationships between medical, amputation-related, and demographic variables and adjustment have been weak or inconsistent; exceptions include post-amputation pain and age at amputation, where greater consistency emerges (Horgan & MacLachlan, 2004; Rybarczyk et al., 2004). A number of studies have linked older age with better adjustment (Behel et al., 2002; Desmond & MacLachlan, 2006b; Dunn, 1996; Phelps et al., 2008; Singh et al., 2009; Williamson et al., 1994). Drawing on lifespan theories of development, explanations for such findings center on proposals that older adults may not react as strongly to amputation as younger individuals because they view changes in functional abilities and body image resulting from limb loss as undesirable but somewhat expected at their age (Horgan & MacLachlan, 2004). As noted previously, persistent post-amputation pain has been highlighted as a significant risk factor for poor adjustment (Gallagher, Allen, & MacLachlan, 2001; Jensen et al., 2002). In keeping with the wider literature on chronic illness and disability, which repeatedly demonstrates that objective measures of physical impairment tend to be poor predictors of psychological well-being, research has failed to support a significant association between level of amputation and adjustment (e.g., Asano et al., 2008; Behel et al., 2002; Unwin et al., 2009). Rybarczyk and colleagues (1997) argue that degree of impairment is too simplistic to serve as an important predictor of overall adjustment and suggest that although physical impairment may have an impact on one's self-concept and related factors, the restrictions it causes in activities of daily living and other life domains are more likely to play a pivotal role in the adaptation process.

Among the psychosocial correlates of adjustment, variables such as hope (Unwin et al., 2009), optimism (Dunn, 1996), perceived control (Dunn, 1996), sense of coherence (Badura-Brzoza, Matysiakiewicz, Piegza, Rycerski, & Hese, 2008), self-esteem (Breakey, 1997; Donovan-Hall et al., 2002), illness perceptions (Callaghan, Condie, & Johnston, 2008), balance confidence (Asano et al., 2008), public self-consciousness (Atherton & Robertson, 2006; Williamson & Schulz, 1995), vulnerability (Behel et al., 2002), and perceived social stigma (Rybarczyk et al., 1995) have been found to be significantly associated with psychosocial adjustment. However, given the small number of studies addressing these domains, further

research is necessary before substantive conclusions may be reached. Coping (e.g., Desmond, 2007; Desmond & MacLachlan, 2006b) and social support (e.g., Asano et al., 2008; Unwin et al., 2009; Williamson et al., 1994) have received most, albeit still relatively limited, research attention. As limb amputation may be considered a major stressful life event characterized by evolving and recurrent stressors that pose significant challenges (Desmond & Gallagher, 2008), a number of studies have adopted a stress–coping framework investigating the types of coping strategies employed in adapting to limb loss (e.g., Desmond & MacLachlan, 2006b; Gallagher & MacLachlan, 1999; Livneh, Antonak, & Gerhardt, 1999; Livneh, Antonak, & Gerhardt, 2000; Oaksford et al., 2005). In accordance with the broader literature on coping, the use of problem-focused and approach coping appears to be more adaptive than emotion-oriented and avoidant strategies in adjusting to amputation (Desmond, 2007; Desmond & MacLachlan, 2006b; Livneh et al., 1999). The importance of meaning-making and meaning-based coping strategies has also emerged in a number of qualitative studies (Gallagher & MacLachlan, 2000b; Oaksford et al., 2005; Saradjian et al., 2007). For an extended review of issues relating to coping with limb amputation see Desmond and Gallagher (2008).

The importance of the support provided by family and friends in the post-amputation recovery process has been emphasized by both rehabilitation specialists and patients alike (Furst & Humphrey, 1983; Schoppen et al., 2003). Social support is likely to help people adapt to limb loss in a number of different ways. First, people with good social resources are likely to benefit from the assistance offered by these relationships in attempting to renegotiate their physical and social environments following amputation. Indeed, Williams and colleagues (Williams et al., 2004) noted that individuals with amputations who had higher levels of social support consistently reported more time out of bed, out of the house, and in their communities, as well as greater participation in social, leisure, vocational, and other meaningful activities. The presence of high-quality social support after amputation is also likely to enhance psychological well-being by providing the person with the emotional support needed to come to terms with this life-changing experience. Perceived social support has been identified as a significant predictor of both physical and mental health outcomes, including depressed affect (Rybarczyk et al., 1995; Williamson et al., 1994),

QOL (Asano et al., 2008; Rybarczyk et al., 1995), and activity restriction (Williamson et al., 1994). Prospective studies indicate that greater perceived social support aids individuals in both physically and psychologically adjusting to their limb loss over time (Bosse et al., 2002; Hanley et al., 2004; Jensen et al., 2002; Unwin et al., 2009; Williams et al., 2004). In a 2-year prospective study of patients with traumatic lower limb amputations, Bosse and colleagues (2002) reported that reduced levels of perceived social support were predictive of poorer self-reported health status. Jensen and colleagues (2002) found that perceived social support at 1 month post-amputation was a significant independent predictor of improvements in pain interference and depression over the following 5 months. Perceived social support on commencement of rehabilitation has also been found to predict both positive affect and general adjustment to amputation 6 months later, making a significant independent contribution in the case of general adjustment (Unwin et al., 2009).

Assessment

A variety of psychometric instruments have been developed to assess psychosocial outcomes specifically associated with lower limb amputation. These include the Trinity Amputation and Prosthesis Experience Scales (TAPES; Gallagher, Franchignoni, Giordano, & MacLachlan, 2010; Gallagher & MacLachlan, 2000a; Gallagher & MacLachlan, 2004), the Prosthesis Evaluation Questionnaire (PEQ; Boone & Coleman, 2006; Legro et al., 1998), the Orthotics and Prosthetics User's Survey (OPUS; Heinemann, Bode, & O'Reilly, 2003), and the Questionnaire for Persons with a Transfemoral Amputation (Q-TFA; Hagberg, Brånemark, & Haag, 2004). Each of these questionnaires assesses a range of psychological, social, and physical functioning outcomes. A recent review recommends that all of the instruments undergo further testing and use, and suggests that "the TAPES seems especially useful for assessing psychosocial adjustment" (Wolfe et al., 2008, p. 84). The TAPES measures psychosocial adjustment, activity restriction, and satisfaction with the prosthesis, as well as severity and frequency of stump and PLP. It has been translated into more than 10 languages, and used with both lower and upper limb amputation and across the age range from the elderly to children. The revised TAPES (TAPES-R; Gallagher et al., 2010) incorporated a Rasch analysis across several datasets to further strengthen its psychometric properties.

(It is freely available to download: http://www.psychoprosthetics.ie/)

As noted above, body image is a salient factor in adjustment for some people post-amputation; various scales have also been developed to assess body image in people with amputations specifically. Although numerous self-report scales exist, a recent comparative review (Wolfe et al., 2008) noted that each had been used in just a few studies, and none had a strong psychometric evidence base. The only assessment with multiple reports providing data for validity and reliability is the Amputee Body Image Scale (Breakey, 1997), and this scale has also recently been submitted to a Rasch analysis to provide further evidence of its psychometric properties (Gallagher et al., 2007). A range of more generic measures may be used to assess QOL, coping styles, cognitive and executive functioning, and affective disorders; these are not specific to people with amputation and are hence beyond the scope of this review. The use of the Hospital Anxiety and Depression Scale is of note, however, as it was designed to avoid conflating the physical symptoms of depression that may be a primary feature of physical illness or disability, such as amputation. Psychometric properties of the HADS have also been reported for people with amputations (Desmond & MacLachlan, 2005). The use of the TAPES-R, ABIS-R, and HADS for people with amputations may provide a reasonably broad assessment of psychosocial, body image, and affective functioning. These self-report measures, which are relatively quickly and easily administered, can be valuable in complementing routine clinical interviews and in monitoring adaptation and the impact of interventions.

Additionally, in light of the prevalence of amputation due to peripheral vascular disease, the systemic nature of this condition, and the noted increase in age at amputation, screening for cognitive impairments should be considered as part of routine clinical practice for rehabilitation psychologists (O'Neill & Evans, 2009; O'Neill, 2008). A routine cognitive screen for mild cognitive impairment or vascular dementia might include assessment of orientation, immediate and delayed visual and verbal memory, new learning, attention, executive functions, expressive and receptive language, and visuospatial abilities.

Role of the Psychologist in the Interdisciplinary Rehabilitation Team

Wegener et al. (2008) outline four principles guiding psychological care of persons with limb loss:

recognizing that there are biological, psychological, and social dimensions of medical conditions and that it is necessary to consider all relevant factors when assessing and treating a patient (Engel, 1977); adopting a *patient-centered care* approach distinguished by empowering patients through increasing self-efficacy and activation; recognizing that many individuals with physical impairments are *resilient* and that mood disturbances or other psychological symptoms are not inevitable; and appreciating that effective assessment and intervention recognizes, capitalizes on, and develops the *patient's strengths*. Within this approach, patients, who have unique abilities, resources, and experiences, are recognized as the *central workers* in the rehabilitation process.

Key areas for psychologists working in interdisciplinary rehabilitation teams with people with limb loss include providing a psychological perspective within the context of the interdisciplinary team at planning, reviews, family meetings, and discharge planning; assessment of psychosocial outcomes, including anxiety, post-traumatic stress symptoms, depression, coping, QOL, body image, and pain; assessment and interpretation of cognitive abilities using appropriately selected screening tools; formulation of the individual's presenting difficulties in the context of a biopsychosocial framework; providing psychological interventions at an individual level to increase coping skills and self-efficacy and to empower the individual to manage his or her adjustment to limb-loss; facilitating group interventions and peer support using cognitive-behavioral and solution-focused approaches with the aim of normalizing the adjustment process, and provision of psychoeducation around mood management; evaluation of the interventions; application of clinical research knowledge to enhance understanding of the experience of limb loss and to increase the evidence base for effective treatments; and systemically working with individuals and their families to enhance family adjustment and support.

Intervention

After limb loss, individuals may require assistance in managing a number of obstacles in their recovery. We have already noted a range of factors that promote psychosocial adjustment to limb amputation. For some individuals, psychological intervention may be designed to promote successful adaptation and growth. For others who develop significant depression, anxiety, or other maladaptive responses, psychologists will need to utilize specific interventions (MacLachlan, 2004). In addition to affective

disturbances, when addressing intrapersonal issues, such as body image adjustment, and interpersonal issues, such as social stigma, intimacy, and sexual functioning (previously discussed), the clinician must be mindful of substance use. Rates of pre- and post-morbid substance abuse among people with limb loss have not been systematically investigated; the potential for substance abuse to contribute to the development of chronic conditions and/or to slow the rate of recovery is clear, and thus appropriate assessment, and intervention where necessary, is warranted (Wegener et al., 2008).

Several classes of interventions may assist persons with limb loss adapt successfully or manage clinical symptoms or syndromes. With rare exceptions, the efficacy of these interventions for persons with limb loss lacks a strong evidence base. Their utilization with this population is based on data in other populations or on clinical judgment rather than rigorous clinical trials; much remains to be researched in the context of amputation rehabilitation. Here, we briefly consider a variety of interventions that are utilized in the rehabilitation of persons with limb loss.

PEER INTERACTIONS AND SELF-MANAGEMENT

Peer interactions and support groups are premised on the idea that through exposure to successful individuals with similar illnesses or injuries, less experienced persons can learn and adopt more effective behaviors and improve social support (Wegener et al., 2008). Support groups can form part of formal rehabilitation programs or may be facilitated via patient advocacy or consumer organizations. The Peer Visitor Program offered by the Amputee Coalition of America (http://www.amputee-coalition.org), a U.S.-based consumer organization, is perhaps the most widely used model in the context of amputation. Although peer support is often welcomed by patients, there are limited reports of improved outcomes, and the appropriate timing of visits and specific benefits to amputation patients have yet to be empirically established (Wegener et al., 2008).

Self-management (SM) interventions incorporate the principles of cognitive- behavioral theory; key elements include knowledge, self-monitoring, skills acquisition, and problem-solving (Lorig & Holman, 2003). Self-management approaches have gained widespread application with chronic conditions in which pain and disability are common (Wegener et al., 2008). Given secondary conditions, such as depression and pain, that accompany limb amputation, interventions that specifically focus on preventing or reducing these have been developed. One such intervention is the Promoting Amputee Life Skills (PALS) self-management course. This intervention consists of eight weekly 90-minute group sessions followed by a booster session 2 weeks later. The groups are led by trained leaders, one of whom is a person with limb loss. Recently, the first randomized controlled trial (RCT) investigating the effectiveness of this SM intervention for people with amputations found that the PALS program improved the outcomes (i.e., less depression, fewer functional limitations, and higher self-efficacy) of people with limb amputations beyond benefits that would have been offered by support group participation (Wegener, Mackenzie, Ephraim, Ehde, & Williams, 2009). There is considerable scope for research to adapt the PALS program and to assess the impact of its implementation in settings other than the United States, where it was originally developed and trialed. Furthermore, there is scope to explore the delivery of such interventions using new and emerging technologies (Wegener et al., 2008).

PSYCHOTHERAPY

Psychotherapy can take many forms and utilize a variety of techniques. Although data support the beneficial effects of psychotherapy for the typical mental health patient (see Kendall & Chambless, 1998), there are no published controlled trials of psychotherapy specifically focused on persons with limb loss. Most, but not all, of the evidence-based treatments to address psychological difficulties use cognitive-behavioral, behavioral, or interpersonal techniques (Chambless, 2005). Data support specific treatment approaches, as well as suggesting that the therapy relationship accounts for much of the treatment outcome (Wampold, 2001). Primary targets of cognitive-behavioral therapy (CBT) interventions are affective problems such as depressive symptoms, anxiety, and anger. Although there is no specific evidence in persons with limb loss, it is likely that social problems, such as dealing with social stigma and increasing social skills, may also be addressed effectively with CBT (Wegener et al., 2008). Interpersonal psychotherapy (IPT; Klerman, Weissman, Rounsaville, & Chevron, 1984) is appropriate for treatment of acute psychological distress, as well as for treatment of prolonged maintenance of symptoms that are mild to moderate in severity. Interpersonal therapy focuses on relationship issues, but also takes into account the biopsychosocial factors that contribute to the problem. The goal of IPT when working with a person with limb loss would be to assist the individual with identifying and changing unhelpful interpersonal interactions, as well with ameliorating depressive symptoms.

COPING SKILLS AND PROBLEM-SOLVING

In general, coping behaviors that are active and goal-oriented are more helpful to the patient (see Desmond & Gallagher, 2008; Elfström, 2007). Interventions focused on building coping skills should include: analysis of the situation and current coping techniques, description of the problem, goal-setting, and modification of the coping strategies. These steps can be accomplished through brief, structured interventions with the patient (Heim, 1995). *Catastrophizing*, a cognitive response to an event that is marked by exaggerated negative expectations and concerns, has been found to predict both self-reported and objective measures of disability in a variety of chronic pain conditions (Sullivan et al., 2001). Among individuals with limb loss and PLP, catastrophizing predicts increased pain interference, depressive symptoms, self-reported disability, and psychosocial dysfunction (Hill, 1993; Hill, Niven, & Knussen, 1995; Jensen et al., 2002). Cognitive-behavioral therapy interventions for catastrophizing focus on monitoring, challenging, and changing negative thoughts, as well as using behavioral activation to increase self-efficacy. Coping strategies such as distraction, positive self-talk, and increasing activity levels are associated with adjustment to chronic pain (Jensen, Turner, Romano, & Karoly, 1991) and may promote psychological health following limb loss. In addition, individuals who can find some positive meaning from the amputation may have less depression and increased activity levels and better adjustment (Dunn, 1996; Gallagher & MacLachlan, 2000b). Therefore, interventions aimed at finding positive meaning, increasing positive self-talk, and stimulating activity may be beneficial in amputation rehabilitation (Ehde & Wegener, 2008; Wegener et al., 2008).

MEDICATIONS

A wide range of medications may offer relief from symptoms of psychological distress associated with amputation; no RCTs provide data for their efficacy specifically in the limb loss population. A comprehensive discussion of medications that may be appropriate is beyond the scope of this chapter; psychologists working in the biopsychosocial model should seek appropriate medical consultation regarding medication as part of a comprehensive treatment approach (Wegener et al., 2008).

PAIN MANAGEMENT

Sherman (1997) reported that despite some 60 different types of treatment being used with PLP—physical, pharmaceutical, or psychological—evidence for their efficacy was lacking. Although some advances have been made in pharmacology and augmented reality treatments, no treatment has well-supported efficacy. Conventional pain management techniques may effectively treat stump pain, but fail to address the confusion and distress that patients may experience as a result of pain or sensation in the part of their body that has been removed. Although there is still no treatment for PLP that is reliably effective, contemporary interventions used by psychologists include transcutaneous nerve stimulation (TENS), biofeedback, relaxation therapy, and hypnotherapy (see Ehde & Wegener, 2008; McIver & Lloyd, 2010). Recently, there has also been considerable interest in the use of mental imagery, and virtual and augmented reality (e.g., Brodie, Whyte, & Niven, 2007; Cole, Crowle, Austwick, & Henderson Slater, 2009; Desmond, O'Neill, de Paor, Mac Darby, & MacLachlan, 2006; Murray, Patchick, Caillette, Howard, & Pettifer, 2006). Based on the assumption that PLP may arise due to a conflict between the visual and proprioceptive experience of an amputated limb, Ramachandran and Rogers-Ramachandran (1996) suggested that illusionary movement of an amputated limb might alleviate pain by aligning experiences, or by helping to replace a remembered image of a painfully twisted limb with an image in a more relaxed posture. They were able to demonstrate pain relief for some patients, but not for others; these results spurred great interest in the area. Although subsequent research has shown some promise (Darnall, 2009; MacLachlan, McDonald, & Waloch, 2004), there have also been reports of the procedure being distressing and painful for some. For instance, Chan et al. (2007) reported that pain reduction was greater in their mirror therapy group, compared with a covered-mirror control group or an imagery comparison group. However, two of the six patients in the mirror therapy group reported brief grief reactions on viewing their "intact amputated limb"; in the covered-mirror group, three of six patients reported worsening pain; and in the imagery group, four of six reported worsening pain. Based on the same principles, the use of augmented reality (using computer simulation) has also had mixed results.

For example, Desmond, O'Neill, de Paor, et al. (2006) found that one of three participants reported a temporary reduction in pain, one no change at all, and one a worsening of pain. In summary, illusory visual representations of missing limb (through imagery, or virtual or augmented reality techniques) appear to have salience for the pain experience of at least some people with PLP. Larger scale studies that report long-term follow-up are needed, but until then clinicians should be aware of the potential for such interventions to cause distress and increase pain for some patients, while offering the possibility of pain relief—although perhaps only transitory—for others. See Ehde and Wegener (2008) for a review of pain management after limb loss.

NEXT STEPS IN TREATMENT

Programs and services that empower patients and consumers to become active participants in their life-long care are needed to meet the increasing demands placed on them by evolving health care systems that hold both consumers and their providers accountable for successful outcomes. Furthermore, development of the continuum of care beyond the acute time period is needed. Several lines of research suggest approaches that may enhance outcomes and expand the continuum of care. The development and evaluation of programs utilizing peer mentors may be helpful in assisting individuals with new impairments to adapt successfully. Motivational interviewing techniques have been developed and shown to be efficacious in increasing participation in a variety of health behaviors (see Rubak, Sandbæk, Lauritzen, & Christensen, 2005, for review). Finally, it is well recognized that computer-based health information and support systems can be used to disseminate information, link people to needed resources, connect people online who are facing similar challenges, and develop communities of individuals with common interests, aspirations, and needs. Although such innovation is relatively recent, these programs and services have the potential to be successfully utilized by patients with a variety of chronic illnesses, including individuals in underserved populations (Wegener et al., 2008).

Conclusion
Future Directions

There is an increasing body of research investigating and describing the consequences and implications of limb amputation from a psychosocial perspective. Nonetheless, relative to other rehabilitation areas, it remains a nascent area of research, and continued efforts are required to advance understanding, influence practice, and improve person-centered care. As noted previously, the efficacy of interventions for persons with limb loss lacks a strong evidence base; randomized controlled interventions with adequate power and long-term follow-up remain scare in the context of amputation.

Given the incidence and prevalence of limb amputation and the concomitant need for prosthetic interventions, optimizing the prescription and use of prosthetic devices is a priority area. For example, two recent parallel studies provided a forum for patients and service providers to voice their opinions on what they believe to be the important predictors and outcomes involved in successful rehabilitation following upper and lower limb loss (NiMhurchadha, 2010; Schaffalitzky, 2010). These factors provide a guide for rehabilitation professionals in appropriately assessing individuals with limb loss/absence and identifying the important core areas to target in rehabilitation with the hope of improving fitting rates and user satisfaction, and reducing the waste of resources. Outcome measurement in prosthetic prescription currently encompasses a number of different outcomes, and measurement is carried out in a number of different ways (see Hebert et al., 2009; Lindner, Nätterlund, & Hermansson, 2010). This makes it difficult to compare and evaluate different interventions and prosthetic components. By identifying the most important outcomes, to both prosthetic users and service providers, we can progress in standardizing outcome measurement to allow comparison and synthesis across studies. Furthermore, we are better equipped in understanding why and when prosthetic technology should be provided (Schaffalitzky et al., 2010).

Despite the potential for increased risk of cognitive impairment following amputation due to associations with vascular disease and older age, and its apparent importance in the rehabilitation process, there is a dearth of research regarding the prevalence and impacts of cognitive impairment among individuals with limb loss. Greater clarity regarding the prevalence of cognitive impairment and which cognitive abilities or limitations are important in determining outcomes should be prioritized (O'Neill & Evans, 2009).

The World Health Organization International Classification of Functioning and Health (ICF; World Health Organization, 2001) is an important framework through which our understanding of the interactions between people and their environment,

participation, and activities can be enhanced (Gallagher et al., 2011). Recognition of the growing importance of the ICF in the field of amputation and prosthetics is evident in the 2011 special edition of *Prosthetics and Orthotics International* and in recent work undertaken to develop a core set, based on the ICF, for persons following an amputation as means of specifying function (Kohler et al., 2009). Continued efforts are required, however, as a greater understanding of the impact of amputation and type of prosthesis on activity, participation, and environmental barriers is important in terms of facilitating improved management and planning at an individual, service, and societal level (Gallagher et al., 2011).

Research on the impact of amputation on families is lacking, although it is clear that families play critical roles and take substantial responsibility in post-amputation care and recovery. Many individuals will experience significant changes in their own lives as a consequence of their family member's amputation. Nonetheless, investigation of the impacts of amputation—be they negative and/ or positive—on the family is lacking. Finally, as noted above, research on sexuality in amputation is severely limited and much needed.

References

Antonak, R. F., & Livneh, H. (1995). Psychosocial adaptation to disability and its investigation among persons with multiple sclerosis. *Social Science and Medicine, 40*(8), 1099–1108.

Asano, M., Rushton, P., Miller, W. C., & Deathe, B. A. (2008). Predictors of quality of life among individuals who have a lower limb amputation. *Prosthetics and Orthotics International, 32*(2), 231–243.

Atherton, R., & Robertson, N. (2006). Psychological adjustment to lower limb amputation amongst prosthesis users. *Disability and Rehabilitation, 28*(19), 1201–1209.

Badura-Brzoza, K., Matysiakiewicz, J., Piegza, M., Rycerski, W., & Hese, R. (2008). Sense of coherence in patients after limb amputation and in patients after spine surgery. *International Journal of Psychiatry in Clinical Practice, 12*, 41–47.

Behel, J. M., Rybarczyk, B., Elliott, T. R., Nicholas, J. J., & Nyenhuis, D. L. (2002). The role of vulnerability in adjustment to lower extremity amputation: A preliminary investigation. *Rehabilitation Psychology, 47*(1), 92–105.

Bhangu, S., Devlin, M., & Pauley, T. (2009). Outcomes of individuals with transfemoral and contralateral transtibial amputation due to dysvascular etiologies. *Prosthetics and Orthotics International, 33*(1), 33–40.

Biddiss, E. A., & Chau, T. (2007a). Upper-limb prosthetics: Critical factors in device abandonment. *American Journal of Physical Medicine and Rehabilitation, 86*(12), 977–987.

Biddiss, E. A., & Chau, T. (2007b). Upper limb prosthesis use and abandonment: A survey of the last 25 years. *Prosthetics and Orthotics International, 31*(3), 236–257.

Biddiss, E. A., & Chau, T. T. (2008). Multivariate prediction of upper limb prosthesis acceptance or rejection. *Disability and Rehabilitation: Assistive Technology, 3*(4), 181–192.

Bishop, M. (2005). Quality of life and psychosocial adaptation to chronic illness and disability. *Rehabilitation Counseling Bulletin, 48*(4), 219–231.

Boone, D. A., & Coleman, K. L. (2006). Use of the Prosthesis Evaluation Questionnaire (PEQ). *Journal of Prosthetics and Orthotics, 18*(1S), 68–79.

Borsje, S., Bosmans, J. C., Van der Schans, C. P., Geertzen, J. H. B., & Dijkstra, P. U. (2004). Phantom pain: A sensitivity analysis. *Disability and Rehabilitation, 26*(14), 905–910.

Bosse, M. J., MacKenzie, E. J., Kellam, J. F., Burgess, A. R., Webb, L. X., Swiontkowski, M. F., et al. (2002). An analysis of outcomes of reconstruction or amputation after leg-threatening injuries. *New England Journal of Medicine, 347*(24), 1924–1931.

Breakey, J. W. (1997). Body image: The lower limb amputee. *Journal of Prosthetics and Orthotics, 9*(2), 58–66.

Brodie, E. E., Whyte, A., & Niven, C. A. (2007). Analgesia through the looking-glass? A randomized controlled trial investigating the effect of viewing a 'virtual' limb upon phantom limb pain, sensation and movement. *European Journal of Pain, 11*(4), 428–436.

Burger, H., & Marincek, C. (2007). Return to work after lower limb amputation. *Disability and Rehabilitation, 29*(17), 1323–1329.

Burger, H., Marincek, C., & Jaeger, R. J. (2004). Prosthetic device provision to landmine survivors in Bosnia and Herzegovina: Outcomes in 3 ethnic groups. *Archives Of Physical Medicine And Rehabilitation, 85*(1), 19–28.

Callaghan, B., Condie, E., & Johnston, M. (2008). Using the common sense self-regulation model to determine psychological predictors of prosthetic use and activity limitations in lower limb amputees. *Prosthetics and Orthotics International, 32*(3), 324–336.

Cavanagh, S. R., Shin, L. M., Karamouz, N., & Rauch, S. L. (2006). Psychiatric and Emotional Sequelae of Surgical Amputation. *Psychosomatics, 47*(6), 459–464.

Chambless, D. L. (2005). Compendium of empirically supported therapies. In G. Koocher, J. Norcross, & S. Hill (Eds.), *Psychologist desk reference* (pp. 183–192). Oxford: Oxford University Press.

Chan, B. L., Witt, R., Charrow, A. P., Magee, A., Howard, R., Pasquina, P. F., et al. (2007). Mirror therapy for phantom limb pain. *New England Journal of Medicine, 357*(21), 2206–2207.

Coffey, L., Gallagher, P., Horgan, O., Desmond, D., & MacLachlan, M. (2009). Psychosocial adjustment to diabetes-related lower limb amputation. *Diabetic Medicine, 26*(10), 1063–1067.

Cole, J., Crowle, S., Austwick, G., & Henderson Slater, D. (2009). Exploratory findings with virtual reality for phantom limb pain; from stump motion to agency and analgesia. *Disability and Rehabilitation, 31*(10), 846–854.

Couture, M., Caron, C. D., & Desrosiers, J. (2010). Leisure activities following a lower limb amputation. *Disability and Rehabilitation, 32*(1), 57–64.

Couture, M., Desrosiers, J., & Caron, C. D. (2011). Cognitive appraisal and perceived benefits of dysvascular lower limb amputation: A longitudinal study. *Archives of Gerontology and Geriatrics, 52*(1), 5–11.

Cutson, T. M., & Bongiorni, D. R. (1996). Rehabilitation of the older lower limb amputee: A brief review. *Journal of the American Geriatric Society, 44*, 1388–1393.

Darnall, B. D. (2009). Self-delivered home-based mirror therapy for lower limb phantom pain. *American Journal of Physical Medicine and Rehabilitation, 88*(1), 78–81.

Desmond, D. M. (2007). Coping, affective distress and psychosocial adjustment among people with traumatic upper limb amputations. *Journal of Psychosomatic Research, 62*(1), 15–21.

Desmond, D. M., & Gallagher, P. (2008). Coping and psychosocial adjustment to amputation. In P. Gallagher, D. M. Desmond, & M. MacLachlan (Eds.), *Psychoprosthetics: State of the knowledge* (pp. 23–31). London: Springer-Verlag.

Desmond, D. M., Gallagher, P., Henderson-Slater, D., & Chatfield, R. (2008). Pain and psychosocial adjustment to lower limb amputation amongst prosthesis users. *Prosthetics and Orthotics International, 32*(2), 244–252.

Desmond, D., & MacLachlan, M. (2002). Psychosocial issues in the field of prosthetics and orthotics. *Journal of Prosthetics and Orthotics, 14*(1), 19–22.

Desmond, D. M., & MacLachlan, M. (2004). Psychosocial perspectives on postamputation rehabilitation: A review of disease, trauma, and war related literature. *Critical Reviews in Physical and Rehabilitation Medicine, 81*(2), 77–93.

Desmond, D. M., & MacLachlan, M. (2005). The factor structure of the Hospital Anxiety and Depression Scale in older individuals with acquired amputations: A comparison of 4 models using confirmatory factor analysis. *International Journal of Geriatric Psychiatry, 20*, 344–349.

Desmond, D. M., & MacLachlan, M. (2006a). Affective distress and amputation-related pain among older men with long-term, traumatic limb amputations. *Journal of Pain and Symptom Management, 31*(4), 362–368.

Desmond, D. M., & MacLachlan, M. (2006b). Coping strategies as predictors of psychosocial adaptation in a sample of elderly veterans with acquired lower limb amputations. *Social Science and Medicine, 62*(1), 208–216.

Desmond, D. M., & MacLachlan, M. (2010). Prevalence and characteristics of phantom limb pain and residual limb pain in the long term following upper limb amputation. *International Journal of Rehabilitation Research, 33*(3), 279–282.

Desmond, D. M., O'Neill, K., de Paor, A., Mac Darby, G., & MacLachlan, M. (2006). Augmenting the reality of phantom limbs: Three case studies using an augmented mirror box procedure. *Journal of Prosthetics and Orthotics, 18*(3), 74–79.

Dijkstra, P. U., Geertzen, J. H. B., Stewart, R., & van der Schans, C. P. (2002). Phantom pain and risk factors: A multivariate analysis. *Journal of Pain and Symptom Management, 24*(6), 578–585.

Dillingham, T. R., & Pezzin, L. E. (2008). Rehabilitation setting and associated mortality and medical stability among persons with amputations. *Archives of Physical Medicine and Rehabilitation, 89*(6), 1038–1045.

Dillingham, T. R., Pezzin, L., & MacKenzie, E. (1998). Incidence, acute care length of stay, and discharge to rehabilitation of traumatic amputee patients: An epidemiologic study. *Archives of Physical Medicine and Rehabilitation, 79*(3), 279–287.

Dillingham, T. R., Pezzin, L. E., & Shore, A. D. (2005). Reamputation, mortality, and health care costs among persons with dysvascular lower-limb amputations. *Archives of Physical Medicine And Rehabilitation, 86*(3), 480–486.

Donovan-Hall, M. K., Yardley, L., & Watts, R. J. (2002). Engagement in activities revealing the body and psychosocial adjustment in adults with a trans-tibial prosthesis. *Prosthetics and Orthotics International, 26*(1), 15–22.

Dougherty, P. J. (2001). Transtibial amputees from the Vietnam War. Twenty-eight-year follow-up. *The Journal Of Bone And Joint Surgery. American Volume, 83-A*(3), 383–389.

Dougherty, P. J. (2003). Long-term follow-up of unilateral transfemoral amputees from the Vietnam War. *Journal of Trauma: Injury, Infection and Critical Care, 54*(4), 718–723.

Dudkiewicz, I., Gabrielov, R., Seiv-Ner, I., Zelig, G., & Heim, M. (2004). Evaluation of prosthetic usage in upper limb amputees. *Disability and Rehabilitation, 26*(1), 60–63.

Dunn, D. (1996). Well-being following amputation: Salutary effects of positive meaning, optimism and control. *Rehabilitation Psychology, 41*(4), 245–302.

Ehde, D. M., Czerniecki, J. M., Smith, D. G., Campbell, K. M., Edwards, W. T., Jensen, M. P., et al. (2000). Chronic phantom sensations, phantom pain, residual limb pain, and other regional pain after lower limb amputation. *Archives of Physical Medicine and Rehabilitation, 81*(8), 1039–1044.

Ehde, D. M., Smith, D. G., Czerniecki, J. M., Campbell, K. M., Malchow, D. M., & Robinson, L. R. (2001). Back pain as a secondary disability in persons with lower limb amputations. *Archives of Physical Medicine and Rehabilitation, 82*(6), 731–734.

Ehde, D. M., & Wegener, S. T. (2008). Management of chronic pain after limb loss. In P. Gallagher, D. M. Desmond, & M. MacLachlan (Eds.), *Psychoprosthetics: State of the knowledge* (pp. 33–51). London: Springer-Verlag.

Elfström, M. L. (2007). Coping and cognitive behavioural models in physical and psychological rehabilitation. In P. Kennedy (Ed.), *Psychological management of physical disabilities* (pp. 40–57). London: Routledge.

Engel, G. (1977). The need for a new medical model: A challenge for biomedicine. *Science, 196*(4286), 129–136.

Ephraim, P. L., Dillingham, T. R., Sector, M., Pezzin, L. E., & MacKenzie, E. J. (2003). Epidemiology of limb loss and congenital limb deficiency: A review of the literature. *Archives of Physical Medicine and Rehabilitation, 84*(5), 747–761.

Ephraim, P. L., Wegener, S. T., MacKenzie, E. J., Dillingham, T. R., & Pezzin, L. E. (2005). Phantom pain, residual limb pain, and back pain in amputees: Results of a national survey. *Archives of Physical Medicine and Rehabilitation, 86*(10), 1910–1919.

Esquenazi, A. (2004). Amputation rehabilitation and prosthetic restoration. From surgery to community reintegration. *Disability and Rehabilitation, 26*(14), 831–836.

Fergason, J., Keeling, J. J., & Bluman, E. M. (2010). Recent advances in lower extremity amputations and prosthetics for the combat injured patient. *Foot and Ankle Clinics of North America, 15*(1), 151–174.

Fisher, K., & Hanspal, R. S. (1998). Body image and patients with amputations: Does the prosthesis maintain the balance? *International Journal of Rehabilitation Research, 21*(4), 355–363.

Fukunishi, I., Sasaki, K., Chishima, Y., Anze, M., & Saijo, M. (1996). Emotional disturbances in trauma patients during the rehabilitation phase: Studies of posttraumatic stress disorder and alexithymia. *General Hospital Psychiatry, 18*(2), 121–127.

Furst, L., & Humphrey, M. (1983). Coping with the loss of a leg. *Prosthetics and Orthotics International, 7*, 152–156.

Gailey, R., Allen, K., Castles, J., Kucharik, J., & Roeder, M. (2008). Review of secondary physical conditions associated with lower-limb amputation and long-term prosthesis use. *Journal of Rehabilitation Research and Development, 45*(1), 15–30.

Gallagher, P., Allen, D., & MacLachlan, M. (2001). Phantom limb pain and residual limb pain following lower limb amputation: A descriptive analysis. *Disability and Rehabilitation, 23*(12), 522–530.

Gallagher, P., Donovan, M. A., Doyle, A., & Desmond, D. (2011). Environmental barriers, activity limitations and participation restrictions experienced by people with major limb amputation. *Prosthetics and Orthotics International, 35*(3), 278–284.

Gallagher, P., Franchignoni, F., Giordano, A., & MacLachlan, M. (2010). Trinity amputation and prosthesis experience scales: A psychometric assessment using classical test theory and Rasch analysis. *American Journal of Physical Medicine and Rehabilitation, 89*(6), 487–496.

Gallagher, P., Horgan, O., Franchignoni, F., Giordano, A., & MacLachlan, M. (2007). Body image in people with lower-limb amputation: A Rasch analysis of the amputee body image scale. *American Journal of Physical Medicine and Rehabilitation, 86*(3), 205–215.

Gallagher, P., & MacLachlan, M. (1999). Psychological adjustment and coping in adults with prosthetic limbs. *Behavioral Medicine, 25*(3), 117–124.

Gallagher, P., & MacLachlan, M. (2000a). Development and psychometric evaluation of the Trinity Amputation and Prosthesis Experience Scales (TAPES). *Rehabilitation Psychology, 45*(2), 130–154.

Gallagher, P., & MacLachlan, M. (2000b). Positive meaning in amputation and thoughts about the amputated limb. *Prosthetics and Orthotics International, 24*(3), 196–204.

Gallagher, P., & MacLachlan, M. (2001). Adjustment to an artificial limb: A qualitative perspective. *Journal of Health Psychology, 6*(1), 85–100.

Gallagher, P., & MacLachlan, M. (2004). The Trinity Amputation and Prosthesis Experience Scales and quality of life in people with lower-limb amputation. *Archives of Physical Medicine and Rehabilitation, 85*, 730–736.

Geertzen, J. H. B., Van Es, C. G., & Dijkstra, P. U. (2009). Sexuality and amputation: A systematic literature review. *Disability and Rehabilitation, 31*(7), 522–527.

Hagberg, K., & Brånemark, R. (2001). Consequences of non-vascular trans-femoral amputation: A survey of quality of life, prosthetic use and problems. *Prosthetics and Orthotics International, 25*(3), 186–194.

Hagberg, K., Brånemark, R., & Haag, O. (2004). Questionnaire for Persons with a Transfemoral Amputation (Q-TFA): Initial validity and reliability of a new outcome measure. *Journal of Rehabilitation Research and Development, 41*(5), 695–706.

Hamill, R., Carson, S., & Dorahy, M. (2010). Experiences of psychosocial adjustment within 18 months of amputation: An interpretative phenomenological analysis. *Disability and Rehabilitation, 32*(9), 729–740.

Hanley, M., Jensen, M., Ehde, D., Hoffman, A. J., Patterson, D. R., & Robinson, L. R. (2004). Psychosocial predictors of long-term adjustment to lower-limb amputation and phantom limb pain. *Disability and Rehabilitation, 26*(14/15), 882–893.

Hebert, J. S., Wolfe, D. L., Miller, W. C., Deathe, A. B., Devlin, M., & Pallaveshi, L. (2009). Outcome measures in amputation rehabilitation: ICF body functions. *Disability and Rehabilitation, 31*(19), 1541–1554.

Heikkinen, M., Saarinen, J., Suominen, V. P., Virkkunen, J., & Salenius, J. (2007). Lower limb amputations: Differences between the genders and long-term survival. *Prosthetics and Orthotics International, 31*(3), 277–286.

Heim, E. (1995). Coping-based intervention strategies. *Patient Education and Counseling, 26*(1–3), 145–151.

Heinemann, A., Bode, R., & O'Reilly, C. (2003). Development and measurement properties of the Orthotics and Prosthetics Users' Survey (OPUS): A comprehensive set of clinical outcome instruments. *Prosthetics and Orthotics International, 27*(3), 191–206.

Hill, A. (1993). The use of pain coping strategies by patients with phantom limb pain. *Pain, 55*, 347–353.

Hill, A., Niven, C. A., & Knussen, C. (1995). The role of coping in adjustment to phantom limb pain. *Pain, 62*(1), 79–86.

Horgan, O., & MacLachlan, M. (2004). Psychosocial adjustment to lower-limb amputation: A review. *Disability and Rehabilitation, 26*(14/15), 837–850.

Ide, M. (2004). Sexuality in persons with limb amputation: A meaningful discussion of re-integration. *Disability and Rehabilitation, 26*(14/15), 939–943.

Jensen, M. P., Ehde, D. M., Hoffman, A. J., Patterson, D. R., Czerniecki, J. M., & Robinson, L. R. (2002). Cognitions, coping and social environment predict adjustment to phantom limb pain. *Pain, 95*(1–2), 133–142.

Jensen, M. P., Turner, J. A., Romano, J. M., & Karoly, P. (1991). Coping with chronic pain: A critical review of the literature. *Pain, 47*, 249–283.

Kendall, P. C., & Chambless, D. L. (1998). Empirically supported psychological therapies. *Journal of Consulting and Clinical Psychology, 66*, 3–167.

Kennedy, P., & Rogers, B. (2000). Anxiety and depression after spinal cord injury: A longitudinal analysis. *Archives of Physical Medicine and Rehabilitation, 81*(7), 932–937.

Klapheke, M. M., Marcell, C., Taliaferro, G., & Creamer, B. (2000). Psychiatric assessment of candidates for hand transplantation. *Microsurgery, 20*(8), 453–457.

Klerman, G. L., Weissman, M. M., Rounsaville, B. J., & Chevron, E. S. (1984). *Interpersonal psychotherapy of depression.* New York: Basic Books.

Kohler, F., Cieza, A., Stucki, G., Geertzen, J., Burger, H., Dillon, M. P., et al. (2009). Developing core sets for persons following amputation based on the international classification of functioning, disability and health as a way to specify functioning. *Prosthetics and Orthotics International, 33*(2), 117–129.

Larner, S., Van Ross, E., & Hale, C. (2003). Do psychological measures predict the ability of lower limb amputees to learn to use a prosthesis? *Clinical Rehabilitation, 17*(5), 493–498.

Legro, M. W., Reiber, G. E., Smith, D. G., del Aguila, M., Larsen, J. A., & Boone, D. A. (1998). Prosthesis Evaluation Questionnaire for people with lower limb amputations: Assessing prosthesis-related quality of life. *Archives of Physical Medicine and Rehabilitation, 79*(8), 931–938.

Lindner, H., Nätterlund, B., & Hermansson, L. (2010). Upper limb prosthetic outcome measures: Review and content comparison based on International Classification of Functioning, Disability and Health. *Prosthetics And Orthotics International, 34*(2), 109–128.

Livneh, H. (2001). Psychosocial adaptation to chronic illness and disability: A conceptual framework. *Rehabilitation Counseling Bulletin, 44*(3), 151–160.

Livneh, H., & Antonak, R. F. (1997). *Psychosocial adaptation to chronic illness and disability.* Gaithersburg, MD: Aspen Publishers.

Livneh, H., Antonak, R. F., & Gerhardt, J. (1999). Psychosocial adaptation to amputation: The role of sociodemographic variables, disability related factors and coping strategies. *International Journal of Rehabilitation Research, 22*(1), 21–31.

Livneh, H., Antonak, R. F., & Gerhardt, J. (2000). Multidimensional investigation of the structure of coping among people with amputations. *Psychosomatics, 41*(3), 235–244.

Lorig, K. R., & Holman, H. (2003). Self-management education: History, definition, outcomes, and mechanisms. *Annals of Behavioral Medicine, 26*(1), 1–7.

MacLachlan, M. (2004). *Embodiment: Clinical, critical and cultural perspectives.* Milton Keynes: Open University Press.

MacLachlan, M., & Gallagher, P. (Eds.). (2004). *Enabling technologies: Body image and body function.* Edinburgh: Churchill Livingstone.

MacLachlan, M., McDonald, D., & Waloch, J. (2004). Mirror treatment of lower limb phantom pain: A case study. *Disability and Rehabilitation, 26*(14/15), 901–904.

McIver, K., & Lloyd, D. (2010). Management of phantom limb pain. In C. D. Murray (Ed.), *Amputation, prosthesis use, and phantom limb pain: An interdisciplinary perspective* (pp. 157–174). London: Springer.

Miller, W., Deathe, A., Speechley, M., & Koval, J. (2001). The influence of falling, fear of falling, and balance confidence on prosthetic mobility and social activity among individuals with a lower extremity amputation. *Archives of Physical Medicine and Rehabilitation, 82*(9), 1238–1244.

Murray, C. D. (2010). Understanding adjustment and coping to limb loss and absence through phenomenologies of prosthesis use. In C. D. Murray (Ed.), *Amputation, prosthesis use, and phantom limb pain: An interdisciplinary perspective* (pp. 81–99). London: Springer.

Murray, C. D., & Fox, J. (2002). Body image and prosthesis satisfaction in the lower limb amputee. *Disability and Rehabilitation, 24*(17), 925–931.

Murray, C. D., Patchick, E. L., Caillette, F., Howard, T., & Pettifer, S. (2006). Can immersive virtual reality reduce phantom limb pain? *Studies in Health Technology and Informatics, 119*, 407–412.

National Amputee Statistical Database. (2009). *The amputee statistical database for the United Kingdom 2006/07.* Edinburgh, Common Services Agency/Crown Copyright 2009.

NiMhurchadha, S. (2010). *Developing consensus on what constitutes "success" following upper limb loss rehabilitation.* Unpublished doctoral thesis, Dublin City University, Dublin, Ireland.

Novotny, M. (1991). Psychosocial issues affecting rehabilitation. *Prosthetics, 2*, 373–393.

O'Neill, B., Moran, K., & Gillespie, A. (2010). Scaffolding rehabilitation behaviour using a voice-mediated assistive technology for cognition. *Neuropsychological Rehabilitation, 20*(4), 509–527.

O'Neill, B. F. (2008). Cognition and mobility rehabilitation following lower limb amputation. In P. Gallagher, D. M. Desmond & M. MacLachlan (Eds.), *Psychoprosthetics* (pp. 53–65). London: Springer-Verlag.

O'Neill, B. F., & Evans, J. J. (2009). Memory and executive function predict mobility rehabilitation outcome after lower-limb amputation. *Disability and Rehabilitation, 31*(13), 1083–1091.

Oaksford, K., Frude, N., & Cuddihy, R. (2005). Positive coping and stress-related psychological growth following lower limb amputation. *Rehabilitation Psychology, 50*(3), 266–277.

Pereira, B. P., Kour, A., Leow, E., & Pho, R. W. H. (1996). Benefits and use of digital prostheses. *Journal of Hand Surgery—American Volume, 21A*(2), 222–228.

Pezzin, L., Dillingham, T., & MacKenzie, E. (2000). Rehabilitation and the long-term outcomes of persons with trauma-related amputations. *Archives of Physical Medicine and Rehabilitation, 81*(3), 292–300.

Phelps, L. F., Williams, R. M., Raichle, K. A., Turner, A. P., & Ehde, D. M. (2008). The importance of cognitive processing to adjustment in the 1st year following amputation. *Rehabilitation Psychology, 53*(1), 28–38.

Ploeg, A. J., Lardenoye, J.-W., Vrancken Peeters, M.-P. F. M., & Breslau, P. J. (2005). Contemporary series of morbidity and mortality after lower limb amputation. *European Journal of Vascular and Endovascular Surgery, 29*(6), 633–637.

Price, E. M., & Fisher, K. (2002). How does counseling help people with amputation? *Journal of Prosthetics and Orthotics, 14*(3), 102–106.

Ramachandran, V. S., & Rogers-Ramachandran, D. (1996). Synaesthesia in phantom limbs induced with mirrors. *Proceedings of the Royal Society of London B: Biological Sciences, 263*(1369), 377–386.

Renzi, R., Unwin, N., Jubelirer, R., & Haag, L. (2006). An international comparison of lower extremity amputation rates. *Annals of Vascular Surgery, 20*(3), 346–350.

Rubak, S., Sandbæk, A., Lauritzen, T., & Christensen, B. (2005). Motivational interviewing: A systematic review and meta-analysis. *British Journal of General Practice, 55*(513), 305–312.

Rybarczyk, B., Edwards, R., & Behel, J. M. (2004). Diversity in adjustment to a leg amputation: Case illustrations of common themes. *Disability and Rehabilitation, 26*(14/15), 944–953.

Rybarczyk, B., Nicholas, J. J., & Nyenhuis, D. L. (1997). Coping with a leg amputation: Integrating research and clinical practice. *Rehabilitation Psychology, 42*(3), 241–256.

Rybarczyk, B., Nyenhuis, D. L., Nicholas, J. J., Cash, S. M., & Kaiser, J. (1995). Body image, perceived social stigma, and the prediction of psychosocial adjustment to leg amputation. *Rehabilitation Psychology, 40*(2), 95–110.

Rybarczyk, B., Nyenhuis, D. L., Nicholas, J. J., Schulz, R., Alioto, R. J., & Blair, C. (1992). Social discomfort and depression in a sample of adults with leg amputations. *Archives of Physical Medicine and Rehabilitation, 73*(12), 1169–1173.

Rybarczyk, B. D., & Behel, J. M. (2008). Limb loss and body image. In P. Gallagher, D. M. Desmond & M. MacLachlan (Eds.), *Psychoprosthetics: State of the knowledge* (pp. 23–33). London: Springer-Verlag.

Saradjian, A., Thompson, A. R., & Datta, D. (2007). The experience of men using an upper limb prosthesis following amputation: Positive coping and minimizing feeling different. *Disability and Rehabilitation, 30*(11), 871–883.

Schaffalitzky, E. (2010). *Optimising the prescription and use of lower limb prosthetic technology: A mixed methods approach.* Unpublished doctoral thesis, Dublin City University, Dublin, Ireland.

Schaffalitzky, E., Gallagher, P., MacLachlan, M., & Ryall, N. (2010). Understanding the benefits of prosthetic prescription. *Disability and Rehabilitation, 33*(15–16), 1314–1323.

Schaffalitzky, E., Ni Mhurchadha, S., Gallagher, P., Hofkamp, S., MacLachlan, M., & Wegener, S. T. (2009). Identifying the values and preferences of prosthetic users: A case study series using the repertory grid technique. *Prosthetics and Orthotics International, 33*(2), 157–166.

Schofield, C. J., Libby, G., Brennan, G. M., MacAlpine, R. R., Morris, A. D., & Leese, G. P. (2006). Mortality and hospitalization in patients after amputation: A comparison between patients with and without diabetes. *Diabetes Care, 29*, 2252–2256.

Schoppen, T., Boonstra, A., Groothoff, J. W., de Vries, J., Goeken, L. N., & Eisma, W. (2003). Physical, mental, and social predictors of functional outcome in unilateral lower limb amputees. *Archives of Physical Medicine and Rehabilitation, 84*(6), 803–811.

Schoppen, T., Boonstra, A., Groothoff, J. W., de Vries, J., Goeken, L. N., & Eisma, W. H. (2001). Employment status, job characteristics, and work-related health experience of people with a lower limb amputation in The Netherlands. *Archives of Physical Medicine and Rehabilitation, 82*(s), 239–245.

Sherman, R. A. (1997). *Phantom pain*. New York: Plenum.

Singh, R., Ripley, D., Pentland, B., Todd, I., Hunter, J., Hutton, L., et al. (2009). Depression and anxiety symptoms after lower limb amputation: The rise and fall. *Clinical Rehabilitation, 23*(3), 281–286.

Sjödahl, C., Gard, G., & Jarnlo, G. B. (2004). Coping after trans-femoral amputation due to trauma or tumour—a phenomenological approach. *Disability and Rehabilitation, 26*(14–15), 851–861.

Smit, G., & Plettenburg, D. H. (2010). Efficiency of voluntary closing hand and hook prostheses. *Prosthetics and Orthotics International, 34*(4), 411–427.

Sullivan, M. J. L., Thorn, B., Haythornthwaite, J. A., Keefe, F., Martin, M., Bradley, L. A., et al. (2001). Theoretical perspectives on the relation between catastrophizing and pain. *Clinical Journal of Pain, 17*(1), 52–64.

Taylor, S. E. (1983). Adjustment to threatening events: A theory of cognitive adaptation. *American Psychologist, 38*(11), 1161–1173.

Unwin, J., Kacperek, L., & Clarke, C. (2009). A prospective study of positive adjustment to lower limb amputation. *Clinical Rehabilitation, 23*(11), 1044–1050.

Unwin, N. (2000). Epidemiology of lower extremity amputation in centres in Europe, North America and East Asia. *British Journal of Surgery, 87*(3), 328–337.

van der Schans, C. P., Geertzen, J. H. B., Schoppen, T., & Dijkstra, P. U. (2002). Phantom pain and health-related quality of life in lower limb amputees. *Journal of Pain and Symptom Management, 24*(4), 429–436.

van der Sluis, C. K., Hartman, P. P., Schoppen, T., & Dijkstra, P. U. (2009). Job adjustments, job satisfaction and health experience in upper and lower limb amputees. *Prosthetics and Orthotics International, 33*(1), 41–51.

van Velzen, J. M., van Bennekom, C. A., Polomski, W., Slootman, J. R., van der Woude, L. H., & Houdijk, H. (2006). Physical capacity and walking ability after lower limb amputation: A systematic review. *Clinical Rehabilitation, 20*(11), 999–1016.

Wampold, B. (2001). *The great psychotherapy debate: Models, methods and findings*. Mahwah, NJ: Erlbaum.

Wegener, S. T., Hofkamp, S. E., & Ehde, D. M. (2008). Interventions for psychological issues in amputation. In P. Gallagher, D. M. Desmond, & M. MacLachlan (Eds.), *Psychoprosthetics: State of the knowledge* (pp. 91–105). London: Springer-Verlag.

Wegener, S. T., Mackenzie, E. J., Ephraim, P., Ehde, D., & Williams, R. (2009). Self-management improves outcomes in persons with limb loss. *Archives of Physical Medicine and Rehabilitation, 90*(3), 373–380.

Whyte, A. S., & Carroll, L. J. (2004). The relationship between catastrophizing and disability in amputees experiencing phantom pain. *Disability and Rehabilitation, 26*(11), 649–654.

Williams, A. C. d. C., Rajput-Ray, M., Lassalle, X., Crombie, I., & Lacoux, P. (2011). Assessing pain and mood in a poorly resourced country in a postconflict setting. *Journal of Pain and Symptom Management, 42*(2), 301–307.

Williams, R., Ehde, D., Smith, D., Czerniecki, J., Hoffman, A., & Robinson, L. (2004). A two-year longitudinal study of social support following amputation. *Disability and Rehabilitation, 26*(14–15), 862–874.

Williamson, G. M., & Schulz, R. (1995). Activity restriction mediates the association between pain and depressed affect: A study of younger and older adult cancer patients. *Psychology and Aging, 10*(3), 369–378.

Williamson, G. M., Schulz, R., Bridges, M. W., & Behan, A. M. (1994). Social and psychological factors in adjustment to limb amputation. *Journal of Social Behavior and Personality, 9*(5), 249–268.

Wolfe, D. L., Hebert, J. S., Miller, W. C., Deathe, A. B., Devlin, M., & Pallaveshi, L. (2008). Psychological adjustment to lower limb amputation: An evaluation of outcome measurement tools. In P. Gallagher, D. M. Desmond, & M. MacLachlan (Eds.), *Psychoprosthetics* (pp. 67–90). London: Springer.

World Health Organization. (2001). *ICF: International classification of functioning, disability and health*. Geneva: World Health Organization.

Ziegler-Graham, K., MacKenzie, E. J., Ephraim, P. L., Travison, T. G., & Brookmeyer, R. (2008). Estimating the prevalence of limb loss in the United States: 2005 to 2050. *Archives of Physical Medicine and Rehabilitation, 89*(3), 422–429.

21 Transplantation

Bruce Rybarczyk, Andrea Shamaskin, Douglas Gibson, *and* Solam T. Huey

Abstract

Solid organ transplantations have become a routine medical procedure, with more than 28,000 performed in the United States alone each year. However, for the individual undergoing a transplant, it is anything but routine. A myriad of psychological challenges are faced by individuals at each stage of the process. This chapter begins with a description of the most common solid organ transplantations: kidney, liver, heart, lung, and heart–lung. It then provides an overview of the potential roles of the psychologist in the different stages of the transplant process and the psychological aspects of the process for the patient: being a candidate for transplant; the waiting period; the transplant surgery and postsurgical period; and, finally, long-term rehabilitation. Case studies are introduced to illustrate the role of psychologists in the pre-transplant evaluation and potential treatments to facilitate adjustment to transplantation. Finally, a discussion on the ethics of organ allocation, with a special emphasis on the role of psychologists, will be provided.

Key Words: Transplantation, solid organ, psychological aspects, pre-transplant evaluation, psychologist, rehabilitation, ethics.

The latter half of the 20th century witnessed the transformation of organ transplantation from a headline grabbing medical miracle to a routine procedure performed on over 28,000 patients in 2009. Since the first successful kidney transplant performed in 1954, and the first successful lung and heart transplants in 1967, the field of transplant medicine has seen substantial breakthroughs in both survival rates and quality of life (QOL) among transplant patients. The watershed event during the early 1980s was the introduction of the immuno-suppressant cyclosporine. Prior to cyclosporine, there was only a 50% survival rate after transplant, and only 10 transplant centers existed worldwide. Within a few years, there were over 1,000 transplant centers worldwide (Calne, 2008). The dramatic rise in liver transplants in Europe in the past 30 years is illustrated in Figure 21.1. In the United States,

both kidney and liver transplants have shown a general increasing trend since 1988, the earliest year that the Organ Procurement and Transplantation Network (OPTN) published data (see Table 21.1). Rates of heart transplant, on the other hand, rose significantly until 1990 and have changed very little since, with the limited number of donor hearts acting as a cap on the number of annual transplants.

Overall, as seen in Table 21.1, in the United States, there are many more patients on the waiting list than the number of transplants completed per year, which demonstrates the problem of demand being much higher than supply. The United States has a moderate rate of organ donation relative to other countries worldwide. Countries with the highest rates usually have an "opt-out" system of organ donation (e.g., Spain), in which individuals are automatically assumed to be willing donors unless they specify otherwise.

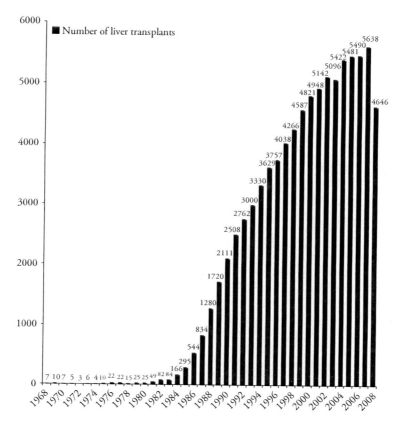

Figure 21.1 Liver transplants in Europe by year.

Even though progress in transplant medicine has been remarkable, any individual fortunate enough to receive an organ still faces formidable physical and psychological challenges in the immediate aftermath of a transplant and the years beyond. Organ transplantation is much more than a surgical procedure, and unique issues arise at each stage of the process, both before and after the transplant. After a review of the types of solid organ transplants considered in this chapter, we will focus on the psychosocial issues that are present in each of the transplant stages and the potential role of psychologists in each of those stages. Case studies will be provided to illustrate these issues and roles, as well as a discussion of unique ethical challenges for psychologists involved in organ allocation decisions.

Types of Solid Organ Transplant
Kidney

Kidney transplants are the most common transplant procedures performed in the United States, with the longest waiting list and average waiting time among solid organ transplants. Patients with advanced and permanent kidney failure may be eligible for a kidney transplant. End-stage renal disease (ESRD) occurs when the kidneys are unable to remove wastes and manage electrolytes in the body, causing harmful wastes to build up in the body (Barry, Jordan, & Conlin, 2007). In the United States, diabetes is the most common cause of end-stage kidney disease, but other causes include high blood pressure, certain autoimmune disorders, or congenital defects of the kidneys, such as polycystic kidney disease. These patients often start dialysis treatment before beginning the transplant process or while they are on the waiting list. Kidney dialysis filters a patient's blood to get rid of harmful waste, excess water, and salt; however, it is a disruptive, time-consuming process and therefore limits QOL (Olbrisch, Benedict, Ashe, & Levenson, 2002).

A donated kidney can come from a living donor (related or unrelated) or a deceased donor. Transplants using living donors are becoming more common as a result of the widespread use of the laparoscopic nephrectomy procedure, which makes the transplant procedure less painful and with a quicker recovery time for the donors. (Brown, Biehl, Rawlins, & Hefty, 2001). An interesting trend in kidney transplant procedures

Table 21.1 United States organ transplant rates from 1988–2009, 1-year survival rates, and patients on waiting lists

	Number of U.S. transplants in 1988	Number of U.S. transplants in 2011	Average survival rates 1 year post-transplant	Number of patients on wait-list as of January 10, 2012
Heart	1,676	1,954	87.5%	3,111
Kidney	8,878	13,931	95.9%	90,488
Liver	1,713	5,288	86.5%	16,079
Lung	33	1,516	83.3%	1,659
Heart–Lung	74	20	67.5%	63

Based on Organ Procurement and Transplantation Network (OPTN) data as of January 6, 2012.

is the increasingly common *never-ending altruistic donor* chain (NEAD). In a NEAD chain, when a recipient's willing donor is found to be incompatible, he or she gives his or her kidney to someone else with whom they are found to be compatible. Next, motivated by altruistic beliefs, that person's willing but incompatible donor can then donate to someone else who is a good match. The longest NEAD chain to date has included 16 kidney transplantations, performed at Georgetown University Hospital, in Washington, D.C. in November of 2010. A simpler pilot program employed with increasing success in the past 3 years employs a national database to arrange swaps of incompatible would-be kidney donors to create matched donor pairs (Bingaman, Wright, & Murphy, 2010). Both methods represent an innovative and creative approach for the future of kidney transplant and, if replicated nationally, may add up to 2,000 live donor transplantations annually in the United states alone (Bingaman et al., 2010; Rees et al., 2009). Although beyond the scope of this chapter, psychologists often play a role in evaluating living donors to confirm that they are not coerced, that they fully understand the risks involved, and that they have the capacity to consent to being a living donor.

LIVER

Patients with end-stage liver disease (ESLD) may be eligible for liver transplant. Liver failure may be acute (fulminant or subfulminant liver failure) or chronic. Chronic liver failure is often the result of decompensated cirrhosis from alcohol abuse or hepatitis. The most common indication today for liver transplant is cirrhosis from chronic hepatitis C infection (Merion, 2010), which is usually associated with alcohol-related liver disease. In the United States, chronic hepatitis B has become a less

common indication for transplant; however, in other areas of the world where hepatitis B is more prevalent, it remains the most common indication for transplant. Patient with certain liver cancers, such as early-stage hepatocellular carcinoma (HCC), can also be considered for liver transplant (Koffron & Stein, 2008). Emergency liver transplants may also occur as a result of suicide attempts that involve acetaminophen overdose (Wiesner, 1996).

End-stage liver disease is the sixth most common cause of death for Americans between the ages of 45 and 54 (Xu, Kochanek, Murphy, & Tejada-Vera, 2010). Patients with liver failure may be placed on the national waiting list, where approximately 12% of those on the list die each year waiting for a liver (Merion, 2010). The large majority of transplanted livers come from deceased donors; however, there was an increasing trend through the 1990s for liver transplants to come from living donors (Merion, 2010). Particularly for younger children (<2 years), living donor graft has the lowest risk of graft failure compared to deceased donor organ sources (Roberts, Hulbert-Shearon, Merion, Wolfe, & Port, 2004). Adult living donor liver transplants, on the other hand, are somewhat risky since the procedure involves splitting the donor's liver and donating a portion to the recipient (the donor's liver regenerates and achieves full volume and function within 2 months). As a result of these risks, the number of living donor transplants in the United States was reduced by half from 2001 to 2007. Within the field of liver transplant, one of the current goals and areas of research is to explore the use and safety of living donors, keeping in mind both the recipient's and donor's health.

HEART

Patients with end-stage heart failure and classified with New York Heart Association class IV heart failure are eligible for heart transplant (HT) consideration. Those with class IV heart failure experience symptoms of cardiac insufficiency even at rest, and these symptoms cannot be managed through standard treatment (Jessup et al., 2009). Common etiologies of heart failure include coronary artery disease, cardiomyopathy, or a congenital heart defect, which is the most common cause of heart failure in children. Patients suffering from heart failure experience symptoms of fatigue, shortness of breath upon exertion, or rapid or irregular heart beat. Prior to a heart transplant, some patients will receive an implantable medical device such as a left ventricular assist device (LVAD). An LVAD helps pump blood from the lower left heart chamber to the rest of the body, and it is often considered a "bridge to transplant" (Slaughter et al., 2009). Research indicates that new improvements in technology and use of continuous flow LVADs improve QOL and functioning for patients (Slaughter et al., 2009). Left ventricular assist devices may also be used as "destination treatment," meaning that the patient would not necessarily be considered for transplantation but may benefit from the device as it can improve QOL and functioning. In other cases, the LVAD can be a temporary treatment that could later be removed as cardiac functioning improves.

LUNG AND HEART–LUNG

Lung transplant may be an option for patients with chronic obstructive pulmonary disease (COPD), pulmonary fibrosis, cystic fibrosis, primary pulmonary hypertension, or congenital heart disease. In the late 1980s and in the 1990s, indication for lung transplant expanded to include parenchymal lung disease (Deuse et al., 2010). The general category of lung transplant includes several different types (National Heart, Lung, and Blood Institute, 2010). A single-lung transplant involves replacing one unhealthy lung in a transplant recipient with a healthy donor lung. A double-lung transplant occurs when a patient requires both lungs to be replaced, which is often the case with cystic fibrosis patients. For both single- and double-lung transplants, the donated organ often comes from a donor who has been pronounced brain dead. A lobe transplant surgery involves a living donor, and the healthy donor provides a lobe or segment of his or her lung to a recipient. Last, heart–lung transplant may be a viable option for patients whose heart and lungs have both been affected by a disease (Olbrisch et al., 2002). For example, patients who have primary pulmonary hypertension or Eisenmenger's complex, a congenital heart defect with an abnormal connection between the heart and lung systems, would be considered for a heart–lung transplant. This is a relatively rare procedure, however, and in 2011 only 24 heart–lung transplant procedures were performed in the United States.

There has been international growth in the number of lung transplant procedures over the last 20 years (Christie et al., 2010). In 2008, there were 2,769 lung transplant procedures reported to the Registry of the International Society for Heart and Lung Transplantation. However, heart–lung transplant rates have been decreasing internationally since the mid-1990s, in a similar fashion to the decreasing trend in the United States.

The Path to Transplantation

In the United States, the transplant process usually begins when patients receive a referral from a physician to contact a transplant center. Patients are given a status code indicating how medically urgent it is for them to receive a transplant. For example, with heart transplant, status 1A patients are critically ill and often stay in intensive care units, status 1B patients need special intravenous medications for their heart but may stay at home if they are medically able, and status 2 patients are not hospitalized nor do they require intravenous medications while they wait. At the transplant center, patients are evaluated by a multidisciplinary team of physicians, nurses, social workers, and psychologists to assess suitability for organ transplant. One purpose of this evaluation is to predict whether the patient will be able to survive the surgery, and to assess how well he or she will adhere to the complex post-transplant medical regimen. If the patient is determined eligible to receive an organ transplant, he or she is placed on the United Network of Organ Sharing (UNOS) national transplant waiting list. As a part of the U.S. Department of Health and Human Services, UNOS monitors every organ allocation and matches donor organs to recipients across the country.

Once on the waiting list, waiting times can vary between patients and are dependent upon numerous factors. One main factor affecting waiting time is patient status code, with higher status codes having highest priority status. For example, status 1A patients are offered first any available donor hearts. Status 1B patients are offered hearts if there no suitable status 1A patients, and, finally, status 2 patients are offered hearts if there are no suitable recipients who are status 1A or 1B. Between 2003 and 2004, the median waiting time was 50 days for heart status 1A patients, 78 days for Heart status 1B patients, and 309 days for heart status 2 patients (OPTN data). Aside from heart status, other factors that can affect waiting list time include blood type, tissue type, height and weight of transplant candidate, size of donated organ, time on the waiting list, distance between recipient's hospital and the potential donor organ, number of donors in the local area over a period of time, and the transplant center's criteria for accepting organ offers. UNOS policies allow patients to register for a transplant at more than one hospital, which is referred to as "multiple listing." Although multiple listing does not guarantee that an organ will become available more quickly, it allows a patient to be considered for donor organs that become available in more than one local area. Each transplant hospital, however, has its own rules about allowing patients to be listed at another hospital, and patients will often have to go through a separate evaluation at each transplant center, even if they are listed at another hospital. One unintended consequence of the multiple listing option is that people who have the finances for the additional travel and evaluations have greater access to organs.

When an organ becomes available, an organ procurement organization (OPO) sends the donor information to UNOS, including organ condition and size, blood type, and tissue type. UNOS creates a list of potential recipient candidates who have profiles that are compatible with the donor. A computer system ranks candidates by their biological information, clinical characteristics, and time spent on the waiting list. A transplant center is then notified if one of their patients appears on the local list. The organ is offered to the transplant team representing a patient, and the team has 1 hour to decide whether to accept or refuse the organ based on organ condition, recipient condition, and availability of the patient and staff, as well as organ transportation. If the transplant team declines the organ, the OPO offers it to other transplant centers until it is accepted.

The path to transplantation can have a large impact on psychological adjustment during the waiting period and beyond, and the pathway can be very different for patients, depending on a number of variables. For example, liver transplantation patients may experience an extensive period of pre-transplantation illness and a downward spiral of health. Many of these patients will not be transplanted until their MELD score (Measure of End-stage Liver Disease) reaches a high enough

level. Although these patients may experience an extensive period of illness, they also have a relatively long period of time to mentally plan and ultimately cope with the situation. In contrast, other liver transplantation patients are seen on a more emergent basis. Fulminant liver failure patients by definition are seen and evaluated while in an acute state. Consequently, they have little if any time to contemplate organ transplantation, and in fact they are frequently unconscious and uninvolved in the decision process. Fulminant liver failure patients often awake to discover they have undergone liver transplantation, and this presents the patient and family with a unique set of adjustment issues.

When there is a lengthy waiting period, the experience can be highly stressful. The experience of waiting for an organ to become available while the disease advances and becomes more life-threatening has been described as a "dance with death" (Kuhn, Davis, & Lippmann, 1988). Patients on the waiting list for heart transplantation, in particular, often have the longest hospitalizations prior to the procedure. It is not unusual for these patients to be confined to a hospital for many months up to a year or longer before undergoing the procedure. These patients can often be treated using newer technology, such as the total artificial heart and or LVAD, which can serve as a bridge to transplant.

Another group that presents with distinct circumstances is the kidney transplantation population. In this population, the procedure is, in a sense, elective, in that patients have the option of hemodialysis. Kidney transplantation patients therefore must decide whether to continue dialysis or undergo transplantation; but, in the end, they have a choice in the matter. Unlike heart and liver transplantation patients, the kidney transplantation population approaches the surgery aware that dialysis is available should transplantation fail. It is increasingly more common for kidney transplants to occur after a living donor has provided a kidney. This situation provides for its own unique set of circumstances, since patients typically receive an organ from a loved one or family member and can often prepare for the process in advance.

Psychologists' Role in Pre-transplant Evaluation and Waiting Period

The goals of the pre-transplant psychological evaluation are to complete a comprehensive psychosocial assessment and to identify potential risk factors that could be contraindicative to post-transplant recovery and long-term treatment success.

Increased risk of noncompliance with medications post-transplant can result in infections, organ rejection, and morbidity. The scarcity of donor organs relative to the number of individuals needing organs and the high cost of organ transplant makes evaluation of each patient's likelihood of success essential (Olbrisch, 1996; Olbrisch et al., 2002). It is imperative to employ a consistent and reliable set of psychosocial selection criteria from which to evaluate patients for organ transplantation in order to ensure that the selection process is not based on unfair, unlawful, or discriminatory practices (Orentlicher, 1996). The primary purpose of utilizing psychosocial assessments is to give access to all patients who meet the criteria and have a reasonable probability for a favorable outcome by placing them on the waiting list to compete for available donor organs (Olbrisch, 1996).

In addition to selecting suitable candidates for organ transplantation, the pre-transplant psychological evaluation also aims to assess patients' current cognitive functioning and vulnerability for developing cognitive impairments, assess patients' knowledge and capacity for consent for transplant, assess patients' capability of handling the stress of transplant surgery and post-transplant recovery, educate patients on the transplant process and prepare them for adhering to a rigorous medical regimen post-transplant, identify any current psychosocial issues that could potentially affect patients' adjustment pre- or post-transplant, assess the support needs of patients and their families through the transplant process, assess any history of or ongoing substance use/abuse and current tobacco use (a contraindication at most transplant centers), and lay the groundwork for effective interventions that might be required at a later time in the transplant process (Collins & Labott, 2007; Olbrisch, 1996). Those who do not meet the selection criteria for organ transplantation at the time of the psychosocial evaluation are given recommendations and opportunities to make the necessary changes in order to meet the selection criteria. Transplant is not refused to individuals unless there is very solid evidence of poor prognosis (Olbrisch, 1996).

A great deal of variation exists among transplant programs in the methods and criteria used for the psychosocial assessment of transplant candidates (Olbrisch et al., 2002). A typical evaluation for psychosocial selection criteria involves a clinical interview and testing to assess each transplant candidate based on five specific domains of potential risk: (1) psychological (i.e., previous psychiatric illness, current psychiatric symptoms, character pathology, coping styles and strategies; psychological strengths); (2) substance use (i.e., past and current tobacco, alcohol, illicit drug use, history of substance abuse and dependence, including prescription drug abuse); (3) transplant knowledge (i.e., understanding of the transplant process, including post-transplant medical regimen and recovery course); (4) social support (i.e., availability of social resources, including primary and alternative sources of practical support post-transplant); and (5) medical adherence (i.e., history of compliance with medications, medical appointments, and treatment recommendations; ability to make sound medical decisions).

Psychological evaluations necessarily rely on interview assessment, but they also include psychological self-report measures such as the Millon Behavioral Medicine Diagnostic instrument (MBMD; Millon, Antoni, Millon, Meagher, & Grossman, 2001), which measures ways in which people cope with health issues on 20 dimensions. Additionally, to be certain that clinicians apply a consistent standard for evaluation, structured interviews are sometimes employed, such as the Structured Interview for Renal Transplant (SIRT; Mori, Gallagher, & Milne, 2000). For some transplant patients with risk factors for cognitive impairment, cognitive screening exams are employed, such as the Repeatable Battery for the Assessment of Neuropsychological Status (RBANS; Randolph, 1998), Wechsler Abbreviated Scale of Intelligence (WASI; Wechsler, 1999), and Trail Making Test Part A and Part B (Reitan & Wolfson, 1985). Cognitive impairment is common among patients with ESLD due to increased risk of developing hepatic encephalopathy, which is a serious complication especially of alcoholic-related cirrhosis (Butterworth, 2003). The use of these clinical and cognitive assessment strategies in the psychological evaluation of transplant candidates has been supported by other authors in the transplant field (Bunzel & Laederach-Hofmann, 2000; Collins & Labott, 2007; Mooney et al., 2007; Olbrisch et al., 2002).

Case #1: Pre-Transplant Psychological Evaluation
Robert is a 52-year-old married Caucasian male with alcohol-related cirrhosis who was referred to a Mid-Atlantic Liver Transplant Program for a pre–liver transplant psychological evaluation to help determine his candidacy for liver transplantation. Medical comorbidities included history of chronic obstructive pulmonary disease (COPD), low back pain, hypertension, and hernias. He has one teenage

child and is currently on disability from his work as a construction worker. He smoked an average of two cigarette packs per day for 30 years prior to his COPD diagnosis 3 years ago, and has continued to smoke five or six cigarettes per day despite learning of the elevated risks of cigarette smoking. He has a 30-year history of alcohol dependence, consuming an average of a fifth of whisky daily until he was diagnosed with cirrhosis. Since his diagnosis, Robert has completed alcohol detoxification and reportedly has not consumed any alcohol during the 2 years prior to his transplant evaluation. Robert indicated experimental use of cocaine 25 years ago and occasionally used cannabis following his diagnosis of cirrhosis to treat symptoms of nausea and vomiting secondary to medical problems. He also admitted to using his narcotic pain medications, oxycodone (15 mg three times daily) and fentanyl patch (25 mcg/hr every 72 hrs), more than prescribed. He denies prior psychiatric history.

Robert's wife is his primary caregiver, and she has a history of alcohol abuse, problems with anger and other psychiatric issues, and a number of medical problems of her own (i.e., COPD, osteoarthritis). She has been resistant to alcohol and mental health treatment and has been noncompliant with many aspects of her own medical care.

Assessment Results

Based on interview, self-report measures, and cognitive screening, the psychologist decided that Robert was not an acceptable candidate for liver transplantation from a psychological perspective at the time of the evaluation. The specific risk factors that were identified include the following:

• *Tobacco and substance use*: Robert's ongoing tobacco use is a contraindication for liver transplantation, which deems him unacceptable for a liver transplant at this time from a behavioral perspective. Preoperative smokers were found to have a significantly worse prognosis than nonsmokers (Nägele, Kalmar, Rödiger, & Stubbe, 1997).

• Although Robert reportedly has not consumed any alcohol over the past 2 years, his significant history of chronic alcohol use and dependence, lack of previous history of alcohol treatment focused on relapse prevention, and his wife's ongoing alcohol abuse problems collectively place him at high risk of alcohol relapse. It has been reported that as high as 63% of alcoholics resume their previous behavior regardless of length of prior abstinence or referral to treatment programs, and current alcohol abuse rapidly

recurs after organ transplantation (Bell & Van Triget, 1991). Bunzel and Laederach-Hofmann's (2000) review of the literature on solid organ transplantation found that patients with alcoholic-related cirrhosis after liver transplantation had relapse rates ranging from 0% to 40%.

• Additionally, Robert is also at an increased risk of drug relapse given his history of cannabis use and suspected current narcotic abuse or dependence. Substance use has been found to be one of the best predictors for post-transplant noncompliance (Shapiro et al., 1995). Overall, Robert's substance use history and social circumstances suggest that he is at high risk for relapse.

• *Social support*: Robert's lack of adequate social support is also a contraindication for liver transplantation, since adequate support from a significant other has been found to be one of the critical factors in predicting the success of organ transplantation (Bunzel & Laederach-Hofmann, 2000). His wife's ongoing alcohol abuse, psychiatric issues, medical problems, and history of noncompliance with medical, alcohol, and mental health treatment make her a poor caregiver to the patient. Collectively, these factors place Robert at high risk of alcohol relapse, noncompliance, and poor post-transplant outcome.

• *Medical compliance*: Robert has exhibited poor medical compliance and questionable health decision-making. He continues to smoke despite having COPD, used cannabis after being diagnosed with cirrhosis, and routinely requests refills for his narcotic pain medications (i.e., oxycodone) prior to the prescribed date for refill. His pain specialist reportedly has declined his request for additional pain medications. The patient also lacks self-sufficiency despite having adequate cognitive abilities and tends to externalize his responsibility by being dependent on his wife to manage his medical treatment. As mentioned, his wife appears to be an unsuitable caregiver who will likely be a barrier to his post-transplant compliance. In organ transplantation, medication compliance and healthy behaviors or lifestyles are vital prerequisites for good graft functioning and retention of the transplanted organ. Poor compliance with post-transplant treatment regimen impairs both the quality of life and the lifespan as it is a major risk factor for graft rejection episodes and is responsible for up to 25% of deaths after the initial recovery period (Dew & Kormos, 1999).

• *Psychiatric symptoms*: Robert's presentation is consistent with mild to moderate depression, as indicated by his verbal report of symptoms and his responses on the MBMD. His MBMD profile also indicates problems with alcohol, smoking, inactivity, somatic concerns, functional deficits, low pain tolerance, pessimistic outlook on his medical problems, and difficulty adjusting to the disease process. Robert may benefit from psychological services if he is willing to engage in such treatment. Psychiatric problems before transplantation are consistently reported to persist after the transplant surgery and are highly associated with noncompliance, and untreated major depression stands out as a predictor of post-transplant noncompliance in patients (Bunzel & Laederach-Hofmann, 2000). Some studies also suggest that patients with pre-transplant psychiatric disorders show higher allograft rejection rates, as well as an increase in post-transplant mortality (Goetzmann et al., 2007).

Recommendations

• Robert must abstain from all tobacco use to be eligible for liver transplantation, as specified by the Liver Transplant Program's pre-transplant criteria. He was educated on the negative effects of smoking following organ transplantation. The available options for smoking cessation treatments (i.e., pharmacological vs. behavioral treatments) were also discussed. Robert expressed his willingness to engage in pharmacological smoking cessation treatments, and this was conveyed to his transplant coordinator and the Liver Transplant Program. Robert will need to have two negative cotinine screenings per his Liver Transplant Program's policy on substance use prior to being considered for organ listing and liver transplantation.

• Random alcohol and drug screenings were recommended, given Robert's significant substance use history and to monitor his current narcotic use. It was recommended that Robert's hepatologist consult with his pain specialist to rule out suspected narcotic abuse and dependence, and to possibly identify alternative effective pain management treatments.

• The Liver Transplant Program's policy on substance use was thoroughly reviewed and signed by Robert. It requires him to quit smoking and to demonstrate abstinence from alcohol and illicit drug use for at least a 6-month period. If Robert is unable to maintain his abstinence from using alcohol or illicit substances, he is to be referred for alcohol or drug treatment to work on relapse prevention.

• Robert will need to demonstrate that he has adequate and reliable social support post-transplant. It was recommended that the liver transplant social worker follow-up with him on social support issues to determine if alternative sources of support are available. Efforts were made to encourage his wife to seek alcohol and mental health treatment.

• Robert can benefit from initiating pharmacological treatment for depression. His depression may partially explain his lack of self-sufficiency for taking responsibility for his medical treatment. Improving his depression and psychiatric symptoms may improve his motivation toward adopting healthier behaviors. Individual psychotherapy following a cognitive-behavioral approach was offered to Robert, but he declined. If depressive symptoms do not improve or if they worsen, a referral to a psychiatrist should be considered.

Ethical Issues in Organ Allocation

Psychologists working in medical settings in general face a myriad of complex issues that go beyond those typically confronted in traditional mental health practice. These issues include honoring confidentiality when interdisciplinary communication is the linchpin for optimal medical care and managing dual relationships when serving as both a team consultant and therapist to the individual patient. Psychologists face even more complex ethical issues when serving as participants in decision-making regarding organ allocation. In this section, we will review the specific ethical issues that psychologists are confronted with at different points in the transplant process.

In the pre-transplant evaluation process, psychological findings often play a role in deciding whether to list someone for transplant. In accordance with the ethical principle of informed consent, psychologists must provide written and verbal disclosure that they are gathering information to make a recommendation as to whether someone is a good candidate to be listed for a transplant. They must make it explicit that they have an ethical obligation to their patients, the transplant team, and the pool of patients awaiting transplants nationally, many of whom will die while on the waiting list. Accordingly, it has been said that when a bad transplant decision has been made and the patient dies as a result of nonadherence, it involves three deaths: the patient, the deceased donor, and the individual who did not get an organ and died while on the waiting list. The gravity of this responsibility for the team cannot be overestimated, and it is the reason why teams typically try to take every measure possible to share the responsibility of making these life-and-death decisions.

Transplant candidates are aware of the "gatekeeper" role that psychologists hold and are frequently anxious that they might "fail" their evaluation, and thus they may not be truthful about issues that they perceive as being viewed as negative factors (Collins & Labott, 2007). Indeed, one study found that approximately 20% of candidates for transplant produced an uninterpretable "fake good" Minnesota Multiphasic Personality Inventory (MMPI) or MMPI-2 profile during evaluation, with half of the cases being individuals who actually appeared to be good candidates based on interview (Olbrisch, Levenson, Sherwin, & Best, 1994). Because of concerns regarding the veracity of self-report, due diligence must be exercised and psychologists must make every effort to employ collateral sources for gathering and confirming critical information. These sources would include family members, who can corroborate alcohol, smoking, and other substance use changes and can also report on cognitive changes and affective disorders that may not be as apparent to the patient (Collins & Labott, 2007). Health care providers who have worked with the patient during the period leading up to the transplant decision can also be queried about the reliability of the patient in keeping appointments and adhering to treatments. To support the evaluation, it can also be necessary to attain consent to release/obtain information from mental health professionals in the community who have or are providing care to the patient. A final concern arises when the psychologist recommends against listing a patient for a transplant due to severe psychopathology. Whether to share the full diagnostic findings with the patient and family is a delicate issue that must be carefully weighed.

Medical ethicists and the public at large generally agree that organ allocation decisions should be made based on predicting who will obtain the maximum health benefit from an organ transplant. In the United States, only factors that relate to chances of success are allowed to be considered. In spite of these agreed-upon principles, precautions must be taken to ensure that evaluations are done fairly and without bias (Olbrisch, 1996). First, it is important that empirically supported objective and consistent criteria are applied across transplant centers to reduce the perception that such decisions are capricious. Second, psychologists must do their part to emphasize to patients, families, and team members that such decisions are not based on value judgments regarding the worthiness of a given individual but, instead, predictions regarding their chances of survival. Third, and related, is the fact that patients and families must be helped to understand that the purpose of the evaluation is not to rank individuals in terms of where they fit on the list based on psychosocial characteristics, but simply to decide whether they have a reasonable chance for survival based on those characteristics. Finally, because of the life-and-death importance of the recommendation to not list a patient, it should be done only in cases in which a clear weight of evidence suggests a low probability of success.

Another psychologist role with ethical implications in the pre-transplant period is in providing informed consent as to the risks and rigors of the transplant process. Although most patients feel that a transplant is their only chance for survival when it comes to liver or heart transplant, this is not the case for kidney transplant. Also, even if patients feel compelled to take the risks, they will presumably cope better with adverse events if they know in advance about the possibility of these events. Yet another ethical challenge for psychologists occurs when the transplant team psychologist is providing services to the patient while he or she is on the waiting list. If it comes to light that the patient has relapsed and used alcohol, tobacco, or illicit drugs, it is imperative that the psychologist inform the team. This limit on confidentiality must be made clear to the patient before beginning the therapy relationship.

A final role that psychologists and all team members can play is to raise awareness of social justice issues by modeling for other team members a constant self-examination of any value judgments or biases that they may bring to their recommendations to list or not list a particular patient. These biases tend to surface for individuals who are convicted felons or who have difficult or unpleasant personalities without frank evidence of poor compliance. Another bias that team members must be vigilant about is the tendency to favor listing patients with the highest chances of success, rather than a reasonable chance, due to the financial and prestige motivation to be a transplant center with a high success rate. Transplant centers essentially compete against each other for potential organ recipients by advertising their survival rates to those who are willing to travel for a transplant or have access to multiple centers in their geographic region.

Another potential bias is the issue of whether older adults should have equal access to donor organs, providing they are in good enough health to survive long term. Each center sets up its own age cutoffs for transplant, and those age limits have been increasing since transplants began in the 1980s, with the mean age of kidney transplant (i.e., ~64 years old) being the highest among organ transplant. Similarly, the percentage of heart transplants provided to adults over the age of 65 rose steadily until the last several years, when it has remained stable at 13% of total transplants. There continues to be debate as to whether older adults have higher rates of mortality and morbidity following heart transplant, with some studies suggesting that older adult recipients have similar survival rates, as well equal or higher QOL, post-transplant relative to younger recipients (Blanche et al., 1996; Coffman et al., 1997; Demers et al., 2003; Shamaskin et al., (in press), Zuckermann et al., 2003). It may be the case that age bias exists well before the team has the opportunity to evaluate a heart transplant candidate in that perhaps fewer physicians or cardiologists recommend their older patients for transplant consideration. One study found that older adults are treated less aggressively in cardiac care and are more likely to be excluded from clinical trials for cardiac treatments relative to younger adults (Bowling, 1999).

Postsurgical and Long-Term Rehabilitation Stages

Initially, in the perisurgical phase, the primary concern is survival. Patients undergo a very lengthy and complicated surgical procedure, and the first several days following transplantation are critical. In most cases, patients are transferred out of the intensive care unit in just 2–3 days and discharged from the hospital in 1–2 weeks. A minority of cases will experience complications that may require a more lengthy hospitalization.

Following discharge from the hospital, the primary focus becomes physical recovery. The patient is still fatigued, in pain, and often decompensated physically, but less ill than prior to the transplant. The expectation is that, over time, the patient will become stronger, the pain will diminish, and his or her level of functioning will improve. For most patients, this is exactly the case. For others, however, complications may arise that could potentially delay the recovery process.

After an initial focus on survival, over time, there is a gradual shift toward rehabilitation and restoring QOL and psychosocial functioning. For some patients, this adjustment is relatively uncomplicated and progresses in a somewhat linear fashion. For many other patients, the rehabilitation process can be quite difficult and marked by continued distress and strife. There is often an assumption by patients, family, and the health care providers themselves that, following transplantation, patients go on to live "happily ever after." In many cases, this turns out to be a false assumption, and the parties involved sometimes learn the hard way that the road to recovery can be quite difficult. These patients often require ongoing psychological follow-up to assist with their transition and recovery. Thus, the role of the transplant psychologist can be crucial.

During rehabilitation, an emphasis is placed on returning to the highest level of functioning possible. Most patients strive to return to their pre-illness level of functioning, although this may not always be realistic. To appreciate the challenge of the rehabilitation process fully, one must look back at the course of illness and factors leading up to transplantation. For example, most patients ultimately stop working because of their illness and many become disabled. Disability often results in significant financial loss, and this may lead to drastic changes in lifestyle. It is not unusual for the patient's physical decompensation, disability, and financial changes to take a toll on other areas of functioning, including sexual functioning, social functioning, and quality of intimate relationships. The effect of chronic illness and physical deterioration is cumulative, with many gradual effects over time. As stated previously, in the earlier phases of transplantation, the primary concern for both patients and family is often mere survival, followed by recovery. Hence, the many areas of functioning beyond survival are often neglected and not addressed until the rehabilitation phase.

The experiences described by patients who return home after the procedure are often akin to those described by soldiers returning home from war. For months and sometimes more than a year after the initial surgery, the primary concern was staying alive. However, following successful transplantation, the patient must rebuild his or her life, much like the returning warrior. The individual is now confronted with a myriad of issues, many of which have been handled by the spouse or other loved ones for a long period of time. For example, many patients have not paid the bills, managed the household, managed the budget, supervised the children, or maintained contact with social networks for quite some time. Other domains, such as sexual functioning, relationships, and social functioning, were also placed on the back burner pending survival. Many patients express feeling overwhelmed with the details of everyday life following transplantation. Like the returning soldier, many state that survival may have been difficult physically, but it kept things simple in terms of having a singular focus to "just live." This readjustment process can be very stressful for both the patient and loved ones. The majority of patients gradually restore most of their roles and re-engage with the day-to-day operations of their lives. For others, this adjustment becomes increasingly difficult and, in many cases, results in significant psychological dysfunction. It is not unusual for these patients to experience depression, anxiety, relapse to drugs and alcohol, post-traumatic stress disorder (PTSD), marital discord, and continued loss of function. These manifestations, if not addressed, can not only inhibit the rehabilitation process, but lead to further deterioration and even death if the patient loses motivation to continue to adhere to the demanding medical regimen.

Post-transplant Regimen and Survival

The extensive regimen for preventing rejection and maintaining health after a transplant is a daunting challenge for most transplant recipients. They must follow a strict medical regimen for the rest of their lives to keep their new organ functioning well and reduce the likelihood of rejection. The regimen includes major lifestyle changes for many patients, including frequent outpatient follow-up, taking up to 40 medications per day, and modifying diet, exercise, and substance use, including smoking and alcohol use. The difficulty of consistently following such recommendations is reflected in research indicating noncompliance rates ranging from 20% to 50% among transplant recipients (Laederach-Hofmann & Bunzel, 2000). Adherence rates can vary greatly depending on the specific health behavior. A study by Bellg and colleagues (2003) indicated that only 9% of heart transplant patients reported difficulty in following their medication regimen, but 80% said they did not follow

prescribed diets, 77% did not follow recommended exercise programs, and 22.2% of previous smokers admitted to still smoking. As a result, it is common for heart transplant patients to be overweight and sedentary, which creates additional health risks for this group.

The importance of post-transplant medical regimen adherence cannot be overestimated; one review found that poor adherence or nonadherence was responsible for up to 25% of patient deaths during the initial recovery period following transplant (Bunzel & Laederach-Hofmann, 2000). Various factors are related to adherence, including levels of social support, patient characteristics (Evangelista, Berg, & Dracup, 2001), and levels of psychological distress (Dew & Kormos, 1999). The Bellg et al. (2003) study found that among long-term heart transplant patients, those who were under the age of 60 were more than twice as likely to not take their medications relative to patients over the age of 60.

As seen in the OPTN online database, survival rates for patients vary by organ, but they typically decrease as more time passes from the date of transplant (see Table 21.2). Other factors affect survival rates as well, including UNOS status at transplant, recipient age, gender, and whether the transplant is a primary or repeat transplant.

For heart transplant in particular, survival rates tend to decrease significantly within the first 6 months after the surgery and continue to decrease at a linear rate for up to 15 years post-transplant (Taylor et al., 2009). The survival rates for adult heart transplant patients have improved over the past 20 years, although it seems that most of the improvement has been within the first year post-transplant. There is some evidence that current survival rates may underestimate the effects of medical advancements on improving outcomes. Since the transplant demographics have changed over the past

Table 21.2 Survival rates by organ and years since transplant

	1 year post- transplant	3 years post-transplant	5 years post-transplant
Heart	87.5%	78.7%	72.2%
Kidney	95.9%	90.7%	84.9%
Liver	86.5%	78.3%	72.3%
Lung	83.3%	62.7%	47.0%
Heart–Lung	67.5%	50.1%	39.2%

Based on Organ Procurement and Transplantation Network (OPTN) data as of January 6, 2012.

several years to include more high-risk recipients and high-risk donors, these patients with higher mortality rates may affect the improvements in transplant outcomes overall. When examining risk-adjusted survival data, which takes these high-risk patients into account, it appears that heart transplant survival rates have improved more than it would seem by looking at overall survival rates, but are being offset by changing transplant demographics (Taylor et al., 2009).

Research on Post-Transplant Psychological Adjustment and Quality of Life

Although short-term improvements in emotional functioning from the waiting list period to post-transplant have been documented (Jones, Taylor, Downs, & Spratt, 1992; Mai, McKenzie, & Kostuk, 1990; Russell, Feurer, Wisawatapnimit, Salomon, & Pinson, 2008), a substantial number of recipients develop new psychological problems in the aftermath of a transplant. The most systematic study to date for heart transplant found that at 3 years after transplant, the cumulative risk of major depressive disorder was 26%, adjustment disorder with anxious mood was 17%, and PTSD related to transplant was 17% (Dew et al., 2000). The first year post heart transplant had the highest rates of psychopathology and PTSD, which occurred almost exclusively during the first year. This initial period appears to be the highest risk period for adjustment difficulties for transplant recipients of all organs, as recipients learn to cope with the rigorous medication regimen, constant medical surveillance, and negative mood effects of immunosuppressive medications (Olbrisch et al., 2002).

In contrast to the higher rates of depression and anxiety disorders in the first year after transplant, these rates in the following years appear to approach the levels found in the general population. Among those who do develop psychological adjustment difficulties, specific risk factors have been identified. In one study (Dew et al., 1994), pre-transplant predictors of anxiety and depression during the first year after heart transplant included a history of psychiatric disorder prior to transplant; younger age; lower social support from their primary family caregiver; exposure to recent major life events involving loss; poor self-esteem; a poor sense of mastery; and use of avoidance coping strategies to manage health problems. In a study examining long-term adjustment to heart transplant (i.e., at least 5 years post-transplant; Rybarczyk et al., 2007), individuals at higher risk for depression were those with significant neurological

side effects (i.e., trouble concentrating, weakness, fatigue, sleep problems), lower recreational functioning, lower satisfaction with emotional support, and a younger age at the time of transplant.

A recent study found that older patients reported better quality of life, psychological adjustment, and adherence five years after heart transplant compared to younger patients (Shamaskin et al., in press). This finding of better adjustment among older transplant recipients in several studies is consistent with evidence of better adjustment among older cancer survivors (Williamson & Schulz, 1994) and individuals with amputations (Dunn, 1997; Livneh, Antonak, & Gerhardt, 1999; Williamson, Shulz, Bridges, & Behan, 1994). It has been theorized that older adults are more resilient in the face of physical decline due to enhance coping skills accrued from cumulative life experiences and the fact that they are more accepting of disability because it is viewed as an "on-time" event that comes with the territory of aging (Neugarten, 1969; Williamson et al., 1994). Older individuals may be more likely to view the hardships of the post-transplant regimen as a tradeoff for the "bonus" time afforded to them by the transplant.

Perceived illness uncertainty has been found to be a predictor of negative affect in chronic medical conditions (Hommel et al., 2003; Sanders-Dewey, Mullins, & Chaney, 2001; Wineman, O'Brien, Nealon, & Kaskel, 1993), particularly in illnesses with less stable and more unpredictable courses, such as epilepsy, cancer, diabetes, and multiple sclerosis (Mishel & Braden, 1988). Perceived illness uncertainty has also been shown to be a factor in negative affect and adjustment in a large sample of patients 5 years post heart transplant (Rybarczyk et al., 2007). There are varied and unpredictable complications after transplant, such as increased risk of serious infections and certain kinds of cancer caused by immunosuppressant medications, as well as overall uncertainty about how many additional years of life will be afforded by the transplant.

A large body of research demonstrates that, overall, patient QOL improves after organ transplantation. Researchers have examined physical and psychological outcomes, as well as explicit self-reported QOL, and found that health, energy, and activity aspects of QOL improved for patients after transplant (Bravata, Olkin, Barnato, Keeffe, & Owens, 1999; Littlefield et al., 1996). In the Littlefield et al. (1996) study, lung transplant patients reported the best improvements in physical, psychological, and social functioning compared to heart or liver transplant recipients. Other studies have demonstrated that functional performance and other QOL features improve significantly for transplant patients within the first 6 months of transplant, as well as up to several years after the surgery (Butler et al., 2003; Grady et al., 2007; Rutherford et al., 2005; Rybarczyk et al., 2007). Data from the International Society for Heart and Lung Transplantation registry indicate that 83% of heart transplant survivors reported no functional limitations at 1 year post-transplant, and studies indicate that these high levels of functional status are sustained for 5 years and longer (Grady et al., 2007; Hetzer et al., 1997).

Several factors have been found to impact the QOL for patients following transplant. In one study, pre-transplant functional performance impacted post-transplant QOL (Butler et al., 2003). Medical regimen adherence, which includes challenging behavioral changes and medication adherence, can impact patients' post-transplant QOL. Another study reviewing the experience of medical symptoms after organ transplant found that symptoms are relatively prevalent and distressing for most kidney, liver, heart, and lung transplant patients (Kugler et al., 2009). The researchers note that the side effects of many immunosuppressive drugs may affect QOL and symptom experience, which in turn may impact rates of nonadherence. They highlight the importance of understanding patients' appraisals of symptoms and immunosuppressive side effects so that clinicians can improve symptom management and reduce risk of nonadherence.

Psychologist's Role During Post-Transplant Rehabilitation

Psychologists both in the community and on the transplant team can play an important role during post-transplant rehabilitation. The experience of receiving a transplant is stressful, sometimes even traumatic, and patients must often deal with specific challenges that may benefit from psychological intervention (Olbrisch et al., 2002). Many patients struggle with accepting their new long-term patient role and adjusting to various losses, including role loss, bodily integrity, privacy, autonomy, and independence. There will likely be stress from financial concerns, since the transplant process can carry large out-of-pocket costs for the patient (Hauboldt, Hanson, & Bernstein, 2008). Patients may have pre-transplant psychiatric issues that are exacerbated after the surgery, or they may experience a new onset of depression, anxiety disorder, or even PTSD (see below) after the transplant.

Although the pre-transplantation psychological evaluation is of great importance in terms of the selection of transplant candidates, post-transplantation psychological evaluation is perhaps of equal importance, given the myriad psychosocial variables involved in recovery and rehabilitation. In addition to assessing for psychiatric illness, the clinician must thoroughly assess treatment compliance and adherence, possible relapse to substance abuse, self-care, motivation, communication with providers, relationship issues, sexual functioning, and overall coping. Neuropsychological testing may also be necessary, especially in cases in which pre-transplantation cognitive dysfunction was evident. The clinician performing such an evaluation may or may not be the treating clinician and often will need to refer the patient to other specialties such as psychiatry, marital counseling, substance abuse counseling, or pastoral care. Additionally, throughout the United States, numerous support groups for transplant recipients and their caregivers can serve a unique capacity in terms of normalizing and sharing the very unique experiences of transplantation, both medically and emotionally.

Various researchers have shown that psychological interventions ranging from cognitive-behavioral therapy to a psychodynamic approach have been beneficial, although an integrative model may be best due to the multidimensional aspects of coping with organ transplant (Reid, 1990). Similarly, Allmon et al. (2010) proposed that multicomponent psychoeducational interventions developed to enhance coping in chronic illness patients would be appropriate for transplant patients, given the overlapping coping and behavioral challenges faced by transplant patients. These interventions typically include cognitive approaches to stress management, relaxation training, problem-solving skills training, communication and assertiveness training, and sometimes sleep hygiene instruction (e.g., Rybarczyk, DeMarco, DeLaCruz, Lapidos, & Fortner, 2001).

In general, similar to those provided to all individuals with chronic illness, interventions for transplant patients should be aimed at reducing *excess disability*. Excess disability is defined as a substantially lower than expected level of physical functioning for a given medical condition that can be attributed to both deconditioning and behavioral factors (i.e., noncompliance, lack of activity). For example, a patient with a heart transplant may completely refrain from strenuous physical activity following a fearful event in which he experienced chest pain after exertion or because he incorrectly believes it is medically advisable to restrict such activity. Psychologists can also play a key role with assisting patients in reducing substance use and abuse, as well as with medical regimen adherence. Motivational interviewing is the most empirically supported mode of intervention for increasing adherence (Rubak, Sandbaek, Lauritzen, & Christensen, 2005). Immunosuppressant drugs often result in an array of aversive side effects, and psychologists may be able to serve as a liaison with the rest of the treatment team in terms of educating patients about the importance of the medication and developing practical strategies for ensuring good adherence. Additionally, several of these medications may have psychological side effects (e.g., mood regulation, body image) that also need to be addressed in therapy.

In addition to the universal issues faced by individuals who must adjust to substantial changes in functioning, transplant recipients may also experience some unique issues related to receiving an organ from a deceased individual. There may be what one author terms "magical thinking" when it comes to incorporating the body part of an unknown person, with negative emotions sometimes related to perceived personality changes or the potential that the donor was a criminal or committed suicide (Vamos, 2010). It may be beneficial to prepare patients for these feelings and encourage their expression, since patients may fear that they will be thought of as "ridiculous or ungrateful if they talk about such misgivings" (Vamos, 2010, p. 886). Other distressing feelings may take the form of survivor guilt for being the fortunate one to receive an organ, or guilt over the fact that while waiting for an organ a recipient may have essentially wished for another individual to die so that their organs could be donated. The latter may be partially addressed by encouraging the recipient to do symbolic things to honor or thank the deceased donor. Many transplant programs have a procedure for corresponding with donor families, proving the donor family is willing, and transplant recipients may find it therapeutic to write a letter expressing their gratitude.

Last, Allmon and colleagues (2010) suggest that an important task for psychologists working with transplant recipients is to assist them in the inevitable process of redefining values, reordering priorities, and finding positive meaning in the adversity they have and will continue to face. Consistent with these therapy goals, Olbrisch and Levenson (1995) indicate that transplant recipients often reorder their priorities after rebounding from what is essentially a terminal illness for heart, lung, and liver transplant patients. They note that patients often refocus on simple goals, such as participating in home life, helping and watching their children and grandchildren grow up, or tending to their gardens. They emphasize that there is often a shift away from goals related to self-actualization in the domain of employment or other achievements. This change in orientation may challenge the transplant team's view, or the public's view, that the optimal outcome of a transplant is to restore someone to a "productive" life. Similarly, some transplant patients may find themselves struggling with larger existential questions such as "What does it mean to have a living or deceased person's organ sustaining my life?" or "How does receiving of the 'gift of life' change the way I have to live my life?"

The following two cases illustrate the range of challenging issues that are faced by patients during the rehabilitation phase post-transplant and how a psychologist provided treatment to help promote adjustment during this phase. Like the previous illustration, these are composites of actual patients treated by authors of this chapter, with identifying information changed to further protect confidentiality.

Case #2: Treatment of Adjustment Problems Following Liver Transplant

William, a 55-year-old married Caucasian male with a history of hepatitis C underwent liver transplantation approximately 2 years ago. Prior to becoming ill, William was an avid fisherman and hunter who enjoyed the outdoors immensely. He worked a great deal as a foreman and enjoyed a middle-class lifestyle. He had no psychiatric history. He enjoyed social alcohol consumption, mainly during Friday happy hour with friends. William discovered his hepatitis C at a routine physical, and by the time it was identified his liver enzymes were already elevated. He became ill soon after and liver biopsy revealed rapidly progressing cirrhosis. Over the ensuing 2 years, William experienced gradual physical deterioration. Eventually, he had to stop working and qualified for disability. His financial status changed drastically as a result. William was listed for transplantation and later underwent the procedure successfully. He was hospitalized for less than 2 weeks before being discharged to his home.

For the first 3–6 months post discharge, William mainly concerned himself with physical recovery. His pain gradually diminished, and his follow-up appointments were eventually tapered as he progressed. At approximately 7 months post discharge, William began feeling bored. He no longer went fishing or hunting, nor did he attend weekly happy hours. He was still unable to work and could not return to his vocation. He was home all day and eventually became the designated baby-sitter to his grandchildren as his daughter worked full-time and was a single mother. Over the next few months, he gradually became more resentful, frustrated, angry, and depressed. He began feeling what he described as useless, hopeless, unfulfilled, and as if he was "going nowhere." He went on to state, "this is not me. This is not my life." Interestingly, William recalled his friends and family constantly reminding him how fortunate he was, while privately he was feeling less than fortunate. William began to sleep during the day, and, as a result, slept poorly at night. His sedentary lifestyle and lack of activity resulted in significant weight gain. His anger and resentment resulted in irritability and frequent arguments with his wife and family. He ultimately began feeling like a "prisoner." This led to feelings of regret regarding his undergoing liver transplantation. William once stated "I gave up pretty much everything I enjoyed. If I had any idea life was going to be like this I would have never ever gotten a liver transplant." William was referred by his physician for psychological evaluation to further assess the situation and attempt to assist in rehabilitation.

Although the primary concern at the time of evaluation was William's depression, other areas of functioning were quickly identified as problematic. In addition to a lengthy interview with William, the clinician also interviewed his wife and members of the transplant team. Of note were William's expectations about transplantation. He stated that he failed to give a great deal of thought to life after the surgery and was therefore "blind-sided" by the many difficulties he experienced getting his life back on track. Assessment of his QOL revealed the very obvious poor level of functioning despite very good medical improvement. William agreed that improving QOL was of the utmost importance. Moreover, he was motivated to engage in treatment. After a discussion with his hepatologist, William was prescribed antidepressant medications, which he agreed to use. A treatment plan that involved weekly or biweekly follow-up sessions was formulated. Using a cognitive-behavioral model, William's beliefs, fears, and expectations were assessed, along with his very negative and sometimes self-destructive self-talk. From a behavioral standpoint, his sleep hygiene, inactivity, diet, and communication skills were assessed for treatment.

William followed-up for approximately 10 visits over the span of 4 months. Through a combination of cognitive restructuring, sleep hygiene, education, communication skills training, anxiety management, and medically supervised exercise, William rapidly made progress. His spouse often attended sessions briefly to give feedback and discuss issues. This caregiver involvement was an important aspect as caregiver burden, stress, and suffering is often overlooked by both the treatment team and patient. His spouse played a pivotal role in his recovery, but she found it very helpful to discuss some of her own challenges and stressors.

William eventually lost over 20 pounds following dietary changes and a daily walking routine. He began to involve his grandchildren and later his spouse in his exercise. He stated that he no longer viewed his role as "baby-sitter," but rather as grandfather and provider. William began fishing once again and also involved his grandchildren and wife in this hobby. Over time, he learned that he was indeed able to engage in many activities but needed to do so with modifications. Although William was unable to return to his old job and did need to remain on disability, he was able to secure part-time employment. The extra income was very helpful, but William stated that the job was more important for his pride and sense of value to his family. William's decreased irritability also resulted in a sharp decrease in marital conflict, and as he became more active and pleasant, his interactions with his family improved. Although William continued to struggle at times in accepting his major changes in life, he gradually made the necessary modifications that, in the end, substantially improved his QOL.

Case #3: Treatment of Post-Traumatic Stress Disorder Following Heart Transplant

Suzanne is a 38-year-old African-American female who, in the course of 1 year, suffered three heart attacks, primarily due to a rare autoimmune disorder. The third heart attack resulted in significant damage, and she was subsequently hospitalized for 3 months. It was later determined that her heart was damaged beyond recovery, and she was deemed a candidate for the total artificial heart. The ultimate goal was for heart transplantation. Suzanne is in the blood group O positive, which resulted in an extensive wait for an available organ. She was on the total artificial heart for another 6 months while awaiting organ transplantation. Following transplantation, she experienced multiple complications that included respiratory failure, renal failure, and the need for intubation. Her health became so poor that she was near death multiple times. Suzanne often watched and listened as her family cried at her bedside and even grieved her impending death. She experienced delirium on multiple occasions as she recovered from her procedure. Following a 10-month hospitalization, Suzanne was discharged to home.

Once home, Suzanne's primary objective remained survival. She began experiencing severe anxiety in response to nearly any symptom. For example, shortness of breath would almost invariably result in a mild panic attack. She stated that virtually all symptoms would lead her to believe she was dying. Suzanne began experiencing nightmares on a regular basis. These often involved terrifying dreams of being intubated, inability to breathe, not being able to talk, the hallucinations and confusion she experienced while in a delirium, and viewing her family at her own funeral. Suzanne would have flashbacks in response to sounds such as beeping or buzzing or when in the presence of health care providers. Suzanne was very anxious and easily startled. Her sleep was poor mainly because she was afraid to fall sleep at night out of concern that she would not awake.

Unlike many transplantation patients who return home, both Suzanne's immediate and long-term concerns involved survival. In other words, she could not be bothered by other concerns, such as household management, bills, lawn care, and even relationships. She was still in survival mode, and the majority of her stress and anxiety revolved around her perceived likelihood of death and dying.

Suzanne was referred for a psychological evaluation and clearly met the criteria for PTSD. Her symptoms were severe and somewhat debilitating. Prior to addressing other areas of concern in her life and setting goals for psychosocial rehabilitation, Her PTSD needed to be immediately addressed. Her physicians prescribed medication for sleep, as well as alprazolam for anxiety, which she took as needed. These medications brought her some mild but immediate relief. Suzanne attended weekly psychotherapy sessions for her PTSD, and the treatment strategy employed involved "prolonged exposure," a validated treatment for the disorder with demonstrated efficacy for women as well as men (Schnurr et al., 2007). While in therapy, Suzanne would share in detail her traumatic experiences. The sessions were recorded and she would listen to them at home as often as possible, as per the treatment protocol. In addition to prolonged exposure, Suzanne was instructed in relaxation training and sleep hygiene and was enrolled in cardiac rehabilitation under the supervision of her physician. Over time, Suzanne's symptoms of reliving the trauma, including the nightmares and flashbacks, began to abate. Her sleep improved significantly, and her anxiety became better managed. She benefited a great deal from cardiac rehabilitation, which capitalized on the fact that, when in her 20s, she was a very athletic and active individual. She also enjoyed the social interaction and time away from home. After termination of therapy, Suzanne remained in contact with the psychologist in case she needed "booster" sessions at a later time point.

Conclusion

In sum, as the literature review and cases illustrate, there are numerous roles for psychologists as part of the interdisciplinary transplant team. In the pre-transplant phase, psychologists screen for risk factors that could contribute to post-transplant recovery; educate potential recipients about the transplant process, including risks and setting realistic expectations about post-transplant recovery; provide targeted interventions for behavioral and psychological risk factors associated with poor outcomes; and work with patients who are on waiting lists to cope with uncertainty and continue compliance with requirements for transplant candidacy (e.g., drug and alcohol abstinence). At post–transplant, psychologists can and should play a role in the provision of consultation and preventive treatment during the crucial initial recovery period and provide targeted interventions during long-term rehabilitation. Treatment interventions are likely to be multimodal as they often include a combination of health, behavioral, psychological, and social aspects.

The scope of this chapter did not include an in-depth discussion of the many issues facing family members who serve as caregivers to individuals who receive transplants. It is a demanding experience for those individuals, and, as in so many other caregiver situations, frequently takes a large toll on emotional health and QOL of the caregiver. Additionally, caregiver burden and distress can affect the quality of support provided to transplant recipients and may adversely affect organ transplant outcomes. Psychologists treating transplant patients should check in frequently with these caregivers and other family members to assess adjustment and make referrals as needed. Also beyond the scope of this chapter is the psychological adjustment issues faced by living donors and/or families who are generous enough to grant permission for an organ to be procured from their loved one when the sometimes difficult-to-comprehend "brain death" has occurred. Those individuals must make a difficult decision during a period of grief and shock and often have to weigh the unstated wishes of their loved one and differing opinions among other family members about the choice of donation. One author poignantly captured the contrasting experiences for donors and recipients by describing transplant as the "gift of life wrapped in mourning" (Holtkamp, 2002).

Organ transplant is a life-altering experience that demands a high level of physical and psychological adaptation. In highlighting the challenges and adjustment difficulties faced by adults who undergo organ transplantation, we run the risk of creating a skewed picture that does not adequately recognize the overwhelming positive impact of transplant on thousands of individuals in the United States alone. Organ transplant has not only extended the lives of countless individuals by up to 20 years, but the majority of these added years are enjoyed at a high QOL. To be a part of this enterprise, on a team that often exceeds more than 100 dedicated health providers for a single patient, is a great privilege for psychologists. It is a front row seat on both a medical miracle, as well as on the unique level of human resiliency that is required to navigate through the experience.

Future Directions

- With the increasing number of organ transplants, more psychologists need to be trained to work with transplantation teams and transplant patients during all stages of the process.
- More research needs to be conducted to further develop standardized measures that predict post-transplant survival and QOL.
- The benefits of providing routine psychoeducational interventions to all transplant patients as a preventive measure should be tested in randomized clinical trials across multiple transplant centers.

References

Allmon, A., Shaw, K., Martens, J., Yamada, T., Lohnberg, J., Schultz, J., et al. (2010). Organ transplantation: Issues in assessment and treatment. *The Register Report*. Retrieved from http://www.e-psychologist.org/index.iml?mdl=exam/show_article.mdl&Material_ID=103.

Barry, J. M., Jordan, M. L., & Conlin, M. J. (2007). Renal transplantation. In A. J. Wein (Ed.), *Campbell-Walsh urology* (9th ed., ch. 40, pp. 1293–1324). Philadelphia: Saunders Elsevier.

Bell, M., & Van Triget, P. (1991). Addictive behavior patterns in cardiac transplant patients. *Journal of Heart and Lung Transplantation, 10,* 158.

Bellg, A., Brady, K., Naftel, D. C., Rybarczyk, B., Young, J., Pelegrin, D., et al. (2003). Patient adherence at 5 to 6 years after heart transplantation. *Journal of Heart and Lung Transplantation, 22,* S127.

Bingaman, A. W., Wright, F. H., & Murphy, C. L. (2010). Kidney paired donation in live-donor kidney transplantation. *New England Journal of Medicine, 363,* 1091–1092.

Blanche, C., Takkenberg, J. J. M., Nessim, S., Cohen, M., Czer, L. S. C., Matloff, J. M., et al. (1996). Heart transplantation in patients 65 years of age and older: A comparative analysis of 40 patients. *The Annals of Thoracic Surgery, 62*(5), 1442–1446.

Bowling, A. (1999). Ageism in cardiology. *British Medical Journal, 319,* 1353–1355.

Bravata, D. M., Olkin, I., Barnato, A. E., Keeffe, E. B., & Owens, D. K. (1999). Health-related quality of life after liver transplantation: A meta-analysis. *Liver Transplantation, 5*(4), 318–331.

Brown, S. L., Biehl, T. R., Rawlins, M. C., & Hefty, T. R. (2001). Laparoscopic live donor nephrectomy: A comparison with the conventional open approach. *Journal of Urology, 165,* 766–769.

Bunzel, B., & Laederach-Hofmann, K. (2000). Solid organ transplantation: Are there predictors for posttransplant noncompliance? A literature review. *Transplantation, 70*(5), 711–716.

Butler, J., McCoin, N. S., Feurer, I. D., Speroff, T., Davis, S. F., Chomsky, D. B., et al. (2003). Modeling the effects of functional performance and post-transplant comorbidities on health-related quality of life after heart transplantation. *The Journal of Heart and Lung Transplantation, 22*(10), 1149–1156.

Butterworth, R. F. (2003). Hepatic encephalopathy—a serious complication of alcoholic liver disease. *Alcohol Research and Health, 27*(2), 143–145.

Calne, R. (2008). *The achievements of organ transplantation and prospects for the future: Ethical dilemmas arising from clinical success.* Retrieved from http://www.thehumanbrainproject.com/sem-roycalne.php

Christie, J. D., Edwards, L. B., Kucheryavaya, A. Y., Aurora, P., Dobbels, F., Kirk, R., et al. (2010). The registry of the International Society for Heart and Lung Transplantation: Twenty-seventh official adult lung and heart-lung transplant report—2010. *The Journal of Heart and Lung Transplantation: The official publication of the International Society for Heart Transplantation, 29*(10), 1104–1118.

Coffman, K. L., Valenza, M., Czer, L. S. C., Freimark, D., Aleksic, I., Harasty, D., et al. (1997). An update on transplantation in the geriatric heart transplant patient. *Psychosomatics, 38*(5), 487–496.

Collins, C. A., & Labott, S. M. (2007). Psychological assessment of candidates for solid organ transplantation. *Professional Psychology: Research and Practice, 38*(2), 150–157.

Demers, P., Moffatt, S., Oyer, P. E., Hunt, S. A., Reitz, B. A., & Robbins, R. C. (2003). Long-term results of heart transplantation in patients older than 60 years. *The Journal of Thoracic and Cardiovascular Surgery, 126*(1), 224–231.

Deuse, T., Sista, R., Weill, D., Tyan, D., Haddad, F., Dhillon, G., et al. (2010). Review of heart-lung transplantation at Stanford. *The Annals of Thoracic Surgery, 90*(1), 329–337.

Dew, M., & Kormos, R. (1999). Early post-transplant medical compliance and mental health predict physical morbidity and mortality one to three years after heart transplantation. *Journal of Heart and Lung Transplantation, 18*(6), 549–562.

Dew, M. A., Simmons, R. G., Roth, L. H., Schulberg, H. C., Thompson, M.E., Armitage, J. M., et al. (1994). Psychosocial predictors of vulnerability to distress in the year following heart transplantation. *Psychological Medicine, 24*(4), 929–945.

Dew, M. A., DiMartini, A. F., Switzer, G. E., Kormos, R. L., Schulberg, H. C., Roth, L. H., & Griffith, B. P. (2000). Patterns and predictors of risk for depressive and anxiety-related disorders during the first three years after heart transplantation. *Psychosomatics, 41*, 191–192.

Dunn, D. S. (1997). Well-being following amputation: Salutary effects of positive meaning, optimism, and control. *Rehabilitation Psychology, 41*, 285–302.

Evangelista, L. S., Berg, J., & Dracup, K. (2001). Relationship between psychosocial variables and compliance in patients with heart failure. *Heart and Lung, 30*(4), 294–301.

Goetzmann, L., Klaghofer, R., Wagner-Huber, R., Halter, J., Boehler, A., Muellhaupt, B., et al. (2007). Psychosocial vulnerability predicts psychosocial outcome after an organ transplant: Results of a prospective study with lung, liver, and bone-marrow patients. *Journal of Psychosomatic Research, 62*(1), 93–100.

Grady, K. L., Naftel, D. C., Young, J. B., Pelegrin, D., Czerr, J., Higgins, R., et al. (2007). Patterns and predictors of physical functional disability at 5 to 10 years after heart transplantation. *The Journal of Heart and Lung Transplantation, 26*(11), 1182–1191.

Hauboldt, R. H., Hanson, S. G., & Bernstein, G. R. (2008). *2008 U.S. organ and tissue transplant cost estimates and discussion.* Brookfield, WI: Milliman, Inc.

Hetzer, R., Albert, W., Hummel, M., Pasic, M., Loebe, M., Warnecke, H., et al. (1997). Status of patients presently living 9 to 13 years after orthotopic heart transplantation. *Annals of Thoracic Surgery, 64*, 1661–1668.

Holtkamp, S. (2002). *Wrapped in mourning: The gift of life and organ donor family trauma.* New York: Brunner-Routledge.

Hommel, K. A., Chaney, J. M., Wagner, J. L., White, M. M., Hoff, A. L., & Mullins, L. L. (2003). Anxiety and depression in older adolescents with long-standing asthma: The role of illness uncertainty. *Children's Health Care, 32*, 51–63.

Jessup, M., Abraham, W. T., Casey, D. E., Feldman, A. M., Francis, G. S., Ganiats, T. G., et al. (2009). 2009 focused update: ACCF/AHA guidelines for the diagnosis and management of heart failure in adults: A report of the American College of Cardiology Foundation/American Heart Association Task Force on Practice Guidelines: Developed in collaboration with the International Society for Heart and Lung Transplantation. *Circulation, 119*(14), 1977–2016.

Jones, B. M., Taylor, F., Downs, K., & Spratt, P. (1992). Longitudinal study of quality of life and psychological adjustment after cardiac transplantation. *The Medical Journal of Australia, 157*, 24–26.

Koffron, A., & Stein, J. A. (2008). Liver transplantation: Indications, pretransplant evaluations, surgery, and post-transplant complications. *The Medical Clinics of North America, 92*, 861–888.

Kugler, C., Geyer, S., Gottlieb, J., Simon, A., Haverich, A., & Dracup, K. (2009). Symptom experience after solid organ transplantation. *Journal of Psychosomatic Research, 66*(2), 101–110.

Kuhn, W. F., Davis, M. H., & Lippmann, S. B. (1988). Emotional adjustment to cardiac transplantation. *General Hospital Psychiatry, 10*, 108–113.

Laederach-Hofmann, K., & Bunzel, B. (2000). Noncompliance in organ transplant recipients: A literature review. *General Hospital Psychiatry, 22*, 412–424.

Littlefield, C., Abbey, S., Fiducia, D., Cardella, C., Greig, P., Levy, G., et al. (1996). Quality of life following transplantation of the heart, liver, and lungs. *General Hospital Psychiatry, 18*, 36–47.

Livneh, H., Antonak, R. F., & Gerhardt, J. (1999). Psychosocial adaptation to amputation: The role of sociodemographic variables, disability-related factors and coping strategies. *International Journal of Rehabilitation Research, 22*, 21–31.

Mai, F. M., McKenzie, F. N., & Kostuk, W. J. (1990). Psychosocial adjustment and quality of life following heart transplantation. *Canadian Journal of Psychiatry, 35*, 223–227.

Merion, R. M. (2010). Current status and future of liver transplantation. *Seminars in Liver Disease, 30*(4), 411–421.

Millon, T., Antoni, M., Millon, C., Meagher, S., & Grossman, S. (2001). *Millon behavioral medicine diagnostic.* Minneapolis, MN: NCS Pearson, Inc.

Mishel, M. H., & Braden, C. J. (1988). Finding meaning: Antecedents of uncertainty in illness. *Nursing Research, 37*, 98–127.

Mooney, S., Hasssanein, T., Hilsabeck, R., Ziegler, E., Carlson, M., Maron, L., et al. (2007). Utility of the repeatable battery for the assessment of neuropsychological status (RBANS) in patients with end-stage liver disease awaiting liver transplant. *Archives of Clinical Neuropsychology, 22*, 175–186.

Mori, D. L., Gallagher, P., & Milne, J. (2000). The Structured Interview for Renal Transplantation—SIRT. *Psychosomatics, 41*, 393–406.

Nägele, H., Kalmar, P., Rödiger, W., & Stubbe, H. M. (1997). Smoking after heart transplantation: An underestimated hazard? *European Journal of Cardio-Thoracic Surgery, 12*(1), 70–74.

National Heart, Lung, and Blood Institute. (2011). *What is a lung transplant?* Retrieved from http://www.nhlbi.nih.gov/health/dci/Diseases/lungtxp/lungtxp_all.html

Neugarten, B. (1969). *Personality in middle and late life.* New York: Atherton Press.

Olbrisch, M. E. (1996). Ethical issues in psychological evaluation of patients for organ transplant surgery. *Rehabilitation Psychology, 41*(1), 53–71.

Olbrisch, M. E., Benedict, S. M., Ashe, K., & Levenson, J. L. (2002). Psychological assessment and care of organ transplant patients. *Journal of Consulting and Clinical Psychology, 70*(3), 771–783.

Olbrisch, M. E., & Levenson, J. L. (1995). Psychosocial assessment of organ transplant candidates: Current status of methodological and philosophical issues. *Psychosomatics, 36*, 236–243.

Olbrisch, M. E., Levenson, J. L., Sherwin, E. D., & Best, A. M. (1994). Validation of psychosocial assessments of cardiac transplant candidates. *Journal of Heart and Lung Transplantation, 13,* S70.

Orentlicher, D. (1996). Psychosocial assessment of organ transplant candidates and the Americans with Disabilities Act. *General Hospital Psychiatry, 18,* 5S–12S.

Randolph, C. (1998). *The Repeatable Battery for the Assessment of Neuropsychological Status (RBANS).* San Antonio: The Psychological Corporation.

Rees, M. A., Kopke, J. E., Pelletier, R. P., Segev, D. L., Rutter, M. E., Fabrega, A. J., et al. (2009). A nonsimultaneous, extended, altruistic-donor chain. *The New England Journal of Medicine, 360,* 1096–1101.

Reid, W. J. (1990). An integrative model for short-term treatment. In R. A. Wells, & V. J. Gianetti (Eds.), *Handbook of the brief psychotherapies* (pp. 55–77). New York: Plenum.

Reitan, R. M., & Wolfson, D. (1985). *The Halstead-Reitan neuropsychological test battery.* Tucson: Neuropsychology Press.

Roberts, J. P., Hulbert-Shearon, T. E., Merion, R. M., Wolfe, R. A., & Port, F. K. (2004). Influence of graft type on outcomes after pediatric liver transplantation. *American Journal of Transplantation, 4*(3), 373–377.

Rubak, S., Sandbaek, A., Lauritzen, T., & Christensen, B. (2005). Motivational interviewing: A systematic review and meta-analysis. *British Journal of General Practice, 55*(513), 305–312.

Russell, R. T., Feurer, I. D., Wisawatapnimit, P., Salomon, R. M., & Pinson, C. W. (2008). The effects of physical quality of life, time, and gender on change in symptoms of anxiety and depression after liver transplantation. *Journal of Gastrointestinal Surgery, 12,* 138–144.

Rutherford, R. M., Fisher, A. J., Hilton, C., Forty, J., Hasan, A., Gould, F. K., et al. (2005). Functional status and quality of life in patients surviving 10 years after lung transplantation. *American Journal of Transplantation, 5*(5), 1099–1104.

Rybarczyk, B., DeMarco, G., DeLaCruz, M., Lapidos, S., & Fortner, B. (2001). A classroom mind-body wellness intervention for older adults with chronic illness: Comparing immediate and one year benefits. *Behavioral Medicine, 27,* 15–27.

Rybarczyk, B., Grady, K. L., Naftel, D. C., Kirklin, J. K., White-Williams, C., Kobashigawa, J., et al. (2007). Emotional adjustment 5 years after heart transplant: A multi-site study. *Rehabilitation Psychology, 52,* 206–214.

Sanders-Dewey, N., Mullins, L., & Chaney, J. M. (2001). Coping style, perceived uncertainty in illness, and distress in individuals with Parkinson's disease and their caregivers. *Rehabilitation Psychology, 46,* 363–381.

Schnurr, P. P., Friedman, M. J., Engel, C. C., Foa, E. B., Shea, M. T., Chow, B. K., et al. (2007). Cognitive behavioral therapy for posttraumatic stress disorder in women: A randomized controlled trial. *Journal of the American Medical Association, 297*(8), 820–830.

Shamaskin, A. M., Rybarczyk, B. D., Wang, E., White-Williams, C., McGee Jr., E., Cotts, W., et al. (in press). Older patients (age 65+) report better quality of life, psychological adjustment, and adherence than younger patients 5 years after heart transplant: A multisite study. *The Journal of Heart and Lung Transplantation.*

Shapiro, P. A., Williams, D. L., Foray, A. T., Gelman, I. S., Wukich, N., & Sciacca, R. (1995). Psychosocial evaluation and prediction of compliance problems and morbidity after heart transplantation. *Transplantation, 60*(12), 1462–1466.

Slaughter, M. S., Rogers, J. G., Milano, C. A., Russell, S. D., Conte, J. V., Feldman, D., et al. (2009). Advanced heart failure treated with continuous-flow left ventricular assist device. *The New England Journal of Medicine, 361*(23), 2241–2251.

Taylor, D. O., Stehlik, J., Edwards, L. B., Aurora, P., Christie, J. D., Dobbels, F., et al. (2009). Registry of the International Society for Heart and Lung Transplantation: Twenty-sixth official adult heart transplant report-2009. *The Journal of Heart and Lung Transplantation, 28*(10), 1007–1022.

Vamos, M. (2010). Organ transplantation and magical thinking. *Australian and New Zealand Journal of Psychiatry, 44*(10), 883–887.

Wechsler, D. W. (1999). *Wechsler Abbreviated Scale of Intelligence (WASI).* San Antonio: The Psychological Corporation.

Wiesner, R. H. (1996). Current indications, contraindications and timing for liver transplantation. In R. W. Busuttil, & G. B. Klintmalm (Eds.), *Transplantation of the liver* (pp. 71–84). Philadelphia: W. B. Saunders.

Williamson, G. M., & Schulz, R. (1994). Activity restriction mediates the association between pain and depressed affect: A study of younger and older adult cancer patients. *Psychology and Aging, 10,* 369–378.

Williamson, G. M., Schulz, R., Bridges, M. W., & Behan, A. M. (1994). Social and psychological factors in adjustment to limb amputation. *Journal of Social Behavior and Personality, 9,* 249–268.

Wineman, N. M., O'Brien, R. A., Nealon, N. R., & Kaskel, B. (1993). Congruence in uncertainty between individuals with multiple sclerosis and their spouses. *Journal of Neuroscience Nursing, 25,* 356–361.

Xu, J. Q., Kochanek, K. D., Murphy, S. L., & Tejada-Vera, B. (2010). Deaths: Final data for 2007. *National Vital Statistics Reports, 58*(19), 1–135.

Zuckermann, A., Dunkler, D., Deviatko, E., Bodhjalian, A., Czerny, M., Ankersmit, J., et al. (2003). Long-term survival (>10 years) of patients >60 years with induction therapy after cardiac transplantation. *European Journal of Cardio-Thoracic Surgery, 24*(2), 283–291.

Diabetes Mellitus

Donita E. Baird *and* David M. Clarke

Abstract

Diabetes mellitus has serious implications for both the individual and society. An understanding of associated psychological processes and interventions is critical in supporting people with diabetes. Factors thought to be important in optimal diabetes management are presented here, and potential difficulties experienced by patients are examined. This chapter deals with the cognitive, emotional, motivational, and psychosocial factors associated with the treatment of people with diabetes. Implications for practice are considered, including health service delivery factors and methods to facilitate self-management and address demoralization. Depression, anxiety, and eating disorders are examined. The *whole person model* is presented as a method of applying a cognitive-behavioral model within a biopsychosocial multidisciplinary framework. The role of clinical psychology in the care of people with diabetes is also considered.

Key Words: Diabetes, depression, cognitive-behavioral therapy, self-management, disease management, demoralization

Diabetes mellitus, more commonly known as *diabetes*, is a group of metabolic diseases with serious implications for both the individual and society. Currently, about 220 million people have diabetes worldwide (World Health Organization [WHO], 2011), and the number is projected to exceed 366 million by 2030 (Wild, Roglic, Green, Sicree, & King, 2004). Worldwide, 7.5 million people are estimated to have died from complications of diabetes in 2000 (Roglic et al., 2005). Living well with diabetes requires active engagement in a treatment regime and making healthy lifestyle choices to minimize the risk of serious complications. Many individuals with diabetes manage the condition well with help from a primary care physician, and these patients experience minimal impact on daily quality of life. Others experience difficulties in effectively managing the condition and develop complications. Understanding psychosocial reactions to illness

is essential, and depression and anxiety are common (Ali et al., 2006; Barnard, Skinner, & Peveler, 2006). Unidentified and untreated psychosocial distress complicates management, and some people will require additional support from specialist clinics or multidisciplinary rehabilitation programs in order to gain the necessary holistic care.

The term *rehabilitation* can be usefully applied to diabetes care, as the aim of such programs is to help patients achieve optimal functioning given the restrictions imposed by this chronic disease. This chapter deals with the cognitive, emotional, motivational, and psychosocial factors associated with the rehabilitation and treatment of people with diabetes. An understanding of associated psychological processes and interventions is critical in supporting people with diabetes mellitus. An overview of diabetes management is presented, as are potential difficulties experienced by patients. Implications for practice are considered. The *whole person model* (WPM) is presented as a method of applying a cognitive-behavioral model within a biopsychosocial multidisciplinary framework.

Understanding Diabetes

In diabetes, the level of blood glucose (blood sugar) is above normal. People with diabetes have problems converting food to energy and maintaining normal blood sugar levels. Normally, when foods containing carbohydrates or simple sugars are digested and absorbed into the blood through the intestines, the hormone insulin helps the body store these nutrients throughout the body for use later as a source of energy. Insulin is essential as it facilitates the entry of glucose into body tissues—particularly the liver, muscles, and fat tissue—for storage (as glycogen) or energy for metabolism. Diabetes is characterized by *hyperglycemia* or high blood sugar. Chronic hyperglycemia of diabetes is associated with serious health consequences. Blood sugar levels can be tested by examining the blood glucose concentration following an overnight fast (fasting blood glucose test) or by an oral glucose tolerance test (the glucose concentration 2 hours after drinking a standard glucose drink). Hemoglobin A_{1c} (HbA_{1c}) gives a measure of the average amount of circulating glucose in the blood over a 120-day period. HbA_{1c} is a widely used marker of chronic glycemia. The American Diabetes Association (ADA, 2010) standards of medical care in diabetes specifies diagnostic criteria and outlines management recommendations. Table 22.1 shows the diagnostic implications of glucose concentrations as measured by the aforementioned tests.

Several pathogenic processes are involved in the development of diabetes; most fundamentally involve the body not producing enough insulin (insulin deficiency) or body tissues not responding normally to the circulating insulin that is produced (insulin resistance), or both. Historically, diabetes has been categorized as either type 1 and type 2. Recently, consideration has also been given to identifying people at risk of developing diabetes, and these are said to have prediabetes.

Prediabetes

Individuals may be considered prediabetic if there are indications of mildly impaired glucose tolerance (IGT); that is, blood glucose levels are higher than normal on the glucose tolerance test (GTT), but below those of a person considered to have diabetes. On a fasting blood glucose test, the levels may be normal or only moderately raised. Impaired glucose tolerance is also often associated with high blood pressure and high low-density lipoprotein (LDL) cholesterol. In 2007, 26.3% of Americans had IGT, and this number is projected to reach 36.8% by 2020 (United Health, 2010). Impaired glucose tolerance is most likely due to a combination of impaired secretion of insulin by the pancreas and insulin resistance. In other words, some insulin is produced, but there is a problem in the tissues ability to drive glucose into the cells. The loss of insulin secretion is the result of malfunctioning pancreatic β cells. At this stage, the person is unlikely to experience any symptoms. However, in the long term, high blood glucose levels are toxic to β cells, leading to further deterioration in β-cell function, reduced insulin production, and higher blood glucose levels. The McMaster University (2005) review reported that the annualized relative risk of a person with IGT progressing to diabetes increased sixfold compared with people with normal glucose tolerance. The relative risk was 12-fold in people with both IGT and abnormal fasting glucose. However, this is not inevitable, as weight loss and increased physical activity can reduce insulin resistance and therefore make insulin more effective. Approximately 30% of individuals with IGT will return to normal glucose tolerance (Soderberg et al., 2004). The ADA (2010) practice guidelines recommend that people with IGT or an HbA_{1c} of 5.7–7.4% are referred to support programs to achieve a weight loss of 5–10% of body weight and an increase in physical activity to at least 150 minutes per week of moderate activity, such as walking. Only about 7% of Americans living with prediabetes today are aware that they have this condition (United Health, 2010). Given the high risk of developing type 2 diabetes from IGT,

Table 22.1 Diagnostic indications of blood glucose readings

Diagnosis	Fasting Blood Glucose	Glucose Tolerance Test (GTT)	HbA_{1c} (reported as % of total Hb)
Normal	99 or below	139 and below	<5.7%
Prediabetic	100 and 125 mg/dL	140 and 199 mg/dL	5.7–6.4%
Diabetes	>126 mg/dL	>200 mg/dL	>6.5%

people with IGT should also be screened for diabetes at regular intervals.

Type 1 Diabetes

Type 1 diabetes (previously known as insulin-dependent or juvenile-onset diabetes) accounts for only 5% to 10% of diabetes cases (ADA, 2010). People with type 1 diabetes have insulin deficiency from a cellular-mediated autoimmune destruction of the pancreatic β cells, with both genetic and environmental factors as major determinants. An abnormally low level of insulin is a serious problem as it leads to high blood glucose levels in the blood, but low levels of glucose available to the tissues. The symptoms of type 1 diabetes—polyuria (excessive excretion of urine), polydipsia (excessive thirst), constant hunger, weight loss, vision changes, and fatigue—appear rapidly over days to weeks, although the damage to the insulin-producing cells has been occurring over years. It is the most common chronic metabolic disorder to affect children. The majority of cases occur before the age of 35, with peak onset during the second decade of life. It is most common in Caucasian populations, especially those in Scandinavia, and is rare in people of Asian or African descent.

The primary aim of treatment is the control of blood glucose, usually termed *glycemic control*. This invariably requires daily injections of insulin, together with well-controlled diet and exercise that regularizes energy intake and expenditure. As a measure of good glycemic control, the ADA (2010) recommend a target for HbA_{1c} of below or around 7%, as this has been shown to be associated with reduced microvascular and neuropathic complications.

Type 2 Diabetes

Type 2 diabetes accounts for 90–95% of cases of diabetes and encompasses individuals who have insulin resistance and usually relative, rather than absolute, insulin deficiency (ADA, 2010). The specific etiologies are not known. However, autoimmune destruction of the β cells does not occur. Instead, insulin is produced, but a problem occurs at the end organs, whereby insulin is unable to have its usual effect of facilitating the transport of glucose into the tissues. This is termed *insulin resistance*. Most patients with this form of diabetes are obese and/or have a predominantly abdominal distribution of fat, and obesity itself causes some degree of insulin resistance. Patients with type 2 diabetes may have insulin levels that appear normal or even elevated; however, it is still a "relative deficiency," as

the high blood glucose levels would result in even higher insulin levels if β-cell function were normal. Thus, for these people, insulin secretion is insufficient to compensate for insulin resistance. Type 2 diabetes frequently goes undiagnosed for many years because hyperglycemia develops insidiously and, during the early stages, is not severe enough for patients to notice any of the classic symptoms. Up to 6.3 million Americans have undiagnosed diabetes (Zhang et al., 2009).

Type 2 diabetes is most common in people over 40 years of age and most prevalent among African Americans, Latinos, Asian-Pacific Islanders, and Native Americans. It is often associated with a strong genetic predisposition, more so than the autoimmune form of type 1 diabetes. However, the genetics of diabetes is not clearly defined (ADA, 2010). The risk of developing type 2 diabetes increases with age, obesity, and lack of physical activity (ADA, 2010). Obesity and physical inactivity are increasing problems in children, and there are indications of increasing prevalence of type 2 diabetes in children. For example, in the United States, a tenfold increase was reported in a New York clinic from 1990 to 2000, with 50% of all new childhood cases of diabetes being type 2 (Grinstein et al., 2003). In Japan, researchers have documented a rise in annual incidence of new cases from 1.73 per 100,000 to 2.76 per 100,000 over the course of 20 years (Urakami et al., 2005). In the United Kingdom, the national incidence of type 2 diabetes in children was found to be 1.3 per 100,000 (Haines, Bararett, Chong Wan, Shield, & Lynn, 2007).

The treatment of type 2 diabetes includes weight management, physical activity, and dietary modification, together with oral glucose-lowering medication. An important recent change to management guidelines for people with type 2 diabetes is the early initiation of medical therapy—at the time of diagnosis rather than later (ADA. 2010). Initiating medical therapy, in conjunction with lifestyle modification, is important for control of blood glucose, which is critical for preventing long-term complications. Achieving an HbA_{1c} level of below or around 7% is recommended (ADA, 2010). At least initially, and often throughout life, these patients do not need insulin treatment for survival, although it may be helpful later to achieve good glycemic control.

Complications of Diabetes

Diabetes, if undetected or poorly controlled, can result in serious long-term health problems and, ultimately, death. The World Health Organization

(WHO, 2011) estimates that 3.4 million people died in 2004 from consequences of diabetes. *Diabetic neuropathy* is damage to the nerves as a result of diabetes and affects up to 50% of people with diabetes (WHO, 2011). Common symptoms are tingling, pain, numbness, or weakness in the hands and feet. Combined with reduced blood flow, neuropathy in the feet increases the chance of foot ulcers and eventual limb amputation. Diabetic retinopathy is an important cause of blindness and occurs as a result of long-term accumulated damage to the small blood vessels in the retina. After 15 years of diabetes, approximately 2% of people become blind, and about 10% develop severe visual impairment. Regular follow-up is required to monitor the status of the disease and to minimize the risk of complications. At a minimum, patients require annual complete physical examination, including a foot examination, dilated eye examination, fasting lipid profile, and serum creatinine levels, as well as a review of any abnormalities. An HbA_{1c} level test should be performed at least once every 6 months in patients who have met glycemic goals and quarterly in others (ADA, 2010).

The WHO (2011) reports that the overall risk of dying among people with diabetes is at least double the risk of those without the disorder. Diabetes is among the leading causes of kidney failure, and 10–20% of people with diabetes die of kidney failure. Diabetes increases the risk of heart disease and stroke. Indeed, 50% of people with diabetes die of cardiovascular disease (primarily heart disease and stroke). Worldwide, 2.9 million deaths per year are directly attributable to diabetes, which is equivalent to 5.2% of world all-cause mortality (Roglic et al., 2005). Excess mortality attributable to diabetes was over 8% in the United States, Canada, and the Middle East (Roglic et al., 2005).

Diabetes is a major contributor to the burden of disease due to disability. In 2003, diabetes was responsible for 5.5% of the total burden of disease and injury in Australia. The burden attributable to diabetes increases to 8.3% if the contribution of the increased risk of coronary heart disease and stroke are considered, thus ranking it fourth out of all diseases (Begg et al., 2007). Type 2 diabetes is projected to be the leading specific cause of disease burden for males and second for females by 2023 (Australian Institute of Health and Welfare [AIHW], 2008).

Managing Diabetes

Diabetes management requires much from the individual. It is more than simply taking medication

and achieving activity and nutritional goals (ADA, 2010). Knowledge and skills are necessary. The National Diabetes Self-Management Education Standards Task force (Funnell et al., 2009) specifies that, at minimum, consumers should have access to education programs that include the following topics:

- Describing the diabetes disease process and treatment options
- Incorporating nutritional management into lifestyle
- Incorporating physical activity into lifestyle
- Using medications safely and for maximum effectiveness
- Monitoring blood glucose and other parameters, and interpreting and using the results for self-management decision-making
- Preventing, detecting, and treating acute complications
- Preventing, detecting, and treating chronic complications
- Developing personal strategies to address psychosocial issues and concerns
- Developing personal strategies to promote health and behavior change

Optimal Diabetes Management

The Task Force concluded that ongoing support is critical and although there is no one "best" education program or approach, those programs incorporating behavioral and psychosocial strategies demonstrate improved outcomes (Funnell et al., 2009). This is consistent with findings by Moos and Holahan (2007), who identified that in order to cope with and adapt to a chronic illness it is necessary to engage in tasks related to the illness and treatment, and tasks related to general psychosocial functioning. For optimal diabetes management, as illustrated in Figure 22.1, a number of other factors may also be relevant. An overview of these components is presented in this section.

MANAGING THE ILLNESS

As indicated previously, ideally, the aim is to achieve HbA_{1c} levels of less than 7.0% (ADA, 2010). Paying attention to HbA_{1c} levels is important because every 1% reduction carries a 14–37% reduction in serious diabetes-related complications such as heart disease, blindness, and kidney disease (Stratton et al., 2000). Setting a target HbA_{1c} is associated with better outcomes in type 1 diabetes (Swift et al., 2010).

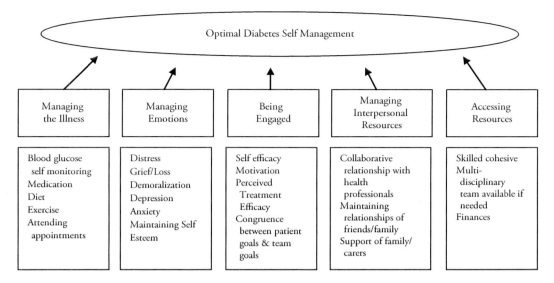

Figure 22.1 Important concepts in optimal diabetes management.

To achieve optimal glycemic control, a daily health regime is necessary. This typically includes:

• Close attention to diet by monitoring carbohydrate intake
• Regular exercise (at least 150 minutes per week of moderate-intensity aerobic activity and, for people with type 2 diabetes, resistance training three times a week)
• Weight management
• Attention to foot care
• Use of medications such as oral glucose-lowering medication and/or subcutaneous insulin injections
• Self-monitoring of blood glucose (SMBG) levels

Self-monitoring of blood glucose using a portable blood glucose machine is the only effective way to manage blood sugar levels in type 1 diabetes. Self-monitoring of blood glucose is also important for type 2 diabetes, although the frequency of monitoring will be determined by a number of individual factors, such as treatment (oral medication vs. insulin), HbA$_{1c}$ levels, and treatment goals. Generally, SMBG needs to be carried out three or more times a day for patients using multiple insulin injections or insulin pump therapy, and sometimes even for patients using less frequent insulin injections or noninsulin therapies (ADA, 2010). Patients need to have the knowledge and skills to appropriately respond to the results (e.g., to consume a glucose drink if readings are low) In addition, as Moos and

Holahan (2007) identified, patients also have to undertake a number of other illness-related tasks, such as adjusting to the hospital environment and medical procedures, including regular injections. It is important to attend appointments regularly and initiate appointments when required. For example, a patient might contact the doctor for an early review if SMBG readings remain high despite taking medication and changing diet as prescribed.

MANAGING EMOTIONS

To effectively manage diabetes, it is also necessary to address the emotional and social consequences of having a chronic medical condition. Assessment of the psychological and social situation should be included as a part of the ongoing medical management of diabetes (ADA, 2010). Illness, like any life event, will elicit an emotional reaction. When the illness is temporary, the emotional reaction passes as the sick role ends (Knight, 1996). A diagnosis of diabetes, however, means adopting a new role. The person does not necessarily feel sick, but he or she does need to manage an ongoing condition, whether he or she views it as an illness or not. When dealing with an illness becomes a matter of years rather than days, the emotional consequences can be very significant (Knight, 1996). The experience of having an ongoing illness increases awareness of the uncertainty of future. This is particularly true when control is difficult or complications begin to set in, and this may give rise to a wide range of emotional responses such as denial, anger, sadness, and fear—sometimes evidenced with clinically significant anxiety or depression. These reactions can be understood by the doctor or psychologist when he or she hears what the illness means for the individual patient. Normalizing fears may help patients understand the need to tolerate some degree of uncertainty.

Moos and Holahan (2007) also identified that learning to control negative feelings, retain a positive outlook, and maintain self-esteem is very important. Grieving for the loss of the healthy self is necessary. For some people, the numerous tasks related to managing their diabetes can be experienced as burdensome. Distress can set in. Patients can become demoralized or feel a failure if their best efforts still do not lead to good control—blood sugars levels are high, weight is increasing. Some people with diabetes feel stigma and a consequential reduction in self-esteem (Tilden, Charman, Sharples, & Fosbury, 2005). Apart from this distress, it must also be realized that when patients become overwhelmed by negative emotions, they find it more difficult to engage in appropriate self-care behaviors. This leads to a downward cycle of poor health.

BEING ENGAGED

The degree to which the patient is engaged in his or her treatment is likely to be mediated by a number of factors. Patients need to have confidence that the treatment can work (perceived treatment efficacy) and confidence in their ability to carry out the required actions (self-efficacy) The literature shows that the more individuals believe that a self-management action will produce a positive outcome and that negative consequences will be absent or minimal, the more likely they are to continue that behavior (Harvey & Lawson, 2009). Behavioral goal setting is integral to this process and has been an effective strategy to support self-management (Funnell et al., 2009). People develop self-efficacy through experiencing success. A patient's perceived ability to control his or her diabetes and the anticipated benefits of this control predict adherence to diet and exercise, other treatments, quality of metabolic control, and overall quality of life (Stenstrom, Wikby, Andersson, & Ryden, 1997). Individuals with greater self-efficacy have more self-motivation and knowledge of their diabetes (Stenstrom et al., 1997) and greater adherence to diet and exercise (King et al., 2010) It is important that a match exists between the patient's goals and the health professional's goals. To succeed, the management plan has to fit the patient's goals, priorities, and lifestyle, as well as their diabetes (Funnell & Anderson, 2004).

The management plan should be collaboratively developed between the patient and the treating team. To remain engaged, the client requires knowledge, skills, and continued support for making lifestyle changes. The Task Force recommends that teaching material be presented in behavioral terms and exemplify the importance of action-oriented behavioral goals and objectives (Funnell et al., 2009). For example, rather than a session simply containing knowledge about "nutrition" and the clients goal being "to eat healthy," the session focuses on how to incorporate nutritional management into the patient's lifestyle; so, the goal may be "each day to eat breakfast, have one serving of vegetables at lunch, and take a piece of fruit to work." Education will only improve outcomes if it results in people behaving differently (Knight, Dornan, & Bundy, 2006).

Clients also require motivation to maintain lifestyle changes. Weinstein (2000) has explored the effect of a person's perception of the *probability* of adverse outcome and the *severity* of the potential outcome on motivation. It turns out that people are surprisingly insensitive to variations in probability of an event when the probability is moderate to high. Furthermore, motivation is worse when the probability is high and the adverse outcome severe. Quite often, in providing information about risk, we assume that if we emphasize a high probability and/or severe adverse outcome people will be motivated to change their health behaviors. Weinstein's study tells us that people ignore differences in probability that are really quite substantial when the probability is in the moderate to high range. It is possible that, at that point, people move into avoidant or passive coping strategies as they believe the adverse outcome is inevitable.

MANAGING INTERPERSONAL RESOURCES
Social Support

Social support is important in coping with any illness. For example, adherence to medical treatment is 1.74 times higher in patients with cohesive families, and 1.53 times lower in patients with families in conflict (DiMatteo, 2004). Management of chronic illness and disability, if and when it occurs, puts a strain on relationships. The patient needs emotional and instrumental support, and a caregiver also needs support. Life goes on; apart from management of the illness there is work to be done, children to look after, friendships to be maintained. Patients and close relatives often need help in maintaining good communications, good health, and mutual relationships. This is important for mental health and well-being and, as we have discussed, good self-care in relation to illness management. Often, behaviors that are good for mental health—such as exercise—are also good for physical health and, if done together, may be good for relational health. It is important for patients to maintain relationships and continue to be engaged in life, despite their illness.

Relationship with Health Professionals

For good management, patients obviously require access to health professionals who are skilled and competent in assisting with all aspects of diabetes management. It is therefore an important skill for patients to be able to relate well and communicate well with health care professionals. Sometimes, patients will need assistance to know how to work collaboratively with health care professionals; sometimes they will need advocacy. For instance, diaries can be helpful in reminding patients of appointments, but they can also be used by patients to keep a record of questions they need to ask the doctor at their next visit.

ACCESSING RESOURCES

Patients may require support, either instrumental or psychosocial, to achieve optimal management. They may not have the financial resources to meet their health needs, such as purchasing medications and fresh food, and paying for specialist appointments. Asking patients about their ability to afford treatment is important (Funnell et al., 2009), as is assisting them to access multidisciplinary care and navigate a complex health system.

Health Service Delivery Factors

The demand that patients with diabetes place on the health care system is significant. The input of multiple health professionals and multiple services will be required; thus, over time, a simple disease becomes a complex illness.

MATCHING SERVICE TO CLIENT NEEDS

The needs of clients differ depending on how long they have had diabetes, the severity of their illness and difficulty of glycemic control, and their self-management capabilities. Newly diagnosed patients may require more support than will those who have had diabetes for 5 years and are experiencing no difficulties with managing the condition. Patients who are experiencing complications may require specialist support over and above the care of their primary

physician. The level of care should be matched to individual client needs and can be moved between levels as required, in a "stepped care" fashion. Many people with type 2 diabetes will spend most of the duration of their disease with suboptimal control (Davis, Davis, & Bruce, 2006).

At the primary care level, clients adequately self-manage with support from a general practitioner (GP) and clinical support services from a diabetes educator or self-management program. Some patients will require secondary care. An example of this would be GP care plus specialist outpatient clinic for clients with multiple morbidities and/or risk of complications or hospital presentation. Tertiary care will be required for patients with chronic and complex needs who require intensive support by diabetes-specific multidisciplinary teams. These patients usually have frequent presentations to a hospital and experience multiple complications.

COORDINATED AND MULTIDISCIPLINARY CARE

Clients with diabetes require the services of a range of health professionals: primary care physicians, endocrinologists, diabetes educators, dieticians, and podiatrists. Depending on patient need, support from psychiatrist, psychologist, physiotherapists, ophthalmologists, and social workers may also be required. Diabetes self-management education programs have been shown to be most effective when delivered by multidisciplinary teams using a comprehensive plan of care (Funnell et al., 2009). Within multidisciplinary teams, team members work independently, consult with one another, and have a shared directive. The DAWN studies (Anonymous, 2004) found the following actions to be important in improving health and quality-of-life for people with diabetes:

• Enhance communications between people with diabetes and their health care providers
• Promote team-based diabetes care
• Promote active self-management
• Overcome emotional barriers to effective therapy
• Enable better psychological care for people with diabetes

Clinical protocols, information systems, and shared medical records can assist in communication between services. Coordinated services are important to ensure patients receive the necessary care and also to avoid duplication.

Health services have a strong influence on client outcome. The Hvidore study group, which investigated metabolic control in large cohorts of adolescents from more than 20 pediatric diabetes centers around the world, demonstrated substantial differences in metabolic outcomes across centers and showed that these differences emerged early in the illness course of newly diagnosed young people and were relatively stable over time. These differences between centers were not accounted for by differences in population demographics or by the presence of interventions targeted to improve outcomes (Danne et al., 2001; De Beaufort et al., 2007). A wide range of psychological, social, and cultural delivery factors were explored in an attempt to understand the differences among these centers. Family dynamics were found to be an important predictor of metabolic outcomes in adolescents, but this effect was relatively consistent across centers and did not account for the between-center differences (Cameron et al., 2008). Swift et al. (2010), however, reported that clear and consistent setting of glycemic targets by diabetes teams was strongly associated with good HbA_{1c} outcomes. A lower target and greater consistency between members of teams within centers were associated with achieving a lower HbA_{1c}. These results point to the importance of team cohesion. As the authors report, the team outcome is strengthened if there is consistency in the targets set between various members of the team. Teams that do not agree on treatment goals do not create confident working relationships with families, and both adolescents and parents recognize these inconsistencies. The better centers, with patients maintaining lower HbA_{1c} levels, were also more successful at educating parents and adolescents in understanding what levels are desirable and also in providing an environment that enabled those targets to be achieved. These findings appear to be the strongest so far uncovered in the search for factors that are responsible for the variation in clinical outcome between centers in the Hvidoere study (Swift et al., 2010).

Implications for Practice

In sum, optimal diabetes management relates to more than the physical management; it includes the psychosocial elements of living with the condition. It is a complex, lifelong process requiring a great deal of effort on the part of the patient. They, more than any health care provider, are key to successful management. It is important that emotional responses are identified and their impact on self-care behavior explored. Interventions aimed at increasing self-efficacy can improve outcomes for

the patient. Creative, patient-centered, experience-based education delivery methods are effective for supporting informed decision-making and behavior change and go beyond the acquisition of knowledge (Funnell et al., 2009). Clinicians may not feel competent in dealing with emotional reactions to the illness and managing psychosocial issues such as financial stress. According to the DAWN study, 50% of clinicians do not feel able to identify psychosocial problems or know what to do once they are identified. Multidisciplinary teams are needed, and health professionals need skills to support clients in being active partners in their health care. Team cohesion is very important, and, for many, this can be a new way of working.

Special Groups to Consider

The optimal diabetes self-management model can be applied to all patients with diabetes. However, it is important to consider the special issues that may apply to certain populations. Here, we briefly overview special issues to consider for young people, older people, and people from a culturally and linguistically diverse (CALD) background.

YOUNG PEOPLE

Children and adolescents have special needs. Diabetes does not simply affect the individual but also the family. Family dynamics have been found to be important predictors of metabolic outcome in adolescents (Cameron et al., 2008; Jacobson, de Groot, & Samson, 1997). As discussed, goal setting is an important part of self-management, and this applies to children and adolescents as well as to adults (Swift et al., 2010). Children and young people can and should be included as active participants in care planning. One of the major tasks of adolescence is identity formation; therefore, the impact of diabetes on identity formation should be considered and the young person supported. Group therapy may be useful to help young people meet and talk with others going through the same experiences. There may also be issues with transitioning from pediatric services to adult services. For some young people, this is a period of uncertainty and upheaval. The young person may have been linked with pediatric services for many years, in the context of which they have been treated as a child, under the care of parents or guardians. The transition to a new part of the service may be experienced as a loss of or rejection from a supporting environment to one in which they have to negotiate their own way and express more autonomy.

OLDER PEOPLE

Almost half the people with diabetes are age 65 or older, and about half of the cases of diabetes in this age group go undiagnosed. To the elderly person, the diagnosis of diabetes may evoke multiple emotions, including dread, fear, and sadness (Caruso & Silliman, 1999). Not only are the complications of diabetes devastating for an older person, since it can lead to functional impairment, but following complex dietary, exercise, medication, and monitoring regimes may be overwhelming. However, older adults who are functional and cognitively intact should receive diabetes care using the same goals developed for younger people (ADA, 2010). For older adults with physical or cognitive impairment, and who require daily functional, nutritional, and medical assistance, it may be necessary to relax glycemic goals using individual criteria (ADA, 2010). Achieving targets may be an issue when patients are socially isolated or may strain relationships with caregivers. It is important to involve patients in their own care as much as possible, and to be sensitive to patients' health-related quality of life. Hyperglycemia leading to symptoms or risk of acute hyperglycemic complications should be avoided in all older patients (ADA, 2010). Exercise offers significant benefits, but it is important that patients are assessed by a physician before commencing an exercise program.

CULTURALLY AND LINGUISTICALLY DIVERSE BACKGROUNDS

As discussed previously, there is a higher incidence of diabetes in certain populations. Much of the published self-management literature is based on participants who have high levels of education, are English speaking, are well-resourced, and have higher socioeconomic status (Walker, Weeks, McAvoy, & NDemetriou, 2005). Recruitment of eligible patients from diverse backgrounds in chronic disease self-management programs has so far been limited (Kennedy, Gately, & Rogers, 2004). A possible contributing factor is the clinician's lack of appropriate skills and confidence to effectively identify and treat psychological distress in CALD clients (Kiropoulos, Blashki, & Klimidis, 2006; Minas, Klimidis, & Tuncer, 2007). Self-management models may need to be tailored to meet the needs of people from CALD backgrounds, and it is recommended that special consideration be given to the meaning of diabetes and illness representations for the client. Some clients may be somewhat reluctant to engage in such discussions for different reasons: some may feel it is disrespectful to share their thoughts with an authority figure, others may fear that their views will be dismissed as not fitting with a Western medical model. In addition, for some populations such as indigenous people in remote communities, social and financial stressors impair the ability to access appropriate services, resources, and even fresh food. Much more research is needed to determine how best to meet the needs of people from CALD backgrounds.

Treatment Adherence

Diabetes management requires a substantial degree of active engagement in treatment. Treatment plans work if they are followed, but often this is hard to do. The challenge for many clients is that neither the potential costs nor benefits of following the treatment plan are immediately observable. This incongruence between intentions and behaviors can cause significant distress. Negative cognitions, such as a perceived failure to do the right thing, can result in lowered self-efficacy and self-esteem. For example, an analysis of participants in a group program targeting people with type 1 diabetes with poor glycemic control found that although self-care behavior was perceived as important, it was accompanied by high levels of diabetes-related emotional distress and low levels of diabetes-specific self-efficacy (van der Ven et al., 2005).

Nonadherence to therapeutic regimes among patients with diabetes has been a continuing problem for health care providers (Nagasawa, Smith, Barnes, & Finchman, 1990; Vermeire, Hearnshway, Van Royen, & Denekens, 2001). Low adherence to prescribed medical interventions is a perennial and complex problem for patients with a chronic illness. It may be reflected in not having a prescription filled at the pharmacy, taking the wrong dose, taking medication at the wrong time, forgetting to take medication, or stopping medication. In type 1 diabetes, 28% of 15- to 18-year-olds do not obtain sufficient insulin from the pharmacy to inject the prescribed dosage (Morris et al., 1997). In type 2 diabetes, only a third of patients on monotherapy obtain at least 80% of their prescribed medication (Donnan, MacDonald, & Morris, 2002). Rates of adequate adherence to diabetes medicines appear low; for example, a specialist clinic in Mexico reported an adherence rate of only 21.6% (Lerman et al., 2004), and a specialist clinic in United States found a rate of 28% (Mann, Poniem, Leventhal, & Halm, 2009). A Cochrane review found that less than 50% of patients adhere to treatment recommendations (Vermeire et al., 2001).

Nonadherence can also apply to the process of seeking, receiving, and engaging with a care plan, as in delaying to seek care, missing appointments, or not following-up referrals to see specialists. It can also include how actively engaged the patient is in his or her relationship with health care professionals. These aspects of adherence are difficult to research.

Glycemic control is a core component of diabetes self-management that lends itself to research. Approximately one-fourth of people on intensive insulin therapy do not achieve and maintain adequate glycemic control (DCCT/EDIC, 2002), even with intensive support (Lorenz et al., 1996). Common reasons for not reaching satisfactory control of blood glucose include the difficulties associated with coping with the many demands of diabetes in daily life (van der Ven et al., 2005). Many patients consider monitoring uncomfortable, intrusive, and unpleasant. Many diligently record their results, but do nothing with them (Heller, 2007). Indeed, an interesting observation from a randomized controlled trial of efficacy of SMBG in 96 patients with newly diagnosed diabetes was that monitoring was associated with a 6% higher score on the depression subscale of a well-being questionnaire, despite a rapid improvement in glycemic control (O'Kane et al., 2008). The authors hypothesized that the negative effect might relate less to feelings of powerlessness in the face of high blood glucose readings, as previously assumed, but rather to the enforced discipline of regular monitoring without tangible gains.

Making and maintaining lifestyle changes can be difficult. The extent to which patients follow lifestyle modification recommendations varies for different areas of self-care. For example, physical activity is often neglected (Pham, Fortin, & Thibaudeau, 1996), and only about half the time do patients report following dietary recommendations (Shultz, Sprague, Branen, & Lambeth, 2001). It has become evident that it is difficult for most people to adhere to every aspect of the regime all of the time (Ruggiero et al., 1997).

UNDERSTANDING NONADHERENCE

There are multiple reasons why a person may not adhere to a treatment regime, both intentional or unintentional. An assumption may be that the person does not understand why it is important to follow a particular recommendation. Although knowledge and skills are important prerequisites for adequate self-management, they do not equate

automatically with behavior change (Coates & Boore, 1996). Traditional diabetes education tends to focus primarily on improvement of knowledge; however, knowledge alone does not result in behavior change or improved glycemic control (Brown, 1999; Clement, 1995, Coates & Boore, 1996; Glasgow, Toobert, & Gillette, 2001; Knight et al., 2006). A guiding principle of the national standards for diabetes self-management education is a move away from primarily didactic education to more theoretically based empowerment models (Funnell et al., 2009).

As indicated previously, perceived treatment efficacy is important in optimal diabetes management. Polonsky and Skinner (2010) argue that this is especially so in type 2 diabetes. As they explain, in type 2 diabetes, patients are asked to regularly engage in a series of complex self-management tasks over the course of years when the chief incentive for those efforts is, essentially, a reduction of risk of developing long-term complications. From the patient's perspective, he is making sacrifices now to protect against something bad happening in the future. From this point of view, there may be little tangible sense of how his efforts are making a positive difference from one day to the next. It is understandable that some people may then choose to ignore the demands of their treatment regime now and take a gamble on the future. These researchers propose that what we typically refer to as "patient noncompliance" in diabetes may be the result of impaired perceived treatment efficacy. If patients do not believe that a recommended action—be it exercise, dietary changes, SMBG, or taking medications—is contributing to an observable, positive short-term impact on their diabetes health, they will not do it. If they believe the prescribed treatments are making it worse, they will be reluctant to cooperate.

Both the ADA standards for medical management (ADA, 2010) and the national diabetes self-management standards (Funnell et al., 2009) stress the importance of eliciting patient beliefs and attitudes. Mann et al. (2009) found that predictors of poor medication adherence were believing you have diabetes only when your sugar is high, saying there was no need to take medicine when the glucose was normal, worrying about side-effects of diabetes medicines, lack of self-confidence in controlling diabetes, and feeling medicines are hard to take. Low self-efficacy is also predictive of poor medication adherence (Mann et al., 2009) and physical activity (Dutton et al., 2009). Horne and Weinman (1999) have noted a distinction between patients' perceptions of the need for taking a specific medication and their beliefs about the potential effects of that medication. These perceptions may also contribute to impaired perceived treatment efficacy.

Emotional reactions may also play a role in nonadherence. Low treatment adherence can be due to a rejection of the "diabetic identity" (Tilden et al., 2005). For patients with persistent poor control, negative feelings toward diabetes may result in poor self-care and consequent poor glycemic control, a negative cycle that may ultimately lead to diabetes burnout (Polonsky, 1999). A meta-analysis of 26 studies found perceived barriers, such as perceived side effects of medication and negative social environment, were correlated with poor adherence (Nagasawa et al., 1990). Depression predicts nonadherence to treatment (Ciechanowski, Katon, Russo, & Hirsch, 2003; Wing, Phelan, & Tate, 2002). Depression decreases client motivation and adherence to treatment strategies such as rehabilitation programs and self-management education. High levels of anxiety decrease the client's self-efficacy to manage symptoms, such as high blood sugar levels, and may result in higher levels of dependence on health professionals and the acute health service. A survey of 445 patients with diabetes and depression found that the relationship between increasing depression severity and worsening of diabetes medication adherence was in part mediated through higher perceived barriers for taking medication (such as forgetfulness, interference of medication-taking with normal life, lack of motivation, family problems) and lower self-efficacy (Chao, Nau, Atkins, & Taylor, 2005).

It is also possible that the patient may be labeled as noncompliant when, in fact, the problem is a joint lack of communication (Parkin & Skinner, 2003). The degree of agreement between patient and health care professional perceptions of consultations were explored in 141 dietitian/nurse specialist consultations. Complete disagreement between patient and professional recall on the issue discussed occurred 19.6% of the time. On the decision made, complete disagreement occurred 20.7% of the time. The authors conclude that this highlights a significant problem in patient–professional relationships: if patients and professionals cannot agree on what they talked about, what does this say for the likelihood that patients will correctly recall and understand any patient education that has taken place? The health professional's communication

skills may play an important role in understanding nonadherence.

In conclusion, if a patient's beliefs about his or her illness, medication, and treatment are inconsistent with a self-management model, the risk of poor medication adherence is greater. These suboptimal beliefs are potentially modifiable and are logical targets for educational interventions to improve diabetes self-management. Addressing any emotional distress and depression will also facilitate adherence. Communication during consultations plays an important role in understanding nonadherence (Parkin & Skinner, 2003).

ENHANCING ADHERENCE

Clients who are experiencing difficulties self-managing require additional support. Many novel and practical approaches have been designed to assist clients in developing and following a treatment plan. A review of interventions for improving adherence to treatment recommendations in people with type 2 diabetes across primary care, outpatient, community, and hospital settings examined 21 studies (Vermeire et al., 2009). Nurse-led interventions, home aids, diabetes education, pharmacy-led interventions, and adaptation of medication dosing and frequency showed a small effect on HbA_{1c}. For example, education classes plus weekly nurse telemedicine home visits over a period of 3 months showed a statistically significant reduction in mean HbA_{1c} level of 0.4%. The reviewers concluded that current efforts to improve or facilitate adherence to treatment recommendations of people with type 2 diabetes do not show significant effects.

As indicated previously, a patient's perceived ability to control his or her diabetes and the anticipated benefits of this control predict adherence to diet and other treatments, quality of metabolic control, and overall quality of life (Stenstrom et al., 1997). Asking clients about their confidence to implement actions at home is a practical way to identify those who have low self-efficacy and may benefit from further support. According to Polonsky and Skinner (2010), it is important to also elicit clients' perceived treatment efficacy and to address low efficacy by focusing on strong indicators of good outcome (i.e., metabolic results). Patients often think that their diabetes health and risk of developing complications is related to how they feel or the number of medications they take. This is not true. What is most predictive of risk of complications is chronically elevated blood glucose, blood pressure, and lipids. Health professionals have an important role in assisting clients in identifying useful markers of treatment efficacy and reframing perceived setbacks. Polonsky and Skinner propose that perceived treatment efficacy can be enhanced by collaborating with patients to develop personalized self-management goals and by providing frequent feedback on outcome (e.g., easy-to-read graphs of metabolic change over time). Devising meaningful home experiments is one way that health professionals and clients can demonstrate how health actions influence outcomes. For example, if a patient is worried about the impact of food choices at breakfast, have him monitor blood glucose before and after breakfast for 7 days. This can assist the client in understanding that the recommended action—be it exercise, dietary changes, SMBG, or taking medications—is contributing to an observable, positive short-term impact on his diabetes health and may enhance motivation to continue the action. By assessing perceived treatment efficacy and addressing it directly, patients may feel more interested and engaged in ongoing diabetes management. Once patients realize which outcomes are most important for them to focus on and how best to achieve those outcomes, the power of perceived treatment efficacy becomes more obvious. This approach makes theoretical sense. However, further research needs to be done to determine whether this approach improves outcome.

Another commonly advocated way to enhance adherence is to improve the quality of the health care professional–patient relationship. To maximize adherence to a treatment plan, it is necessary to establish a shift in attitude from an expectation of passive compliance from the patient to one of shared decision-making. The patient's goals and the health professional's goals should match as closely as possible. To illustrate, in centers that achieved better outcomes for adolescents with type 1 diabetes, high agreement existed between team members about the importance of setting a lower target HbA_{1c} (Swift et al., 2010). Kuijer and Ridder (2003) found that a large discrepancy between the importance and attainability of health-related goals was negatively associated with psychological well-being among people with chronic illness. For example, a patient may experience distress if he or she thought it was important to lose weight but felt it was impossible. Self efficacy was found to mediate this relationship: low self-efficacy reflected the inability to achieve a desired outcome. This study points to the importance of tailoring the goals to the client. In a concordance approach, the treatment regime is tailored to

what is manageable and attainable for the particular patient (Vermeire et al., 2009). The national standards for self-management education also recommend measuring the attainment of patient-defined goals (Funnell et al., 2009).

To support the client in self-management, it is helpful if the health professional takes into account the client's beliefs about his or her condition, medication, and treatment recommendations (ADA, 2010). The relationship between the patient and health professional must be characterized by cooperation, partnership, and shared decision-making. A meta-analysis of 26 studies indicates that the psychological factors, such as emotional stability, internal and external motivations, perceived benefit, and supportive structure, are associated with better adherence to diabetes medicines (Nagasawa et al., 1990). Similarly, Stewart's (1995) review of communication studies on health outcomes indicates the importance of simply asking patients about their understanding of their problems, concerns, expectations, and perceived impact of their illnesses. Exploring and supporting these factors in clinical practice is of benefit to clients. Observations of consultations have found that the greater the support for patient autonomy, the greater the reported levels of motivation (Parkin & Skinner, 2003).

Diabetes and Mental Health

As discussed previously, the presence of multiple morbidities, including mental health conditions, increases the complexity of an illness and its management. There is an increased prevalence of psychiatric disorders in people with type 1 and type 2 diabetes, and it is estimated that up to a third of patients with diabetes have a psychiatric disorder and/or a psychological problem (Smith, 2005). In this section, depression, anxiety disorders, and eating disorders are considered.

Depression and Diabetes

Depression is more common in people with type 2 diabetes than in the general population. Rates of depression are reported at between 9% and 27% of patients, depending on the population studied and method of assessment used (Gavard, Lustman, & Clouse, 1993; Lustman, Freedland, Griffiths, & Clouse, 2000b; Peyrot & Rubin, 1997; Young et al., 2010). The prevalence rate of depression is about twice as high in people with type 1 and 2 diabetes as in nonclinical populations (Anderson, Freedland, Clouse, & Lustman, 2001; Sacco & Yanover, 2006). Nouwen et al. (2010), in a systematic review, found a 24% greater level of incident depression in people with diabetes compared to those without. However, in a recent study of 824 people with newly diagnosed type 2 diabetes, no increase in the rate of depressive symptoms was reported (Skinner et al., 2010). At 12 months, 5% of the sample had clinical levels of depression, with no evidence of symptom remission. This suggests that the observed elevated rates of depressive symptoms reported elsewhere develop later in the course of illness.

OVERVIEW OF DEPRESSION

It makes intuitive sense that depression may play an important role in the development and worsening of diabetes. Depression is a whole body disorder. As well as experiencing low mood and/or anhedonia (loss of pleasure), people with depression may experience poor concentration, altered sleep patterns, and appetite disturbance. Feelings of helplessness and hopelessness may also occur. All of these symptoms could adversely influence the patient's ability to engage in self-management and make lifestyle changes. For example, depression may reduce the ability of patients to carry out the complex tasks required for diabetes self-care (Leichter & See, 2005). Although it is evident that an association exists between depression and diabetes, the direction of the association is unclear. Depression may occur as a consequence of having diabetes, but may also be a risk factor for developing diabetes.

DEPRESSION AS A RISK FACTOR

There are indications that depression is an independent risk factor for the development of type 2 diabetes (Talbot & Nouwen, 2000). The existence and severity of depression correlates positively with the severity of insulin resistance in patients at risk of developing diabetes (Timonen et al., 2005). A meta-analysis of nine longitudinal studies concluded that depressed adults have a 37% increased risk of developing type 2 diabetes, compared to those who are not depressed or have few depressive symptoms (Knol et al., 2006). The mechanism for this is not definitively known. Clearly, behavioral factors contribute. Depressed people are more likely to be overweight (Luppino et al., 2010) and to smoke (Wilhelm, Wedgwood, Niven, & Kay-Lambkin, 2006) than are nondepressed persons. People with depression and a medical comorbidity are three times as likely to not adhere to treatment recommendations (DiMatteo, Lepeprs, & Crogha, 2000). However, the relationship between depression and diabetes persists even after these behavioral factors are taken into account.

Other researchers have proposed that the association can be explained by a direct pathophysiological effects of depression acting via the hypothalamic-pituitary-adrenal axis or sympathetic nervous system (Aikens, Wallander, Bell, & Cole, 1992; Goetsch, 1989) resulting in the increased release of cortisol and the catecholamines adrenaline and noradrenaline. Cortisol is a stress hormone that stimulates glucose production, increases lipolysis and circulating free fatty acids, decreases insulin secretion from beta cells, and decreases sensitivity to insulin (Bjorntorp, 2001). A chronically high cortisol level is a feature of about 50% of depressed patients and leads to obesity, insulin resistance, and type 2 diabetes. Furthermore, depression is associated with increased activity of the proinflammatory pathway, and inflammation is also associated with insulin resistance (Shoelson, Lee, & Goldfine, 2006). Other hypotheses include the dysregulation of the immune system or low intake/impaired metabolism of polyunsaturated fatty acids.

The risk factors for diabetes are the same as the risk factors for heart disease, and these are often referred to collectively as the *metabolic syndrome*. The International Diabetes Federation (Ford, 2005) defines the metabolic syndrome by the presence of:

- Central obesity, measured by waist circumference or body mass index (BMI)
  plus two of:
- Raised triglycerides
- Reduced high-density lipoprotein (HDL) cholesterol
- Raised blood pressure
- Raised fasting blood glucose

Depression is associated with the metabolic syndrome (Dunbar et al., 2008) and, therefore, with both diabetes and heart disease, and the mechanisms for depression are both behavioral and biological, as illustrated in Figure 22.2 and described earlier.

DEPRESSION AS A MODERATOR

There are a number of mechanisms by which depression may contribute to a poorer outcome in people with already established diabetes. Behavioral mechanisms, such as low adherence with routine blood sugar monitoring, diet, and other aspects of treatment, could be an underlying link between depression and glycemic control in diabetes (de Groot, Jacobson, Samson, & Welch, 1999). Even low levels of depressive symptoms have been shown

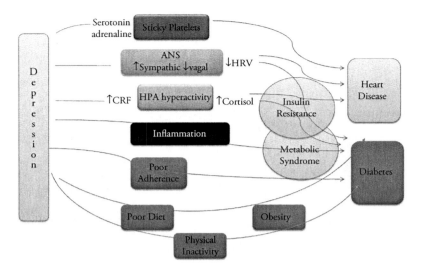

Figure 22.2 Association among depression, diabetes, and heart disease.

to be associated with nonadherence to diabetes self-care (Gonzalez, Safren, Cagliero, Wexler, & Delahanty, 2007). Studies show that depression reduces patients' ability to cope with their diabetes-related self-care needs (Lin et al., 2004; Williams et al., 2004). This relationship may be further mediated by a number of factors, including the complexity of self-care regime (Surwit, van Tilburg, Parekh, Lane, & Feinglos, 2005) or lack of social support (Sacco & Yanover, 2006).

Other researchers have proposed that depression exerts an influence via personal illness representations that, in turn, act to impair physical functioning. Hampson et al. (2000) found that illness beliefs (perceived seriousness of diabetes, beliefs about treatment effectiveness, and perceived control) were independently associated with HbA$_{1c}$, eating patterns, physical functioning, and mental health in patients with type 1 and type 2 diabetes. Anxiety and depression only predicted the mental health aspects of quality of life. Similarly, in a cross-sectional study, anxiety and depression were associated with more negative appraisals of diabetes, more perceived symptoms, greater anticipated duration of illness, more adverse consequences, and less control over type 2 diabetes (Paschalides et al., 2004). At present, it is not clear whether negative illness representations result in anxiety or depression or vice versa.

However, a number of studies indicate that the association between depression and diabetes cannot be solely explained by behavioral mechanisms. For example, a study by Katon et al. (2004) illustrates

how depression may influence risk factors in patients with diabetes. Patients with depression and diabetes were more likely to smoke than were patients without depression; however, in addition, these patients were more likely to have an HbA$_{1c}$ of over 8%, a BMI of greater than 30 kg/m^2, and a serum triglyceride level of over 400 mg/dL. These factors all increase the risk for serious complications. Lustman et al. (2005) examined depressive symptoms and diabetes self-care in a sample of 188 patients with type 1 diabetes. Depression was found to predict HbA$_{1c}$ level independently of weight and insulin dose. Adding diabetes self-care to the regression model did not significantly alter the effect of depression. The authors therefore concluded that, although adherence to diabetes self-care does influence metabolic control, self-care behaviors did not explain the additional hyperglycemia associated with depression.

DEPRESSION IS ASSOCIATED WITH A POOR OUTCOME

The coexistence of depression in people with diabetes is associated with an adverse effect on functioning and quality of life (Jacobson et al., 1997; Lustman, Griffiths, Gavard, & Clouse, 1992). A World Health Organization (WHO) study found the greatest decrements in self-reported health were observed in those with depression and diabetes, more so than in those with depression and other chronic conditions, such as arthritis or asthma (Moussavi et al., 2007). A systematic review of the literature found that depressive symptoms markedly impaired health-related quality of life on both generic and diabetes-specific domains (Ali et al., 2010). Furthermore, the presence of depression is associated with an increased cost of diabetes care by 50%, more than the 11% increased cost of persistently elevated HbA_{1c} (Gilmer et al., 2005).

Depression is associated with higher blood glucose levels (Ciechanowski et al., 2003; Wing et al., 2002), greater insulin resistance (Musselman, Beta, Larsen, & Phillips., 2003), and impaired metabolic control (Hanninen, Takala, & Keinanen-Kiukaannemi, 1999; Katon et al., 2004; Lustman et al., 1992). This, in turn, may result in more diabetes-related medical complications and higher mortality. A study by Akimoto et al. (2004) found that depressed patients had less optimal glycemic control than did nondepressed patients following a 2-week education program and that the worse glycemic control was related to poorer self-care behaviors. Significantly, depression was found to predict worsening of glycemic control at the 2-year follow-up. Other researchers have found that although depression was associated with worse self-care behaviors, it was not associated with hyperglycemia (Lin et al., 2004; Williams et al., 2004). These conflicting results may be due to differences in sampling or perhaps due to generally low HbA_{1c} values in the study samples (Leichter & See, 2005). The meta-analysis by Lustman et al. (2000a) indicates that depression is significantly associated with hyperglycemia ($p < 0.001$), with a small effect size of 0.17. This means that depression accounts for 3% of the variance in HbA_{1c}. This is important because small, persistent elevations in HbA_{1c} significantly increase the risk of major complications, and a decrease in HbA_{1c} of 1.0% (from 9.5 to 8.5%) is associated with a 33% reduction in the progression rate of retinopathy (Lustman et al., 2000a). At present, the underlying mechanisms for the association between depression and hyperglycemia is not certain, although a number of possible biological intermediaries have been discussed. Depression may be a cause or consequence of hyperglycemia, and the mechanism may vary over time, between episodes, and between and within individuals (Lustman et al., 2000a).

Of great concern is that, in people with diabetes, depression is associated with more diabetes-related medical complications and higher mortality. Egede et al. (2005) found that people diagnosed with both diabetes and depression were 2.5 times more likely to die during the subsequent 8-year period than were those diagnosed with either disorder alone.

Similarly, Young et al. (2010), in Pathway, a longitudinal prospective study of the impact of depression outcomes among people with diabetes treated in primary care, found that, over a 5-year period, major depression was associated with a three times greater risk of mortality among people with stage 5 chronic kidney disease.

Treatment of Depression

Effective treatments are available for depression. Well-known approaches include antidepressant medication, cognitive-behavioral therapy (CBT), and interpersonal therapy. Research has explored the effectiveness of psychological interventions in people with diabetes. For example, the Diabetes Education and Self-Management of Ongoing and Newly Diagnosed (DESMOND) randomized controlled trial for people with newly diagnosed type 2 diabetes found that the program resulted in less depressive symptomatology in the intervention group, this effect being achieved by 4 months (Davies et al., 2008). It is interesting to note that there were no significant differences between the intervention group and the control group in terms of weight loss or HbA_{1c}. The Sequenced Treatment of Alternatives to Relieve Depression (STAR*D) Study, a pragmatic controlled trial of 2,876 depressed outpatients, found that a diagnosis of diabetes had no impact on treatment effectiveness for major depression (Bryan et al., 2010). Furthermore, when treated with a selective serotonin reuptake inhibitor (SSRI), patients with diabetes had fewer side effects compared to other participants. The authors stated that this may indicate that depressed patients with diabetes may be excellent candidates for more aggressive SSRI dosing (Bryan et al., 2010). This study did not examine if remission of depression had any impact on the diabetes. The results are interesting and promising.

IMPACT OF DEPRESSION TREATMENT ON DIABETES

Given the association between depression and poor glycemic control, an important research question to consider is whether effective treatment of depression can result in improved glycemic control. Lustman et al. (2000a) report that, if extrapolated, the data suggest that treatment of depression could potentially increase the proportion of subjects in good control from 41% to 58% in a diabetic population. Randomized controlled intervention trials have shown that treatment with either CBT or antidepressant medication can improve both mood and glycemic control (Delamater et al., 2001). Lustman et al.'s (1998) randomized controlled trial of CBT in people with depression and type 2 diabetes found related improvements in glycemic control and in depression. Furthermore, a randomized controlled trial of the antidepressant medication nortriptyline in people with type 1 and type 2 diabetes found an association between depression improvement and glycemic control, although it was independent of treatment status (Lustman et al., 1997). Interestingly, a subsequent randomized controlled trial using the antidepressant fluoxetine found a small beneficial effect on HbA_{1c}, but this effect was independent of changes in depression score (Lustman et al., 2000b).

Winkley et al. (2006), in a meta-analysis of 21 trials involving psychological interventions in people with type 1 diabetes, showed that psychological interventions were associated with significant improvements in glycemic control in children and adolescents, but not in adults. The pooled absolute reduction in glycated hemoglobin was 0.5%. It is suggested that this is of sufficient magnitude to reduce the risk of development and progression of diabetic microvascular complications. Further research is necessary to better understand the impact of depression treatment on glycemic control, especially in adults with type 1 diabetes.

Implications for Practice

Many patients with diabetes also suffer from depression. Whether depression is considered as a risk factor for developing diabetes or as part of the complexity of the illness itself, the impact of depression on glycemic control, quality of life, and mortality is the same, highlighting the importance of integrating nonpharmacological, evidence-based treatment for depression into disease management. Psychological morbidity in people with diabetes poses huge challenges for clinical practice (Nouwen et al., 2010). Clinical priority should be given to the effective identification and treatment of coexisting affective disorders.

Treating depression in people with diabetes requires specialist knowledge. Ali et al. (2010) propose that approaches that focus on facets of health-related quality of life could potentially be effective. Psychological interventions that include an understanding of the personal significance of diabetes for the patient are likely to have a greater impact than are treatments focusing on relief of depression alone. Future prospective studies are warranted to confirm the direction of causation, as well as the degree to which interventions for depression can improve health-related quality of life outcomes and vice versa.

Despite the high prevalence of depression, affective disorders are often unrecognized and inadequately treated (Katon, 2008). Katon (2008) estimates that depression remains unrecognized and untreated in approximately two-third of patients with diabetes. Many health care systems do not adequately provide an integrated approach for physical and mental health care (Ivbijaro, 2010), and an individual often receives mental health care from one organization and physical health care from another. In some cases, one condition may be treated while the other is not. The reasons for this are many. Consumer, provider, and system factors all contribute to poor quality of care (Ganju, 2010). Consumers and family members may not recognize or correctly identify symptoms or may be reluctant to seek care (Ganju, 2010). Clients who are receiving treatment at a diabetes outpatient clinic may not consider their depressed mood to be relevant to their diabetes treatment. Clinicians may also not seek out this information. The perception may exist among clinicians that psychological issues are less important than medical concerns in people with diabetes (Katon, 2008), or the providers may not have the right training or support to provide appropriate interventions (Ganju, 2010). As both clients and clinicians may be reluctant to explore signs of psychosocial distress, it may be useful to employ screening measures and to have protocols in place to ensure that depressive symptoms are addressed; such screening tools are considered later in the chapter. Finally, systems may include constraints and limitations related to financing, availability, and access to mental health treatment (Ganju, 2010). (At the end of the chapter, a model for integrating cognitive-behavioral principles into diabetes care is presented.)

Special Issue: Depression, Distress, or Demoralization?

A very important issue to consider is the nature of depression and the different types of depression. Although there is a tendency to speak of depression as if it were a singular thing, it clearly is not. A person who is depressed after going through a divorce and separation is going through a somewhat different thing than is the person trapped in a spiral of increasing ill health or an untreatable cancer. The man experiencing the shame of erectile dysfunction is different from the woman losing her vision. Although depression is clearly important, recent interest has emerged around other aspects of distress—such as hopelessness, demoralization, and diabetes-specific distress.

Hopelessness is neither a necessary nor sufficient criterion for a clinical diagnosis of depression. Hopelessness correlates weakly with standard depressions scales and therefore may deserve study in its own right (Everson et al., 1996). Pedersen et al. (2009) investigated the impact of co-occurring diabetes and hopelessness on 3-year prognosis in cardiac patients undergoing percutaneous procedures. The incidence of 3-year death or nonfatal myocardial infarction was highest in patients with diabetes and hopelessness (15.9%). Participants who were high in hopelessness without diabetes had a higher rate (11.2%) than did those with diabetes alone (8.2%) or people with neither (3.5%). These results remained after adjusting for baseline characteristics (age, multivessel disease), clinical risk factors (hypertension, dyslipidemia, current smoking, and use of angiotensin-converting enzyme inhibitors), and depressive symptoms. It is noteworthy that hopelessness had an impact on prognosis above and beyond depressive symptoms at baseline. This study has important implications for proactive management; for example, enhancing partner support and patients' perceptions of this support may increase a sense of optimism and reduce hopelessness (Gustavsson-Lilius, Julkunen, & Heitanen, 2007). This study also points to the importance of the clinician instilling hope of change in patients. Pedersen et al. (2009) recommend that future studies investigate whether or not addressing hopelessness improves clinical outcomes and quality of life.

Clarke and colleagues have intensively studied depression occurring in the medically ill and were able to differentiate the experiences of demoralization, characterized by helplessness and hopelessness; grief, characterized by a feeling of loss, pangs of grief, and a pining after the lost object; and an anhedonic depression, characterized by loss of joy in things that would normally bring pleasure (Clarke, Kissane, Trauer, & Smith, 2005; Clarke, Mackinnon, Smith, McKenzie, & Herrman, 2000). The latter is the hallmark of traditional melancholic depression (Rush & Weissenburger, 1994). Demoralization and hopelessness can be associated with despair and loss of the will to live, and it arises when a person feels unable to resolve his predicament or to extricate himself from it (Clarke & Kissane, 2002). Problem-solving therapy may be helpful here, if the problem is solvable. Offering patients assistance in ways that

increase their sense of mastery and self-efficacy, and which reduce their feelings of helplessness, is most important. For people in the terminal stages of illness, when disease control is greatly diminished and hope for a bright future seems to be fading, psychotherapeutic techniques to explore meaning and purpose become important (Griffiths & Gaby, 2005). Interestingly, very many people with physical illness have some experience of loss—loss of health, loss of relationship, loss of hope, loss of a future. The treatment for this "grief" component of depression is quite specific—support, expression of emotion, challenging denial, planning for the future—and should be a part of any psychological intervention.

With any illness, of course, disease-specific aspects exist. The DESMOND study provides interesting data on the course of depressive symptoms and an opportunity to explore the role of diabetes-specific distress on depressive symptomatology (Skinner et al., 2010). A post-hoc analysis of the whole sample showed that, at the end of the first year of living with diabetes, 5% of the sample had clinical depression and, for a significant proportion, diabetes-specific distress remained. Of particular concern, 10% of participants reported struggling with guilt and anxiety when going off their diabetes plan, 12% were worrying about future complications, and 2% reported being constantly concerned about food and eating. Diabetes-specific distress was found to contribute to depressive symptomatology over and above ongoing depressive symptoms. Skinner et al. (2010) raise the possibility that these persistent depressive symptoms are in fact a realistic appraisal of the likely course of these patients' diabetes, given that these participants had substantially higher BMI. This is an example of demoralization, and the treatment of it warrants further thought and investigation.

IMPLICATIONS FOR PRACTICE

Diabetes-specific distress, hopelessness, and demoralization frequently contribute to depression and are issues worthy of intervention themselves, even when a formal diagnosis of clinical depression is not made. Skinner et al. (2010) argue that it may be possible to prevent depression in people with diabetes by targeting those diabetes-specific issues that are causing people to experience diabetes distress. Addressing diabetes-specific distress in depression treatments may improve the effectiveness of current interventions. Exploring both negative beliefs about diabetes (particularly symptom burden, consequences, and control) and emotional factors is likely to optimize health-related quality of life in people with diabetes. It may be productive to establish structured approaches to managing distress and depression in this population, especially if the clients are overweight, since attempts at weight loss are unlikely to be successful without addressing an individual's depressive symptoms, which are a known barrier to patient motivation and ability to self-manage (Skinner et al., 2010).

Anxiety Disorders and Diabetes

Anxiety is a normal reaction to any illness and can be an important lead-in to depression or demoralization if not addressed. In terms of disease management, anxiety becomes problematic when it leads to avoidance and impacts on functioning. A systematic review found that generalized anxiety was present in 14% of patients with diabetes, and elevated anxiety symptoms occurred in 40% of patients with diabetes participating in clinical trials (Anderson et al., 2002). Recent results from the World Mental Health Surveys indicate an increased risk of anxiety disorders (odds ratio = 1.20) in patients with diabetes compared with persons without (Lin & Von Korff, 2008). There is a high comorbidity between depression and anxiety. Various levels of anxiety, mild through to severe, are a part of the distress and demoralization previously described. Anxiety disorders are associated with poor glycemic control (Lloyd, Dyer, & Barnett, 2000). In diabetes, specific anxiety disorders, such a needle phobias and fear of hypoglycemic attack (Green, Feher, & Catalan, 2000; Mollema, Snoek, Heine, & van der Ploeg, 2001), create special problems but can be successfully handled if recognized and treated with standard cognitive-behavioral techniques.

Eating Disorders and Diabetes

Controversy exists regarding whether there is an increased prevalence of eating disorders in people with diabetes (Young-Hyman & Davis, 2010). For example, in adolescent females with diabetes, eating disorders have been shown to be 2.5 times more common than in similar nondiabetic subjects (10% vs. 4%) (Smith, 2005). A literature review by Young-Hyman and Davis (2010) found estimates of diagnosable eating disorders in adolescent and young adult females with type 1 diabetes ranging from 3.8% to 27% for patients classified as bulimic or having binge eating disorder, and 38% to 40% when insulin omission is considered a type of purging behavior. Adolescents and young women frequently report using insulin omission or dose reduction as an easy method for weight management via glycosuria

(excretion of glucose in the urine) (Young-Hyman & Davis, 2010). Type 1 diabetic cohorts studied have been significantly heavier than clients without eating disorders, with the average BMI above the normal range (Young-Hyman & Davis, 2010). In a 5-year prospective study, BMI was the strongest predictor of eating disorders (Colton, Olmstead, Daneman, Rydall, & Rodin, 2007).

Weight increases can occur as glycemic control improves and is a common side effect of successful treatment with insulin (Young-Hyman & Davis, 2010). Increasing weight can require increasing doses of insulin or growth hormone to control blood glucose, which can in turn lead to hypoglycemia, increased hunger, and increased dietary intake. Destruction of β cells results in an inability to secrete insulin, contributing to dysregulation of appetite and satiety. Diagnosed eating disorders have been associated with poorer health in individuals with type 1 diabetes and poorer glycemic control (Young-Hyman & Davis, 2010).

Little is known about binge eating disorder in type 2 diabetes; however, it is thought that the incidence (5%) is similar to that seen in obese people in the general population (2%) (Smith, 2005). A multicenter study by Herpertz et al. (2000) of people with type 2 diabetes found about 10% of the sample had an eating disorder characterized by binge eating. All the participants with an eating disorder were overweight. No relationship was observed between glycemic control and eating disorders.

When diabetes and eating disorders co-occur, it creates enormous difficulties for management. As well as the more obvious cases of diagnosable eating disorders, it is important to look for subclinical disordered eating behavior, which is also associated with poor health in people with type 1 diabetes. In type 2 diabetes, eating-related problems, especially a sense of restraint in eating and lack of control, and body awareness-related problems increase with weight gain (Herpertz et al., 2000). These patients lack self-esteem and show considerably more depressive symptoms. In a 5-year prospective study of diabetes patients, the rate of subclinical disordered eating ranged up to 26%, depending on the threshold of behaviors used (Colton et al., 2007). Cognitive-behavioral therapy is an effective treatment for eating disorders and disordered eating and can be used in patients with diabetes (Fairburn, 2008).

Cognitive-Behavioral Therapy

Cognitive-behavioral therapy is increasingly being adopted as an intervention in the management of chronic disease. Cognitive-behavioral therapy uses the therapeutic alliance between patient and therapist to explore the patient's problems in terms of emotions, cognitions, and behaviors. A person's interpretation of an event and associated mood changes are explored. Strategies may include:

- Behavioral analysis
- Goal setting
- Activity scheduling
- Problem solving
- Relaxation training
- Identifying and expressing emotions
- Cognitive restructuring

Typically, as CBT is a specialist treatment, it is often not readily accessible to all diabetes patients and is applied only to clients with affective or eating disorders. Furthermore, if a client is referred for CBT, the treating clinicians are usually not integrated within a diabetes team. External clinicians may not have in-depth knowledge of the impact of diabetes on clients in the manner we have described above.

A cognitive-behavioral framework can be helpful in understanding responses to an illness. The skills and benefit from a cognitive model could be of benefit to all clients with diabetes, regardless of diagnosable depression. For example, an awareness of thinking styles may prevent normal reactions to illness from developing into depression or anxiety. It can also allow early intervention for clients with low mood, anxiety symptoms, and diabetes-related distress. The WPM is a method of applying a cognitive-behavioral framework that can be used in an interdisciplinary context.

The Whole Person Model: An Integrated Approach to the Care of People with Diabetes

The WPM (Figure 22.3) integrates disease self-management and emotional management through a cognitive-behavioral framework. As can be seen from Figure 22.3, the body is explicitly included in the model to enable exploration of responses to symptoms. In traditional CBT, less emphasis is placed on the physical components, and when this component is discussed, it is usually limited to somatic symptoms of anxiety. The mindfulness-based cognitive therapy approach illustrates the importance of body awareness and how closely this is linked with emotional responses (Segal, Williams, & Teasdale, 2002). Similarly, for effective self-management of diabetes or other chronic illnesses, monitoring of physical symptoms and insight is essential (Newman, Steed, & Mulligan, 2004). The WPM is a structure for the patient to use in thinking about how he or she will approach the management of his or her health.

The WPM approach to self-management provides a tool to enable consumers and health professionals to engage in discussions about all aspects of diabetes management. In addition to providing information about the condition and management strategies, it talks about how to put these into place, anticipates potential barriers, and looks at

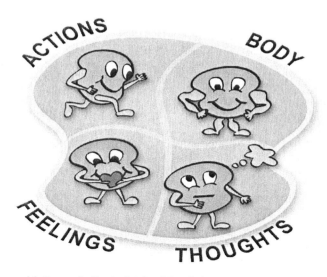

Figure 22.3 Whole person model. Concept by Donita Baird and David Clarke.

the emotional impact of the condition. It is client-centered and client-driven. It can provide a useful vehicle for addressing the problem of diabetes management from the client's perspective. It can be used to explore emotional responses to diabetes and is also a method of identifying diabetes-related distress, depression, anxiety, or other disorders. The WPM approach to self-management is a good model for addressing both the physical and psychosocial components of optimal management, and promotes active participation. It is a structure that can flex up or down to meet client needs.

Case Example

M is a 67-year-old married man of Latino background. Approximately 5 years ago, he visited his doctor because he was experiencing a cold. His doctor noted that M was overweight. He conducted a thorough physical examination, including blood tests. He informed M that he was prediabetic and explained that, due to a history of diabetes in M's family, it was important to lose weight and make lifestyle changes. He gave M a referral to see a dietician and a specialist nurse for education.

When M returned home, his wife asked what had happened at the doctor's appointment. M said, "I went for a cold, and now he's trying to tell me I might get diabetes. I feel fine. He said to lose weight." For a few weeks, M made some effort to lose weight but soon lost interest. He did not follow-up on the referrals.

The next time M visits the doctor, he is diagnosed with diabetes. The doctor states that his HbA_{1c} levels mean that he will have to begin medication. He recommends a self-management program, including a diabetes educator and dietician. M does not follow-up on referrals, as he "doesn't want to be in a group with old people." However, he does regularly monitor his blood sugar, reduces his sugar consumption, and starts going for walks once a week. M takes the prescription, has it filled, but only takes the medication when he feels he has had too much sugar. At the next appointment, the doctor reviews M's medication and is about to write another prescription. M declines, as he has "enough medicine at home." The doctor recommends that he see the diabetes educator because clearly he is not adhering to the treatment plan.

M visits the diabetes educator. He said he was embarrassed that the doctor "caught him out" not taking the medication. The diabetes educator introduces the WPM model and examines how it may apply to taking the medication. Table 22.2 is presented to M.

M identifies with person 3 by saying, "I don't think I need that medication. It's a waste of money. I know I've failed at losing weight, but I'll try a bit harder and I won't need the medication." The diabetes educator acknowledges his *feelings* of anger, "It sounds like there is some frustration there, or even anger?" This statement prompts M to expand further: "Yeah, it is frustrating. I don't drink. I don't

Table 22.2 Example of whole person model

Consider this situation: "I need to take medication to improve my glycemic control (*Body*). But I don't like taking so many medications (*Actions*). What if I get side effects? (*Thoughts*)"

Person	Thoughts What might you think in this situation?	Feelings What feelings are likely?	Actions What is likely to happen following these thoughts and feelings?
1	"There are huge benefits for me if I take my medications. We will deal with it if it happens."	*Determined*	Stick with action plan and take medication. Will speak to the doctor if side effects happen.
2	"I know I'm going to get all the side effects and I won't be able to cope. It will be awful."	*Anxious*	Will look out for side effects and stop the medications at the first indication of any problem.
3	"These medications cost a fortune. It's a scam."	*Angry*	Might not get the prescription filled.
4	"What's the use? It won't make a difference. I'm never going to be the same. Why bother?"	*Helpless and sad*	Likely not to stick with action plan.

smoke. So I like my food. Now I have diabetes and have to spend a fortune on medication, appointments, and even on what I eat. My wife wants me to buy all this expensive food now. And for what? I feel fine." The diabetes educator acknowledges the fact that treatment and medications can be expensive and gently challenges the *thinking* by asking questions like:

- What are the benefits of the medication?
- What are your concerns about taking medication?
- How likely do you think it is that side effects occur?

These questions start a discussion that shows how *thoughts* and *feelings* affect illness behavior (*actions*), which in turn affects disease outcomes. The diabetes educator enabled a discussion about M's beliefs (*thoughts* and *feelings*) about medication and the nature of diabetes, and explained that, for the medication to work, it needs to be taken daily—not just when his sugar is high. This started a process for M to understand that the best measure of how he is progressing with his diabetes is his blood glucose levels, not the way he *feels*. Together, they came up with a behavioral experiment to test out M's ideas about medication. M charted his blood glucose levels for a week after taking medication daily and for a week taking them as he had been. This made the link between feelings and thoughts, actions, and physical outcome. Using such an approach reduces the likelihood of a client feeling like a "success" or a "failure" at self-management. The WPM model enables clients to understand the impact of black-and-white thinking on mood and to understand how thoughts and feelings impact on their behaviors and their disease. Instead, actions are seen as opportunities to learn more about the nature of the situation, related thoughts, feelings, barriers, and helpful actions. In subsequent sessions, M and the diabetes educator apply the WPM to losing weight.

At next review, M is walking three times a week and is taking his medication regularly. His doctor tells M that his HbA_{1c} has reduced by 1.0%. M understands that this reduces his risk of complications. He returns from the doctor's appointment and tells his wife "I got a good report. These changes are paying off."

The Importance of Collaborative Care

The WPM easily fits within a collaborative care model. The key components of collaborative care include enhanced patient education using books and video tapes; monitoring of outcomes, side-effects, and adherence to treatment; and stepped-care approaches that provide incremental increases in levels of treatment for people with persistent symptoms or comorbidities (Katon & Seelig, 2008; Katon, Unutzer, Wells, & Jones, 2010). Extensive evidence across 37 randomized trials has shown the effectiveness of collaborative care versus usual primary care in enhancing the quality of treatment for depression and in improving depressive outcomes for up to 2 to 5 years (Katon et al., 2010). Collaborative care leads to a twofold greater adherence to antidepressant medication over the first 6 months of treatment and improved depressive outcomes often lasting for at least 2 years (Gilbody, Bower, Fletcher, Richards, & Sutton, 2006). A collaborative care model for diabetes requires the involvement of diabetes specialists (endocrinologists, diabetes educators) and mental health specialists skilled in techniques of behavioral medicine.

The Role of Psychology

The growing body of literature suggests the need for integrating psychosocial and physical health care, and that the inclusion of clinical psychology into a diabetes care team is desirable (Leichter, Dreelin, & Moore, 2004). Indeed, the ADA Standards of Medical Care in Diabetes (2010) specify:

- Assessment of psychological and social situation should be included as an ongoing part of diabetes management.
- Psychosocial screening and follow-up should include, but is not limited to, attitudes about the illness, expectations for medical management and outcomes, affect/mood, general and diabetes-related quality of life, resources (financial, social, and emotional), and psychiatric history.
- Screen for psychosocial problems such as depression and diabetes-related distress, anxiety, eating disorders, and cognitive impairment when self-management is poor.

In the United Kingdom, the National Institute for Health and Clinical Excellence (NICE, 2009) has made similar explicit recommendations for provision of psychological care in people with diabetes.

Clinical psychologists enable better psychological care for people with diabetes in a number of ways: assisting with screening and detection of distress, providing secondary consultation to a multidisciplinary team, providing specialist assessment for nonadherence or complex cases, and training staff in health belief models and behavioral activation.

Psychology also has a role in facilitating reflective practice to increase knowledge of interpersonal processes and group dynamics. As clinicians, our perception of our practice and our clients' experiences may differ. We may think we have been empathic, engaging, and collaborative, but the client may have a different experience. The study by Parkin and Skinner (2003) highlights a significant problem in patient–professional relationships—a huge gap between health professionals' recollection of consultations and the clients' experiences. Professionals' communication skills need to be developed to ensure that these discrepancies are minimized. Skills to provide greater patient autonomy and support in the consultation will enhance the process and improve outcome (Parkin & Skinner, 2003).

The observations of Swift et al. (2010) have important implications for the role of psychology. Target setting appears to be an import facet of center success, based not so much on the treatment regimes themselves, but on the team attitudes and behaviors directed toward best clinical outcomes (Swift et al., 2010). In other words, these teams were most cohesive. Psychology has a role in improving team cohesion and communication processes to ensure that a team approach and agreement in approach exists for clients.

Although many courses are available covering the potential content of the consultation, there is little on how to work together with the patient on resolving these problems (Ross, Bower, & Sibbald, 1994) and little on how to work together as a multidisciplinary team. In a survey of diabetes centers, psychological input into teams was associated with improved training in psychological issues for team members, perceptions of better skills in managing more complex psychological issues, and increased likelihood of having psychological care pathways (Nicholson, Taylor, Gosdent, Trigwell, & Ismail, 2009).

Gaps in Psychological Care Still Exist

Sadly, not all services have access to clinicians who can provide the aforementioned services. A national survey of U.K. diabetes centers ($n = 464$) explored the availability of psychological services and compliance with national guidelines. Less than one-third of responding centers ($n = 182$) had access to specialist psychological services. Over two-thirds of centers had not implemented the majority of national guidelines, and only 2.6% met all

guidelines (Nicholson et al., 2009). Centers that do not have a psychologist feel the gap. The DAWN studies found that many clinicians do not feel confident in addressing the emotional aspects of the illness (Anonymous, 2004). Even diabetes services that have expert providers of psychological care feel the strain of meeting the demand for service. The median number of sessions (half days) for psychological care was 2.5 (range 0.25–11) per week per team (Nicholson et al., 2009). Most (81%) expert providers interviewed by telephone felt they were under-resourced to meet the psychological needs of their population (Nicholson et al., 2009).

Screening Measures

Clinicians should screen patients with any clinical suggestion of depression and ensure that effective treatment is offered (ADA, 2010; Leichter & See, 2005; NICE, 2009). Examples of validated measures include the Hospital Anxiety Depression Scale (Zigmond & Snaith, 1983), Beck Depression Inventory-2 (Beck, Steer, & Brown, 1996), and the Depression Anxiety Stress Scale 21 (Lovibond & Lovibond, 1995).

As discussed previously, it may also be worthwhile to consider other signs of distress. Hopelessness can be screened by a one-item measure "Have you experienced a feeling of hopelessness recently?" as used by Pedersen et al. (2009).

A range of scales are available to measure education outcomes. Eigenmann et al. (2009) identify three as useful and valid: the Problem Area in Diabetes scale, Summary of Diabetes Self-Care Activities, and the Appraisal of Diabetes. A diabetes eating problems survey (Markowitz et al., 2010) includes questions regarding insulin adjustment specifically for the purposes of weight reduction and couches questions in terms of diabetes care. The Patient Assessment of Chronic Illness (Glasgow, Whitsides, Nelson, & King, 2005) care may be useful tool to examine a client's experience of behavioral counseling. This helps to identify gaps in service.

Conclusion

The central role of psychological and behavioral factors in diabetes management is evident. There is significant benefit in integrating psychosocial support into all levels of diabetes care to assist patients in achieving adequate glycemic control and, at the same time, maintaining a satisfactory quality of life. Achieving self-management is a challenge for many clients with diabetes. An understanding of the psychosocial aspects of managing the condition for each client can assist in reaching concordance and developing an achievable plan. A cognitive-behavioral framework such as the WPM can be used to address psychosocial responses (thoughts, feeling, and actions) to diabetes, combining both knowledge and skills in implementing a treatment plan. It is a method of engaging a client in a discussion about his or her thoughts and feelings about living with diabetes. This allows for early identification of clients who are feeling demoralized. These strategies can be used by all clinicians working with patients with diabetes. It is important to identify the presence of depression, anxiety, and disordered eating and to ensure that clients receive appropriate treatment. These conditions are associated with poor outcomes. A growing literature exists on the effectiveness of psychosocial interventions incorporated into stepped and collaborative care models to underpin the medical care of people with diabetes.

Future Directions

These questions present future directions for the field, difficult problems to be solved, or topics that remain to be addressed:

- What is the direction of causal association between depression and diabetes?
- How do we best support clients with diabetes distress, hopelessness, or demoralization?
- Does addressing hopelessness improve clinical outcomes and quality of life?
- How do we increase collaborative care models in diabetes?

References

Aikens, J. E., Wallander, J. L., Bell, D. S. H., & Cole, J. A. (1992). Daily stress variability, learned resourcefulness, regimen adherence and metabolic control in type 1 diabetes mellitus: Evaluation of a path model. *Journal Consulting Clinical Psychology, 6,* 113–118.

Akimoto, M., Fukunishi, I., Kanno, K., Oogai, Y., Horikawa, N., Yamazaki, T., et al. (2004). Psychosocial predictors of relapse among diabetes patients: A 2-year follow-up after inpatient diabetes education. *Psychosomatics, 45,* 343–349.

Ali, S., Stone, M., Skinner, T.C., Roberston, N., Davies, M., & Khunit, K. (2010). The association between depression and health-related quality of life in people with type 2 diabetes: A systematic literature review. *Diabetes/Metabolism Research and Reviews, 26,* 75–89.

Ali, S., Stone, M. A., Peters, J. L., Davies, M. J., & Khunti K. (2006). The prevalence of co-morbid depression in adults with type 2 diabetes a systematic review and meta-analysis. *Diabetic Medicine, 23,* 1165–1173.

American Diabetes Association (ADA). (2010). Executive summary: Standards of medical care in diabetes—2010. *Diabetes Care, 33,* S4–S11.

Anderson, R. J., Freedland, K. E., Clouse, R. E., & Lustman, P.J. (2001). The prevalence of comorbid depression in adults with diabetes: A meta-analysis. *Diabetes Care, 24,* 1069–1078.

Anderson, R. J., Grigsby, A. B., Freedland, K. E., de Groot, M., McGill, J. B., Clouse, R. E. (2002). Anxiety and poor glycemic control: A meta-analytic review of the literature. *International Journal of Psychiatry Medicine, 32,* 235–247.

Anonymous. (2004). The 2nd DAWN International Summit November 5, 2003, London, UK: A call to action to improve psychosocial care for people with diabetes. *Practical Diabetes International, 21,* 201–208.

Australian Institute of Health and Welfare (AIHW). (2008). *Australia's Health 2008.* Canberra: Australian Institute of Health and Welfare.

Barnard, K. D., Skinner, T. C., & Peveler, R. (2006). The prevalence of co-morbid depression in adults with type 1 diabetes: Systematic literature review. *Diabetic Medicine, 23,* 445–448.

Beck, A. Steer, R. A, & Brown, G. K. (1996). *Manual for the Beck Depression Inventory—II.* Antonio, Texas: Psychological Corporation.

Begg, S., Vos, T., Barker B., Stevenson, C., Stanley, L., & Lopez, A. D. (2007). *The burden of disease and injury in Australia 2003.* AIHW cat no. PHE 82. Canberra: AIHW.

Bjorntorp, P. (2001). Do stress reactions cause abdominal obesity and comorbidities. *Obesity Review, 2,* 73–86.

Brown, S. A. (1999). Interventions to promote diabetes self-management: State of the science. *Diabetes Educator, 25,* 52–61.

Bryan, C., Songer, T., Brooks, M., Rush, J., Thase, M., Gaynes, B., et al. (2010). The impact of diabetes on depression treatment outcomes. *General Hospital Psychiatry, 22,* 33–41.

Cameron, F. J., Skinner, T. C., de Beufort, C. E., Hoey, H., Swift, P. G., Aanstoot, H., et al. (2008). Are family factors universally related to metabolic outcomes in adolescents with type 1 diabetes? *Diabetes Medicine, 25,* 463–468.

Caruso, L. B., & Silliman, R. A. (1999). Diabetes mellitus in the elderly patient. In J. J. Gallo, J. Busby-Whitehead, P. V. Rabins, R. A. Silliman, J.B. Murphy (Eds.), *Reichel's Care of the Elderly: Clinical Aspects of Aging* (5th ed., pp. 503–524). Baltimore: Lippincott Williams & Wilkins.

Chao, J., Nau, D. P., Atkins, J. E., & Taylor, S. D. (2005). The mediating role of health beliefs in the relationship between depressive symptoms and medication adherence in persons with diabetes. *Research in Social and Administrative Pharmacy, 1,* 508–525.

Ciechanowski, P., Katon, W., Russo, J., & Hirsch, I. (2003). The relationship of depressive symptoms to symptom reporting, self-care and glucose control in diabetes. *General Hospital Psychiatry, 25,* 246–252.

Clarke, D. M., & Kissane, D. W. (2002). Demoralisation: Its phenomenology and importance. *Australian New Zealand Journal of Psychiatry, 36,* 733–742.

Clarke, D. M., Kissane, D. W., Trauer, T., & Smith, G. (2005). Demoralisation, anhedonia and grief in patients with severe physical illness. *World Psychiatry, 4,* 96–105.

Clarke, D. M., Mackinnon, A. J., Smith, G. C., McKenzie, D. P., & Herrman, H. E. (2000). dimensions of psychopathology in the medically ill: A latent trait analysis. *Psychosomatics, 41,* 418–425.

Clement, S. (1995). Diabetes self-management education. *Diabetes Care, 16,* 1204–1214.

Coates, V. E., & Boore, J. R. P. (1996). Knowledge and diabetes self management. *Patient Education Counselling, 29*, 99–108.

Colton, P. A., Olmsted, M. P., Daneman, D., Rydall, A. C., & Rodin, G. M. (2007). Five-year prevalence and persistence of disturbed eating behavior and eating disorders in girls with type 1 diabetes. *Diabetes Care, 30*, 2861–2863.

Danne, T., Mortensen, H. B., Hougaard, P., Lynggard, H., Aanstoot, H. J., Chiarelli, F., et al. (2001). Persistent differences among centers over the 3 years in glycemic control and hypoglycemia in a study of 3,805 children and adolescents with type 1 diabetes. *Diabetes Care, 24*. 1342–1347.

Davies, M. J., Heller, S., Skinner, T. C., Campbell, M. J., Carey, M. E., Cradock, S. et al. on behalf of the Diabetes Education and Self Management for Ongoing and Newly diagnosed with Type 2 diabetes. (2008). A cluster randomised controlled trial of the DESMOND programme. *British Medical Journal, 336*, 491–495.

Davis, T. M. E., Davis, W. A., & Bruce, D. G. (2006). Glycemic levels triggering intensification of therapy in type 2 diabetes in the community: The Fremantle Diabetes Study. *Medical Journal of Australia, 184*, 325–328.

DCCT/EDIC Research Group. (2002). Effect of intensive therapy on microvascular complications of type 1 diabetes mellitus. *Journal of American Medical Association, 287*, 2563–2569.

De Beaufort C. E., Skinner, T. C., Swift, P. G. F., Aanstoot, H. J., Aman, J., Cameron, F., et al. for the Hvidore study group on childhood diabetes. (2007). Continuing stability of center differences in pediatric diabetes care: Do advances in diabetes treatment improve outcome? *Diabetes Care, 30*, 2245–2250.

de Groot, M., Jacobson, A. M., Samson, J. A., & Welch, G. (1999). Glycemic control and major depression in patients with type 1 and type 2 diabetes mellitus. *Journal Psychosomatic Research, 46*, 425–435.

Delamater, A. M., Jacobson, A. M., Anderson, B., Cox, D., Fisher, L., Lustman, P., et al. (2001). Psychosocial therapies in diabetes: Report of the psychosocial therapies working group. *Diabetes Care, 24*, 1286–1292.

DiMatteo, M. R. (2004). Social support and patient adherence to medical treatment: A meta-analysis. *Health Psychology, 23*, 207–218.

DiMatteo, M. R., Lepeprs, H. S., & Crogha, T. W. (2000). Depression is a risk factor for noncompliance with medical treatment: meta-analysis of the effects of anxiety and depression on patient adherence. *Archives Internal Medicine, 160*, 2101–2107.

Donnan, P. T., MacDonald, T. M., & Morris, A. D. (2002). Adherence to prescribed oral hypoglycemic medication in a population of patients with Type 2 diabetes: A retrospective cohort study. *Diabetic Medicine, 19*, 279–284.

Dunbar, J. A., Reddy, P., David-Lameloise, N., Philpot, B., Laatikainen, T., Kilkkinen, A., et al. (2008). Depression: An important comorbidity with metabolic syndrome in a general population. *Diabetes Care, 31*, 2368–2373.

Dutton, G. R., Tan, F., Provost, B. C., Sorenson, J. L., Allen, B., & Smith, B. (2009). Relationship between self-efficacy and physical activity among patients with type 2 diabetes. *Journal of Behavioral Medicine, 32*, 270–277.

Egede, L. E., Nieter, P. J., & Zheng, D. (2005). Depression and all-cause and coronary heart disease mortality among adults with and without diabetes, *Diabetes Care, 28*, 1339–1345.

Eigenmann, C. A., Colagiuri, R., Skinner, T. C., & Trevena, L. (2009). Are current psychometric tools suitable for measuring outcomes of diabetes education? *Diabetic Medicine, 26*, 425–436.

Everson, S. A., Goldberg, D. E., Kaplan, G. A., Cohen, R. D., Pukkala, E., Tuomilehto, J., et al. (1996). Hopelessness and risk of mortality and incidence of myocardial infraction and cancer. *Psychosomatic Medicine, 58*, 113–121.

Fairburn, C. G. (2008). *Cognitive behavior therapy and eating disorders.* New York: Guilford Press.

Ford, E. S. (2005). Prevalence of the metabolic syndrome defined by the International Diabetes Federation among adults in the U.S. *Diabetes Care, 28*, 2745–2749.

Funnell, M. M., & Anderson, R. M. (2004). Empowerment and self-management of diabetes. *Clinical Diabetes, 22*, 123–127.

Funnell, M. M., Brown, T. L., Childs, B. P., Haas, L. B., Hosey, G. M., Jensen, B., et al. (2009). National standards for diabetes self-management. *Diabetes Care, 32*(Supp), S87–S94.

Ganju, V. (2010). *Mental health and chronic physical illnesses: The need for integrated care.* Woodbridge: World Federation for Mental Health. Accessed October 1, 2010, at www.WFMH.org

Gavard, J. A., Lustman, P. J., & Clouse, R. E. (1993). Prevalence of depression in adults with diabetes: An epidemiological evaluation. *Diabetes Care, 16*, 1167–1178.

Gilbody, S., Bower, P., Fletcher, J., Richards, D., & Sutton, A. J. (2006). Collaborative care for depression: A cumulative meta-analysis and review of longer term outcomes. *Archive Internal Medicine, 166*, 2314–2321.

Gilmer, T. P., O'Connor, P. J., Rush, W. A., Crain, A. L., Whitebird, R. R., Hanson, A. M., et al. (2005). Predictors of health care costs. *Diabetes Care, 28*, 59–64.

Glasgow, R. E., Toobert, D. J., & Gillette, C. D. (2001). Psychosocial barriers to diabetes self-management and quality of life. *Diabetes Spectrum, 14*, 33–41.

Glasgow, R. E., Whitsides, H., Nelson, C. C., & King, D. K. (2005). Use of the patient assessment of chronic illness care (PACIC) with diabetic patients. *Diabetes Care, 22*, 2655–2661.

Goetsch, V. L. (1989). Stress and blood glucose in diabetes mellitus: A review and methodological commentary. *Annals Behavioral Medicine, 11*, 102–107.

Gonzalez, J. S., Safren, S. A., Cagliero, E., Wexler, D. J., & Delahanty, L. (2007). Depression, self-care, and medication adherence in type 2 diabetes: Relationships across the full range of symptom severity. *Diabetes Care, 30*, 2222–2227.

Green, L., Feher, M., & Catalan, J. (2000). Fears and phobias in people with diabetes. *Diabetes/Metabolism Research and Reviews, 16*, 287–293.

Griffiths, J. L., & Gaby, L. (2005). Brief psychotherapy at the bedside: countering demoralization from medical illness. *Psychosomatics, 46*, 109–116.

Grinstein, G., Muzumdar, R., Aponte, L., Vuguin, P., Saenger, P., DiMartino-Nardi, J. (2003). Presentations and 5-year follow-up of type 2 diabetes mellitus in African-American and Caribbean-Hispanic adolescents. *Hormone Research, 60*, 121–126.

Gustavsson-Lilius, M., Julkunen, J., Y., & Heitanen, P. (2007). Quality of life in cancer patients: The role of optimism, hopelessness and partner support. *Quality of Life Research, 16*, 75–87.

Haines, L, Bararett, T. G., Chong Wan, K., Shield, J. P. H., & Lynn, R. (2007). Rising incidence of type 2 diabetes in children in the U.K. *Diabetes Care, 20*(5), 1097–1101.

Hampson, S. E., Glasgow, R. E., & Strycker, L. A. (2000). Beliefs versus feelings: A comparison of personal models and depression for predicting multiple outcomes in diabetes. *British Journal Health Psychology, 5,* 27–40.

Hanninen, J. A., Takala, J. K., & Keinanen-Kiukaannemi, S. M. (1999). Depression in subjects with type 2 diabetes: predictive factors and relation to quality of life. *Diabetes Care, 22,* 997–998.

Harvey, J. N., & Lawson, V. L. (2009). The importance of health belief models in determining self-care behavior in diabetes. *Diabetes Medicine, 26,* 5–13.

Heller, S. R. (2007). Self monitoring of blood glucose in type 2 diabetes: Clinicians should stop patients doing this if it has no benefit. *British Medical Journal, 335,* 105–106.

Herpertz, S., Albus, C., Lichtblau, K., Kohle, K., Mann, K., Senf, W. (2000). Relationship of weight and eating disorders in type 2 diabetic patients: A multicenter study. *International Journal of Eating Disorders, 28,* 68–77.

Horne, R. & Weinman, J. (1999). Patients' beliefs about prescribed medicines and their role in adherence to treatment in chronic physical illness. *Journal of Psychosomatic Research, 47,* 555–567.

Ivbijaro, G. (2010). The role of primary care in improving access to care for persons with mental health problems and chronic illness. In V. Ganju (Ed.), *Mental Health and Chronic Physical Illnesses the need for integrated care* (pp. 25–88). Woodbridge: World Federation for Mental Health. Accessed October 1, 2010 at: www.WFMH.org.au

Jacobson, A. M., de Groot, M., & Samson, J. A. (1997). The effects of psychiatric disorders and symptoms on quality of life in patients with type I and type II diabetes mellitus. *Quality of Life Research, 6,* 11–20.

Katon, W. J. (2008). The comorbidity of diabetes mellitus and depression. *The American Journal of Medicine, 121,* S8–S15.

Katon, W. J., Von Korff, M., Lin, E. H., Simon, G., Ludman, E., Russo, J., et al. (2004). The pathways study: A randomized control trial of collaborative care in patients with diabetes and depression. *Archives General Psychiatry, 61,* 1042–1049.

Katon, W. J., Lin, E. H., Russo, J. Von Korff, M., Ciechanowski, P., Simon, G., et al. (2004). Cardiac risk factors in patients with diabetes and major depression. *Journal General Internal Medicine, 19,* 1192–1199.

Katon, W. J., & Seelig, M. (2008). Population-based care of depression: Team care approaches to improving outcomes. *Journal Occupation Environment Medicine, 50,* 459–467.

Katon, W. J., Unutzer, J., Wells, K., & Jones, L. (2010). Collaborative depression care: history, evolution and ways to enhance dissemination and sustainability. *General Hospital Psychiatry, 32,* 456–464.

Kennedy, A., Gately, C., & Rogers, A. (2004). *National evaluation of the expert patients programme.* Manchester, UK: National Primary Care Research and Development Center.

King, D. K., Glasgow, R. E, Toobert, D. J., Strycker, L. A., Estabrooks, P. A., Osuna, D. et al. (2010). Self-efficacy, problem solving and social-environmental support are associated with diabetes self-management behaviors. *Diabetes Care, 33,* 751–753.

Kiropoulos, L., Blashki, G., & Klimidis, S. (2006). Managing mental illness in patients from CALD backgrounds. *Australian Family Physician, 34,* 259–264.

Knight, B. G. (1996). *Psychotherapy with older adults* (2nd edition). Newbury Park, California: Sage Publications.

Knight, K. M., Dornan, T., & Bundy, C. (2006). The diabetes educator: Trying hard, but must concentrate more on behavior. *Diabetic Medicine, 23,* 485–501.

Knol, M. J., Twisk, J. W. R., Beckman, A. T. F., Heine, R. J., Snoek, F. J., et al. (2006). Depression as a risk factor for the onset of type 2 diabetes mellitus. A meta-analysis. *Diabetologia, 49,* 837–845.

Kuijer, R. G., & de Ridder, D. (2003). Discrepancy in illness-related goals and quality of life in chronically ill patients: The role of self-efficacy. *Psychology and Health, 18,* 313–330.

Leichter, S. B., Dreelin, E. D., & Moore, S. (2004). Integration of clinical psychology in the comprehensive diabetes care team. *Clinical Diabetes, 22,* 129–131.

Leichter, S. B., & See, Y. (2005). Problems that extend visit time and cost in diabetes care: 1. How depression may affect the efficacy and cost of care of diabetic patients. *Clinical Diabetes, 23,* 53–54.

Lerman, I., Lozano, L., Villa, A. R., Hernadez-Jimenez, S., Weinger, K., et al. (2004). Psychosocial factors associated with poor diabetes self-care management in a specialized center in Mexico City. *Biomedical Pharmacotherapy, 58,* 566–570.

Lin, E. H., Katon, W., Von Korff, M., Rutter, C., Simon, G. E., Oliver, M., et al. (2004). Relationship of depression and diabetes self-care, medication adherence, and preventative care. *Diabetes Care, 27,* 343–349.

Lin, E. H., & Von Korff, M. (2008). Mental disorders among persons with diabetes—Results from the World Mental Health Surveys. *Journal of Psychosomatic Research, 65,* 571–580.

Lloyd, C. E., Dyer, P. H., & Barnett, A. H. (2000). Prevalence of symptoms of depression and anxiety in a diabetes clinic population. *Diabetes Medicine, 17,* 198–202.

Lorenz, R., Bubb, J., Davis, D., Jacobson, A., Jannasch, K., et al. (1996). Changing behavior: Practical lessons from the diabetes control and complications trial. *Diabetes Care, 19,* 648–652.

Lovibond, S. H., & Lovibond, P. F. (1995). *Manual for the Depression Anxiety Stress Scales* (2nd ed.). Sydney: Psychology Foundation.

Luppino, F. S., de Wit, L. M., Bouvy, P. F., Stijnen, T., Cuijpers, P., et al. (2010). Overweight, obesity, and depression: A systematic review and meta-analysis of longitudinal studies. *Archives General Psychiatry, 67,* 220–229.

Lustman, P. J., Anderson, R. J., Freedland, K. E., de Groot, M. D., Carney, R. M., & Clouse, R. E. (2000a). Depression and poor glycemic control. A meta-analytic review of the literature. *Diabetes Care, 23,* 934–942.

Lustman, P. J., Clouse, R. E., Ciechanowski, P. S., Hirsch, I. B., & Freedland, K. E. (2005). Depression-related hyperglycemia in type 1 diabetes: A mediational approach. *Psychosomatic Medicine, 67,* 195–199.

Lustman, P. J., Freedland, K. E., Griffiths, L. S., & Clouse, R. E. (2000b). Fluoxetine for depression in diabetes: a randomised double blind, placebo-controlled trial. *Diabetes Care, 23,* 618–623.

Lustman, P. J., Griffiths, L. S., Clouse, R. E., Freedland, K. E., Eisen, S. A., et al. (1997). Effects of nortriptyline on depression and glucose regulation in diabetes: Results of a double-blind, placebo controlled trial. *Psychosomatic Medicine, 59,* 241–250.

Lustman, P. J., Griffiths, L. S., Freedland, K. E., Kissell, S. S., & Clouse, R. E. (1998). Cognitive behavioral therapy for depression in type 2 diabetes: A randomized controlled trial. *Annals Internal Medicine, 129,* 613–621.

Lustman, P. J., Griffiths, L. S., Gavard, J. A., & Clouse, R. E. (1992). Depression in adults with diabetes. *Diabetes Care, 15,* 1631–1639.

Mann, D. M., Poniem, D., Leventhal., H., & Halm, E. A. (2009). Predictors of adherence to diabetes medication: The role of disease and medication beliefs. *Journal of Behavioural Medicine, 32,* 278–284.

Markowitz, J. T, Butler, D. A., Bolkening, L. K., Antisdel, J. E., Anderson, B. J., et al. (2010). Brief screening tool for disordered eating in diabetes: Internal consistency and external validity in a contemporary sample of pediatric patients with type 1 diabetes. *Diabetes Care, 33,* 495–500.

McMaster University Evidence-based Practice. (2005). Diagnosis, prognosis, and treatment of impaired glucose tolerance and impaired fasting glucose. *Evidence Report/Technology Assessment. Number 128.* Accessed October 10, 2011, at www.ahrq.gov

Minas, I., Klimidis, S., & Tuncer, C. (2007). Illness causal beliefs in Turkish immigrants. *BMC Psychiatry, 7,* 34.

Mollema, E. D., Snoek, F. J., Heine, R. J., & van der Ploeg, H. M. (2001). Phobia of self-injecting and self-testing in insulin-treated diabetes patients: Opportunities for screening. *Diabetic Medicine, 18,* 671–674.

Moos, R. H., & Holahan, C. J. (2007). Adaptive tasks and methods of coping with illness and disability. In E. Martz & H. Liven (Eds.), *Coping with chronic illness and disability* (pp.107–126). New York, NY: Springer.

Morris, A. D., Boyle, D. I., McMahon, A. D., Greene, S. A., MacDonald, T. M., et al. (1997). Adherence to insulin treatment, glycemic control, and ketoacidosis in insulin-dependent diabetes mellitus. *Lancet, 350,* 1505–1510.

Moussavi, S., Chatterji, S., Verdes, E., Tandon, A., Patel, V., et al. (2007). Depression chronic diseases and decrements in health: Results from the World Health Surveys. *Lancet, 379,* 851–858.

Musselman, D. L., Beta, E., Larsen, H., & Phillips, L. S. (2003). Relationship of depression to diabetes types 1 and 2: Epidemiology, biology, and treatment. *Biological Psychiatry, 1*(45), 317–329.

Nagasawa, M., Smith, M., Barnes, J. J., Jr., & Finchman J. E. (1990). Meta-analysis of correlates of diabetes patients' compliance with prescribed medications. *The Diabetes Educator, 16,* 192–200.

National Institute for Health and Clinical Excellence (NICE). (2009). *Depression in adults with a chronic physical health problem: Treatment and management.* NICE clinical guideline 91. Accessed October 1, 2011, at: www.nice.org.uk

Newman, S., Steed, L., & Mulligan, K. (2004). Self-management in chronic illness. *Lancet, 394*(9444), 1523–1537.

Nicholson, T. R. J., Taylor, J. P., Gosdent, C., Trigwell, P., & Ismail, K. (2009). National guidelines for psychological care in diabetes: How mindful have we been? *Diabetic Medicine, 26,* 447–450.

Nouwen, A., Winkey, J., Twisk, C. E., Lloyd, M., Peyrot, M., et al. (2010). Type 2 diabetes mellitus as a risk factor for the onset of depression: A systematic review and meta-analysis. *Diabetologia, 53,* 2480–2486.

O'Kane, M. J., Bunting, B., Copeland, M., Coates, V., et al. (2008). Efficacy of self monitoring of blood glucose in patients with newly diagnosed type 2 diabetes (ESMON study) randomized control trial. *British Medical Journal, 336,* 1174–1177.

Parkin, T., & Skinner T. C. (2003). Discrepancies between patient and professionals recall and perception of an outpatient consultation. *Diabetic Medicine, 20,* 909–914.

Paschalides, C., Wearden, A. J., Dunkerlye, C., Bundy, R. Davies, C. M., & Dickens, C. M. (2004). The associations of anxiety, depression and personal illness representations with glycemic control and health-related quality of life in patients with type 2 diabetes mellitus. *Journal of Psychosomatic Research, 57,* 557–564.

Pedersen, S. S., Denollet, J., Erdman, R. A. M., Serruys, P. W., & von Domburg, R. T. (2009). Co-occurrence of diabetes and hopelessness predicts adverse prognosis following percutaneous coronary intervention. *Journal Behavioural Medicine, 32,* 294–301.

Peyrot, M., & Rubin, R. R. (1997). Levels and risks of depression and anxiety symptomatology among diabetic adults. *Diabetes Care, 20,* 585–590.

Pham, D., Fortin, F., & Thibaudeau, M. (1996). The role of the health belief model in amputees' self evaluation of adherence to diabetes self-care behaviors. *Diabetes Educator, 22,* 126–132.

Polonsky, W. H. (1999). *Diabetes burnout: What to do when you can't take it anymore* Alexandria, VA: American Diabetes Association.

Polonsky, W. H., & Skinner, T. C. (2010). Perceived treatment efficacy: An overlooked opportunity in diabetes care. *Clinical Diabetes, 28,* 89–92.

Roglic, G., Unwin, N., Bennett, P. H., Mathers, C., Tuomilehto, J., et al. (2005). The burden of mortality attributable to diabetes. *Diabetes Care, 8,* 2130–2135.

Ross, F. M., Bower, P. J., & Sibbald, B. S. (1994). Practice nurses: Characteristics, workload and training needs. *British Journal General Practice, 44,* 15–18.

Ruggiero, L., Glasgow, R. E., Dryfoos J. M., Rossi, J. S. Proschaska J. O., Orleans, C. T., et al. (1997). Diabetes self-management: Self-reported recommendations and patterns in a large population. *Diabetes Care, 20,* 568–576.

Rush, A. J., & Weissenburger, J. E. (1994). Melancholic symptoms features and DSM-IV in medical patients. *American Journal of Psychiatry, 151,* 489–498.

Sacco, W. P., & Yanover, T. (2006). Diabetes and depression: The role of social support and medical symptoms. *Journal of Behavioral Medicine, 29,* 523–531.

Segal, Z. V., Williams, M. G., & Teasdale, J. D. (2002). *Mindfulness-based cognitive therapy for depression: a new approach to preventing relapse.* New York: Guilford Press.

Shoelson, S. E., Lee, J., & Goldfine, A. B. (2006). Inflammation and insulin resistance. *Journal of Clinical Investigation, 116,* 1793–1801.

Shultz, J. A., Sprague, M. A., Branen, L. J., & Lambeth, S. (2001). A comparison of views of individuals with type 2 diabetes mellitus and diabetes education about barriers to diet and exercise. *Journal Health Communication, 6,* 99–115.

Skinner, T. C., Carey, M. E., Cradock, S., Dallossot, M., Daly, H., et al. (2010). Depressive symptoms in the first year from diagnosis of type 2 diabetes: Results from the DESMOND trial. *Diabetic Medicine, 27,* 965–967.

Smith, M. (2005). Psychology in diabetes: Identifying and meeting the need. *Practical Diabetes International, 22,* 181–184.

Soderberg, S., Zimmet, P., Tuomilehto, J., de Courten, M., Dowse, G. K., Chitson, P., et al. (2004). High incidence of type 2 diabetes and increasing conversion rates from impaired fasting glucose and impaired glucose tolerance to diabetes in Mauritius. *Journal of Internal Medicine, 256*, 37–47.

Stenstrom, U., Wikby, A., Andersson, P. O., & Ryden, O. (1997). Relationship between locus of control beliefs and metabolic control in insulin dependent diabetes mellitus. *British Journal of Health Psychology, 2*, 15–25.

Stewart, M. A. (1995). Effective physician-patient communication and health outcomes: A review. *Canadian Medical Association Journal, 152*, 1423–1433.

Stratton, I. M., Adler, A. L., Neil, H. A., Matthews, D. R., Manley, S. E., et al. (2000). Association of glycemia with macrovascular and microvascular complications of type 2 diabetes (UKPDs 35): Prospective observational study. *British Medical Journal, 321*, 405–412.

Surwit, R. S., van Tilburg, M. A. L., Parekh, P. I., Lane, J. D., & Feinglos, M. N. (2005). Treatment regimen determines the relationship between depression and glycemic control. *Diabetes Research and Clinical Practice, 69*, 78–80.

Swift, P. G. F., Skinner, T. C., de Beaufort, C. E., Cameron, F. J., et al. (2010). Target setting in intensive insulin management is associated with metabolic control: The Hvidoere Childhood Diabetes Study Group Center Differences Study 2005. *Pediatric Diabetes, 11*, 271–278.

Talbot, F., & Nouwen, A. (2000). A review of the relationship between depression and diabetes in adults: Is there a link? *Diabetes Care, 23*, 1556–1562.

Tilden, B., Charman, D., Sharples, J., & Fosbury, J. (2005). Identity and adherence in a diabetes patient: Transformations in psychotherapy. *Qualitative Health Research, 15*, 312–324.

Timonen, M., Laakso, M., Jokelainen, J., Rajala, U., Meyer-Rochow, V. B., et al. (2005). Insulin resistance and depression: cross sectional study. *British Medical Journal, 330*, 17–18.

United Health. (2010). *The United States of Diabetes: Challenges and opportunities in the decade ahead Working Paper 5. November 2010.* Minnetonka, MN: UnitedHealth Center for Health Reform & Modernization. Accessed October 1, 2010, at www.unitedhealthgroup.com/reform

Urakami, T., Kubota, S., Nitadori, Y, Harad, K., Owada, M., et al. (2005). Annual incidence and clinical characteristics of type 2 diabetes in children as detected by urine glucose screening in the Tokyo metropolitan area. *Diabetes Care, 28*, 1876–1881.

van der Ven, N. C. W., Lubach, C. H. C., Hogeneslt, M. H. E., van Iperen, A., Tromp-Wever, A. M. E., Vriend, A., et al. (2005). Cognitive behavioral group training for patients with type 1 diabetes in persistent poor glycemic control: Who do we reach? *Patient Education and Counselling, 56*, 313–322.

Vermeire, E., Hearnshway, H., Van Royen, P., & Denekens, J. (2001). Patient adherence to treatment: Three decades of research. A comprehensive review. *Journal of Clinical Pharmacy and Therapeutics, 26*, 331–342.

Vermeire, E., Wens, J., Van Royen, P., Biot, Y., Hearnshway, H., et al. (2009). Interventions for improving adherence to treatment recommendations in people with type 2 diabetes mellitus (review). *The Cochrane Library, 1*, 1–140.

Walker, C., Weeks, A., McAvoy, B., & Demetriou, E. (2005). Exploring the role of self-management programs in caring for people from culturally and linguistically diverse backgrounds in Melbourne, Australia. *Health Expectations, 8*, 315–323.

Weinstein, N. D. (2000). Perceived probability, perceived severity, and health-protective behavior. *Health Psychology, 19*, 65–74.

Wild, S., Roglic, G., Green, A., Sicree, R., & King, H. (2004). Global prevalence of diabetes: Estimates for the year 2000 and projections for 2030. *Diabetes Care, 27*, 1047–1053.

Wilhelm, K., Wedgwood, L., Niven, H., & Kay-Lambkin, F. (2006). Smoking cessation and depression: current knowledge and future directions. *Drug Alcohol Review, 25*, 97–107.

Williams, J. W., Katon, W., Lin, E. H. B., Noel, P. H., Worchel, J., et al. (2004). The effectiveness of depression care management on diabetes related outcomes in older persons. *Annals Internal Medicine, 140*, 1015–1024.

Wing, R. R., Phelan, S., & Tate, D. (2002). The role of adherence in mediating the relationship between depression and health outcomes. *Journal of Psychosomatic Research, 53*, 877–881.

Winkley, K., Landau, S., Eisler, I., & Ismail, K. (2006). Psychological interventions to improve glycaemic control in patients with type 2 diabetes: Systematic review and meta-analysis of randomised controlled trials. *British Medical Journal, 333*, 65–70.

World Health Organization (WHO). (2011). *Diabetes Fact Sheet. No. 312.* Geneva: World Health Organization.

Young-Hyman, D. L., & Davis, C. L. (2010). Disordered eating behavior in individuals with diabetes. *Diabetes Care, 33*, 683–689.

Young, B. A., von Korff, M., Heckber, S. R., Ludman, E. J., Rutter, C., et al. (2010). Association of major depression and mortality in stage 5 diabetic chronic kidney disease. *General Hospital Psychiatry, 32*, 119–124.

Zhang, Y., Dall, T. M., Mann, S. E., Chen, Y., Martin, J., et al. (2009). The economic costs of undiagnosed diabetes. *Population Health Management, 12*, 95–101.

Zigmond, A. S., & Snaith, R. P. (1983). The Hospital Anxiety and Depression Scale. *Acta Psychiatrica Scandinavica, 67*, 361–370.

PART 3

Professional Issues and Future Challenges

Education and Training in Rehabilitation Psychology

William Stiers *and* Kathryn Nicholson Perry

Abstract

Issues of education and training are fundamental to the conceptualization and development of the specialty of applied rehabilitation psychology, as they are in all areas of professional health service psychology. A specialty is shaped by the preparation of its practitioners, including its selection of trainees, the structures and processes of its training programs, and the competencies expected of successful trainees. In considering education and training in rehabilitation psychology, this chapter discusses a *conceptual space*, based on the definition of the specialty and its relevance to important world health issues; *conceptual elements*, based on existing training guidelines and expected practitioner competencies; and data about what actually occurs in preparing practitioners for work in rehabilitation psychology.

Recommendations are made for improving education and training in rehabilitation psychology.

Key Words: Rehabilitation psychology, rehabilitation, psychology, education, training, specialty, specialization.

In the United States, rehabilitation psychology has existed as a formally organized specialty for over 50 years, In contrast, in the United Kingdom, Ireland, Europe, and Australia, rehabilitation psychology is not always recognized as a specialty by that name, and psychologists working with persons with disabilities may have completed formal training in other specialties of psychology, even though they may do specialized work that would be called rehabilitation psychology in the United States. Stevens and Wedding (2004) describe that in India, Japan, Iran, Turkey, and Israel, areas of psychology practice called "rehabilitation psychology" are similar in focus to the U.S. and Canada concepts. However, in Russia, China, Egypt, and Pakistan, activities related to what is called "rehabilitation psychology" have to do with prisoners, but may also include substance abuse rehabilitation, as in Poland, Indonesia, and the Philippines. In some countries,

the word "rehabilitation" is used only in regard to persons with primary mental health problems. This chapter is focused on rehabilitation psychology as it applies to persons with physical disability, and not on rehabilitation psychology as it may apply to persons with primary mental health impairments or primary substance use disorders, or to prisoners within criminal or political correctional systems.

Discussion of education and training in rehabilitation psychology is complex because significant differences exist among countries in the education and training of all types of psychology health care providers, including in the overall structure of training and the organization of specialties and subspecialties. The basic structure of training for practitioners differs widely across countries. For example, they may be trained at the elementary school, secondary school, associate, bachelor, master, or doctoral level. In some countries, the training of psychology health care providers follows an apprenticeship model, providing basic general education and then on-the-job training. In other countries, psychology practitioners may receive a formal psychological education and then independent work experience, whereas in still others they may specialize through advanced formal educational preparation and supervised work experience. In addition, in some countries, the practice of psychology and the term "psychologist" are protected by legislation, whereas in others practitioners may perform psychological work and call themselves psychologists without legal specification or regulation, or may perform work that is psychological in nature without calling themselves psychologists. For the purposes of this chapter, psychology practitioners working with persons with physical disabilities will be referred to as *rehabilitation psychologists* when their level of education, training, and licensure is appropriate for their geographic, cultural, and legal setting.

Conceptualizing the Specialty of Rehabilitation Psychology

The definition of rehabilitation psychology and its relevance to current world health problems can provide a conceptual space within which issues related to education and training in this specialty can be fruitfully discussed. In regard to definition, each psychological health care specialty is defined and differentiated from other specialties by its specific *populations*, *problems*, and *procedures* (American Psychological Association, 2004). The history of rehabilitation psychology originates from the mid-20th century. In the 1940s, during the World War II era, health professionals in the United States developed specialized concepts and practices to optimize the application of their professions to injuries sustained during the conflicts. Physicians developed the concepts and practices of *rehabilitation medicine*, psychologists developed the concepts and practices of *rehabilitation psychology*, and nurses developed the concepts and practices of *rehabilitation nursing*. As rehabilitation psychologists worked alongside the emerging fields of rehabilitation medicine and nursing, early theorists and practitioners studied persons with physical and cognitive impairments, and conducted the early research on individual, interpersonal, and social reactions to changes in persons' appearance and functional capacity, as well as on the social psychology of stereotyping and prejudice related to disability (e.g., Barker, Wright & Gonick, 1946; Barker & Wright, 1952; Dembo, Leviton, & Wright, 1956). Rehabilitation

psychology researchers and health care providers focused on the specific problems and procedures that defined the specialty.

Applied rehabilitation psychology developed as a health care specialty that applies psychological knowledge and skills on behalf of individuals with disabilities and chronic health conditions in order to maximize their health and welfare, independence and choice, functional abilities, and social role participation, and to minimize secondary health complications. This includes services to individuals with disability and chronic illnesses and to their families, as well as to rehabilitation teams and institutions. Because disability is a person–task–environment interaction, consideration is given to the network of biological, psychological, social, cultural, physical, and political environments in which the individual exists, and to addressing barriers in these areas (Stiers & Stucky, 2008).

Rehabilitation psychologists have specialized knowledge regarding a number of types of disabilities and chronic conditions and their effects upon physical, psychological, and social functioning (specialized *populations*). These disabilities include, among others, spinal cord injury, brain injury, stroke, amputations, burns, multiple traumatic injuries, chronic pain, cancer, heart disease, multiple sclerosis, neuromuscular disorders, AIDS, developmental disorders, and impairments in sensory functioning. Although a number of psychology specialists may work with such individuals, rehabilitation psychology is defined by its focus on specific *problems* and *procedures*, and is distinct from other specialties in addressing these issues within a disability-specific body of theory and research (Dunn & Elliott, 2005; Shontz & Wright, 1980; Gold, Meltzer, & Sherr, 1982). The specific *problems* include:

- Impairments in body functions and structures, and associated changes in physical functioning that can result in changes in self-concept, body image, and self-perceived attractiveness and value
- Limitations in activity and associated changes in task functioning that can result in changes in self-control, personal choice, independence, autonomy, and privacy
- Restrictions in social participation and associated changes in social functioning that can result in disruption of family, community, vocational, and recreational role sets from which individuals derive self-esteem

- Reactions by others to changes in appearance and functional ability involving negative stereotypes, negative halo effects, and prejudice
- Abuse and exploitation of persons with disability
- Effects of developmental age transitions on disability
- Physical, social, and policy environments that can restrict participation by persons with disability

Rehabilitation psychologists have developed essential skills and procedures associated with this specialty. The specific *procedures* are focused on:

- Assessment and treatment of individual and family physical, cognitive, emotional, and social adaptation and compensation to injury, illness, and disability
- Assessment and treatment of cognitive, emotional, and behavioral dysfunction in persons with disability
- Psychological and neuropsychological evaluation of persons with sensory and motor impairments
- Evaluation and enhancement of self-care and independent living skills
- Evaluation and enhancement of educational, vocational, social, and recreational participation
- Assessment and enhancement of health self-management and prevention of secondary complications
- Assessment and enhancement of caregiver status and functioning, including caregiver knowledge and skills, social support, and self-care
- Facilitation of interdisciplinary rehabilitation team functioning
- Facilitation of appropriate selection and use of assistive technology and personal assistance services
- Working with health professionals, educational and vocational agencies, service agencies, and policy-makers on disability rights, and physical and social accessibility

In regard to relevance, training in rehabilitation psychology is important because it is the pipeline to a health care career that is applicable to a number of important world health problems. It is estimated that 10% of the world population experience some form of disability—approximately 650 million people. It is estimated that worldwide each year there are:

- 160 million persons with work-related injuries (WHO(c))

- 50 million persons injured and 1.2 million killed from road traffic crashes (Peden et al., 2001)
- 2 million persons with war injuries (Peden, McGee, & Krug, 2002; WHO(d)), including civilians experiencing mutilation and limb amputation as a form of organized terrorism (Krug et al., 2002)
- 15,000–25,000 persons injured or killed by land mines (Krug, Dahlberg, Mercy, Zwi, & Lozano, 2002)
- Episodes involving hundreds to thousands of persons injured by earthquakes (Rathore et al., 2008)

The number of persons with disability is growing as a result of population growth, medical advances that sustain life into older age, and increases in chronic diseases and motor vehicle use (WHO(a), WHO(b)). As disability and chronic health conditions place the greatest demand on health care services, and the number and percentage of persons with chronic impairments is increasing (Hoffman, Rice, & Sung, 1996), issues related to improving individual function, enhancing caregiver ability, decreasing secondary health complications, and enhancing community integration are increasingly important.

The definition of rehabilitation psychology and its relevance to world health needs can help shape education and training goals and objectives in this specialty. Clearly, it is important that rehabilitation psychology training includes supervised work experience and didactic education involving persons with disability; that it be focused on assessing and treating the psychological and social difficulties that arise with disability, with the goal of improving functional abilities and social role participation; and that it involve services to individuals, families, and rehabilitation teams and institutions. It is also important that such training emphasizes that disability is a person–task–environment interaction, and that appropriate assessment and treatment of difficulties may occur at the person level, the task level, or the environment level (including the physical, social, cultural, and political environments in which the individual exists).

Existing Rehabilitation Psychology Training Guidelines and Expected Practitioner Competencies

Existing rehabilitation psychology training guidelines and expected practitioner competencies can provide conceptual elements for the discussion of education and training in this specialty. In regard to training guidelines, the specialized populations, specialized problems, and specialized procedures with which rehabilitation psychologists work define the field of rehabilitation psychology. The unique aspects of training in rehabilitation psychology practice have been discussed for many decades. In 1982, Gold, Meltzer, and Sherr described how psychological training in physical rehabilitation settings differs from psychological training in mental health settings. First, the patient population is made up mostly of persons without significant pre-existing mental health issues who have experienced dramatic changes in physical integrity. Second, the structure of the service delivery system is based on team functioning, and psychologists are expected to focus their efforts toward specific rehabilitation goals that mesh with those of other providers. Third, specialized knowledge is required of specific injury and disease states and their effects upon physical, cognitive, and emotional functioning, activity and task performance, and social interactions. Fourth, trainees are confronted with their own feelings of physical vulnerability and their emotional reactions to persons with disability. Fifth, trainees must deal with unfamiliar issues, such as bowel and bladder incontinence, and at times must provide physical assistance to patients. Gold, Meltzer, and Sherr (1982) recommended didactic and experiential training in the physical and medical aspects of disability (specialized populations), the psychological and social issues of persons with disabilities (specialized problems), and the relevant diagnostic and intervention techniques for this population (specialized procedures). However, they did not discuss specific ways in which this type of training might be operationalized.

In 1995, Patterson and Hanson published the first postdoctoral training guidelines for rehabilitation psychology. These guidelines discussed trainee entrance criteria, length of training, overall curriculum model, service provision, supervision, client populations, training content areas, program characteristics, and trainee and program evaluation (Table 23.1).

These guidelines generally focus on the structural and process elements of training programs, rather than on any specific competencies acquired by their trainees. However, they do specify that teaching and practice should be focused on persons with disability and chronic health conditions.

The American Board of Rehabilitation Psychology (ABRP) is another source of guidance about

Table 23.1 Patterson and Hanson 1995 guidelines for postdoctoral training in rehabilitation psychology

- Trainees are accepted only from programs approved by the national psychological association
- The minimum length of training is 1 year
- There are a minimum of two supervisors during training
- The curriculum includes supervised practice, seminars, and coursework
- The patient populations and didactics are related to disabilities and chronic health conditions
- There is a minimum of 2 hours of didactics per week
- There is a minimum of 2 hours of supervision per week
- All trainees are funded
- There are written objectives for the training program
- Formal trainee evaluations occur at least twice a year
- Program evaluations occur annually

the practice of rehabilitation psychology. The ABRP confers specialty designation (referred to as *board certification*) on psychologists who demonstrate by written work and verbal examination a list of expected competencies (Table 23.2).

In regard to practitioner competencies, a number of evidenced-based rehabilitation psychology

Table 23.2 American Board of Rehabilitation Psychology expected competencies

- The ability to provide assessment and treatment related to:
  ○ Adjustment to disability
  ○ Cognitive functioning
  ○ Personality functioning
  ○ Family/couples functioning
  ○ Social environments and social functioning
  ○ Educational, vocational, and recreational functioning
  ○ Sexual functioning
  ○ Substance abuse
  ○ Pain
- The ability to participate in interprofessional collaboration and consultation
- Knowledge of ethical, legal, and professional issues including:
  ○ Laws related to persons with disability
  ○ Laws related to the practice of psychology
  ○ Psychological ethical principles
- Knowledge of research, and treatment and program evaluation methods, and the ability to apply research findings to one's patients and to evaluate one's practice
- Knowledge of and attention to diversity and cultural issues

treatments are important for practitioners to know and be able to implement, and these can help guide education and training.

Individual Coping and Adjustment

Supportive, interpersonal, and psychodynamic psychotherapy can help individuals experiencing changes in self-concept, changes in self-control, disruption of existing interpersonal systems, and negative stereotypes. Individuals can be helped to shift their emotional, cognitive, and behavioral emphasis from impaired role sets to unimpaired role sets, such as decreasing reliance on physical abilities and increasing reliance on cognitive abilities and personality characteristics as sources of self-esteem and social participation (Keany & Glueckauf, 1993; Wright, 1983). In addition, helping the family and community make such shifts in emotional, cognitive, and behavioral emphasis can also serve to reduce disability by allowing improved access to the physical and social environments.

Activity and participation behaviors are closely associated with perceived quality of life (QOL). Behavioral approaches involving principles of classical and operant conditioning can increase task activity and social participation (Fordyce, 1976; Ince, 1980), including the use of baseline measurement, and gradually increasing quotas to build capacity and tolerance (Patterson & Ford, 2000).

Cognitive-behavioral therapy and coping effectiveness training can develop, enhance, and support coping and problem-solving behaviors, and effective coping and problem-solving behaviors are associated with better outcomes in persons with disability (Elliott, Godshall, Herrick, Witty, & Spruell, 1991a; Elliott, Whitty, Herrick, & Hofman, 1991b). Such behaviors are associated with increased hope and self-efficacy and decreased catastrophizing appraisals (Gonzalez, Goeppinger, & Lorig, 1990; McLaughlin & Zeeberg, 1993). Coping effectiveness training for persons with spinal cord injury (Kennedy, Duff, Evans, & Beedie, 2003; King & Kennedy, 1999; Mohr & Hart, 2007) has been shown to reduce affective distress and increase adaptive cognitions and behaviors.

Self-Management

Disease self-management strategies can improve disease-specific control and decrease secondary health complications (Lorig et al., 2008; Marks, Allegrante, & Lorig 2005a,b). These interventions have been shown to decrease symptoms; improve health behaviors, self-efficacy, and satisfaction with the health care system; and reduce health care utilization. Effective models may involve internet-based educational materials and the use of peer educators to increase disease-management expertise in individuals and their caregivers, as well as to increase caregiver self-care behaviors.

Cognitive Rehabilitation

Rehabilitation psychologists have developed specialized psychological and neuropsychological assessment instruments and procedures for persons with sensory and/or motor impairments that do not allow standardized test procedures (Caplan & Shechter, 1995; Dowler et al., 1997; Richards, Brown, Hagglund, Bua, & Reeder, 1988). These involve tests of intellectual and cognitive function that do not require usual motor or speech abilities and that are standardized for populations with physical impairments.

Rehabilitation psychologists have also developed many of the principles and practices of cognitive rehabilitation (Ben-Yishay & Diller, 1993; Cicerone et al., 2008). Comprehensive rehabilitation involving integrated treatment of cognitive, interpersonal, and functional skills within a therapeutic environment has been shown to result in greater improvements in self-regulation of cognitive and emotional processes, community integration, employment, and QOL as compared to standard discipline-specific neurorehabilitation treatment. Community-based transitional living programs and community teams are especially effective in improving long-term social integration of persons with brain injury (Malec & Ponsford, 2000).

Meta-analyses have shown that some types of cognitive deficits respond better to restorative efforts to improve the underlying function, whereas other types of cognitive deficits respond better to compensatory efforts to accommodate the problem (Cicerone et al., 2000, 2005). There can be substantial benefit from cognitive-linguistic therapies for persons with aphasia after left hemisphere stroke, and substantial benefit from visual-spatial therapies for persons with impaired spatial awareness after right hemisphere stroke. It appears that these underlying focal abilities can be substantially improved through rehabilitation. However, more generalized problems with attention and memory do not respond as well to therapies focused on remediation. Although there may be improvement in attentional or memory tasks with training, these improvements often do not generalize well to other activities. Instead, the use of *cognitive orthoses* to compensate for the underlying attention or memory problems appears to work better (Cicerone et al., 2000, 2005).

Cognitive orthoses can be considered in three categories. *Internal orthoses* include the use of contextual self-cueing to initiate behavior, mnemonics to organize behavior, associative memory to link behavioral steps, and repetition to develop procedural learning. *Environmental orthoses* include the use of visual flags to direct and engage attention, written labels to identify objects and locations, pill boxes to organize medications, and written instructions to guide specific task performance. *External orthoses* include the use of timer alarms to cue behavioral initiation or cessation, calendars to organize and cue activities, and memory books to record and retrieve important information. One technological improvement in external prompting and guidance is the use of text messages delivered by cell phones or pagers at predetermined times. This can be done internally within some cell phones or personal digital assistants, or by internet computer services that send specified messages at specified times.

Physical Rehabilitation

Injury and disuse can lead to *learned nonuse*, in which, for example, an individual immediately following stroke experiences paralysis on one side of his body and learns that he must use the less impaired side to accomplish activities. This then becomes a habit, and this nonuse can continue even after there has been some recovery in function. Constraint-induced therapy, in which the more functional limb is restrained and individuals are forced to use their less functional limb, can result in dramatic increases in function, even years after initial injury (Taub & Uswatte, 2000), by changing nonuse patterns and by generating use-dependent cortical reorganization, in which uninjured areas of the cerebral cortex develop new connections to take over control of important functions from injured areas (Celnik & Cohen, 2004; Nudo, Plautz, & Frost, 2001).

Rehabilitation Teams

Rehabilitation psychologists have also developed specialized knowledge and practices in regard to working with rehabilitation teams and programs (Farmer, Clippard, Luehr-Wiemann, Wright, & Owings, 1996; Frank, 2001; Malec & Ponsford, 2000; Rohe, 1998), and the concept of team has been broadened to include patients and caregivers, as well as individuals involved in community, school, and work relationships (Farmer, Marien,

Clark, Sherman, & Selva, 2004; Farmer, Clark, & Sherman, 2003; Farmer & Muhlenbruck, 2000). Family caregivers are at risk for numerous physical, mental, emotional, social, and financial problems, and helping caregivers obtain and utilize social supports is helpful in maintaining caregiver health and well-being, and thus improving patient outcomes (Elliott & Pezent, 2008; Grant, Elliott, Giger, & Bartolucci, 2001; Lim & Zebrack, 2004).

Ethics and Disability

There is a tendency in the general population to assume that persons experiencing disability cannot have meaningful QOL, and this introduces biases into policies and practices regarding decisions about providing or withholding health care and other services. However, many persons experiencing disability do have satisfactory QOL (Chun & Lee, 2008). Rehabilitation psychologists have developed specific ethical principles related to persons with disability and chronic health conditions, including persons with diminished decision-making capacity (Hanson, Guenther, Kerkhoff, & Liss, 2000; Kerkhoff, Hanson, Guenther, & Ashkanazi, 1997); that acknowledge their independence and choice, and do not impose biased and inaccurate assumptions by persons who are outsiders to the disability experience.

It is also important to recognize that children and adults with disabilities are more likely to be victims of sexual and physical abuse than are individuals without disability (Grossman & Lundy, 2008; Oliván Gonzalvo, 2005; Sanghera, 2007). The rate of abuse of persons with disabilities may be from three to ten times greater than in the general population (Kvam, 2000; Waldman, Swerdloff, & Perlman, 1999). They are more likely to be abused by family members, attendants, and health care providers; are more likely to suffer injury from the abuse; and are more likely to experience repeated abuse. Higher levels of disability are associated with increased risk of abuse and less likelihood of disclosing the abuse (Hershkowitz, Lamb, & Horowitz, 2007; Kvam, 2000). Rehabilitation psychologists should be aware of the importance of explicit assessment of abuse and abuse potential.

Assistive Technology

Assistive technology (AT) refers to anything that is used to maintain or increase functional capabilities. AT can include mobility devices, such as walkers and wheelchairs; self-care devices, such as reachers/grabbers; dressing aids, such as sock donners, button hooks, or holding clamps; environmental control devices to operate lights, doors, and telephones; reminder and alarm systems for eating, taking medication, and other daily activities; and computer hardware, software, and peripherals that assist in use of computer-based products. More recent assistive technology includes direct auditory and optic cortex stimulation, computer-controlled muscle activation, and even computer-detected cortical activity to control devices.

However, matching a person with an assistive device is complex. Person–technology mismatches can waste resources, frustrate and disappoint users and providers, and perpetuate functional limitations (Scherer, Sax, Vanbiervliet, Cushman, & Scherer, 2005; Scherer, 2005). The best match of consumer and device is based upon evaluating users' physical, sensory, and cognitive abilities, as well as their needs, expectations, preferences, motivation, and reactions to technologies, and matching these factors with the appropriate AT (Scherer et al., 2005). In addition, the perceptions and attitudes of others in the family and community are important factors in individuals' acceptance and use of AT (Scherer, 2005; Scherer & Cushman, 2002).

Rehabilitation psychologists study perceptions and attitudes of users and others toward particular technologies, and determine how technologies fit within their activities and contribute to their abilities in daily life. Individuals are more likely to use AT when the device meets their personal preferences and expectations, they were involved in the selection, they have realistic expectations, the device provides perceived value and benefit, and there is informed caregiver support (Scherer et al., 2005). Given the uniqueness of the disability experience for any given individual, it is crucial that rehabilitation psychologists be included on the AT selection team.

Existing rehabilitation psychology training guidelines and expected practitioner competencies can provide conceptual elements for the discussion of education and training in this specialty. Clearly, it is important that rehabilitation psychology education and training involve the specialized populations, specialized problems, and specialized procedures with which rehabilitation psychologists work. In addition, it is important that trainees be familiar with those existing evidenced-based rehabilitation psychology treatments that are known to be effective.

Survey Data About Current Rehabilitation Psychology Training

Survey data describing what actually occurs in psychology doctoral, internship, and postdoctoral training programs related to rehabilitation psychology can provide valuable information for this current discussion. There are existing survey data from the United States and Canada, the United Kingdom, and Australia.

Stiers and Stucky (2008) surveyed psychology training sites involving rehabilitation populations in the United States and Canada and found that only 36% reported providing training in rehabilitation psychology, and less than half of those had a complete rehabilitation focus. Despite working with rehabilitation patient populations, the psychology supervisors rarely specialized in rehabilitation psychology.

Stiers and Stucky (2008) used an evaluation research approach to examining these training programs. This approach considered the program structures, processes, and outcomes. Program structures (the "who" and "where" of the program) consist of the setting (hospital, clinic, private practice), the subsetting (departments within settings), the funding source for training activities, faculty and trainee characteristics (numbers, preparation, specialization), patient populations, and the philosophy, goals, and curricula of the training program. Program processes (the "when" and "how" of the program) consist of the numbers and types of patients encountered, the numbers and types of classes attended, the frequency and type of supervision, and the frequency and type of program and trainee evaluations. Program outcomes (the "what" of the program) consist of the extent to which trainees went on to additional training; became licensed and board certified; were employed in teaching, research, or practice jobs; and were employed in rehabilitation settings. Because these were survey data, and most training programs did not have information available regarding measurement of trainee competencies, actual knowledge and skill outcomes could not be included.

In this U.S. and Canadian survey, most rehabilitation psychology training sites had been in existence from 15–20 years. Training sites were almost always based in a hospital setting, and many were affiliated with a medical school. Within the hospital setting, the psychology group was most often part of a larger department rather than an independent department, and most were part of psychiatry or physical medicine and rehabilitation. Psychology faculty were equally likely to be classified as medical staff or allied health staff.

Most rehabilitation psychology training sites had about four faculty, two to four interns, and one to three postdoctoral trainees. The most common patient populations treated were individuals with brain injury, neurologic disorders, and pain. Other common conditions included spinal cord injury, psychiatric disorders, orthopedic problems, substance abuse, cardiovascular conditions, and cancer. Less common conditions included congenital conditions, developmental disorders, blindness, burns, and HIV/AIDS.

Most sites had a written mission/vision statement. Most sites also had specific written goals and objectives for trainees, including a specific level of achievement required for successful completion of the training program. Only about two-thirds of the sites had a written curriculum for didactics.

Length of training was universally 1 year for interns. For residents, length of training was almost equally either 1 year or 2 years. Most sites provided 2–4 hours of supervision per week, and 2–5 hours of didactics per week.

Frequency of evaluations in most programs was two to four times per year. Almost all sites relied on written evaluations by supervisors to examine trainee progress. A significantly smaller group of sites used knowledge/skill/behavior checklists, ratings of patient–trainee observation, and written evaluations by peers and staff to examine trainee progress. Very few sites used patient satisfaction ratings, oral or written examinations, measurement of patient outcomes, or ratings of written vignettes or simulated patients as means of examining trainee progress.

In regard to the Patterson and Hanson 1995 guidelines for postdoctoral training in rehabilitation psychology, all sites met the following recommendations: the length of training was a minimum of 1 year; the curriculum included activities such as supervised work with patients, and seminars and coursework; populations and didactics involved disabilities and chronic health conditions; and at least two evaluations were given during the training period. Almost all sites provided at least 2 hours per week of didactic training, provided at least 2 hours per week of individual supervision, had at least 2 supervisors involved in rehabilitation psychology training, provided funding, and had written objectives.

Postdoctoral training sites were asked about their provision of training in the specific ABRP core competencies, and whether training in each area was provided formally (didactics, journal clubs, conferences, or seminars), informally (during supervision and involvement with rehabilitation

teams and disability groups), or not at all. These training sites most often provided formal training in diversity issues, cognitive functioning, and ethical principles. Other areas in which programs often provided formal training were state laws of practice, adjustment to disability, pain, substance abuse, personality functioning, and research. These sites less often provided formal training in social and environmental functioning, sexual functioning, and laws related to the Americans with Disabilities Act (ADA). Topics that were most often taught informally were social functioning, family/couple functioning, educational/vocational/recreational functioning, and interprofessional collaboration. Topics that were most often not taught at all, either formally or informally, were laws related to ADA, sexual functioning, and educational/vocational/recreational functioning.

In regard to interns, 95% of sites were able to report some type of outcome data regarding interns who had completed their training programs. After intern training, sites reported that their interns predominantly went on to practice jobs, with some going on to postdoctoral training or teaching positions. Only an average of 29% of interns were subsequently employed in rehabilitation settings, ranging from 0% to 100% in different programs.

In regard to residents, 87% of sites were able to report some type of outcome data regarding residents who had completed their training programs. Residents took the U.S. or Canadian national psychology licensing exam either prior to or during the program or within 1 year of completing the program. Postdoctoral trainees became state licensed either prior to or during the program or within 1 year of completing the program. Only an average of 15% proceeded to board certification within 5 years, and this was most often in neuropsychology, with few in rehabilitation psychology, clinical psychology, or health psychology. Sites reported that their post-postdoctoral trainees mostly went on to practice jobs, with fewer going to teaching positions and research positions. An average of 63% were subsequently employed in rehabilitation settings, ranging from 0% in some programs to 100% in others.

A survey of training in rehabilitation psychology in Australia (Nicholson Perry & Kerin, 2010) examined the availability of professional practice placements with rehabilitation populations and the rehabilitation psychology content in taught components within psychology doctoral training programs. Forty-three percent of course directors responded to the survey, primarily from clinical psychology training programs, with some responses from organizational, forensic, sport and exercise, and health psychology. Master's degree programs comprised 41% of the courses for which data were available, with 30% professional doctorate and 30% Ph.D. programs.

The most common patient populations treated were substance dependence and abuse, psychiatric impairment, and developmental intellectual disorders. Less common patient populations included neurologic disorders, pain, brain injury, and cancer. Very few or no trainees worked with patient populations involving orthopedic and musculoskeletal conditions, spinal cord injury, burns, and amputations.

In comparison to U.S. and Canadian training programs, training programs in Australia had dramatically fewer professional practice placement opportunities for work with persons with amputation, burns, spinal cord injury, orthopaedic and musculoskeletal problems, and acquired brain injury. This demonstrates more emphasis placed on the traditional areas for psychological practice—that is, persons with mental health, substance abuse, and developmental disorders—and limited opportunity for work with the core populations of persons receiving rehabilitation services.

Australian psychology training course providers were also asked about their provision of training in the specific ABRP core competencies, and whether training in each area was provided formally (didactics, journal clubs, conferences, or seminars), informally (during supervision and involvement with rehabilitation teams and disability groups), or not at all. These data revealed that these courses most often provided formal training in substance abuse, cognitive functioning, pain, adjustment to disability, injury and disability legal frameworks, compensation systems, and interdisciplinary/multidisciplinary interaction. Other areas in which formal training was often provided were common rehabilitation populations, personality functioning, social environments, and study and return to work. The least common areas of formal training were family/couple functioning, recreational functioning, and sexual functioning in injury and illness.

In comparison to U.S. and Canadian training programs, training programs in Australia were similar in their inclusion of teaching related to adjustment to disability, substance abuse, cognitive functioning, pain, and injury and disability legal frameworks and compensation systems. They were also similar in that they were less likely to include teaching related to personality functioning in injury/illness, family/couple functioning in injury and illness, sexual functioning in injury and illness, social environments, and interprofessional collaboration. This appears to demonstrate more emphasis being placed on the individual factors associated with disability, and less emphasis on the environmental, interpersonal, and social aspects of disability, similar to U.S. and Canadian training programs.

A survey of training in rehabilitation psychology in the United Kingdom (A. Kuemmel, personal communication, September 9, 2010) also examined the availability of professional practice placements with rehabilitation populations and the rehabilitation psychology content in taught components within psychology doctoral training programs. Thirty percent of programs responded to the survey. The most common patient populations treated were developmental intellectual disorders, amputation, spinal cord injury, and psychiatric impairments. Slightly less common patient populations included neurologic disorders, acquired brain injury, and pain. Few trainees worked with patient populations involving burns, orthopedic and musculoskeletal problems, HIV/AIDS, congenital conditions, cancer, and cardiovascular conditions.

In comparison to U.S. and Canadian psychology training programs, training programs in the United Kingdom placed more emphasis on one of the traditional areas for psychological practice—that is, persons with developmental disorders—but offered slightly fewer professional practice placement opportunities for work with persons with brain injury, neurologic disorders, orthopedic problems, cardiovascular conditions, and cancer. There were practice opportunities for work with persons with amputation and spinal cord injury. Thus, the psychology training programs in the United Kingdom provided more training opportunities to work with some traditional rehabilitation populations than did programs in Australia, although not quite as many as in the United States and Canada.

Psychology training course providers in the United Kingdom were also asked about their provision of training in the specific ABRP core competencies, and whether training in each area was provided formally (didactics, journal clubs, conferences, or seminars), informally (during supervision and involvement with rehabilitation teams and disability groups), or not at all. These data revealed that these courses most often provided formal training in common rehabilitation population, adjustment to disability, cognitive functioning, personality functioning, pain, and interdisciplinary interaction. They less often provided training in substance abuse, legal frameworks related to injury and disability, family/couple functioning, social environments and social functioning, recreational functioning, and sexual functioning.

As with the U.S./Canadian and Australian psychology training programs, training programs in the United Kingdom were similar in less often providing formal training in family/couple functioning, recreational functioning, and sexual functioning in injury and illness. In all of these countries, this again demonstrates more emphasis being placed on the individual factors associated with disability, and less emphasis on the environmental, interpersonal, and social aspects of disability.

Survey data describing psychology doctoral, internship, and postdoctoral training related to rehabilitation psychology, although limited to the United States, Canada, the United Kingdom, and Australia, can provide valuable information for this discussion. It appears that psychology training could be improved in all of these countries by increasing the availability of formal training involving sexual functioning, family/couple functioning, educational/vocational/recreational functioning, social and environmental functioning, laws related to persons with disability, and interprofessional collaboration to trainees wishing to specialize in rehabilitation psychology. In addition, it is important to increase professional practice placement opportunities in Australia for work with persons with amputation, spinal cord injury, acquired brain injury, orthopaedic and musculoskeletal problems, cardiovascular conditions, cancer, and burns.

Conclusion

This chapter focused on rehabilitation psychology as it applies to persons with physical disability. Within that context, the definition of the specialty of rehabilitation psychology and its relevance to world health needs suggest that it is important that education and training in rehabilitation psychology involve teaching and supervised work experience involving individuals with disability, their rehabilitation teams and institutions, and their families and communities, in order to maximize health, functional abilities, and social role participation, and to minimize secondary health complications. Because disability is a person–task–environment interaction, it is important to address barriers in the social,

cultural, physical, and political environments in which the individual exists.

Existing training guidelines and expected practitioner competencies can provide conceptual elements for the consideration of education and training in rehabilitation psychology. The 1995 Patterson and Hanson guidelines for rehabilitation psychology training reflect the general guidelines of the American Psychological Association for postdoctoral training in any specialty, and therefore should be considered as essential for rehabilitation psychology training programs in the United States. However, given the wide global variation that exists in the education and training of psychologists in general, as well as for rehabilitation psychologists, these specific guidelines may require modification in non-U.S. training programs. Clearly, it is important that rehabilitation psychology education and training involve the specialized populations, specialized problems, and specialized procedures with which rehabilitation psychologists work. In addition, it is important that trainees be familiar with the existing evidenced-based rehabilitation psychology treatments that are known to be effective.

Regardless of location and context, it is important that teaching and supervised work experience in rehabilitation psychology develop competencies related to assessment of and intervention with cognitive, emotional, behavioral, and interpersonal adjustment; physical and cognitive task functioning; self-care and independent living skills; educational, vocational, social, and recreational participation; health self-management; caregiver, team, and community service/agency functioning; selection and use of AT and personal assistance services; and physical and social accessibility. Additional issues involving pain, substance use, and disability-related ethics are also relevant. It is important that rehabilitation psychology trainees be familiar with the application of psychotherapy and behavior therapy in persons with disability, coping effectiveness training, disease self-management strategies, psychological and neuropsychological assessment of persons with sensory and/or motor impairments, comprehensive cognitive rehabilitation, working with rehabilitation teams and programs, helping caregivers obtain and utilize social supports, specific ethical principles related to persons with disability, explicit assessment of abuse and abuse potential, and matching persons with assistive technology.

Psychology training for individuals wishing to specialize in rehabilitation psychology could be improved by increasing the availability of formal training involving sexual functioning, family/couple functioning, educational/vocational/recreational functioning, social and environmental functioning, laws related to persons with disability, and interprofessional collaboration. In addition, professional practice placement opportunities in Australia and the United Kingdom for work with persons with acquired brain injury, orthopedic and musculoskeletal problems, cardiovascular conditions, cancer, and burns could be improved. In Australia, professional practice placement opportunities for work with persons with amputation and spinal cord injury are especially important areas for improvement.

An essential aspect of any professional training program is periodic evaluation of the program and the use of evaluation findings for program improvement. This includes evaluation of both trainee competencies and program functioning. Because evaluation requires the comparison of intended goals with the actual goals achieved, it is essential that rehabilitation psychology training programs have a written mission/vision statement, written goals and objectives for trainees, and a written curriculum for didactics. It is also essential that regular supervision and didactics occur, and that formal evaluations of trainees occur periodically. Clearly, it is important to develop measurement tools and procedures for evaluation of trainee competencies in this specialty.

Future Directions

Issues of education and training are fundamental to the conceptualization and development of the specialty of applied rehabilitation psychology, as they are in all areas of professional health service psychology. A specialty is shaped by the preparation of its practitioners, including its selection of trainees, the structures and processes of its training programs, and the competencies expected of successful trainees. In looking to the future of the profession, a number of particular issues need to be addressed; these include providing adequate numbers of appropriately trained rehabilitation psychologists to meet relevant public health needs, enhancing methodologies for assessing training outcomes, and developing improved training guidelines that include important issues such as cultural competence training and user involvement in practitioner training.

MEETING WORKFORCE DEMAND

Rehabilitation psychology is relevant to the estimated 650 million individuals in the world who live with a disability. However, there does not appear to be enough specialty workforce capacity to best respond to these important growing world health priorities (Stiers & Stucky, 2009), and therefore there is a need for increased rehabilitation psychology training. In the United States, there are currently approximately 20 psychology postdoctoral training programs with a primary focus on rehabilitation psychology, and an additional 26 training programs with a partial focus on rehabilitation psychology. The U.S. government has recently allocated $7 million to support psychology training, and some of this may be available to increase rehabilitation psychology training. In general, it is clear that government support is important for health care workforce development. In this context, it is necessary for rehabilitation psychologists to educate policy-makers about the increase in the numbers of persons with disability and chronic health conditions, the significant extent to which such persons require health care resources, and the importance of this specialty in increasing independent living, reducing secondary health conditions, and reducing health care costs for this population.

Training programs in the United Kingdom and Australia had dramatically fewer professional practice placement opportunities for work with primary rehabilitation populations, and tend to emphasize work with persons with mental health, substance abuse, and developmental disorders—the more traditional mental health practice areas for psychology. Rather than rely on continuing education and on-the-job training, training programs in these countries could better expand their ability to provide rehabilitation psychology–specific training and experience for interested trainees.

Enhancing Assessment Methodologies in Rehabilitation Psychology Training

It is essential that formal evaluations of trainees occur periodically and that appropriate measurement of trainee competencies is used to improve program functioning. However, psychology in general has not yet developed specific tools to measure and improve trainee competencies. In the United States, almost all training programs relied on written evaluations by supervisors to examine trainee progress. Few programs used knowledge/skill/behavior checklists, observational ratings of patient–trainee interactions, and written evaluations by peers and staff, and only a very few used patient satisfaction ratings or measurements of patient outcomes.

The currently practical means of assessing trainee competence in rehabilitation psychology postdoctoral fellowship training programs include:

- *Knowledge* may be assessed through 360-degree evaluation, including self-assessment, peer ratings, supervisor ratings, collateral professional ratings, and patient satisfaction, with an accompanying knowledge-oriented checklist.
  - *Skills* may be assessed through:
    - 360-degree evaluation
    - Live patient observation
    - Videotape reviews
    - Record/chart review
    - With an accompanying skills-oriented behavior checklist
  - *Attitudes/values* may be assessed through
    - 360-degree evaluation
    - Ongoing association of faculty with the trainee, and observation of their interactions with patients and other professionals
    - With an accompanying attitudes/values-oriented behavior checklist

Other possible means of assessing trainee competence are not currently practical in rehabilitation psychology postdoctoral fellowship training programs:

- Some professions have developed standardized written and oral examinations for trainees, but these do not exist in rehabilitation psychology, as they do not for other specialty areas in professional health service psychology. In the United States, the mechanism for evaluation of such specialty competencies is through examination for board certification (e.g., ABRP) following the completion of training.
- Although one might consider written topic essays and literature reviews, these are usually not required at advanced-practice clinical training sites, and, in addition, many trainees have already completed dissertations or other formal written products relevant to their area of specialization.
- Standardized patient examinations, including written vignettes, simulated patients, and computerized simulations, have not been well developed in rehabilitation psychology, as they have not in other specialty areas in professional health service psychology. However, the development of standardized clinical vignettes is an area that may be fruitful for further work.

The use of 360-degree evaluation (including self-assessment, peer ratings, supervisor ratings, collateral professional ratings, and patient satisfaction)

with accompanying knowledge, skills/abilities, and attitudes/values behavior checklists appears sufficient to ensure trainee competency, is within the means of training programs, and reflects the current state of the art in professional health service psychology. This combination of multitrait evaluations (knowledge, skills/abilities, and attitudes/values) and multimethod evaluations (360 degree ratings, observation of live patient encounters, and ongoing association during the course of professional activities) increases the reliability and validity of the evaluation process.

Theories of professional competence are important, and do exist for psychology, as well as for medicine and nursing. However, medical and nursing education have developed important measurement tools of trainee competencies, which psychology has not yet done. An important type of tool is *structured clinical observation*; that is, the use of behavioral checklists completed by supervisors observing patient–trainee interactions. These may include items such as:

- Introduced him- or herself
- Gave patient time to express concerns
- Asked logical sequence of questions one at a time
- Conducted a thorough and proficient examination
- Explained diagnosis and recommendations in words patient understood
- Asked for questions
- Asked if patient was willing and able to follow the recommendations
- Discussed and planned for return visit

Useful supervisor evaluations should be as concrete as possible, and may also include items such as:

- Demonstrated professional appearance
- Proficiently administered and scored psychological testing relevant to the referral question
- Interpreted test results accurately and reached appropriate diagnostic conclusions
- Wrote a well-organized, concise psychological report with relevant and detailed recommendations
- Identified appropriate treatment goals in collaboration with the patient
- Presented interventions that are well-timed and consistent with empirically supported data.

IMPROVING TRAINING GUIDELINES

Rehabilitation psychology would benefit from the development of a clear set of training pathways and guidelines. It is important that rehabilitation psychology training programs have a written mission/vision statement, written goals and objectives for trainees, and a written curriculum for didactics. However, survey data from the United States and Canada showed that postdoctoral training sites formally taught an average of 69% of the ABRP competencies, and only 21% of the sites formally taught 100% of the competencies (Stiers & Stucky, 2009). It appears that many rehabilitation psychology training sites do not have sufficient resources to develop these curricular materials, and the field would benefit from the development and availability of such. In particular, training related to sexual functioning, family/couple functioning, educational/vocational/recreational functioning, and interprofessional collaboration, all important areas of rehabilitation psychology, should be improved.

In some other areas of professional psychology training, as well as in the practice of rehabilitation psychology, new areas of competency are being identified and developed that will need to be integrated into future versions of training guidelines. Cultural issues present a range of challenges to the rehabilitation psychologist, including pragmatic questions such as the appropriate selection of assessment tools, as well as the more subtle influence of cultural beliefs about health, disability, and the role of health professionals (Niemeier, Burnett, & Whitaker, 2003). A good example of the way in which such issues are being addressed within the rehabilitation field is the Center for International Research Information & Exchange's project "Culture in the Curriculum" (http://cirrie.buffalo.edu/curriculum/index.php), which has developed teaching materials for prequalification university training courses for health professions related to rehabilitation, such as physical therapy and rehabilitation counseling. Although the literature on the effectiveness of different approaches to teaching cultural competence to pre- or postqualification health professionals is limited (Chipps, Simpson, & Brysiewicz, 2008), the importance of the area is such that attention should be drawn to it by specifically including it within the guidelines for rehabilitation psychology training programs.

Another important area is the issue of user involvement in the development and management of services, as well as in the training of health professionals. This has flourished in the area of mental health in the past three decades (Crawford et al., 2002). As an example, policy development in the United Kingdom has stressed the importance of user involvement in all aspects of service design and delivery, including the selection and training of clinical psychology trainees. Although there is a strong tradition of the involvement of users in rehabilitation services in many settings (for a recent example, see Jalovcic & Pentland, 2009), the competencies for collaborating with users in program development and operation are currently not included in training guidelines for rehabilitation psychology, and this will also form an important part of future development.

Although there are limits to how many different topics can be included in rehabilitation psychology training, it may be important to consider some training focus on population and public health issues. Relevant topics might include the epidemiology of common disabling conditions, as well as issues related to injury prevention and health promotion.

In summary, rehabilitation psychology could benefit from the development of specialty-specific training guidelines and curricular resources, increased opportunities for trainees to work with rehabilitation populations, and collaboration with medicine and nursing in developing program and trainee evaluation instruments and procedures. Users could certainly add valuable input in training development. In addition, emphasis on developing understanding and practice competencies related to differing cultural attitudes and beliefs about health, individuals with disabilities, and the role of health professionals is important.

References

American Board of Rehabilitation Psychology. *Examination manual*. Rochester, MN: Author. Retrieved August 30, 2010 from http://www.abpp.org/files/page-specific/3361%20Rehab/15_ABRP_Candidate_Manual.pdf

American Psychological Association Council of Credentialing Organizations in Professional Psychology. (2004). *A conceptual framework for specialization in the health service domain of professional psychology*. Washington, DC: Author.

Barker, R., & Wright, B. (1952). The social psychology of adjustment to physical disability. In J. Garrett (Ed.), *Psychological aspects of physical disability* (pp. 18–32). Washington, DC: U.S. Government Printing Office (Office of Vocational Rehabilitation, Rehabilitation Services Series No. 210).

Barker, R., Wright, B., & Gonick, M. (Eds.). (1946). *Adjustment to physical handicap and illness: A survey of the social psychology of physique and disability*. New York: Social Science Research Council.

Ben-Yishay, Y., & Diller, L. (1993). Cognitive remediation in traumatic brain injury: Update and issues. *Archives of Physical Medicine and Rehabilitation, 74*(2), 204–213.

Caplan, B., & Shechter, J. (1995). The role of nonstandard neuropsychological assessment in rehabilitation: History, rationale, and examples. In L. Cushman, & M. Scherer (Eds.), *Psychological assessment in medical rehabilitation* (pp. 359–391). Washington, DC: American Psychological Association.

Celnik, P., & Cohen, L. (2004). Modulation of motor function and cortical plasticity in health and disease. *Restorative Neurology and Neuroscience, 22*(3–5), 261–268.

Chipps, J. A., Simpson, B., & Brysiewicz, P. (2008). The effectiveness of cultural-competence training for health professionals in community-based rehabilitation: A systematic review of literature. *Worldviews on Evidence-Based Nursing, 5*(2), 85–94.

Chun, S., & Lee, Y. (2008). The experience of posttraumatic growth for people with spinal cord injury. *Quality Health Research, 18*(7), 877–890.

Cicerone, K., Dahlberg, C., Kalmar, K., Langenbahn, D., Malec, J., Bergquist, T., et al. (2000). Evidence-based cognitive rehabilitation: Recommendations for clinical practice. *Archives Physical Medicine and Rehabilitation, 81*, 1596–1615.

Cicerone, K., Dahlberg, C., Malec, J., Langenbahn, D., Felicetti, T., Kneipp, S., et al. (2005). Evidence-based cognitive rehabilitation: Updated review of the literature from 1998 through 2002. *Archives of Physical Medicine and Rehabilitation, 86*(8), 1681–1692.

Cicerone, K., Mott, T., Azulay, J., Sharlow-Galella, M., Ellmo, W., & Paradise, S. (2008). A randomized controlled trial of holistic neuropsychologic rehabilitation after traumatic brain injury. *Archives of Physical Medicine and Rehabilitation, 89*(12), 2239–2249.

Crawford, M. J., Rutter, D., Manley, C., Weaver, T., Bhui, K., Fulop, N., & Tyrer, P. (2002). Systematic review of involving patients in the planning and development of health care. *British Medical Journal (Clinical Research Ed.), 325*(7375), 1263.

Dembo, T., Leviton, G., & Wright, B. (1956). Adjustment to misfortune-a problem of social-psychological rehabilitation. *Artificial Limbs, 3*(2), 4–62.

Dowler, R., Herrington, D., Haaland, K., Swanda, R., Fee, F., & Fiedler, K. (1997). Profiles of cognitive functioning and chronic spinal cord injury and the role of moderating variables. *Journal of the International Neuropsychological Society, 3*, 464–472.

Dunn, D., & Elliott, T. (2005). Revisiting a constructive classic: Wright's physical disability: A psychosocial approach. *Rehabilitation Psychology, 50*(2), 183–189.

Elliott, T., Godshall, F., Herrick, S., Witty, T., & Spruell, M. (1991a). Problem-solving appraisal and psychological adjustment following spinal cord injury. *Cognitive Therapy Research, 15*, 387–398.

Elliott, T., Whitty, T., Herrick, S., & Hoffman, J. (1991b). Negotiating reality after physical loss: Hope, depression, and disability. *Journal of Personality and Social Psychology, 61*, 608–613.

Elliott, T., & Pezent, G. (2008). Family caregivers of older persons in rehabilitation. *NeuroRehabilitation, 23*(5), 439–446.

Farmer, J., Clark, M., & Sherman, A. (2003). Rural versus urban social support seeking as a moderating variable in traumatic brain injury outcome. *Journal of Head Trauma Rehabilitation, 18*(2), 116–127.

Farmer, J., Clippard, D., Luehr-Wiemann, Y., Wright, E., & Owings, S. (1996). Assessing children following traumatic brain injury: Promoting school and community reentry. *Journal of Learning Disabilities, 29*, 532–548.

Farmer, J., Marien, W., Clark, M., Sherman, A., & Selva, T. (2004). Primary care supports for children with chronic health conditions: Identifying and predicting unmet family needs. *Journal of Pediatric Psychology, 29*(5), 355–367.

Farmer, D., & Muhlenbruck, L. (2000). Pediatric neuropsychology. In R. Frank, & T. Elliott (Eds.), *Handbook of rehabilitation psychology* (pp. 377–397). Washington, DC: American Psychological Association.

Fordyce, W. (1976). *Behavioral methods for chronic pain and illness.* St. Louis: Mosby.

Frank, R. (2001). Rehabilitation. In A. Baum, T. Revenson, & J. Singer (Eds.), *Handbook of health psychology* (pp. 581–590). Mahwah, NJ: Lawrence Erlbaum Associates, Inc.

Gold, J., Meltzer, R., & Sherr, R. (1982). Professional transitions: Psychology internships in rehabilitation settings. *Professional Psychology, 13*, 397–403.

Gonzalez, V., Goeppinger, J., & Lorig, K. (1990). Four psychosocial theories and their application to patient education and clinical practice. *Arthritis Care and Research, 3*,132–143.

Grant, J., Elliott, T., Giger, J., & Bartolucci, A. (2001). Social problem-solving telephone partnerships with family caregivers of persons with stroke. *International Journal of Rehabilitation Research, 24*(3),181–189.

Grossman, S., & Lundy, M. (2008). Double jeopardy: A comparison of persons with and without disabilities who were victims of sexual abuse and/or sexual assault. *Journal of Social Work Disability and Rehabilitation, 7*(1), 19–46.

Hanson, S., Guenther, R., Kerkhoff, T., & Liss, M. (2000). Ethics: Historical foundations, basic principles, and contemporary issues. In R. Frank, & T. Elliott (Eds.), *Handbook of rehabilitation psychology* (pp. 629–643). Washington, DC: American Psychological Association.

Hershkowitz, I., Lamb, M., & Horowitz, D. (2007). Victimization of children with disabilities. *American Journal of Orthopsychiatry, 77*(4), 629–635.

Hoffman, C., Rice, D., & Sung, H. (1996). Persons with chronic conditions: Their prevalence and costs. *Journal of the American Medical Association, 266*, 1473–1479.

Ince, L. (1980). *Behavioral psychology in rehabilitation medicine.* Baltimore: Williams and Wilkins.

Jalovcic, D., & Pentland, W. (2009). Accessing peers' and health care experts' wisdom: A telephone peer support program for women with SCI living in rural and remote areas. *Topics in Spinal Cord Injury Rehabilitation, 15*(1), 59–74.

Keany, K., & Glueckauf, R. (1993). Disability and value change: An overview and reanalysis of acceptance of loss theory. *Rehabilitation Psychology, 38*, 199–210.

Kennedy, P., Duff, J., Evans, M., & Beedie, A. (2003). Coping effectiveness training reduces depression and anxiety following traumatic spinal cord injuries. *British Journal of Clinical Psychology, 42*(Pt 1), 41–52.

Kerkhoff, T., Hanson, S., Guenther, R., & Ashkanazi, G. (1997). The foundation and application of ethical principles in rehabilitation psychology. *Rehabilitation Psychology, 42*(1), 17–30.

King, C., & Kennedy, P. (1999). Coping effectiveness training for people with spinal cord injury: Preliminary results of a controlled trial. *British Journal of Clinical Psychology, 38*(Pt 1), 5–14.

Krug, E., Dahlberg, L., Mercy, J., Zwi, A., & Lozano, R. (2002). *World report on violence and health.* Geneva: World Health Organization.

Kvam, M. (2000). Is sexual abuse of children with disabilities disclosed? A retrospective analysis of child disability and the likelihood of sexual abuse among those attending Norwegian hospitals. *Child Abuse and Neglect, 24*(8), 1073–1084.

Lim, J., & Zebrack, B. (2004). Caring for family members with chronic physical illness: A critical review of caregiver literature. *Health Quality of Life Outcomes, 17*(2), 50.

Lorig, K., Ritter, P., Dost, A., Plant, K., Laurent, D., & McNeil, I. (2008). The expert patients programme online, a 1-year study of an Internet-based self-management programme for people with long-term conditions. *Chronic Illness, 4*(4), 247–256.

Malec, J., & Ponsford, J. (2000). Postacute brain injury. In R. Frank, & T. Elliott (Eds.), *Handbook of rehabilitation psychology* (pp. 417–439). Washington, DC: American Psychological Association.

Marks, R., Allegrante, J., & Lorig, K. (2005a). A review and synthesis of research evidence for self-efficacy-enhancing interventions for reducing chronic disability: Implications for health education practice (part II). *Health Promotion Practices, 6*(2), 148–156.

Marks, R., Allegrante, J., & Lorig, K. (2005b). A review and synthesis of research evidence for self-efficacy-enhancing interventions for reducing chronic disability: Implications for health education practice (part I). *Health Promotion Practices, 6*(1), 37–43.

McLaughin, J., & Zeeberg, I. (1993). Self-care and multiple sclerosis: A view from two cultures. *Social Science and Medicine, 3*, 315–329.

Mohr, D., Hart, S., & Vella, L. (2007). Reduction in disability in a randomized controlled trial of telephone-administered cognitive-behavioral therapy. *Health Psychology, 26*(5), 554–563.

Nudo, R., Plautz, E., & Frost, S. (2001). Role of adaptive plasticity in recovery of function after damage to motor cortex. *Muscle and Nerve, 24*, 1000–1009.

Nicholson Perry, K., & Kerin, F. (2010). *Professional psychology training in Australia: How does it prepare psychologists for practice with rehabilitation populations?* Paper presented at the International Congress of Applied Psychology, Melbourne, Australia.

Niemeier, J. P., Burnett, D. M., & Whitaker, D. A. (2003). Cultural competence in the multidisciplinary rehabilitation setting: Are we falling short of meeting needs? *Archives of Physical Medicine and Rehabilitation, 84*(8), 1240–1245.

Oliván Gonzalvo, G. (2005). What can be done to prevent violence and abuse of children with disabilities? *Annals of Pediatrics (Barc), 62*(2),153–157.

Patterson, D., & Hanson, S. (1995). Joint Division 22 and ACRM guidelines for post-doctoral training in rehabilitation psychology. *Rehabilitation Psychology, 40*, 299–310.

Patterson, D., & Ford, G. (2000). Burn injuries. In R. Frank, & T. Elliott (Eds.), *Handbook of rehabilitation psychology* (pp. 145–162). Washington, DC: American Psychological Association.

Peden, M., Krug, E., Mohan, D, Hyder, A., Norton, R., MacKay, M., & Dora, C. (2001). *Five-year WHO strategy on road traffic injury prevention*. Geneva: World Health Organization. Retrieved March 15, 2009 from http://whqlibdoc.who.int/hq/2001/WHO_NMH_VIP_01.03.pdf

Peden, M., McGee, K., & Krug, E. (Eds.). (2002). *Injury: A leading cause of the global burden of disease, 2000*. Geneva, World Health Organization. Retrieved March 15, 2009 from http://www.who.int/violence_injury_prevention/publications/other_injury/injury/en/index.html

Rathore, F., Farooq, F., Muzammil, S., New, P., Ahmad, N., & Haig, A. (2008). Spinal cord injury management and rehabilitation: Highlights and shortcomings from the 2005 earthquake in Pakistan. *Archives of Physical Medicine and Rehabilitation, 89*(3), 579–585.

Richards, J., Brown, L., Hagglund, K., Bua, G., & Reeder, K. (1988). Spinal cord injury and concomitant traumatic brain injury: Results of a longitudinal investigation. *American Journal of Physical Medicine and Rehabilitation, 67*, 211–216.

Rohe, D. (1998). Psychological aspects of rehabilitation. In J. DeLisa, & B. Gans (Eds.), *Rehabilitation medicine: Principles and practice* (3rd ed., pp. 189–212). Philadelphia: Lippincott-Raven.

Sanghera, P. (2007). Abuse of children with disabilities in hospital: issues and implications. *Paediatric Nursing, 19*(6), 29–32.

Scherer, M. (2005). Assessing the benefits of using assistive technologies and other supports for thinking, remembering and learning. *Disability and Rehabilitation, 27*(13), 731–739.

Scherer, M., & Cushman, L. (2002). Determining the content for an interactive training programme and interpretive guidelines for the Assistive Technology Device Predisposition Assessment. *Disability and Rehabilitation, 24*(1–3), 126–130.

Scherer, M., Sax, C., Vanbiervliet, A., Cushman, L., & Scherer, J. (2005). Predictors of assistive technology use: The importance of personal and psychosocial factors. *Disability and Rehabilitation, 27*(21), 1321–1331.

Shontz, F., & Wright, B. (1980). The distinctiveness of rehabilitation psychology. *Professional Psychology, 11*(6), 919–924.

Stevens, M., & Wedding, D. (Eds.). (2004). *Handbook of international psychology*. New York: Brunner-Routledge.

Stiers, W., & Stucky, K. (2008). A survey of training in rehabilitation psychology practice in the United States and Canada: 2007. *Rehabilitation Psychology, 53*(4), 536–543.

Taub, E., & Uswatte, G. (2000). Constraint-induced movement therapy based on behavioral neuroscience. In R. Frank, and T. Elliott (Eds.), *Handbook of rehabilitation psychology* (pp. 475–496). Washington, DC: American Psychological Association.

Waldman, H., Swerdloff, M., & Perlman, S. (1999). A "dirty secret": The abuse of children with disabilities. *ASDC Journal of Dentistry for Children, 66*(3), 197–202.

World Health Organization (a). *World report on disability and rehabilitation*. Geneva: World Health Organization. Retrieved March 15, 2009 from http://www.who.int/disabilities/Concept%20NOTE%20General%202008.pdf

World Health Organization (b). *Disability, including prevention, management and rehabilitation*. Geneva: World Health Organization. Retrieved March 15, 2009 from http://www.who.int/nmh/a5817/en/

World Health Organization (c). (2004). *Occupational health and safety in the African region: Situation analysis and perspectives*. Geneva: World Health Organization. Retrieved March 15, 2009 from http://www.google.com/url?sa=t&rct=j&q=%22Occupational+health+and+safety+in+the+African+region%22&source=web&cd=1&ved=0CDoQFjAA&url=http%3A%2F%2Fwww.afro.who.int%2Findex.php%3Foption%3Dcom_docman%26task%3Ddoc_download%26gid%3D1872&ei=iXoYT6D7D-H30gH6koXQCw&usg=AFQjCNHi_dUEn0GIluQAibtroNNe5F19og

World Health Organization (d). (2002). *Collective violence*. Geneva: World Health Organization. Retrieved March 15, 2009 from http://www.who.int/violence_injury_prevention/violence/world_report/factsheets/en/collectiveviolfacts.pdf

Wright, B. (1983). *Physical disability: A psychological approach*. New York: Harper and Row.

Ethics in Psychology: Expanding Horizons

Thomas R. Kerkhoff *and* Stephanie L. Hanson

Abstract

This chapter considers ongoing challenges in applied health care ethics from an international perspective. The nature of these challenges focuses upon fundamental ethical processes such as clinical and surrogate decision-making and informed consent, considers duty to provide care in difficult circumstances, discusses issues involved in health care research, and moves into the realm of applying technological advances. Additionally, consideration of cultural diversity presents serious issues of relevance in attempting to apply ethical concepts within the Western philosophical tradition. Finally, we consider the emerging professional competence movement within psychology and the role of ethics in developing and maintaining functional practice competencies.

Key Words: Ethics, rehabilitation, diversity, cultural factors.

In a 2010 communication from Dr. Normal Anderson, President of APA, he noted that the passage of the Patient Protection and Affordable Care Act (P.L. 111–148) and Health Care and Education Reconciliation Act of 2010 (P.L. 111–152) has created significant opportunity for the expansion of psychology research and practice in the United States. For example, as reported in the American Psychological Association (APA)'s Update on Health Care Reform (an e-mail commentary to the APA membership on the newly signed legislation) Dr. Andersonannounced inclusion of psychologists on primary health care and home health care interdisciplinary teams. A planned increase in funded research related to developing methodology to reduce mental health disparities and improving preventative services, health care delivery and outcomes, and the process of treatment decision-making will support implementation of this new legislation. Planned health care infrastructure improvements include creating a task force to organize best practices across health professions and

modifying graduate training funding/loan repayment programs. These welcome developments recognize that psychology has contributed significantly to both the clinical and research health enterprises. Nonetheless, the dramatic debate surrounding health care reform legislation reflects residual social uncertainties regarding the structure of an optimal health care system in terms of quality health services, creative research, and economic sustainability. The role of psychology remains to be played out, given this dramatic shift in health care policy. As the drama unfolds, psychologists will become immersed in ethical domains that had been the traditional purview of medical and other health professionals. It is this broadening professional opportunity that drives the future-oriented content of this chapter.

The purposes of the chapter are fourfold. First, we will discuss ethical challenges in health care practice (sampled from multinational sources) and will present opportunities for psychology engagement. Second, we will discuss emerging ethical issues related to health research and technological advances. Third, we will explore special challenges nested within our moral obligation to increase awareness of and sensitivity toward cultural and ethnic diversity. Finally, we will discuss the evolution of professional competencies within a Western cultural framework and highlight the importance of global networking.

Ethical Challenges in Health Care
Clinical Decision-Making

The manner in which ethically driven clinical decision-making occurs, whether at the level of the individual health care professional (HCP) or the interdisciplinary treatment team, is critical to consequent outcomes. Ethical analysis supports combining the best available research evidence, clinical expertise, and patient values, consistent with evidence-based practice. This approach implies taking the time necessary to partner with the patient, a process consistent with user-centered care and one that underlies the autonomous decisional process. Partnering with the patient has also been shown to positively impact professional job satisfaction and longevity (Geller, Bernhardt, Carrese, Rushton, & Kolodner, 2008; Terry, 2007; Thornton, 2006).

User-centered care can be framed as the "smallest unit of life is the whole person," in which the whole person is comprised of contextual factors within the immediate physical and social environment (Thornton, 2006, p. 10). In contrast, psychology practice by algorithm (i.e., based on rigid application of research-based practice standards without considering the collective contributions of experience, tacit knowledge, and patient-centered factors) diminishes the value and relevance of a clinical decision for both the patient and clinician, independent of its accuracy (Nilsson & Pilhammar, 2009). Contextual factors clearly play a critical role in bedside decision-making in particular. Psychology has the opportunity to integrate all of these factors, especially within the scientist-practitioner model, thus demonstrating the discipline's undeniable value to the health care team in the form of clinicians and role models for balanced biopsychosocial advocacy.

Beyond direct clinical care, an integrative approach can be helpful when psychologists take advantage of the opportunity to serve on health care ethics committees. Psychologists are particularly well-suited as members of ethics consultation teams because they bring to the table well-honed critical thinking skills that enhance decision-making performance in challenging situations. In the emotionally pressured health care environment, the clinical decision-making process can become mired in such complex issues as communicative dynamics surrounding a dying patient, disagreements between patients and HCPs or among treatment team members about assessment and treatment options, uncertainty about treatment goals, treatment refusal, and requests for futile treatment. These situations sometimes trigger requests for assistance in the form of ethics consults. However, there are significant hurdles to overcome when considering ethics consultation.

We can relate the findings of the Hurst et al. (2005) survey of physicians to all HCPs who find themselves in the position of decision-maker. A key result of this study showed that the clinician decision-maker's strongest desire was to protect their integrity. This proved to be a cluster concept comprised of integration of personality into a harmonious whole, holding true to one's commitments, regarding one's own judgment as one that should matter to others, and acting morally. The other major finding was the HCP's desire to avoid conflict. The Hurst et al. study found that conflict avoidance was best accomplished when there was only one opinion on the table. The possibility of a consultant raising additional ethical considerations was believed to unnecessarily complicate decision-making, contribute to conflict avoidance, and trigger a response of protective exclusion of outsiders from the clinical environment. Additionally, team members can be perceived as "breaking ranks" when initiating an ethics consult in response to conflicting values. Retention of power and authority is a predictable by-product of hierarchical organizational structures, erecting attitudinal barriers against ethics consultation.

By way of contrast, consider the insightful perspectives regarding improving complex decision-making and performance in health care put forth by Gawande (2009). In his view, when confronted by complex, nonroutine problems, "you push the power of decision making out to the periphery and away from the center" (p. 73). The challenge of establishing a tradition of open and effective communication among a team of professionals in any given setting is a necessary step in reducing procedural errors and improving organizational efficiency once complex tasks have been codified in checklists (to ensure consistent, thorough, stepwise performance). Gawande's critique of the health care arena focuses upon changing the hierarchical leadership structure of health institutions to foster team-integrated problem-solving, as has occurred successfully in other professions.

Knowledge of interpersonal and organizational dynamics in the health care environment prepares the ethics consultation team to adaptively deflect peripheral process issues and model decentralized communication while focusing upon the central ethical theme(s) of the consult. A situation-relevant, value-added approach on the part of ethics consultation teams can effectively reduce barriers to consultation service utilization. Broadly considered, the fundamental value of collaborative ethics committee consultations is realized within the social dynamic of an interdisciplinary health care treatment team—experienced colleagues bringing an applied ethics perspective to assist the treatment team in difficult clinical decisions or situations. A hallmark of well-functioning health care organizations is the seamless integration of ethics consultation and general ethics education into daily operation—consonant with the collaboration-based practice of psychology in the health care environment.

A functionally healthy ethics committee's activities permeate organizational cultures, providing relevancy when addressing practice competence. Consider the critical issue of medical errors, first brought center stage by an Institute of Medicine study Corrigan Kohn & Donaldson, (1999). Kaldjian et al. (2007) found that a substantial gulf existed between providers' opinions about disclosing errors in hypothetical case scenarios (93–97% faculty/trainee support disclosure of major and minor errors to patients/families) versus actual error disclosure (5–41% disclosure of major and minor errors). Interestingly, experience with malpractice litigation was unrelated to either hypothetical or actual error disclosure. One potential explanation for this finding may be institutional culture. An institutional climate of defensively blaming culpable HCPs for practice errors can create a potential cadre of dysfunctional "second victims" (Wu, 2000), in addition to any patient harmed. Indeed, when circumstances dictate, shared responsibility for errors is a concept worthy of consideration. An adaptive role for psychologists in assigning responsibility for error identification and disclosure is highlighted in a paper by Buetow and Elwyn (2006). These authors argue an intriguing position—that personal moral responsibility for errors on the part of patients, through inadvertent nonadherence or forgetfulness (being a fallible human being), should be supported. Reflexively blaming the health care system and its staff members for errors related to patient behaviors can deprive individuals of personhood within their social context. Thus, personal responsibility facilitates the opportunity for HCPs and patients to partner in a process of resolution to reduce errors. In a complementary manner, psychologists, armed with sophisticated communication skills, can operationalize such adaptive and corrective partnerships per incident in the clinical practice setting and, more broadly, in error prevention via participant action research methods.

The commonalities among the issues discussed above lie in adhering to the tenets of patient-centered care, in which values relevant to the person served hold sway when problems with or disagreements about health service delivery occur. Health care practice settings reflect parallel social dynamics—interplay among health care team members and the focused interaction of the team with the person served. When difficult decisions must be made, psychologists can fulfill the valued role of mediator, offering measured balance astride the precarious line between provider and advocate.

Technology Issues

Technological advances in health care over the past century have increased the efficiency and effectiveness of diagnosis and treatment, as well as opened new arenas of theoretical and applied investigation. Indeed, a new area of ethics—neuroethics—has developed in response to the need for establishing ethical guidelines to keep abreast of the rapid pace of scientific discovery and technological applications. Technology has almost become synonymous with quality health care in the United States. It is often employed because of its perceived inherent value. However, it is the involvement of the patient in technology utilization decisions that can temper ill-considered enthusiasm. This point is emphasized in Rizzieri et al.'s (2008) study of left ventricular assist devices (LVAD). The authors discuss the ethical and biopsychosocial implications of U.S. Food and Drug Administration (FDA) approval of the LVAD as a destination device, as opposed to a bridging strategy employed while awaiting heart transplantation (an admittedly scarce resource). This strategic decision has created significant quality-of-life problems (chronic infections, neurologic complications, device malfunction, financial burden, emotional problems, and social restrictions) for some patients being implanted with such devices and for their families. The authors argue for multidisciplinary team intervention that involves both the patient and family in detailed informed consent and counseling, including topics like end-of-life trajectories and timing of device deactivation.

Similar ethical risks exist in mental health. In one study, patients and HCPs who were presented with a predictive scenario of using functional magnetic resonance imaging (fMRI) in diagnosing major affective disorder (MDD) responded differently to its perceived benefit (Illes, Lombera, Rosenberg, & Arnow, 2008). Patients focused upon the generalized acceptance of the technology. Those positively disposed toward the technology believed that such information would be beneficial (increased knowledge of MDD biology and better family understanding of the condition—social acceptance). Patients negatively disposed toward the technology had correspondingly lower expectations of benefit regarding outcome. The relatively uniform attitudes of HCPs toward the use of fMRI focused on improved patient adherence with medication treatment. Patients, on the other hand, were evenly distributed across consideration of different treatment options (medications and psychotherapy). The implications of this study suggest caution regarding HCP assumptions that universal benefit accrues simply from expanding knowledge of physiological functions underlying health conditions via a specific technology. The psychosocial consequences of providing such information to patients and families require further inquiry.

Another emerging area of interest, based upon the tacit assumption that technology is socially desirable, surrounds human genome sequencing and its psychosocial implications for genetic counseling (Pina-Neto, 2008; Rantanen et al., 2008; Shostak & Ottman, 2006). No matter the level of involvement of psychologists in this process (e.g., genetics clinic team member, genetics counselor, researcher, treating professional in the community), predictive knowledge of genetic risks is a complex and emotionally laden area of concern for any individual recipient. The literature reflects the field of genetic counseling racing headlong to catch up with technological advances in human genome sequencing, as illustrated in the development of internationally recognized practice guidelines (see Bazell, 2010). The development of international guidelines is even more important now that individuals can purchase some form of individualized genetic risk profile. In addition, over 1,000 single-gene tests already exist (Scully, 2008). While the totality of genetic information will ultimately include advantageous genetic traits, the potential for conflict among beneficence, nonmaleficence, and social justice in the near term is apparent as human genome sequencing businesses are available within free market economies to identify pathological risks. In addition, the goals of specific genetics research are not necessarily congruent with the goals of those advocating for its scientific progression (Scully, 2008).

Research to date has generally focused upon funding agency-prioritized genetic disease entities, necessarily skewing the available information toward pathology. Offering sequencing data in the form of illness risk profiles to anyone with the funds to pay for such information, without adequately accounting for the emotional risks attendant to access to such information, invites contentious, justified social criticism. Scully discusses this criticism in detail, as well as support for the use of genetics knowledge, which comes from the disability movement.

As research progresses, the breadth and accuracy of genetic predictions will increase along with availability (as prices decline with higher volume utilization). Likewise, the influential nature of this probabilistic information will increase for those with access (for example, "designer" offspring). The issue of social injustice inherent in unbalanced economic access to genetic sequencing information aside, when does intimate individualized genetic information about which we have traditionally been ignorant become a burden, as opposed to simply an unknown? Will genetic probabilities regarding different physical conditions traditionally related to disability lead to discrimination in family planning?

What is lost in these discussions is that genetic markers do not define most disabilities, and happiness is not defined by the absence of disability. As Scully asks, "What constitutes the disadvantage of a disability?" Our species has never before been confronted with these conundrums. Given individual access to personal, detailed genetic information, implications for the conduct of daily life activities, life planning, decisions regarding procreation, etc. are profound and demand careful consideration. Leaving such values-laden issues open to the purely economic forces of the free market to determine post-hoc ethical benefits versus burdens borders upon capriciousness. Scully strongly advocates representation by people with disabilities on ethics and policy panels and more accurate communication with the public regarding the often ambiguous links between genes and disabilities, which are commonly shaped as much by sociocultural considerations as they are by genetic considerations.

The issues raised in the genetics debate, such as socioeconomically defined value, can also be seen in the use of other technology. We have witnessed the increasing use of internet-based communications in the field of tele-health for several decades (e.g., Glueckauf, 2007; Lustria, Cortese, Noar, & Glueckauf, 2009; Pickett et al., 2007). Internet-based telecommunication technology has allowed individuals with physical disabilities in rural communities access to health maintenance and treatment services via direct (often patient-to-HCP) contact. However, our final topic for consideration in this section reflects the continuing evolution of the internet as a social-interactive medium (e.g., gaming, social networks, simulated worlds, etc.).

Hoffman et al. (2000) exemplify the focused therapeutic use of virtual world technology. These authors have designed and demonstrated the efficacy of a virtual world immersion protocol that facilitates cognitive-behavioral pain management in adolescents with burn injuries. However, on a broader scale, we wish to consider the ethical implications of distance communication as a substitute for face-to-face interaction. Gorini et al. (2008) pose psychological, social, and ethical challenges regarding this burgeoning facet of social behavior. The authors describe potential ethical risks regarding venturing into cyberspace with the intention of creating therapeutic initiatives: the social challenges created by substituting cyberspace-based relationships for face-to-face interaction; that fact that anonymity offers more potential freedom of expression, but that the credibility and intentions of the interactive parties remain uncertain, and personal protection codes are likely required to ensure privacy; and psychotherapists needing to become facile with alternative forms of treatment. For example, different and variable sets of system-specific operating rules apply in virtual treatment but existing standards of care are based solely upon traditional health care service models. These synthetic environments will require creation of a whole new set of operational professional standards. As artificial intelligence engines become more sophisticated, virtual world characters could potentially function as autonomous beings, dramatically changing the rules of social engagement. The willingness of the technologically sophisticated members of varied societies to not only accept, but crave constant new developments in electronic social networking and internet applications demands that we consider possible ethical implications of this social evolution. Acknowledging this social trend toward

regular interaction within a virtual world(s), the challenge has been put forth to explore an ethically sound operational platform from which psychologists could engage, evaluate, and treat individuals by means of virtual world technology.

Surrogate Decision-Making

The complex issue of surrogate/proxy decision-making extends beyond the senior population. Psychologists in acute health care settings routinely work with surrogate decision-makers, given that many serious illnesses and injuries and/or their early treatments can result in delirium and accompanying waxing and waning cognition. Since the adoption of the advance directive as a legally supported concept in the United States in the 1990s and its promulgation within the health care system (the Patient Self-Determination Act), the traditional dyad of HCP and patient as decision-makers has been expanded to include the surrogate. The gold standard of surrogate decision-making is *substituted judgment*—the surrogate's role is to accurately reflect the preferences of the incapacitated party, as that person would have decided when capacitated (Beauchamp & Childress, 2009). The alternative, *patient best interests*, is fraught with risk of provider paternalism, family conflict, and issues related to litigation. However, the deliberative process for substituted judgment requires detailed communication about health care preferences between the patient and delegated surrogate prior to an incapacitating illness or injury—a process that rarely occurs in actuality. In addition, even when patients and families or other surrogates communicate, the surrogate still often ineffectively represents the patient's wishes. Ang and colleagues (2009) remind us that surrogates (in the absence of carefully documented patient preferences) are often inaccurate in predicting patients' preferences even when capacitated (approximately 68% accuracy), and the reality of surrogates imposing their own values on decisions based on disagreeing with patient preferences biases decisions.

Berger, DeRenzo, and Schwartz (2008) detail the problems that arise when surrogates find themselves in a critical health care decisional role. Surrogates vary from substituted judgment when considerations extend beyond narrow medical and patient-centered factors, family dynamics add stress to the role, psychological processes intervene bias toward overtreatment in opposition to patient preferences, and surrogate values and needs differ from those of the patient. Schwab (2006) warns about the mistaken assumption that, outside relatively extreme conditions, people make good decisions. Indeed, the author states that people are inconsistent in making instrumentally rational decisions. He posits that decisions are significantly affected by the conditions under which they are made, including limited amounts of available information, unawareness of decisional criteria, time constraints, and inconsistent memory for relevant details pertinent to the decision. Surrogates will often revert to heuristics (intuition, short cuts, rules of thumb) when faced with emotionally laden situations in which decisions may impact life, death, or level of independence, thus abrogating their intended role and compromising substantive or effective respect for patient autonomy.

Reed, Mikels, and Simon (2008) offer a similar position with respect to aging research. When choice is excessive (too many alternatives to consider), the subjective quality of decisions may be impaired, satisfaction with decisions reduced, and motivation to choose sapped. One possible reason may be an enhanced sense of personal responsibility for poor outcomes. Additionally, preference for choice can decline with age, resulting in receipt of less information and more reliance on heuristics for decisions because these intuitive choices are perceived as more emotionally meaningful.

Reed and colleagues offer recommendations for HCPs facilitating the decision-making process. These include assisting the surrogate by presenting alternatives/consequences to help calibrate judgment; assisting patients in filling out advance directives that indicate what role the surrogate should play (binding, weighty but not binding, merely informative); being both inclusive and exclusive regarding who can participate in decisions; and attempting to elicit specific wishes when assisting patients. Time spent on the front end of such discussions will minimize later confusion and surrogate burden. Messinger-Rapport, Baum, and Smith (2009) advocate HCP discussions with patients regarding advance directives be spread out over multiple brief episodes. They also advise that patients should seek *durable power of attorney* as a legal instrument that is more versatile and broader in scope than power of attorney for health care.

When interacting with surrogates, Braun, Naik, and McCullough (2009) suggest explaining that the role often involves giving a report from the patient, de-emphasizing making a decision. However, when genuine decisions need to be made, the HCP's obligation is to remain engaged with the surrogate, proactively identifying relevant alternatives, negotiating

treatment goals, and attempting to evaluate the surrogate's sense of burden. Ang et al. (2009) advocate use of a "Ulysses Contract" in the presence of mental health conditions, or by extension, progressively debilitating neurological conditions—making a declaration of wishes during times of relative decisional clarity, in anticipation of future incapacity. Such statements are reversible, not legally binding, and not designed to protect autonomy, but can be reviewed to remind a patient of earlier stated preferences in light of current decisional factors.

The complexity of the decisional process under duress of serious health risk requires that the HCP's ethical focus be directed toward preserving effective autonomous choice by the patient (whether capacitated or not). HCPs presenting prognosis and viable treatment/nontreatment alternatives (and consequences for each), and supporting the patient and/or surrogate during the stressful process will facilitate goal achievement in this regard. HCPs are discerning, trained decision-makers with expertise and knowledge of health care research who provide a decisional rationale. Stepping away from this position of authority in order to honor a patient's wishes (which may modify or even reject professional opinion) requires courage and a firm ethical grounding reflective of our Western societal values surrounding respect for autonomy. HCPs modeling such a stance for surrogates can provide needed counsel for them under decisional duress.

Clinical Care Issues

In this section, we use the example of chronic pain service delivery to consider social bias impeding our moral obligation to beneficially treat persons in need. Failure to adequately treat pain is related to a variety of cultural, attitudinal, educational, political, religious, and logistical reasons. Although this example illustrates potential bias in decisions regarding a specific chronic health issue, social bias can affect other challenging subpopulations, such as individuals who smoke (Glantz, 2007) or who are obese (Schutte et al., 2007).

Brennan, Carr, and Cousins (2007) provide a compelling rationale supporting pain management as a fundamental human right. Inadequate pain treatment has major physiological, psychological, economic, and social ramifications for patients, families, and society. Undertreated pain can result in physiological effects, such as increased heart rate, systemic vascular resistance, and circulating catecholamines (increasing risk for myocardial infarction and stroke); in acute conditions, it elicits neural alterations (i.e., peripheral and central neuronal sensitization that evolve into chronic pain). Chronic pain also represents a functional decrease in itself, resulting in decreased mobility and strength, disturbed sleep, immune impairment, dependence on medication, and codependence with family members and other caregivers. The World Health Organization indicated that patients whose pain is undertreated are four times more likely to be depressed or anxious, and have decreased concentration and increased social isolation. Despite this evidence, the Emergency Medical Treatment and Labor Act (EMTALA) does not mandate chronic pain treatment (McGrew & Giordano, 2009).

Peppin (2009) terms the type of social attitudinal response often seen in chronic pain *marginalization*—to relegate to an unimportant or powerless position within a society or group. He states that cognitive changes are often reflexively considered a response to opioids, without carefully ruling out alternative explanations. Clinicians' fears of substance abuse, addiction, and concerns with regulatory oversight should not negatively bias treatment decisions, especially if the patient has a negative history for these outcomes. In fact, McGrew and Giordano (2009) decry their colleagues' failure to offer proper care. They cite acute treatment statistics indicating that 33–50% of all cases presenting to emergency rooms (ERs) include reports of chronic pain of severe intensity, which remains unrelieved in more than 30% of patients at discharge (Todd, Sloan, Chen, Eder, & Wamstad, 2002). Convention holds that most ERs are not equipped to provide chronic pain care, yet many uninsured and underinsured patients use emergency services as their primary care site. McGrew and Giordano also state that the Drug Enforcement Agency (DEA) has prosecuted less than one-tenth of 1% of licensed prescribers in the past 10 years for regulatory violations. The authors conclude by stating that failure to provide chronic pain management consultations to ERs constitutes an ethical violation (contravening beneficence and nonmaleficence).

Brennan and colleagues based their ethical assertions of a fundamental right to treatment upon four core ethical principles. *Beneficence* obligates HCPs to relieve pain and suffering, providing sufficient justification for pain management services. In addition, adequate pain management can contribute to enhanced quality of life (facilitates good). *Nonmaleficence* cautions the HCP not to abandon patients in chronic pain through inadequate treatment. *Autonomy* is contravened if the HCP fails to assess repeated requests for pain control, as severe pain can negatively affect one's capacity to exercise unfettered choice. *Justice* is involved secondary to massive resource discrepancies, with pain control problems arising from health disparities. A human right exists because there is a preexisting obligation on the part of the HCP to help alleviate the pain and suffering. Giordano and Schatman (2008) criticize the health care system for lack of uniformity in basic health care services based on clinical effectiveness (not just cost) of treatments for chronic pain. Along with this need, they state that the inclusion of the multidisciplinary treatment team approach within the biopsychosocial model of care should be resurrected, properly supported, and funded to meet individualized patient needs.

Research Issues

Ethical issues in research tend to cluster, with some exceptions, around the issues of populations at risk and informed consent. We will therefore present these issues in some detail. Enoch et al. (2009) call into question ethical formulations related to applied health research when they raise the following question regarding alcoholism treatment. Can benefits to society outweigh risks to individuals if treatment protocols call for inducing alcohol craving or providing alcohol to abstinent individuals seeking treatment? This question is put into sharper focus when we consider that current research typically limits use of alcohol challenges to non–treatment seeking people. Importantly, the recidivism literature reports only 20–30% of treatment-seeking people remain abstinent after 1 year. It appears that treatment-seeking individuals have a different clinical course than do non–treatment seekers, thus severely limiting generalization from current research to clinical application. A partial technical solution offered is to more finely discriminate the heterogeneous pool of non–treatment seeking people to find a subpopulation that overlaps with treatment-seekers.

Kim et al. (2005) present survey data regarding sham surgery (placebo-controlled groups) related to this kind of technical issue. Researchers were surveyed in response to recent false-positive research findings in patients with Parkinson disease for gene therapies. The majority of researchers surveyed favored the use of sham surgery control. However, potential participants were not surveyed regarding risks related to sham surgery. The proposed ethical solution was to inform participants that, should the procedure be deemed effective, they would be administered the treatment. This proposal does not adequately address informed consent regarding risks and therapeutic misconception (preservation of hope for a cure in the face of disconfirming information). Both sets of authors call for HCPs familiar with applied health care ethics to assist with crafting technical recommendations toward resolution.

This call for proactive application of ethical thinking to the research setting is echoed by Fischback and Fischback (2004) who, in the midst of the moratorium on human stem cell research, decried what they saw as a dangerous trend in the public debate surrounding the question of when life begins. They feared "offering religious opinions cloaked in the language and veneer of science (e.g., using systems theory to justify the belief that life begins at conception)" (p. 1369). These issues speak to the ongoing need for ethical direction regarding the specifics of evolving scientific methodology and overarching research policy in the context of prevailing social-political-religious values.

In an interesting twist on the issue of the validity of a storied ethical research concept, the validity of *clinical equipoise* (uncertainty about research outcome) is challenged in a paper by Fries and Krishnan (2004) describing the current state of science regarding randomized controlled drug studies. The authors reviewed abstracts accepted for the 2001 American Academy of Rheumatology meeting that reported randomized controlled trials (RCTs), acknowledged drug company sponsorship, and had clinical endpoints ($n = 45$). They then examined the proportion of studies that favored the registration or marketing of the sponsor's drug. All forty-five studies selected for presentation met these criteria, suggesting that simply citing sponsorship could have predicted the outcomes. They contend that clinical equipoise is routinely violated and should be considered an outmoded ethical concept in current drug research parlance. Researchers routinely employ *design bias*—extensive preliminary data are used to design studies with a high likelihood of positive outcomes. In place of equipoise, the authors propose the "principle of positive expected outcomes." They contend that by offering the potential participant ample information about known facts of the drug under investigation and applying the participant's personal values (including altruism and utility assignment) in the context of expected outcomes and risks, reasonable and sufficient autonomous informed consent should be expected.

Informed Consent

The issue of informed consent in research is a multifactorial challenge for the researcher, the participant, and governance bodies tasked with oversight of the research enterprise. Ethical requirements for sufficient understanding involve capacity to understand, voluntariness, disclosure, understanding (free choice and content), decision-making, and authorization. Participants need to be adequately, but not fully, informed to satisfy their own needs to participate (Beauchamp & Childress, 2009). Signing a release form without discussion of the above content does not constitute informed consent. Blackmer (2003) listed several unique ethical challenges that must be accounted for prior to and during the research consenting process with individuals with disabilities: decision-making capacity under conditions of variable cognitive function, communication limitations, potential participant overuse (limited numbers of participants in a given setting), timing of recruitment (different phases of the recovery course introduce different biases), hope for a cure/therapeutic misconception biasing participation agreement, and the nature of the provider–participant relationship in the context of research. In an effort to be inclusive, informed consent documents have become a complex challenge for potential participants to understand research projects and participant roles, risks, and benefits.

Although the formal informed consent procedure as outline above may be a forthright process in the laboratory, extra- and intraindividual factors can impede consenting. Helgesson, Ludvigsson, and Gustafsson-Stolt (2005) raise an interesting conundrum regarding informed consent in a longitudinal study. What if some participants want less information than the consent specifies? Complex studies often overwhelm participants, lessening understanding of their role and increasing the chance of rejecting study participation. The authors reason that the study specifics required vary across individuals by virtue of varying needs among participants. Lack of understanding may be voluntary (choosing not to process all of the information provided) or involuntary (beyond comprehension). Helgesson and collaborators make a case for providing "relevant information" tailored to each participant during the consent process, thus boosting authenticity for the participant and enhancing the participant's trust in the researcher. Beskow and Dean (2008) also found in a survey study that declining participation in biorepository research was significantly related to mistrust of the researcher or the research process.

Knifed et al. (2008) report participant satisfaction with the consent process in neuro-oncology trials, although participants inaccurately understood and recalled risks associated with participation—a reiteration of therapeutic misconception. Individuals will minimize or dismiss risks in hopes of receiving a curative treatment, even if the purpose of the study does not address that issue (see related comments, Stenson et al., 2010). Of related interest, Hampson et al. (2006), in a survey study of participants in cancer research trials, found that a significant majority of patients were unconcerned about potential conflicts of interest created by researcher support from drug companies sponsoring the study. Further, participants believed that an unspecified oversight mechanism existed to offer protection. Again, we have participants involved in what are perceived as beneficial research experiments agreeing to tolerate potentially biasing researcher–sponsor relationships in service of a chance at a cure.

Keefe et al. (2008) cite a placebo pain study by Chung et al. (2007) as a model of presenting placebo as a treatment and not a deception during the consent process. Robinson, a co-author of the study, remarked in a personal communication (April 13, 2010), "Previous ethical objections were based on deception as being harmful, not for the good of the patient. We found that placebo is a well-characterized physiological and psychological phenomenon that is as potent as exogenous drugs." Keefe and colleagues state that presenting placebos in a straightforward manner to participants during consent emphasizes the role of positive expectations on clinical regulatory pain response. This open approach may also strengthen the trust relationship between the participant and researcher.

The complexities of ethical concerns in research require some rethinking of basic assumptions regarding technical aspects of study design, as well as the critical informed consent process. It may be time for HCPs well-versed in applied ethics to partner with the research community to proactively craft approaches to difficult scientific questions that combine solid methodology with ethical protections for participants representing diverse populations. The next section will focus upon those challenges to ethical thought and application.

Diversity Issues

We have come to think of diversity in the context of sensitivity and respect toward varied cultural/ethnic beliefs and values across multiple subpopulations accessing the health care system (e.g., Hanson & Kerkhoff, 2007; Hanson, Kerkhoff, & Bush, 2005). Yet, a broader consideration of diversity includes societal values influencing the components of service delivery within different health care systems around the world. Attempting to apply predominantly Western conceptions of historical ethical principles to Eastern cultures can result in a fundamental disconnect when it comes to conducting research and providing clinical service. For example, a study by Tekola et al. (2009) revealed that social stigma was a significant barrier to receiving treatment for podoconiosis (mossy foot) in Ethiopia. This condition had been traditionally considered untreatable, and even reflective of problematic family heritage. A Western focus on preserving patient autonomy was altered to accommodate family and community education and to secure approval of both groups prior to individuals being approached for consent to treat (see National Institutes of Health, 2008, Protecting Human Research Participants).

Bridging the gap in applied ethics between traditional or indigenous "ways of knowing" and scientific method is the subject of a paper by Cochran et al. (2008). Rather than considering traditional belief systems and values of indigenous Alaskans as antithetical to science, health researchers are urged to consider participant action research methods as a mechanism to incorporate traditional systems of belief into applied health care research. The rationale for such an approach spans the spectrum from practical (obtaining more willing and knowledgeable participants) to philosophical (standard methodologies may fail to match needs and customs of populations under study). The authors offer the concept of creating translational entities (e.g., Alaska Native Science Commission—ANSC) as a way of addressing this critical public health problem.

Westra, Willems, and Smit (2009) discuss religious-cultural barriers to clinical service provision in which the assumption of transcultural neutrality for the four core ethical principles is called into question. They cite the example of Islamic parents asked by nonreligious pediatricians to consent to end-of-life decisions for their children—often resulting in refusal. Islamic law forbids all actions that may harm life. Similarly, autonomy-based informed consent is rendered superfluous by the notion of respect for the patient's (or in this case, the parents') belief that Allah decides such matters. By way of resolution for potential impasses, the authors suggest extra time be provided for reflective decisions as the will of Allah or Nature runs its course. This strategy leaves room for hope within the defined limits of what the HCP can do. It is apparent that the Western frameworks for unnecessary suffering and quality of life do not necessarily translate across cultures.

Hedayat, Shooshtarizadeh, and Raza (2006) present another example of religious dictates shaping both clinical decision-making and access to the health care system. In Iran, ethical decision-making cannot be parsed out from religious doctrine, the driving mechanism of the social-governmental structure. Indeed, the broad view of Shiite Muslim thought regarding health care decision-making is one that differs significantly from Western respect for autonomy. It is not based upon the rights of the individual, but concentrates instead upon a homogenous community-based mindset in which the individual is but a subset of the larger community, which is, in turn, bound by religiously prescribed life procedures.

In a very real sense, the varied health systems of the industrialized world reflect the social mores and values of those countries or socioeconomic conglomerates (e.g., European Union) in which they evolved, thus necessarily impacting application of ethical principles and concepts as construed by Western philosophical tradition. The validity of applied ethical principles is challenged by conflict with social and spiritual values and belief systems reflected in the constructs of varied health systems in which individuals living their everyday lives. Table 24.1 summarizes recent studies challenging the application of traditional ethical principles and concepts to dynamic problems nested within specific social situations and health care systems across different societies.

Petrova, Dale, and Fulford (2006) posit a values-based practice model that critiques the current application of ethics in a rigid, legalistic manner, as well as the narrow algorithm-based application of evidence-based health care practice. Strict adherence to core ethical principles has resulted in the development of rules, regulations, and codes of practice in health care (which the authors consider legalistic). The authors argue that the mainstream ethics approach is too limited. For example, autonomy—strongly cherished by Western cultures—does not have a comparable priority in more collectivist societies. The same goes for beneficence and nonmaleficence—what is considered good in one culture may be unacceptable or harmful in another.

Patient-centered care is the foundation of values-based practice, an approach that focuses upon the individual's values within the broader environmental context, including the values of HCPs, caregivers and family, health care organizations, society, values embedded in research, and within health care delivery systems and policy. Petrova et al. criticize some aspects of evidence-based practice. They cite its limited usefulness for the unique, individual patient, and its overly narrow definition of acceptable evidence. The alternative evidentiary model offered includes integrating the best research evidence, clinical expertise, and patient values. Types of evidence include quantitative-personal, quantitative-general, qualitative-personal, and qualitative-general. When evidence clashes with a person's values, their approach suggests that the HCP focus upon bringing the two conflicting sets of values closer together, thus increasing personal relevance for the individual making a health decision.

Professional Competency

Given the significant momentum around operationalizing practice competence in the United States, in this section we will first review some of this literature and then discuss its intersection with an increasingly global society that necessitates cross-cultural competence.

As the psychology profession has expanded its scope of practice and as expectations of accountability for one's products and services has become embedded in the U.S. social fabric, an evolutionary process has been under way to define professional practice competence. Significant historical work laid the foundation for the contemporary focus on competency-based approaches to education and training. The Boulder Conference was a historic event in which was born the scientist-practitioner framework for the professional practice of psychology in the United States. It was not until 34 years later, however, that a policy statement articulating the scientist-practitioner model was published (Belar & Perry, 1992). As a significant precursor to the competence movement, this policy statement highlighted the interlocking nature of core training components, such as assessment and intervention, and emphasized that the professional development of knowledge, skills, and attitudes facilitates the scientific approach to practice.

The evolution away from content-based assessment and toward assessment of outcomes based on competence has taken significant shape in the last two decades (see, for example, Sumerall et al., 2000). The National Council of Schools and Programs of Professional Psychology (NCSPP) identified six

Table 24.1 Diversity in ethical challenges across health care systems

Year Published	Author(s)	Ethical Issues	Health Care System
2009	Nilsson & Pilhammar	Clinical decision-making	Sweden
2008	Cochran et al. Dunn, Clare, & Holland Halpern, Halpern, & Doherty Humayun et al. Li et al. Murphy Pina-Neto Plu et al. Rydvall & Lynde Valdez et al.	Indigenous peoples Surrogate decision-making Torture vs. interrogation Patient perception vs. actual informed consent Disclosure and HIV Family involvement in health care decisions Genetic counseling models, legal discrimination Informed consent in health care networks Withholding and withdrawing treatment Analysis of HCP values	Canada England/Wales United States India China Australia China France Sweden Mexico
2007	Li et al. Maden Mamhidir et al. Roberts et al. Song et al. Tillyard	Mandatory HIV testing Mental Capacity Act of 2005, rationale Elder care and high-level decision-makers Rural health care in New Mexico, Alaska End-of-life, homeless Mental Capacity Act, Advance Directives in U.S. vs. LPA in UK	China England/Wales Sweden United States United States England/Wales
2006	Kostopolou & Katsouyanni Secker et al. Ziebland et al.	Truth-telling in health care Regionalizing rehabilitation services Assisted suicide, euthanasia	Greece Canada European Union
2005	Breslin et al. Dodds Eastman & Starling Fiscella & Franks Giordano Grill & Hansson Liegeois & Van Audenhove	Public views re: Top Ten Ethical Challenges Gender, aging injustice in health care, a feminist view Mental Capacity Act, confidentiality Social-ethnic disparities in health care Use of cadavers in health education Paternalism re: health care risks, right to know Community mental health	Canada Australia England/Wales United States England/Wales England/Wales European Union

core competencies (e.g., relationship, assessment, intervention, research and evaluation, consultation and education, and management and supervision) that integrate science and practice, and that reflect the shift in thinking about psychology education (Peterson, Peterson, Abrams, & Stricker, 1997). The council stated that "evolving curricula...combine practical and scientific knowledge with professional skills and attitudes to produce the outcome goal of a particular competency...The competencies develop together and often remain inextricably intertwined" (p. 380). These concepts would be echoed again in the last decade, during which competencies became more clearly defined.

The 2002 Association of Psychology Postdoctoral and Internship Centers (APPIC) Competencies Conference represented a pivotal contribution to the early paradigm shift. The purpose of the Competencies Conference was not only to characterize competency domains, training, and assessment, but to do so by bringing broad psychology constituencies together. By fostering this broad collaboration, psychology training could be defined in a less fragmented manner, ultimately resulting in better service to and protection of the public, consistent with sound ethical practice. Although hosted in the United States by APPIC, the conference was unique in that it included delegates from Canada,

Mexico, and the United States and was co-sponsored by a variety of organizations, such as the Canadian Council of Professional Psychology Programs, the National Latino Psychological Association, and multiple APA divisions. Kaslow et al. (2004) provide a description of the conference process, the outcome of which was the identification of several themes: competencies include knowledge, skills, and attitudes; cross-cutting competencies (e.g., ethical practice and cultural diversity) exist across developmental levels; educational processes should be developmentally appropriate and reflect the scientist-practitioner model, including evidence-based practice; a respectful, facilitative learning environment in which effective mentoring can occur is critical and can also facilitate lifelong learning; "matching assessment strategies to training goals is essential" (p. 707); assessment should involve multiple approaches and be sensitive to diversity; and evaluating assessment methods is critical before they become core components of credential preparation (e.g., licensure).

The conference provided a framework to move forward to more clearly delineate competency subcomponents. *Competence* was defined as the person's overall ability (i.e., the person is qualified and capable), whereas *competencies* represented the components comprising competence. To characterize the competencies, the cube model was proposed, including *foundational competencies* (i.e., core knowledge, skills, and attitudes that lay the groundwork for functional competencies) and *functional competencies* (i.e., knowledge, skills, and values critical to action—to what psychologists do—including specialty work in which psychologists engage). The model was conceptualized as three-dimensional, with the first axis representing the foundational competencies (e.g., self-assessment, ethical and legal standards), the second axis representing functional competencies (e.g., diagnosis, intervention, consultation), and the third axis representing professional developmental stages (e.g., doctoral student, internship, postdoctoral supervision). The cube components were envisioned as interconnected rather than mutually exclusive. Any changes in external contingencies and scope of practice would first be represented in foundational domains, which would then impact functional competencies, such as new skill acquisition. Rodolfa and colleagues (2005) discuss three domain levels—competencies relevant to all psychologists, to narrower practice areas (e.g., clinical psychology), and to specialty focus (e.g., rehabilitation psychology, health psychology). However,

foundational and functional competencies were not meant to change to specializations under the application of the cube model. Instead, changes are seen in the settings, populations, professional orientation, and challenges faced within the specific context of practice.

The cube model was a significant step forward in the shifting psychology paradigm from a curricular focus toward a competency-based conceptualization of education and training. This work was further extended in 2006, when the Assessment of Competency Benchmark Work Group was organized (APA, 2007). This work group developed benchmarks (i.e., performance measures) for the 12 competency areas identified in the cube model using a developmental framework. The group defined four developmental levels: readiness for practicum, internship, entry level practice, and advanced training. The outcome was the refinement of the competence domains, the creation of behavioral anchors associated with the essential components of each competency area at each developmental level, and recommended assessment methods. For example, one behavioral anchor for knowledge about ethical and legal standards at the practicum level was understanding ethical decision-making models; at the internship level, an example was being able to discuss the "ethical implications of professional work" (p. 25), and at the entry level, it was being aware of the need to confront colleagues about ethical violations.

The work group's efforts served as a springboard for the subsequent creation of a competency assessment toolkit that describes specific methods for assessing the acquisition of competence (Kaslow et al., 2009). The toolkit offers a critique of specific assessment methods (e.g., case presentations, consumer surveys, professional reviews, exams) and a discussion of the relevance of these tools in assessing each competency domain at different developmental levels. A driving point is that competency assessment must be multimodal across time, in order to maximize its validity. In addition, determining which methods match best with each competency area and developing subsequent national standardization and training on the use of tools are critical future steps. Otherwise, assessment of competence cannot be done in a systematic, reliable, and valid manner on a large scale.

To further advance the competency movement, Kenkel (2009) argues four points: that the competency model of education requires the endorsement of organizations involved in psychology training;

that when competencies are achieved, and who teaches and assesses these, must be clarified; that assessment tools must be available; and that organizational and cultural support is important for implementing a competency-based model of psychology training. Endorsement of competence-based models for education and training is becoming a reality in the United States. The American Board of Professional Psychology specialty boards are in the process of aligning their advanced training requirements within the competence domains. For example, Hibbard and Cox (2010) have delineated the application of foundational and functional competencies to rehabilitation psychology. They provide a comprehensive list of core topics within each competency domain, such a sexual functioning and pain assessment under the assessment domain, and cognitive retraining and group therapy for disability adjustment under the intervention domain. Clinical health psychology has also been actively adapting the competence framework for multiple levels of training (France et al., 2008; Kerns, Berry, Frantsve, & Linton, 2009; Masters, France, & Thorn, 2009). However, as Kenkel (2009) notes, acceptance of the model must occur at multiple levels, and even with that acceptance, buy-in is not enough. If we do not have appropriate evaluative systems to determine who is minimally competent in what areas and at which point in time, and if we cannot evaluate and educate trainees in a cost-effective manner over a reasonable period of time, the competency movement will fall far short of its aspirations. Masters et al. (2009) try to address at least one of these concerns by offering advice regarding competency engagement in financially constrained programs (e.g., use of adjuncts; internship selection to address weaknesses).

Donovan and Ponce (2009) highlight other challenges, including the need to broaden the model's focus to reflect our multicultural societies and to give serious consideration to the sociocultural point of view reflected in the competencies. The first point is influenced by at least two factors: the U.S. population is clearly shifting to a broader multiethnic society, and technology has expanded our capacity to reach across the world through travel, relocation, and the internet. Therefore, consumers are more diverse and psychologists' skill sets must incorporate a multicultural perspective. Although the APA has established multicultural guidelines that include education and training, Forrest (2010) has eloquently raised concerns about the U.S. focus upon competencies' development, highlighting the lack of participation by scholars from outside the United States and the lack of evaluation of competency efforts in other countries. This is problematic if history holds and the competencies design is exported from the United States to other nations because its application may be ill-matched. Conversely, critical competence components or measures may have been overlooked because of this narrow view. Forrest argues that unintentional harm could occur if U.S. standards and values unduly influence competencies established in other countries. How relevant are professional standards promulgated in the United States to practice standards in other countries? Arnett (2008) has highlighted this problem in psychological research: research is largely published on U.S. samples who represent only 5% of the world's population, thus neglecting 95% of the world when drawing conclusions.

Part of the issue is whether we view competence standards applied to U.S. psychologists as relevant to psychology in other parts of the world and vice versa. Although intuitively we might want to answer with certainty, the data do not exist with which to make an affirmative claim regarding the utility of the competencies across borders, particularly considering the variability with which psychology is defined and regulated in different countries (Forrest, 2010). Even within the United States, once psychologists are in practice, requirements for licensure have historically varied across states, and continuing professional education requirements related to lifelong learning differ by more than 20 credit hours biannually depending upon where one practices.

That said, there are significant advantages to shared competency standards, including increased mobility for psychologists, both within the United States and abroad, and increased consumer confidence in the quality of services delivered. Forrest (2010) views this lack of common standards as an issue of social justice. If some psychologists can practice across borders and other cannot, both the psychologist and consumer are constrained, despite increasingly mobile lifestyles. Although we do not know if the specific competency standards will work cross-culturally (a point to which we return later), we do know that practice standards embedded in psychology training, such as adherence to the APA Ethics Code, are relevant. At the 2008 APA Leadership Conference on Internationalizing Psychology Education, Shullman summarized statistics revealing that over 8,000 international students were studying in the United States in 2006 and that 10% of the Ph.D. degrees in psychology awarded in the United States were to non-U.S. citizens. Forrest similarly indicated that over 3,000 APA members live outside the United States. Regardless of one's position on competence, the fact is undeniable that psychology is operating in a global environment, and existing U.S. education and training models are being exported and adapted for application in other countries, regardless of the ease with which this adaptation has occurred in a specific cultural context.

To be truly mobile, however, one must be multicultural. As Belar (2009) has stated, we must ensure culturally competent training. The 2002 APA Ethics Code clearly added emphasis in this regard when the 1992 Code was amended. This evolution of thought on being culturally competent is reflected in the foundational competency domain of individual–cultural development, as well as in the behavioral anchors proposed for multiple other foundational competencies. Examples include respecting others' cultures (interpersonal relationships domain), tolerating uncertainty (affective skills), articulating beliefs toward diverse others (reflective practice), and monitoring one's own cultural identity (self-awareness). However, Marsella et. al. (2008), like Forrest, reminds us that U.S. psychology has its own cultural context; in essence, it represents a cultural product. Therefore, the competencies reflect a Western viewpoint (e.g., linear, individualistic). Cross-border competencies would require us to work at the macro level as a "globally focused learning partner" in order to develop psychology education and training policy (Shullman et. al. 2008).

So, what progress has been made? Clearly, significant efforts have been made by the APA to support more culturally sensitive guidelines that intersect with competence both in terms of recognition of diversity and multiculturalism. The changes to the 2002 APA Ethics Code, the 2002 Multicultural Guidelines, and the 2008 Executive Leadership Conference referenced earlier represent a few such efforts. The Division of International Psychology (Division 52) has also grown and undertaken educational efforts regarding the international scope of practice. Similarly, the APA established the Office of Ethnic Minority Affairs and more recently the Office of International Affairs, and the Board of Educational Affairs established a task force on international quality assurance (QA) in 2007. It was charged with surveying current QA systems around the globe and making recommendations regarding the APA's role in international QA procedure,

policy, and program development and implementation. This was, in part, a response to the fragmented approach being used to address mobility inquiries by individuals, agencies, and other governments. This task force received QA information about other countries from an ad hoc international advisory group with members from 16 countries. The task force recommendations were as important for what the APA should not do as for what it should do. The task force clearly stated that the APA should not be an international accreditor of programs. Instead, it should exchange information and collaborate on shared QA goals and policy development that facilitate review of psychology credentials. The APA should also self-evaluate its international efforts based on knowledge acquired from collaborating with other countries. Shullman describes a framework for consideration of a cross-border QA program that includes core values (e.g., inclusion, respect), operating principles (e.g., opportunities for mutual learning, integrating diverse cultural contexts, promoting local development), and roles/actions (the APA will learn from QA examples elsewhere, and work as a learning partner to develop international policy for psychology education and training).

To make real progress on mobility, the discipline as a whole must address international standards for education and training, including competencies, or continue to advance reciprocity recognition. As Cole (2006) suggests, we are more culturally conditioned than we might appreciate in our interpretations of psychological processes and outcomes. In competence, we should take a page out of the QA meeting and the International Union of Psychological Sciences, which has developed an international network of contributors committed to advancing research (Cole, 2006). We need to be humble, yet engaged. The challenges are great, but our ability to create culturally relevant competency standards partly hinges on our ability to reach beyond borders. We need to continue the dialog by understanding how other societies define and assess competence. The 2002 Competencies Conference began this work, but much remains to be done. We must cast a broader net.

Consider the work of the British Psychological Society in the United Kingdom, the European Union, and Canada. The United Kingdom has been engaged in debate around the concept of competence, similarly to the debate seen in the United States. Until 2002, the British Psychological Society used a model of education that focused on the acquisition of experience, at which point the focus shifted to learning outcomes. Beinart, Llewelyn, and Kennedy (2009) summarize these outcomes and list the specific competencies now used in the United Kingdom. As in the United States, the authors conceptualize competence as the integration of knowledge, skills, and attitudes (as well as diligence) and competencies as its components. They also offer perspective on the evolution of competency-based approaches, which they view as more aspirational, and that thus emphasize its developmental nature. While similar to the United States in many respects, they highlight the collaborative nature of clinical psychology's work, discuss the importance of meta-knowledge (what you do and do not know, a component of which is self-awareness), and suggest that, like competence, capability (i.e., the ability to apply skills to new challenges and to adapt and learn over time) requires assessment. Similar to the United States, they struggle with the current lack of understanding about which educational components facilitate competence and how to assess these. This work suggests much overlap and opportunity for collaborative thought among potential Western partners.

The European Union has created the European Certificate in Psychology (known as the EuroPsy) (Batram 2008) to allow mobility of psychologists. The creation of the EuroPsy was based on the belief that consumers should be able to access psychological services anywhere in the European Union, and that a common certificate informs the public that a psychologist has gained appropriate competencies and is committed to ethical standards of practice. The EuroPsy defines competence as the "ability to adequately fulfill a professional role" and includes the primary competence (mastering content) and enabling competence (rendering services effectively). The specific competencies defining these two categories are presented in Table 24.2. Similar to the cube model, the EuroPsy model includes knowledge, skills, and attitudes as critical components and conceptualizes competence as context-specific. Although a developmental framework is also presented for conceptualizing the acquisition of competence, its assessment structure places more emphasis on whether supervision is required to perform a task competently (i.e., level 1—basic knowledge/skill, but not sufficiently competent; level 2—competent under supervision; level 3—competent on basic tasks without supervision; level 4—competent in complex situations without guidance). This aligns very loosely with

Table 24.2 Psychology competencies reflected in regional mobility agreements

Mutual Recognition Agreement (Canada)	EuroPsy (European Union)
Core Competencies	**Primary Competencies**
Interpersonal relationships	Goal specification
Assessment and evaluation	Assessment
Interpersonal relationships	Development
Intervention and consultation	Intervention
Research	Evaluation
Ethics and standards	Communication
General knowledge (not a specific core competency)	**Enabling Competencies**
	Professional strategy
	Continuing professional Development
	Professional relations
	Research and development
	Marketing and sales
	Account management
	Practice management
	Quality assurance
	Self-reflection

the developmental levels used by the Benchmark Work Group (i.e., readiness for practicum, internship, etc.). However, the timeframes do not directly correspond to internships (potentially earlier in European training) or completion of the degree. Another difference is that the EuroPsy includes levels of skill (individual, group, organizational, situational), not just types of skills.

A second major effort to increase psychologists' mobility has been realized in the establishment of the Mutual Recognition Agreement of the Regulatory Bodies for Professional Psychologists in Canada. This agreement again identifies core competencies, including specific knowledge and skills, that Canadian psychologists must demonstrate to move from one province or territory to another and continue to practice. The core competencies are noted in Table 24.2.

These efforts recognize that mobility across borders requires that a psychologist clearly demonstrate his or her competence. What a rich opportunity we have to continue the dialog on competence by engaging our global partners! Shullman (2008) commented that, despite the variability in psychology education around the world, we all share the following beliefs: psychology should be recognized as an independent profession, the discipline needs to be flexible and mobile, and we must ensure competent services.

The Universal Declaration of Ethical Principles for Psychologists may also provide some guidance regarding a more global approach to competence development. The declaration, adopted by both the Assembly of the International Union of Psychological Science and the Board of Directors of the International Association of Applied Psychology (2008), established four ethical principles as a moral framework to guide the worldwide psychology community. These principles include *respect* for the dignity of persons and peoples, *competent caring* for the well-being of persons and peoples, *integrity*, and *professional and scientific responsibilities* to society. The document was meant to serve as a framework for developing and evaluating the relevance of ethics codes, for encouraging global thinking that remains "sensitive and responsive to local needs and values" (p. 1), and for presenting one unified voice when ethical concerns arise.

Similar to the Universal Declaration of Ethical Principles for Psychologists, we believe there are universal ideals and principles that can "speak with a collective voice" (p. 1) regarding competence. Fundamental to the principle of competent caring is the "application of knowledge and skills that are appropriate for the nature of the situation as well as the social and cultural context" (p. 2). For example, competence in one culture may support comprehensive disclosure of information, whereas in another culture it does not. One culture may support working primarily with the patient; another demands work with the family or elders. Therefore, in order to make a declaration of competence salient, such a declaration would not define specific structures or formats for education, similar to the principle used in the creation of the EuroPsy. Instead, a universal declaration of competence would serve to establish common core competencies (e.g., assessment, intervention, self-reflection, commitment to professional development), frame psychologists'

responsibilities, and delineate the values associated with those professional responsibilities that ensure competence. Pettifor and Sawchuk (2006) found that competence was the third most highly rated troubling ethical area among psychologists representing nine countries. This would suggest that there is common ground upon which to build such a declaration. Like ethical behavior, competence requires an integration of components—"a collective whole." Although one can learn individual skills (e.g., administering a test), to be a competent psychologist requires the integration of knowledge, skills, beliefs, and values. We believe there are several universal principles upon which competence can be shaped across borders:

• Competence is critical to the safety and welfare of consumers.
• Competence is an ongoing professional commitment; what is competent practice today is not necessarily competent practice tomorrow.
• All psychologists have competence limits.
• Self-awareness is important but not sufficient to judge one's competence.
• Competence is viewed through a sociocultural lens that requires ongoing environmental adjustment and adaptation for each individual's circumstance.
• Ethical behavior underpins competent practice.

In addition, one of the best competence practices one can undertake is to seek collegial input and support to evaluate competence concerns. The internet allows us the opportunity to rethink our access to colleagues, who can literally live across the world.

This brings us back to a fundamental issue with the competency movement. Are we, in the United States, limited by the Western focus upon competence, thereby narrowing our cultural lens and ultimately our value as a discipline? Have we limited our view of what cultural sensitivity might or should be, given our increasingly global society? Global issues will continue to be a significant driver of the needs of psychology consumers—immigration, health disparities, environmental vulnerabilities, and the changing roles of families/status of women are just a few issues that will create shifts in service needs and thus impact the training needs of our students to become competent providers. Being competent to understand and respond to these needs will be critical to the relevance of psychology as a profession. As the Task Force on Quality Assurance learned, the APA needs to widen its lens, listen to our global partners, and enrich our competency efforts in a manner consistent with our evolution toward truly becoming culturally competent at all levels of our profession.

We are all enriched by understanding the values and practices of other cultures as we seek to expand our own worldview and understand what it means to be culturally competent. Sowmini and De Vries (2009) provide an example of how two different cultures (the Netherlands and Kerala in Southern India) that are trying to address dementia can promote better care by leaning from each other's practices despite vastly different care models and needs. It is also very important to note that understanding similarities and differences as we view other countries is not the only window on culture. Each person has interconnected cultural identities woven into the different facets of her or his life. A civilian psychologist practicing in the military is one example (see Reger, Etherage, Reger, & Gahm, 2008, for a discussion of cultural competence related to this issue). Multiculturalism is really about our ability to effectively serve our clients by considering their individual characteristics in an informed, self-reflective manner. Significant literature offers the reader insight into potential conflicts among training, practice, and ethical expectations regarding culture in American psychology and includes examples of how to improve cultural competence (Chen, Kakkad, & Balzano, 2008; Gallardo, Johnson, Parham, & Carter, 2009; Stuart, 2004; Sullivan, Harris, Collado, & Chen, 2006; Zhou & Siu, 2009).

Although the work to date has been a herculean undertaking, American psychology is early in its paradigm shift—we are really only at a point of taking baby steps along this competency path. Where we are reflects our developmental process, which began with what is familiar to us. Thus, a Western framework was set in motion. We have a growing awareness of the need to define, characterize, and evaluate competencies so that we can successfully instill these in the intellectual and emotional psyche of our students. The competency benchmark model represents a significant step forward in grappling with what it means to be a competent psychologist in America. However, the flexibility of a cube model is in its details. We would not expect the behavioral anchors and measures delineated by the work group to be the same in different cultural circumstances. For example, the relative value of customs and indigenous practices to assessment, intervention, and consultation, and the use of quantitative versus qualitative measures, would likely vary. If we can incorporate cross-cultural considerations and can partner to shape the shared components of competence, we will ultimately facilitate the mobility of psychologists in reaching consumers across the globe. The ultimate realization of this goal will occur when a set of universal principles of competence is created. Successfully delivering competent care across cultural boundaries will be the outcome metric. Cultural immersion will allow attainment of cross-cultural competence in the context of common ideals, values, and practices that uphold ethical and competent standards of care.

Conclusion

It is evident that the global health care enterprise, in all its iterations, continues to challenge the status quo regarding ethical issues. It is also clear that ethically grounded psychologists must play a proactive role in the professional arenas of clinical practice; and engage in active involvement in discovering the operational components of health care organizations, research, education, and training, and in creating culturally relevant competency models in partnership with colleagues across the world. The lightning pace of technological evolution demands proactive person-centered perspectives in developing applications. The cultural "melting pot" that characterized America in the past is becoming increasingly diverse, in new and exciting ways that challenge our traditional Western values and beliefs. Within the context of this rapidly changing—sometimes chaotic—socioculturally and economically interrelated world, the next chapter in the biopsychosocial development of psychology will be written.

Future Directions

In looking to the future of health and systems of health care, we see several important questions that have yet to be adequately addressed. First, what fundamental structural model(s) can be applied to Western philosophical-ethical traditions to broaden their applicability across varied cultures? A goal of this process could certainly be the creation of a values-sensitive method of unambiguous cross-cultural communication regarding provision of competent health care, international collaborative health care policy development, and health-related research.

Second, the pace of technological advances in health care seems to have moved ahead of biopsychosocial-ethical considerations regarding its impact upon consumers. We must ask the inevitable question regarding potential conflict of interest between business models of health care, and access to and benefits versus risks related to the application of health technology. Crafting ethical considerations into cost–benefit analyses of such technological advances prior to implementation may cast a different light upon health care resource allocation and expenditure.

Finally, we ask an important question regarding the preservation of personal autonomy on both sides of the health provision interface—the HCP and the person served. Movement toward algorithmic data-based decisions in clinical care provides a tempting lure of the perception of a "truth-added" benefit to the treatment recipient. However, if the cost of data-laden decision-making is truncated clinical judgment and inadequate consideration of the patient's personal values, what have we gained?

References

American Psychological Association (2002). Ethical principles of psychologists and code of conduct. *American Psychologist, 57*(12), 1060–1073.

Ang, A., Loke, P. C. W., Campbell, A. V., & Chong, S. A. (2009). Live or let die: Ethical issues in a psychiatric patient with end-stage renal disease. *Annals of Academic Medicine Singapore, 38*(4), 370–373.

Arnett, J. J. (2008). The neglected 95%. Why American psychology needs to become less American. *American Psychologist, 63*(7), 602–624. doi: 10.1037/0003-066x.63.7.602

Assessment of Competency Benchmarks Work Group. (2007). *A development model for the defining and measure competence in professional psychology*. Retrieved May 15, 2010, from http://wsm.ezsitedesigner.com/share/scrapbook/50/502062/Benchmark_Competencies_Document_-_Feb_2007.pdf

Bazell, R. (2010). Fears surround over-the-counter genetic tests. *The Washington Post*, accessed from http://www.msnbc.msn.com/id/37076766/ns/health_more_health-news/TwHe7TWXRZA 5/11/2010

Bartram, D., Bamberg, E., Bräuner, B., Georgas, J., Jern, S., Job, R., et al. (2008). *EuroPsy—The European certificate in psychology*. Retrieved from Italian Network Psychologists Association website http://www.inpa-europsy.it/nuovi.docum.2008/EuroPsy_english.pdf

Beauchamp, T. L., & Childress, J. F. (2009). *Principles of biomedical ethics* (6th ed.). New York: Oxford University Press.

Beinart, H., Llewelyn, S., & Kennedy, P. (2009). Competency approaches, ethics and partnership in clinical psychology. In H. Beinart, P. Kennedy, & S. Llewelyn (Eds.), *Clinical psychology in practice* (pp. 18–32). Leicester, UK: British Psychological Society.

Belar, C.D. (2009). Advancing the Culture of Competence. *Training and Education in Professional Psychology, 3*(4, Suppl) S63–S65.

Belar, C. D., & Perry, N. W. (1992). National conference on scientist-practitioner education and training for the professional practice of psychology. *American Psychologist, 47*(1), 71–75.

Berger, J. T., DeRenzo, E.G., & Schwartz, J. (2008). Surrogate decision making: Reconciling ethical theory and clinical practice. *Annals of Internal Medicine, 149*(1), 48–53.

Beskow, L. M., & Dean, E. (2008). Informed consent for biorepositories: Assessing prospective participants' understanding and opinions. *Cancer Epidemiological Biomarkers Preview, 17*(6), 1440–1451. doi: 10.1158/1055-9965.EPI-08-0086

Blackmer, J. (2003). The unique ethical challenges of conducting research in the rehabilitation medicine population. *BMC Medical Ethics, 4*, 2. doi: 10.1186/1472-6939-4-2

Braun, U. K., Naik, A. D., & McCullough, L. B. (2009). Reconceptualizing the experience of surrogate decision-making: Report vs. genuine decisions. *Annals of Family Medicine, 7*(3), 249–253. doi: 10.1370/afm.963

Brennan, F., Carr, D. B., & Cousins, M. (2007). Pain management: A fundamental human right. *Pain Medicine, 105*(1), 205–221. doi: 10.1213/01.ane.0000268145.52345.55

Breslin, J. M., MacRae, S. K., Bell, J., & Singer, P. A. (2005). University of Toronto Joint Centre for Bioethics Clinical Ethics Group, Top 10 health care ethics challenges facing the public: Views of Toronto bioethicists. *BMC Medical Ethics, 6*(5), 49–56. doi: 10.1186/1472-6939-6-5

Buetow, S., & Elwyn, G. (2006). Are patients morally responsible for their errors? *Journal of Medical Ethics, 32*, 260–262. doi: 10.1136/jme.2005.012245

Chen, E. C., Kakkad, D., & Balzano, J. (2008). Multicultural competence and evidence-based practice in group therapy. *Journal of Clinical Psychology: In Session, 64*(11), 1261–1278. doi: 10.1002/jclp.20533

Chung, S. K., Price, D. D., Verne, G. N., & Robinson, M. E. (2007). Revelation of a personal placebo response: Its effects on mood, attitudes and future placebo responding. *Pain, 132*, 281–288. doi: 10.1016/j.pain.200701.034

Cochran, P. A., Marshall, C. A., Garcia-Downing, C., Kendall, E., Cook, D., McCubbin, L., & Glover, R. M. (2008). Indigenous ways of knowing: Implications for participatory research and community. *American Journal of Public Health, 98*, 22–27. doi: 10.2105/AJPH.2006.093641

Cole, M. (2006). Internationalism in psychology: We need it now more than ever. *American Psychologist, 61*(8), 904–917. doi: 10.1037/0003-066X.61.8.904

Corrigan, J., Kohn, L. T., & Donaldson, M. S. (1999). *To err is human: Building a safer health system*. Washington, DC: Institute of Medicine.

Dodds, S. (2005). Gender, ageing, and injustice: Social and political context of bioethics. *Journal of Medical Ethics, 31*(5), 295–298. doi: 10.1136/jme.2003.006726

Donovan, R. A., & Ponce, A. N. (2009). Identification and measurement of core competencies in professional psychology: Areas for consideration. *Training and Education in Professional Psychology, 3*(4, Suppl), S46–S49. doi:10.1037/a0017302

Dunn, M. C., Clare, I. C., & Holland, A. J. (2008). Substitute decision-making for adults with intellectual disabilities living in residential care: Learning through experience. *Health Care Analysis, 16*(1), 52–64. doi: 10.1007/s10728-007-0053-9

Eastman, N., & Starling, B. (2005). Mental disorder ethics: Theory and empirical investigation. *Journal of Medical Ethics, 32*(2), 94–99. doi: 10.1136/jme.2005.013276

Enoch, M. A., Johnson, K., George, D. T., Schumann, G., Moss, H. B., Kranzler, H. R., & Goldman, D. (2009). Ethical considerations for administering alcohol or alcohol cues to treatment-seeking alcoholics in a research setting: Can the benefits to society outweigh the risks to the individual? *Alcohol Clinical Experimental Research, 33*(9), 1508–1512. doi: 10.1111/j.1530-0277.2009.00988.x

Fiscella, K., & Franks, P. (2005). Is patient HMO insurance or physician HMO participation related to racial disparities in primary care? *American Journal of Managed Care, 11*(6), 397–402.

Fischback, G. D., & Fischback, R. L. (2004). Stem cells: Science, policy and ethics. *Journal of Clinical Investigation, 114*(10), 1364–1370. doi: 10.1172/JCI2004423549

Forrest, L. (2010). Linking international psychology, professional competence, and leadership: Counseling psychologists as learning partners. *The Counseling Psychologist, 38*(1), 96–120. doi: 10.1177/0011000009350585

France, C. R., Masters, K. S., Belar, C. D., Kerns, R. D., Klonoff, E. A., Larkin, K. T., et al. (2008). Application of the competency model to clinical health psychology. *Professional Psychology: Research and Practice, 39*(6), 573–580. doi: 10.1037/0735-7028.39.6.573

Fries, J. F., & Krishnan, E. (2004). Equipoise, design bias, and randomized controlled trials: The elusive ethics of new drug development. *Arthritis Research and Theory, 6*(3), R250–R255. doi: 10.1186/ar1170

Gallardo, M. E., Johnson, J., Parham, T. A., & Carter, J. A. (2009). Ethics and multiculturalism: Advancing cultural and clinical responsiveness. *Professional Psychology: Research and Practice, 40*(5), 425–435. doi: 10.1037/a0016871

Gawande, A. (2009) *The checklist manifesto: How to get things right.* New York: Metropolitan Books, Henry Holt & Co. LLC.

Geller, G., Bernhardt, B. A., Carrese, J., Rushton, C. H., & Kolodner, K. (2008). What do clinicians derive from partnering with their patients? A reliable and valid measure of "personal meaning in patient care." *Patient Education Council, 72*(2), 293–300. doi: 10.1016/j.pec.2008.03.025

Giordano, S. (2005). Is the body a republic? *Journal of Medical Ethics, 31*(8), 470–475. doi: 10.1136/jme.2004.009944

Giordano, J., & Schatman, M. E. (2008). A crisis in chronic pain care: An ethical analysis. Part three: Toward an integrative, multi-disciplinary pain medicine built around the needs of the patient. *Pain Physician Journal, 11*(6), 775–784. ISSN 1533-3159

Glantz, L. (2007). Should smokers be refused surgery? *British Medical Journal, 334*(7583), 21. doi: 10.1136/bmj.39059.532095.68

Glueckauf, R. L. (2007). Telehealth and older adults with chronic illness: New frontiers for research and practice. *Clinical Gerontologist, 31*, 1–4. doi: 10.1300/J018v31n01_01

Gorini, A., Gagglioli, A., Vigna, C., & Riva, G. (2008). A second life for eHealth: Prospects for the use of 3-D virtual worlds in clinical psychology. *Journal of Medical Internet Research, 10*(3), e21. doi: 10.2196/jmir.1029

Grill, K., & Hansson, S. O. (2005). Epistemic paternalism in public health. *Journal of Medical Ethics, 31*, 648–653. doi 10.1136/jme.2004.010850

Halpern, A. L., Halpern, J. H., & Doherty, S. B. (2008). "Enhanced" interrogation of detainees: Do psychologists and psychiatrists participate? *Philosophy, Ethics and Humanities in Medicine,open access http://www.peh-med.com/content/3/1/21 pdf, 3*(21). doi: 10.1186/1747-5341-3-21

Hampson, L. A., Agarwal, M., Joffe, S., Gross, C. P., Verter, J., & Emanuel, E. J. (2006). Patients' views on financial conflicts of interest in cancer research trials. *New England Journal of Medicine, 355*(22), 2330–2337.

Hanson, S. L., Kerkhoff, T. R., & Bush, S. S. (2005). *Health care ethics: A casebook for psychologists.* Washington, DC: APA Press.

Hanson, S. L., & Kerkhoff, T. R. (2007). Ethical decision-making in rehabilitation: Consideration of Latino cultural factors. *Rehabilitation Psychology, 52*(4), 409–420. doi: 10.1037/0090-5550.52.4.409

Hedayat, K. M., Shooshtarizadeh, P., & Raza, M. (2006). Therapeutic abortion in Islam: Contemporary views of Muslim Shiite scholars and the effect of recent Iranian legislation. *Journal of Medical Ethics, 32*(11), 652–657. doi: 10.1136/jme2005.0156289

Helgesson, G., Ludvigsson, J., & Gustafsson-Stolt, U. (2005). How to handle informed consent in longitudinal studies when participants have a limited understanding of the study. *Journal of Medical Ethics, 31*(11), 670–673. doi: 10.1136/jme.2004.009274

Hibbard, M. R., & Cox, D. R. (2010). Competencies of a rehabilitation psychologist. In R. G. Frank, M. Rosenthal, & B. Caplan (Eds.), *Handbook of rehabilitation psychology* (2nd ed., pp. 467–475). Washington, DC: American Psychological Association.

Hoffman, H. G., Doctor, J. N., Patterson, D. R., Carrougher, G. J., & Furness III, T. A. (2000). Virtual reality as an adjunctive pain control during burn wound care in adolescent patients. *Pain, 85*(1–2), 305–309. doi: 10.1016/S0304-3959(99)00275-4

Humayun, A., Fatima, N., Naqqash, S., Hussain, S., Rasheed, A., Imtiaz, H., & Imam, S. Z. (2008). Patients' perception and actual practice of informed consent, privacy and confidentiality in general medical outpatient departments of two tertiary care hospitals of Lahore. *BMC Medical Ethics, 9*, 14. doi: 10.1186/1472-6939-9-14

Hurst, S. A., Hull, S. C., DuVal, G., & Danis, M. (2005). How physicians face ethical difficulties: A qualitative analysis. *Journal of Medical Ethics, 31*(1), 7–14. doi: 10.1136/jme.2003.005835

Illes, J., Lombera, S., Rosenberg, J., & Arnow, B. (2008). In the mind's eye: Provider and patient attitudes on functional brain imaging. *Journal of Psychiatric Research, 43*(2), 107–114. doi: 10.1016/j.jpsychires.2008.02.008

International Association of Applied Psychology. (2008). *Universal declaration of ethical principles for psychologists.* Retrieved from http://www.am.org/iupsys/resources/ethics/univdecl2008.html

Kaldjian, L. C., Jones, E. W., Wu, B. J., Forman-Hoffman, V. L., Levi, B. H., & Rosenthal, G. E. (2007). Disclosing medical errors to patients: Attitudes and practices of physicians and trainees. *Society of General Internal Medicine, 22*(7), 988–996. doi: 10.1007/s11606-007-0227-z

Kaslow, N. J., Borden, K. A., Collins, F. L. Jr., Forrest, L., Illfelder-Kaye, J., Nelson, P. D., & Rallo, J. S. (2004). Competencies conference: Future directions in education and credentialing in professional psychology. *Journal of Clinical Psychology, 60*(7), 699–712. doi: 10.1002/jclp.20016

Kaslow, N. J., Grus, C. L., Campbell, L. F., Fouad, N. A., Hatcher, R. L., & Rodolfa, E. R. (2009). Competency assessment toolkit for professional psychology. *Training and Education in Professional Psychology, 3*(4, Suppl), S27–S45. doi: 10.1037/a0015833

Keefe, F., Abernethy, A. P., Wheeler, J., & Affleck, G. (2008). Don't ask, don't tell? Revealing placebo responses to research participants and patients. *Pain, 135*(3), 213–214. doi: 10.1016/j.pain.2008.01.009

Kenkel, M. B. (2009). Adopting a competency model for professional psychology: Essential elements and resources.

Training and Education in Professional Psychology, 3(4, Suppl), S59–S62. doi: 10.1037/a0017037

Kerns, R. D., Berry, S., Frantsve, L. M. E., & Linton, J. C. (2009). Life-long competency development in clinical health psychology. *Training and Education in Professional Psychology, 3*(4), 212–217. doi: 10.1037/10016753

Kim, S. Y., Frank, S., Holloway, R., Zimmerman, C., Wilson, R., & Kieburtz, K. (2005). Science and ethics of sham surgery: A survey of Parkinson Disease clinical researchers. *Archives of Neurology, 62*(9), 1357–1360.

Knifed, E., Lipsman, N., Mason, W., & Bernstein, M. (2008). Patients' perceptions of the informed consent process for neurooncology clinical trials. *Neuro-Oncology, 10*(3), 348–354. doi: 10.1215/15228517-2008-007

Kostopoulou, V., & Katsouyanni, E. (2006). The truth-telling issue and changes in lifestyle in patients with cancer. *Journal of Medical Ethics, 32*(12), 693–697. doi: 10.1136/jme.2005.01.5487

Li, L., Lin, C., Wu, Z., Lord, L., & Wu, S. (2008). To tell or not to tell: HIV disclosure in family members in China. *Developing World Bioethics, 8*(3), 235–241. doi: 10.1111/j.1471-8847.2007.00220.x

Li, L., Wu, Z., Wu, S., Lee, S. J., Rotheram-Borus, M. J., Detels, R., Jia, M., & Sun, S. (2007). Mandatory HIV testing in China: The perception of health-care providers. *Journal of STD AIDS, 18*(7), 476–481. doi: 10.1258/095646207781147355

Liegeois, A., & Van Audenhove, C. (2005). Ethical dilemmas in community mental health care. *Journal of Medical Ethics, 31*(8), 452–456. doi: 10.1136/jme.2003.006999

Lustria, M. L., Cortese, J., Noar, S. M., & Glueckauf, R. L. (2009). Computer-tailored health interventions delivered over the web: Review and analysis of key components. *Patient Education and Counseling, 74*, 156–173. doi: 10.1016/j.pec.2008.08.023

Maden, A. (2007). England's new Mental Health Act represents law catching up with science: A commentary on Peter Lepping's ethical analysis of the new mental health legislation in England and Wales. *Philosophy, Ethics and Humanities in Medicine*, open access http://www.peh-med.com/content/2/1/16 pdf 1–3 2(16). doi: 10.1186/1747-5341-2-16

Mamhidir, A. G., Kihlgren, M., & Sorkie, V. (2007). Ethical challenges related to elder care: High-level decision-makers' experiences. *BMC Medical Ethics, 8*(3). doi: 10.1186/1472-6939-8-3

Marsella, A.J., Johnson, J.L., Watson, P., Gryczynski, J. (Eds.) (2008). *Ethnocultural Perspectives on Disaster and Trauma: Foundations, Issues, and Applications*. New York: Springer SBM Publishers.

Masters, K. S., France, C. R., & Thorn, B. E. (2009). Enhancing preparation among entry-level clinical health psychologists: Recommendations for "best practices" from the first meeting of the Council of Clinical Health Psychology Training Programs (CCHPTP). *Training and Education in Professional Psychology, 3*(4), 193–201. doi: 10.1037/a0016049

McGrew, M., & Giordano, J. (2009). Whence tendance? Accepting the responsibility of care for the chronic pain patient. *Pain Physician Journal, 12*(3), 483–485.

Messinger-Rapport, B. J., Baum, E. E., & Smith, M. L. (2009). Service care planning: Beyond the living will. *Cleveland Clinic Journal of Medicine, 76*(5), 276–285. doi: 10.3949/ccjm.76a.07002

Murphy, B. F. (2008). What has happened to clinical leadership in futile care discussions? *Medical Journal of Australia, 188*(7), 418–419.

National Institutes of Health (NIH). (2008). *Protecting human research participants. NIH Office of Extramural Research.* Retrieved from http://phrp.nihtraining.com/index.php

Nilsson, M. S., & Pilhammar, E. (2009). Professional approaches in clinical judgments among senior and junior doctors: Implications for medical education. *BMC Medical Education*, open access http://www.biodedcentral.com/1472–69201/9/24 pdf 1–9, 9(25). doi: 10.1186/1472-6920/9/25

Patient Self-Determination Act of 1990. Cited: Koch, K. A. (1992) *Journal of the Florida Medical Association, 79*(4), 240–243.

Peppin, J. F. (2009). The marginalization of chronic pain patients on chronic opioid therapy. *Pain Physician Journal, 12*(3), 493–498. ISSN 1533–3159

Peterson, R. L., Peterson, D. R., Abrams, J. C., & Stricker, G. (1997). The national council of schools and programs of professional psychology educational model. *Professional Psychology: Research and Practice, 28*(4), 373–386. doi: 10.1037/12068-001

Petrova, M., Dale, J., & Fulford, B. K. (2006). Values-based practice in primary care: Easing the tensions between individual values, ethical principles and best evidence. *British Journal of General Practice, 56*, 703–709. PMCID: PMC1

Pettifor, J. L., & Sawchuk, T. R. (2006). Psychologists' perceptions of ethically troubling incidents across international borders. *International Journal of Psychology, 41*(3), 216–225. doi: 10.1080/00207590500343505876638

Pickett, T. C., Fritz, S. L., Ketterson, T. U., Glueckauf, R. L., Davis, S. B., Malcolm, M. P., & Light K. E. (2007). Telehealth and constraint-induced movement therapy (CIMT): An intensive case study approach. *Clinical Gerontologist, 31*, 5–20. doi: 10.1013/J018v31n01_03

Pina-Neto, J. M. (2008). Genetic counseling. *Jornal de Pediatria, 84*(4, Suppl), 520–526. doi: 10.2223/JPED.1782

Plu, I., Purssell-Francois, I., Moutel, G., et al. (2008). Ethical issues arising from the requirement to sign a consent form in palliative care. *Journal of Medical Ethics, 34*, 279–280. doi: 10.1136/jme.2006.019075

Rantanen, E., Hietala, M., Kristoffersson, U., Nippert, I., Schmidtke, J., Sequeiros, J., & Kaarianen, H. (2008).What is ideal genetic counseling? A survey of current international guidelines. *European Journal of Human Genetics, 16*, 445–452. doi: 10.1038/sj.ejhg.5201983

Reed, A. E., Mikels, J. A., & Simon, K. I. (2008). Older adults prefer less choice than younger adults. *Psychology of Aging, 23*(3), 671–675. doi: 10.1037/a0012772

Reger, M. A., Etherage, J. R., Reger, G. M., & Gahm, G. A. (2008). Civilian psychologists in an army culture: The ethical challenge of cultural competence. *Military Psychology, 20*, 21–35. doi: 10.1080/08995600701753144

Rizzieri, A. G., Verheijde, J. L., Rady, M. Y., & McGregor, J. L. (2008). Ethical challenges with the left ventricular assist device as a destination therapy. *Philosophy, Ethics and Humanities in Medicine, 3*(20), 1–15. doi: 10.1186/1747-5341-3-20

Roberts, L. W., Johnson, M. E., Brems, C., & Warner, T. D. (2007). Ethical disparities: Challenges encountered by multidisciplinary providers in fulfilling ethic standards in the care of rural and minority people. *Journal of Rural Health, 23*(suppl.), 89–97. doi: 10.1111/j.1748-0361.2007.00130.x

Rodolfa, E., Bent, R., Eisman, E., Nelson, P., Rehm, L., & Ritchie, P. (2005). A cube model for competency development: Implications for psychology educators and regulators. *Professional Psychology: Research and Practice, 36*(4), 347–354. doi: 10.1037/0735-7028.36.4.347

Rubin, N. J., Bebeau, M., Leigh, I. W., Lichtenberg, J. W., Nelson, P. D., Portnoy, S., et al. (2007). The competency movement within psychology: An historical perspective. *Professional Psychology: Research and Practice, 38*(5), 452–462. doi: 10.1037/0735-7028.38.5.452

Rydvall, A., & Lynde, N. (2008). Withholding and withdrawing life-sustaining treatment: A comparative study of the ethical reasoning of physicians and the general public. *Critical Care open access http://ccforum.com/content/12/1/R13, 12*(R13). doi: 10.1086/cc6786

Schutte, P. A., Wagner, G. R., Ostry, A., Blanciforti, L. A., Cutlip, R. G., Krajnak, K. M., et al. (2007). Work, obesity and occupational safety and health. *American Journal Of Public Health, 97*, 428–436. doi: 10.2105/AJPH.2006.086900

Scully, J. L. (2008). Disability and genetics in the era of genomic medicine. *Nature Reviews Genetics, 9*, 797–802. doi: 10.1038/nrg2453

Schwab, A.P. (2006). Formal and effective autonomy in health-care. *Journal of Medical Ethics, 32*, 575–579. doi: 10.1136/jme.2005.013391

Scully, J. L. (2008). Science and society. Disability and genetics in the era of genomic medicine. *Nature Reviews Genetics, 9*, 797–802. doi: 10.1038/nrg2453

Secker, B., Goldenberg, M. J., Gibson, B. E., Wagner, F., Parke, B., Breslin, J., et al. (2006). Just regionalization: Rehabilitating care for people with disabilities and chronic illnesses. *BMC Medical Ethics, 7*, 9. doi: 10.1186/1472-6939-7-9

Shostak, S., & Ottman, R. (2006). Ethical, legal and social dimensions of epilepsy genetics. *Epilepsia, 47*(10), 1595–1602. doi: 10.1111/j1528-1167.2006.00632.x

Shullman, S. (2008), "Psychologist as Learning Partners: Some Reflections on Globalization and Psychology" (lecture, 2008 APA Education Leadership Conference, Washington, DC, September, 6, 2008).

Song, J., Bartels, D. M., Ratner, E. R., Alderton, L., Hudson, B., & Ahluwalla, J. S. (2007). Dying on the streets: Homeless persons' concerns and desires about end of life care. *Journal of Internal General Medicine, 22*, 435–441. doi: 10.1007/s11606-006-0046-7

Sowmini, C. V., & De Vries, R. (2009). A cross cultural review of the ethical issues in dementia care in Kerala, India and The Netherlands. *International Journal of Geriatric Psychiatry, 24*, 329–334. doi: 10.1002/gps.2127

Stenson, K., Chen, D., Tansey, K., Kerkhoff, T. R., Butt, L., Gallegos, A. J., & Kirschner, K. L. (2010). Informed consent and phase 1 research in spinal cord injury. *Archives of Physical Medicine and Rehabilitation, 2*, 664–670.

Stuart, R. B. (2004). Twelve practical suggestions for achieving multicultural competence. *Professional Psychology: Research and Practice, 35*(1), 3–9. Doi: 10.1037/0735-7028.35.1.3

Sullivan, M. A., Harris, E., Collado, C., & Chen, T. (2006). Noways tired: Perspectives of color on culturally competent crisis intervention. *Journal of Clinical Psychology: In Session, 62*(8), 987–999.

Sumerall, S., Lopez, S. J., & Oehlert, M. E. (2000). *Competency-based education and training in psychology*. Springfield, IL: Charles C Thomas.

Tekola, F., Bull, S., Farsides, B., Newport, M. J., Adeyemo, A., Rotimi, C. N., & Davey, G. (2009). Impact of social stigma on the process of obtaining informed consent for genetic research on podoconiosis: A qualitative study. *BMC Medical Ethics, 10*, 13. doi: 10.1186/1472-6939-10-3

Terry, P. B. (2007). Informed consent in clinical medicine. *Chest, 131*, 563–568. doi: 10.1378/chest.06–1955

Thornton, T. (2006). Tacit knowledge as the underlying factor in evidence based medicine and clinical judgment. *Philosophy, Ethics and Humanities in Medicine, 1*(2), 1–10. doi: 10.1186.1747-5341-1-2

Tillyard, A. R. (2007). Ethics review: "Living wills" and intensive care—an overview of the American experience. *Critical Care, 11*, 219. doi: 10.1186/cc5945

Todd, K., Sloan, E., Chen, C., Eder, S., & Wamstad, K. (2002). Survey of pain etiology, management practices and patient satisfaction in two urban emergency departments. *Canadian Journal of Emergency Medicine, 4*(4), 252–256

Valdez-Martinez, E., Lavielle, P., Bedolla, M., & Squires, A. (2008). Ethical behaviours in clinical practice among Mexican health care workers. *Nursing Ethics, 15*(6), 729–744. doi: 10.1177/0969733008095384

Westra, A. E., Willems, D. L., & Smit, B. J. (2009). Communicating with Muslim parents: "The four principles" are not as culturally neutral as suggested. *European Journal of Pediatrics, 168*, 1383–1387. doi: 10.1007/s00431-009-0970-8

Wu, A. (2000). Medical error: The second victim. *British Journal of Medicine, 320*, 726–727. doi: 10.1136/bjm.320.7237.726

Zhou, Z., & Siu, C. R. (2009). Promoting cultural competence in counseling Asian American children and adolescents. *Psychology in the Schools, 46*(3), 290–298. doi: 10.1002/pits.20375

Ziebland, A., McPherson, A., & Herxheimer, A. (2006). What people close to death say about euthanasia and assisted suicide: A qualitative study. *Journal of Medical Ethics, 32*, 706–710. doi: 10.1136/jme.2006.015883

Vocational Rehabilitation, Inclusion, and Social Integration

Carol Blessing, Thomas P. Golden, Sukyeong Pi, Susanne M. Bruyère, *and* Sara Van Looy

Abstract

People are social beings and as such have a right to personal dignity, social security, citizenship, and full participation in civil and social activities as a member of society. Active engagement in social roles enables each individual to have a sense of connection and acceptance through interacting with other people, build his or her self-esteem by contributing to the society; and, consequently, improve his or her overall quality of life. Paid work is a core factor in one's ability to contribute fully to society. This is important for all people, but can be particularly important for people with disabilities, who often experience social isolation. Vocational training is a means to achieve the desired goal of paid employment in an integrated setting and full community participation as a resulting outcome, and is one that rehabilitation psychologists should not overlook in their services. This chapter begins with the importance of community citizenship and valued roles for people with disabilities and examines the positive impact of social integration and inclusion on quality of life. In addition to an overview of the historical and philosophical roots and evolution of related employment and disability policy, we discuss the importance of vocational training and related services that can lead to successful employment outcomes. Following a discussion of current issues and concerns in vocational training and social integration, we conclude with the implications for rehabilitation psychology practice, training, and research.

Key Words: Social inclusion, social integration, people with disabilities, vocational rehabilitation, vocational training.

This chapter focuses on the important connection between the vocational rehabilitation (VR) and vocational training of individuals who negotiate life with a disability, and meaningful paid employment as a means for achieving community reintegration and social inclusion. *Social exclusion* refers to the dynamic process of being shut out, fully or partially, from any of the social, economic, political, and cultural systems that determine the social integration of the person in society (Walker & Walker, 1997). The best safeguard against social exclusion and poverty (the result of economic exclusion) is a quality job for those who can work, because it then leads

to adequate income support and social participation (Lister, 2000).

Vocational rehabilitation is the provision of a particular set of services aimed at enhancing the employability of people whose lives have been impacted by a disabling physical or psychological condition. Physical disabilities, chronic diseases, congenital problems, and mental health concerns often create overwhelming obstacles to the full inclusion and participation of individuals in their communities (Elliott & Leung, 2005). This is especially true in the realm of employment, where a gap of 40 percentage points exists between the employment rates of people with and without disabilities (Erickson, Lee, & von Schrader, 2010a). Employment data published by the United Nations Department of Information (United Nations Enable, 2007) indicates that in developing countries, 80–90% of persons with disabilities of working age are unemployed. In industrialized countries, the figure is between 50% and 70%. This employment disparity results in significant economic disparities between people with disabilities and those without. These disparities will be discussed in further detail later in this chapter.

Given the major role that work plays in human life, the implications of being without meaningful work are staggering (Waters & Moore, 2002). In addition to providing a source of income, work holds important social value, creates the opportunity to develop community networks, and contributes to an individual's healthy sense of identity and self-esteem. Work is only one part of being valued and respected within society, but it is an important means of social inclusion (Evans & Repper, 2000). Work is a key to economic and social independence, self-respect, and opportunities for achievement (Harman, 1997, as cited in Lister, 2000). Indeed, a premise of this chapter is that paid work is at the heart of needed efforts to build a more inclusive society, one that contributes not only to the economic self-sufficiency and independence of the individual, but also enables that individual to contribute to the social and economic fabric of his or her own community. We see vocational training as a component of community-based rehabilitation that is necessary to achieving paid employment in an integrated setting and with full community inclusion.

In this chapter, we begin by discussing the importance of community citizenship and valued roles for people with disabilities and the positive impact of social integration and inclusion on quality of life. Next, we provide an overview of the historical and philosophical roots and evolution of related employment and disability policy and discuss the importance of vocational training and related services that can lead to successful employment outcomes, identify current issues of focus in VR, describe the population affected by those programs, and discuss measurement of outcomes. We follow that with an overview of social inclusion and identify current issues and concerns in vocational training and social integration. Finally, we discuss implications of these concepts for rehabilitation psychology practice, training, and research.

Community Citizenship and Valued Roles

Membership within typical communities is vital to the well-being of people with disabilities (Ludlum, 2002). Being a welcomed and accepted part of a community provides a sense of belonging and the chance to make valuable contributions for the greater benefit. Full community membership carries with it the expectation of citizenship (Ludlum, 2002). To be a citizen, one is expected to uphold certain rights and responsibilities—to strive toward the betterment of the whole community through economic participation, public service, and other such efforts to build a healthy, sustainable community. Yet, quite often, people who experience a disability are denied or excused from this expectation. In Cambodia, for example, people with disabilities are among the most vulnerable and poorest groups in that society. There is very limited access to basic services that offer education, vocational training, and job placement, thus deepening the level of poverty and stigma surrounding those with disabilities (San, 2005).

Social interactions between people with disabilities and members of their community without disabilities are often distorted by cultural attitudes and by the societal norm to avoid honest feedback to people with disabilities in social settings (Rohe, 1998). Attitudes toward disability differ across different cultures. In Turkey (Gunduz, Erhan, & Nur Bardak, 2010), and among many Indian people, disability is thought to be a consequence of destiny from God. In areas of China, disability is viewed as punishment for sins of the person's—or the person's parents—past life (Zhang Liu, 2005). Western countries have built a complex socioeconomic and political infrastructure around disability that is defined solidly in medical terms. Universally, people with disabilities are provided center-based or home-based care removed from the mainstream of community life.

Employment holds a primary valued social role in American culture (Luecking, Fabian, & Tislon, 2004). Initial introductions between people generally start with what one "does" for a living. Gunduz et al. (2010) cite data that suggest that the return to work or becoming employed after acquiring a spinal cord injury (SCI) is one of the most important outcomes of reintegration into society. This study further posits that positive expectations regarding returning to work, job counseling, and vocational services are important indicators of successful reintegration to work.

Work provides people with a positive identity, social status, and a meaning to life. It is critical that rehabilitation psychologists integrate the expectation of obtaining or returning to meaningful employment and other important roles of community membership into individualized treatment planning. Optimally, planning will encompass a holistic approach to the rehabilitation process by identifying specific functional support needs, including the identification of accommodations and assistive technologies that will enable the person to successfully navigate and overcome barriers to social inclusion (Luecking et al., 2004). Attention must be paid to the interests and needs of the person across each of the domains of community living, inclusive education, and integrated employment throughout the rehabilitative process so that existing skills, capacities, and interests can be built upon even as the person addresses the issues that surround the impact of his or her disability. This calls for a person-centered or whole-person approach to self-determined community-based rehabilitation intervention. The Joint Positions Paper from the International Labor Organization, the United Nations Education, Scientific, and Cultural Organization (UNESCO), and the World Health Organization (World Health Organization [WHO], 2004) defines community-based rehabilitation as a "strategy within general community development for rehabilitation, equalization of opportunities and social inclusion of all people with disabilities." It is a model designed to change the way in which traditional services are created and executed, and is implemented in more than 90 countries to facilitate capacity building, empowerment, and community mobilization of people with disabilities and their families (http://www.who.int/disabilities/publications/cbr/en/index.html). It is a strategy for providing more equal opportunities to people with disabilities while at the same time protecting their human rights (Helander, 1999).

Developing countries such as Cambodia, the Philippines, Bangladesh, and Nigeria have been experimenting with community-based rehabilitation (CBR) models to raise public awareness of disability issues at multiple levels and to address core barriers to accessing appropriate rehabilitation supports. A pilot project for community-based VR launched in 1991 in the southwestern region of Nigeria, claims that the model has been very effective in facilitating the inclusion of people with disabilities into the mainstream of society through the gainful and sustained employment of 90% of its 155 beneficiaries (Alade, 2004). In Bangladesh, the CBR model has been seen as the most effective rehabilitation approach to reaching millions of people with disabilities residing primarily in rural areas of the country (Jahurul Alam, Bari, & Abedin Khan, 2005). In the Philippines, the CBR model became a priority in the 2003–2012 National Plan of Action for the Philippine Decade of Persons with Disabilities and was used as an effective strategy for empowering people with disabilities and for forming collaborations among multidisciplinary sectors and community members (Jarhurul Alam et al., 2005).

The concept of social roles and social inclusion provides a way to best configure community-based rehabilitation supports and interventions that maximize the person's opportunities for making meaningful contributions. The identification of the social roles a person is likely to perform in community settings, with relevant and appropriate support, provides a clear measure of social integration (O'Brien, 2006). The idea of community inclusion carries with it the assumption that people with disabilities are living and working in nonmedical, noncustodial settings. In the realm of community living, an individual would be recognized for his or her active participation in household work and neighborhood life (Ludlum, 2002). The person might hold valued community roles, such as home-owner, tenant, neighbor, customer, or club member. His or her family roles could be wife, husband, son, daughter, brother, sister, uncle, aunt, partner, or grandparent.

For education to be integrated and inclusive, individuals with disabilities should experience the same learning environments and opportunities that are available to individuals who do not have disabilities, rather than limited access to education in segregated and specialized programs. In this domain, the person engages in study for a purpose. Learning activities offer a clear path to a goal that the person has identified as being meaningful. It may be formal or informal, and it may be based purely on interest or to acquire specific information and/or skills. In this milieu, valued roles would include those of teacher, mentor, trainer, tutor, guide, student, and learner.

A person who experiences social integration and inclusion through employment will be paid a competitive wage through work that reflects his or her interests, preferences, skills, and abilities in ordinary or typical places of business (O'Brien, 2006). He or she will be provided opportunities to build on existing and learn new skills that offer the potential for advancement. In addition to a particular job title associated with the role of employee, an individual may also be valued in the role of colleague, co-worker, team member, apprentice, intern, owner, supervisor, or employer.

Impact of Social Integration and Inclusion

Individuals whose lives are interrupted by disability may find their sense of self suddenly and dramatically challenged (Crocker & Major, 1989). They may experience significant changes in their social and familial relationships and feel at a loss for reconciling their current situation with what once was (Rohe, 1998). It is vital that rehabilitation practitioners work holistically with people to identify and quickly address these concerns.

Discussion of community integration of individuals with SCI has been addressed by several researchers. Gorden and Brown (1997) present research indicating that, following initial rehabilitation, 92% of individuals with SCIs were discharged to private residences in their community. In looking at vocational roles, the research clearly states that the completion of a VR program as a component of the overall rehabilitation experience increases the likelihood of returning to work. According to Gorden and Brown, a primary barrier to returning to work and active involvement in the community is the lack of encouragement or assistance in developing a new set of hopes and aspirations.

Rohe and Athelstan (1982, 1985) and Rohe and Krause (1998) have shown that SCI does not change a person's interests, including vocational interests, and that after their injuries, people with SCI experience frequent barriers in continuing to access communities and employment opportunities that reflect those interests. More recent research focused on health status, community integration, and economic risk factors for mortality after SCI and found that measures of community integration and economic status indicators had small but statistically significant effects on the likelihood of dying during the year after SCI (Krause, DeVivo, & Jackson, 2004). Krause and Terza (2006) also found that there are substantial differences in the likelihood of post injury employment as a function of gender, race, and having less than a college degree.

Evidence suggests that the degree to which people with chronic stroke conditions participate in regular community interactions is determined by the interaction between physical function and the perception of self as being capable of typical skills in traditional community settings (Pang, Eng, & Miller, 2007). The data confirm that rehabilitation services that offer balanced self-efficacy treatment to people who have had a stroke promote more successful and satisfying community integration.

After acquiring a traumatic brain injury, people experience high incidences of unemployment, decreased independence, and diminished access to social networks, leading to an increase in loneliness and a reduction in participation in leisure activities (Doctor et al., 2005). Community inclusion provides an alternative to isolation and loneliness by affording people the opportunity to actively participate in a broad range of community involvements, especially in the realm of building relationships and having something to do (Sander, 2006).

At the Community Reintegration Summit: Service Members and Veterans Returning to Community Life held in 2009 in Washington, D.C., stakeholders identified six core inter-related issues, including rehabilitation, that are vital to the successful return of service members, veterans and their families to work, school, and community. "The roots of successful reintegration begin at the community level." (Booz Allen Hamilton, 2009, p.5).

The process of intentional social and community integration of people with disabilities provides a framework through which rehabilitation psychologists can work with individuals to develop and increasingly build capacity for interpersonal connectedness and citizenship. These skills can be effectively developed as part of typical rehabilitative care and practice (Ware, Hopper, Tugenberg, Dickey, & Fisher, 2008). Rehabilitation efforts that focus on capacity building for social integration that results in practical community contribution will also likely increase an individual's awareness of the level at which he or she is able to function with responsibility, accountability, imagination, empathy, judgment, and advocacy in his or her community. Rehabilitation psychologists would do well to create the occasions through which these capacities are exercised and further developed (Ware et al., 2008) through the establishment of clear, concrete goals that effectively lead the person back into being an active community member.

Overview of Vocational Rehabilitation
Definition of Vocational Rehabilitation, Historical and Philosophical Roots

Gobelet, Luthi, Al-Khodairy, and Chamberlain (2007) define VR as a "multidisciplinary intervention in a process linked to the facilitation of return to work or to the prevention of loss of work." According to the International Labor Organization (1998), VR is the continued and coordinated process of rehabilitation, which involves the provision of those vocational services (e.g., vocational guidance, vocational training, and selective placement) designed to enable a person with disabilities to secure and retain suitable employment. In other words, VR services can prepare a qualified applicant to achieve a lifestyle of independence and integration within the workplace, family, and community (Luecking et al., 2004).

To better understand VR services aimed at social integration of people with disabilities through economic self-sufficiency and community participation, policies related to financial aids (benefits) and human rights issues (disability discrimination), as well as the services a country adopts for people with disabilities should be reviewed. It can be readily observed that VR or disability policies are different among countries, for example even between Europe and North American, especially the nature of the programs that govern who gets VR services. For example, VR is a right in Austria, France, Germany, and Poland, whereas people with disabilities in the United States, where policies are more targeted to people with severe disabilities, can only receive VR services after application submission and eligibility determination. In terms of the timing of VR services, vocational intervention starts early and is implemented promptly before, during, or after the medical rehabilitation process in Germany and Sweden, whereas people with disabilities receive VR services only after long-term sickness in Canada, Mexico, and the United States (Organization for Economic Cooperation and Development [OECD], 2003).

In Germany, a country with long history of disability policies, all people with disabilities have a right to the assistance necessary "to avert, eliminate, or ease the disability, prevent its aggravation or to reduce its effects and to secure a place in the community, in particular in working life" (Thornton & Lunt, 1997). Stressing the concepts of rehabilitation and compulsory employment, legislation to employ victims of war and of accidents appeared in 1919 and wes extended in 1924 to certain other groups of disabled people. In 1953, Germany set a quota requiring employers with at least seven workers in the public sector and the banking and insurance industries have at least 10% of the workforce be people with disabilities (the quota was 6% for private industry). These quotas

were changed in 1961 to a single quota of 6% for all employers. As the basis of current compulsory employment policy, the Severely Disabled Persons Act (*Schwerbehindertergesetz*) of 1974 extended the quota. Continuously, before the Growth and Employment Act was passed in 1997, all people with disabilities were able to claim VR services with no waiting period requirement to demonstrate difficulty in securing employment (OECD, 2003; Thornton & Lunt, 1997).

In the United States, VR is delivered through a state and federal VR partnership formula grant program and discretionary grant program. It is federally administered by the Department of Education's Rehabilitation Services Administration to individual state VR agencies (§34 CFR Part 361). Individual state agencies, in turn, maintain a statewide network of vendors and contractors for delivery of services and supports to consumers. The VR program exclusively serves individuals with significant disabilities who meet stringent eligibility criteria. Services and supports authorized under the Rehabilitation Act are provided by a highly skilled cadre of credentialed personnel whose development is monitored and tracked through each state's Comprehensive System of Personnel Development.[1] The state and federal VR program serves over 1.2 million individuals with disabilities a year, placing close to a quarter of a million consumers into competitive employment. The VR program has grown exponentially from its $3.5 million appropriation in 1935 to over $2.8 billion in 2009 (Bruyère, Van Looy, & Golden, 2010). The following sections will further review historical aspects of U.S. policy on VR services for people with disabilities, the scope of services, and VR outcomes.

Evolution of U.S. Employment and Disability Policy Pertaining to Vocational Rehabilitation

The earliest pieces of disability policy legislation in the United States emerged from the workers compensation and veterans programs passed at the turn of the 20th century. In 1908, the Federal Worker's Compensation program was established, with compensation extended to civilians in 1916 (Obermann, 1965). The early compensation programs acknowledged the utility of restoring workers to the workplace. In recognition of the importance of vocational education and need for vocational training of injured veterans from World War I, the Fess-Smith Civilian Vocational Rehabilitation Act extended the program to civilians as well, creating the current federal and state partnership for VR in 1920.

The earliest VR programs focused almost exclusively on the physical restoration of individuals who had suffered some sort of physical trauma or impairment. That focus continued through the 1940s, although an increased national emphasis was placed on employment of people with disabilities. The 20-year span between 1950 and 1970 saw an increased focus on the needs of individuals with disabilities other than physical impairments (Wright, 1980). Public conscience regarding disability and social inclusion was growing, as evidenced by the passage of the Architectural Barriers Act of 1968, the Rehabilitation Act of 1973, the Education for All Handicapped Children Act of 1975, and the 1975 Developmental Disability Bill of Rights. These created the foundation for contemporary disability policies in the United States.

The Rehabilitation Act of 1973 made serving persons with severe disabilities a key priority, and affirmative action programs were established under certain titles and sections of the Act. The law required development of an Individual Written Rehabilitation Program (IWRP) (later renamed an IPE or Individualized Plan for Employment) to ensure the enhanced involvement of the consumer in developing a rehabilitation plan of action. The most recent amendments to the Act (1992 and 1998) detailed the intent of Congress to ensure consumer choice in career opportunities, with competitive employment as the preferred outcome (WIA; P.L. 105–220).

As important as the 1950s and 1960s were in advancing civil rights and deinstitutionalization, the 1970s and 1980s advanced theories of normalization, protection and advocacy, and empowerment. The independent living moving mantra "Nothing About Us Without Us" (Charlton, 1998) provided momentum toward removal of architectural and transportation barriers in the 1970s, followed by expansion of accessible telecommunication technologies in the 1980s, and, ultimately, passage of the Americans with Disabilities Act in 1990 (U.S. Department of Justice, 2005). The last few decades have seen a considerable shift in the U.S. mindset, from a medical model of rehabilitation to a social construct of disability, and the identification and expansion of evidence-based practices leading to more positive employment outcomes for people with disabilities have taken center stage. Demand-driven employment programs, such as the Ticket to Work and Self-Sufficiency Program, created under the Ticket to Work and Work Incentives Improvement Act of 1999 (TWWIA), have handed the consumer control over access to employment services and other supports needed to go to work.

The U.S. Congress passed the Workforce Investment Act (the WIA; PL 105–220) in 1998 as an attempt to consolidate various federally administered employment and job training programs into statewide partnerships for a workforce development system. The integration of these diverse and separate programs into the respective titles of the Workforce Investment Act was to primarily consolidate, coordinate, and improve employment, training, literacy, and VR programs in the U.S. (U.S. Department of Labor, 2007).

Consolidation of Employment and Job Training Programs

As referenced above, the current Workforce Investment System is a combination of adult education, literacy, vocational and job training, and other job retraining programs targeted toward the general public. Although the WIA consolidated this array of programs, some of which serve targeted populations, the local One-Stop Centers in each state were established with the charge of operationalizing the Act and its intent. One-Stop Centers were created to reduce the previous fragmentation problems that occurred in the employment and training realm by serving every job seeker through a central location that provides access to multiple services, programs, and supports (Imel, 1999). Founded on the precept of inclusion and integration, the One-Stop approach was developed to make all core workforce development services available to everyone; to allow customers to drive the selection of services based on their unique needs and interests; to collapse all workforce development services provided by local, state, and federal programs into a centralized location; and to create accountability via an outcomes-based funding formula (Imel, 1999).

Vocational rehabilitation and the One-Stop systems have struggled with how best to turn the WIA's policies into practices. The public VR program is a mandatory partner in the universal workforce development system. However, Title IV of the Act maintains the Rehabilitation Act of 1973 as amended intact, with minimal definition and attention given in statute for how to effectively interface the broader workforce development system and the specific VR system in a meaningful way that results in positive employment outcomes for individuals with disabilities (Imel, 1999).

One primary challenge faced by the merged systems is the recognition that individuals served by the VR system require specific and specialized expertise, as mentioned earlier in this chapter, in regard to the Comprehensive System for Personnel Development (CSPD). The broader workforce development system does not have a commensurate CSPD requirement, which creates a tension between the workforces of the two systems. As an approach to ameliorating this tension, the Social Security Administration (SSA) and Department of Labor (DOL) created Disability Program Navigators (DPN) within the national network of One-Stop Career Centers (U.S. Department of Labor, 2009). Navigators link people with disabilities who visit One-Stop Centers with employers, state VR and other providers, and other employment supports needed to prepare for, attach to, and advance in work. In addition, Navigators also provide critical information on SSA's work incentives and return-to-work initiatives, including the Ticket to Work Program.

The movement toward a unified, universally accessible workforce development system was a bold and important step toward integrating employment and disability policy (National Collaborative on Workforce and Disability, 2009). It is critical for rehabilitation psychologists to recognize the interface between these two distinct systems if they are to maximize employment outcomes. Often, consumers being served could benefit from services in one or both systems. It is important for the rehabilitation psychologist to understand the specific scopes of services provided by the VR program that might prove most beneficial to their consumers and create linkages and partnerships to ensure access to these services and supports.

Scope of Vocational Rehabilitation Training Services and Supports

The Rehabilitation Act clearly states that all programs, projects, and activities receiving assistance under the Act are to be carried out in a manner consistent with the following core principles: respect for individual dignity, personal responsibility, self-determination, and pursuit of meaningful careers based on the informed choice of individuals with disabilities; respect for the privacy, rights, and equal access (including the use of accessible formats) of the individuals; inclusion, integration, and full participation of the individuals; support for the involvement of an individual's representative if an individual with a disability requests, desires, or needs such support; and support for

individual and systemic advocacy and community involvement.

The Rehabilitation Act of 1973, as amended, defines VR services as any services, whether provided directly by state VR programs or facilitated by the state VR program through their network of community rehabilitation programs. These services must be described in an individualized plan for employment necessary to assist an individual with a disability in preparing for, securing, retaining, or regaining an employment outcome that is consistent with the strengths, resources, priorities, concerns, abilities, capabilities, interests, and informed choice of the individual (Section §103). The types of services provided by VR agencies are listed in Table 25.1.

As the first civil rights act for people with disabilities, the Act not only stipulates several types of VR services but also emphasizes the manner in which they are to be carried out according to the core principles listed above.

Vocational Rehabilitation Impact and Outcomes

Numerous studies have examined the effectiveness of VR services. These studies have used the RSA 911 data, a VR administrative dataset that contains individual demographic information (e.g., race, level of education), service-related information in the VR system (e.g., types of services received, cost of services), and outcome-related variables (e.g., type of closure, wages, hours worked) of consumers who exited the VR agency during a fiscal year. Each year, around 600,000 consumers exit the VR system in the United States, and about a third of them have achieved an employment outcome at the time of closure. Although there were some variations in terms of strength of relationships, previous studies concluded that provision of two VR services—job placement assistance and on-the-job supports—increased the probability of achieving an employment outcome, regardless of type of disability (Bolton, Bellini, & Brookings, 2000; Boutin & Wilson, 2009; Cantalano, Pereira, Wu, Ho, & Chan, 2006; Chan, Cheing, Chan, Rosenthal, & Chronister, 2006; Dutta, Gervey, Chan, Chou, & Ditchman, 2008).

For example, Table 25.2 shows the same results drawn from an analysis of 2008 RSA-911 data. Of consumers with their own IPE, 64% received VR counseling and guidance services. Of those recipients, 60% exited the VR agency with a successful employment outcome. Rehabilitation technology, on the job supports, and job placement services

Table 25.1 Type of services recorded in the RSA-911 Data System

Type of Services	Descriptions
Assessment Services	Assessment means services provided and activities performed to determine an individual's eligibility for vocational rehabilitation (VR) services, to assign an individual to a priority category of a state VR agency that operates under an order of selection, and/or to determine the nature and scope of VR services to be included in the Individualized Plan for Employment (IPE). Include here trial work experiences and extended evaluation.
Diagnosis and Treatment Services	Diagnosis and treatment for mental and emotional disorders and treatments for medical or medically related rehabilitation services (e.g., corrective surgery, dentistry, physical therapy).
Vocational Rehab Counseling and Guidance Services	Vocational rehabilitation counseling and guidance means discrete therapeutic counseling and guidance services that are necessary for an individual to achieve an employment outcome. This service is distinct from the general counseling and guidance relationship that exists between the counselor and the individual during the entire rehabilitation process.
College or University Training Services	Full-time or part-time academic training above the high school level leading to a degree (associate, baccalaureate, graduate, or professional), a certificate, or other recognized educational credential.
Occupational/Vocational Training Services	Occupational, vocational, or job skill training provided by a community college and/or business, vocational/trade or technical school to prepare students for gainful employment in a recognized occupation, not leading to an academic degree or certification.
On-the-job Training	Training in specific job skills by a prospective employer. Generally, the individual is paid during this training and will remain in the same or a similar job upon successful completion. Also includes apprenticeship-training programs conducted or sponsored by an employer, a group of employers, or a joint apprenticeship committee representing both employers and a union.
Basic Remedial or Literacy Services	Literacy training or training provided to remediate basic academic skills that are needed to function on the job in the competitive labor market.
Job Readiness Training Services	Training to prepare an individual for the world of work (e.g., appropriate work behaviors, getting to work on time, appropriate dress and grooming, increasing productivity).
Augmentative Skills Training Services	Disability-related augmentative skills training includes but is not limited to: orientation and mobility; rehabilitation teaching; training in the use of low vision aids; Braille; speech reading; sign language; and cognitive training/retraining.
Miscellaneous Training Services	Any training not recorded in one of the other categories listed, including GED or high school training leading to a diploma.
Job Search Assistance Services	Job search activities support and assist a consumer in searching for an appropriate job. Job search assistance may include help in resume preparation, identifying appropriate job opportunities, developing interview skills, and making contacts with companies on behalf of the consumer.
Job Placement Assistance Services	Job placement assistance is a referral to a specific job resulting in an interview, whether or not the individual obtained the job.
On-the-job Supports Services	Support services provided to an individual who has been placed in employment in order to stabilize the placement and enhance job retention. Such services include job coaching, follow-up and follow-along, and job retention services.

(continued)

Table 25.1 (Continued)

Type of Services	Descriptions
Transportation Services	Transportation, including adequate training in the use of public transportation vehicles and systems, means travel and related expenses that are necessary to enable an applicant or eligible individual to participate in a VR service.
Maintenance Services	Maintenance means monetary support provided for those expenses such as food, shelter, and clothing that are in excess of the normal expenses of the individual, and that are necessitated by the individual's participation in an assessment for determining eligibility and VR needs or while receiving services under an IPE.
Rehabilitation Technology Services	Rehabilitation technology means the systematic application of technologies, engineering methodologies, or scientific principles to meet the needs of, and address the barriers confronted by individuals with disabilities in areas that include education, rehabilitation, employment, transportation, independent living, and recreation.
Reader Services	Reader services are for individuals who cannot read print because of blindness or other disability.
Interpreter Services	Interpreter services are sign language or oral interpretation services for individuals who are deaf or hard of hearing and tactile interpretation services for individuals who are deaf-blind.
Personal Attendant Services	Personal attendant services are those personal services that an attendant performs for an individual with a disability such as bathing, feeding, dressing, providing mobility and transportation, etc.
Technical Assistance Services	Technical assistance and other consultation services provided to conduct market analyses, to develop business plans, and to provide resources to individuals in the pursuit of self-employment, telecommuting, and small business operation outcomes.
Information and Referral Services	Information and referral services are provided to individuals who need services from other agencies (through cooperative agreements) not available through the VR program.
Other Services	This category is for all other VR services that cannot be recorded elsewhere. Included here are occupational licenses, tools and equipment, initial stocks and supplies. Medical care for acute conditions arising during rehabilitation and constituting a barrier to the achievement of an employment outcome is also included in this category.

From Rehabilitation Services Administration. (2009). *Reporting manual for the case service report (RSA-911)*. Washington, DC: U.S. Department of Education, Office of Special Education and Rehabilitation Services.

were the top three services related to successful employment outcomes, which is consistent with prior research findings. However, only 10% of the consumers received rehabilitation technology services, so a careful interpretation is necessary in terms of generalizability of the results. Odds ratios for three types of services show their association with the VR outcomes, which indicates that provision of rehabilitation technology, job placement services, and on-the-job supports increased the likelihood of obtaining a successful employment outcome at closure for VR consumers by 2.7 times, 1.9 times, and 1.7 times, respectively. Note that seven types of services were utilized by less than 5% of

the consumers with an IPE, excluded for the binary logistic regression analysis.

It is also interesting to see that receiving transportation and job readiness services were less related to an employment outcome, which does not imply that transportation and job readiness services are not necessary to achieve a successful outcome. As shown in the Rehabilitation Act, as amended, VR services are designed to help people with disabilities to obtain or retain employment based on their strengths and needs. This rather suggests that people with transportation problems have a lower probability of achieving employment than do people without transportation problems. Thus, providing

Table 25.2 Percentages of consumers who received vocational rehabilitation services and achieved a successful employment outcome

	Percent of Consumers with IPE who Received Services	Percent of Consumers with a Successful Employment Outcome	Odds Ratio
Vocational Rehabilitation Counseling and Guidance Services	64.4%	60.0%	1.20
Assessment Services	63.8%	57.8%	.97
Diagnosis and Treatment Services	43.8%	62.9%	1.41
Job Placement Assistance Services	34.3%	66.8%	1.86
Transportation Services	32.8%	56.5%	.77
Other Services	29.3%	61.1%	1.09
Job Search Assistance Services	27.3%	62.3%	0.92
On-the-job Supports Services	18.1%	67.9%	1.68
Information and Referral Services	17.0%	61.7%	1.11
Maintenance Services	15.8%	64.5%	1.42
College or University Training Services	14.3%	53.9%	.90
Job Readiness Training Services	14.3%	58.1%	.84
Occupational/Vocational Training Services	12.9%	57.1%	1.05
Miscellaneous Training Services	11.9%	61.3%	1.05
Rehabilitation Technology Services	10.0%	76.4%	2.70
Technical Assistance Services	3.3%	68.1%	–
On-the-job Training	3.1%	70.9%	–
Augmentative Skills Training Services	3.1%	66.6%	–
Basic Remedial or Literacy Services	1.6%	57.5%	–
Interpreter Services	1.3%	63.6%	–
Reader Services	0.3%	63.6%	–
Personal Attendant Services	0.3%	59.0%	–

From 2008 RSA 911 data; IPE, Individualized Program for Employment

transportation or job readiness services is important, which indicates that an individualized and consumer-driven approach is crucial. In fact, VR participants with individual placement plans tend to be more successful, have more realistic expectations of the VR process, and find placements that match their skills and desires more quickly (Fraser, Vandergoot, Thomas, & Wagner, 2004).

Job placement assistance is defined as a referral to a specific job resulting in an interview, whether or not the individual obtained the job. On-the-job support is designed to stabilize the placement and enhance job retention through job coaching, follow-up and follow-along, and job retention services (Rehabilitation Services Administration, 2009). In other words, help finding a job and the provision of continuous supports at the workplace based on an individual's needs are crucial for people with disabilities to obtain and retain employment.

Current Issues and Focus in Employment Initiatives

Employment is a vital pathway for all individuals to help achieve full social inclusion and increase participation in the community, yet people with disabilities continue to encounter multiple barriers to this pathway. Leff and Warner (2006) identified two major obstacles to employment for persons with disabilities: disincentives to work due to the disability benefits system and the lack of suitable work opportunities. In this section, we will discuss two new efforts and strategies to overcome these obstacles: Partnership Plus and Customized Employment.

Supports for Social Security Beneficiaries

Numerous studies and public reports have documented major discrepancies in employment outcomes and quality of employment between Social Security beneficiaries and nonbeneficiaries (Boutin & Wilson, 2009; Cantalano et al., 2006; Chan et al., 2006; Dutta et al., 2008; Stapleton & Erickson, 2005). According to FY 2008 RSA-911 data on VR consumers at the time of closure, 31% of Social Security beneficiaries attained employment as compared to 44% of nonbeneficiaries. The average weekly earnings were $321 (median = $180) for beneficiaries, as compared to $403 (median = $340) for nonbeneficiaries. Mean hourly income showed a $2.14 difference between beneficiaries ($9.37) and nonbeneficiaries ($11.51). These disparities speak to the potential barrier of the SSA disability standard and the unintended consequence of public policies that do not support a common work agenda.

The Ticket to Work, the Work Incentives Improvement Act of 1999, and the Workforce Investment Act (PL 105–220) were passed to address these gaps and to provide more opportunities for SSA beneficiaries to work in the community and achieve self-sufficiency with less risk of losing their current benefits. Under the original Ticket regulations, a beneficiary was not able to use a Ticket to receive services from more than one employment network (EN) agency since the SSA adopted the Cost Reimbursement (CR) program, designed to make payments to either a state VR agency or another EN. The Ticket to Work program recently created a new service delivery model, Partnership Plus, to expand the scope of services for Social Security beneficiaries. Under the new regulations, VR agencies no longer need a Ticket assignment to submit a CR claim. Thus, Partnership Plus allows a beneficiary to receive VR services to meet his or her intensive, up-front service needs and, after the VR case is closed, assign his or her Ticket to an EN for ongoing support services or job retention services. This program also creates opportunities for state VR agencies to partner with approved ENs to meet the service and support needs of beneficiaries after they go to work (Social Security Administration, 2008).

Customized Employment

The Rehabilitation Act of 1973 established a priority to serve people with severe disabilities. For persons with severe disabilities, supported employment has frequently been implemented as an alternative strategy (Wehman & Kregel, 1992). However, there have been some issues regarding supported employment. Wehmeyer (2001) found that individuals who were placed using supported employment services were earning less than minimum wage and more likely placed in group settings rather than in individualized placements. In addition, people with severe disabilities were more often placed in jobs driven by the local labor market rather than in negotiated positions based on the individuals' preferences and choices (Inge, 2006).

In 2002, the Department of Labor's Office of Disability Employment Policy (ODEP) developed the concept of customized employment to better serve people with disabilities through the One-Stop delivery system. This was established to provide universal access to comprehensive services, information, and resources to improve the employment and career advancement of people with disabilities.

This consumer-directed service usually starts with the development of an employment plan based on a person's interests, dreams, and passions related to living and working in the community. Next, one or more potential employers, consistent with the employment goals, are identified. A preliminary proposal is developed for presentation to the employer, which should meet both the employment needs of the applicant and the employer's actual business needs. Based on the negotiation, the staff develops the plan and assists the consumer throughout the hiring process. Follow-up services are offered, when appropriate (Inge, 2007; Revell & Inge, 2007). Customized employment assumes the provision of reasonable accommodations and supports necessary for the individual to perform the functions of the job, and these are individually negotiated and developed (Federal Register, June 26, 2002, Vol. 67. No. 123 pp. 43154 -43149).

Since 2002, customized employment has been utilized as an employment option by many states and different agencies in collaboration with the One-Stop centers across the nation (Griffin, Hammis, Geary, & Sullivan, 2008). As most of the outcomes were anecdotal and qualitative using small size of samples without a control group (Citron et al., 2008; Elinson, Frey, Li, Palan, & Horne, 2008; Luecking, Cuozzo, Leedy, & Seleznow, 2008; Phillips et al., 2009), it seems premature to draw conclusions about its effectiveness. However, a study conducted by Roger, Lavin, Tran, Gantenbein, and Sharpe (2008) appears to show promising impact on a range of customized employment strategies. Thus, better designed research with well-established protocols will be necessary. Based on the current prevailing philosophy and concept, however, people with disabilities would benefit from this consumer-directed approach to increase their participation in the world of work and their community, especially those with newly acquired disabilities.

Importance of Population of Focus and Employment Issues
National Prevalence Rates of People with Disabilities

To successfully deliver rehabilitation services, it is important to understand the characteristics of people with disabilities and the personal and environmental factors that may influence their employment outcomes. Currently, the Census Bureau-administered Current Population Survey (CPS) and American Community Survey (ACS), the National Health Interview Survey (NHIS), and the Survey of Income Program Participation (SIPP) all collect information on disability via questions about functional limitations, sensory disabilities, mental disabilities, limitations in activities of daily living (ADLs), limitations in instrumental activities of daily living (IADLs), and work limitations, although definitions vary (Burkhauser & Houtenville, 2010; Burkhauser, Houtenville, & Wittenburg, 2003; She & Stapleton, 2006).

Employment Participation Rates of People with Disabilities

These datasets also provide national comparison statistics on workforce participation and document the significant employment disparity between people with disabilities and their nondisabled peers.

According to ACS data, in 2008, an estimated 39.5% of noninstitutionalized working age (21–64) people with a disability, regardless of gender, race, ethnicity, or education level, were employed, compared to 79.9% for those without disabilities. In the United States, in 2008, the median annual household income of households that included any working age (ages 21–64) people with a disability was $39,600, compared to $61,200 for households without any person with disability. This translates to a significantly higher percentage of Americans with disabilities living below the poverty rate and with lower overall household incomes, compared to their nondisabled peers. In the United States, in 2008, an estimated 25.3% of noninstitutionalized persons aged 21–64 years with a disability were living below the poverty line, compared to 9.6% of those without disabilities (Erickson, Lee, & Von Schrader, 2010a,b).

Need for Enhanced Measures of Employment Outcomes

These statistics are a dramatic documentation of the continuing economic disparities for people with disabilities, and they make a compelling argument for the consideration of vocational training and efforts to maximize social inclusion for people with disabilities. This continuing disparity also highlights the additional need to refine the definitions of quality indicators of employment outcomes for people with disabilities. Historically, the VR system used placement in a job lasting at least 90 days as its indicator of success. In 2000, the Rehabilitation Services Administration (RSA) moved to establish performance indicators for the VR program that included outcome and related measures of program performance (U.S. Department of Education, 2000).

Vocational rehabilitation's effect on employment is measured by three primary indicators of successful outcomes: placement in competitive employment (percent of employment outcomes that are competitive employment), the significance of the disability (percentage of persons with competitive employment outcomes who had significant disabilities), and earnings ratio (the ratio of the average hourly wage of VR client service recipients to the average state hourly wage). Further refinement of ways to measure the quality of an employment outcome are needed, so that outcomes can be compared not only across the state VR system, but also across other employment service systems for people with disabilities.

One tool frequently discussed as a possibility for measuring rehabilitation outcomes is the

International Classification of Functioning, Disability, and Health (ICF; Bruyère, 2005; Bruyère, Van Looy, & Peterson, 2005; Fedeyko & Lollar, 2003; Iezzoni & Greenberg, 2003; Peterson, 2005; Üstün, Chatterji, Kostansjek, & Bickenbach, 2003). The ICF is the World Health Organization framework for measuring health and disability at both individual and population levels. The ICF consists of four main areas: body function, body structures, activities and participation, and environmental factors. This classification system aims to provide a standard definition of health and health conditions that can be used in any discipline or any nation, and it moves those definitions away from a medically oriented, diseased-based classification toward identifying "components of health." By shifting the focus from causes to impacts, it places all health conditions on an equal footing, allowing them to be compared using a common metric. The ICF includes not only functional components, but also contextual factors that allow the ICF to be used to record the impact of the environment on an individual's functioning (Peterson & Rosenthal, 2005; World Health Organization, 2001). These areas include vocational training along with apprenticeship, acquiring, keeping, and terminating a job, and both remunerative and nonremunerative employment (WHO, 2001).

Participation is a major theme of the ICF, providing a framework that can be used to include social integration and inclusion factors in an assessment of employment outcomes. Participation can be seen in people's support and relationships; in the attitudes of their acquaintances, peers, colleagues, and neighbors; in the attitudes of people in authority over the person; and in the attitudes of their subordinates. This can be a most useful tool for rehabilitation psychology practice when measuring rehabilitation outcomes along the dimensions of employment and community inclusion and social participation.

The ICF model might be applied as a schema to refine our understanding of the success of the job placement process in attaching the individual to the labor force and his or her employment and community/social context. Indicators of successful employment participation that fit into ICF categories would allow fields and programs related to employment to speak a common language and to draw connections to the other components of the ICF, such as body functions, body structures, environmental factors, or the other categories and chapters of the activities and participation component.

Consideration of the individual's social participation in the workforce leads us to a discussion of workplace culture and the environmental factors reflected in the ICF model. The usefulness of this model to rehabilitation psychology might be more fully realized by including in the framework (in addition to remuneration and long-term job security) the social and cultural context of the work environment. The environmental factors to be considered could be as straightforward as the health and safety considerations of the work environment (standards established through occupational safety and health), or, they might also be cultural and qualitative in nature, such as relationships with supervisor and co-workers (Bruyère, 2005).

Overview of Social Inclusion
Definition of Social Inclusion and Historical and Philosophical Roots

People experience psychological, physical, and emotional benefits when they can see that they are making contributions to the greater community (Wolfensberger, 1972). Social integration and inclusion is the means through which people interact, form connections, and give and receive validation (Wolfensberger, 1998). Community inclusion and community integration are constructs that challenge ideologies that promote the exclusion and marginalization of people who are vulnerable to stigma and discrimination (Wolfensberger, 1998). Practical application of the new paradigm of social inclusion may seem to many practitioners to be out of reach, but it is not. Continued striving toward this outcome is imperative.

Contemporary trends in the field of rehabilitation are placing emphasis on discovering and capitalizing on the unique strengths, skills, interests, and capacities of individuals with disabilities (Metts, 2000).

Contributing Trends in U.S. Legislation and Policy Evolution Over Time

The earliest disability policies in developed countries focused heavily on a medical model of disability (Blessing, Golden, & Bruyère, 2009). These policies fostered resource allocation that supported restorative technologies, community participation, and citizenship for certain groups. Disability groups that would not benefit from a medical/restorative approach, such as individuals with developmental disabilities and mental illness, were institutionalized and not afforded the same rights and privileges to community living (Blatt, 1965). Such policies perpetuated a segregated infrastructure of services and supports more focused at managing risk and protecting the public from these populations of people.

The deinstitutionalization movement of the 1960s was in response to the significant human rights violations experienced by people in institutions. It was also recognized that the current paradigm of disability did not value full community participation and citizenship for all. Unfortunately, the movement of people out of large institutions was the whole of the agenda, without much planning for meaningful community-based alternatives. The result was a proliferation of smaller but nevertheless segregated programs and services (Blessing et al., 2009). These efforts continued to be guided by a medical approach that established a continuum-based paradigm of services and supports that established a path from segregation to integration that was rarely, if ever, traveled. The medical model, based on an assumption that disability is an intrinsic characteristic of the individual, was first challenged by Nagi (1965, 1991), and his alternate model has grown in acceptance, as reflected in the ICF model (WHO, 2001, 2002). In Nagi's model, disability is represented as a movement through four stages: pathology (presence of a physical or mental condition), impairment (physiological, anatomical, or mental loss of functional capacity), functional limitation (limitation in the performance or completion of a fundamental activity), and disability (limitation in performance of expected social activities). This creates a social construct that views disability as an interaction between a person's health condition and the physical and social environment—making disability a function of society. Hahn (1986) describes a "socio-political definition of disability," which recognizes that improvements in the status of people with disabilities will require alterations to the environment, more so than any changes to their physical or economic skills. This model "implies that disability stems from the failure of a structured social environment to adjust to the needs and aspirations of citizens with disabilities rather than from the inability of a disabled individual to adapt to the demands of society" (Hahn, 1986, p. 132).

With the increasing cultural acceptance of this construct of disability has come growing discontent with the existing institutional nature of the human service delivery system and awareness of the need for substantive reform (Humphrey, 2000; McConnell, 1999; Oliver, 1996). Influencing this growing movement for change was the work of Wolf Wolfensberger and his principle of normalization (Nirje, 1980; Wolfensberger, 1972), and, later, the introduction of his theory of social role valorization (Wolfensberger, 1998). Wolfensberger's work set an important tone for the evolution of human services, recognizing that the existing paradigm of services and supports was static and did nothing to ensure that people with disabilities were seen in valued community roles commensurate with their nondisabled peers. The pairing of the social construct model with the underlying principles of Wolfensberger's work created a platform for provoking widespread change in the field of disability rehabilitation. His theory of social role valorization held that acquiring such valued social roles would require much greater emphasis on discovering and amplifying individuals' competence and leveraging their unique innate abilities to make a valued contribution in their community.

Current Issues and Focus in Social Inclusion

Pressure from federal and state governmental agencies for community-based, person-centered programs and services has been steadily increasing over the past two decades (National Council on Disability, 1986; New Freedom Commission on Mental Health, 2005). Individuals with disabilities, their families, and advocates are raising their expectations for, at best, primary or at least equal authority in the making of decisions that affect their lives (Mount, 1990).

The disability rights movement has done much to advance the field of rehabilitation services for individuals with a disability. It has successfully embedded into the disability culture key concepts of self-determination, people-first language, and individualized support that are essential to enhancing the quality of life experienced by people who live with disability and disability-related circumstances. Yet, despite good intentions, the past 20 years or more has made little advancement in devising innovative strategies and resource allocations that promote and sustain the authentic social integration and inclusion of individuals with disabilities within the mainstream community.

The shift from a traditional service delivery model to a model of social inclusion that emphasizes self-determination and self-direction will require a multidimensional shift in the role that rehabilitation plays in enhancing the quality of life experienced by people with a disability. At the core level, basic quality of life domains include life satisfaction and psychological well-being, physical wellness, social and interpersonal well-being, financial and material well-being, employment and productivity, and functional ability (Bishop, 2005). At a much deeper level, attention must be paid to ensuring that the individual is at the forefront of hope-inspired decision-making around aspirations such as where and with whom to live, meaningful employment, purposeful education, health and wellness management, personal relationships, community inclusion, and financial management.

Over the past 100 years of disability and rehabilitation policy, the U.S. system has been built on five pillars that have remained relatively constant—culture, policy, infrastructure, payment, and quality (Golden et al., 2008). The first two pillars serve to create the conditions under which the other three pillars are defined. Our disability *culture* has been primarily defined over the past few decades by the struggles we have faced in trying to move away from a medical/expert model and establish the civil rights of people with disabilities. Disability *policy* continues to reflect the current tone of culture and creates the structure or systems by which our services and supports are designed and implemented. *Infrastructure* is the vehicle by which we operationalize policy and includes the sanctioned organizations charged with service and support delivery, as well as the designated agencies responsible for policing implementation (Golden et al., 2008). We define *payment* as the package of incentives provided to put the infrastructure in motion. The final pillar, *quality*, has typically been defined by the extent to which we have achieved compliance with statute or policy. Figure 25.1 presents the current paradigm across the five pillars. Whereas culture and policy have evolved over time, little has changed across infrastructure, payment, and quality, thus creating an increasing tension between the two factions.

Our values, beliefs, and underlying principles regarding the importance of empowerment, choice, integration, and valued community roles have made only incremental progress over the past few decades toward realigning "systems" to "people" across the latter three pillars. This figure illustrates that people with disabilities, although increasingly engaged as part of the culture and policy pillars, still have played too modest a role in the designing and defining of needed infrastructure, payments, and employment quality.

Interestingly, as one looks back over time, the infrastructure, payment, and quality pillars have remained relatively constant. Although, through the decades of the 1970s and 1980s, we saw culture and policy support the development of the independent living and empowerment movement—as well as innovations in integrated employment models such as supported employment, inclusive, and mainstreamed education, and person-centeredness—these efforts merely served as enhancements to our current paradigm and were simply layered onto the existing infrastructure, payment, and quality pillars. People with disabilities are no more integrated into society today than they were 20 years ago.

Further complicating these issues is the fact that, over time, service delivery structures and

CULTURE	POLICY	INFRA-STRUCTURE	PAYMENT	QUALITY
☐ Demand for civil rights ☐ Desire for full community participation and citizenship ☐ Growing consumer voice although often outweighed by other interest	☐ Civil rights & disability non-discrimination legislation ☐ Desire for full community participation and citizenship ☐ National agenda for disability reform	☐ Medical model ☐ Expert-controlled ☐ System-focused and responsive ☐ Care and control of consumers	☐ Payment for services and products not outcomes ☐ Guided by voucher for services and supports ☐ Limited incentives to both consumer and provider for change	☐ Statutory and regulatory compliance ☐ Limited consumer feedback regarding overall satisfaction with services and input regarding continuous quality
PUBLIC		SYSTEM		

Figure 25.1 The five pillars of the disability system. From Golden, T. P., Blessing, C., & Bruyere, S.M. (2008). *Recommendations to advance person-centered adult day services and supports in Ireland: An international review of progressive policies and innovative practices.* Report to the Health Services Executive on behalf of the National Working Group on the review of Adult Day Services for People with Disabilities. Ithaca, NY: Cornell University, ILR School, Employment, and Disability Institute.

organizations become embedded, eroding the competitive edge and demand-driven nature of services and supports provided. Across the board, the disability paradigm is deeply entrenched in the system side of the five pillars—they are the foundation upon which it has been built. Part of the challenge faced by change advocates is recognizing that the system was created because the public side of the five pillars demanded it. This expression and investment of the public often is the primary obstacle to real change. When opportunity for change presents itself, the current system and the proposed reforms are measured against one another, and more times than not a choice is made to not jeopardize what exists for what could be—even when our values and principles are more aligned with the proposed reform. This typically results in a compromise whereby we minimize the reform and settle for potential enhancements to the existing system. Recognizing this behavior, the key then becomes creating a vehicle for the public to express its values and preferences (culture), so that policy makers can reflect them in changed infrastructure, payment, and quality.

The experience of modernizing human services toward more person-centered approaches starts with the best of intentions, usually initiated through a public edict, executive order, or statutory or legislative requirement. It is not enough, however, to simply articulate the principles and values from which it is hoped systems change will miraculously flow. This approach, although well-intentioned, does nothing to change the level of entrenchment that exists in the current service delivery paradigm. While practitioners and consumers alike embrace the general themes and values being touted, little to no effort goes into truly transforming the system-driven paradigm into an individual-driven one. Services and supports are still demanded by culture, designed through policy, delivered through infrastructure, and incented through payment, and success is still gauged by compliance with statute.

As rehabilitation psychologists consider the implications of the current state of the system and their role in promoting a construct of social inclusion, it is important to recognize that it is not enough to merely provide each consumer of rehabilitation psychology services the opportunity to develop an individualized plan. Rehabilitation psychologists must develop accessible, affordable, and locally relevant service and support strategies that empower individuals throughout the stages of their life to put those plans into action, be supported in making choices about the services and support they feel they need to achieve their goals and aspirations, and have quality defined by their lack of satisfaction with outcomes achieved as a result of their efforts.

Conclusion
Implications for Rehabilitation Psychologists

Work holds important social value and creates an opportunity to connect with community networks and develop an individual's healthy sense of self as a contributing person in society. Being without meaningful work carries far more than economic implications. Work is only one part of being valued and respected within society, but it is an important route to social inclusion. The disability statistics on prevalence rates of people with disabilities, as well as documentation of their continuing disparity in employment and household income rates, confirm the compelling need to focus on and thereby improve economic outcomes for this significant part of the American, as well as global population. This chapter has focused on the critical connection between vocational training, meaningful paid work, and the ability of a person with a disability to achieve community integration and social inclusion, thereby leading to these desired economic and social outcomes. We here summarize the implications of these principles and recommend systems and individual professional practice approaches for rehabilitation psychology practice, training, and research.

Rehabilitation Psychology Practice

Our premise is that the process of intentional social inclusion and community integration of people with disabilities provides a framework through which rehabilitation psychologists can work with individuals to develop and build capacity for interpersonal connectedness and citizenship. We have provided information about the principles of social inclusion and community participation, their historical evolution, and contemporary execution to inform rehabilitation psychology practice and advocacy on behalf of individuals with disabilities and thereby encourage inclusion.

The principles of self-determination, client-centered planning, and empowerment must now be the undergirding philosophy of every segment of rehabilitation psychology service delivery. When we ourselves as practitioners adopt such a philosophy, we not only convey the dignity of choice and belief in inherent value upon the individual, but also demonstrate the importance of this stance to family members and others on the rehabilitation team, as well as to community members that we interface with on behalf of the individual. Social inclusion and community participation does not start at the hospital or intermediate care facility exit, but rather as a philosophy that must permeate the entire rehabilitation experience of the individual and his or her family.

In addition, the return-to-community planning process should include an expectation for a return to work or initiation of real vocational outcomes for each rehabilitation psychology service recipient to the maximum extent possible. It is critical that rehabilitation psychologists integrate the expectation of obtaining or returning to meaningful employment and other important roles of community membership into their individualized treatment planning. Rehabilitation psychologists must develop service and support strategies that empower individuals throughout the stages of their life to put those plans into action, provide support to service recipients in their making choices about the services and support they feel they need to achieve their goals and aspirations, and have quality of outcomes defined by their satisfaction, or lack thereof, with the outcomes that their efforts produce. This consumer-directed service usually starts with the development of an employment plan based on a person's interests, dreams, and passions related to living and working in the community. Such a plan must also identify specific functional support needs, including the identification of accommodations and assistive technologies that will enable the person to successfully navigate barriers that would otherwise prevent full participation in work and the other key areas that constitute social inclusion.

A plan that will lead to successful employment outcomes needs to also take into consideration the reality of local communities, and the next step is to identify one or more potential employers consistent with these employment goals. As discussed, individualized or customized employment may be the necessary approach for an individual with significant disabilities. Information on the state-federal VR system, as well as that of the workforce development system, has been provided in an effort to familiarize rehabilitation psychologists with the current governmental infrastructure in place to move people with disabilities toward economic independence. To support improved vocational outcomes among people with disabilities, it is important for rehabilitation psychologist practitioners to understand the specific scope of services provided by the VR program that

might prove most beneficial to their service consumers, in order to create linkages and partnerships that ensure access to these services and supports. An important nexus to effective return to community and vocational productivity in this process is in partnering with local agencies, service providers, and individual rehabilitation counseling professionals.

Rehabilitation Psychology Training

Both the tenets of social inclusion and community participation *and* the importance of vocational training and employment outcomes must be a part of both rehabilitation psychology pre-service and post-service training. Increasingly, we see the importance of empowerment discussed in textbooks for rehabilitation psychology, but vigilance to assure integration into coursework in a meaningful way is needed. Since many rehabilitation psychology practitioners are either fully immersed in or tangentially influenced by the field and professions of our medical and health practitioner colleagues, we have an opportunity to assist in transcending the medical model and conceptualization of disability to a more empowering and individually centered approach that will systemically change systems and philosophies while empowering individuals.

Continuing education opportunities for rehabilitation psychologists should also include a focus on the importance of seeking meaningful vocational outcomes as a part of the rehabilitation planning process. These courses may be very specific, such as vocational assessment approaches to help clarify vocational interests and abilities and targeted interview techniques. But more general courses in the importance of work to the individual's well-being and related community services and supports that can enhance the identification, securing, and maintenance of successful work outcomes should also be a part of the focus.

Rehabilitation Psychology Research

Finally, there is a role for rehabilitation psychology in many of the remaining questions about quality of outcomes in vocational goals for people with disabilities. Further refinement of ways to measure the quality of an employment outcome are needed, so that outcomes can be compared not only across the state VR system, but also across other employment service systems for people with disabilities. Another area for consideration is how our profession might apply the ICF model as a schema to refine our understanding of the success of the job placement process by attaching the individual to the labor force and his or her employment and community/social context. The usefulness of this model to rehabilitation psychology might be more fully realized by including in the framework—in addition to remuneration and long-term job security—the social and cultural context of the work environment. There is much work to be conducted here, and rehabilitation psychologists' expertise and experience will be most critical allies in this search for new knowledge in these areas.

Notes

1. 34 CFR 361.18 mandates a comprehensive system of personnel development requiring that each state vocational rehabilitation agency must complete a state plan that describes the procedures and activities the state agency will undertake to establish and maintain a comprehensive system of personnel development designed to ensure an adequate supply of qualified rehabilitation personnel, including professionals and paraprofessionals, for the designated state unit.

References

Alade, E. (2004). Community-based vocational rehabilitation (CBVR) for people with disabilities: Experiences from a pilot project in Nigeria. *British Journal of Special Education, 31*(3), 143–149.

Bishop, M. (2005). Quality of life and psychosocial adaptation to chronic illness and acquired disability: A conceptual and theoretical synthesis. *Journal of Rehabilitation, 71*(2), 5–13.

Blatt, B. (1965). *Christmas in purgatory.* Syracuse, NY: Syracuse University, Center on Human Policy.

Blessing, C., Golden, T., & Bruyère, S. (2009). Evolution of U.S. employment and disability policies and practices: Implications for global implementation of person-centered planning. In C. Marshall, E. Kendall, M. Banks, & R. Gover (Eds.), *Disability: Insights from across fields and around the world, : Vol. 3. Responses: Practice, Legal, and Political Framework.* (pp. 1–16). Westport, CT: Praeger.

Bolton, B. F., Bellini, J. L., & Brookings, J. B. (2000). Predicting client employment outcomes from personal history, functional limitations, and rehabilitation services. *Rehabilitation Counseling Bulletin, 44*(1), 10–21.

Booz Allen Hamilton (2009). The path to healthy homecomings: Findings from the Community Reintegration Summit: Service members returning to civilian life. McLean, VA: Author. Retrieved from http://www.boozallen.com/media/file/Path_To_Healthy_Homecomings.pdf

Boutin, D. D., & Wilson, K. (2009). An analysis of vocational rehabilitation services for consumers with hearing impairments who received college or university training. *Rehabilitation Counseling Bulletin, 52*, 156–166.

Bruyère, S. (2005). Using the International Classification of Functioning, Disability, and Health (ICF) to promote employment and community integration in rehabilitation. *Rehabilitation Education, 19*(2 & 3), 105–117.

Bruyère, S., Van Looy, S., & Golden, T. (2010). Legislation and rehabilitation service delivery. In S. Flanagan, H. Zaretsky, & A. Moroz (Eds.), *Medical aspects of disability: A handbook for the rehabilitation professional* (4th ed., pp 669–686). New York: Springer Publishing.

Bruyère, S., Van Looy, S., & Peterson, D. (2005). The International classification of functioning, disability and health (ICF): Contemporary literature overview. *Rehabilitation Psychology, 50*(2), 113–121.

Burkhauser, R., & Houtenville, A. (2010). Employment among working age people with disabilities: What the latest data can tell us. In E. Szymanski, & R. Parker (Eds.), *Work and disability: Contexts, issues, and strategies for enhancing employment outcomes for people with disabilities* (pp. 49–86). Austin, TX: Pro-Ed.

Burkhauser, R.V., Houtenville, A. J., & Wittenburg, D. (2003). A user guide to current statistics on the employment of people with disabilities. In R. V. Burkhauser, & D. Stapleton (Eds.), *The decline in the employment of people with disabilities: A policy puzzle* (pp. 23–86). Kalamazoo, MI: W. E. Upjohn Institute for Employment Research.

Cantalano, D., Pereira, A., Wu, M., Ho, H., & Chan, F. (2006). Service patterns related to successful employment outcomes of persons with traumatic brain injury in vocational rehabilitation. *NeuroRehabilitation, 21*, 279–293.

Chan, F., Cheing, G., Chan, J. Y. C., Rosenthal, D. A., & Chronister, J. (2006). Predicting employment outcomes of rehabilitation clients with orthopedic disabilities: A CHAID analysis. *Disability and Rehabilitation, 28*(5), 257–270.

Charlton, J. (1998). *Nothing about us without us: Disability oppression and empowerment.* Berkley, CA: University of California Press.

Citron, T., Brooks-Lane, N., Crandell, D., Brady, K., Coopers, M., & Revell, R. (2008). A revolution in the employment process of individuals with disabilities: Customized employment as the catalyst for system change. *Journal of Vocational Rehabilitation, 28*, 169–179.

Crocker, J., & Major, B. (1989). Social stigma and self-esteem: The self-protective properties of stigma. *Psychological Review, 96*(4), 608–630.

Doctor, J. N., Castro, J., Temkin, N. R., Fraser, R. T., Machamer, J. E., & Dikmen, S. S. (2005). Workers' risk of unemployment after traumatic brain injury. *Journal of the International Neuropsychological Society, 11*, 747–752.

Dutta, A., Gervey, R., Chan, F., Chou, C., & Ditchman, N. (2008). Vocational rehabilitation services and employment outcomes for people with disabilities: A United States study. *Journal of Occupational Rehabilitation, 18*, 326–334.

Elinson, L., Frey, W., Li, T., Palan, M., & Horne, R. (2008). Evaluation of customized employment in building the capacity of the workforce development system. *Journal of Vocational Rehabilitation, 28*, 141–158.

Elliott, T., & Leung, P. (2005). Vocational rehabilitation: history and practice. In W. B. Walsh & M. Savickas (Eds.), *Handbook of Vocational Psychology* (3rd ed., pp. 319–343). New York: Lawrence Erlbaum Press.

Erickson, W., Lee, C., & von Schrader, S. (2010a). *2008 Disability status report: The United States.* Ithaca, NY: Cornell University Rehabilitation Research and Training Center on Disability Demographics and Statistics. Retrieved from www.disabilitystatistics.org

Erickson, W., Lee, C., & von Schrader, S. (2010b). *Disability statistics from the 2008 American Community Survey (ACS) and Current Population Survey (CPS).* Ithaca, NY: Cornell University Rehabilitation Research and Training Center on Disability Demographics and Statistics (StatsRRTC). Retrieved Aug 04, 2010 from www.disabilitystatistics.org

Evans, J., & Repper, J. (2000). Employment, social inclusion and mental health. *Journal of Psychiatric and Mental Health, 7*, 15–24.

Fedeyko, H., & Lollar, D. J. (2003). Classifying disability data: A fresh, integrative perspective. Using survey data to study disability: Results from the NHIS Survey on Disability. *Social Science and Disability, 3*, 55–72.

Fraser, R., Vandergoot, D., Thomas, D., & Wagner, C. (2004). Employment outcomes research in vocational rehabilitation: Implications for rehabilitation counselor (RC) training. *Journal of Vocational Rehabilitation, 20*, 135–142.

Gobelet, C., Luthi, F., Al-Khodairy, A. T., & Chamberlain, M. A. (2007). Vocational rehabilitation: A multidisciplinary intervention. *Disability and Rehabilitation, 29*(17), 1405–1410.

Golden, T. P., Blessing, C., & Bruyère, S. M. (2008). *Recommendations to advance person-centered adult day services and supports in Ireland: An international review of progressive policies and innovative practices.* Report to the Health Services Executive on behalf of the National Working Group on the review of Adult Day Services for People with Disabilities. Ithaca, NY: Cornell University, ILR School, Employment and Disability Institute.

Gorden, W., & Brown, M. (1997). Community integration of individuals with spinal cord injuries. *American Rehabilitation, 23*(1), 11–14.

Griffin, C., Hammis, D., Geary, T., & Sullivan, M. (2008). Customized employment: Where we are, where we're headed. *Journal of Vocational Rehabilitation, 28*, 135–139.

Gunduz, B., Erhan, B., & Nur Bardak, A. (2010). Employment among spinal cord injured patients living in Turkey: A cross-sectional study. *International Journal of Rehabilitation Research, 33*(3), 193–282.

Hahn, H. (1986). Public support for rehabilitation programs: The analysis of U.S. disability policy. *Disability and Society, 1*(2), 121–137.

Harman, H. (1997). *Speech to mark the launch of the Centre for Analysis of Social Exclusion.* London School of Economics, Nov. 13, 1997.

Helander, E. (1999). *Einar Helander: Prejudice and dignity. An introduction to community-based rehabilitation.* New York: United Nations Development Program.

Humphrey, J. (2000). Researching disability politics: Some problems with the social model in practice. *Disability and Society, 15*(1), 63–85.

Iezzoni, L., & Greenberg, M. (2003). Capturing and classifying functional status information in administrative databases. *Health Care Financing Review, 24*(3), 61–76.

Imel, S. (1999). *One stop career centers.* (ERIC Digest No. 208). Columbus, OH: ERIC Clearinghouse on Adult, Career, and Vocational Education. (ERIC Document Reproduction Service, NO. ED434244).

Inge, K. (2006). Customized employment: A growing strategy for facilitating inclusive employment. *Journal of Vocational Rehabilitation, 24*, 191–193.

Inge, K. (2007). Demystifying customized employment for individuals with significant disabilities. *Journal of Vocational Rehabilitation, 26*, 63–66.

International Labor Organization. (1998). *Vocational rehabilitation and the employment of disabled persons.* Geneva: Author.

Jahurul Alam, K., Bari, N., & Abedin Khan, M. (2005). *Community-based rehabilitation practices and alleviation of poverty of people with disabilities in Bangladesh.* Paper presented at the Workshop on Community-Based Rehabilitation (CBR) and Poverty Alleviation of Persons with Disabilities. Bangkok, July 5, 2005. Retrieved from http://www.dpiap.org/national/pdf/Community_Based_Rehabilitation.pdf

Krause, J., DeVivo, M., & Jackson, A. (2004). Health status, community integration, and economic risk factors for mortality after spinal cord injury. *Archives of Physical Medicine and Rehabilitation, 85*, 1764–1773.

Krause, J., & Terza, J. (2006). Injury and demographic factors predictive of disparities in earnings after spinal cord injury. *Archives of Physical Medicine and Rehabilitation, 87*, 1318–1326.

Leff, J., & Warner, R. (2006). *Social inclusion of people with mental illness.* Cambridge: University Press.

Lister, R. (2000). Strategies for social inclusion: Promoting social cohesion or social justice? In P. Askonsas, & A. Stewart (Eds.), *Social inclusion: Possibility and tensions* (pp. 37–54). New York: St. Martin's Press, Inc.

Ludlum, C. (2002). *One candle power: Seven principles that enhance lives of people with disabilities and their communities.* Toronto, ON: Inclusion Press International.

Luecking, R., Cuozzo, L., Leedy, M., & Seleznow, E. (2008). Universal one-stop access: Pipedream or possibility? *Journal of Vocational Rehabilitation, 28*, 181–199.

Luecking, R. G., Fabian, E. S., & Tilson, G. P. (2004). *Working relationships: Creating career opportunities for job seekers with disabilities through employer partnerships.* Baltimore: Paul H. Brookes Publishing Company.

McConnell, R. (Ed.). (1999). *Disability policy: Issues and implications for the new millennium: The disability paradigm.* A report on the 21st Mary E. Switzer Memorial Seminar, September 27–29, 1999, East Lansing, MI.

Metts, R. L. (2000). *Disability issues, trends and recommendations for the World Bank.* Washington, DC: World Bank, Disability and Development Team.

Mount, B. (1990). *Making futures happen: A manual for facilitators of personal futures planning.* St. Paul, MN: Metropolitan Council's DD Case Management Project.

Nagi, S. (1965). Some conceptual issues in disability and rehabilitation. In M. B. Sussman (Ed.), *Sociology and rehabilitation.* Washington, DC: American Sociological Association.

Nagi, S. (1991). Disability concepts revisited: Implications to prevention. In A. M. Pope, & A. R. Tarlove (Eds.), *Disability in America: Toward a national agenda for prevention* (pp. 309–327). Washington, DC: National Academy Press.

National Collaborative on Workforce and Disability. (2009). *Universal design for the workforce development system.* Boston: Institute for Community Inclusion.

National Council on Disability. (1986). *Toward independence: An assessment of federal laws and programs affecting persons with disabilities-with legislative recommendations.* A report to the President and to the Congress of the United States. Washington, DC: Author.

New Freedom Commission on Mental Health. (2005). *Subcommittee on evidence-based practices: Background paper* (DHHS pub. No. SMA-05–4007). Rockville, MD: DHHS.

Nirje, B. (1980). The normalization principle. In R. J. Flynn, K. E. Nitsch (Eds.), *Normalization, social integration and community services.* Baltimore: University Park Press.

Obermann, C. E. (1965). *A history of vocational rehabilitation in America.* Minneapolis: T. S. Denison.

O'Brien, J. (2006). *Reflecting on social roles: Identifying opportunities to support personal freedom and social integration.* Lithonia, GA: Responsive Systems Associates, Inc.

Oliver, M. (1996). *Understanding disability: From theory to practice*. London: Macmillan.

Organization for Economic Cooperation and Development (OECD). (2003). *Transforming ability into disability*. Retrieved from http://www.oecd.org/document/14/0,3343,en_2649_34747_35290126_1_1_1,00&&en-USS_01DBC.html

Pang, M., Eng, J., & Miller, W. (2007). Determinants of satisfaction with community reintegration in older adults with chronic stroke: Role of balance self-efficacy. *Physical Therapy, 87*(3), 282–291. Retrieved from http://ptjournal.apta.org/content/87/3.toc

Peterson, D. B. (2005). International Classification of Functioning, Disability and Health (ICF): An introduction for rehabilitation psychologists. *Rehabilitation Psychology, 50*, 105–112.

Peterson, D. B., & Rosenthal, D. (2005). The International Classification of Functioning, Disability and Health (ICF): A primer for rehabilitation educators. *Rehabilitation Education, 19*(2 & 3), 105–117.

Phillips, W., Callahan, M., Shumpert, N., Puckett, K., Retrey, R., Summers, K., & Phillips, L. (2009). Customized transition: Discovering the best in us. *Journal of Vocational Rehabilitation, 30*, 49–55.

Rehabilitation Services Administration. (2009). *Reporting manual for the case service report (RSA-911)*. Washington, DC: U.S. Department of Education, Office of Special Education and Rehabilitation Services.

Revell, W., & Inge, K. (2007). Customized employment Q and A: Funding consumer-directed employment outcomes. *Journal of vocational Rehabilitation, 26*, 123–127.

Roger, C., Lavin, D., Tran, T., Gantenbein, T., & Sharpe, M. (2008). Customized employment: Changing what it means to be qualified in the workforce for transition-aged youth and young adults. *Journal of Vocational Rehabilitation, 28*, 191–207.

Rohe, D. E. (1998). Psychological aspects of rehabilitation. In J. A. DeLisa, & B. Gans (Eds.), *Rehabilitation medicine: Principles and practice* (3rd ed., pp. 189–212). Philadelphia: Lippincott-Raven.

Rohe, D. E., & Athelstan, G. T. (1982). Vocational interests of persons with spinal cord injury. *Journal of Counseling Psychology, 29*(3), 283–291.

Rohe, D. E., & Athelstan, G. T. (1985). Change in vocational interests after disability. *Rehabilitation Psychology, 30*(3), 131–143.

Rohe, D. E., & Krause, J. S. (1998). Stability of interests after severe physical disability: An 11-year longitudinal study. *Journal of Vocational Behavior, 52*, 45–58.

San, N. (2005). Poverty reduction community based work with people with disabilities in Cambodia. Paper presented at the Workshop on Community-Based Rehabilitation (CBR) and Poverty Alleviation of Persons with Disabilities, July 5, 2005, Bangkok.

Sander, A. M. (2006). *Novel approaches to community integration following traumatic brain injury*. Lecture presented at the Contemporary Forums Brain Injury Conference, San Antonio, Texas. (R1, R3, T4).

She, P., & Stapleton, D. (2006). *A review of disability data for the institutional population*. Ithaca, NY: Cornell University, Employment and Disability Institute, Rehabilitation Research and Training Center on Disability Demographics and Statistics.

Social Security Administration. (2008). *Partnership plus*. Retrieved July 30, 2010 from http://www.socialsecurity.gov/work/documents/SSA-63–034%20Partner%20Plus11_7_08.pdf

Stapleton, D. C., & Erickson, W. A. (2005). *Characteristics or incentives: Why do employment outcomes for the SSA beneficiary clients of VR agencies differ, on average, from those of other clients?* Ithaca, NY: Cornell University.

Thornton, P., & Lunt, N. (1997). *Employment policies for disabled people in eighteen countries: A review*. Social Policy Research Unit, University of York. Retrieved from http://digitalcommons.ilr.cornell.edu/cgi/viewcontent.cgi?article=1158&context=gladnetcollect

United Nations Enable. (2007). *Fact Sheet 1: Employment of persons with disabilities*. United Nations Department of Public Information—DPI/2486—November.

U.S. Department of Education. (2000). *Evaluation of programs: Evaluation standards and performance indicators for the vocational rehabilitation services program*. Retrieved July 3, 2005 from http://www.ed.gov/rschstat/eval/rehab/standards.html

U.S. Department of Justice. (2005). *A guide to disability rights laws*. Washington, DC: Civil Rights Division.

U.S. Department of Labor. (2007). *2007 Workforce investment act of 1998*. Retrieved October 8, 2007 from http://www.doleta.gov/usworkforce/wia/wialaw.txt

U.S. Department of Labor. (2009). *Disability program navigator fact sheet*. Washington, DC: Employment and Training Administration.

Ustun, T., Chatterji, S., Kostansjek, N., & Bickenbach, J. (2003). WHO's ICF and functional status information in health records. *Health Care Financing Review, 24*(3), 77–88.

Walker, A., & Walker, C. (Eds.). (1997). *Britain divided: The growth of social exclusion in the 1980s and 1990s*. London: Child Poverty Action Group.

Ware, N., Hopper, K., Tugenberg, T., Dickey, B., & Fisher, D. (2008). A theory of social integration and quality of life. *Psychiatric Services, 59*(1), 27–33.

Waters, L. E., & Moore, K. A. (2002). Self-esteem, appraisal and coping: A comparison of unemployed and reemployed people. *Journal of Organizational Behaviour, 23*, 593–604.

Wehman, P., & Kregel, J. (1992). Supported employment: Growth and impact. In P. Wehman, P. Sale, & W. Parent (Eds.), *Supported employment: Strategies for integration of workers with disabilities* (pp. 3–28). Boston: Andover Medical Publishers.

Wehmeyer, M. (2001). Self-determination and mental retardation. In L. Glidden (Ed), *International review of research in mental retardation* (Vol. 24). San Diego: Academic Press.

Wolfensberger, W. (1972). *The principle of normalization in human services*. Toronto: National Institute on Mental Retardation.

Wolfensberger, W. (1998). *A brief introduction to social role valorization: A high- order concept for addressing the plight of societally devalued people, and for structuring human services*. Syracuse, NY: Training Institute for Human Service Planning, Leadership and Change Agent (Syracuse University).

Workforce Investment Act of 1998, 29 U.S.C. § 1320 et seq.

World Health Organization. (2001). *International Classification of Functioning, Disability and Health: ICF*. Geneva: Author.

World Health Organization. (2002). *Toward a common language for functioning, disability and health. The International Classification of Functioning, Disability and Health*. Retrieved July 14, 2008 from http://www.who.int/classifications/icf/site/icftemplate.cfm

World Health Organization. (2004). *CBR: a strategy for rehabilitation, equalization of opportunities, poverty reduction and social inclusion of people with disabilities: Joint position paper*. International Labour Organization, United Nations Educational, Scientific and Cultural Organization and the World Health Organization. Retrieved from http://www.who.int/disabilities/publications/cbr/en/index.html

Wright, G. N. (1980). *Total rehabilitation*. Boston: Little, Brown, & Co.

Zhang Liu, G. (2005). Best practices: Developing cross-cultural competencies from a Chinese perspective. In J. H. Stone (Ed.), *Culture and disability: Providing culturally competent services* (pp. 65–85). Thousand Oaks, CA: Sage Publications, Inc.

Resilience in People with Physical Disabilities

Ashley Craig

Abstract

Historically, research into the nature of resilience was applied mostly to children and adolescents exposed to problems such as ill-treatment in the family or drug abuse, and this resilience research employed a risk and protective factors model. Protective factors included attributes that minimize risk or act as a buffer by cushioning the person against negative outcomes, and included environmental, interpersonal, and individual personal factors. Being resilient, therefore, described a process that involved someone who had assets and resources that enabled him or her to self-protect and thus overcome the adverse affects of risk exposure. It is concerning that the model for research most often used when investigating outcomes for physical disabilities has been a risk-deficit model that focuses more upon factors, such as negative mood states, that may prevent a person from adjusting adaptively to his or her disability. Few studies have concentrated on both risk and resilience factors. In this chapter, *resilience* is defined as a process involving a person maintaining stable psychological, social, and physical functioning when adjusting to the effects of a physical disability and subsequent impairment. Research that has investigated protective factors in physical disability will be explored and implications for the management of these conditions discussed.

Key Words: Disability, resilience, risk, rehabilitation, protective factors, self-efficacy.

Adjusting adaptively in the face of trauma, overcoming the odds, or prevailing over adversity are all phrases that describe a process in which a person with resilient assets and resources adapts to adverse life events. Synonyms for "resilience" include *hardiness, robustness, durability of spirit, stamina, endurance,* and *resoluteness.* The term "resilience" attempts to capture not only the idea of surviving but also thriving, so that, if I am a resilient person, it is presupposed that I have the capability of coping adaptively and resolutely with life risks I may be exposed to. However, given the abundance of resilience terminology, it is important that "resilience" be defined in a scientifically meaningful way. This chapter explores the definitions of resilience developed by researchers and clinicians in the field, and

examines models of resilience that have been used to investigate attributes that protect people from risk. Resilience research with children and adolescents will then be briefly reviewed. We will then examine resilience related to physical disability by providing a selective review of research that has investigated protective factors in the area of physical disability. Resilience measures will then be discussed and implications for the treatment and management of physical disability will be reviewed.

Definition and Nature of Resilience

Early studies of children with mothers who had schizophrenia were crucial in the emergence of the study of childhood resilience as a major area in the quest to discover why and how people cope and adjust to adversity (Garmezy & Masten, 1991; Luthar, Cicchetti, & Becker, 2000). The finding that many of these children survived and coped despite the risks they faced led to increasing research into individual differences in reactions to adversity. Some grief researchers and theorists believed that the relative absence of grief following severe loss or trauma was a form of psychopathology; that is, that the absence of grief symptoms will eventually result in delayed grief reactions (Bonanno & Mancinni, 2008). However, there is no compelling evidence for this belief, and a growing body of evidence now shows that many people display resilient behavior through the experience of severe adversity and grief, and that resilience is a consequence of "normal" adjustment processes (Bonanno & Mancinni, 2008). Furthermore, the work of Wortman and Silver (1989) into adjustment following loss, and their contention that depressive mood was not an inevitable outcome following serious loss, also contributed to this quest to learn how people adjust to adversity. Wortman and Silver (1989) contended that in attempts to deal adaptively with their loss, individuals need not become depressed to preserve their mental health. For instance, a person who loses mobility following a traumatic spinal cord injury (SCI) or a person who loses substantial cognitive capacity following traumatic brain damage can adjust positively without becoming depressed (Middleton & Craig, 2008). Pollard and Kennedy (2007) studied adjustment following SCI, and showed that many people with SCI were able to adjust to their injuries without developing significant levels of psychopathology. Their findings, did suggest, however, that the coping strategies used by those who successfully adjust were complex. Also, the large individual differences in the responses of people to adversity (e.g., only a proportion of people suffering adversity become depressed) raised the strong possibility that protective factors operate over and beyond negative life events (Rutter, 1985). For instance, personality (hardiness) and attitudinal factors (sense of mastery) interact with environmental and genetic factors to serve as a protection against negative outcomes when faced with adversity. Thus, the search began for those internal and external factors that served as buffers against adversity and for those risks that made people susceptible (Rutter, 1985).

Resilience research in physical disability should therefore be about the detection of a range of interactive factors that allow a person to adjust positively in the face of difficulties arising from disability impairment. This chapter provides an opportunity to evaluate factors that contribute to and determine resilient responses, such as coping adaptively with loss and adjusting constructively to difficult and challenging problems. Unfortunately, limited research has been conducted to investigate directly resilience associated with physical disability. An exception is Wright's early work in rehabilitation psychology (1983), who discussed concepts similar to those in the risk and protective factors model. Wright (1983) discussed many examples of risk and protective factors, such as the relationship between self-esteem and acceptance of the disability. If one accepts one's disability, then self-esteem can be boosted. If one rejects or attempts to hide the disability, Wright believed that self-esteem may suffer. Another example she emphasized were the differences between coping with and succumbing to disability. Factors such as the person's assets and positive psychology factors, such as hope, were viewed as crucial for positive coping and adjustment. Wright (1983) also questioned simple approaches to adjustment: for instance, the idea that a person with a mild disability would be much more likely to cope in a superior manner compared to someone with a severe disability. Wright (1983) argued for the primary role of factors such as self-esteem and other positive psychosocial factors in the adjustment process. Furthermore, this assumption that adjustment is determined by disorder severity is not supported by recent research literature (Middleton & Craig, 2008). Notwithstanding the above, findings from resilience research in other fields will first be explored to provide clues for how people with a physical disability may cope in a resilient manner.

Earliest resilience research involved the study of risk in children and adolescents who were disadvantaged in some way (e.g., poverty, exposure to abuse). As this research progressed, a shift gradually occurred from an almost exclusive focus on risk factors and personal deficits to a model that focused on both protective factors and risk factors (Fergus & Zimmerman, 2005). Consequently, a number of definitions of resilience have emerged over the years arising from the child and adolescent studies that examined healthy development in the context of risk exposure and risk minimization (Fergus & Zimmerman, 2005). Historically, the concept of resilience has emerged from risk and protective factors models, in which "resilience" referred to a process involving an ability to overcome negative effects of risk exposure, resulting in effective coping with stressful events and avoiding negative outcomes

(Luthar et al., 2000; Rutter, 1985; Werner, 1993). "Risk" reflected the possibility of adverse or negative outcomes in response to stressors, and risk factors were described as either internal or external threats that can result in increased vulnerability to negative outcomes, such as poor adjustment and maladaptive coping (Fergus & Zimmerman, 2005). Luthar et al. (2000) defined resilience as: "a dynamic process encompassing positive adaptation within the context of significant adversity" (p. 543).

Luthar et al. (2000) point out that two critical conditions are required for this definition: exposure to significant threat or severe adversity is necessary, and the achievement of positive adaptation needs to occur despite the major adversity faced. However, Luthar et al. (2000) have raised several concerns about the concept of resilience that need consideration. First, there are numerous definitions of resilience in existence that are based on variable conditions, such as different types of adversity and varying approaches to what adjustment means. However, Luthar et al. (2000) agree that "research in the area of resilience appears to be in good standing" (p. 547) if these conditions are standardized. Second, differences exist in the conceptualization of resilience as either a personal trait or as a process. Luthar et al. (2000) believe that some researchers use these two concepts of resilience interchangeably. However, resilience should always be conceived of as a process and not as a personal trait. Therefore, in this chapter, resilience has been conceptualized as a dynamic process in which Luthar et al.'s (2000) definition is satisfied. Third, when using the concept of resilience, Luthar et al. (2000) make the valid point that "it is unrealistic to expect any group of individuals to exhibit consistently positive or negative adjustment across multiple domains that are conceptually unrelated" (p. 549). This means, by way of example, that a person with SCI may well be resilient when adjusting to pain, but not be resilient when coping with studying for examinations. Therefore, researchers must specify the particular context to which their resilience data apply. For example, in physical disability, it will be important that reference is made to emotional resilience when studying mood and anxiety, vocational resilience when studying performance in employment contexts, and perhaps physical resilience when referring to the ability to manage infections.

Zimmerman and Arunkumar (1994) defined resilience as "those factors and processes that interrupt the trajectory from risk to problem behavior or psychopathology and thereby result in adaptive

outcomes even in the presence of challenging and threatening circumstances" (p. 4). Garmezy and Masten (1991) described resilience as an ability to adapt successfully despite challenging and threatening circumstances. Others came to view resilience as a transactional process in which outcomes are related to the interaction of genetic, biological, psychological, and sociological factors in the context of environmental support (Egeland, Carson, & Sroufe, 1993). Egeland et al. (1993) suggested that both personal and environmental factors have the potential to become either risk or protective agents, thus making it important that they be identified as the interaction of factors that can act to shape health behavior and health outcomes. Examples of protective factors in the child and adolescent field included internal psychological factors such as self-esteem, competence, coping skills, and a sense of mastery or self-efficacy. Other protective factors included those external to the person, including things like parental support, community support, and employment (Fergus & Zimmerman, 2005). Bonanno and Mancinni (2008), when discussing which factors help people cope and thrive through trauma and adversity, suggest that the following factors are protective: adaptive flexibility (the capacity to modify behavior to meet the demands of a stressful life event), adaptive exposure to adverse stimuli, older age, a higher level of education, social support, employment, and successful management of past stressors.

When applied to physical disability, these resilience definitions apply appropriately to the study of how people adaptively adjust to disability. Specifically, for the purposes of this chapter on resilience in people with physical disability, a working definition of resilience was developed:

> Resilience is the process of maintaining stable psychological, social, and physical functioning when adjusting to the effects of a physical disability and subsequent impairment.

Resilience Research in Children and Adolescents Without a Physical Disability

Resilience research with children and adolescents has been associated with areas such as child welfare (Festinger, 1984), juvenile justice (Vigil, 1990), and substance abuse (Werner & Smith, 2001). When exposure to risk is high, evidence suggests that most children and adolescents experience some type of problem or developmental difficulty (Cicchetti & Rogosch, 1997). First, however, it is not the presence of a disability that totally determines risk and negative outcome. Morrison and Cosden (1997) found that the presence of a learning disability did not in itself always predict positive or negative outcomes. Morrison and Cosden (1997) reported that a number of risk factors acted to increase the chances of negative outcomes in children and adolescents with a learning disability. These included premature birth, socioeconomic disadvantage, elevated anxiety and depressive mood states, low parental expectations, overprotection, and poor impulse control. A number of protective factors were also isolated that decreased the chances of negative outcomes, and these included supportive and cohesive family functioning, high self-esteem, parental emotional stability, and a capability to form positive attachments. Risk and protective factors have been found to interact in the presence of a learning disability to facilitate or impede adjustment (Morrison & Cosden, 1997).

Egeland et al. (1993) found factors related to resilience in a longitudinal study of children in high-risk families. These included the quality of the relationship between mother and child (secure attachments reduced negative outcomes), a responsive home environment despite high stress, and the provision of a role model for positive coping (usually a parent). Their research highlighted the importance of an interaction of factors in determining outcomes, thus emphasizing the need for longitudinal studies with comprehensive assessment. Rew and Horner (2003) presented a framework for reducing risk behavior in adolescents, and they recognized a number of protective factors found in the research literature; these included a sense of humor, the competence level of the child, the presence of adaptive coping styles, the level of social support available, and an acceptable level of knowledge of risks and skills needed to resolve problems. Werner (1993) studied the developmental paths of a cohort of children who had been exposed to perinatal stress, poverty, and parental psychopathology. They found five clusters of protective factors from the children judged to be resilient, as assessed by success in their adult life. Cluster 1 included temperament factors in the children that allowed them to react positively. Cluster 2 included skills and values that assisted them to use their abilities efficiently. Cluster 3 included parental caregiving styles. Cluster 4 consisted of available social support such as parents, grandparents, elder mentors, youth leaders, and members of church groups. Cluster 5 consisted of factors such as the opening of opportunities at

major life transitions. Masten, Best, and Garmezy (1990) had similar findings to Werner (1993). They found that children who experienced chronic adversity were more resilient when they had a constructive relationship with an adult, had problem-solving skills, were engaged with other people in a constructive way, had a proficient level of competence, and were equipped with a sense of mastery or self-efficacy over their life. The above studies into resilience in children and adolescents provide significant insight into resilience factors that may operate in people with physical disabilities.

Protective Versus Risk Factors

Examples of protective factors that have been found to operate in children and adolescents in the face of adversity are listed in Table 26.1, and these are based on research conducted outside the field of physical disability (Connor & Davidson, 2003; Egeland et al., 1993; Fergus & Zimmerman, 2005; Masten et al., 1990; Morrison & Cosden, 1997). There are numerous potential protective factors operating, so the list in Table 26.1 is not exhaustive. Likewise, risks that someone is likely to face are also numerous, and examples are listed in Table 26.2. The question is whether these factors determined from children and adolescents without a physical disability also operate in people with a physical disability. This question will be addressed later, when select resilience-related research in the area of physical disability is presented.

Additionally, the lists in Tables 26.1 and 26.2 illustrate the complexity of the issue. For example, there is a potential for a protective factor to slide into a risk factor, depending on the strength of the protection available at any one time. As a case in point, a strong sense of mastery (or self-efficacy, internal locus of control, perceived optimism etc.) over one's life and future is the degree to which a person believes he or she can influence his or her behavior and life direction (Bandura, 1989). Strong self-efficacy is considered a protective factor. However, when this sense of mastery is lacking or declines as a result of a particular challenging event or due to a toxic context, self-efficacy fails to be protective and results in potentially maladaptive responses, such as a sense of helplessness or hopelessness. However, the negative of a protective factor is not automatically a risk factor. Consider hospitalization. Frequent hospitalization may be a risk, given that the person with a disability may require constant medical attention and thus may be exposed to the negative affects of being hospitalized frequently (e.g., being

Table 26.1 Possible protective factors that may operate in a person

Protective factors		
Environmental	Social and interpersonal	Psychological and physical
Community resources	Stable family support	Robust self-esteem
Healthy environment	Available affection	A sense of self mastery
Secure housing	Employment	Physically healthy
Available finances	Being socially active	Problem solving skills
Education opportunities	Positive attachments formed	Adequate social skills
Community cohesion	Friends support	Stable mood states
Access to recreation	Access to social networks	Adequate coping skills

dehumanized or institutionalized). Nevertheless, a lack of hospitalization will be a serious risk factor if medical attention is essential and the person is in danger of experiencing negative health outcomes. Even a strong sense of mastery can become a risk factor if the person believes he has so much self-control that he has no need for medical or psychological assistance and thus avoids contact with health professionals.

This protective–risk factor complexity illustrates the importance of conducting comprehensive assessments for people with physical disability, so that any protective factors and risk factors operating are known and evaluated, and the best help can be provided (Craig & Nicholson Perry, 2008). The New South Wales Spinal Cord Injury Service (Australia) is currently conducting controlled research into developing a sensitive and comprehensive assessment regimen that can be used at strategic times during SCI rehabilitation, with the goal of detecting and monitoring risk and protective factors and adjusting treatment accordingly (Craig & Nicholson Perry, 2008).

Models of Resilience

Three models of resilience have been proposed: the *compensatory model*, the *protective factor model*, and the *challenge model* (Fergus & Zimmerman, 2005). These three models attempt to explain how resilience factors protect the person (Rutter, 1985). First, the compensatory model involves a protective factor counteracting in some way the negative influence of a risk factor. For example, a person with multiple sclerosis (MS) who also suffers from persistent fatigue may be more likely to suffer from a depressive mood state than is someone with MS who does not suffer severe fatigue (Schwartz, Coulthard-Morris, & Zeng, 1996). However, if a person with

Table 26.2 Possible risk factors that may operate in a person

Risk factors		
Environmental	Social and interpersonal	Psychological and physical
No community access	No family support	Elevated anxiety
Unhealthy environment	Poor social networks	Sense of helplessness
Secure housing	Unemployed	Elderly
Poor finances	Avoids activities	Poor insight
Little education	Single	Lack of communication skills
Stressful living context	Frequent hospitalization	Depressive mood
		Significant cognitive deficits

MS has a high sense of mastery concerning her MS symptoms, she will be likely to take adaptive steps to counter her fatigue. The person's sense of mastery or self-efficacy will compensate for the negative effects of fatigue (Schwartz et al., 1996).

In the protective factor model, a protective factor directly reduces the effects of a particular risk factor. For instance, if a person with MS has a partner dedicated to care for him, the caregiver's social support operates as a protective factor because it restrains and reduces the negative risks faced by the person with MS (Chwastiak & Ehde, 2007).

The challenge model (Fergus & Zimmerman, 2005) suggests that the association between a risk factor and an outcome is not always linear, in that successful or resilient outcomes are dependent on various levels of risk exposure. For instance, a person with a physical disability who is exposed to moderate levels of a particular risk (e.g., low to moderate persistent pain) can be motivated to learn how to deal with the pain. Dealing with her pain successfully strengthens her capability to deal successfully with any additional risks she faces over time. Conversely, if she were exposed to severely debilitating levels of pain, it may well become totally overwhelming and result in negative outcomes, such as feeling hopeless and distressed, as when someone with chronic pain catastrophizes about her pain (Sullivan, Stanish, Waite, Sullivan, & Tripp, 1998). The challenge model therefore suggests that some manageable level of risk exposure could be beneficial because it provides an opportunity to employ protective resources. The challenge model also suggests that very low levels of risk may not always be beneficial as the person may ignore acting adaptively to remedy the situation (Fergus & Zimmerman, 2005). The model may also offer insight into a person's capacity to become more resilient as he or she ages and matures. The model predicts that the continual exposure to adversity that is dealt with successfully may enhance one's capacity to deal successfully with risks in the future.

Resilience, Adjustment, and Coping

Fergus and Zimmerman (2005) point out that resilience should not be confused with the concept of adjustment or coping. Although adjustment and coping are obviously related to resilience, they should be considered distinct processes. Adjustment that is adaptive is an outcome of a resilient process. When a physically disabled person copes in a positive manner with a challenging life event (e.g., comes to accept his impairment or his traumatic

injury and begins to take adaptive action to deal with it), he has begun to demonstrate resilience. The alternative negative response is to adjust poorly by becoming depressed, avoiding social activity and friends, and abusing alcohol. Adjusting adaptively is a resilient outcome, and the process of being able to overcome the risk of not effectively coping and adjusting is due to one's attributes that contribute to resilience, some of which are no doubt listed in Table 26.1. The resilience process can also involve avoiding a negative outcome (such as purposely not blaming others for the injury or disability). Fergus and Zimmerman (2005) also point out that resilience should be distinguished from attributes such as competence, and constructs such as intelligence/emotional intelligence should also be considered as distinct entities, although obviously crucial to the process of being resilient. For instance, an emotionally intelligent person with a physical disability may be expected to be more likely to adjust to her disability than is someone with low emotional intelligence. Clearly, however, personal/psychological factors are just one type of contributor to the process of being resilient, and the importance of environmental, interpersonal, and social factors must not be underestimated.

Adjustment is distinct from the resilience process and is considered to be the desirable goal following serious injury and resultant disability. However, it has rarely been operationally defined for a physical disability, such as a SCI (Middelton & Craig, 2008), although it has been defined for people with SCI as "the act of bringing something into conformity with external requirements" and "harmony achieved by modification or alteration of a position" (Trieschmann, 1982, p. 3). These definitions fall short as working definitions for adjustment to disability. Middelton and Craig (2008) addressed the lack of a working definition for adjustment following SCI, and their definition has been slightly adapted to make it more relevant to disability generally:

> Adjustment occurs when a person with a physical disability responds adaptively by modifying their behavior, thinking, and personal circumstances in relation to the many factors associated with the disability and impairment, with a goal of achieving a satisfactory quality of life (QOL).

This definition of adjustment is clearly distinguished from the definition of resilience in that it emphasizes a process of modifying behavior and thinking, whereas the resilience definition emphasized a process involving adversity in which a person demonstrates a capacity to change in a positive way. Coping must also by nature be highly related to resilience, and it was defined by Middleton and Craig (2008) as "any effort expended by a person with a physical disability to solve challenges and difficulties experienced, with the goal of mastering or minimizing their problems or conflicts."

Middleton and Craig (2008) have emphasized the importance of viewing adjustment and coping as a continuing nonlinear process of adapting to the problems arising from a physical disability. Linear models of adjustment, such as a stage theory, alluded to by Wortman and Silver (1989), do not take into account the unpredictability and complexity of adjusting to the impairment associated with severe physical disability, such as a SCI. Adjustment can be viewed as a cyclical process that occurs over many years (Krause & Broderick, 2005), involving periods of negative adjustment (such as feeling sad or depressed) and adaptive positive adjustment (such as feeling in control and vital), which, in turn, may be followed by a further period of difficulty, so that adjustment is composed of peaks and troughs. A cyclical approach to adjustment has been described as a gradual process of learning (continuous life transition) to tolerate a set of very difficult and challenging circumstances (Kendall & Buys, 1998). A model of adjustment relevant to severe physical disability has been developed by Middleton and Craig (2008) that describes the major processes involved when someone attempts to adjust. It assumes that many factors contribute to the process of adjustment, and thus resilience, including a combination of biological, psychological, and social factors. The model also incorporates appraisal and reappraisal in the adjustment process and posits that behavioral and mental actions are contingent on this appraisal and reappraisal process. The model attempts to explain how maladaptive coping occurs, leading to poor adjustment and dysfunctional outcomes. It also explains how adaptive coping and adjustment can occur, leading to resilient behavior and thinking. It is highly desirable that research in the physical disabilities investigate the process of resilience, beginning by employing working definitions of resilience that can be assessed in a meaningful way. Of equal importance, the nature and working definitions of adjustment and coping should be developed and agreed upon. The above definitions do allow the meaningful assessment of resilience, adjustment, and coping.

Resilience and Stress

Southwick, Vythilingam, and Charney (2005) completed a review on psychosocial factors related to the process of resilience when experiencing severe stress and unstable depressive mood states. They found that psychosocial factors associated with positive outcomes included optimism, humor, having a strong faith, social support, positive role models, positive coping styles, appropriate exercise, and a history and capacity of recovering from negative events. Lyons (1991) conducted a systematic review searching for protective factors that enhance the capacity to deal positively with traumatic experiences, such as combat, serious accidents, assault, and so on. Lyons made the point that, in most cases, the dysfunctional subset who have coped poorly, such as those who develop post-traumatic stress disorder (PTSD), have been examined for associated risks. Those who have coped well with trauma have been largely ignored. Based on a systematic review, Lyons (1991) proposed that the following factors protect against adverse reactions associated with trauma: a less severe trauma, an experience in resolving trauma and life stressors, a better level of education, a capacity to re-experience trauma with a high degree of self-control, a capacity to find meaning in the cause of the trauma, and the quality of social support networks available. Farber, Schwartz, Schaper, Moonen, and McDaniel (2000) studied factors related to dealing with the stress of symptomatic HIV disease and AIDS in 200 people. Employing a series of standard multiple regression analyses, they isolated protective factors that they believed enhanced the capacity to deal with the stress associated with the disease. Resiliency or "high hardiness" was significantly related to lower psychological distress levels, higher perceived QOL in physical health, stable mental health, positive personal beliefs, a higher sense of self-worth, and a sense of commitment to self help.

Resilience in People with Physical Disability

The risk and resilience research conducted on children and adolescents provides a guide for a better understanding of protective factors that may contribute to the process of resilience in people with physical disability. One of the first attempts to apply the results of this earlier resilience research to adults at risk of psychiatric disorder was published in the *British Journal of Psychiatry* by Rutter (1985), who proposed a number of protective factors that have the potential to modify, alter, or cushion a person from the negative consequences of adversity. These factors included having a constructive understanding of events, taking adaptive action, having robust self-esteem and a strong sense of mastery or self-efficacy, being adaptable when faced with change, having problem-solving skills, having a sense of humor when faced with stressful events, dealing successfully with problems in the past, accepting responsibility when dealing with problems, and having quality social support. Most of Rutter's (1985) protective factors are similar to those listed in Table 26.1. Researchers have supported a number of these possible protective factors. For example, Jang, Haley, Small, and Mortimer (2002) showed that a higher sense of self-mastery and a greater satisfaction with social support and social networks cushioned the adverse impact of disability in older people by lowering rates of depression. In other words, those elderly people who had age-related disabilities were protected from depressive mood if they had higher levels of self-efficacy and greater levels of social resources. Moghadam (2006) studied resilience factors in 133 young adults with disabilities and showed that self-efficacy and an optimistic outlook were independent predictors of resilience.

Although there is a paucity of resilience research conducted in the field of physical disability, and even less with adults with a physical disability (White, Driver, & Warren, 2008), this section will nevertheless examine a selection of studies that have investigated physical disability using a resilience model or a model that at least has attempted to predict positive outcomes in people with physical disabilities. The physical disabilities will be discussed in no particular order.

Burns

Dealing with a severe burn is a seriously challenging experience. Anzarut, Chen, Shankowsky, and Tredget (2005) found that adults receiving severe burns (burn size more than 50% of total body surface area) had substantially lowered QOL. However, they showed that perceived levels of social support were associated with improved outcomes and therefore, social support is a potential factor for enhancing resilience in people with serious burns (Anzarut et al., 2005). Several studies have examined factors that assist children to be more resilient to the stress of burn injury. Sheridan, Hinson, Liang, Nackel, Schoenfeld, Ryan, et al. (2000) studied survivors of massive burns (more than 70% of the body

surface burned) in children aged less than 18 years when injured. As perhaps expected, they found that many had lower physical functioning QOL scores than similar community norms. However, they also found that a functional family and better pre-burn health served to protect the children from negative outcomes following the burn. Byrne, Love, Browne, Brown, Roberts, and Streiner (1986) also studied the adjustment of children who received severe burns and found that children who adjusted in a superior manner had the following resources and assets: a more adaptive and active family, greater access to participation in social and recreational activities, a higher socioeconomic status, a larger number of family members, a mother who viewed her child's injury and adjustment more positively, greater time since the burn injury, and surprisingly, a more severe burn. Clearly, the quality of the child's family functioning is a primary protective factor in young burn victims.

Chronic Pain

Chronic or persistent pain has been found to be associated with debilitating levels of anxiety, depression, and social/occupational dysfunction, and is obviously a severe test for adaptive adjustment (Sullivan et al., 1998). In a systematic review, McCracken and Turk (2002) evaluated the efficacy of cognitive-behavioral therapy (CBT) for chronic pain and identified predictors of successful treatment outcome. Cognitive-behavioral therapy was found to reduce the distress associated with pain, modified successfully pain-related behaviors, and improved daily functioning. Factors associated with successful management of pain included improved emotional responses to pain and improved adaptive attitudes toward pain, such as decreased perceived disability and increased perceived self-control. Catastrophizing about one's pain has been found to be a risk factor for maladjustment and, therefore, most likely poor resilience, whereas the opposite has been found. Reduced catastrophizing about pain predicted better adjustment to pain and conceivably improved resilience in people with chronic pain, such as occurs in rheumatoid arthritis (Keefe, Brown, Wallston, & Caldwell, 1989; Sullivan et al., 1998). It is assumed that reduced catastrophizing involves dynamics such as improved self-efficacy and perceived self-control. In our laboratory, we have recently conducted preliminary search for resilience factors in 41 people with SCI who have been living in the community for some years and who experience chronic pain. Factors explored included demographic and injury-related factors, community integration, personality factors, and the SCI participants' sense of mastery or self-efficacy over aspects of their injury. A multiple regression analysis isolated those factors that contributed to low levels of pain. Five factors were found to contribute significantly to low pain levels, and these were, in order of strength of contribution, a sense of mastery over factors related to their injury, emotional stability, an open and candid personality, longer time since the injury, and a relaxed and patient nature. It is believed that these five factors in combination may make a major contribution to a persons' ability to be resilient when faced with chronic pain, a life event that can be very disruptive and distressing.

Traumatic Brain Injury

Challenges such as fatigue and depressive mood are common and disabling sequelae in people with traumatic brain injury (TBI). Fatigue is present in up to 70% of people with TBI. Interestingly, fatigue has not been found to be related to severity of the head injury or time since injury (Belmont, Agar, Hugeron, Gallais, & Azouvi, 2006), meaning that fatigue is a serious risk regardless of the severity of the injury. Mental health problems, such as depression, are also common (Schwartz, Taylor, Drotar, Yeates, Wade, & Stancin, 2003). Dumont, Gervais, Fougeyrollas, and Bertrand (2004) explored resiliency factors related to social participation in 53 people with TBI. Although fatigue was found to be one of the greatest risks for integrating socially, two factors that improved reintegration accounted for 51% of the variance in social participation. These factors included a positive mental state, like optimism, and strong self-efficacy or a sense of mastery. Schwartz et al. (2003) studied long-term behavioral problems in children with TBI up to a mean of 4 years after the injury. Predictors of poor adjustment included severe TBI, socioeconomic disadvantage, pre-injury behavioral problems, poor adaptive behavioral skills, and problematic family dynamics. Although Schwartz et al. (2003) determined risks of poor outcome following TBI and did not attempt to determine protective factors, arguably, in this case, there is some credibility to taking the reverse of the risk to isolate resilience enhancing factors. If we do this, then protective factors for adjusting to TBI would include less severe cognitive damage, socioeconomic advantage, stable pre-injury behavior, adaptive behavioral skills, and stable family dynamics.

Multiple Sclerosis

Multiple sclerosis (MS) is a prevalent chronic disabling disease of the central nervous system and its course can be extremely distressing and unpredictable, with common symptoms including fatigue, weakness, visual loss, incontinence, cognitive impairment, and depression. Persons who have MS have a high risk of psychiatric disorders with, for instance, a 23% lifetime prevalence of major depressive disorder and up to a 40% risk of any anxiety disorder (Chwastiak & Ehde, 2007). Clearly, however, many do not become depressed or clinically anxious, maintaining their daily functioning in the face of the adversity associated with MS. However, little research has been conducted in this area on resilience factors (Chwastiak & Ehde, 2007). In fact, Chwastiak and Ehde (2007) have called for future research to "take into account not only what goes 'wrong' after the onset of MS, but perhaps more importantly, on what goes 'right,' and the risk and protective factors predicting both" (p. 812). Barnwell and Kavanagh (1997) studied resilience factors in 71 people with MS. Their specific hypothesis was whether self-efficacy predicted improved social activity and better mood control. They found that self-efficacy did significantly contribute to positive mood control and social activity. Their study provides strong support for the value of employing self-efficacy as a predictor of positive outcomes in MS. Similar to research in other areas of disability and adversity, self-efficacy continues to be isolated as an important resilience and protective factor.

Diabetes

Type 1 (insulin-dependent diabetes mellitus) and type 2 (non–insulin dependent diabetes mellitus) diabetes are chronic diseases that can result in severe challenges to a person's physical and mental health (Bradshaw et al., 2007). Peyrot, McMurry, and Kruger (1999) examined the interaction of biological vulnerability and psychosocial risk factors to see whether people with type 1 and type 2 diabetes had greater responsiveness to psychosocial risk factors. They found that those with type 1 or type 2 diabetes who were emotionally stable demonstrated better glycemic control than did those who were emotionally less stable. Psychosocial factors such as a better level of education, being married, and having positive coping styles were associated with improved chronic glycemic control, and thus can be considered to be resilience factors. Yi, Vitaliano, Smith, Yi, and Weinger (2008) investigated the influence of resilience factors on two outcomes in

111 people with diabetes in the face of rising diabetes-related distress. The outcomes consisted of the participants' glycosylated hemoglobin (HbA_{1c}) and their self-care behaviors. Resilience was assessed using an algorithm consisting of a combination of self-esteem, self-efficacy, and optimism, and, based on the algorithm, participants were divided into three groups: those with low, moderate, and high resilience potential. Their findings proved interesting. Those with low and moderate resilience potential were found to have a strong association between increased stress and worsening HbA_{1c} across time. In contrast, this association was not found for those with high resilience levels. In other words, the people with high resilience potential had improved self-care behavior and better HbA_{1c} levels. Mednick, Cogen, Henderson, Rohrbeck, Kitessa, and Streisand (2007) studied factors that help protect against the experience of psychological distress in mothers of children aged 2 to 5 years with type 1 diabetes. They selected hope as a potential resilience factor and anxiety as a risk factor. Even after controlling for the influence of significant medical and demographic variables, hope still contributed a significant positive influence on maternal anxiety. The authors suggested that hope serves as a protective factor against psychological distress in mothers of very young children with diabetes. Bradshaw et al. (2007) demonstrated the importance of resiliency training in boosting adjustment levels in people with diabetes. Participants were randomly assigned to either a treatment-as-usual group ($n = 37$) or a resiliency treatment group ($n = 30$). Outcome variables included physiological measures (glycosylated hemoglobin, waist measurement, dietary and exercise habits) and psychosocial measures (self-efficacy, social support, and purpose in life). Bradshaw et al. (2007) showed that the resiliency treatment group had significantly improved psychosocial outcome measures, whereas HbA_{1c} and waist measurement improved, but not significantly. This study illustrates the importance of developing resilience interventions that may enhance and boost resilience in people with diabetes.

Spinal Cord Injury

Spinal cord injury poses one of the greatest emotional and physical adversities to face a human being. It involves a potentially devastating loss of control and mobility, uncertainty about the future, and altered physical functioning that threatens independence, limits social participation, and reduces QOL (Middleton & Craig, 2008). A person with SCI has to cope and adjust to the many potential adverse outcomes following the injury such as chronic neuropathic pain, depressive mood, social avoidance, and unemployment, and up to 40% are not successful in achieving positive adjustment (Craig, Tran, & Middleton, 2009). Inspection of the research literature reveals that few studies have explored SCI using a risk and protective factor model. However, some studies have attempted to predict risks to achieving positive outcomes. For instance, Martz, Livneh, Priebe, Wuermser, and Ottomanelli (2005) isolated risk factors associated with poor adjustment outcomes in 313 people with SCI living in the community. They found depressive mood, elevated anxiety, maladaptive coping styles (e.g., disengagement-type coping such as denial and avoidance), and the severity and impact of disability were related to lower levels of adaptation to the SCI. Although this study did not isolate protective factors, there is a reasonable case to accept the reverse of the risks as potential resilience factors. Craig, Hancock, and Chang (1994a) showed that effective psychological treatment delivered during SCI rehabilitation was significantly associated with enhanced perceptions of control (or self-efficacy) 2 years after the treatment. Given that self-efficacy has been found to be a strong resilience factor, this study showed the benefit of effective treatment in enhancing resiliency factors such as self-efficacy in severe physical disability. Craig, Hancock, and Chang (1994b) predicted long-term (2 years) adverse outcomes (depressive mood) in people with SCI. They found the primary and most significant predictors were poor self-efficacy and high pain severity. Kennedy, Marsh, Lowe, Grey, Short, and Rogers (2000) prospectively investigated psychological factors associated with adverse outcomes in 87 people who had suffered a traumatic SCI. At various times following the injury, positive adjustment (i.e., a nondepressed status) was predicted by the use of coping strategies such as acceptance, positive reinterpretation in growth, active coping, planning, and social support. Interestingly, variables such as functional independence, sex, age, and income were not found to be related to the resilience process. Kennedy, Frankel, Gardner, and Nuseibeh (1997) explored factors related to pain (an adverse outcome) in people with SCI. They found perceived pain, depressive mood, and anxiety were the most significant factors predicting outcomes. Berry, Elliott, and Rivera (2007) have conducted one of the few resilience-based studies in people with SCI. They studied 199 persons with SCI and used the NEO Five-Factor

Inventory to assess resilience-related personality factors when these patients were admitted to an inpatient medical rehabilitation program. Employing a cluster analysis of the NEO personality data, they identified a cluster that was believed to characterize a resilient group compared to other clusters believed to be more related to people with negative adjustment. Findings indicated that the resilient group was better adjusted than those showing negative adjustment (e.g., undercontrolling type). The resilient group had lower levels of depressive mood at admission and higher acceptance of their disability at discharge. Furthermore, the resilient group at admission was associated with the most effective social problem-solving abilities at discharge. This study suggests that resilience factors do protect a person with severe SCI.

Measures of Resilience

Several attempts have been made to measure resilience or hardiness using psychometric approaches (Hull, Van Treuren, & Virnelli, 1987; Kobasa, 1979; Wagnild & Young, 1993). However, these earlier scales have not had wide usage (Connor & Davidson, 2003). Connor and Davidson (2003) view resilience as a measure of a person's ability to cope with stress, and they have developed a resilience scale called the Connor-Davidson Resilience Scale (CD-RISC). It is comprised of 25 items, with each item rated on a 5-point scale, with higher scores reflecting greater levels of resilience. The CD-RISC has demonstrated reliability and validity. The scale measures aspects of hardiness or tenacity ("Not easily discouraged by failure"); positive acceptance of change ("Past success gives confidence for new challenge"), social support and relationships ("Close and secure relationships"), sense of mastery or self-control ("You can achieve your goals"), tolerance of negative emotions("Can handle unpleasant feelings"), and so on. As such, it attempts to measure resilience in terms of personal attributes rather than as a process, so that, in this case, resilience may be more properly a "protective factor." Nevertheless, the CD-RISC has been used to assess the capacity to be resilient. Campbell-Sills and Stein (2007) have attempted to improve the factor structure of the CD-RISC scale.

Recently, Smith, Dalen, Wiggins, Tooley, Christopher, and Bernard (2008) have developed a brief measure of resilience called the Brief Resilience Scale (BRS). They defined resilience as the ability to bounce back or recover from stress, and the scale was designed to assess an ability to recover and adapt. The BRS has been shown to be reliable and to be a unitary construct. It was found to be related to personal characteristics, social relations, coping, and health in all samples tested. The authors contend that the BRS is a reliable and valid means of assessing the ability to bounce back or recover from adversity. The BRS also measures protective factors related to resilience. Friborg, Hjemdal, Rosenvinge, and Martinussen (2006) developed a resilience scale designed to measure "the presence of protective resources that promote adult resilience" (p. 65). The scale consists of 45 items covering five dimensions, including personal competence, social competence, family coherence, social support, and personal structure; it is called the Resilience Scale for Adults (RSA). The RSA was shown to be test–retest reliable and to have acceptable construct and discriminate validity. This scale provides a psychometric tool to measure protective factors involved in the resilience process. Clauss-Ehlers (2008) has provided evidence that the resilience process is affected by culture. Clauss-Ehlers showed that adversity influenced children and adolescents differently depending on their diverse cultural backgrounds. She explored aspects of cultural resilience (e.g., adaptive coping and sociocultural support) in 305 college-aged women. Results suggest that cultural factors were related to measures of aspects of resilience. Stressors were experienced differently by people from various ethnic and social backgrounds, supporting a proposal that cultural factors affect the development of resilience. This work by Clauss-Ehlers (2008) raises an important assessment issue: resilience assessment should take account of cultural differences when considering a person's capacity to be resilient.

Summary

The dynamics of the human capacity to adjust and cope with adversity and trauma has been explored in this chapter, with specific application to people with physical disability. This dynamic is called "resilience" (Rutter, 1985), and research into resilience contrasts significantly with research that concentrates only on determining risks and deficits associated with adversity and trauma. The benefits of studying both risk and protective factors have been argued and recognized (Bonanno & Mancinni, 2008; Rutter, 1985). An approach that involves determining both risk and protective factors associated with a particular adversity should be accepted as an essential and innovative procedure for the study of outcomes in people who have a physical disability. Studying both risks and protective factors conforms to a resilience model, specifically, a risk and protective factors model (Luthar et al., 2000). It is critical that health professionals in the physical disability field explore in a comprehensive and dynamic way the risks and protective factors operating in people with a physical disability, simply because an approach that explores the risks of coping badly, as well as factors that protect a person, has rarely been used in the physical disability area; and the findings from this type of research that employs a risk and protective factor model will very likely expand substantially our understanding of the psychological, social, and environmental processes involved in positive adjustment, and this information will be central to the better management of the consequences of disability and chronic disease.

Table 26.3 provides a list of some protective factors shown to be operating in people with a physical disability. Risk factors have not been included in Table 26.3 as protective factors have been taken from the risk factors found in many of the studies shown in Table 26.3. In these cases, the protective factor has been deduced from the risk factor (e.g., if the risk factor was found to be unstable mood, then the protective factor was assumed to be stable mood). Other studies have sought predictors of positive outcomes, and these factors have been assumed to be protective factors. Table 26.3 provides details of each selected study (i.e., primary author, type of physical disability involved, and protective factors that may be operating). It is evident from an inspection of Table 26.3 that a large overlap occurs between protective factors operating in children and adolescents facing adversity without a physical disability (see Table 26.1) and children and adults with a physical disability. For example, quality social support and self-efficacy were frequently found to be protective factors in children facing adversity, and this was also found to be the case for adults with a severe injury or disability. The main protective factors found to be operating in the resilience process will now be briefly discussed.

Self-efficacy

Self-efficacy has been found to be an important factor that mediates between an adverse life event and adjustment to that adversity (Craig et al., 2009). Maciejewski, Prigerson, and Mazure (2000) showed self-efficacy was a very significant predictor of depressive symptom severity. They also showed that having a higher level of self-efficacy resulted in fewer depressive mood symptoms in adults, and that self-efficacy mediates around 40% of the effects of stressful life events on depressive mood. They concluded that maintaining healthy self-efficacy—that is, a strong sense of control over one's life and environment—serves to protect a person from psychopathology, perhaps by ameliorating the negative effect of stressful life events (Maciejewski et al., 2000). Rutter (1985) recognized that stressful life events may serve to precipitate psychopathology. Self-efficacy and similar constructs, such as fighting spirit, have also been found to influence outcomes significantly following SCI (Craig et al., 1994a,b), and toxic life experiences such as chronic pain have also been found to be mediated by levels of self-efficacy (Arnstein, Caudill, Mandle, Norris, & Beasley, 1999). Arnstein et al. (1999) conducted research with chronic pain patients attending a pain clinic and found that disability partially mediated the relationship between pain intensity and depression. When they added self-efficacy to the regression model they were using to determine unique contributors, they found self-efficacy was a stronger mediator than disability. This suggested that support for disability as a mediator of depression was a secondary finding, and that both pain intensity and self-efficacy contributed substantially to the development of disability and depression in patients with chronic pain. Arnstein et al. (1999) concluded that the lack of belief in one's ability to cope with pain and function despite persistent pain is a significant predictor of the extent to which individuals with chronic pain become disabled and depressed. Middleton, Tran, and Craig (2007) conducted research with over 100 persons with SCI living in the community and found that low self-efficacy was associated with reduced QOL across all SF-36 domains, above and beyond the effect of any physical impairment (Middleton et. al., 2007). Importantly, the association with poor QOL and low self-efficacy was equal to the association between severe pain and poor QOL (Middleton et al., 2007). Self-efficacy was found to be an important protective factor in the young (Moghadam, 2006) and elderly (Jang et al., 2002) with disability, in people with chronic pain (McCracken & Turk, 2002), in TBI (Dumont et al., 2004), diabetes (Yi et al., 2008), and SCI (Craig et al., 1994b). Clearly, in the management of people with a physical disability, interventions should be developed to contain a resilience-enhancing component that is known to boost self-efficacy (Craig et al., 1994a).

Social Support

Supportive social relationships are also known to act as a protective buffer against distress and

Table 26.3 Protective factors isolated from physical disability research and trauma

Study	Physical disability	Protective factors
Jang et al., 2002	Disability in the elderly	Self-efficacy; social support
Moghadam 2006	Disability in young adults	Self-efficacy, optimism
Anzarut et al., 2005	Adults with severe burns (>50%)	Perceived social support
Sheridan et al., 2000	Children aged <18 years with severe burns (>70%)	Functional family, good pre-burn health,
Byrne et al., 1986	Children with burns	Functional family, social networks, recreational activity, higher socioeconomic status, caring mother, greater number of family members
McCracken & Turk, 2002	Chronic pain	Stable emotional responses to pain, self-efficacy, positive attitude
Keefe et al., 1989	Chronic pain due to rheumatoid arthritis	Reduced catastrophization about pain
Dumont et al., 2004	People with traumatic brain injury	Optimism, self-efficacy
Schwartz et al., 2003	People with traumatic brain injury	Stable family, stable pre-injury behavior, higher socioeconomic status, less cognitive damage, adaptive behavioral skills
Barnwell & Kavanagh, 1997	Multiple sclerosis	Self-efficacy
Peyrot et al., 1999	Diabetes	emotionally stable, higher level of education, marital partner, positive coping skills
Yi et al., 2008	Diabetes	Self-esteem, self-efficacy, optimism
Mednick et al., 2007	Diabetes	Hope
Martz et al., 2005	People with SCI	Stable mood, low anxiety, adaptive coping skills, low severity of injury
Craig et al., 1994a	People with SCI	Self-efficacy
Craig et al., 1994b	People with SCI	Self-efficacy, lower levels of pain
Kennedy et al., 2000	People with SCI	Adaptive coping skills, social support
Kennedy et al., 1997	People with SCI	Stable mood, adaptive perceptions of pain
Berry et al., 2007	People with SCI	Problem-solving skills, stable mood, acceptance of disability
Southwick et al., 2005	Severe stress	Optimism, humor, social support, faith, positive role models, positive coping style, exercise, history of recovery
Lyons, 1991	Trauma and PTSD	Less severe trauma, history of recovery, well-educated, adaptive coping, finds meaning in trauma, social support
Farber et al., 2000	Stress and disease (HIV)	Stable mood, self-worth, high perceived quality of life, lower anxiety, commitment

psychopathology (Kendler, Myers, & Prescott, 2005; Kessler, Price, & Wortman, 1985). Rutter (1985) argued that social support will only buffer against adversity when the quality of the support is helpful and the person in question makes use of the available support. Social support is believed to be beneficial because it augments a person's sense of belonging and well-being. For example, when a person has a social network that provides quality emotional support, he perceives that he has access to assistance in difficult times, and this most likely boosts his mood and resilience (Kessler et al., 1985). Bloom (1990) suggested that social networks act as a protective factor in a direct manner by providing access to information or by enhancing motivation to engage in adaptive behaviors. She also suggested it could influence a person indirectly, by encouragement to adhere to treatment recommendations, maintain health-promoting behaviors such as exercise and a regular and balanced diet, or provide support such as giving a ride to someone who needs to keep a medical appointment or shop for food. Bloom concluded that "integration within the social network and the ability to draw resources from this network can maintain health and, in the event of illness, facilitate physical recovery" (Bloom, 1990, p. 635). Social support was found to be protective in the young with disability (Moghadam, 2006), in those with severe burns (Anzarut et al., 2005; Byrne et al., 1986), in those with SCI (Kennedy et al., 2000), and in those with severe stressors and trauma (Lyons, 1991; Southwick et al., 2005). In the management of people with a physical disability, strong emphasis must continue to be placed on enhancing social resources and networks, such as introducing the person to employment resources; providing counseling, if necessary, for caregivers; and introducing potential recreation resources.

Stable and Caring Family Factors

A number of studies found that family factors provided protection against adverse events. Functional family dynamics were found to protect people who are elderly and who also have a disability (Jang et al., 2002), those with severe burns (Byrne et al., 1986; Sheridan et al., 2000), and people with TBI (Schwartz et al., 2003). Having a caring marital partner protects people with diabetes from maladaptive outcomes (Peyrot et al., 1999), and having positive role models protects people experiencing severe stress from negative outcomes (Southwick et al., 2005). Presumably, role models would include family members, as well as friends and neighbors. Functional family factors certainly have a large protective influence on children and adolescents facing adversity (Morrison & Cosden, 1997), and from the limited resilience research conducted with physical disability, a functional family has an important influence also, and this is true also in adults. A challenge in the physical disability field will be to research comprehensively the protective influence of the function of families and partners in specific physical disabilities.

Positive Emotional States

Stable and positive emotions states such as self-esteem, optimism, hope, faith, and humor are known protections against adversity (Rutter, 1985). This was found in young people with a disability (Moghadam 2006), in people with severe chronic pain (McCracken & Turk, 2002), in people with TBI (Dumont et al., 2004), in people with diabetes (Mednick et al., 2007; Peyrot et al., 1999; Yi et al., 2008), in people with SCI (Berry et al., 2007; Martz et al., 2005), and in people coping with severe stress (Farber et al., 2000; Southwick et al., 2005). This chapter supports the conclusion that treatments that promote positive emotions will assist in enhancing resilience behavior and help to prevent problems associated with negative emotions such as anxiety, depression, aggression, anger, and other stress-related health problems (Tugade, Frederickson, & Barrett, 2004). Furthermore, some evidence exists that enhancing positive emotions such as hope and optimism can also protect against the development of disease, such as diabetes (Richman, Kubzansky, Maselko, Choo, & Bauer, 2005). Treatment strategies need to continue to draw upon known interventions, such as cognitive restructuring in CBT, that reduce negative mood states (Craig et al., 2009). However, they also need to develop strategies that simultaneously improve the person's level of optimism, hope, humor, and self-esteem, and perhaps even the person's ability to forgive (for instance, to forgive themselves if they had an accident in which they may have been partly to blame, and in which they suffered a severe injury). Research has recently shown forgiveness (a mixture of empathy, sympathy, and compassion) is a protective factor that improves resilience in the face of extreme stress (Worthington & Scherer, 2004). Blaming and not forgiving self or others is associated with negative emotions such as anxiety, anger, and depressive mood (Worthington & Scherer, 2004).

Adaptive Coping Skills

Coping effectively with adversity is a characteristic of resilience (Rutter, 1985). Kennedy (2008) argued that effective coping improves outcomes associated with disability and helps the person to regulate his or her emotional responses to the adversity. In coping skills training with people with SCI, as developed by Kennedy (2008) and colleagues, the person with a SCI is trained to become competent in coping skills (e.g., problem-solving, changing negative thinking and catastrophizing, organizing pleasant events, controlling stress levels through relaxation, and so on). Coping strategies that they found to be associated with positive adjustment included accepting the reality of an injury or disability, accessing quality social support and social networks, engaging in positive reappraisal, and employing problem-solving techniques (Kennedy, 2008). Maladaptive coping strategies found to be associated with poor adjustment included behavioral and mental disengagement, substance abuse, denial, social avoidance, underuse of social networks, and becoming angry with others and self (Kennedy, 2008). Turner and Clancy (1986) used coping skills training with chronic low back pain clients. Increased use of adaptive coping skills (e.g., decreased catastrophizing about the pain, distraction, reappraisal, problem-solving) was associated with decreases in pain intensity, as well as with decreases in physical and psychosocial impairment. The acquisition of adaptive coping skills was found to be protective in people with TBI (Schwartz et al., 2003), in people with diabetes (Peyrot et al., 1999), in people with SCI (Berry et al., 2007; Kennedy et al., 2000; Martz et al., 2005), and in people with severe stress (Lyons, 1991; Southwick et al., 2005).

Conclusion
Challenges for Work with Physical Disability

Many challenges remain for resilience research in people with physical disabilities. Very few studies have been conducted that employ a risk and protective factors model, with most studies to date employing either a risk deficit model or an outcome prediction model. However, the recent challenge presented in a paper by Wood and Tarrier (2010) to investigate both positive and negative functioning in clinical psychology research is an encouraging move in the direction of a risk and resilience research model. Wood and Tarrier (2010) emphasize the importance of studying positive characteristics (e.g., optimism and flexibility) as well as negative factors (e.g., anxiety, mood disorder) if we are to best understand psychological disorder. Similar to the research from the risk and resilience model research, Wood and Tarrier (2010) also suggest that positive characteristics have the capacity to "buffer the impact of negative life events" (p. 819). Future research in rehabilitation science should aim at investigating both risks for poor adjustment and those factors related to protection that result in positive adjustment. Rutter (1987) discussed four processes that should be addressed when exploring resilience: the reduction of risks; the reduction of cycles of failure; the establishment and maintenance of protective factors, such as self-esteem and self-efficacy; and opening up of opportunities. "Opportunities" need to be explored in physical disability research. For example, vocation opportunities are most likely important protective factors. Werner (1993) found that mothers of resilient children were more likely to be employed than were mothers of nonresilient children. Employment status is one of the strongest predictors of QOL in people with SCI, and those people with SCI who are employed report higher levels of psychological and physical health, as well as reduced use of health facilities (Murphy & Young, 2008). Family dynamics and social support still need to be more fully explored in relation to their resilience value. There is an urgent need to explore other potential protective factors in people with physical disability, such as the value of community integration and mobility, hospitalization dynamics, the severity of the disability and resilience, the influence of past successes in managing adversity, and perhaps the development of a comprehensive model that can encompass and explain the dynamics involved in how people of any age can demonstrate resilient behavior when they have a severe injury.

Future Directions

The following questions suggest further avenues for research:

• Is resilience best conceived as a process or a personal attribute?

• How best can the risk and protective factors model be applied to physical disability research?

• What are the benefits of applying a risk and protective factors model to physical disabilities such as a SCI or MS?

• What is an appropriate working definition for the resilience process that can be applied to the physical disabilities?

References

Anzarut, A., Chen, M., Shankowsky, H., & Tredget, E. (2005). Quality-of-life and outcome predictors following massive burn injury. *Plastic and Reconstructive Surgery, 116,* 791–797.

Arnstein, P., Caudill, M., Mandle, C. L., Norris, A., & Beasley, R. (1999). Self efficacy as a mediator of the relationship between pain intensity, disability and depression in chronic pain patients. *Pain, 80,* 483–491.

Bandura, A. (1989). Human agency in social cognitive theory. *American Psychologist, 14,* 1175–1184.

Barnwell, A. M., & Kavanagh, D. J. (1997). Prediction of psychological adjustment to multiple sclerosis. *Social Science and Medicine, 45,* 411–418.

Belmont, A., Agar, N., Hugeron, C., Gallais, B., & Azouvi, P. (2006). Fatigue and traumatic brain injury. *Annales de Réadaptation et de Médecine Physique, 49,* 370–374.

Berry, J. W., Elliott, T., R., & Rivera, P. (2007). Resilient, undercontrolled, and overcontrolled personality prototypes among persons with spinal cord injury. *Journal of Personality Assessment, 89,* 292–302.

Bloom, J. R. (1990). The relationship of social support and health. *Social Sciences Medicine, 30,* 635–437.

Bonanno, G. A., & Mancini, A. D. (2008). The human capacity to thrive in the face of potential trauma. *Pediatrics, 121,* 369–375.

Bradshaw, B. G., Richardson, G. E., Kumpfer, K., Carlson, J., Stanchfield, J., Overall, J., et al. (2007). Determining the efficacy of a resiliency training approach in adults with Type 2 diabetes. *The Diabetes Educator, 33,* 650–659.

Byrne, C., Love, B., Browne, G., Brown, B., Roberts, J., & Streiner, D. (1986). The social competence of children following burn injury: A study of resilience. *Journal of Burn Care and Rehabilitation, 7,* 247–252.

Campbell-Sills, L., & Stein, M. B. (2007). Psychometric analysis and refinement of the Connor–Davidson Resilience Scale (CD-RISC): Validation of a 10-item measure of resilience. *Journal of Traumatic Stress, 20,* 6, 1019–1028.

Chwastiak, L. A., & Ehde, D. M. (2007). Psychiatric issues in multiple sclerosis. *Psychiatric Clinics of North America, 30,* 803–817. N

Cicchetti, D., & Rogosch, F. A. (1997). The role of self-organization in the promotion of resilience in maltreated children. *Development and Psychopathology, 9,* 787–815.

Clauss-Ehlers, C. S. (2008). Sociocultural factors, resilience, and coping: Support for a culturally sensitive measure of resilience. *Journal of Applied Developmental Psychology, 29,* 197–212.

Connor, K. M., & Davidson, J. R. T. (2003). Development of a new resilience scale: The Connor-Davidson Resilience Scale (CD-RISC). *Depression and Anxiety, 18,* 76–82.

Craig, A. R., Hancock, K., & Chang, E. (1994a). The influence of spinal cord injury on coping styles and self-perceptions two years after the event. *Australian and New Zealand Journal of Psychiatry, 28,* 307–312.

Craig, A. R., Hancock, K. M., & Dickson, H. (1994b). Spinal cord injury: A search for determinants of depression two years after the event. *British Journal of Clinical Psychology, 33,* 221–230.

Craig, A., & Nicholson Perry, K. (2008). *Guide for health professionals on the psychosocial care for people with spinal cord injury.* Sydney: New South Wales State Spinal Cord Injury Service.

Craig, A., Tran, Y., & Middleton, J. (2009). Psychological morbidity and spinal cord injury: A systematic review. *Spinal Cord, 47,* 108–114.

Dumont, C., Gervais, M., Fougeyrollas, P., & Bertrand, R. (2004). Toward an explanatory model of social participation for adults with traumatic brain injury. *Journal of Head Trauma Rehabilitation, 19,* 431–444.

Egeland, B., Carson, E., & Sroufe, L. A. (1993). Resilience as process. *Development and Psychopathology, 5,* 517–528.

Farber, E. W., Schwartz, J. A. J., Schaper, P. E., Moonen, D. J., & McDaniel, J. S. (2000). Resilience factors associated with adaptation to HIV disease. *Psychosomatics, 41,* 140–146.

Fergus, S., & Zimmerman, M. A. (2005). Adolescent resilience: A framework for understanding healthy development in the face of risk. *Annual Reviews of Public Health, 26,* 399–419.

Festinger, T. (1984). *No one ever asked us: A postscript to the foster care system.* New York: Columbia University Press.

Friborg, O., Hjemdal, O., Rosenvinge, J. H., & Martinussen, M. (2006). A new rating scale for adult resilience: What are the central protective resources behind healthy adjustment? *International Journal of Methods in Psychiatric Research, 12,* 65–76.

Garmezy, N., & Masten, A. S. (1991). The protective role of competence indicators in children at risk. In E. M. Cummings, A. L. Greene, & K. H. Karraker (Eds.), *Life-span developmental psychology: Perspectives on stress and coping* (pp. 151–174). Hillsdale, NJ: Lawrence Erlbaum Publishers.

Hull, J. G., Van Treuren, R. R., & Virnelli, S. (1987). Hardiness and health: A critique and alternative approach. *Journal of Personality Social Psychology, 53,* 518–530.

Jang, Y., Haley, W. E., Small, B. J., & Mortimer, J. A. (2002). The role of mastery and social resources in the associations between disability and depression in later life. *The Gerontologist, 42,* 807–813.

Keefe, F. J., Brown, G. K., Wallston, K. A., & Caldwell, D. S. (1989). Coping with rheumatoid arthritis pain: Catastrophizing as a maladaptive strategy. *Pain, 37,* 51–56.

Kendall, E., & Buys, N. (1998). An integrated model of psychosocial adjustment following acquired disability. *Journal of Rehabilitation, 64,* 16–21.

Kendler, K. S., Myers, J., & Prescott, C. A. (2005). Sex differences in the relationship between social support and risk for major depression: A longitudinal study of opposite-sex twin pairs. *American Journal of Psychiatry, 162,* 250–256.

Kennedy, P. (2008). Coping effectively with spinal cord injuries. In A. Craig, & Y. Tran (Eds.), *Psychological dynamics associated with spinal cord injury rehabilitation: New directions and best evidence* (pp. 55–70). New York: Nova Science Publishers.

Kennedy, P., Frankel, H., Gardner, B., & Nuseibeh, I. (1997). Factors associated with acute and chronic pain following traumatic spinal cord injuries. *Spinal Cord, 35,* 814–817.

Kennedy, P., Marsh, N., Lowe, R., Grey, N., Short, E., & Rogers, B. (2000). A longitudinal analysis of psychological impact and coping strategies following spinal cord injury. *British Journal of Health Psychology, 5,* 157–172.

Kessler, R. C., Price, R. H., & Wortman, C. B. (1985). Social factors in psychopathology: Stress, social support and coping processes. *Annual Reviews Psychology, 36,* 531–572.

Kobasa, S. C. (1979). Stressful life events, personality, and health: An inquiry into hardiness. *Journal of Personality Social Psychology, 37,* 1–11.

Krause, J. S., & Broderick, L. (2005). A 25-year longitudinal study of the natural course of aging after spinal cord injury. *Spinal Cord, 43*, 349–356.

Luthar, S. S., Cicchetti, D., & Becker, B. (2000). The construct of resilience: The construct of resilience: A critical evaluation and guidelines for future work. *Child Development, 71*, 543–562.

Lyons J. (1991). Strategies for assessing the potential for positive adjustment following trauma. *Journal of Traumatic Stress, 4*, 93–111.

Maciejewski, P. K., Prigerson, H. G., & Mazure, C. M. (2000). Self-efficacy as a mediator between stressful life events and depressive symptoms. *British Journal of Psychiatry, 174*, 373–378.

Martz, E., Livneh, H., Priebe, M., Wuermser, L. A., & Ottomanelli, L. (2005). Predictors of psychosocial adaptation among people with spinal cord injury or disorder. *Archives Physical Medicine Rehabilitation, 86*, 1182–1192.

Masten, A. S., Best, K. M., & Garmezy, N. (1990). Resilience and development: Contributions from the study of children who overcome adversity. *Development and Psychopathology, 2*, 425–444.

McCracken, L., & Turk, D. (2002). Behavioral and cognitive-behavioral treatment for chronic pain: Outcome, predictors of outcome, and treatment process. *Spine, 27*, 2564–2573.

Mednick, L., Cogen, F., Henderson, C., Rohrbeck, C. A., Kitessa, D., & Streisand, R. (2007). Hope more, worry less: Hope as a potential resilience factor in mothers of very young children with Type 1 diabetes. *Children's Health Care, 36*, 385–396.

Middleton, J., & Craig, A. (2008). Psychological challenges in treating persons with spinal cord injury. In A. Craig, & Y. Tran (Eds.), *Psychological dynamics associated with spinal cord injury rehabilitation: New directions and best evidence* (pp. 3–53). New York: Nova Science Publishers.

Middleton, J., Tran, Y., & Craig, A. (2007). Relationship between quality of life and self-efficacy in persons with spinal cord injuries. *Archives of Physical Medicine and Rehabilitation, 88*, 1643–1648.

Moghadam, M. A. (2006). *Predictors of resilient successful life outcomes in persons with disabilities: Towards a model of personal resilience.* Unpublished doctoral dissertation: The George Washington University.

Morrison, G. M., & Cosden, M. A. (1997). Risk, resilience, and adjustment of individuals with learning disabilities. *Learning Disability Quarterly, 20*, 43–60.

Murphy, G. C., & Young, A. E. (2008). Vocational achievement following traumatic spinal cord injury. In A. Craig, & Y. Tran (Eds.), *Psychological dynamics associated with spinal cord injury rehabilitation: New directions and best evidence* (pp.197–214). New York: Nova Science Publishers.

Peyrot, M., McMurry, Jr., J. F., & Kruger, D. F. (1999). A biopsychosocial model of glycemic control in diabetes: Stress, coping and regimen adherence. *Journal of Health and Social Behavior, 40*, 141–158.

Pollard, C., & Kennedy, P. (2007). A longitudinal analysis of emotional impact, coping strategies and post-traumatic psychological growth following spinal cord injury: A 10-year review. *British Journal of Health Psychology, 12*, 347–362.

Rew, L., & Horner, S. D. (2003). Youth resilience framework for reducing health-risk behaviors in adolescents. *Journal of Pediatric Nursing, 18*, 379–388.

Richman, L. S., Kubzansky, L., Maselko, J., Choo, P., & Bauer, M. (2005). Positive emotion and health: Going beyond the negative. *Health Psychology, 24*, 422–429.

Rutter, M. (1985). Resilience in the face of adversity. Protective factors and resistance to psychiatric disorder. *British Journal of Psychiatry, 147*, 598–611.

Rutter, M. (1987). Psychosocial resilience and protective factors. *American Journal of Orthopsychiatry, 57*, 316–331.

Schwartz, C. E., Coulthard-Morris, L., & Zeng, Q. (1996). Psychosocial correlates of fatigue in multiple sclerosis. *Archives Physical medicine Rehabilitation, 77*, 165–170.

Schwartz, L., Taylor, H. G., Drotar, D., Yeates, K. O. Wade, S. L., & Stancin, T. (2003). Long-term behavior problems following pediatric traumatic brain injury: Prevalence, predictors, and correlates. *Journal of Pediatric Psychology, 28*, 251–263.

Sheridan, R. L., Hinson, M. I., Liang, M. H., Nackel, A. F., Schoenfeld, D. A., Ryan, C. M., et al. (2000). Long-term outcome of children surviving massive burns. *Journal of the American Medical Association, 283*, 69–73.

Smith, B. W., Dalen, J., Wiggins, K., Tooley, E., Christopher, P., & Bernard, J. (2008). The Brief Resilience Scale: Assessing the ability to bounce back. *International Journal of Behavioral Medicine, 15*, 194–200.

Southwick, S. M., Vythilingam, M., & Charney, D. S. (2005). The psychobiology of depression and resilience to stress: Implications for prevention and treatment. *Annual Reviews Clinical Psychology, 1*, 255–291.

Sullivan, M. J. L., Stanish, W., Waite, H., Sullivan, M., & Tripp, D. A. (1998). Catastrophizing, pain, and disability in patients with soft-tissue injuries. *Pain, 77*, 253–260.

Trieschmann, R. B. (1982). *Spinal cord injuries. Psychological, social and vocational adjustment.* New York: Pergamon Press.

Tugade, M. M., Fredrickson, B. L., & Barrett, L. F. (2004). Psychological resilience and positive emotional granularity: Examining the benefits of positive emotions on coping and health. *Journal of Personality, 72*, 1161–1190.

Turner, J. A., & Clancy, S. (1986). Strategies for coping with chronic low back pain: Relationship to pain and disability. *Pain, 24*, 355–364.

Vigil, J. D. (1990). Cholos and gangs: Culture change and street youth in Los Angeles. In R. Huff (Ed.), *Gangs in America: Diffusion, diversity, and public policy* (pp. 142–162). Thousand Oaks, CA: Sage.

Wagnild, G. M., & Young, H. M. (1993). Development and psychometric validation of the Resilience Scale. *Journal of Nursing Measurement, 1*, 165–178.

Werner, E. E. (1993). Risk, resilience, and recovery: Perspectives from the Kauai Longitudinal Study. *Development and Psychopathology, 5*, 503–515.

Werner, E. E., & Smith, R. S. (2001). *Journeys from childhood to the midlife: Risk, resilience, and recovery.* New York: Cornell University Press.

White, B., Driver, S., & Warren, A. M. (2008). Considering resilience in the rehabilitation of people with traumatic disabilities. *Rehabilitation Psychology, 53*, 9–17.

Wood, A. M., & Tarrier, N. (2010). Positive clinical psychology: A new vision and strategy for integrated research and practice. *Clinical Psychology Review, 30*, 819–829.

Worthington, E. L., & Scherer, M. (2004). Forgiveness is an emotion-focused coping strategy that can reduce health risks and promote health resilience: Theory, review, and hypotheses. *Psychology and Health, 19*, 385–405.

Wortman, C. B., & Silver, R. C. (1989). The myths of coping with loss. *Journal of Consulting and Clinical Psychology, 57*, 349–357.

Wright, B. (1983). *Physical disability: A psychosocial approach* (2nd ed.). New York: Harper-Collins Publishers, Inc.

Yi, J. P., Vitaliano, P. P., Smith, R. E., Yi, J. C., & Weinger, K. (2008). The role of resilience on psychological adjustment and physical health in patients with diabetes. *British Journal of Health Psychology, 13*, 311–325.

Zimmerman, M. A., & Arunkumar, R. (1994). Resiliency research: Implications for schools and policy. *Social Policy Report: Society for Research in Child Development, 8*, 1–17.

The Expert Patient and the Self-Management of Chronic Conditions and Disabilities

Michelle A. Meade *and* Linda A. Cronin

Abstract

Expert patient refers to the inherent knowledge that individuals living with disabilities or chronic conditions have about their condition, its impact on their life, and what decisions they feel comfortable making. Self-management refers to the ability of these individuals to manage their health and its physical and psychosocial consequences. However, just because an individual has a chronic condition or disability does not imply that they have expertise in dealing with it, and, in fact, some chronic conditions result from difficulty in performing health management behaviors. This chapter reviews some of the theories, programs, components, and issues that inform or support the development of self-management skills. At the end, the various roles that rehabilitation psychologists may take in supporting the development and application of self-management skills are discussed.

Key Words: Self-management, health behavior, disabilities, chronic health conditions.

Expert patient is a term that is used to acknowledge the role of an individual with a disability or chronic condition in managing his or her health and life. It came into common use in 2001, as part of an initiative by the United Kingdom's Department of Health to improve national health status by shifting management of chronic disease from health care professionals to the individuals with the chronic conditions or disabilities (Department of Health, U.K., 2001; Donaldson, 2003). The primary aspects of this initiative were (a) to recognize that patients have expertise about their illness/impairments and how it impacts their lives (including social circumstances) and that their values, preferences, and attitudes are critical in disease management decisions; and (b) to provide them with the education, support, skills, and structure to take a primary role in disease management activities (Badcott, 2005). The term and concept of the *expert patient* provide important recognition for the idea that, although health care providers can provide information, medication,

and specific treatments, ultimately health is based on the individual's ability (e.g., knowledge, motivation, independence resources) to perform behaviors (e.g., eating a healthy diet, taking medications, getting out of bed, exercising) consistently. Individuals with disabilities can and should expect to be able to form relationships, be part of their community, and engage in activities that are fulfilling and meaningful. However, for this to really work, they first need the skills to manage their health and its consequences.

Self-management refers to the ability of an individual with a chronic condition or disability to manage his or her health and its physical and psychosocial consequences (Barlow, Wright, Sheasby, Turner, & Hainsworth, 2002). In 2003, *self-management support* was defined by the Institute of Medicine (IOM) as "systematic provision of education and supportive interventions by health care staff to increase patients' skills and confidence in managing their health problems, including regular assessment of progress and problems, goal setting, and problem solving support" (Institute of Medicine [IOM], 2003; Pearson, Mattke, Shaw, Ridgely, & Wiseman, 2007). Self-management skills, then, are thought to enhance an individual's ability to make decisions and lifestyle choices that will optimize functioning and allow for greater participation in family, social, community, and vocational roles and environments (Creer & Holroyd, 2006).

Self-management is an evidence-based approach to managing chronic illness. It provides education and skill-building related to self-monitoring, communication, problem-solving, and relaxation. Self-management approaches have been proven effective for improving health status and health behaviors, increasing self-efficacy, improving compliance with medication regimens, decreasing pain, and lowering health care costs (Bodenheimer, Lorig, Holman, & Grumbach, 2002; Holman & Lorig, 2004; Lorig, 1982, 2003; Lorig & Holman, 2003; Lorig, Ritter, Laurent, & Plant, 2006; Lorig, Ritter, Villa, & Armas, 2009; Lorig, Sobel, Ritter, Laurent, & Hobbs, 2001; Lorig et al., 1999; Newman, Steed, & Mulligan, 2004; Steed, Cooke, & Newman, 2003), and protocols have been effectively tailored to meet the needs and concerns of minority populations (Carbone, Rosal, Torres, Goins, & Bermudez, 2007; Lorig, Ritter, & Gonzalez, 2003; Lorig, Ritter, & Jacquez, 2005; Lorig, Ritter, Villa, & Piette, 2008; Rosal et al., 2005; Vincent, Clark, Zimmer, & Sanchez, 2006; von Goeler, Rosal, Ockene, Scavron, & De Torrijos, 2003).

Theory

Self-management interventions are typically based on four theoretical constructs or techniques (either individually or combined): social cognitive theory, stress and coping models, the transtheoretical model, and/or cognitive-behavioral therapy (CBT; Newman et al., 2004); however, additional theories and models are useful for fully understanding the process and purposefully modifying behaviors. For example, the health behavior model can be used to understand health behavior change, whereas self-regulation theory and the International Classification of Functioning, Disability, and Health (otherwise known as the ICF) provide insight into the interaction with the environment and larger social contexts.

Social cognitive theory states that health behavior is influenced by relationships with people and the social environment, and that people's behavior in turn influences both (Bandura, 1995; Baranowski,

Perry, & Parcel, 2002). Self-efficacy, together with expectations, mediates behavior. That is, an individual is more likely to perform an action if he is confident that he will be able to accomplish it successfully. As a result, components of self-management programs focus on the acquisition of skills such as problem-solving and goal-setting. With regard to rehabilitation, social cognitive theory can provide insight into empowerment, self-regulation, and understanding the relationships between people, places, and abilities. People with strong self-efficacy may perceive their disabilities as less severe (Seeman, Unger, & McAvay, 1999).

Stress and coping models posit that health will be affected by an individual's ability to deal with stresses associated with her condition. Stress, within the various models, can be conceptualized as a stimulus, a response, or an interaction between a person and her environment. As a stimulus, stress is the physical and/or psychological burden of an event or series of events. As a response, stress is the three-stage physiological sequence consisting of alarm, resistance, and exhaustion (at least as proposed in Selye's *general adaptation syndrome* (GAS; Selye, 1950) that occurs when an individual is exposed to a noxious stimulus. It can have direct consequences to both physical and psychological health, including decreases in immune functioning, depression, and post-traumatic stress disorder. The *transactional model of stress and coping* posits that during an individual's *primary appraisal*, he develops a judgment about the significance of an event (i.e., controllable, threatening, irrelevant), whereas a *secondary appraisal* occurs when the person assesses his own coping resources and options about what he can do about the situation (Cohen, 1988; Lazarus & Folkman, 1984). Stress, then, is based on the imbalance between perceived demands and evaluation of coping resources. *Coping efforts* are the actual strategies used to mediate primary and secondary appraisals. In general, these fall into two broad categories: problem management strategies, directed at changing a stressful situation; and emotional regulation, aimed at changing the way one thinks or feels about a stressful situation (Glanz, Rimer, & Lewis, 2002). These theories support the instruction of stress-management techniques, such as relaxation, meditation, and guided imagery, to alter physiological status and support emotional regulation, as well as cognitive-based strategies to improve problem management and promote coping responses.

Cognitive-behavioral therapies provide some of the tools to assist people with disabilities and chronic conditions in influencing appraisals of the situation or event, as well as their own resources. Self-management programs often address how people think about their conditions and themselves and the inter-relationship between thoughts, feelings, and behaviors. In particular, therapies and techniques have worked to identify negative or irrational cognitions. For example, a self-management program may address the erroneous assumption that individuals with disabilities cannot work or that they cannot effectively parent a child and then explore how that assumption has impacted behavior. *Problem-solving therapy* is one type of CBT that has been empirically validated for both adolescents and adults with various clinical presentations ranging from medical conditions to depression, obesity, and schizophrenia (D'Zurilla & Nezu, 2007). Problems and psychopathology are viewed as the consequences of unsuccessful attempts to deal with stressful events. The role of the therapist is to facilitate a positive attitude while promoting rational problem-solving techniques. Its five basic steps include: (1) problem orientation, (2) problem definition and formulation, (3) generation of alternative solutions, (4) decision-making; and (5) solution implementation and evaluation (D'Zurilla & Nezu, 2007). Once problems and the goal of treatment have been identified, these steps are used to address attitudes, beliefs, negative emotions, and behaviors that maintain problems, as well as how these can be changed to find solutions.

The *health belief model* discusses four key concepts—perceived susceptibility or vulnerability, perceived severity of a condition, perceived benefits of treatment, and perceived barriers—and posits that people will not change their behaviors unless they see themselves as susceptible, view the condition as sufficiently severe, and feel that taking action will make a difference. In these contexts, *health behavior change* can be defined as the switch from risky or unhealthy behaviors to healthy or positive behaviors (Nieuwenhuijsen, Zemper, & Miner, 2006). The health belief model also involves cues for action that can lead to behavior modification, such as increased pain or increasing knowledge of a condition (Janz, Champion, & Strecher, 2002). *Self-efficacy* is also important in this model; since healthy behaviors are difficult to practice, a person must believe that a healthy lifestyle is possible (Strecher & Rosenstock, 1997).

The *transtheoretical model (TTM) of behavior change* is a stage theory that refers to how prepared individuals are to make changes to their behaviors.

In order to change a health-related behavior, individuals progress through six stages of change, including pre-contemplation (in which the patient is not currently considering change), contemplation (ambivalent about change; considers making it eventually), preparation (planning to act within the next month), action (actively practicing the new behavior), maintenance (continued commitment to sustaining behavior), and termination or relapse (resumption of old behavior) (Prochaska & Velicer, 1997). Research on TTM has identified activities or processes that are used to progress people through stages, including five experiential processes (increasing awareness, dramatic relief, social reappraisal, environmental opportunities, and self-reappraisal) and five behavioral processes (stimulus control, helping relationship, counter conditioning, rewarding, and committing) (Velicer, Prochaska, Fava, Norman & Redding, 1998). The TTM can be used to inform program recruitment, assist with retention of participants, understand progress through stages, inform intervention processes, and, ultimately, facilitate outcomes. In particular, by applying techniques that match stage of change with intervention components, researchers have increased the number of individuals who join and complete programs and those who successfully change behavior.

The self-regulation model and the ICF acknowledge and discuss the role of environmental factors in health. Self-regulation is a type of social cognitive theory that emphasizes the continual and reciprocal processes that allow an individual to be observant and make judgments based on observation (rather than automatically or based on biases), then alter their own behavior as needed to achieve desired goals, with goal importance influencing the effort put into the self-regulation process. Both intrapersonal and external factors influence and modify the judgments, observations, and reactions that influence the use of management strategies. Intrapersonal factors may include knowledge, attitudes, feelings, and beliefs, whereas external factors include role models, technical advice and service, social support, and money and material resources (Clark, Gong, & Kaciroti, 2001). Management strategies for both disease control and prevention (i.e., the behaviors that an individual performs to keep the disease and its effects under control) lead to the various endpoints, including personal goals, physiological status, functioning, and health care use, which in turn influence both external and intrapersonal factors, thus leading to the aforementioned continuous cycle.

The *common-sense model* (CSM) of self-regulation (also referred to as the *illness representation model* or the *personal model of illness*) proposed by Howard Leventhal and colleagues (Hale & Treharne, 2007; Leventhal & Cameron, 1987; Leventhal & Diefenbach, 1991; Leventhal, Meyer, & Nerenz, 1980; Meyer, Leventhal, & Guttman, 1985; Spafford, 2004) views the patient as an active and motivated participant in his own health who perceives the illness, disease, or impairment as a threat that he then attempts to respond to. This response is a three-stage self-regulatory process that involves illness representations (i.e., personal or "common sense" models of disease/impairment), coping behaviors, and evaluation of coping effectiveness (appraisal). People construct these "common sense" models to understand their illness or impairment around five components: *identity* (beliefs about the illness/disability label and associated symptoms), perceived *cause* of the condition (based on personal somatic cues and experiences, as well as information gathered from health professionals, media sources, and influential others within the social and/or cultural environment), *time-line or course* (expectations about length or course of the condition), *consequences* of the condition (including its physical and social impact), and *curability/controllability* (beliefs about whether the condition can be controlled or kept in check and the degree to which the individual plays a role in this). Each component is influenced by both internal and external factors and each build on and influences the others. In addition, each of these components evolves and is reevaluated over time, impacting how an individual regulates or manages his condition and his health. An individual with a sudden-onset traumatic injury might initially focus on full recovery and eventually, then after living with the condition and interacting with both health care professionals and individuals with disabilities, gradually shift his focus to managing the impairment and maintaining wellness.

In addition, the CSM posits both cognitive and emotional processing of the three stages (illness representation, coping, and appraisal) and states that information processing can occur independently or dynamically on one or both pathways. As such, fear, anxiety, and other emotional responses are given weight equal to biomedical information in understanding motivation and health behaviors. Finally, the CSM recognizes that health behaviors occur within home and community environments, not the health care system, and that procedural actions rather than words determine behavior in everyday

life (Levanthal, Leventhal, & Breland, 2011). Health and self-management strategies based on CSM, then, take into account patients' current and past experiences and focus on issues that patients see as important (Harvey & Lawson, 2009). More importantly, they attempt to modify illness representation and coping responses by addressing both cognitive and emotional factors that influence behavior and suggest the collaborative development of action plans by patients and health care providers (Leventhal, Leventhal, & Halm, 2010).

Self-regulation theory, as interpreted by Clark and colleagues (Clark et al., 2001), recognizes that patient self-management occurs within the context of external influences consisting most proximally of family involvement and moving more distally to include clinical expertise, work/school support, community awareness, support and action, and community-wide environmental control measures, and finally ending with conducive policies (Clark et al., 2001). As such, interventions may engage and educate people in various settings to promote or support more positive health behaviors.

The ICF is an international classifications model developed by the World Health Organization (World Health Organization [WHO], 2001) and endorsed by the Institute of Medicine (Field & Jette, 2007), the World Health Assembly, and the North American Collaborating Center (NACC) for use in research, surveillance, and reporting (WHO, 2001). Although health conditions are classified primarily in ICD-10, the ICF classifies functioning and disability to describe how people *live with* their health condition. Functioning is described at three levels (see Figure 27.1): the level of the body (functions and structures), the level of the person (activities), and at the level of society (participation in life situations). Negative functioning at these three levels is represented by impairments, activity limitations (or disability), and participation restrictions. For example, an individual with arthritis may experience pain

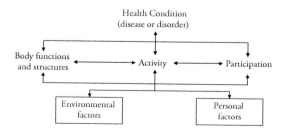

Figure 27.1 The International Classification of Functioning, Disability, and Health model.

(impairments in body functions and structures) that leads to severe difficulty in walking (mobility disability), which may restrict his or her involvement in life situations, such as meeting with close friends (participation restriction). Interventions that provided information and social support to increase exercise, then, would use personal and environmental factors to modify activity levels and promote improved health.

The ICF model (WHO, 2001) acknowledges the importance of environmental and personal factors in modifying the consequences of impairments for activities or participation. Specifically, in the ICF, environmental factors "make up the physical, social and attitudinal environment in which people live and conduct their lives" (p. 232). These factors are classified under five broad headings: products and technology, supports and relationships, attitudes and stereotypes, public/private services or policies, and natural and human-made environments. A complete review of the specific factors is beyond the scope of this chapter; however, the two key points to realize are that these environmental factors influence both behavior and health and that they are often modifiable, and so can be addressed or optimized through self-management and other strategies.

Self-Management Programs

Self-management programs, whether or not they carry that specific title, have been developed for many conditions commonly treated by rehabilitation psychologists. There are general programs and skills training approaches that can be used with individuals with many types of disabilities, as well as tailored approaches for specific disease populations. A defining characteristic is the positioning of the program or intervention within the health care system; that is, the extent to which the program is managed and administered within or outside of a patient's primary or tertiary health care setting (Pearson et al., 2007). Generally, programs external to the health care system are designed to be administered by laypersons whereas those within a primary health care setting are delivered by health care professionals. Programs facilitated by laypersons are generally administered in group formats by other individuals with disabilities, while those administered by health care professionals are more varied with regard to composition and implementation.

The most widely known and studied self-management program is the Chronic Disease Self-Management Program (CDSMP) developed by Kate Lorig and associates at Stanford University, in which lay trainers teach self-management skills to classes of individuals with a range of risk factors and chronic diseases (Lorig, Ritter et al., 2001). Trainers go through a certification process and have, themselves, a chronic condition or disability. Classes are participatory but highly structured and based on a manualized curriculum designed to be administered in over a series of six 2.5-hour classes held 1 day a week in a community setting. The program covers the topics of communication, nutrition and meal planning, exercising, appropriate use of medications, and evaluating new treatments and making informed decisions, and teaches techniques for dealing with common problems such as frustration, fatigue, pain, and isolation. Randomized clinical trials using variations of this program have shown improvements in self-rated health, coping skills, and reductions in disability and health care costs (Lorig, Hurwicz, Sobel, Hobbs, & Ritter, 2005; Lorig, Mazonson, & Holman, 1993; Lorig, Ritter et al., 2001; Lorig, Ritter, Dost et al., 2008). The program has been adapted into Spanish and for web-based administration (Lorig et al., 2006; Lorig, Ritter, Villa et al., 2008).

As used in the United Kingdom under the auspices of the Expert Patient Programme (EPP), Primary Care Trusts (PCTs) organize and deliver an adapted version of CDSMP to individuals who have self-identified as having a long-term condition. Although program coordinators are supported under the PCTs, the courses themselves are conducted by a volunteer workforce of laypersons who themselves have chronic conditions. Results from a randomized control trial on the outcomes of the program found moderate improvements in participant self-efficacy, smaller but significant improvements in energy and psychological well-being, and some reduction in overnight hospital stays, although not in general health service utilization. Overall, it was reported that the EPP was likely to be cost-effective (Rogers et al., 2006). However, it was noted that there were significant issues with administering the program and that individuals who participated were not necessarily representative of those with long-term conditions; rather, those likely to attend EPP courses were white, middle-class, well-educated individuals who were already committed to self-managing.

Problem-solving training is more standardized version of problem-solving therapy (previously described) that has been used and adapted extensively to promote health in a variety of populations with disabilities and chronic conditions (D'Zurilla & Nezu, 2007). Participants are taught a positive problem orientation and to systematically follow four steps when solving disability-related (or caregiving-related) problems: (1) identify and define the problem, (2) decide what needs to be accomplished and list possible solutions to the problem, (3) choose and test the best solution(s), and (4) evaluate the outcomes of problem-solving (Grant, Elliott, Weaver, Bartolucci, & Giger, 2002). Training can be administered to individuals or in groups in a variety of settings, and facilitators are generally health care providers. After the initial training session, follow-up contacts review and encourage continued application of the problem-solving approach. Problem-solving training has been found to be effective for improving problem-solving skills, increasing preparedness, and improving vitality, social functioning, mental health, and role limitations related to emotional problems (D'Zurilla & Nezu, 2007).

Living Well with a Disability is a wellness intervention for individuals with mobility impairments designed to promote health and reduce secondary conditions and health care costs (Ravesloot, Seekins, & White, 2005). The program is administered by individuals with disabilities in a community setting for 2 hours each week over an 8-week period. Facilitators review and work with participants to complete exercises from the associated program workbook. The program reflects the independent living philosophy and is based around social cognitive models and the health behavior change theories to encourage goal pursuit and health behavior change. Topics addressed in the program include goal setting, problem-solving, attribution training, depression, communication, information-seeking, nutrition, physical activity, advocacy, and maintenance. An interrupted time series design with randomized assignment found reductions in limitations from secondary conditions, symptom days, and health care utilization (Ravesloot et al., 2005).

Lifestyle Redesign is an occupational therapy intervention developed by Florence Clark and colleagues at the University of Southern California (USC) to enhance the health and psychosocial well-being of various populations, including the well elderly, individuals with spinal cord injury, college students, and individuals with multiple sclerosis (University of Southern California, 2010). This professionally facilitated program combines education with peer exchange and personal experience and exploration in order to promote positive attitudes and health-promoting behaviors while addressing practical considerations of transportation, finances, and safety (Horowitz & Chang, 2004; Jackson, Carlson, Mandel, Zemke, & Clark, 1998). Research has shown the intervention to be effective in enhancing physical and mental health, occupation, and life satisfaction (Clark et al., 1997)

Examples of disease-specific programs are provided in Table 27.1. This is not meant to be an exhaustive list, but rather to provide both a flavor and a reference for how self-management techniques have been applied to specific conditions.

Components

As previously noted, basic components of self-management include self-monitoring, problem-solving, communication strategies, and stress management/reduction. Sometimes information about nutrition and diet, exercise, use of community resources, and managing psychological responses to illness/disability are also included (Lorig et al., 1996). Programs are structured to combine information about a disease and its management with the development and/or reinforcement of associated skills and behaviors.

Self-management programs and protocols almost always start by providing information and education about a specific disease or chronic condition. Most disease-specific programs help the individual with disability understand, in clear and simple terms, what is going on and what can be done to help address the condition. Information is also provided about what treatment recommendations are and why they are given. If this is done as part of a provider-led program or intervention, these recommendations should be discussed with the patient and related to his or her long or short-term goals, and patients should have the opportunity to provide input based on their priorities and experiences.

Self-monitoring involves observing and recording information about oneself and ones' health. It is critical to the performance of all other self-management skills, as it provides the data that is used to make decisions. Within self-management programs, people may be taught to track or monitor information about emotions, sleep patterns, pain levels, dietary intake, or a host of other factors. Once a patient is able to identify when she felt a certain way or experienced a symptom, she can begin asking "How intense was that?" "What was going on at the time?" And, ultimately, "Why did I experience this?" Monitoring can be a matter of internal reflection, of observing behaviors or actions, or keeping track of physiological responses. Patients can monitor themselves or rely on various devices and

Table 27.1 Examples of disease-specific self-management programs

Condition	Administered by	Components	Other
Brain Tumors (Locke et al., 2008)	Psychology professional (either master's or Ph.D. level)	Cognitive-rehabilitation interventions consisting of 12 sessions with two specific foci—one on cognitive-rehabilitative technique (teaching the use of formatted calendar as external cognitive aid) and one focusing on problem-solving training	Intervention sessions provided to patient–caregiver dyads concurrently with radiation therapy over 2-week period
Breast Cancer: Taking CHARGE (Cimprich et al., 2005)	Co-facilitated by an oncology nurse and a health educator trained in the Taking CHARGE program	Two small group and sessions and two individual telephone sessions providing opportunity to share experiences and self-management strategies, develop self-regulation skills, and receive tailored education related to managing symptoms and functional wellness; personal strategic planning encouraged	Individual telephone and in-person small-group sessions; review of Taking CHARGE workbook; (CHARGE, Choose a concern; Have the information; Assess the situation; Record the plan, Gain confidence and insight; and Evaluate your progress)
Diabetes A New DAWN (Diabetes Awareness & Wellness Network) (Samuel-Hodge et al., 2006)	Diabetes advisors or peer counselors recruited from congregations to be part of the intervention team and assist with administering intervention, which also included dietician and health care professionals	One individual counseling visit, 12 group sessions, three postcard messages from participants' diabetes care provider, and 12 monthly telephone calls from a diabetes advisor. Educational sessions cover diet, exercise, and self-monitoring and stress management components; health behaviors practiced during each session; goal setting and social support integrated into process	Culturally sensitive, church-based diabetes self-management education programs
Epilepsy (Dilorio et al., 2008)	Individually accessed, unfacilitated, interactive web-based program	Daily log/behavioral journal, online discussion board; educational resources; modules in medication, stress and sleep; goal planning	

Limb Loss: Promoting Amputee Life Skills Program (PALS) (Wegener, Mackenzie, Ephraim, Edhe, & Williams, 2009)	Community-based program delivered by trained volunteer leaders	Nine, 90-minute group sessions introducing self-management skills, including knowledge, skill acquisition, problem-solving, and self-monitoring	Topics addressed include pain management, building positive mood, managing negative mood, interacting with family and friends, working with health care team/community resources, building health habits, relapse prevention, and maintaining progress
Migraine (Merelle, Sorbi, van Doornen, & Passchier, 2008)	Lay individuals with migraine, who received training and supervision	Seven, 2-hour sessions over a 10-week period; primary components were identification and modification of triggers and application in physiological and cognitive-behavioral relaxation skills	Written manual with diary ratings; organizer with homework assignments and self-evaluations; CD-ROM with relaxation
Multiple Sclerosis (Bombardier et al., 2008)	Care manager trained in motivational interviewing and receiving ongoing supervision from a clinical psychologist	Single in-person motivational interview plus five telephone counseling sessions to facilitate improvement in one of six possible areas	Possible areas of behavior change included exercise, fatigue management, communication and/or social support, anxiety and/or stress management, and reducing alcohol or drug use
Spinal Cord Injury (SCI): Coping Effectiveness Training (Kennedy, Duff, Evans, & Beedie, 2003)	Inpatient group for individuals with new SCI facilitated by psychologist	Seven, 60- to 75-minute sessions run twice a week; session content included education related to stress and stress reactions, appraisal and coping skills, problem-solving, cognitive reframing, stress management, and increasing social support	

equipment to provide data. All this information or data can then be used by either the patient or her healthcare provider to determine how to optimize her health. Basically, the patient should be taught to monitor for information (or data) that can then be used to make choices about actions or behavior.

Communication typically involves learning the skills and approaches to communicate effectively and appropriately with health care professionals, as well as with family members and significant others. Practical exercises for this component might include asking questions, acting assertively, and advocating for oneself. Standardized self-management programs tend to review approaches or provide suggestions for communicating with specific people—such as health care providers—whereas individual interventions may focus on identifying the goals of the interaction, then developing a strategy for achieving that outcome. For example, self-management programs may help encourage patients to keep a list of problems and questions to bring to medical appointments.

Problem-solving is a frequent component of self-management programs, as well as cognitive-behavioral interventions and coping skills training, as the ability of an individual to solve problems is seen as a central component of successful chronic disease self-management (Bodenheimer et al., 2002; Glasgow, Fisher, Skaff, Mullan, & Toobert, 2007; Glasgow, Toobert, Barrera, & Strycker, 2004). Research has found that problem-solving ability and a positive problem-solving orientation are associated with improved health and wellness behavior (Barkley, Edwards, Laneri, Fletcher, & Metevia, 2001; Dreer, Elliott, Shewchuk, Berry, & Rivera, 2007; Dreer, Elliott, & Tucker, 2004; Glasgow et al., 2004, 2007; Hill-Briggs, 2003). Problem-solving is based around providing detailed information about a problem, brainstorming possible solutions, then evaluating and ranking those solutions, and finally implementing the best solution and evaluating its effectiveness.

Cognitive restructuring involves identifying negative or irrational thoughts or beliefs in order to facilitate health and relieve depression (Safren, Gonzalez, & Soroudi, 2008). Once identified, alternative but realistic thoughts are generated to replace them. In particular, cognitive distortions, such as all-or-nothing thinking, overgeneralization, and catastrophizing, are explained and identified. Thought records may be implemented as a way of tracking automatic thoughts, how they related to mood, and rational responses that may be taken to replace them.

Self-management programs often encourage participants to *set a goal* or target and work through the necessary *action planning* steps in order to reach it. Such goals may include exercising, eating a more nutritious diet, or smoking cessation. In structured group programs with multiple sessions, participants are generally encouraged to develop short-term goals that can be accomplished between sessions. Action plans are then developed that operationalize specific behaviors that will occur or change, with attention to detail encouraged. Research has shown that developing a realistic action plan with increasing degrees of specificity about what will occur, when it will occur, and how often it will occur is associated with increased likelihood of positive behavior (Creer, Caplin, & Holroyd, 2005). In addition, by writing an action plan or sharing it with others, patients then have the opportunity to evaluate its effectiveness and modify it as needed to improve outcomes.

Self-management programs may also include sections designed to promote the development of confidence and *self-efficacy*. Factors that influence self-efficacy include experiencing a sense of mastery, social learning or vicarious experience, and social persuasion. In particular, discussion of coping strategies and comparison with peers within a group framework can increase confidence in performing specific behaviors (Rogers et al., 2006). Physiological factors can also play a role. When people are trying to determining how they feel and how likely they are to accomplish something, they look for cues. Signs of nervousness and distress—including shaking, upset stomach, pain, fear, etc.—are often taken as evidence that they are not prepared and will not succeed. Changing the association between the response and its implications can change its ability to mediate self-efficacy.

Age and Developmental Stage in the Self-Management Process

For decades, self-management programs have been created for both children and adults with chronic conditions. In the development and implementation of these programs and models, the characteristics, issues, and skills of each of these life stages need to be considered.

Childhood

Childhood encompasses many developmental stages and tasks, and a full discussion of which are beyond the scope of this chapter. However, key issues and tasks revolve around the development of trust, autonomy, initiative, and industry (Erikson, 1950). Programs that facilitate the development of these characteristics are likely to encourage more age-appropriate behavior and interactions.

When working with a pediatric population, self-management skills are generally associated with the ability of the caregiver to manage the child's condition and interact with the health care system. Although the child himself may have a role in learning information about his condition and medications or specific behaviors to perform or avoid, it is usually the caregiver who works to make sure that information provided by the physician is translated into simple, concrete actions that can be easily followed. Information should be developed in formats that are accessible to both children and adults and written at a level that is understandable to individuals at a wide variety of reading levels. Rehabilitation psychologists may want to collaborate with disease organizations to develop child- and parent-friendly materials, as it will be much easier for parents to have the child comply if the child understands why it's necessary.

As suggested by the self-regulation model, training and interventions to support self-management skills among children should encompass not only the patient but also family and school environments. Education about disease, disability, or health condition should be provided to parents, aunts and uncles, and cousins, as well as to teachers, principals, and coaches, in order to reinforce medical recommendations as well as to dispel any myths or misconceptions. Behavioral contingencies and reward-based systems may be used in such settings to shape specific behaviors, such as medication adherence, improvements in knowledge about medication, or communication with the pediatric rehabilitation team.

Adolescence

Our primary task during adolescence is developing identity, defining who we are by what we do and how we interact with others. With regard to self-management, the focus is on transitioning to management of health and direction of health behaviors by the adolescent as opposed to his or her parents or caregivers. Teaching and education needs to occur with both the adolescent and the family. Adolescents and family members should learn about medications, associated health recommendations, and activity and behavioral limitations. In addition, parents and older adolescents need to learn about insurance and what resources may be available to them. It is important that members of the health care team develop relationships with both the adolescent and his or her family and that the adolescent is seen individually in order to build rapport and promote a sense of respect and responsibility between the adolescent and the team, which may promote adherence (Rianthavorn, Ettenger, Malekzadeh, Marik, & Struber, 2004; Rianthavorn & Ettenger, 2005).

Self-management programs that assist adolescents in developing social supports and networks may be an important function of encouraging appropriate health behaviors (Melzer, Leadbeater, Reisman, Jaffe, & Lieberman, 1989). Group therapy and peer support can improve social skills, social networks, and self-esteem while decreasing feelings of isolation among teenagers with disabilities and chronic conditions (Furr, 1998; LePontois, Moel, & Cohn, 1987; Walker, 1985). Group therapy, in particular, appears most successful when arranged in conjunction with preexisting medical appointments. Summer camps may also provide a good opportunity to integrate healthy behaviors while increasing social networks, gaining independence, and interacting with health care providers in a more casual setting (Leumann, Mueller, & Leumann, 1989).

Adulthood

From a developmental perspective, the tasks of adulthood are intimacy, affiliation, and generativity (Erikson, 1950). Adults are seen as successful to the extent that they are able to develop relationships, connect to others, find meaningful work, and contribute to society. Self-management programs and interventions need to acknowledge and incorporate these goals and priorities while recognizing the social environment of the patient, including his or her practical, financial, and emotional resources. Identification and utilization of community supports and resources may be an important aspect of program and interventions.

Older Adults

Self-management programs for older adults should recognize and address the multiple health conditions and complex treatment regimens that this population is likely to face. Research shows that, as people age, they have an increasing number of chronic conditions and correspondingly more complex and involved health care regimens. At age 70, the average adult in the United Kingdom has two or three chronic conditions; by age 75, 90% have some clinical diagnosis, and by age 85, 30%

of the population has Alzheimer disease (Hartree, 2010). Self-management abilities, though, appear more associated with frailty as opposed to age, where *frailty* is defined as the risk for adverse outcomes due to losses in different domains of functioning, including cognitive functioning, physical functioning, social functioning, and psychological functioning (Schuurmans, Steverink, Lindenberg, Frieswijk, & Slaets, 2004).

In a needs assessment of older adults with heart disease, Clark and her colleagues (1988) identified six problem areas discussed by participants: accepting activity limitations, following physician recommendations, monitoring body signals and issues of activity pacing, handling fear and anxiety, maintaining optimism and taking pride in what can be done given disease constraints, and assisting family members in being calm and helpful instead of worrying (Clark et al., 1988). Each of these, they proposed, needs to be evaluated and assessed by the provider for self-management programs to be effective.

Within the framework of health care systems, geriatric evaluation and management protocols that take a comprehensive approach to identifying and addressing health and functioning have been intermittently found to be effective in preventing disability and reducing health care costs in older adults (Boult et al., 2001; Cohen et al., 2002). Such programs generally involve comprehensive evaluation, including history taking, physical examination, and assessment of patient's functional, cognitive, affective, nutritional status, social situation, and caregiver capabilities, by a multidisciplinary intervention team consisting (at minimum) of a geriatrician, social worker, and nurse. This evaluation results in a plan of care, including coordinated preventive and management services, with an emphasis on maintaining functional status and specific follow-up protocol. It is possible that such structured protocols can be used in conjunction with chronic disease management programs to promote motivation, adherence, and changes toward healthy behaviors.

Finally, self-management programs and interventions aimed at older adults need to consider and be prepared to address age-related changes that occur in cognition and sensory functioning. It is estimated that between 25% and 50% of individuals older than 65 years have significant hearing loss that affects understanding of commands and questions, as well as self-expression. By age 65, approximately 50% of people have cataracts, and by age 75, 92% of people have lost some ability to focus on near objects (presbyopia). Both visual and auditory impairments increase the risk of social isolation, withdrawal, depression, anxiety, and safety issues. In addition, aging is linked to declines in fluid cognitive abilities such as speed, executive function, and working and episodic memory (Hassing & Johansson, 2005; Lustig, Shah, Seidler, & Reuter-Lorenz, 2009; Raz & Rodrigue, 2006), and so self-management programs may want to build in supports to assist with retaining information and planning decision-making.

Modality

Most self-management interventions and programs use multiple modalities, usually combining in-person sessions and written material. However, alternative methods of interventions are becoming increasingly common, at least within research studies. These include telephone interventions, as well as electronic, internet-, and web-based formats. Current evidence appears to suggest that telephone-based programs may be just as effective as in-person settings and that participants generally are able to connect with facilitators and view them as supportive and empathic (Bombardier et al., 2008).

However, it cannot be assumed that all educational programs, contents, or interventions are equally engaging or useful; this is particularly true of print and technology-based modalities. Although facilitators of in-person interventions can assess how much the person in front of them is paying attention, use and engagement may be more difficult to establish as distance from the facilitator increases or when the facilitator disappears entirely. In these cases, the characteristics of these materials or formats become important, particularly as they are tailored to become relevant to various groups. Ritterband and colleagues (2009) provide a behavior change model for internet interventions that posits that users approach electronic interventions with a set of individual characteristics (such as gender, education, self-efficacy, etc.) influenced by (and reciprocally influencing) environmental factors. These user characteristics, together with website characteristics (i.e., content, appearance, message) and provided support, impact use of the application; website use then influences behavior change via various mechanisms that lead to symptom improvement. This model is inclusive of behavioral change theories, acknowledging a wide variety of mechanisms for changing behavior and leading to symptom improvement, but adds a recognition of user characteristics and their influence on website (application/intervention) use (and adherence) as precursors that allow for behavior change. That is, an individual must access and use the web, internet, or self-management application in order for it to influence behavior change, and the extent of use can influence the degree of behavior change, at least within certain limits. Users with different characteristics, then, are going to have different reactions to the same website or game application (Ritterband, Thorndike, Cox, Kovatchev, & Gonder-Frederick, 2009). In particular, as adolescents and young adults who are members of the millennial generation expect a high degree of interactivity, technological sophistication, and visual impact (Oblinger & Oblinger, 2005; Ritterband et al., 2009), the degree to which these expectations are met will directly influence the individual's engagement and enjoyment and, ultimately, use of the program.

Role of the Rehabilitation Psychologist

Rehabilitation psychologists can play a critically important role in the development and implementation of self-management skills and should play a prominent role in the health management process for individuals with disabilities and chronic diseases. An individual provider's expertise in child development, education, vocational issues, neuropsychology, or marital and family therapy can benefit both patients and other health care providers (North & Eminson, 1998) in identifying learning disorders and cognitive difficulties, facilitating academic advancement, working with school systems or employers to address concerns and facilitate productivity and achievement, or systematically addressing issues within social environments. Their expertise has also been found useful in research, program development, health care administration, and system design, guiding the management of specific situations and providing an objective and informed perspective on difficult cases.

Assessment

One of the many skills that rehabilitation psychologists can contribute to the area of self-management is in the assessment of knowledge, cognitions, skills, and behaviors that support the ability of an individual to manage his or her health condition or impairment. At the most basic level, this may include assessment of intelligence, developmental stage, or disease-specific knowledge, but assessment can quickly to be expanded to include evaluation of those factors that influence an individual's performance of specific behaviors. Although many measures are used to assess the impact or efficacy of research interventions, comprehensive assessment of those components that effect self-management skills appears to be less common.

Depending on the patient or disease population, measures of cognitive status and impairment may be important to include. A review of neuropsychological assessment measures is beyond the scope of this chapter; however, it is fairly easy to ascertain how cognitive ability may impact self-management skills: attention problems can interfere with both the acquisition of new skills and the demonstration of previously acquired skills (Gerson et al., 2006), whereas problems with immediate and delayed memory can limit retention of information. Both of these difficulties can lead to impaired functional performance and affect adherence to medical regimen. Once cognitive strengths and impairments have been identified, patients, family members, and health care providers can begin to build self-management regimens and treatment plans that address difficulties and use compensatory strategies and assistive devices and techniques.

Implied in the concepts of self-management and self-regulation are recognition of the changes, issues, and challenges associated with a chronic condition or disability. If an individual with traumatic brain injury does not recognize the cognitive impairments associated with her condition, she will not take active steps to compensate for deficits or reorganize her environment to improve functioning. Measures that examine awareness or varying perspectives may provide important information for program design and implementation. One such measure is the Self-Regulation Skills Inventory (SRSI), a clinical tool designed to measure the self-regulatory skills essential for planning, monitoring, and evaluating one's own progress. It has three factors (Awareness, Readiness to Change, and Strategic Behavior) and has been shown to be effective in detecting change resulting from a group support program for individuals with acquired brain injury (Ownsworth, McFarland, & Young, 2000a,b).

Measurement of current coping strategies and problem-solving ability may also provide important data to inform an intervention or program. One general measure is the Social Problem Solving Inventory-Revised (SPSI-R), which provides information about problem orientation (positive and negative problem orientation), as well as specific problem-solving styles (rational problem solving, impulsive/careless style, and avoidance style; D'Zurilla, Nezu, & Maydeay-Olivares, 2002). Disease-specific measures of problems-solving, such as the Diabetes Problem-Solving Inventory (DPSI; Glasgow et al., 2004) may provide more precise information about how an individual may handle disease-related situations. In addition, measures that provide information about general approaches to coping and dealing with stress can assist in informing or tailoring interventions or assessing the effectiveness of programs.

Level of emotional distress and self-efficacy can both inform interventions and serve as outcome measures. Although general measures of self-efficacy exist, the concept is most often assessed using disease-specific measures that ask about confidence performing a variety of tasks associated with the condition. These measures use self-report formats, which is appropriate considering the inclusion of self-perception as a core aspect of the concept. However, to the extent that these measures are not validated against actual behaviors or outcomes, they lose potential benefit.

Finally, it may be useful to be able to conceptualize overall skill level or competency with self-management. Even after people are taught self-management skills, they will not automatically use them. Developing and applying these skills takes practice, so individuals with disability will have different levels of skill or competency in managing their conditions and the physical and psychosocial consequences. Many factors influence the level of self-management skills and competency; age, education, and cognitive capacity all play a role. Preexisting experience in using the skills in other contexts (i.e., to succeed in school or manage tasks at home or work) also contributes to current level. Finally, level of adjustment and mental health status influence both ability and motivation to take on the responsibility of actively managing health. A proposed scheme of five levels of self-management competency is provided in Table 27.2, along with suggestions for how providers or facilitators may want to tailor their approach based on these levels.

Psychotherapy/Clinical Treatment of Patients

A key role for rehabilitation psychologists within a self-management paradigm is to work with individuals with disabilities and chronic conditions in individual, group, or marital/family therapy settings to identify and address barriers to health and assist them in developing positive health behaviors and building a good quality of life. Rehabilitation psychologists can help patients identify their long-term goals, recognize the importance of specific activities

in improving enjoyment or happiness, identify cognitions and their role in behaviors and emotions, translate recommendations into specific actions or behaviors, integrate behaviors into life or regimen, increase motivation, address adherence, and facilitate adjustment to disability. They can also work with patients to facilitate the development of specific skills, such as pain management, relaxation, and communication/negotiation/assertiveness.

Specific techniques, such as motivational interviewing, may be used to assist patients in identifying goals and target behaviors. Strategies and techniques are well described by Rollnick in his book *Health Behavior Change: A Guide for Practitioners* (Rollnick, Mason, & Butler, 1999), as well as in other training material. Rehabilitation psychologists can ask patients about what they expect to encounter and help them to anticipate common barriers and challenges. Once potential problems are identified, providers can promote the use of problem-solving strategies to address them. They should encourage the individual with disability to stop, think, gather information, and make informed decisions. The action plan also should provide the individual with disability with information about steps that he or she should take should certain things occur. *Planning for decision-making* will help the patient create an action plan beforehand. Planning can reduce patient's anxiety by instructing him or her on which signs to monitor and what action to take if particular symptoms arise.

Group therapy is an important and powerful medium to provide information, facilitate the development of self-management skills, and encourage peer support. However, it can be a challenge to implement outside of a residential or inpatient setting. Specialized disease-specific programs may provide oversight and services to a large geographic area, thus making group interventions that require travel problematic. Sessions should be scheduled to provide minimal interference with already stressed work and school schedules (Meade, Creer, & Mahan, 2003). Increasingly, web-based intervention may be used to fulfill the same role—however, in-person interactions between clients are still recommended to facilitate actual (rather than virtual) social networks.

Educating Health Care Providers

One of the primary roles that rehabilitation psychologists perform is in working with other health care providers on interdisciplinary and multidisciplinary teams. Research indicates that a key

Table 27.2 Levels of self-management competence

Self-Management Level	Patient Skills and Issues	Suggestions for Providers
0	The individual with disability probably has little information or little real understanding about his condition and how it may affect his life. He may feel overwhelmed and not sure of what to do or where to start or even what questions to ask.	Health care providers and/or facilitators can assist by providing him with a framework for what is going on and a map of where he is, where he is heading, and the likely steps to get there.
1	An individual at this level has a rough idea of what is going on and what is ahead. He may have basic information about disability and know what he is supposed to do to manage his condition and achieve specific short-term goals. He is probably able to follow directions and suggestions, but his knowledge may not be well integrated, and figuring out how he is going to follow all the recommendations in everyday life may still be hard.	Health care providers and/or facilitators may want to check the patient's level of understanding, before either providing more details or corrections. Concrete examples and assistance with planning, organizing, and integrating information into home life is generally very helpful. In addition, patients may need assistance in identifying reasonable and realistic long-term goals.
2	Individuals have good general knowledge about their condition/impairment. They know what they have to do and why, and are able to adapt recommendations and guidelines to fit their own life or situation.	Providers and facilitators need to recognize and respect this increased level of knowledge. They should work to engage the individual with disability in problem-solving and agenda setting.
3	At level 3, individuals with disability know their bodies and have a lot of information about their condition. They are familiar with recommendations, but also have a good idea of what is reasonable in different situations. Individuals at this level are able to plan ahead and consider how to manage new environments given their abilities. Competency at this level requires realistic understanding of disease process and functional limitations; in addition, a good attitude is critical.	For facilitators and health care providers, it is important to remember that individuals at this level have good skills and good judgment and are generally able to manage their condition. Serving as a consultant may be of most benefit to the individual with disability—providing feedback to help him modify his behavior or management strategies.
4	This is the expert level. The individual with disability is an expert about his body and about his condition. He knows what things influence his functioning and why. Individuals at this level are great self-regulators and readily adapt what they do based on feedback from their body, from the environment, or from important others (spouses, health care providers, caregivers, etc.). Of primary importance is the high degree of problem-solving skills, as well as cognitive flexibility and ability to make adjustments when faced with new information and environments; attitude, adjustment, and mental health are all good to excellent. The individual with disability is definitely the one managing his health (as well as his environment) and has learned to communicate effectively with health care providers to get what he needs.	Rehabilitation psychologists and other health care providers should work with patients to help them evaluate information and refine self-regulation skills given new situations.

aspect of influencing patient health behavior is the patient's relationship with his or her health care provider. Rehabilitation psychologists can help other health care providers identify barriers and strengths in communication styles and teach them to work more collaboratively with their patients. In a collaborative relationship, the health care provider is the expert on the condition, the patient is the expert on his or her own life, and decisions are made through the efforts of both parties. If a patient and physician do collaborate, the provider learns more about the patient's lifestyle and beliefs and so can make better decisions about the best treatment (Arbuthnott & Sharpe, 2009).

Among the possible areas of discussion may be encouraging providers to examine their expectations and assumptions about quality of life and living with a disability, as well as issues of health, gender, race, and motivation. Research has revealed that relatively few health care providers (only 18%) believed that they would be glad to be alive after a severe disability (in contrast to 92% of people with disability), and only 17% believed their quality of life would be average or above average after disability (compared to 86% of people who already have disability). These opinions can impact the decisions physicians make in treating disability and also what they tell the families of injured patients about critical care decisions and options (Gerhart, Koziol-McLain, & Lowenstein, 1994). If a health care provider does not believe that an individual with a disability can have an active and fulfilled life, he or she is less likely to address issues such as education, vocation, sexuality, or parenting, or to help patients see these as long-term goals.

Health care providers can also be taught to build steps into their educational strategies to help patients increase confidence and self-efficacy by having them demonstrate the behavior during an appointment or session; this provides the patient with the opportunity to practice and receive feedback about the technique or skill. Providers need to be sure to praise success and, to the extent possible, reinforce successive approximations. They should affirm the person and point out successes, even small ones, and reframe "failures" as intermediate successes whenever possible.

As previously mentioned, developing an action plan has also been shown to be associated with increases in positive behavior. Within the context of a health care environment, individuals with disability and their health care providers should discuss the goals that each has and wants to see achieved. The patient should determine his or her long-term goals, with the health care provider helping break it into manageable steps, working as a testing board as to whether it is likely or achievable, or providing information about what aspects appear feasible within the limits of modern medicine or existing resources. Although long-term goals may need to be reframed or modified, the patient is the one who should be in charge of selecting a goal, because whether or not he will make the agreed-upon change or achieve the goal is dependent on his behavior. This process of setting long-term goals and building short-term goals to support the patient's priorities and preferences may require negotiation between the two parties. Once the goals have been established, a contract and action plan should be developed to improve the likelihood of success.

Developing Programs for Patients

Because of their dual training in both science and practice, rehabilitation psychologists are primed to take on lead roles in developing self-management interventions for specific patients or in creating programs tailored to specific condition or population groups. By using the aforementioned theories and existing research findings, they can develop evidence-based programs and interventions that fit within the context of both the health care system and people's lives. In particular, interventions may be based on a stepped approach to care in which the broadest and most cost-effective programs are provided to the widest group, with increasingly specialized programs and expertise available to meet the needs of more complex patients (Creer, 2007; Von Keorff & Tiemens, 2000).

Advocacy

As a philosophy, self-management is about recognizing and valuing the goals and expertise of the individual with the disability or chronic condition. Rehabilitation psychologists act to empower individuals with disabilities while also working to improve the environment in which they live. Rehabilitation psychologists provide education at all levels to improve understanding and dispel misconceptions about the physical and psychosocial impact of chronic conditions and disabilities, as well as about the steps that can be taken to facilitate health and functioning. They serve as policy advisors, educators, lobbyists, and coaches. By conducting research and implementing evidence-based approaches, they refine the state-of-the-art in practice. Primarily, though, rehabilitation psychologists ensure that the voices of individuals with disabilities and chronic conditions are listened to and that their concerns are incorporated into all aspects of programs, policies, and intervention.

Conclusion

Hopefully, this chapter has made it obvious that self-management is an approach, a philosophy, and a science—all of which have at their core the self-determination and empowerment of the individual with the disability or chronic condition. Self-management programs and interventions can be applied at varying points in the health care system to address broad issues of health management or specific aspects of conditions. The role of rehabilitation psychologists within this paradigm, then, is to facilitate the expertise of patients and improve their functioning. For this task, we are armed with theory, research evidence, and clinical experience.

Future Directions

Self-management approaches are becoming increasingly integrated into health service delivery; however, many areas still demand an evidence-based perspective to facilitate implementation. In particular, as more individuals find themselves living with chronic diseases, learning and applying self-management skills becomes increasingly important, and the questions of *how*, *where*, and *who* arise and demand attention.

• How, and/or how well, is self-management integrated into existing health systems? What are the best methods for building collaborative relationships between patients and health care providers?

• Where can self-management programs be useful? How might they be tailored for health care systems and health conditions in developing countries?

• Who has responsibility for developing and funding self-management programs?

References

Arbuthnott, A., & Sharpe, D. (2009). The effect of physician patient collaboration on patient adherence in nonpsychiatric medication. *Patient Education and Counseling, 77*(1), 60–67.

Badcott, D. (2005). The expert patient: Valid recognition or false hope? *Medicine, Health Care Philosophy, 8,* 173–178.

Bandura, A. (1995). *Self-efficacy in changing societies,* Cambridge University Press.

Baranowski, T., Perry, C. L., & Parcel, G. S. (2002). How individuals, environments and health behavior interact—social cognitive theory. In K. Glanz, B.K. Rimer & F.M. Lewis (Eds.), *Health behavior and health education: Theory, research, and practice* (pp. 165–184). Jossey-Bass, San Francisco.

Barkley, R. A., Edwards, G., Laneri, M., Fletcher, K., & Metevia, L. (2001). The efficacy of problem-solving communication training alone, behavior management training alone, and their combination for parent-adolescent conflict in teenagers with ADHD and ODD. *Journal of Consulting and Clinical Psychology, 69*(6), 926–941.

Barlow, J., Wright, C., Sheasby, J., Turner, A., & Hainsworth, J. (2002). Self-management approaches for people with chronic conditions: A review. *Patient Education and Counseling, 48,* 177–187.

Bodenheimer, T., Lorig, K., Holman, H., & Grumbach, K. (2002). Patient self-management of chronic disease in primary care. *Journal of the American Medical Association, 288*(19), 2469–2475.

Bombardier, C. H., McCunniffe, M., Wadhwani, R., Gibbons, L., Blake, K., & Kraft, G. (2008). The efficacy of telephone counseling for health promotion in people with multiple sclerosis: A randomized controlled trial. *Archives of Physical Medicine and Rehabilitation, 89,* 1849–1856.

Boult, C., Boult, L., Morishita, L., Dowd, B., Kane, R., & Urdangarin, C. (2001). A randomized clinical trial of outpatient geriatric evaluation and management. *Journal of the American Geriatric Society, 49,* 351–359.

Carbone, E. T., Rosal, M. C., Torres, M. I., Goins, K. V., & Bermudez, O. I. (2007). Diabetes self-management: Perspectives of Latino patients and their health care providers. *Patient Education and Counseling, 66*(2), 202–210.

Cimprich, B., Janz, N. K., Northouse, L., Wren, P., Given, B., & Given, C. (2005). Taking charge: A self-management program for women following breast cancer treatment. *Psycho-oncology, 14,* 704–717.

Clark, F., Azen, S. P., Zemke, R., Jackson, J., Carlson, M., Mandel, D., et al. (1997). Occupational therapy for independent-living in older adults: A randomized control trial. *Journal of the American Medical Association, 278,* 1321–1326.

Clark, N., Gong, M., & Kaciroti, N. (2001). A model of self-regulation for control of chronic disease. *Health Education and Behavior, 28*(6), 769–782.

Clark, N. M., Rakowski, W., Ostrander, L., Wheeler, J. R., Oden, S., & Keteyian, S. (1988). Development of self-management education for elderly heart patients. *Gerontologist, 28,* 491–494.

Cohen, H. J., Feussner, J. R., Weinberger, M., Carnes, M., Hamdy, R. C., Hsieh, F., et al. (2002). A controlled trial of inpatient and outpatient geriatric evaluation and management. *New England Journal of Medicine, 346*(12), 905–912.

Cohen, S. (1988). Psychosocial models of the role of social support in the etiology of physical disease. *Health Psychology, 7*(3), 269–297.

Creer, T. L. (2007). A modest proposal: Universal self-management training for all. Retrieved November 29, 2010 from http://www.manageyourillness.com/archives/2007/06/chronic_diseases_and_their_man.php Creer, T. L., Caplin, D. A., & Holroyd, K. A. (2005). A self-management program for adult asthma: Part IV, analysis of context and patient behaviors. *Journal of Asthma, 42*(6), 455–462.

Creer, T. L., & Holroyd, K. A. (2006). Self-management of chronic conditions: The legacy of Sir William Osler. *Chronic Illness, 2*(1), 7–14.

D'Zurilla, T. J., & Nezu, A. M. (2007). *Problem-solving therapy: A positive approach to clinical intervention* (3rd ed.). New York: Springer Publishing Company.

D'Zurilla, T. J., Nezu, A. M., & Maydeay-Olivares, A. (2002). *Manual for the Social Problem-Solving Inventory-Revised (SPSI-R)*. North Tonawanda, NY: Multi-Health Systems.

Department of Health, U. K. (2001). *The expert patient: A new approach to chronic disease management for the 21st century*. London: Department of Health,.Available at http://www.dh.gov.uk/en/Publicationsandstatistics/Publications/PublicationsPolicyAndGuidance/DH_4006801

Dilorio, C., Escoffery, C., McCarty, F., Yeager, K. A., Henry, T. R., Koganti, A., et al. (2008). Evaluation of WebEase: An epilepsy self-management Web site. *Health Education Research, 24*(2), 185–197.

Donaldson, L. (2003). Expert patients usher in a new era of opportunity for the NHS. *British Journal of Medicine, 326*, 1279.

Dreer, L. E., Elliott, T. R., Shewchuk, R., Berry, J. W., & Rivera, P. (2007). Family caregivers of persons with spinal cord injury: Predicting caregivers at risk for probable depression. *Rehabilitation Psychology, 52*(3), 351–357.

Dreer, L. E., Elliott, T. R., & Tucker, E. (2004). Social problem-solving abilities and health behaviors among persons with recent-onset spinal cord injury. *Journal of Clinical Psychology in Medical Settings, 11*(1), 7–13.

Erikson, E. H. (1950). *Childhood and society*. New York: Norton.

Field, M.J. & Jette, A.M. (2007). The Future of Disability in America. Washington, DC: The National Academies Press.

Furr, L. A. (1998). Psycho-social aspects of serious renal disease and dialysis: A review of the literature. *Social Work in Health Care, 27*(3), 97–118.

Gerhart, K. A., Koziol-McLain, J., & Lowenstein, S. R. (1994). Quality of life following spinal cord injury: Knowledge and attitudes of emergency care providers. *Annals of Emergency Medicine*, 807–812

Gerson, A., Butler, R., Moxey-Mims, M., Wentz, A., Shinnar, S., Lande, M., et al. (2006). Neurocognitive outcomes in children with chronic kidney disease: Current findings and contemporary endeavors. *Mental Retardation and Developmental Disabilities Research Reviews, 12*(3), 208–215.

Glanz, K., Rimer, B. K., & Lewis, F. M. (2002). *Health behavior and health education: Theory, research and practice*. San Francisco: Wiley & Sons.

Glasgow, R. E., Fisher, L., Skaff, M., Mullan, J., & Toobert, D. J. (2007). Problem solving and diabetes self-management: Investigation in a large, multiracial sample. *Diabetes Care, 30*(1), 33–37.

Glasgow, R. E., Toobert, D. J., Barrera, Jr., M., & Strycker, L. A. (2004). Assessment of problem-solving: A key to successful diabetes self-management. *Journal of Behavioral Medicine, 27*(5), 477–490.

Grant, J. S., Elliott, T. R., Weaver, M., Bartolucci, A. A., & Giger, J. N. (2002). Telephone intervention with family caregivers of stroke survivors after rehabilitation. *Stroke, 33*, 2060–2065.

Hale, E. D., & Treharne, G. J. K., Kitas, G. D. (2007). The common-sense model of self-regulation of health and illness: How can we use it to understand and respond to our patients' needs? *Rheumatology, 46*, 904–906.

Hartree, N (2010). *Disability in older people*. Patient.co.uk. Retrieved November 30, 2010, from http://www.patient.co.uk/doctor/Disability-in-Older-People.htm

Harvey, J. N., & Lawson, V. L. (2009). The importance of health belief models in determining self-care behavior in diabetes. *Diabetic Medicine, 26*, 5–13.

Hassing, L. B., & Johansson, B. (2005). Aging and cognition. *Nordisk Psykologi, 57*(1), 4–20.

Hill-Briggs, F. (2003). Problem solving in diabetes self-management: A model of chronic illness self-management behavior. *Annals of Behavioral Medicine, 25*(3), 182–193.

Holman, H., & Lorig, K. (2004). Patient self-management: A key to effectiveness and efficiency in care of chronic disease. *Public Health Rep, 119*(3), 239–243.

Horowitz, B. P., & Chang, P. -F. J. (2004). Promoting well-being and engagement in life through occupational therapy lifestyle redesign: A pilot study within adult day programs. *Topics in Geriatric Rehabilitation, 20*(1), 46–58.

Institute of Medicine. (2003). *Priority areas for national action: Transforming health care quality*. Washington, DC: The National Academies Press.

Jackson, J., Carlson, M., Mandel, D., Zemke, R., & Clark, F. (1998). Occupation in lifestyle redesign: The WII elderly study occupational therapy program. *The American Journal of Occupational Therapy, 52*(5), 326–336.

Janz, N. K., Champion, V. L., & Strecher, V. J. (2002). The health belief model. In K. Glanz, B.K. Rimer, & F.M. Lewis (Eds.), *Health behavior and health education: Theory, research, and practice* (pp.45–66). Jossey-Bass, San Francisco.

Kennedy, P., Duff, J., Evans, M., & Beedie, A. (2003). Coping effectiveness training reduces depression and anxiety following traumatic spinal cord injuries. *British Journal of Clinical Psychology, 42*, 41–52.

Lazarus, R. S., & Folkman, S. (1984). *Stress, appraisal and coping*. New York: Springer.

LePontois, J., Moel, D. I., & Cohn, R. A. (1987). Family adjustment to pediatric ambulatory dialysis. *American Journal of Orthopsychiatry, 57*, 78–83.

Leumann, C., Mueller, U., & Leumann, E. (1989). Insights gained from dialysis camps. *International Journal of Adolescent Medicine and Health, 4*(1), 29–34.

Leventhal, H., Leventhal, E.A., & Breland, J.Y. (2011). Cognitive science speaks to the "common-sense" of chronic illness management. *Annals of Behavioral Medicine, 41*(2), 152–163.

Leventhal, H., & Cameron, L. (1987). Behavioral theories and the problem of compliance. *Patient Education and Counseling, 10*, 117–138.

Leventhal, H., & Diefenback, M. (1991). Illness cognition: Using common sense to understand treatment adherence and affect cognition interactions. *Cognitive Therapy and Research, 16*, 143–163.

Leventhal, H., Leventhal, E., & Halm, E. (2010). *Improving chronic illness management among the elderly*. Center for the Study of Health Beliefs and Behaviors, Rutgers University, New Brunswick. Retrieved December 14, 2010, from http://emotion-research.net/projects/humaine/ws/summerschool2/Leventhal-color.pdf

Leventhal, H., Meyer, D., & Nerenz, D. (1980). The common sense representation of illness danger. In S. Rachman (Ed.), *Medical psychology* (Vol. 2). New York: Pergamon.

Locke, D., Cerhan, J., Wu, W., Malec, J., Clark, M., Rummans, T., et al. (2008). Cognitive rehabilitation and problem-solving to improve quality of life of patients with primary brain tumors: A pilot study. *Journal of Supportive Oncology, 6*(8), 383–391.

Lorig, K. (1982). Arthritis self-management: A patient education program. *Rehabilitation Nursing, 7*(4), 16–20.

Lorig, K. (2003). Self-management education: More than a nice extra. *Medical Care, 41*(6), 699–701.

Lorig, K., & Holman, H. (2003). Self-management education: History, definition, outcomes, and mechanisms. *Annals of Behavioral Medicine, 26*(1), 1–7.

Lorig, K., Hurwicz, M. L., Sobel, D., Hobbs, M., & Ritter, P. L. (2005). A national dissemination of an evidence-based self-management program: A process evaluation study. *Patient Education and Counseling, 59*(1), 69–79.

Lorig, K., Mazonson, P. D., & Holman, H. R. (1993). Evidence suggesting that health education for self-management in patients with chronic arthritis has sustained health benefits while reducing health care costs. *Arthritis and Rheumatism, 36*(4), 439–446.

Lorig, K., Ritter, P., Stewart, A. L., Sobel, D. S., Brown, B. W., Jr., Bandura, A., et al. (2001). Chronic disease self-management program: 2-year health status and health care utilization outcomes. *Medical Care, 39*(11), 1217–1223.

Lorig, K., Ritter, P. L., Dost, A., Plant, K., Laurent, D. D., & McNeil, I. (2008). The Expert Patients Programme online, a 1-year study of an internet-based self-management programme for people with long-term conditions. *Chronic Illness, 4*(4), 247–256.

Lorig, K., Ritter, P. L., & Gonzalez, V. M. (2003). Hispanic chronic disease self-management: A randomized community-based outcome trial. *Nursing Research, 52*(6), 361–369.

Lorig, K., Ritter, P. L., & Jacquez, A. (2005). Outcomes of border health Spanish/English chronic disease self-management programs. *Diabetes Educator, 31*(3), 401–409.

Lorig, K., Ritter, P. L., Laurent, D. D., & Plant, K. (2006). Internet-based chronic disease self-management: A randomized trial. *Medical Care, 44*(11), 964–971.

Lorig, K., Ritter, P. L., Villa, F., & Piette, J. D. (2008). Spanish diabetes self-management with and without automated telephone reinforcement: Two randomized trials. *Diabetes Care, 31*(3), 408–414.

Lorig, K., Ritter, P. L., Villa, F. J., & Armas, J. (2009). Community-based peer-led diabetes self-management: A randomized trial. *Diabetes Educator, 35*(4), 641–651.

Lorig, K., Sobel, D. S., Ritter, P. L., Laurent, D., & Hobbs, M. (2001). Effect of a self-management program on patients with chronic disease. *Effective Clinical Practice, 4*(6), 256–262.

Lorig, K., Sobel, D. S., Stewart, A. L., Brown, B. W., Jr., Bandura, A., Ritter, P., et al. (1999). Evidence suggesting that a chronic disease self-management program can improve health status while reducing hospitalization: a randomized trial. *Medical Care, 37*(1), 5–14.

Lorig, K., Stewart, A., Ritter, P., Gonzalez, V., Laurent, D., & Lynch, J. (1996). *Outcome measures for health education and other health care interventions.* Thousand Oaks, CA: Sage Publications.

Lustig, C., Shah, P., Seidler, R., & Reuter-Lorenz, P. (2009). Aging, training, and the brain: A review and future directions. *Neuropsychology Review, 19*, 504–522.

Meade, M. A., Creer, T. L., & Mahan, J. D. (2003). A self-management program for adolescents and children with renal transplantation. *Journal of Clinical Psychology in Medical Settings, 10*(3), 165–171.

Melzer, S. M., Leadbeater, B., Reisman, L., Jaffe, L. R., & Lieberman, K. V. (1989). Characteristics of social networks in adolescents with end-stage renal disease treated with renal transplantation. *Journal of Adolescent Health Care, 10*(4), 308–312.

Merelle, S., Sorbi, M., van Doornen, L., & Passchier, J. (2008). Lay trainers with migraine for a home-based behavioral training: A 6 month follow-up study. *Headache, 48*, 1311–1325.

Meyer, D., Leventhal, H., & Guttman, M. (1985). Common-sense models of illness: The example of hypertension. *Health Psychology, 4*, 115–135.

Newman, S., Steed, L., & Mulligan, K. (2004). Self-management interventions for chronic illness. *Lancet, 364*(9444), 1523–1537.

Nieuwenhuijsen, E. R., Zemper, E., & Miner, K. (2006). Health behavior change models and theories: Contributions to rehabilitation.

North, C., & Eminson, M. (1998). A review of a psychiatry-nephrology liaison service. *European Child and Adolescent Psychiatry, 7*(4), 235–245.

Oblinger, D. G., & Oblinger, J. L. (2005). Is It Age or IT: First Steps Toward Understanding the Net Generation. In D. G. Oblinger and J. L. Oblinger (Eds.), *Educating the Net Generation.* Washington, DC: E-book available online at www.educause.edu/educatingthenetgen.

Ownsworth, T. L., McFarland, K., & Young, R. M. (2000a). Development and standardization of the Self-Regulation Skills Interview (SRSI): A new clinical assessment tool for acquired brain injury. *The Clinical Neuropsychologist, 14*(1), 76–92.

Ownsworth, T. L., McFarland, K., & Young, R. M. (2000b). Self-awareness and psychosocial functioning following acquired brain injury: An evaluation of a group support programme. *Neuropsychological Rehabilitation, 10*(5), 465–484.

Pearson, M. L., Mattke, S., Shaw, R., Ridgely, M. S., & Wiseman, S. H. (2007). *Patient self-management support programs: An evaluation.* Santa Monica, CA: Agency for Healthcare Research and Quality.

Prochaska, J. O., & Velicer, W. F. (1997). The transtheoretical model of health behavior change. *American Journal of Health Promotion, 12*(1), 38–48.

Ravesloot, C., Seekins, T., & White, G. W. (2005). Living well with a disability health promotion intervention: Improved health status for consumers and lower costs for health care policymakers. *Rehabilitation Psychology, 50*(3), 239–245.

Raz, N., & Rodrigue, K. M. (2006). Differential aging of the brain: Patterns, cognitive correlates and modifiers. *Neuroscience and Biobehavioral Reviews, 30*(6), 730–748.

Rianthavorn, P., & Ettenger, R. B. (2005). Medication non-adherence in the adolescent renal transplant recipient: A clinician's viewpoint. *Pediatric Transplantation, 9*(3), 398–407.

Rianthavorn, P., Ettenger, R., Malekzadeh, M., Marik, J., & Struber, M. (2004). Noncompliance with immunosuppressive medications in pediatric and adolescent patients receiving solid organ transplants. *Transplantation, 77*(5), 778–782.

Ritterband, L. M., Thorndike, F. P., Cox, D. J., Kovatchev, B. P., & Gonder-Frederick, L. A. (2009). A behavior change model for internet interventions. *Annals of Behavioral Medicine, 38*, 18–27.

Rogers, A., Bower, P., Cardner, C., Gately, C., Kennedy, A., Lee, V., et al. (2006). *The national evaluation of the pilot phase of the expert patients programme: Final report.* UK Department of Health.

Rollnick, S., Mason, P., & Butler, C. (1999). *Health behavior change: A guide for practitioners.* China: Churchill Livingstone.

Rosal, M. C., Olendzki, B., Reed, G. W., Gumieniak, O., Scavron, J., & Ockene, I. (2005). Diabetes self-management among low-income Spanish-speaking patients: A pilot study. *Annals of Behavioral Medicine, 29*(3), 225–235.

Safren, S. A., Gonzalez, J. S., & Soroudi, N. (2008). *Coping with chronic illness: A cognitive-behavioral therapy approach for adherence and depression.* Oxford: Oxford University Press.

Samuel-Hodge, C. D., Keyserling, T. C., France, R., Ingram, A., Johnston, L. F., Pullen Davis, L., et al. (2006). A church-based diabetes self-management education program for African Americans with type 2 diabetes. *Preventing Chronic Disease, 3*(3), 1–16.

Schuurmans, H., Steverink, N., Lindenberg, S., Frieswijk, N., & Slaets, J. P. J. (2004). Old or frail: What tells us more? *Journal of Gerontology: Medical Sciences, 59A*(9), 936–965.

Seeman, T. E., Unger, J. B., & McAvay, G. (1999). Self-efficacy beliefs and perceived declines in functional ability: MacArthur studies of successful aging. *Journal of Gerontology: Psychological Sciences, 54B* (4), 214–222.

Selye, J. (1950). Stress and the general adaption syndrome. *British Medical Journal, 4667*, 1383–1392.

Spafford, P. A. (2004). *The role of illness representations in the coping and adjustment of children with asthma and their parents.* University of Western Australia. Unpublished thesis. Accessed December 14, 201. Available online at http://theses.library.uwa.edu.au/adt-WU2005.0046/public/04chapter3.pdf

Steed, L., Cooke, D., & Newman, S. (2003). A systematic review of psychosocial outcomes following education, self-management and psychological interventions in diabetes mellitus. *Patient Education and Counseling, 51*(1), 5–15.

Strecher, V.J., & Rosenstock, I. M. (1997). The health belief model In K. Glanz, F.M. Lewis & B.K. Rimer (Eds.), *Health behavior and health education: Theory, research, and practice* (pp.41–59). Jossey-Bass, San Francisco.

University of Southern California. (2010). *Center for occupation and lifestyle redesign.* Retrieved November 20, 2010, from http://ot.usc.edu/about-us/center/

Velicer, W. F, Prochaska, J. O., Fava, J. L., Norman, G. J., & Redding, C. A. (1998). Smoking cessation and stress management: Applications of the Transtheoretical Model of behavior change. *Homeostasis, 38*, 216–233.

Vincent, D., Clark, L., Zimmer, L. M., & Sanchez, J. (2006). Using focus groups to develop a culturally competent diabetes self-management program for Mexican Americans. *Diabetes Educator, 32*(1), 89–97.

von Goeler, D. S., Rosal, M. C., Ockene, J. K., Scavron, J., & De Torrijos, F. (2003). Self-management of type 2 diabetes: A survey of low-income urban Puerto Ricans. *Diabetes Educator, 29*(4), 663–672.

Von Keorff, M., & Tiemens, B. (2000). Individualized stepped care of chronic illness. *Culture and Medicine, 172*, 133–137.

Walker, L. (1985). Adolescent dialysands in group therapy. *Social Casework, 66*, 21–29.

Wegener, S. T., Mackenzie, E. J., Ephraim, P., Edhe, D., & Williams, R. (2009). Self-management improves outcomes in persons with limb loss. *Archives of Physical Medicine and Rehabilitation, 90*, 373–380.

World Health Organization. (2001). *International Classification of Functioning, disability and health (ICF).* Geneva: World Health Organization.

Health Legislation and Public Policies

Nancy Cheak-Zamora, Stephanie A. Reid-Arndt, Kristofer J. Hagglund, *and* Robert G. Frank

Abstract

As demographics shift to include more elderly populations and those living with chronic medical conditions, costs for health care services continue to escalate. As a result, health care systems around the world increasingly struggle to provide cost-effective, coordinated, and quality health care to those they serve. Significant policy, procedural, and practice changes are essential in solving these growing problems. With experience in interdisciplinary teams, rehabilitation psychologists and other psychological providers have a clear vantage point from which to help guide movement toward an integrated health care model that values health promotion, prevention, and collaborative care. Psychologists can be an integral part of this new "interdisciplinary team," but, as a profession, we must advocate for this inclusion and position ourselves to take on this new role through education and training.

Key Words: Rehabilitation psychology, health care legislation, health care policy, national health services, Patient Protection and Affordable Care Act, medical home, cardinal symptom model, primary care.

The practice of rehabilitation psychology, like much of health care, will experience considerable change in the next decade. Aging populations, variable quality in health care delivery, and unsustainable cost increasingly threaten the health care systems in the United States, Britain, and much of the rest of the European Union. Health policy leaders in the United States and Europe are taking policy steps to improve and, in the case of the United States, expand health delivery systems. The magnitude of challenges surrounding the financing and delivery of health care assures significant change will occur. If rehabilitation psychology actively and creatively participates in policy development, it may find its role and utility in health care delivery systems expanded. If rehabilitation psychologists hold to traditional practices and fail to engage in the political and policy process, the field may find itself marginalized.

Compared to other industrialized nations, the United States faces multiple hurdles in the management and delivery of health care. In addition to an aging population and cost and quality challenges, the United States experiences the additional burden of poor access to care: data from 2010 indicate that approximately 52 million U.S. citizens are uninsured (U.S. Bureau of the Census, 2010). The Patient Protection and Affordable Care Act (PPACA; PL 111–148) signed into law by President Barack Obama in 2010 aims to address this issue. It focuses on improving access to care by expanding public insurance programs and overhauling the private health insurance sector. This law is arguably the most significant health policy legislation in the United States since the passage of Medicare and Medicaid in 1965.

The U.S. Medicare program was implemented at the end of the baby boom generation (those born in the years 1946–1964) to provide financial and health security for the baby boomers' grandparents. These same baby boomers are now reaching age 65, and they are relying on Medicare to provide access to health care and avoid possible health-related financial catastrophe as much as, or more, than the first generation of Medicare recipients. The first baby boomers reached the age of 65 in 2011 and will begin to retire in staggering numbers over the next 20 years. In the United States, the number of people aged 65 years or older is expected to increase from approximately 40 million in 2010 to 72 million by 2030 (U.S. Census Bureau, 2010b). This population will retire in relatively good health, but many will have chronic, frequently disabling conditions (National Center for Health Statistics, 2010). The prevalence of activity limitations from chronic illnesses rises rapidly from age 55 to age 85. Approximately 28% of those aged 85 years and older experience activity limitations from arthritis and musculoskeletal conditions, heart and circulatory conditions, vision and hearing limitations, and progressive dementias (National Center for Health Statistics, 2010). Another study revealed that 26% of adults 65–74 years old and 36% of those 75–84 years old had significant activity limitations (National Center for Health Statistics, 2010). The baby boom generation's size and its anticipated health care needs threaten the financial solvency of Medicare and strain the health care systems in the United States and Europe.

Activity limitations due to chronic medical conditions are not only a concern among the elderly, however, as a growing proportion of society is being diagnosed with chronic medical conditions (Reed & Tu, 2002). Conservative estimates suggest that 72 million working-age Americans are currently living with one or more chronic conditions (Druss, Marcus, Olfson, & Taniellian, 2001; Hwang, Weller, Ireys, & Anderson, 2001; Partnership for Solutions, 2004; Tu & Cohen, 2009; Tu & Reed, 2002). By 2020, it is projected that more than 150 million people in the United States will have one or more chronic conditions and that more than 81 million will have multiple chronic conditions (Bodenheimer, Chen, & Bennett, 2009).

Across age groups, having a chronic medical condition severely jeopardizes a person's health, level of functioning, and financial stability (Cohen & Krauss, 2003; Davies, 2004; Druss et al., 2001). Individuals with chronic medical conditions have complex medical needs and rely on care from multiple medical professionals. They also require

disproportionately more high-dollar health-related services than the average consumer (Anderson & Knickman, 2001; Stanton, 2006; Wagner, Austin, Davis, Hindmarsh, Schaefer, & Bonomi, 2001). As with older persons, there is a concerning growth in the number of younger adults (aged 50–64 years) needing help with personal care activities (Martin, Freedman, Schoeni, & Andreski, 2010).

These high-cost services associated with chronic health conditions engender significant health spending that burdens individuals and society. A small proportion of the population is accountable for the majority of health care expenditures: between 50% and 78% of all health care spending in the United States is used by persons with one or more chronic conditions (Anderson & Horvath, 2004; Anderson & Knickman, 2001; Stanton, 2006; Wagner et al., 2001). Medicare beneficiaries with four or more chronic health conditions generated health care costs of more than $468 billion in 2008, accounting for 80% of all Medicare spending (Boult, Counsell, Leipzig, & Berenson, 2010). Coverage for these chronic conditions, and the expectation of health services, has driven health care spending and has played a large role in the significant cost containment problem facing the United States. Data regarding health care in the United States prior to the PPACA revealed that the nation spent $2.5 trillion on health care services in 2009, representing 17.6% of its gross domestic product (Martin, Lassman, Whittle, & Catlin, 2011).

To continue to provide adequate care and make strides in improving systems of care, European and North American countries must better control health care costs. In the United States, cost control and consistent quality have been historically pushed aside by fee-for-service payment systems. Fee-for-service reimbursement exacerbates cost escalation and quality problems because it rewards providers for volume instead of quality of care or health outcomes of patients (Fisher, Bynum, & Skinner, 2009; Franzini, Mikhail, & Skinner, 2010). The recent health reform law provides for experimentation with restructuring primary care, using bundled payment mechanisms, and the development of Accountable Care Organizations, however. The goals of these approaches are to lower costs and improve health care quality through coordinated, efficient care that focuses on prevention (Orszag & Emanuel, 2010).

Widespread application of bundled payment methods, medical homes, accountable care organizations, and similar reimbursement models that incorporate quality and provider accountability will force a major shift in health care providers' practices, including those in psychology and rehabilitation. Rehabilitation psychology may effectively use its aggregate experience and expertise in the biopsychosocial model, interdisciplinary teamwork, and long-term outcomes emphasis to expand its participation in the health care system under new reimbursement and delivery systems. Medical homes designed for the elderly and those with chronic conditions and/or disabilities would benefit from rehabilitation psychologists who can provide such services as cognitive and neuropsychological assessment, behavioral and environmental interventions to promote adherence to treatment regimens, individual and family interventions to facilitate independent functioning and living, therapy to promote mental health, and consultation with team members to maximize effective care coordination.

Models of Health Care

Although the United States continues to have a fragmented system for financing and delivering health care services, many industrialized nations have long operated under systems wherein the government funds, manages, and/or regulates the health care system. A 2010 review of 13 industrialized nations (Commonwealth Fund, 2010) revealed that the governments of eight countries both fund and manage health care services (Australia, Canada, Denmark, England, Italy, New Zealand, Norway, and Sweden). The French government also manages its health insurance system, but individuals' insurance is funded through payroll and central taxes. In several of these countries (e.g., New Zealand, Denmark, Australia, Canada, and France), a substantial portion of individuals (33–90%) also have private insurance, typically for noncovered services.

Although retaining the ideal of universal coverage, several other countries rely on a system of competing private health insurance providers in the health care market. For example, health insurance in Germany is also funded through payroll taxes, yet insurance providers are competing nongovernmental insurers. Additionally, approximately 10% of Germans choose private insurance rather than the statutory insurance system. Citizens in the Netherlands and Switzerland are also required to purchase insurance, which is provided through private insurance markets in both countries; a majority of persons in the Netherlands also have complementary private insurance.

In contrast with these systems, the United States does not have a centralized, organized system, but rather relies on numerous private and government-based institutions and programs for health care services. Data from 2010, prior to the full implementation of the PPACA, indicate that approximately 50% of the population has insurance funded by payroll taxes, 25% receive insurance through government-managed programs (e.g., Medicare, Medicaid), and 5% pay for insurance themselves. Approximately 15% of the U.S. population does not currently have health insurance (Commonwealth Fund, 2010). The new health law will dramatically reduce the number of uninsured in the United States, but its effect on costs and access to coordinated care is less clear.

Several studies have examined how variations between countries affect the utilization of health care services and the health of the residents within each country. In 2010, a telephone survey of adults in 11 industrialized countries was undertaken to examine how access to health care may be affected by the health insurance system and respondents' income (Schoen et al., 2010). In general, respondents from the United States were significantly more apt to report problems with health care affordability, as they were more likely to have gone without care due to costs, to have spent more than $1,000 out-of-pocket for health care services, and to have had problems paying medical bills in the previous year (20% of U.S. respondents vs. 9% or less in other countries). In contrast, those in the United Kingdom had the lowest reported out-of-pocket costs. Also notable is France's public health insurance system: in addition to resulting in one of the lowest out-of-pocket expense rates per capita (Commonwealth Fund, 2010), it includes a program that eliminates out-of-pocket costs for people with 30 specified chronic medical conditions.

The barrier that health care costs presents to access to care in the United States relative to other countries becomes even greater when considering the effects of income level. Schoen and colleagues (2010) found that rates of discrepancy in health care access and affordability based on income were the highest in the United States and the lowest in the United Kingdom. Compared to other countries, the United States had the greatest percentage of low-income respondents reporting that they experience access barriers due to cost, out-of-pocket spending exceeding $1,000 annually, and being unable to afford to pay accrued medical bills. Findings from an 11-country survey of primary care physicians (Schoen et al., 2010) mirrored these concerns: U.S. physicians were more likely than physicians in other countries to report concerns that their patients have problems paying for medications and/ or medical care.

Cost of care is additionally troublesome for persons living with chronic medical conditions. Schoen and colleagues (2009a) conducted a survey designed to examine care provided to adults in eight industrialized countries (Australia, Canada, France, Germany, Netherlands, New Zealand, England, and the United States) with chronic medical conditions including hypertension, heart disease (and heart attack), diabetes, arthritis, lung ailments (asthma, emphysema, and chronic lung obstruction), cancer, and depression. Compared to respondents from all other countries, U.S. respondents consistently reported the greatest cost-related barriers in access to care (e.g., 54% reported skipping medications due to costs). Moreover, this problem was magnified among those without health insurance. Twenty-nine percent of U.S. respondents indicated they had been uninsured during the year; of these, 82% reported not receiving recommended care (e.g., filling a prescription, seeing a physician when ill) due to costs (Schoen et al., 2009a).

Although insurers cover citizens regardless of their demographic characteristics in other countries surveyed, the United States remains the only country to divide population into different insurance programs depending on age and income. Schoen et al. (2010) reported that lower income U.S. adults under age 65 were at greatest risk for lacking health insurance: 27% of survey respondents from the United States. The PPACA is designed to help address this income-related discrepancy in health care benefits, as it will expand eligibility for Medicaid recipients to people at 133% of the federal poverty level. Additionally, the PPACA includes provisions to subsidize premiums for individuals earning up to 400% of the poverty level and for cost sharing for people up to 250% of the poverty level. Because the United States has separate insurance programs for individuals with lower incomes (i.e., Medicaid) and is the only country in which providers are paid according to patient income, the willingness of providers to provide care is influence by patient income (Schoen et al., 2010). The PPACA will increase the rates of reimbursement for providers caring for Medicaid patients, but it is unclear if this will influence providers' willingness to treat all patients.

Chronic Care Services

Providing appropriate access to affordable health care may be particularly challenging for persons with chronic medical conditions. The frequency and intensity of care required is often higher in this population. Persons with chronic illnesses and disabilities often require sophisticated and coordinated care from multiple providers to manage their conditions, maximize function, and maintain independent living, yet a majority of industrialized nations' health care systems continue to emphasize an acute care model, which focuses on single episodes of care. As a result, patients and their families are given the responsibility of coordinating care. Given the complexities of illness management associated with multiple chronic conditions, many patients/ families do not succeed in managing their care over the long term.

Additionally, the provision of care coordination and transitional services as persons traverse between inpatient and outpatient health care services is a critical component of care for individuals with chronic illnesses. It has been suggested that up to 75% of hospital readmissions of chronically ill patients may be preventable with appropriate follow-up care post discharge (Medicare Payment Advisory Commission, 2007). In a 2008 international survey (Schoen et al., 2009a), the United States received higher marks than other countries for transitional services and care coordination efforts following hospitalization. For example, the United States had the lowest rate of reported deficiencies in hospital discharge instructions (38%), whereas France had the highest (71%). In addition, respondents from the United States were the most likely to report involvement in treatment goal/priority setting and follow-up care. However, even with these achievements, the U.S. government spends $17 billion on unplanned hospital readmission costs annually (Jencks, Williams, & Coleman, 2009). The costs associated with a health care system based on an acute care model are great for all countries, and are largely shouldered by public payers. For example, in the United States during 2005–2006, nearly half of ambulatory care and more than 60% of hospital care for chronic conditions was paid by Medicare or Medicaid (Decker, Schappert, & Sisk, 2009).

The liabilities of the acute care model have been widely recognized and lamented (e.g., Cortese & Korsmo, 2009). Forward thinking leaders within the field of rehabilitation psychology have suggested other models, such as the *cardinal symptom model* (Frank, Hagglund, & Farmer, 2004). In the United States, coordinated, continuous models of care exist, but are the exception. Institutions such as the Mayo Clinic, Kaiser Permanente, Group Health, and Geisenger Health Systems are at the forefront of emerging models of coordinated approaches to care (e.g., Larson, 2009; Nichols, 2010). Similarly, smaller models of coordinated care systems are in place for specific populations and have demonstrated success, although relatively few benefit because eligibility is limited (e.g., the Program of All-Inclusive Care of the Elderly [PACE], which is restricted to those who are certified as eligible for nursing home care; Berenson & Horvath, 2003; National PACE Association, 2011). Unfortunately in the United States, as in many countries, the acute care approach is further reinforced by the predominance of fee-for-service reimbursement.

Although many agree that integrated health care delivery models are needed to adequately provide health care for those with chronic conditions and/or disabilities, including a substantial portion of the growing elderly population, few nations have implemented such systems or examined how their reimbursement model exacerbates the problem. Converting to integrated care models has been made even more difficult in recent years because most nations are now facing financial crises in their health care systems due to incessantly rising health care costs and the most recent "great recession."

Health Care Legislation Trends

Health care legislation in the past several decades has had a significant impact in industrialized nations. These efforts have been most apparent in the United Kingdom and United States.

National Health Service

Since 1998, parliament has been transforming the U.K. National Health Service (NHS) to use a systematic approach to the management of chronic care and to provide quality incentives to providers (Campbell et al., 2007; Schoen et al., 2009b). One component of this process was the 1999 establishment of the National Institute for Health and Clinical Excellence (NICE), which has three core functions to promote consistent, widely disseminated, high-quality health care in the United Kingdom (see Table 28.1; Chalkidou, 2009). At the same time, the Health Care Commission (HCC; transformed into the Care Quality Commission [CQC] in April 2009) was created to monitor the performance of NHS providers for adherence to best practice guidelines and other standards established by NICE. Government funding was also deemed necessary to promote quality and access. In 2000, NHS funding was increased from 6.7% of the gross

Table 28.1 National Institute for Health and Clinical Excellence (NICE) core objectives

- Increase consistency of practice throughout the United Kingdom via development and dissemination of best practice standards.
- Encourage rapid dissemination and adoption of medical innovations.
- Monitor investment into the National Health System to ensure health benefit to citizens.

From Chalkidou, K. (July 2009). Comparative Effectiveness Review Within the U.K.'s National Institute for Health and Clinical Excellence. The Commonwealth Fund. Retrieved December 20, 2010, from http://www.commonwealthfund.org/~/media/Files/Publications/Issue%20Brief/2009/Jul/Chalkidou/1296_Chalkidou_UK_CER_issue_brief_717.pdf

domestic product (GDP) to 8%, the European average at that time (Doran & Roland, 2010).

Patient Protection and Affordable Care Act

In the United States, the PPACA seeks to dramatically overhaul the health care system by expanding coverage for individuals with preexisting health conditions (high-risk pool), guaranteeing coverage for dependents under age 26, expanding eligibility for Medicaid (federal and state social insurance program for low-income individuals) to those under 134% of the federal poverty level, instituting individual and employer mandates for insurance coverage, and decreasing provider reimbursement by Medicare (Sisko et al., 2010). By 2014, the PPACA will provide insurance coverage to more than 32 million previously uninsured Americans and make comprehensive insurance affordable for millions of currently underinsured Americans. In addition, the PPACA will fund numerous federal, state, and local demonstration projects to develop new health care delivery and reimbursement methods, structural changes, and new methods of utilizing health care services, particularly for the elderly and those with chronic medical conditions or disabilities. The PPACA provides funding for research and innovation grants to promote patient-centered care and community health initiatives and develop new strategies of care for patients with complicated medical conditions like chronic pain and depression. The new legislation will also increase the number of health care providers, especially those providing care in underserved areas.

In addition to increasing the number of those with access to health insurance, the PPACA expands what is covered within each health insurance plan. By 2014, all qualified health plans must offer the essential health benefits package. Benefits in the essential benefits plan must include ambulatory, emergency, hospitalization, laboratory, and rehabilitative and habilitative care; maternity, newborn and pediatric care; mental health and substance use disorder services; preventative and wellness services, as well as chronic disease management care; and prescription medication coverage (House Committee on Ways and Means, 2010).

Mental Health Access

Building on the Wellstone and Domenici Mental Health Parity and Addiction Equality Act of 2008, the PPACA mandates the inclusion of mental health and substance abuse services in all qualified health packages on par with medical and surgical benefits (American Psychological Association, 2010; Sundararaman, 2009). Both medical and mental health services must be covered in all basic health insurance plans (individual and group), and the amount, duration, and cost of services must be comparable between service types (American Psychological Association, 2010; House Committee on Ways and Means, 2010; Sundararaman, 2009). The PPACA does not address the use of behavioral health *carve-out programs*, a method of contracting out behavioral health benefits to managed care organizations to save cost and reduce risk (Sundararaman, 2009). Carve-out programs continue to be used by insurance companies despite concerns by medical providers that they hinder communication and collaboration between medical and behavioral health providers. However, the growing emphasis on coordinated care plans and the integration of primary and specialty services may discourage the practice (Sundararaman, 2009).

Changing Reimbursement Methods

In Europe and North America, governments are revising reimbursement methods for their health care systems in attempts to control costs and improve quality of care. Broadly speaking, the principal objective of most governments is to reward integrated, continuous care, thereby reducing costs and increasing quality and prevention. In the United States, these shifts away from the current acute care model represent a more dramatic change than those taking place in Europe.

United Kingdom's Quality Incentives

Interest in improving quality of care while maximizing efficiency is widespread throughout industrial countries, yet the implementation of incentives

to achieve these goals is variable. One study (Schoen et al., 2009b) indicated that physicians from the United Kingdom were most likely to report the existence of incentives to improve quality and reduce costs (89% of sample), whereas relatively few surveyed physicians from Sweden and the United States reported availability of quality incentives (10% and 36%, respectively).

As detailed by Doran and Roland (2010), incentives to improve quality of care in the United Kingdom were specified in a Quality Outcomes Framework (Roland, 2004) that was a component of the practice contract between the U.K. Department of Health and the British Medical Association, implemented in 2004. Per the original Quality Outcomes Framework, physician practices earned points based on clinical indicators. The indicators included both processes, such as measuring blood pressure, and short-term outcomes, such as maintaining acceptable blood pressure levels. Because this disincentivised the provision of care to the most ill, the framework was revised in 2009 (e.g., emphasis on successful achievement of short-term outcomes was reduced; Doran & Roland, 2010).

This pay for performance model has remained controversial in the United Kingdom. Critics expressed concerns that physicians may focus more on financial targets than patient care goals. Doran and Roland (2010) argue that this system has resulted in the development of practices that currently meet criteria for patient-centered medical homes, a model currently under examination in the United States. In addition, Doran and Roland (2010) suggest that some of the positive outcomes include an increase in the number of general practitioners in the United Kingdom to better meet demand, increased morale of U.K. providers (British Medical Association, 2007), an increase in the number of nurses, and a higher than expected percentage of quality indicators being met by physicians.

U.S. Strategies
ACCOUNTABLE CARE ORGANIZATIONS

The development of accountable care organizations (ACOs) is one way in which the PPACA is working to reduce the burden on the individual patient and health care system by enhancing quality and coordination of care and decreasing cost. Within the PPACA, ACOs may replace the Medicare fee-for-service payment model, and pilot programs will be used to expand them in Medicaid, pediatric care, and private insurance settings (PPACA, PL 331–337).

Accountable care organizations are groups of medical providers that join forces to provide coordinated and collaborative care to a designated group of patients in an effort to improve quality while reducing duplication and cost (PPACA; PL 331–337). All providers within the ACO accept legal responsibility to care for patients within their network and share the payment derived from care. Each ACO must demonstrate the utilization of evidence-based medicine and patient engagement protocols, such as tele-health and the use of electronic health records (EHR) to monitor patient performance. Further, ACOs must meet patient-centeredness criteria, such as the development and utilization of individual care plans. Accountable care organizations serving Medicare beneficiaries are responsible for the provision of both Part A and B services, which includes all primary and hospital care, as well as psychological and rehabilitative services (Winslow, 2010).

Similar to the United Kingdom's system, providers within the ACO receive additional incentive payments if they meet quality and cost standards set by the Secretary of Health and Human Services under the PPACA. The coordinated system of payment should encourage efficiency and integration by promoting an environment of information sharing and the distribution of services to appropriate providers. This will likely reduce testing and procedural duplication, procedural uncertainty, and medical errors (Shortell, Casalino, & Fisher, 2010). Accountable care organizations may also decelerate the growing primary care physician shortage as providers may be able to care for more patients through an effective team-based practice (Shortell et al., 2010). As all nations are aspiring to do, the ACO initiative within the PPACA initiates a fundamental shift from the current acute care model to one emphasizing preventive and collaborative care and provides financial incentives for service provision that treats the whole person.

In order for the ACO model to be successful and improve care within all disciplines, the PPACA provisions must be flexibly implemented, with constant multilevel evaluation and a continual feedback loop that corrects internal issues and shares accomplishments and challenges externally. Not all provider networks wishing to become an ACO will have a well-developed infrastructure to promote coordinated collaborative care. For those networks, Shortell, Casalino, and Fisher (2010) advise a tiered system of entry in which less-developed networks receive a more flexible implementation and

evaluation timeline, as well as additional technical assistance.

Thorough, consistent, and applicable performance measures are an integral part the overall provision. Measures must include quality of care provided; outcomes of care; level of patient, provider, and system engagement; patient satisfaction; and cost of care. Measurement tools must be consistent within and among ACOs and must be implemented at each stage of the development and care process. Electronic health records within all ACOs may improve the collection and immediate utilization of performance data. When evaluating this data, analysts should consider the structural, leadership, care process, and environment within which each ACO functions to determine the effect that these characteristics have on outcome measures and networks success (Shortell et al., 2010).

To promote the success of these programs, state and federal Medicare agencies and individual ACOs should maintain close communication that allows them to share achievements, difficulties, and lessons learned without fear of retribution. The better the communication, the lower the risk of numerous ACOs experiencing the same challenges and the more likely a universal structure for effective ACO development and practice can be generated. In addition, the United States should examine the incentive models used by the United Kingdom and other nations to learn from their achievements and challenges.

CENTER OF MEDICARE AND MEDICAID INNOVATION

The Center of Medicare and Medicaid Innovation (CMI) will test payment and service delivery models that reduce program expenditures and increase quality patient-centered care. Models will likely focus on several key initiatives (see Table 28.2). The Medicaid Global Payment System Demonstration Project will fund five states to replace the fee-for-serve payment mechanism with a global capitated model of payments for eligible safety-net hospital networks. Each initiative promises innovative mechanisms for system improvement, patient involvement, and cost containment. The CMI will evaluate each project's spending and ability to provide quality health care. Following each evaluation, the Secretary of Health and Senior Services will provide Congress with CMI and Global Payment reports detailing the project outcomes and making specific recommendations for future implementation. These findings

Table 28.2 The Center of Medicare and Medicaid Innovation (CMI) initiatives

- Promotion of primary care medical home models for high-risk patients replacing fee-for-service payments with comprehensive or salary-based payment methods.
- Development and utilization of geriatric assessment and comprehensive care plans for patients with serious and comorbid conditions.
- Utilization of health information and tele-health technology to support care coordination.
- Development of community-based health teams to aid small practice medical homes with implementing chronic care management and health promotion activities.
- Promotion and improvement of continuing care hospitals with rehabilitation services to address post acute care issues.
- Development and implementation of models that eliminate requirements for physician referrals.

and recommendations can then be used to develop national delivery and reimbursement methods that more effectively care for those with special health care needs as well as the general public.

HOME-BASED CARE INITIATIVES

The Health Home Initiative is a Medicaid state plan option that allows recipients to specify a health professional as their health home if they have two or more chronic conditions, one condition and are at risk of developing another, or one serious and persistent mental health condition (American Psychological Association, 2010; PPACA, PL 248–252). Health home services include comprehensive care management, care coordination and health promotion, comprehensive transitional care, patient and family support, referral to community and social support services, and use of health information technology (PPACA, PL 248–252). This utilizes the principles of the medical home model to empower providers and patients with the tools necessary to take an active role in the management of these complex conditions.

Similarly, the Independence at Home Medical Practice Demonstration program is another initiative that will test payment and service delivery models utilizing physician- and nurse practitioner–directed home-based primary care teams to provide home-based care (PPACA, PL 324–328). These programs are essential in allowing individuals with disabilities or severe conditions to remain in their homes and thus inhibit the increasing utilization of nursing home services for this population.

In general, services provide quality coordinated care, in-home medical visits, and 24-hour access to medical assistance. This bundle of in-home services aims to reduce preventable hospitalizations, readmissions, and emergency room visits, thereby reducing expenditures and improving health outcomes and patient satisfaction. Physician and nurse practitioner teams may include any provider affiliated with the practice and integral to the rehabilitation and care process (PPACA, PL 324–328). These, along with other initiatives, will promote interdisciplinary interprofessional health teams and an overall environment that promotes collaboration and coordination of services.

EXPANSION OF PSYCHOLOGICAL SERVICES

Specifically relevant to rehabilitation psychology services, the PPACA designates $50 million in grants for demonstration projects that co-locate primary and specialty care services in community-based mental and behavioral health settings. The addition of primary care services to mental health settings will enhance the coordination and integration of services for adults with mental illness and other co-occurring physical conditions. Additional funding streams were developed to provide mental and behavioral health education to health care providers and the general public.

Value-Based Insurance

In addition to testing system-based changes, minimizing overconsumption of health services by individuals is another approach to reducing health care costs. Among the more controversial but widespread methods to influence the consumption of health services is to adjust the financial contribution required of patients to obtain health services: patient cost sharing. Cost sharing is most typically achieved through insurance deductibles, co-insurance, and co-payments. Studies have shown that changing required cost sharing directly affects patients' health service choices (Choudhry, Rosenthal, & Milstein, 2010) and can be used to minimize the problem of "moral hazard" or overconsumption of health services because of insurance. In countries using co-payments or co-insurance, the amount of patient cost sharing can be manipulated to impact health practices. This practice, labeled *value-based insurance design*, is gaining more attention as it can be used to influence patient's decisions to use low- or high-value medical services (Robinson, 2010). Although having the potential to reduce unnecessary care, high levels of cost sharing also may reduce consumption of high-value health care services (Newhouse, 1996). For example, Choudhry, Rosenthal, and Milstein (2010) note that doubling co-payments for managed care recipients reduced their use of cholesterol lowering medication by 10%. The elimination of co-payments can also influence selection of other services, such as hospitals (with no co-payment requirement) or reduce use of low-value services (Choudhry et al., 2010). In the future, insurance systems are likely to channel patients to high-value services, providers, or products through co-payment (Robinson, 2010). Use of critical preventive services and medication regimens can be enhanced by reducing co-payments as well. The PPACA will put these principles into action by eliminating co-payments for all preventive services used by Medicare and Medicaid recipients.

Primary Care

Many health care restructuring proposals utilize the primary care model as a basis for change. Primary care is a system of care defined by its common characteristics. One approach defines primary care by the specialty of the individual providing care. Most often this includes general pediatricians, general internists, family medicine providers, nurse practitioners, or other generalists. Specifically excluded from this approach are specialty base practitioners, regardless of their experience or service. This approach suggests that an individual's training defines his or her style of practice (Friedberg, Hussey, & Schneider, 2010). A second approach to defining primary care identifies primary care as a set of functions provided to patients. Patients who receive first-contact, comprehensive, coordinated care over the long-term receive primary care services. The emphasis in this approach is upon coordination and integration of health care services. A provider's training is not defining in this approach; specialists, especially those providing comprehensive, integrated care to individuals with chronic health conditions, would be viewed as primary care providers (Friedberg et al., 2010). A third definition of primary care focuses on system-levels analysis of the ratios of primary care providers to patients and specialty physicians (Friedberg et al., 2010).

Enhanced outcomes associated with primary care have led many nations to implement primary care as the backbone of health reform efforts. The PPACA, the proposed changes in the NHS in the United Kingdom, and concerns for escalating health care costs around the world have once again refocused interest on primary care systems able to provide more affordable, efficient health care. Although U.S. citizens traditionally utilize primary care as the first point of contact, the decentralized referral system in the United States often results in poorly coordinated care. Most other advanced health systems rely on general practice/family practice physicians to serve as the hub of health care service provision (Borkan, Eaton, Novillo-Ortiz, Corte, & Jadad, 2010; Schoen et al., 2009b). Examination of models of health care in industrialized nations reveals that strong, well-integrated primary care systems are associated with better health care and lower costs (Starfield, Shi, & Macinko, 2005; WHO, 2008). For example, persons with chronic illnesses report better access to needed health care in the Netherlands and the United Kingdom relative to other countries with less-advanced primary care infrastructure (Schoen et al., 2009b).

In the United Kingdom, a radical reform of the 62-year-old National Health System will hand control of most budgeted services to family doctors (Timmins, 2010). In the proposed model, general practitioners, in addition to providing primary care services, will be part of commissioning consortia that will purchase hospital services for their patients (Timmins, 2010).

Legislation in the Netherlands created after-hours physician cooperatives that provide a system for accessing primary care services 24 hours a day (Schoen et al., 2009b), thereby lessening the use of emergency room care for nonemergency after-hours medical needs. Other nations' policies focused on primary care have led to improved health information technology capacity (e.g., in Australia, the Netherlands, New Zealand; Schoen et al., 2009b), also associated with more efficient care and better health outcomes.

Given the strong advocacy, and the belief that primary care services cost less and produces better outcomes, surprisingly few outcomes studies have examined the concept. Primary care providers are more likely to perform recommended care processes. Specialists, in contrast, are more likely to use new treatments and technologies lacking demonstrated efficacy. Individuals with chronic conditions who identified primary care physicians had lower 5-year mortality than did those identifying specialists as their providers (Friedberg et al., 2010).

Overall, although the evidence is inconclusive, the structure of the system of primary care practices may improve outcomes, quality, and the cost of care (Friedberg et al., 2010). At the policy level, encouragement of systems of care that provide uninterrupted care between the patient and provider may be the most effective (Friedberg et al., 2010). In the United States, several models of integrating care have been proposed, including the medical home model and the cardinal symptom model.

Medical Home Model

Medical homes, a clinical entity that coordinates all care for an individual, were initially proposed to serve children with special needs (Fields, Leshen, & Patal, 2010). They have since attracted interest from health policy advocates and others, who have suggested they are a vehicle for coordinating IT and EHR, differing disease states, and new payment models (Fields et al., 2010). Medical homes were thus incorporated into the PPACA as a tool that can modify cost while increasing quality (Fields et al., 2010).

Fields, Leshen, and Patal (2010) evaluated seven existing medical homes and interviewed experts to identify critical components of the medical home. They identified four "value-generating" elements. The first element was effective coordinated care facilitated by dedicated nonphysician providers. The second element they identified was expanded access to providers. Communication between provider and patients should assure care is not sought in emergency rooms or other high-cost venues and should include face-to-face, e-mail, and phone contact. The third element was accessible, real-time data that provides predictive modeling and allows the identification of high-risk individuals based on population-based observations. The last element identified in successful medical home implementation projects is the availability of incentives for providers that enhance adoption of care coordination mechanisms.

Cardinal Symptom Model

Central to the concept of the medical home is the provision of coordinated, team care. Team care is defined as care delivered by teams of providers working with a primary care provider (Bates & Bitton, 2010). Bates and Bitton (2010) note the importance of effective information tools that facilitate communication among providers in patient-centered medical homes. They also suggest that effective communication among team providers through use of a functional EHR is vital to creating an effective health care team.

Although there is clear recognition within primary care that interdisciplinary teams can enhance treatment outcomes, there has been little recognition that teams have been the underpinning of rehabilitation treatment since the inception of the field. Howard Rusk, a pioneer in rehabilitation, was an early advocate for interdisciplinary teams in rehabilitation (Butt & Caplan, 2010). In both rehabilitation and primary care, effective team functioning is challenged by pressure upon physician's time, thus requiring the team to focus more on supporting the physician than upon the patient's needs (Chesluk & Holmboe 2010). Effective teams, whether in rehabilitation or primary care, require patient-centered care rather than physician-centered support (Butt & Caplan, 2010, Chesluk & Holmboe, 2010).

Although primary care has been found to enhance health outcomes, improve cost effectiveness, and increase access to care, traditional primary care systems are not designed to treat chronic or debilitating health conditions (Frank et al., 2004; Starfield, 2000). In addition, the traditional "patient" is becoming a "health consumer," who researches different conditions, treatments, and outcomes and expects more services from health providers (Frank et al., 2004). In particular, individuals with chronic conditions will seek: "(a) education to manage their conditions, (b) individualized programs supported by professional collaborators, and (c) continuity of care" (Frank et al., 2004, p. 269). These new health consumers, aided by a wealth of information, will seek an active role in their care, choice of providers, and place of service.

Frank and colleagues (2004) noted that traditional primary care systems are designed to treat acute illness, not individuals with chronic conditions that require coordinated, integrated care in addition to education, responsiveness, and timeliness. In addition to more frequent appointments and the need for integrated care across medical services, individuals with chronic health conditions require routine assessment of clinical, behavioral, and psychological factors (Frank et al., 2004). The medical home concept addresses some of these concerns, but not all.

As health consumers become more sophisticated, they will seek integration of health services, pharmaceutical, nutrition, exercise, and social systems. More informed consumers would seek practitioners with more expertise in the conditions most limiting their activities. Primary care providers have traditionally provided a relatively narrow spectrum of care that does not integrate all of these services and therefore may not meet their patients' expectations. Rather, a model of care utilizing the integrated information systems and continuity of care demanded by the medical home with rehabilitation-type team and education programs system appears to meet many of the demands of the future health consumer.

This approach, labeled the *cardinal symptom model* (Frank, 1997; Frank et al., 2004), recognizes that specialists manage many chronic health conditions that limit health and function. For many individuals with chronic disease, this primary condition dominates their life and activities. The primary premise of the cardinal symptom model is that individuals are followed by specialists who offer unique expertise relevant to their chief complaints. Fundamental to this model, as with the medical home, is the universal development of EHR that allow the coordination and integration of clinical care. The second premise of the cardinal symptom model, as with the medical home, is the management of chronic illness by an integrated team of health professionals including physician, psychologist, physical and occupational therapists, and other disciplines. Care is coordinated by a care manager who can be a nurse, rehabilitation counselor, or other health professional.

Although the medical home proposes changes to routine care to make primary care specialties more effective in managing chronic health conditions, the cardinal symptom model recognizes that most patients want health care from medical specialists knowledgeable in the condition that limits their health and activities. Thus, a person with cardiac dysfunction seeks care from a cardiologist or an individual with spinal cord injury seeks care from a physiatrist.

One of the ironies of the move toward a medical home is the higher cost associated with this level of care. As in all of health care, increased levels of care are associated with higher costs. Although the coordinated, integrated care associated with the medical home may prevent complications, enhance quality of life, and/or improve function, it is also the case that increased care increases cost. During the last 20 years, rehabilitation services have come under extensive cost scrutiny that has pushed the provision of services away from reliance upon interdisciplinary teams (Ashkanazi, Hagglund, Lee, Swaine, & Frank, 2010). The move away from interdisciplinary teams within rehabilitation has diminished coordinated, continuous care facilitated by the rehabilitation model. Thus, rehabilitation has moved away from many traits of the cardinal symptom approach. As the United States explores payment models that promote coordinated, long-term care, however,

rehabilitation may be rewarded for moving back to interdisciplinary treatment approaches.

Conclusion

The issues of cost containment, coordination, and quality of care are affecting the effectiveness of health care systems around the world and the solvency of each. It appears clear that legislative, procedural, and practice changes must be implemented to resolve these ever-growing problems. Previous experiences have provided lessons on how to make health care systems more productive and avoid ineffective utilization of the system. These lessons indicate the importance of providing access to basic health care services for all; implementing incentives for medical providers to monitor and promote quality care; eliminating fee-for-service payment systems that incentivize volume over quality of patient care; implementing effective cost-sharing practices for those utilizing the health care system; and centering medical care around medical home and cardinal care models, particularly for individuals with chronic medical conditions and/or disabilities. Implementation of these lessons will be arduous and require long-term, coordinated efforts from individual governments, health care providers, educators, and citizens alike. Fortunately, as the cost of providing health care services is straining the budgets of most nations, few have the option to remain stagnate.

Psychologists, and specifically rehabilitation psychologists, need to move away from the traditional model of considering mental and behavioral health care services as separable from medical care. Instead, we must work toward a model of integrated health care, incorporating psychology services into standard medical care (Frank, 1999). Exciting opportunities in integrated primary care, emphasizing co-location and shared patient care between psychologists and primary care physicians (DeLeon, Giesting, & Kenkel, 2003), have recently been highlighted by health care reform legislation in the United States. In health care systems of the future, psychologists will have the opportunity to increase their presence in primary care settings, addressing behavioral health factors that contribute to poor physical health (e.g., smoking, weight management), as well as basic mental health care needs, a large percentage of which may be missed by primary care physicians (Brody, 2003).

As a field, we must continue to emphasize that mental and behavioral health care needs are a significant public health issue, as stressed by a Surgeon

General report revealing that one in five U.S. adults experience a mental disorder each year (Health Resources and Services Administration, 2002; U.S. Department of Health and Human Services, 1999). We should build upon increasing awareness of the role of behavioral health issues in physical wellness and primary care, as noted in a 2004 study documenting that the leading causes of death in 2000 were all behavior-related: tobacco use, poor diet, physical inactivity, and alcohol consumption (Mokdad, Marks, Stroup, & Gerberding, 2004). Moreover, we must highlight the fact that rehabilitation, pain management, oncology, and a variety of other specialty services commonly include psychologists as an integral part of the interdisciplinary team. By building upon this team approach to health care, already embraced by our field in both theory and practice, rehabilitation psychologists will be positioned to remain critical partners in the provision of health care services in the future.

Future Directions

Changes in the nature of health care management and provision brought on by difficult economic times and shifting demographics (e.g., a growing number of elderly) bring opportunities as well as uncertainties. The United States, in particular, is on the threshold of monumental changes to its health care system with the signing of the PPACA in 2010. Questions remain regarding how the PPACA will unfold, and the myriad of ways that it may affect the U.S. health care system have yet to be answered. Consistent analysis, adaptation, and improvement are instrumental in all reform efforts, but how will these processes be implemented to influence the efficiency and effectiveness of the health care system and success of the reform?

During this time of opportunity for behavioral/mental health care providers, it remains to be seen how rehabilitation psychology and other psychological services will be affected and how they will affect health care reform in the United States and internationally. By capitalizing on a growing awareness of the value of psychological and behavioral health services to mental and physical health, and by making documentation of psychology workforce issues a top priority, we and our membership organizations can lead the field in efforts to increase funding for psychology training that will enable our profession to meet the ever-expanding psychological and behavioral health needs in the United States. Yet, will psychology and rehabilitation psychology embrace this changing health care model

and become actively involved in efforts to become integral members of the team approach to health care that is gaining momentum?

Moreover, how will psychologists ensure that future professionals in our field are equipped to cope with changes in the health care system? It has been argued that training opportunities must evolve to meet the changing mental and behavioral health care needs within the United States if psychologists are to stay relevant in the cardinal symptom approach and the future system of care (DeLeon, Dubanoski, & Oliveira-Berry, 2005; Reid-Arndt, Stucky, Cheak-Zamora, DeLeon, & Frank, 2010). Will the field be successful in overcoming barriers to achieving this goal? Evidence of creative thinking and determined effort by leaders in health care in general, and rehabilitation psychology in particular, give rise to cautious optimism about potential gains that may result from health care reform for the field of psychology and the people we serve.

References

American Psychological Association. (2010). *The Patient Protection and Affordable Care Act: New protections and opportunities for practicing psychologists*. Retrieved November 24, 2010 from http://www.apapracticecentral.org/advocacy/reform/patient-protection.aspx

Anderson, G., & Horvath, J. (2004). The growing burden of chronic disease in America. *Public Health Report, 119*, 263–269.

Anderson, G., & Knickman, J. R. (2001). Changing the chronic care system to meet people's needs. *Health Affairs, 20*(6), 146–161.

Ashkanazi, G. S., Hagglund, K. J., Lee, A., Swaine, Z., & Frank, R. G. (2010). Health Policy 101: Fundamental issues in health care reform. In R. G. Frank, M. R. Rosenthal, & B. Caplan (Eds.), *Handbook of rehabilitation psychology* (2nd ed., pp. 439–449). Washington, DC: American Psychological Association.

Bates, D. W., & Bitton, A. (2010). The future of health information technology in the patient centered medical home. *Health Affairs, 29*(4), 614–621.

Berenson, R. A., & Horvath, J. (2003). Confronting the barriers to chronic care management in medicare. *Health Affairs, W3*, 37–53.

Bodenheimer, T., Chen, E., & Bennett, H. D. (2009). Confronting the growing burden of chronic disease: Can the U.S. health care workforce do the job? Health Affairs, *28*(1), 64–74.

Borkan, J., Eaton, C. B., Novillo-Ortiz, D., Corte, P. R., & Jadad A. R. (2010). Renewing primary care: Lesson learned from the Spanish health care system. *Health Affairs, 29*(8), 1432–1440.

Boult, C., Counsell, S. R., Leipzig, R. M., & Berenson, R. A. (2010). The urgency of preparing primary care physicians to care for older people with chronic conditions. *Health Affairs, 29*(5), 811–818.

British Medical Association. (2007). *National survey of GP opinion*. London: British Medical Association. Retrieved

December 20, 2010 from http://www.bma.org.uk/images/NationalsurveyGP2007_tcm41–144622.pdf

Brody, D. S. (2003). Improving the management of depression in primary care: Recent accomplishments and ongoing challenges. *Disease Management Health Outcomes, 11*, 21–31.

Butt, L., & Caplan, B. (2010). The rehabilitation team. In R. G. Frank, M. R. Rosenthal, & B. Caplan. *The handbook of rehabilitation psychology* (2nd ed., pp. 451–457). Washington, DC: American Psychological Association.

Campbell, S., Reeves, D., Kontopantelis, E., Middleton, E., Sibbald, B., & Roland, M. (2007). Quality of primary care in England with the introduction of pay for performance. *New England Journal of Medicine, 357*(2), 181–190.

Chalkidou, K. (2009). *Comparative effectiveness review within the U.K.'s National Institute for Health and Clinical Excellence. The Commonwealth Fund.* Retrieved December 20, 2010 from http://www.commonwealthfund.org/-/media/Files/Publications/Issue%20Brief/2009/Jul/Chalkidou/1296_Chalkidou_UK_CER_issue_brief_717.pdf

Chesluk, B. J., & Holmboe, E. S. (2010). How teams work- or don't- in primary care: A field study of internal medicine practices. *Health Affairs, 29*(5), 874–879.

Choudhry, N. K., Rosenthal, M. B., & Milstein, A. (2010). Assessing the evidence for value-based insurance design. *Health Affairs, 20*(11), 1988–1994.

Cohen, J. W., & Krauss, N. A. (2003) Spending and service use among people with the fifteen most costly medical conditions, 1997. *Health Affairs, 22*(2), 129–138.

Commonwealth Fund. (2010). International profiles of health care systems. Retrieved December 20, 2010 from http://www.commonwealthfund.org/-/media/Files/Publications/Fund%20Report/2010/Jun/1417_Squires_Intl_Profiles_622.pdf

Cortese, D., & Korsmo, J. O. (2009). Health care reform: Why we cannot afford to fail. *Health Affairs, 28*(2), W173–W176.

Davies, P. (2004, Aug. 25). Fifteen diseases named as drivers of health costs. *Wall Street Journal (Eastern ed.).* p. D3.

Decker, S. L., Schappert, S. M, & Sisk, J. E. (2009). The use of medical care for chronic conditions. *Health Affairs, 28*(1), 26–35.

DeLeon, P. H., Dubanoski, R., & Oliveira-Berry, J. M. (2005). An education for the future. *Journal of Clinical Psychology, 61*(9), 1105–1109.

DeLeon, P. H., Giesting, B., & Kenkel, M. S. (2003). Community health center: Exciting opportunities for the 21st century. *Professional Psychology: Research and Practice, 34*(6), 579–585.

Doran, T., & Roland, M. (2010). Lessons from major initiatives to improve primary care in the United Kingdom. *Health Affairs, 29*(5), 1023–1029.

Druss, B. G., Marcus, S. C., Olfson, M., & Taniellian, T. (2001). Comparing the national economic burden of five chronic conditions. *Health Affairs, 20*(6), 233–241.

Fields, D., Leshen, E., & Patel, K. (2010). Driving quality gains and cost savings through adoption of medical homes. *Health Affairs, 29*(5), 819–826.

Fisher, E. S., Bynum, J. P., & Skinner J. S. (2009). Slowing the growth of health care costs—lessons from regional variation. *New England Journal of Medicine, 360*(9), 849–852.

Friedberg, M. W., Hussey, P. S., & Schneider, E. C. (2010). Primary care: A review of the evidence on quality and costs of health care. *Health Affairs, 29*(5), 766–772.

Frank, R. G. (1997). Lessons from the great battle: Health care reform, 1992–1994. John Stanley Coulter lecture. *Archives of Physical Medicine and Rehabilitation, 76*(2), 120–124.

Frank, R. G. (1999). Rehabilitation psychology: We zigged when we should have zagged. *Rehabilitation Psychology, 44*(1), 36–51.

Frank, R. G., Hagglund, K. J., & Farmer, J. E. (2004). Chronic illness management in primary care: The cardinal symptom model. In R. G. Frank, S. McDaniel, J. Bray & M. Heldring (Eds.), *Primary care psychology* (pp. 259–271). Washington, DC: American Psychological Association Press.

Franzini, L., Mikhail, O. I., & Skinner, J. S. (2010). McAllen and El Paso revisited: Medicare variations not always reflected in the under-sixty-five population. *Health Affairs, 29*(12), 2302–2309.

Health Resources and Services Administration (HRSA). (2002). *Second annual report to the secretary of Department of Health and Human Services and to the Congress, review and recommendations > interdisciplinary, community- based linkages, Title VII, Part D Public Health Services Act.* Retrieved February 16, 2011 from http://www.hrsa.gov/advisorycommittees/bhpradvisory/acicbl/Reports/secondreport.pdf House Committees on Ways and Means, Energy and Commerce, and Education and Labor. (2010). *Affordable health care for America: Health insurance reform at a glance guaranteed benefits.* Retrieved November 20, 2010 from http://docs.house.gov/energycommerce/GUARANTEED_BENEFITS.pdf

Hwang, W., Weller, W., Ireys, H., & Anderson, G. (2001). Out-of-pocket medical spending for care of chronic conditions. *Health Affairs, 20*(6), 267–278.

Jencks, S. F., Williams, M. V., & Coleman E. A. (2009). Rehospitalization among patients in the Medicare Fee-for-Service program. *New England Journal of Medicine, 360*(7), 1418–1428.

Larson, E. B. (2009). Group Health Cooperative—one coverage-and-delivery model for accountable care. *New England Journal of Medicine, 361*, 1620–1622.

Martin, L. G., Freedman, V. A., Schoeni, R. F., & Andreski, P. M. (2010). Trends in disability and related chronic conditions among people ages fifty to sixty-four. *Health Affairs, 29*(4), 725–731.

Martin, A., Lassman, D., Whittle, L., & Catlin, A. (2011). Recession contributes to slowest annual rate of increase in health spending in five decades. *Health Affairs, 30*(1), 11–22.

Medicare Payment Advisory Commission. (2007). *Report to the Congress: Promoting greater efficiency in medical care.* Retrieved December 20, 2010 from http://www.medpac.gov/documents/jun07_entirereport.pdf

Mokdad, A. H., Marks, J. S., Stroup, D. F., & Gerberding, J. L. (2004). Actual causes of death in the United States, 2000. *The Journal of the American Medical Association, 291*(10), 1238–1245.

National Center for Health Statistics. (2010). *Health, United States, 2009: With special feature on medical technology.* Hyattsville, MD: Department of Health and Human Services.

National PACE Association. (2011). *What is PACE?* Retrieved January 24, 2011 from http://www.npaonline.org/website/article.asp?id=12

Newhouse, J. P. (1996). *Free for all? Lessons from the Rand health insurance experiment.* New Haven, CT: Harvard University Press.

Nichols, L. (2010). Be not afraid. *New England Journal of Medicine, 362*(e30). Epub 2010 Feb 24.

Orszag, P. R, & Emanuel, E. J. (2010). Health care reform and cost control. *New England Journal of Medicine, 363*(7), 601–603.

Partnership for Solutions, Johns Hopkins University, & Robert Wood Johnson Foundation. (2004). Chronic conditions: Making the case for ongoing care. Retrieved Jan. 25, 2007 from www.partnershipforsolutions.org

Reid-Arndt, S. A., Stucky, K., Cheak-Zamora, N. C., DeLeon, D. H. & Frank, R. G. (2010). Investing in our future: Unrealized opportunities for funding graduate psychology training. *Rehabilitation Psychology, 55*(4), 321–330.

Reed, M. C., & Tu, H. T. (2002). *Triple jeopardy: Low income, chronically ill and uninsured in America* (Issue Brief 49 ed.). Washington, DC: Center for Studying Health System Change.

Robinson, J. C. (2010). Applying value-based insurance design to high-cost services. *Health Affairs, 29*(11), 2009–2015.

Roland, M. (2004). Linding physicians' pay to the quality of care—A major experiment in the United Kingdom. *New England Journal of Medicine, 351*, 1448–1454.

Schoen, C., Osborn, R., Squires, D., Doty, M. M., Pierson, R., & Applebaum, S. (2010). How health insurance design affects access to care and costs, by income, in eleven countries. *Health Affairs, 29*(12), 2323–2334.

Schoen, C., Osborn, R., How, S. K. H., Doty, M. M., & Peugh, J. (2009a). In chronic condition: Experiences of patients with complex health care needs, in eight countries, 2008. *Health Affairs, 28*(1), w1–w16.

Schoen, C., Osborn, R., Doty, M. M., Squires, D., Peugh, J., & Applebaum, S. (2009b). A survey of primary care physicians in eleven countries, 2009: Perspectives on care, costs, and experiences. *Health Affairs, 28*(6), w1171–w1183.

Sisko, A. M., Truffer, C. J., Keenhan, S. P., Poisal, J. A., Clemens, M. K., & Madison, A. J. (2010). National health spending projections: The estimated impact of reform through 2019. *Health Affairs, 29*(10), 1933–1941.

Shortell, S. M., Casalino, L. P., & Fisher, E. S. (2010). How the Center for Medicare and Medicaid Innovation should test accountable care organizations. *Health Affairs, 29*(7), 1293–1298.

Stanton, M. W. (2006). *The high concentration of U.S. health care expenditures.* Research in Action, Issue 19. (Publication No. 06–0060). Rockville, MD: Agency for Healthcare Research and Quality. Retrieved January 25, 2007 from http://www.ahrq.gov/research/ria19/expendria.htm

Starfield, B. (2000). Is U.S. health really the best in the world? *New England Journal of Medicine, 284*, 483–485.

Starfield, B., Shi, L., & Macinko, J. (2005). Contribution of primary care to health systems and health. *The Milbank Quarterly, 83*(3), 457–502.

Sundararaman, R. (2009). *Behavioral health care in health care reform legislation.* Congressional Research Service Report for Congress. Retrieved November 20, 2010 from ahttp://www.nami.org/Template.cfm?Section=Issue_Spotlights&template=/ContentManagement/ContentDisplay.cfm&ContentID=91887

Timmins, N. (2010). Letter from Britain: Across the pond, giant new waves of health reform. *Health Affairs, 29*(12), 2138–2141.

Tu, H. T., & Cohen, G. R. (2009). *Financial and health burdens of chronic conditions grow* (Tracking Report No. 24). Washington, DC: Center for Studying Health System Change.

Tu, H. T., & Reed, M. C. (2002). *Options for expanding health insurance for people with chronic conditions* (Issue Brief 50 ed.). Washington, DC: Center for Studying Health System Change.

U.S. Bureau of the Census. (2010a). *Income, poverty, and health insurance coverage in the United States: 2009.* Current Population Reports, 60–233. Washington, DC: U.S. Government Printing Office.

U.S. Census Bureau. (2010b). *Projections of the population by selected age groups and sex for the United States: 2010 to 2050.* Retrieved January 3, 2011, from http://www.census.gov/population/www/projections/summarytables.html

U.S. Department of Health and Human Services. (1999). *Mental health: A report of the surgeon general.* Rockville, MD: U.S. Department of Health and Human Services, Substance Abuse and Mental Health Services Administration, Center for Mental Health Services, National Institutes of Health, National Institute of Mental Health.

Wagner, E. H., Austin, B. T., Davis, C., Hindmarsh, M., Schaefer, J., & Bonomi, A. (2001). Improving chronic illness care: Translating evidence into action. *Health Affairs, 20*(6), 64–78.

Winslow, T. (2010). *What does the Patient Protection and Affordable Care Act say about alignment?* Winslow Medical Group. Retrieved February 14, 2012 from http://winslowmedical.com/2010/10/26/what-does-the-patient-protection-and-affordable-care-act-pp-aca-pl-111–148-say-about-alignment/

World Health Organization. (2008). *The World Health Report 2008: Primary care now more than ever.* Geneva, Switzerland: WHO.

Disease Prevention Through Lifestyle Interventions

Stephen D. Anton *and* Michael G. Perri

Abstract

Many chronic diseases are now recognized to be related to an individual's lifestyle behaviors. This chapter focuses on the critical role that eating and exercise behaviors have in the prevention of cardiovascular disease and type 2 diabetes. We also review empirically supported treatment approaches for modifying unhealthy eating and exercise behaviors. In addition to directly increasing risk of cardiovascular disease and type 2 diabetes, excessive caloric intake and physical inactivity may also elevate disease risk by increasing body weight. In line with this, obesity is recognized as a significant risk factor for cardiovascular disease and type 2 diabetes. Fortunately, there is now strong evidence that comprehensive lifestyle programs that involve dietary modification, physical activity, and weight loss can reduce risk factors for cardiovascular disease and type 2 diabetes. Although change may be difficult, health care professionals who are trained in behavioral techniques can greatly facilitate healthy lifestyle changes in their patients.

Key Words: Obesity, diet, exercise, physical activity, cardiovascular disease, diabetes, lifestyle.

In 50 AD, Seneca the Younger stated "Having good health is very different from only being not sick." In line with this famous quote, the World Health Organization defined health as "a state of total physical, mental and social well-being, not merely the absence of disease." Although the contribution that factors from many domains have in influencing health has been accepted for many years, most traditional treatment paradigms have not considered the important role lifestyle and psychological factors have in health promotion. For much of the 20th century, disease processes were thought to be due to physiological imbalances, and the contribution of lifestyle or psychological factors to health conditions was not recognized. This paradigm, termed the *biomedical model*, was based on the Cartesian division between the body and mind, in which disease processes were thought to originate from imbalances within the body or soma. This

symptom-oriented approach has been very effective in treating the major health challenges of our past, namely infectious and communicable diseases. However, a symptom-oriented approach is less effective for treating many of today's chronic diseases that are directly related to unhealthy lifestyle behaviors, as well as psychological and environmental conditions.

Due to the increasing recognition of the complex interplay that psychological, behavioral, and social factors have in affecting an individual's health status and disease risk, a new model for understanding the development of disease was proposed in the 1970s. This was termed the *biopsychosocial model* (Engel, 1977; Schwartz, 1982). An important implication of the biopsychosocial model is that behavioral, psychological, and social factors (including environmental conditions), as well as their interactions, are viewed as having a central role in affecting an individual's health status. A number of studies support the biopsychosocial model for disease prevention, as well as its use in informing lifestyle intervention approaches (e.g., Coyne & Downey, 1991; Lin et al., 2009).

In line with the biopsychosocial model, the fields of health psychology and rehabilitation psychology are disciplines of psychology concerned with understanding how biology, behavior, and social context interact to influence health and illness. The field of health psychology applies its knowledge base toward the promotion and maintenance of health, and the prevention and treatment of disease, as well as the identification of etiological factors for disease and dysfunction (Matarazzo, 1980). Therefore, the field of health psychology is distinct from more biological approaches because it recognizes the important contribution that behavioral and psychosocial factors have in health promotion and disease prevention. The field of rehabilitation psychology focuses on the application of psychological knowledge to help individuals with chronic, traumatic, or congenital injuries and illnesses, which may have resulted in physical, sensory, neurocognitive, emotional, and/or developmental disabilities manage and maximize all areas of their lives including their health, functional abilities, and independence.

In this chapter, we provide an overview of how dietary and physical activity behaviors contribute to chronic health conditions, as well as describe interventions that have demonstrated efficacy in reducing disease burden and chronic disease risk. Specifically, this chapter focuses on the critical role that eating and exercise behaviors have in contributing to two of today's top health challenges, cardiovascular disease (CVD) and type 2 diabetes. We also review empirically supported approaches for modifying these behaviors to reduce known disease risk factors (e.g., obesity, hypertension, etc.), as well as disease progression. Finally, we review the important role that health care providers can have in reducing their patient's risk for CVD and type 2 diabetes by assisting them in making healthy lifestyle changes.

Health Problems Related to Unhealthy Lifestyle

Many chronic diseases are now recognized to be directly caused by (or related to) an individual's lifestyle behaviors. Some experts have even argued that daily habits (e.g., smoking, physical activity, dietary intake, and alcohol use) contribute to the development of virtually all of the major causes of morbidity and mortality in the United States and other industrialized nations (McGinnis & Foege, 1993). In support of this, numerous studies have found that dietary intake (excess consumption), physical inactivity, smoking, and alcohol abuse directly contribute to an individual's risk for a number of chronic health conditions including CVD, type 2 diabetes, and cancer (Frazao, 1999).

In addition to directly increasing risk of specific disease conditions, excessive caloric intake and physical inactivity may also increase risk of chronic health conditions through their effects on body weight (Hill & Peters, 1998; Horgen & Brownell, 2002; Poston & Foreyt, 1999). The prevalence of obesity (defined as a body mass index [BMI] ≥ 30 kg/m^2) in the United States has increased at an alarming rate during the past few decades, with current estimates indicating that approximately 33% of the population are classified as obese and an additional 33% are considered overweight (Ogden et al., 2006). In addition, in England, approximately 24% of men and 25% of women are classified as obese, whereas 42% of men and 32% of women are considered overweight (NHS Information Centre, 2010). Of significant concern, obesity has been found to substantially increase risk for hypertension, hyperlipidemia, and high blood glucose, and as a consequence substantially elevate risk for CVD and diabetes (Dumitrescu & Cotarla, 2005; Freedland, 2005; Gregg et al., 2005; Lowenfels, Sullivan, Fiorianti, & Masionneuve, 2005; Mokdad et al., 2001). Moreover, secular trend data suggest that weight increases with age in young and middle-aged adults (Lewis et al., 2000), and the potential impact of these trends on morbidity and mortality are likely to be greater in the upcoming years than at present. Thus, prevention efforts are urgently needed to assist individuals in maintaining healthy body weights.

Health Consequences of Excessive Caloric Intake

Dietary intake is a major factor influencing patients' health and body weight. A number of studies have linked excessive caloric intake to increased risk of CVD and type 2 diabetes (Frazao, 1999). Epidemiological studies indicate that per capita energy intake increased by approximately 300 kcal per day from 1985 to 2000 (Finkelstein, Ruhm, & Kosa, 2005). Assuming energy expenditure remained constant during this time, this increase in caloric intake would be expected to lead to a 2- to 3-lb weight gain per month. A number of alarming health trends appear to be linked to higher caloric intakes, including the dramatic rise in the rates of obesity and type 2 diabetes during the past few decades (Briefel & Johnson, 2004). Moreover, a number of risk factors for CVD (e.g., high blood cholesterol), the number one cause of death in the United States, can be modified through changes in dietary intake (Frazao, 1999).

Health Consequences of Sedentary Lifestyle

Physical inactivity is currently the most common behavioral risk factor in the United States. The majority of adults in the United States do not engage in even the minimum physical activity recommendations, and there is a trend for individuals to engage in less activity with increasing age through life (Pleis, Schiller, & Benson, 2003; Prevalence of physical activity, including lifestyle activities among adults—United States, 2000–2001, 2003). Moreover, 40% of adults engage in no leisure-time physical activity, according to the most recent report by the Centers for Disease Control and Prevention (Prevalence of self-reported physically active adults—United States, 2007, 2008). This is of significant concern because sedentary lifestyle has been identified as one of the most important modifiable risk factors for cardiovascular morbidity and mortality (Prasad & Das, 2009). As compared to physically active individuals, sedentary individuals have double the risk of developing coronary artery disease. A sedentary lifestyle is known to increase the risk of developing type 2 diabetes mellitus (Hayes & Kriska, 2008) and is also a major contributor to the increasing obesity epidemic (Chaput & Tremblay, 2009). In 2000, physical inactivity and poor dietary intake combined were responsible for 16.6% of the deaths in America (Mokdad et al., 2004).

Disease Prevention Through Healthy Lifestyle

Health improvements and reduced risk of many chronic diseases have been documented when patients follow lifestyle changes recommended in behavioral health interventions (e.g., reductions in dietary intake, increased physical activity, smoking cessation [Cutler & Miller, 2005]). For example, in the Nurses' Health Study, which followed 84,129 healthy women for 14 years, women who reported adhering to lifestyle guidelines related to diet, exercise, and smoking abstinence had the lowest risk of coronary heart disease (CHD) (Stampfer, Hu, Manson, Rimm, & Willett, 2000). Moreover, a progressive decrease in coronary disease risk was associated with engagement in each recommended

lifestyle change. In addition to decreasing risk of many disease conditions, health behavior change has also been found to be a critical element of chronic disease management (Wagner et al., 2001). Thus, the effectiveness of future prevention efforts and treatments may greatly depend on the extent to which healthy individuals and patients actively participate in prevention efforts by changing their health habits. Specific dietary approaches and physical activity guidelines for promoting health and wellness are described in the next sections.

Health Benefits of Calorically Balanced Diet

Against the backdrop of the increasing obesity epidemic, studies across numerous species have demonstrated the benefits of calorie restriction (CR) without malnutrition for improving health, maintaining function, and increasing mean and maximum lifespan (Weindruch & Walford, 1988). Adaptations elicited by long-term CR in human subjects appear to resemble those observed in animal models. For example, inhabitants of Okinawa Island, whose traditional diet contains approximately 20% and 40% fewer calories compared to inland Japan and the U.S., respectively, have the longest disability-free lifespan and the greatest percentage of centenarians in the world.

Apart from this case of naturally occurring CR, a large body of evidence indicates that dietary restriction results in significant improvements in traditional cardiovascular risk factors (e.g., blood pressure, blood glucose, lipids, body composition) among overweight and obese subjects (Ashida, Ono, & Sugiyama, 2007; Fontana et al., 2007; Hammer et al., 2008; McTigue, Harris, & Hemphill, 2003; Racette et al., 2006; Wing & Jeffery, 1995), as well as in lean individuals (Meyer et al., 2006; Fontana, Klein, Holloszy, & Premachandra, 2006; Fontana, Weiss, Villareal, Klein, & Holloszy, 2008). For example, 6 months of CR (25% of baseline energy requirements) was found to improve CVD risk factors and biomarkers of longevity in healthy, overweight adults (Heilbronn et al., 2006). Caloric restriction was also found to improve whole-body insulin sensitivity (Larson-Meyer, 2008), enhance skeletal muscle mitochondrial biogenesis (Civitarese et al., 2007), and produce favorable changes in systemic inflammation, coagulation, lipid, and blood pressure (Larson-Meyer et al., 2008; Lefevere et al., 2009). In another recent study, 12 months of CR (20% of baseline energy requirements) improved glucose tolerance (Weiss et al., 2006) and reduced

DNA and RNA oxidative damage in both healthy normal and overweight persons aged 50–60 years (Hofer et al., 2008). It is currently unknown if all humans benefit from adopting a CR lifestyle; however, extensive research has shown that overweight and obese individuals receive numerous health benefits following weight loss achieved through CR (Goldstein, 1992).

Beyond the potential health benefits of reducing dietary intake for overweight and obese individuals, studies have demonstrated a strong protective effect of an increased intake of antioxidants and folic acid, both of which are found in many fruits and vegetables, on the risk of developing CVD (Plotnick, Corretti, & Vogel, 1997; Riddell, Chisholm, Williams, & Mann, 2000). An effective approach to reducing caloric intake and improving diet quality is increasing the consumption of fruits and vegetables (Rolls, Ello-Martin, & Tohill, 2004). Fruits and vegetables are low in energy density but high in nutrient density, and may also decrease energy intake by promoting satiety because they are high in fiber, nutrients, and water (Rolls, Roe, & Meengs, 2004).

In recognition of the central role that diet plays in health promotion and disease prevention, the Dietary Guidelines for Americans (Dietary Guidelines), which were first published in 1980, have been put forth to provide science-based advice to promote health and to reduce risk for chronic diseases through diet and physical activity (U.S. Department of Health and Human Services/U.S. Department of Agriculture, 2005). The key dietary recommendations of the 2005 Dietary Guidelines for Americans are for adults to (1) consume a variety of nutrient-dense foods and beverages within and among the basic food groups while choosing foods that limit the intake of saturated and trans fats, cholesterol, added sugars, salt, and alcohol; and (2) meet recommended intakes within energy needs by adopting a balanced eating pattern, such as the U.S. Department of Agriculture (USDA) Food Guide or the DASH Eating Plan. To accomplish these goals, individuals need to pay special attention to portion sizes, which have increased significantly over the past two decades. Additional information on the increase in portion sizes over the past few decades can be found on the following National Institutes of Health (NIH) website (http://hin. nhlbi.nih.gov/portion/index.htm). Recent studies suggest that larger portion sizes are associated with both increased energy intake and weight gain (Berg et al., 2009; Kelly et al., 2009). Thus, reducing

portion sizes may help individuals limit calorie intake, particularly when eating calorie-dense foods (Rolls, Roe, & Meengs, 2006).

To promote health, psychological well-being, and a healthy body weight, the 2005 Dietary Guidelines recommend balancing calories from foods and beverages with calories expended. The guidelines also recommend that adults engage in at least 30 minutes of moderate-intensity physical activity, above usual activity, at work or home, on most days of the week and reduce sedentary activities. To help manage body weight and prevent gradual, unhealthy body weight gain in adulthood, the Dietary Guidelines recommend that adults engage in approximately 60 minutes of moderate- to vigorous-intensity activity on most days. For weight loss, the guidelines recommend that adults achieve a slow, steady weight loss by decreasing calorie intake while maintaining an adequate nutrient intake and increasing physical activity levels. For guidance on helping patients improve the quality of their diet while also reducing their caloric intake, a number of nutrition resources specifically designed for health professionals can be accessed at another Centers for Disease Control (CDC) website (http://www.cdc. gov/nutrition/index.html).

Health Benefits of Physical Activity

To properly understand the health benefits associated with regular physical activity, it may be useful to first define the terms *physical activity, exercise*, and *physical fitness*. The following definitions of these terms have been provided by the American Heart Association (Thompson et al., 2003): "*Physical activity* is any bodily movement produced by skeletal muscles that results in energy expenditure beyond resting expenditure. *Exercise* is a subset of physical activity that is planned, structured, repetitive, and purposeful in the sense that improvement or maintenance of physical fitness is the objective. *Physical fitness* includes cardiorespiratory fitness, muscle strength, body composition, and flexibility."

The health benefits of engaging in regular physical activity have been demonstrated in numerous studies. A graded, inverse relationship between total physical activity and mortality from all causes has been documented. Moreover, vigorous-intensity activities have also been associated with longevity (Lee, Hseih, & Paffenbarger Jr., 1995). Regular engagement in physical activity also leads to improvements in many of the established risk factors for CVD (Thompson et al., 2003; Thompson & Lim, 2003). Specifically, physical activity has been shown to reduce blood pressure, serum triglycerides, low-density lipoprotein (LDL) and total cholesterol, and glucose intolerance, as well as increase insulin sensitivity and high-density lipoprotein (HDL)-cholesterol (Thompson et al., 2003). Recent analyses of the dose–response relation between physical activity and CVD affirm an inverse and generally linear relationship between physical activity levels and CVD morbidity and mortality (Blair, Cheng, & Holder, 2001; Kesaniemi et al., 2001). If CVD does develop in active or fit individuals, it occurs at a later age and tends to be less severe (U.S. Public Health Service, 1996). Moreover, lower physical activity levels have been shown to precede the development of CVD rather than to occur as a result of CVD (Thompson et al., 2003).

Physical activity can also play a significant role in body weight regulation. Although findings from meta-analyses indicate that exercise interventions only produce modest weight losses (i.e., 1- 3 kg; Kelley & Kelley, 2008; Kelley, Kelley, & Tran, 2005; Richardson et al., 2008), some studies suggest there is a dose–response relation between quantity of physical activity and weight loss (Jakicic, Marcus, Gallagher, Napolitano, & Lang, 2003). Based on findings such as these, many experts recommend high amounts of daily physical activity (i.e., 60–90 minutes) for weight loss (Jakicic & Otto, 2006). Physical activity has also been found to be an important behavioral factor for enhancing long-term weight loss and minimizing weight regain (Jakicic, 2009). Other evidence demonstrating the key role of physical activity in weight loss maintenance comes from the National Weight Control Registry, as the majority of individuals who have maintained significant weight loss (i.e., >10% of initial body weight) reported expending more than 2,400 kcal per week in various physical activities.

There also appears to be a dose–response relation between level and intensity of physical activity with enhanced aerobic capacity, as well as improvements in muscular function and strength (Hornig, Maier, & Drexler, 1996). Since many of the health benefits associated with regular engagement in physical activity (e.g., reduced risk of CVD) are mediated by improvements in cardiorespiratory fitness, the amount and intensity of aerobic exercise needed to improve cardiorespiratory fitness represents an important research and clinical question. Findings from studies to date suggest that even moderate-intensity physical activity can significantly improve fitness in low fit, sedentary individuals. Engagement in vigorous-intensity physical activities, however,

appears to produce the largest improvements in cardiorespiratory fitness (Kesaniemi et al., 2001). Of note, changes in cardiorespiratory fitness typically improve quality of life for most people, as well as increase self-confidence, lower stress, and decrease anxiety levels (Myers, Atwood, & Froelicher, 2003).

Due to the many beneficial effects (both acute and chronic) of physical activity, the most recent Physical Activity Guidelines for Americans (Physical activity guidelines for Americans, 2008) recommend that adults engage in at least 150 minutes (2 hours and 30 minutes) per week of moderate-intensity aerobic activity (i.e., brisk walking), or 75 minutes (1 hour and 15 minutes) of vigorous-intensity aerobic activity (i.e., jogging or running), as well as muscle-strengthening activities on 2 or more days a week. For additional and more extensive health benefits, the 2008 Physical Activity Guidelines recommend adults increase their moderate-intensity aerobic physical activity to 300 minutes (5 hours) or engage in 150 minutes (2 hours and 30 minutes) a week of vigorous-intensity aerobic physical activity. The guidelines also state that additional health benefits are gained by engaging in physical activity beyond this amount. In addition to providing specific recommendations regarding the frequency, duration, and intensity of physical activity, these guidelines provide specific recommendations on how to put them into practice. For more information on promoting physical activity, health care providers can access the 2008 Physical Activity Guidelines for Americans on the U.S. Department of Health and Human Services' website (www.health.gov/paguidelines).

Assessment and Diagnostic Issues

The findings described above highlight the critical role that dietary intake and physical activity patterns play in both health promotion and disease prevention. An important implication of this large body of research is that health care professionals should routinely assess their patients' health habits and current behavioral patterns in addition to their physical state of health. Health care professionals should also attempt to understand their patients' motivations and decision-making processes, as well as the antecedents and consequences of particular behaviors. Therefore, preventive health efforts require health care professionals to engage patients, at times, in potentially difficult conversations about their current lifestyle behaviors and reasons that they may be engaging in unhealthy behaviors (e.g., physical inactivity). Although these conversations may be challenging, health care professionals should openly communicate with patients about these topics since full cooperation from the patient is key to developing successful interventions.

A number of assessment tools can aid clinicians in evaluating or understanding their patients' current behavioral patterns related to diet and physical activity. For example, many self-report measures may be clinically useful for assessing physical activity levels, such as the International Physical Activity Questionnaire, which has shown a high degree of reliability and validity based on a study conducted by 14 centers in 12 countries. This measure can be easily accessed online (http://www.ipaq.ki.se/ipaq.htm) (Craig et al., 2003). If a more objective measure of physical activity is desired, relatively low-cost options include pedometers (step counters) and accelerometers (Babor, Sciamanna, & Pronk, 2004). Of these, accelerometers provide substantially more information about overall physical activity patterns and the intensity levels of various physical activities, but the time needed to obtain this information may offset the potential benefits of the additional information provided by accelerometers.

A number of brief screening measures have also been designed to detect unhealthy eating patterns and dietary habits (Babor et al., 2004; Briefel & Johnson, 2004). For example, self-report scales, such as the Weight, Activity, Variety and Excess (WAVE) and the Rapid Eating and Activity Assessment for Patients (REAP), can be clinically useful tools to quickly obtain information about patients' dietary and physical activity patterns. The WAVE (Soroudi, Wylie-Rosett, & Mogul, 2004) is designed to numerically evaluate an individual's reported caloric intake and caloric expenditure and can also provide feedback to patients. The REAP is a brief questionnaire that evaluates both dietary intake and physical activity levels (Gans et al., 2003). Both the REAP and the WAVE are accompanied by a Physician Key to help facilitate nutrition assessment and counseling in the provider office. Another validated instrument that can provide a quick assessment of a patient's food intake, portion size, and frequency of intake is the Meat, Eggs, Dairy, Frying foods, In baked goods, Convenience foods, Table fats, and Snacks (MEDFICTS) instrument, developed as an expansion of Meat, Egg yolks, Dairy, Invisible fat, Cooking/table fats, Snacks (MEDICS) instrument (Kris-Etherton et al., 2001).

Potential clinical manifestations of excessive caloric intake include obesity, high levels of serum LDL and total cholesterol, high levels of serum triglycerides, and high blood pressure. Thus, serum cholesterol may be used if a more objective measure of dietary intake of saturated fat and dietary cholesterol is desired (Kendall & Jenkins, 2004). When seeing patients with any of these conditions, physicians and other health care professionals should consider using one or more of the measures described above.

The extent to which health care professionals and patients can work together in changing unhealthy lifestyle habits may directly influence the effectiveness of future prevention efforts. Patients should be taught to see themselves as active participants in their health care and recognize the central role they have in improving their health status through their lifestyle habits. Although change may be difficult, health care professionals can greatly facilitate the behavior change process for their patients. By adopting theory-driven approaches, particularly those that have been empirically supported, health care professionals can greatly assist their patients in successfully modifying their current lifestyle behaviors. Fortunately, numerous psychological models, which are briefly reviewed in the next section, have been put forth that can aid health care professionals in understanding the complex interactions that factors from multiple domains have in contributing to the etiology and maintenance of habitual behavior patterns.

Theoretical Basis of Lifestyle Interventions

The theoretical basis for current lifestyle interventions is derived largely from cognitive-behavioral models, particularly *social cognitive theory* (Bandura, 1986, 1997). This theory describes how personal factors (i.e., cognitions, emotions) and aspects of the social and physical environment influence behavior and how a person's behavior in turn may have a reciprocal influence on these personal and environmental factors. According to social cognitive theory, the initiation and maintenance of behavioral changes involve four sets of constructs:

- *Health knowledge.* The individual's awareness of how a specific behavior affects health.
- *Beliefs regarding self-efficacy and outcome expectancies.* The individual's belief in his or her ability to perform a specific behavior in a particular situation, and the individual's belief that performing a specific behavior will have a particular outcome.
- *Self-regulatory skills.* The ability of the individual to exert control over his or her behavior,

cognitions, and environment. This process entails several subcomponents: (a) *performance standards*, the goals by which the individual judges his/her behavior; (b) *self-observation*, the awareness of internal and external influences on one's behavior; (c) *self-judgment*, the comparison of one's behavior to a performance standard; and (d) *self-reaction*, one's cognitive, behavioral, or environmental response to self-observations and self-judgments.

• *Barriers to change.* Perceived personal or environmental impediments to performing a specific behavior.

Lifestyle interventions target the key constructs of social cognitive theory: by increasing health knowledge regarding the influence of diet and physical activity on weight and risk for disease; by enhancing self-efficacy and positive outcome expectancies through the promotion of a series of successful experiences in changing eating and exercise behavior; by improving self-regulatory skills through the use of goal setting, written self-monitoring, self-reinforcement, stimulus control, and cognitive restructuring strategies; and by overcoming impediments to change through problem-solving of barriers to the initiation or maintenance of change.

Chronic Care Model

The *chronic care model* (CCM), which was originally proposed by Wagner in 1998, was designed to improve the quality of chronic illness care, prompting more proactive health care systems (Wagner, 1998). The CCM focuses on making patient-centered, evidence-based care easier to accomplish by optimizing six interrelated system changes: effective health care organization, delivery system design that proactively addresses health needs, clinical information systems that provide patient data access, evidence-based decision support for clinicians, self-management support for patients to be involved in managing their own care, and community resource linkages to facilitate care outside of the clinical setting (Coleman, Austin, Brach, & Wagner, 2009; Hung et al., 2008; Strickland et al., 2010). Although the extent of CCM integration often varies, studies examining the relationship between CCM elements and quality of care found that the implementation of multiple CCM components was associated with improved levels of patient care (Coleman et al., 2009; Flemming, Silver, Ocepek-Welikson, & Keller, 2004; Si et al., 2005).

Some concerns raised about the model include its complexity, cost, and time consumed in transforming the operation of a practice (Health Technology News, 2009). Despite these concerns, there have been promising research results supporting the utility of the CCM in patient care. For example, one recent study showed that congestive heart failure patients were more knowledgeable, more often on the recommended therapy, and had 35% fewer hospital days when treated by providers actively participating in a congestive heart failure collaborative that promoted the CCM as opposed to control patients without collaborative providers (Asch et al., 2005). Further, a study focusing on adolescent asthma care in different health care organizations showed that patients cared for by CCM-integrated intervention sites (vs. control sites) reported significantly higher ratings of general health-related quality of life, as affected by appropriate distribution of asthma medication and appropriate asthma treatment (Mangione-Smith et al., 2005). Hung et al. (2008) assessed CCM implementation in 57 nationwide practices and found that utilization of different CCM features were increased over time, suggesting increased awareness of the model's benefits. In further support of its utility, the CCM has been successfully applied to a behavioral health care program (Community Treatment and Rehabilitation) and was found to bring about better delivery of mental health services, as well as greater success/recovery outcomes for clients (Blakely & Dziadosz, 2008). Even low levels of CCM integration have been found to have beneficial effects in diabetes care (i.e., increased assessment/treatment of glycated hemoglobin, lipids, and blood pressure, as well as increased levels of physical activity counseling for overweight patients) (Strickland et al., 2010). Taken as a whole, the results of studies conducted to date support the implementation of this model for improving the treatment of individuals with chronic illnesses.

Theory of Planned Behavior

The *theory of planned behavior* (Ajzen, 1985) proposes that intentions are the primary determinants of whether a person will engage in a particular behavior. Intention to perform a behavior is primarily determined by two factors: the person's attitude toward the behavior (i.e., beliefs about perceived control and the outcomes of the behavior, as well as the value of the outcomes) and perceptions of social norms (i.e., beliefs about what other people think the person should do and motivation to comply with opinions of others). The relative influence of each of these components may vary for each individual, as well as by the behavior undergoing change (Clark & Becker, 1998).

In contrast to other models, sociodemographic factors are thought to influence engagement in health behaviors solely through their influences on the determinants of behavioral intention, which is viewed as the direct mediator of behavior. Reviews (Godin & Kok, 1996) have found the theory of planned behavior to be very useful in predicting behavioral intentions. Most studies indicate that intentions are generally good predictors of short-term (<1 month), but not long-term behavior change (Maddux & DuCharme, 1997). However, positive attitude, or the belief that a specific behavior will lead to a desired outcome, has generally been associated with better adherence to health regimens (Godin & Shephard, 1985; Godin, Valois, & Lepage, 1993). Health locus of control has also been found to predict adherence to supervised exercise programs (Oldridge & Streiner, 1990; Sallis et al., 1989).

COMMONALITIES OF BEHAVIOR CHANGE MODELS

The strong similarities among the various health behavior models and theories suggest that overlap exists in many of the basic concepts and that the models may differ more in their nomenclature than in their actual conceptual underpinnings (Maddux & DuCharme, 1997). For example, perceived behavioral control in the theory of planned behavior is highly similar to self-efficacy, a construct that has been incorporated in the social cognitive model (Courneya, 1995). Each of the behavior change models described above also views behavior as being influenced by multiple factors that likely interact with each other. In particular, social cognitive theory views an individual's behavior as being influenced by his or her previous behavior, cognitions, and other personal factors (Bandura, 1986). These determinants are also theorized to influence each other bidirectionally. In the following sections, we review various strategies that health care providers can utilize to encourage healthy behavior change in their patients.

Treatment Approaches That Facilitate Behavior Change

The important role that correctly administered behavioral health treatments can have in improving patients' health and quality of life has been demonstrated in studies conducted over the past few decades (Smith, Kendall, & Keefe, 2002). For example, the Multiple Risk Factor Intervention Trial (MRFIT), a large-scale trial designed to evaluate the effects of a 7-year multi-factor intervention program on mortality from coronary heart disease among high-risk men, demonstrated that diet and smoking cessation interventions significantly reduced risk of all-cause mortality, as well as mortality from coronary heart disease at 10.5- and 16-year follow-up visits (Kuller, Tracy, Shaten, & Meilahn, 1996). In another prospective, randomized controlled trial, a comprehensive lifestyle change program involving a low-fat diet, aerobic exercise, stress management, and social support was found to reduce the progression of coronary atherosclerosis in 82% of patients with documented coronary heart disease (CHD), versus 42% of patients in a usual-care control group. Additionally, patients with the highest adherence levels showed the most regression of atherosclerosis (Ornish et al., 1998). Findings such as these indicate that lifestyle interventions can have potent effects in reducing both disease risk in high-risk populations and disease progression in patients with chronic health conditions.

In addition to directly affecting disease progression, lifestyle interventions can also reduce disease risk by decreasing body weight. The beneficial effects of lifestyle-based weight loss interventions on a variety of health parameters have been documented in numerous studies conducted over the past few decades National Heart, Lung, and Blood Institute, 1998; Perri 1998; Powell, Calvin, & Calvin Jr., 2007; Pi-Sunyer et al., 2007; Wadden, Brownell, & Foster, 2002). Lifestyle-based weight loss interventions are typically delivered in weekly group sessions over 4–6 months and usually produce reductions in body weight of 5–10 kg (i.e., approximately 5–10% reductions in body weight). Weight losses of this magnitude generally result in clinically significant improvements in CVD and metabolic disease risk factors (i.e., blood pressure, blood glucose, and lipid profiles). The clinical significance of 5–10% reductions in body weight, however, may ultimately be determined by long-term rather than short-term outcomes. Thus, weight loss maintenance is likely the critical factor in determining whether health improvements are sustained. If health care providers are interested in acquiring further training on obesity treatment, the LEARN Institute for Lifestyle Management offers certification programs in behavioral weight management techniques developed by experts in the field.

Similar to weight loss treatments, the health benefits of other lifestyle-based treatments are likely only sustained as long as adherence to lifestyle recommendations is maintained. Unfortunately, the majority of patients have difficulty making and sustaining healthy behavior changes related to dietary intake and physical activity. A large number of studies now indicate that sustained behavior change, particularly in dietary intake and physical activity, is very challenging for most individuals. Rates of nonadherence to chronic illness treatment regimens have been reported to be as high as 30–60% and up to 50–80% for preventive regimens (Christensen, 2004). Findings from the behavioral therapy literature also suggest that most individuals have difficulty maintaining healthy behavior changes, with reports of premature drop-out ranging from 30% to 60% (Christensen, 2004; Cleemput, Kesteloot, & DeGeest, 2002; Garfield, 1994; Reis & Brown, 1999). Thus, most patients who desire to make healthy behavior changes need assistance in initiating and maintaining these changes. In the following sections, we review various strategies that health care providers can utilize to encourage healthy behavior change in their patients.

Strategies to Promote Adherence

Health care professionals can play a key role in facilitating healthy lifestyle changes in their patients, particularly if they have training in behavior modification and knowledge about the role that lifestyle behavior can have in contributing to health and disease. Since treatments may become more challenging once a chronic health condition has developed, early prevention efforts may be critical to improving the health of many patients, as well as the public at large. To this end, behavioral or lifestyle evaluations should routinely be incorporated into health assessments to identify at-risk patients, even if no overt signs of disease are present. If a patient's behavioral or lifestyle pattern would suggest that he or she is at increased risk for a chronic health condition, then health care providers should initiate behaviorally oriented interventions as early as possible.

Health care providers can facilitate the behavior change process by first attempting to understand the circumstances (or perceptions) that lead their patients to engage in unhealthy behavior patterns (e.g., physical inactivity) and then exploring the perceived costs and benefits associated with behavior change for their patients. For example, a patient may report that he or she is not motivated to engage in a particular behavior (e.g., increasing physical activity) because he or she views the "cons" of the behavior change as exceeding the "pros." In this circumstance, health care providers can facilitate the

behavior change process by exploring the perceived costs and benefits of behavior change. The goal of this interaction is to increase the patient's motivation for behavior change by helping him or her recognize the importance of the benefits obtained from a healthy lifestyle change and minimizing the perceived costs. For further information about these strategies, an excellent reference is *Motivational Interviewing in Health Care: Helping Patients Change Behavior,* by Stephen Rollnick, William R. Miller, and Christopher C. Butler (2008).

Health care providers should also remember that patients are more likely to open up and express concerns, fears, frustrations, and problems they have encountered when they are approached in a friendly, collaborative, and nonjudgmental manner, rather than in a hierarchical, coercive manner. The more comfortable patients feel talking with their health care provider the more likely they are to view themselves as active collaborators, rather than passive recipients, in determining the best path toward improving their health. Related to this, health care providers should remember that patients are more likely to be persuaded by their own arguments (i.e., what they hear themselves say) than by what they are told to do. Thus, health care providers should encourage patients to develop solutions to their health challenges rather than directly offer solutions or tell them what they should or should not do. If patients appear to need assistance in coming up with possible solutions, health care providers should ask patient's permission before offering potential solutions. For further reading into how this can be achieved through the technique of motivational interviewing, a classic reference is Miller and Rollnick (1991).

Health care providers can also encourage healthy lifestyle changes in their patients by teaching them behavior skills and strategies that have a long-standing record of success in facilitating healthy behavior change and adherence to lifestyle recommendations. Common elements of behavioral health promotion programs and lifestyle obesity treatments include self-monitoring, goal setting, problem-solving, stimulus control, cognitive restructuring, stress management, social support, and relapse prevention (Brownell, 2004; Knowler et al., 2002; Perri et al., 2011). This list should be thought of as a tool set that health care professionals can use to assist their patients in making healthy behavior changes related to dietary intake and physical activity. For more information about the use of these strategies in clinical practice, see Pearce and Wardle (1989) and Stunkard (1982). In the following section, we provide a brief description of these eight frequently utilized empirically supported behavioral skills.

Behavior Change Strategies

SELF-MONITORING

Self-monitoring can be described as the systematic observation and recording of target behaviors (e.g., number of days exercised). A number of studies indicate that self-monitoring is one of the most important tools in behavior modification (Germann, Kirschenbaum, & Rich, 2007). For example, self-monitoring of the types, amounts, and caloric content of foods consumed increases awareness of eating habits, which in itself can lead to healthy behavior changes (Pierce & Gunn, 2007).

GOAL SETTING

Goals are critical to the success of any behavior change program since they provide targets for behavior change. A good goal is specific, achievable, clear, and measurable (Wing, Phelan, & Tate, 2002). Setting a limited number of goals can also help increase patients' confidence that they can make desired behavior change. Shaping, or the reinforcement of successive approximations of the goal behavior, can also be used to encourage healthy behavior changes.

PROBLEM-SOLVING

The ability to solve problems involves a specific process, which can be learned and applied to any obstacle encountered during the behavior change process (Nezu & Perri, 1989; Nezu & Ronan, 1985; Perri et al., 2001). Most individuals have difficulty developing effective solutions to challenges that occur during the behavior change process; thus, problem-solving represents a key skill that can be used to help patients overcome obstacles encountered during this process.

COGNITIVE RESTRUCTURING

Cognitive restructuring is a process in which individuals learn to identify maladaptive thought patterns and replace these with more adaptive thoughts (Beck, Rush, Shaw, & Emery, 1979; Beck, 1995). Negative thought patterns can lead to negative emotional states, which have been associated with unhealthy lifestyle behaviors in previous studies (Anton & Miller, 2005; Beck, 1995).

STIMULUS CONTROL

Stimulus control involves identifying and modifying cues that are associated with unhealthy behavior patterns and replacing these with cues that facilitate healthy behaviors (Ferster, Nurnberger, & Levitt, 1996). For example, certain foods can be eliminated from the environment (e.g., remove high-fat, calorically dense foods from home) to remove cues for unhealthy eating.

STRESS MANAGEMENT

Perceived stress has been associated with food consumption and engagement in a sedentary lifestyle (Greeno & Wing, 1994; Lattimore, 2001; Oliver & Wardle, 1999; Roemmich, Wright, & Epstein, 2002). Although eating in response to stress may provide immediate relief, it does not ultimately aid in stress management (Oliver, Wardle, & Gibson, 2000). Teaching patients healthy stress management tools may reduce the likelihood that they will engage in unhealthy behavior patterns due to perceived stress.

SOCIAL SUPPORT

Social support can be an important component of both weight loss and other health promotion programs. A number of studies indicate that significant others within one's social network can either support or hinder a patient's efforts to change their lifestyle (Wing & Jeffery, 1999).

RELAPSE PREVENTION

Slips or relapses are common occurrences during weight loss and other healthy lifestyle programs (Wing et al., 2002). Most individuals occasionally slip or temporarily return to their old habits during the behavior change process. Thus, patients should be taught relapse prevention tools. Specifically, patients should be coached to anticipate the occasional slip, as well as develop a plan for getting back on track when this inevitably occurs.

Program Components That Facilitate Long-Term Change

The obesity treatment literature provides a rich source of information to inform treatment approaches that may be effective in facilitating healthy dietary and physical activity changes. A review of multi-component lifestyle interventions with follow-ups of at least 2 years concluded that, "There is consistent and strong evidence that lifestyle interventions for obesity can produce modest but clinically significant reductions in weight with minimal risk" (Powell et al., 2007). In another recent review (Perri, Foreyt, & Anton, 2008), an interesting pattern of findings was observed regarding program components that improve long-term weight loss outcomes. Specifically, extending treatment beyond 6 months through the use of weekly or biweekly sessions and providing multicomponent programs with ongoing patient–therapist contact were found to improve the maintenance of lost weight. Potential reasons why extended treatment and multicomponent programs improve weight loss outcomes include increased accountability and social support, as well as increased opportunities for patients to learn problem-solving sills (e.g., Perri, McAdoo, Spevak, & Newlin, 1984; Wing & Jeffery, 1999). Other strategies that appear to facilitate weight loss maintenance include supplying patients with no-cost, portion-controlled meals and utilizing home-based exercise programs (Perri et al., 2008), as well as the use of cognitive coping skills (Dohm, Beattie, Aibel, & Striegel-Moore, 2001).

PRACTICAL APPLICATIONS

Health care professionals can use the constructs proposed in the various models to tailor the approach taken with specific patients. For example, health care professionals can first assess an individual's awareness of how a specific behavior affects his or her health. They should next evaluate the individual's level of *self-efficacy* (i.e., belief in ability to perform a specific behavior in a particular situation), as well as *outcome expectations* (i.e., belief that performing a specific behavior will have a particular outcome). If discussions with a patient reveal that he or she views a behavior change (e.g., decreasing caloric intake) as important for improving his or her health but does not believe that he or she is capable of making this change, then the health care provider may attempt to increase the patient's sense of self-efficacy.

In addition to evaluating a patient's self-efficacy and outcome expectations related to a particular behavior change, the health care provider should also evaluate the patient's self-regulatory skills (i.e., ability to exert control over his or her behavior, cognitions, and environment). As described above, this process entails several subcomponents: *performance standards, self-observation, self-judgment,* and *self-reaction*. For more information on strategies that health care professionals can use to increase their patient's level of self-efficacy for making healthy behavior changes, see Bandura (1997). Finally, health care providers should also assess perceived personal or environmental impediments to performing a specific behavior and assist individuals in developing solutions to these perceived barriers.

Treatment Dissemination

Most work to date within preventive medicine has been done in the context of efficacy studies, which are typically conducted on middle-class, white participants by experts working in academic medical centers. The results of these studies demonstrate that lifestyle interventions involving diet, exercise, and behavior modification produce clinically significant weight reductions (e.g., Knowler et al., 2002; Pi-Sunyer et al., 2007). Additionally, some studies indicate that lifestyle-based interventions can be effective in preventing disease onset in high-risk populations. For example, the Diabetes Prevention Program, which targeted a 7% weight loss through healthy lifestyle change, found the lifestyle intervention reduced the incidence of diabetes by 58% as compared with a placebo control group in overweight persons at risk for diabetes (Knowler et al., 2002; Diabetes Prevention Program Research Group, 2002). The findings of this study are noteworthy in that they clearly illustrate the potential of weight-loss interventions to prevent disease onset.

Few studies, however, have translated efficacious interventions, such as the Diabetes Prevention Program, into clinical settings or to medically underserved individuals (Kerner, Rimer, & Emmons, 2005; Zerhouni, 2005). Thus, relatively little is known about the effectiveness of these types of interventions in clinical and community-based settings. A key objective of the National Institutes of Health Roadmap initiative is to translate findings derived from efficacy trials to community-based practices, thus this represents an important focus of future research (Zerhouni, 2005). One study that can serve as an example of this type of translational research is the Treatment of Obesity in Underserved Rural Settings (TOURS) Trial (Perri et al., 2008), which examined the effectiveness of different weight loss interventions in medically underserved rural individuals. Specifically, the TOURS study examined the comparative effectiveness of delivering extended lifestyle-based programs through telephone counseling versus face-to-face sessions.

The TOURS study utilized treatment programs derived from the Diabetes Prevention Program, but incorporated a few changes based on previous efficacy studies. First, the TOURS study utilized group-based treatments rather than individual therapy since previous studies have found group interventions produce greater weight loss than individual therapy, even among participants who express a preference for individual treatment (Renjilian et al., 2001). Second, the TOURS study incorporated a home-based rather than supervised group training program based on previous findings that home-based exercise programs facilitate long-term exercise participation, as well as greater weight losses, compared to group programs (Perri, Martin, Leermakers, Sears, & Notelovitz, 1997). Finally, the TOURS study evaluated the effectiveness of different modalities of delivering problem-solving approaches for the maintenance of behavior change.

The primary findings of the TOURS study were that delivering extended lifestyle treatment via telephone counseling was equally effective but less costly than providing face-to-face sessions. Thus, the TOURS study represents the first randomized controlled trial to demonstrate the effectiveness of telephone counseling for the long-term management of obesity in rural communities. These findings highlight the benefits of extended-care interventions (Wadden, Butryn, & Wilson, 2007) and indicate that telephone counseling may be a useful and cost-effective approach in the long-term management of obesity. Because distance represents a major barrier to medical care in rural areas (Eberhardt, Ingram, & Makuc, 2001; Gamm, Hutchison, Dabney, & Dorsey, 2003; Phillips & McLeroy, 2004), the availability of a treatment modality that does not require time, travel costs, or attendance at clinic visits represents a potentially important approach to providing ongoing care to rural residents.

Another unique aspect of the TOURS study is that the intervention was delivered through the existing infrastructure of the Cooperative Extension Service (CES) (U.S. Department of Agriculture, 2007). With offices in almost all 3,100 counties of the United States, the CES represents a potentially effective and efficient means for translating findings from efficacy studies into rural communities with limited access to preventive health services (Eberhardt et al., 2001; Gamm et al., 2003). Thus, utilization of already existing infrastructures may represent an effective approach for disseminating lifestyle-based interventions to community settings. Moreover, this type of approach may also be effective in reducing geographic disparities in access to preventive health services, an objective of high national priority as detailed in Healthy People 2010 (U.S. Department of Health and Human Services, 2000).

Self-management programs may also have potential to be translated to broader community settings. For example, a recent study found a 6-week Arthritis Self-Management Course (ASMC) was effective in improving health status as marked by reported reductions in levels of pain, fatigue, and health distress at 6 months and 2 years (Osborne, Wilson, Lorig, & McColl, 2007). The majority of participants also reported increasing their engagement in aerobic exercise, and the percentage of participants who reported no activity decreased by 8% (Osborne et al., 2007). Other studies by Lorig and colleagues that utilized either the ASMC or general Chronic Disease Self-Management Program (CDSMP) have shown that these programs are effective in reducing physician visits (Lorig et al., 2001; Lorig, Mazonson, & Homan, 1993), as well as hospitalizations (Lorig et al., 1999), among participants with chronic disease conditions.

Self-management techniques have been demonstrated to be effective for both induction and maintenance of weight loss as well (Latner, 2001). Indeed, the most common way that people attempt to lose weight is through self-managed efforts of their eating and activity patterns (Jeffery, Adlis, & Forster, 1991). For example, 45% of individuals in the National Weight Control Registry (NWCR) who have lost and maintained 30 pounds or more for at least 1 year report that they achieved this loss through self-management strategies (Wing & Hill, 2001). Almost all of these individuals report using three key weight management strategies: regularly consuming a low-calorie, low fat diet (i.e., <1,400 kcal/day), regularly engaging in high levels (about 1 hour) of moderate-intensity physical activity (e.g., brisk walking), and regularly monitoring their body weight. In line with self-regulation theory (Kanfer & Gaelick-Buys, 1991; Wing, Tate, Gorin, Raynor, & Fava, 2006), which emphasizes the integral role of vigilance (i.e., self-monitoring) in behavior change, the majority of individuals on the weight loss registry also report keeping track of their food intake on a daily basis (Wing & Hill, 2001).

Research Implications

Strong evidence now supports that comprehensive lifestyle programs involving diet, exercise, and weight loss can reduce risk factors for CVD and type 2 diabetes. An emerging literature also suggests that lifestyle interventions may be able to prevent disease onset and progression in some cases. More research is needed, however, to demonstrate the efficacy of lifestyle interventions in disease prevention among individuals at risk for CVD and/or type 2 diabetes. Moreover, most work to date has been conducted in the context of efficacy studies, and there remains a strong need for trials testing the effectiveness of efficacious lifestyle interventions in clinical and community settings treating underserved populations.

There is increasing empirical support for many of the components of behavior change derived from theoretical frameworks. Nevertheless, some experts have argued that more rigorous testing of existing behavior change models and theories is needed because previous research on behavior change and maintenance has not been sufficiently theory-based (Ockene & Zapka, 2000). By rigorously testing existing theories and models of health behavior change and maintenance, future research may inform about ways of refining or revising these theories and models. Interdisciplinary research examining the influence of biomedical, behavioral, psychological, and environmental factors on the individual's health behaviors may also provide a more complete understanding of the dynamic processes involved in behavior change, maintenance, and relapse. These research efforts may also facilitate the development of new models or expanded versions of previous models, which could lead to breakthroughs in the understanding of health behavior change, as well as inform about approaches that may be particularly successful in facilitating long-term adherence. Therefore, future research should focus on understanding the multiple factors that influence health behavior change, as well as on identifying the specific lifestyle intervention components that can favorably modify these factors.

Clinical Implications

An important implication of recent translational research findings is that interventions that have demonstrated efficacy in research studies may be successfully applied in clinical or community settings. For example, findings from recent trials (e.g., TOURS study) indicate that lifestyle interventions can be successfully delivered in community settings through the use of existing infrastructures, such as the CES (U.S. Department of Agriculture, 2007). Thus, utilization of already existing infrastructures may represent an effective approach for disseminating lifestyle-based interventions to community settings. Self-management programs also appear to have significant potential to be translated to broader community settings.

Future health promotion interventions may also be improved by increasing the amount of time devoted to teaching cognitive coping skills during treatment (Dohm et al., 2001). Since negative thought patterns can lead to negative emotional states and potentially maladaptive behavior patterns, cognitive coping skills can be a critical component to weight loss treatments, as well as other health promotion interventions. As noted above, cognitive coping skills teach individuals how to identify and replace unrealistic, negative thought patterns with more positive, but realistic thoughts (Beck 1998). By helping individuals identify maladaptive thought patterns (i.e., thought processes that contribute to negative emotional states and unhealthy behavioral patterns) and replace these with more adaptive thought processes (i.e., thought processes that encourage positive emotional states and healthy behaviors), cognitive coping skills can assist individuals in adopting and maintaining healthy behavior changes. By extending treatment length and providing individuals with more extensive training in cognitive coping skills, in addition to behavioral self-management skills, we believe future treatments may be more effective in helping individuals maintain healthy lifestyle changes over the long-term.

The biopsychosocial model has been well supported by research conducted over the past few decades and is taught in undergraduate and graduate education; however, it has not yet been successfully integrated into clinical medicine, at least on a broad scale. Although some progress has been made, such as the development of integrated care models in pain clinics and medical psychiatric units, more progress is needed. For this model to be integrated and successfully applied in medical practice, physicians and other health care professionals will likely need to change their views on the causes of health and diseases, as well as increase their knowledge of those factors that influence human behavior. As Engel noted over 30 years ago, "Nothing will change unless or until those who control resources have the wisdom to venture off the beaten path of exclusive reliance on biomedicine as the only approach to health care."

Conclusion

The focus of this chapter has been on the central role that eating and exercise patterns have in health promotion and disease prevention. Obesity, one of the major contributors to today's chronic disease conditions, is a clear example of how eating and exercise behaviors can have a significant influence on a person's health. Extensive evidence demonstrates that lifestyle interventions involving modification of dietary and physical activity patterns are effective in producing clinically significant weight losses in obese individuals. In addition to reducing risk factors for CVD and type 2 diabetes, accumulating research suggests that lifestyle interventions may be capable of preventing disease onset and progression in some cases; large-scale studies have demonstrated the ability of weight loss interventions to prevent the onset of type 2 diabetes. Moreover, the efficacy of lifestyle interventions in preventing the progression of heart disease has recently been documented. The effectiveness of future prevention and treatment efforts, however, may greatly depend on the extent to which patients actively participate in prevention efforts related to healthy lifestyle change. Although change may be difficult, health care professionals, who have a theoretical understanding of the multiple factors that can influence an individual's health behavioral choices, can greatly facilitate the behavior change process for their patients.

Future Directions

These questions are related to topics that remain to be addressed by future research:

• What types of study designs or methodological improvements to previous studies are needed to more rigorously test existing behavioral theories and models of health behavior change?

• How can interdisciplinary research projects be designed to better identify the biomedical, behavioral, psychological, and environmental factors that affect an individual's health behavior choices?

• How can trials be designed to test the effectiveness of interventions that have demonstrated efficacy in research studies in clinical and community settings?

References

Ajzen, I. (1985). From intentions to actions: A theory of planned behavior. In J. Kuhl, & J. Beckmann (Eds.), *Action control: From cognition to behavior* (pp. 11–39). New York: Springer-Verlag.

Anton, S. D., & Miller, P. M. (2005). Do negative emotions predict alcohol consumption, saturated fat intake and physical activity in older adults? *Behavior Modification, 29*(4), 677–88.

Asch, S. M., Baker, D. W., Keesey, J. W., Broder, M., Schonlau, M., Rosen, M., et al. (2005). Does the collaborative model improve care for chronic heart failure? *Medical Care, 43*(7), 667–675.

Ashida, T., Ono, C., & Sugiyama, T. (2007). Effects of short term hypocaloric diet on sympatho-vagal interaction assessed by spectral analysis of heart rate and blood pressure variability during stress tests in obese hypertensive patients. *Hypertension Research, 30*, 1199–1203.

Babor, T. F., Sciamanna, C. N., & Pronk, N. P. (2004). Assessing multiple risk behaviors in primary care. Screening issues and related concepts. *American Journal of Preventive Medicine, 27*(2 Suppl), 42–53.

Bandura, A. (1986). *Social foundations of thought and cognition: A social-cognitive theory.* Englewood Cliffs, NJ: Prentice Hall.

Bandura, A. (1997). *Self-efficacy: The exercise of control.* New York: W. H. Freeman and Co.

Beck, A. T., Rush, A. J., Shaw, B. F., & Emery, G. (1979). *Cognitive therapy of depression.* New York: The Guilford Press.

Beck, C. K. (1998). Psychosocial and behavioral interventions for Alzheimer's disease patients and their families. *American Journal of Geriatric Psychiatry, 6*(Suppl 1), S41–S48.

Beck, J. S. (1995). *Cognitive therapy: Basic and beyond.* New York: The Guilford Press.

Berg, C., Lappas, G., Wolk, A., Stranghagen, E., Toren, K., Rosengran, A., et al. (2009). Eating patterns and portion size associated with obesity in a Swedish population. *Appetite, 52*, 21–26.

Blair, S. N., Cheng, Y., & Holder, J. S. (2001). Is physical activity or physical fitness more important in defining health benefits? *Medicine and Science in Sports and Exercise, 33*(6 Suppl), S379–S399, discussion S419–S420.

Blakely, T. J., & Dziadosz, G.M. (2008). The chronic care model for behavioral health care. *Population Health Management, 11*(6), 341–346.

Briefel, R. R., & Johnson, C. L. (2004). Secular trends in dietary intake in the United States. *Annual Review of Nutrition, 24*, 401–431.

Brownell, K. D. (2004). Obesity and managed care: A role for activism and advocacy? *American Journal of Managed Care, 10*(6), 353–354.

Chaput, J. P., & Tremblay, A. (2009). Obesity and physical inactivity: The relevance of reconsidering the notion of sedentariness. *Obesity Facts, 2*, 249–254.

Christensen, A. J. (2004). *Patient adherence to medical treatment regimens: Bridging the gap between behavioral science and biomedicine.* New Haven, CT: Yale University Press.

Civitarese, A. E., Carling, S., Heilbronn, L. K., Hulver, M. H., Ukropcova, B., Deutsch, W. A., et al. (2007). Calorie restriction increases muscle mitochondrial biogenesis in healthy humans. *PLos Medicine, 4*(3), e76.

Clark, N. M., & Becker, M. H. (1998). Theoretical models and strategies for improving adherence and disease management. In S. A. Shumaker, E. B. Schron, J. K. Ockene, & W. L. McBee (Eds.), *The handbook of health behavior change* (2nd ed., pp. 5–32). New York: Springer Publishing Co.

Cleemput, I., Kesteloot, K., & DeGeest, S. (2002). A review of the literature on the economics of noncompliance. Room for methodological improvement. *Health Policy, 59*, 65–94.

Coleman, K., Austin, B. T., Brach, C., & Wagner, E. H. (2009). Evidence on the Chronic Care Model in the new millennium. *Health Affairs, 28*(1), 75–85.

Courneya, K. S. (1995). Understanding readiness for regular physical activity in older individuals: An application of the theory of planned behavior. *Health Psychology, 14*, 80–87.

Coyne, J. C., & Downey, G. (1991). Social factors and psychopathology: Stress, social support, and coping processes. *Annual Review of Psychology, 42*, 401–425.

Craig, C. L., Marshall, A. L., Sjostrom, M., Bauman, A. E., Booth, M. L., Ainsworth, B. E., et al. (2003). International physical activity questionnaire: 12-country reliability and validity. *Medicine and Science in Sports and Exercise, 35*(8), 1381–1395.

Cutler, D., & Miller, G. (2005). The role of public health improvements in health advances: The twentieth-century United States. *Demography, 42*(1), 1–22.

Diabetes Prevention Program Research Group. (2002). Reduction in the incidence of type 2 diabetes with lifestyle intervention or metformin. *New England Journal of Medicine, 346*(6), 393–403.

Dohm, F. A., Beattie J. A., Aibel C., & Striegel-Moore R. H. (2001). Factors differentiating women and men who successfully maintain weight loss from women and men who do not. *Journal of Clinical Psychology, 57*, 105–117.

Dumitrescu, R. G., & Cotarla, I. (2005). Understanding breast cancer risk: Where do we stand in 2005? *Journal of Cellular and Molecular Medicine, 9*, 208–221.

Eberhardt M. S., Ingram D. D., & Makuc D. M. (2001). *Urban and rural health chartbook: Health, United States, 2001.* Hyattsville, MD: National Center for Health Statistics.

Engel, G. L. (1977). The need for a new medical model: A challenge for biomedicine. *Science, 196*(4286), 129–136.

Ferster, C. B., Nurnberger, J. I., & Levitt, E. B. (1996). The control of eating (reprinted from *Journal of Mathetics, 1*, 87–109, 1962). *Obesity Research, 4*, 401–410.

Finkelstein, E. A., Ruhm, C. J., & Kosa, K. M. (2005). Economic causes and consequences of obesity. *Annual Review of Public Health, 26*, 239–257.

Flemming, B., Silver, A., Ocepek-Welikson, K., & Keller, D. (2004). The relationship between organizational systems and clinical quality in diabetes care. *American Journal of Managed Care, 10*(12), 934–944.

Fontana, L. Klein, S., Holloszy, J. O., & Premachandra, B. N. (2006). Effect of long-term calorie restriction with adequate protein and micronutrients on thyroid hormones. *Journal of Clinical Endocrinology and Metabolism, 91*, 3232–3235.

Fontana, L., Villareal, D. T., Weiss, E. P., Racette, S. B., Steger-May, K., Klein, S., & Holloszy, J. O. (2007). Calorie restriction or exercise: Effects on coronary heart disease risk factors. A randomized controlled trial. *American Journal of Physiology - Endocrinology and Metabolism, 293*, E197–E202.

Fontana, L., Weiss, E. P., Villareal, D. T., Klein, S., & Holloszy, J. O. (2008). Long-term effects of calorie or protein restriction on serum IGF-1 and IGFBP-3 concentration in humans. *Aging Cell, 7*, 681–687.

Frazao, E. (Ed.). (1999). *American's eating habits: Changes and consequences.* Agriculture Information Bulletin No. (AIB750), 484. Retrieved from PubMed database, http://www.ers.usda.gov/publications/aib750/

Freedland, S. J. (2005). Obesity and prostate cancer: A growing problem. *Clinical Cancer Research, 11*, 6763–6766.

Gamm, L. D., Hutchison, L. L., Dabney, B. J., & Dorsey, A. M. (Eds.). (2003). *Rural healthy people 2010: A companion document to healthy people 2010* (Vol. 1–3). College Station: Texas A&M University System Health Science Center, School of Rural Public Health, Southwest Rural Health Research Center.

Gans, K. M., Ross, E., Barner, C. W., Wylie-Rosett, J., McMurray, J., & Eaton, C. (2003). REAP and WAVE: new tools to rapidly assess/discuss nutrition with patients. *Journal of Nutrition, 133*(2), 556S–562S.

Garfield, S. L. (1994). Research on client variables in psychotherapy. In A. E. Bergin, & S. L. Garfield (Eds.), *Handbook of psychotherapy and behavior change* (4th ed., pp. 190–228). New York: Wiley.

Germann, J. N, Kirschenbaum, D. S., & Rich, B. H. (2007). Child and parental self-monitoring as determinants of success in the treatment of morbid obesity in low-income minority children. *Journal of Pediatric Psychology, 32*(1), 111–121.

Goldstein, D. J. (1992). Beneficial health effects of modest weight loss. *International Journal of Obesity and Related Metabolic Disorders, 16*, 397–415.

Godin, G., & Kok, G. (1996). The theory of planned behavior: A review of its applications to health-related behaviors. *American Journal of Health Promotion, 11*, 87–98.

Godin, G., & Shephard, R. J. (1985). A simple method to assess exercise behavior in the community. *Canadian Journal of Applied Sport Science, 10*, 141–146.

Godin, G., Valois, P., & Lepage, L. (1993). The pattern of influence of perceived behavioral control upon exercising behavior: An application of Ajzen's theory of planned behavior. *Journal of Behavior Medicine, 16*, 81–102.

Greeno, C. G., & Wing, R. R. (1994). Stress-induced eating. *Psychological Bulletin, 115*, 444–464.

Gregg, E. W., Cheng, Y. J., Cadwell, B. L., Imperatore, G., Williams, D. E., Flegal, K. M., et al. (2005). Secular trends in cardiovascular disease risk factors according to body mass index in US adults. *Journal of the American Medical Association, 293*, 1868–1874.

Hammer, S., Snel, M., Lamb, H. J., Jazet, I. M., van der Meer, R. W., Pijl, H., et al. (2008). Prolonged caloric restriction in obese patients with type 2 diabetes mellitus decreases myocardial triglyceride content and improves myocardial function. *Journal of the American College of Cardiology, 52*, 1006–1012.

Hayes, C., & Kriska, A. (2008). Role of physical activity in diabetes management and prevention. *Journal of the American Dietetic Association, 108*(4 Suppl 1), S19–S23.

Health Technology News. (2009). *Chronic care: Wagner's chronic care model.* Retrieved from http://news.avancehealth.com

Heilbronn, L. K., de Jonge, L., Frisard, M. I., DeLany, J. P., Larson-Meyer, E., Rood, J., et al. (2006). Effect of 6-month calorie restriction on biomarkers of longevity, metabolic adaptation, and oxidative stress in overweight individuals: A randomized controlled trial. *Journal of the American Medical Association, 295*, 1539–1548.

Hill, J. O., & Peters, J. C. (1998). Environmental contributions to the obesity epidemic. *Science, 280*, 1371–1374.

Hofer, T., Fontana, L., Anton, S. D., Weiss, E. P., Villareal, D., Malayappan, B., & Leeuwenburgh, C. (2008). Long-term effects of caloric restriction or exercise on DNA and RNA oxidation levels in white blood cells and urine in humans. *Rejuvenation Research, 11*, 793–799.

Horgen, K. B., & Brownell, K. D. (2002). Confronting the toxic environment: Environmental public health actions. In T. A. Wadden, & A. J. Stunkard (Eds.), *Handbook of obesity treatment* (pp. 95–106). New York: Guilford Press.

Hornig, B., Maier, V., & Drexler, H. (1996). Physical training improves endothelial function in patients with chronic heart failure. *Circulation, 93*(2), 210–214.

Hung, D. Y., Glasgow, R. E., Dickinson, L. M., Froshaug, D. B., Fernald, D. H., Balasubramanian, B. A., & Green, L. A. (2008). The Chronic Care Model and relationships to patient health status and health-related quality of life. *American Journal of Preventive Medicine, 35*(5), S398–S406.

Jakicic, J. M. (2009). The effect of physical activity on body weight. *Obesity, 17*, S34–S38.

Jakicic, J. M., Marcus, B. H., Gallagher, K. I., Napolitano, M., & Lang, W. (2003). Effect of exercise duration and intensity on weight loss in overweight, sedentary women: A randomized trial. *Journal of the American Medical Association, 290*(10), 1323–1330.

Jakicic, J. M., & Otto, A. D. (2006). Treatment and prevention of obesity: What is the role of exercise? *Nutrition Review, 64*(2 Pt 2), S57–S61.

Jeffery, R. W., Adlis, S. A., & Forster, J. L. (1991). Prevalence of dieting among working men and women: The healthy worker project. *Health Psychology, 10*(4), 274–281.

Kanfer, F. H., & Gaelick-Buys, L. (1991). Self-management methods. In F. H. Kanfer, & A. P. Goldstein (Eds.), *Helping people change: A textbook of methods* (4th ed., pp. 305–360). New York: Pergamon Press.

Kelley, G. A., & Kelley, K. S. (2008). Effects of aerobic exercise on non-HDL-C in children and adolescents: A meta-analysis of randomized controlled trials. *Progress in Cardiovascular Nursing, 23*, 128–132.

Kelley, G. A., Kelley, K. S., & Tran, Z. V. (2005). Exercise, lipids, and lipoproteins in older adults: A meta-analysis. *Preventive Cardiology, 8*(4), 206–214.

Kelly, M. T., Wallace, J. M., Robson, P. J., Rennie, K. L., Welch, R. W., Hannon-Fletcher, M. P., et al. (2009). Increased portion size leads to a sustained increase in energy intake over 4d in normal-weight and overweight men and women. *British Journal of Nutrition, 102*, 470–477.

Kendall, C. W., & Jenkins, D. A. (2004). A dietary portfolio: Maximal reduction of low-density lipoprotein cholesterol with diet. *Current Atherosclerosis Reports, 6*, 492–498.

Kerner, J., Rimer, B., & Emmons, K. (2005). Introduction to the special section on dissemination:dissemination research and research dissemination: How can we close the gap? *Health Psychology, 24*(5), 443–446.

Kesaniemi, Y. K., Danforth, E. Jr., Jensen, M. D., Kopelman, P. G., Lefebvre, P., & Reeder, B. A. (2001). Dose-response issues concerning physical activity and health: An evidence-based symposium. *Medicine and Science in Sports and Exercise, 33*, S351–S358.

Knowler, W. C., Barrett-Connor E., Fowler, S. E., Hamman, R. F., Lachin, J. M., Walker, E. A., & Nathan, D. M. (2002). Reduction in the incidence of type 2 diabetes with lifestyle intervention or metformin. *New England Journal of Medicine, 346*(6), 393–403.

Kris-Etherton, P., Eissenstat, B., Jaax, S., Srinath, U., Scott, L., Rader, J., & Pearson, T. (2001). Validation for MEDFICTS, a dietary assessment instrument for evaluating adherence to total saturated fat recommendations of the National Cholesterol Education Program Step 1and Step2 diets. *Journal of the American Dietetic Association, 101*, 81–86.

Kuller, L. H., Tracy, R. P., Shaten, J., & Meilahn, E. N. (1996). Relation of C-reactive protein and coronary heart disease in the MRFIT nested case-control study. Multiple Risk Factor Intervention Trial. *American Journal of Epidemiology, 144*, 537–547.

Larson-Meyer, D. E., Newcomer, B. R., Heilbronn, L. K., Volaufova, J., Smith, S. R., Alfonso, A. J., et al. (2008). Effect of 6-month calorie restriction and exercise on serum and liver lipids and markers of liver function. *Obesity, 16*, 1355–1362.

Latner, J. D. (2001). Self-help in the long-term treatment of obesity. *Obesity Review, 2*(2),87–97.

Lattimore, P. J. (2001). Stress-induced eating: An alternative method for inducing ego-threatening stress. *Appetite, 36*, 187–188.

Lee, I. M., Hsieh, C. C., & Paffenbarger, Jr., R. S. (1995). Exercise intensity and longevity in men. The Harvard Alumni Health Study. *Journal of the American Medical Association, 273*(15), 1179–1184.

Lefevere, M., Redman, L. M., Heilbronn, L. K., Smith, J. V., Martin, C. K., Rood, J. C., et al. (2009). Calorie restriction alone with exercise improves CVD risk in healthy non-obese individuals. *Atherosclerosis, 203*, 206–213.

Lewis, C. E., Jacobs Jr., D. R., McCreath, H., Kiefe, C. I., Schreiner, P. J., Smith, D. E., & Williams, O. D. (2000). Weight gain continues in the 1990s: 10-year trends in weight and overweight from the CARDIA study. Coronary Artery Risk Development in Young Adults. *American Journal of Epidemiology, 151*(12), 1172–1181.

Lin, E. H., Heckbert, S. R., Rutter, C. M., Katon, W. J., Ciechanowski, P., Ludman, E. J., et al. (2009). Depression and increased mortality in diabetes: Unexpected causes of death. *Annals of Family Medicine, 7*(5), 414–421.

Lorig, K. R., Mazonson, P. D., & Holman, H. R. (1993). Evidence suggesting that health education for self-management in patients with chronic arthritis has sustained health benefits while reducing health care costs. *Arthritis Rheum, 36*(4), 439–446.

Lorig, K. R., Ritter, P., Stewart, A. L., Sobel, D. S., Brown Jr., B. W., Bandura, A., et al. (2001). Chronic disease self-management program: 2-year health status and health care utilization outcomes. *Medical Care, 39*(11), 1217–1223.

Lorig, K. R., Sobel, D. S., Stewart, A. L., Brown, B. W. Jr., Bandura, A., Ritter, P., et al. (1999). Evidence suggesting that a chronic disease self-management program can improve health status while reducing hospitalization: A randomized trial. *Medical Care, 37*(1), 5–14.

Lowenfels, A. B., Sullivan, T., Fiorianti, J., & Maisonneuve, P. (2005). The epidemiology and impact of pancreatic diseases in the United States. *Current Gastroenterology Reports, 7*, 90–95.

Maddux, J. E., & DuCharme, K. (1997). Behavioral intentions in theories of health behavior. In D. S. Gochman (Ed.), *Handbook of health behavior research* (pp. 133–152). New York: Plenum.

Mangione-Smith, R., Schonlau, M., Chan, K. S., Keesey, J., Rosen, M., Louis, T. A., & Keeler, E. (2005). Measuring the effectiveness of a collaborative for quality improvement in pediatric asthma care: Does implementing the Chronic Care Model improve processes and outcomes of care? *Ambulatory Pediatrics, 5*(2), 75–82.

Matarazzo, J. D. (1980). Behavioral health and behavioral medicine: Frontiers for a new health psychology. *American Psychologist, 35*(9), 807–817.

McGinnis, J. M., & Foege, W. H. (1993). Actual causes of death in the United States. *Journal of the American Medical Association, 270*(18), 2207–2212.

McTigue, K. M., Harris, R., Hemphill, B., Lux, L., Sutton, S., Bunton, A. J., & Lohr, K. N. (2003). Screening and interventions for obesity in adults: Summary of the evidence for the U.S. Preventative Services Task Force. *Annals of Internal Medicine, 139*, 933–949.

Meyer, T. E., Kovacs, S. J., Ehsani, A. A., Klein, S., Holloszy, J. O., & Fontana, L. (2006). Long-term caloric restriction ameliorates the declines in diastolic function in humans. *Journal of the American College of Cardiology, 47*, 398–402.

Miller, W. R., & Rollnick, S. (1991). *Motivational interviewing: Preparing people to change addictive behavior.* New York: The Guilford Press.

Mokdad, A. H., Bowman, B. A., Ford, E. S., Vinicor, F., Marks, J. S., & Koplan, J. P. (2001). The continuing epidemics of obesity and diabetes in the United States. *Journal of the American Medical Association, 286*(10), 1195–1200.

Mokdad, A. H., Giles, W. H., Bowman, B. A., Mensah, G. A., Ford, E. S., Smith, S. M., & Marks, J. S. (2004). Changes in health behaviors among older Americans, 1990 to 2000. *Public Health Report, 119*(3), 356–361.

Myers, J., Atwood, J. E., & Froelicher, V. (2003). Active lifestyle and diabetes. *Circulation, 107*(19), 2392–2394.

National Heart, Lung, and Blood Institute. (1998). Obesity education initiative expert panel on the identification, evaluation, and treatment of overweight and obesity in adults. *Obesity Research, 6,* 51–209.

Nezu, A. M., & Perri, M. G. (1989). Social problem-solving therapy for unipolar depression- an initial dismantling investigation. *Journal of Consulting and Clinical Psychology, 57,* 408–413.

Nezu, A. M., & Ronan, G. F. (1985). Life stress, current problems, problem-solving, and depressive symptoms- an integrative model. *Journal of Consulting and Clinical Psychology, 53,* 693–697.

NHS Information Centre. (2010). *Statistics on obesity, physical activity and diet.* Leeds: NHS Information Centre, Lifestyles Statistics.

Ockene, J. K., & Zapka, J. G. (2000). Provider education to promote implementation of clinical practice guidelines. *Chest, 118,* 33S–39S.

Ogden, C. L, Carroll, M. D, Curtin, L. R., McDowell, M. A., Tabak, C. J., & Flegal, K. M. (2006). Prevalence of overweight and obesity in the United States, 1999–2004. *Journal of the American Medical Association, 295,* 1549–1555.

Oldridge, N. B., & Streiner, D. L. (1990). The health belief model: Predicting compliance and dropout in cardiac rehabilitation. *Medicine and Science in Sports and Exercise, 22,* 678–683.

Oliver, G., & Wardle, J. (1999). Perceived effects of stress on food choice. *Physiology and Behavior, 66,* 511–515.

Oliver, G., Wardle, J., & Gibson, E. L. (2000). Stress and food choice: A laboratory study. *Psychosomatic Medicine, 62,* 853–865.

Ornish, D., Scherwitz, L. W., Billings, J. H., Brown, S. E., Gould, K. L., Merritt, T. A., et al. (1998). Intensive lifestyle changes for a reversal of coronary heart disease. *Journal of the American Medical Association, 280,* 2001–2007.

Osborne, R. H., Wilson, T., Lorig, K. R., & McColl, G. J. (2007). Does self-management lead to sustainable health benefits in people with arthritis? A 2-year transition study of 452 Australians. *Journal of Rheumatology, 34*(5), 1112–1117.

Pearce, S., & Wardle, J. (1989). *The practice of behavioural medicine.* Oxford: BSB Books with Oxford University Press.

Perri, M. G. (1998). The maintenance of treatment effects in the long-term management of obesity. *Clinical Psychology: Science and Practice, 5,* 526–543.

Perri, M. G., Foreyt, J. P., & Anton, S. D. (2011). Preventing weight regain after weight loss. In G. A. Bray, & C. Bouchard (Eds.), *Handbook of obesity treatment: Clinical applications* (3rd ed., pp. 249–268). New York: Informa Healthcare.

Perri, M. G., Limacher, M. C., Durning, P. E., Janicke, D. M., Lutes, L. D., Bobroff, L. B., et al. (2008). Extended-care programs for weight management in rural communities: The treatment of obesity in underserved rural settings (TOURS) randomized trial. *Archives of Internal Medicine, 168,* 2347–2354.

Perri, M. G., Martin, A. D., Leermakers, E. A., Sears, S. F., & Notelovitz, M. (1997). Effects of group- versus home-based exercise in the treatment of obesity. *Journal of Consulting and Clinical Psychology, 65,* 278–285.

Perri M. G., McAdoo W. G., Spevak P. A., & Newlin, D. B. (1984). Effect of a multi-component maintenance program on long-term weight loss. *Journal of Consulting and Clinical Psychology, 52,* 480–481.

Perri, M. G., Nezu, A. M., McKelvey, W. F., Shermer, R. L., Renjilian, D. A., & Viegener, B. J. (2001). Relapse prevention training and problem-solving therapy in the long-term management of obesity. *Journal of Consulting and Clinical Psychology, 69*(4), 722–726.

Phillips, C. D., & McLeroy, K. R. (2004). Health in rural America: Remembering the importance of place. *American Journal of Public Health, 94*(10), 1661–1663.

Physical activity guidelines for Americans. (2008). *Oklahoma Nurse, 53*(4), 25.

Pierce, D., & Gunn, J. (2007). GPs' use of problem solving therapy for depression: A qualitative study of barriers to and enablers of evidence based care. *BMC Family Practice, 8,* 24.

Pi-Sunyer, X., Blackburn, G., Brancati, F. L., Bray, G. A., Bright, R., Clark, J. M., et al. (2007). Reduction in weight and cardiovascular disease risk factors in individuals with type 2 diabetes: One-year results of the look AHEAD trial. *Diabetes Care, 30*(6), 1374–1383.

Pleis, J. R., Schiller, J. S., & Benson, V. (2003). Summary health statistics for U.S. adults: National Health Interview Survey, 2000. *Vital Health Statistics, 10,* 215, 1–132.

Plotnick, G. D., Corretti, M. C., & Vogel, R. A. (1997). Effect of antioxidant vitamins on the transient impairment of endothelium-dependent brachial artery vasoactivity following a single high-fat meal. *Journal of the American Medical Association, 278*(20), 1682–1686.

Poston, W. S., & Foreyt, J. P. (1999). Obesity is an environmental issue. *Atherosclerosis, 146,* 201–209.

Powell, L. H., Calvin, J. E., & Calvin Jr., J. E. (2007). Effective obesity treatments. *American Psychologist, 62,* 234–246.

Prasad, D. S., & Das, B. C. (2009). Physical inactivity: a cardiovascular risk factor. *Indian Journal of Medical Science, 63,* 33–42.

Prevalence of physical activity, including lifestyle activities among adults—United States, 2000–2001. (2003). *MMWR Morbidity and Mortality Weekly Report, 52*(32), 764–769.

Prevalence of self-reported physically active adults—United States, 2007. (2008). *MMWR Morbidity and Mortality Weekly Report, 57*(48), 1297–1300.

Racette, S. B., Weiss, E. P., Villareal, D. T., Arif, H., Steger-May, K., Schechtman, K. B., et al. (2006). One year of caloric restriction in humans: Feasibility and effects on the body composition and abdominal adipose tissue. *Journals of Gerontology Series A: Biological Sciences and Medical Sciences, 61,* 943–950.

Reis, B. F., & Brown, L. G. (1999). Reducing psychotherapy dropouts: Maximizing perspective convergence in the psychotherapy dyad. *Psychotherapy: Theory/Research/Practice/Training, 36*(2), 123–136.

Renjilian, D. A., Perri, M. G., Nezu, A. M., McKelvey, W. F., Schein, R. L., & Anton, S. D. (2001). Individual versus group therapy for obesity: Effects of matching participants to their treatment preferences. *Journal of Clinical and Consulting Psychology, 69,* 717–721.

Richardson, C. R., Newton, T. L., Abraham, J. J., Sen, A. A., Jimbo, M., & Swartz, A. M. (2008). A meta-analysis of pedometer-based walking interventions and weight loss. *Annals of Family Medicine, 6*(1), 69–77.

Riddell, L. J., Chisholm, A., Williams, S., & Mann, J. I. (2000). Dietary strategies for lowering homocysteine concentrations. *American Journal of Clinical Nutrition, 71*(6), 1448–1454.

Roemmich, J. N., Wright, S. M., & Epstein, L. H. (2002). Dietary restraint and stress-induced snacking in youth. *Obesity Research, 10*, 1120–1126.

Rollnick, S., Miller, W.R. & Butler, C.C. (2007). *Motivational Interviewing in Health Care: Helping Patients Change Behavior.* New York: Guilford.

Rolls, B. J., Ello-Martin, J. A., & Tohill, B. C. (2004). What can intervention studies tell us about the relationship between fruit and vegetable consumption and weight management? *Nutrition Reviews, 62*(1), 1–17.

Rolls, B. J., Roe, L. S., & Meengs, J. S. (2004). Salad and satiety: Energy density and portion size of a first-course salad affect energy intake at lunch. *Journal of the American Dietetic Association, 104*(10), 1570–1576.

Rolls, B. J., Roe, L.S., & Meengs, J. S. (2006). Reductions in portion size and energy density of foods are additive and lead to sustained decreases in energy intake. *American Journal of Clinical Nutrition, 83*, 11–17.

Sallis, J. F., Hovell, M. F., Hofstetter, C. R., Faucher, P., Elder, J. P., Blanchard, J., et al. (1989). A multivariate study of determinants of vigorous exercise in a community sample. *Preventive Medicine, 18*, 20–34.

Schwartz, G. E. (1982). Testing the biopsychosocial model: The ultimate challenge facing behavioral medicine? *Journal of Consulting and Clinical Psychology, 50*(6), 1040–1053.

Si, D., Bailie, R., Connors, C., Dowden, M., Stewart, A., Robinson, G., et al. (2005). Assessing health care systems for guiding improvement in diabetes care. *BMC Health Services Research, 5*, 56.

Smith, T. W., Kendall, P. C., & Keefe, F. J. (2002). Behavioral medicine and clinical health psychology: Introduction to the special issue, a view from the decade of behavior. *Journal of Consulting and Clinical Psychology, 70*(3), 459–462.

Soroudi, N., Wylie-Rosett, J., & Mogul, D. (2004). Quick WAVE Screener: A tool to address weight, activity, variety, and excess. *Diabetes Educator, 30*, 616–628.

Stampfer, M. J., Hu, F. B., Manson, J. E., Rimm, E. B., & Willett, W. C. (2000). Primary prevention of coronary heart disease in women through diet and lifestyle. *New England Journal of Medicine, 343*(1), 16–22.

Strickland, P. A. O., Hudson, S. V., Piasecki, A., Hahn, K., Cohen, D., Orzano, A. J., et al. (2010). Features of the Chronic Care Model (CCM) associated with behavioral counseling and diabetes care in community primary care. *Journal of the American Board of Family Medicine, 23*(3), 295–305.

Stunkard, A. J. (1982). Obesity. In A. S. Bellack, M. Hersen, & A. E. Kazdin (Eds.), *International handbook of behavior medicine and therapy* (pp. 535–573). New York: Plenum Press.

Thompson, P. D., Buchner, D., Pina, I. L., Balady, G. J., Williams, M. A., Marcus, B. H., et al. (2003). Exercise and physical activity in the prevention and treatment of atherosclerotic cardiovascular disease: A statement from the council on Clinical Cardiology (Subcommittee on Exercise, Rehabilitation, and Prevention) and the Council on Nutrition, Physical Activity, and Metabolism (Subcommittee on Physical Activity). *Circulation, 107*(24), 3109–3116.

Thompson, P. D., & Lim, V. (2003). Physical activity in the prevention of arthrosclerotic coronary heart disease. *Current Treatment Options in Cardiovascular Medicine, 5*(4), 279–285.

U.S. Department of Agriculture, Cooperative State, Research, Education, and Extension Service. (2007). United States Department of Agriculture; National Institute of Food and Agriculture. Retrieved from http://www.csrees.usda.gov/qlinks/extension.html.

U.S. Department of Health and Human Services. (2000). *Healthy people 2010: Understanding and improving health and objectives for improving health.* Washington, DC: US Government Printing Office.

U.S. Department of Health and Human Services and U.S. Department of Agriculture. (2005). *Dietary guidelines for Americans* (6th ed.). Washington, DC: U.S. Government Printing Office.

U.S. Public Health Service. (1996). *Physical activity and health: A report of the surgeon general.* Atlanta, GA: U.S. Department of Health and Human Services, Centers for Disease Control and Prevention, National Center for Chronic Disease Prevention and Health Promotion.

Wadden, T. A., Brownell, K. D., & Foster, G. D. (2002). Obesity: Responding to the global epidemic. *Journal of Consulting and Clinical Psychology, 70*, 510–525.

Wadden, T. A., Butryn, M. L., & Wilson, C. (2007). Lifestyle modification for the management of obesity. *Gastroenterology, 132*(6), 2226–2238.

Wagner, E. H. (1998). Chronic disease management: what will it take to improve care for chronic illness? *Effective Clinical Practice, 1*(1), 2–4.

Wagner, E. H., Austin, B. T., Davis, C., Hindmarsh, M., Schaefer, J., & Bonomi, A. (2001). Improving chronic illness care: Translating evidence into action. *Health Affairs (Millwood), 20*(6), 64–78.

Weindruch, R., & Walford, R. L. (1988). *The retardation of aging and disease by dietary restriction.* Springfield, IL: Charles C. Thomas Publisher.

Weiss, E. P., Racette, S. B., Villareal, D. T., Fontana, L., Steger-May, K., Schechtman, K. B., et al. (2006). Improvements in glucose tolerance and insulin action induced by increasing energy expenditure or decreasing energy intake: A randomized controlled trial. *American Journal of Clinical Nutrition, 84*, 1033–1042.

Wing, R. R., & Jeffery, R. W. (1995). Effect of modest weight loss on changes in cardiovascular risk factors: Are there differences between men and women or between weight loss and maintenance? *International Journal of Obesity and Related Metabolic Disorders, 19*, 67–73.

Wing, R. R., & Jeffery, R. W. (1999). Benefits of recruiting participants with friends and increasing social support for weight loss and maintenance. *Journal of Consulting and Clinical Psychology, 67*, 132–138.

Wing, R. R., & Hill, J. O. (2001). Successful weight loss maintenance. *Annual Review of Nutrition, 21*, 323–341.

Wing, R. R., Phelan, S., & Tate, D. (2002). The role of adherence in mediating the relationship between depression and health outcomes. *Journal of Psychosomatic Research, 53*, 877–881.

Wing, R. R., Tate, D. F., Gorin, A. A., Raynor, H. A., & Fava, J. L. (2006). A self-regulation program for maintenance of weight loss. *New England Journal of Medicine, 355*(15), 1563–1571.

Zerhouni, E. A. (2005). Translational and clinical science: Time for a new vision. *New England Journal of Medicine, 353*(15), 1621–1623.

Aspects of Culture Influencing Rehabilitation and Persons with Disabilities

Elias Mpofu, Julie Chronister, Ebonee T. Johnson, *and* Geoff Denham

Abstract

Disability is largely defined by the sociocultural context in which it is perceived and in relation to the atypicality with which a person identified as having a disability participates in ordinary activities of daily living. The ways in which social others perceive the category of disability influences access to resources for participation, so that some disabilities may result in more restrictions to participation than others. Rehabilitation interventions for people with disabilities seek to maximize quality of daily life in typical community settings. Communities as participation environments differ in the extent to which they are structured to enable the full inclusion of others who may have disabilities. Concepts rooted in a human rights perspective to disability enable checks on assumptions on which opportunities for community participation are configured and distributed to accommodate the full range of human attributes, thus making it likely for changes to occur toward disability-inclusive sociocultural systems. Culturally safe contexts for participation are those that enable those with a disability to have the same access to resources for activities of daily living as those without disability. Research is needed on sociocultural systems to determine full community participation of people with disabilities and how this can best be implemented.

Key Words: Disability, culture, cultural safety, participation, human rights.

Sociocultural understanding influences how those with disabilities are categorized and the nature of the services they are provided. This understanding occurs because disability and associated rehabilitation services are phenomena defined by social actors who share a value system regarding participation facilitators or enablers in a specific cultural context (Mpofu, Bishop, Hirschi, & Hawkins, 2010). *Participation facilitators* are resources for enacting a preferred life situation or activity (World Health Organization [WHO], 2001a). Those perceived to access activities and to participate differently or in atypical ways, presumably because of their bodily or mental impairments, are likely to be considered to have a disability. Thus, disability in itself is not a diagnosis, but a category applied to others who may

be different in the ways that they transact with their environment. Disability is often defined in reference to the presence of actual or perceived limitations in functioning by an individual in a sociocultural environment in comparison with the functioning of typical others from the same or a similar environment. Effective interventions to meet needs ascribed to a disability-related difference may be designed to be responsive to the sociocultural context in which health care resources are appropriated.

This chapter briefly considers the major cultural-historical influences on rehabilitation practice systems and the role of culture in the construction of disability and, in particular, to the influence of perceived difference in the ascription of disability. It also briefly surveys rehabilitation philosophies as cultural representations that influence the nature of rehabilitative services provided to people identified as having a disability. Finally, the chapter reviews pertinent best practices in providing rehabilitative services to people with disabilities and the research evidence for the influence of culture on rehabilitation service outcomes

International Cultural Historical Influences on Rehabilitation Practices

Rehabilitation practices are formulated and enacted in a cultural-historical context aligned to the development of health care services in the particular jurisdiction. In general, countries with more developed health and social services tend to have more complex rehabilitation policies, education, and training programs than those with less developed health care and social service systems. As health care systems evolve, health care and other social services (e.g., education) first become more widely available to the general population, followed by the development of formal rehabilitation services (Mpofu et al., 2007). Developmentally, early-stage rehabilitation services have a medical emphasis whereas later-stage programs combine both medical and social models (Dell Orto, 2003). The development of rehabilitation services in particular geographical regions is also explained by culture, including major political events (e.g., colonialism/foreign occupation, wars, international conventions) the developmental needs of the socioculturally contiguous region (Llewellyn et al., 2010), and national disability policy priorities (Madden, Glozier, Mpofu, & Llewellyn, 2010; Mpofu & Harley, 2002). For instance, major disability and rehabilitation program development in Western nations have followed the two major world wars, and the programs were put in place first to serve war veterans, with subsequent devolution to the civilian population. The rehabilitation models developed in Western countries have tended to be exported to developing countries mostly by international development agencies and with varying degrees of adaptation.

In designing and implementing rehabilitation services for the general population, issues of culture have achieved prominence, particularly with the increasing emphasis on the provision of community-based rehabilitation (CBR) services. Community-based rehabilitation is defined as "a strategy for rehabilitation, equalization of opportunities, poverty reduction and social inclusion of people with disabilities" (ILO, UNESCO & WHO, 2004, p. 2). By nature, successful CBR would provide culturally responsive services for the participation of those with disabilities. Recently, the realization by United Nations member states that sustainable development and the attainment of Millennium Development goals was likely to be achieved with disability-inclusive development strategies, has resulted in a variety of initiatives to map the cultural determinants of disability in development (Llewellyn et al., 2010).

Overlying these international trends in the conceptualization of rehabilitation services is the influence and maturation of disability and human rights advocacy movements (Chimedza & Peters, 1999; Mpofu & Harley, 2002). As noted later in the chapter, pro-disability and rehabilitation United Nations conventions have created an international lingua franca for communicating about and understanding disability and rehabilitation in ways that impact how rehabilitation services can be delivered in cultural settings while upholding basic human rights. The importance of patients' rights is recognized in the current emphasis on patient-oriented care (Hwang & Mpofu, 2010). Major disparities in health care quality by race/ethnicity have been observed, but with less attention paid to the cultural and systemic aspects influencing health service delivery systems. For instance, racial minority patients in the United States were less satisfied with their physicians and trusted them less than did white patients after controlling for socioeconomic and health status (Blanchard & Lurie, 2004; Haviland, Morales, Dial, & Pincus, 2005). U.S. Hispanic and Asian patients were less satisfied with their interpersonal interactions with physicians than were white patients (Merrill & Allen, 2003). Patient-oriented care necessarily includes addressing the cultural aspects of health care.

Cultural Influences

Culture is a major prism through which social perceptions are formed and applied onto others, which in turn, categorizes persons on a single or few qualities. For instance, a medically identified impairment may translate into a disability in the absence of sociocultural resources that allow access to activities and participation by atypical others. Conversely, the availability of sociocultural resources (i.e., for full access and community inclusion), may result in an impairment not resulting into a disability. Therefore, although medical diagnoses can contribute to the understanding of impairments associated with disability, the ascription of the label of disability is the result of a constellation of conditions, of which the specific impairment may be only one and not necessarily the most significant barrier to participation in desired life situations (WHO, 2001a). Perceived difference and the undervaluing of other barriers are keys to understanding how disability is constructed.

Perceived Difference

Disability is most often a label of (in)convenience that, when applied to others, reflects a perceived difference attributed to an impairment in the context of a sociocultural environment. The World Health Organization (WHO)'s ICF model (WHO, 1999, 2001a) provides an integrative conceptual framework for understanding disability as category or service status. It proposes that disability may result from the interactions between bodily impairment or functions, and environmental and personal factors to influence opportunities for participating in life situations. Environmental factors are underpinned by culture, whereas personal qualities important for living with a disability are a product of both individual and environmental influences. Nonetheless, disability is only one of numerous human characteristics "and on its own does not necessarily constrain an individual's opportunities or choices" (Mpofu, Thomas, & Thompson, 1998, p. 211). For example, two people with objectively the same level of impairment may have have very different participation outcomes depending on their personal circumstances (e.g., age, social class, education) and the sociocultural environment in which they live (e.g., rural subsistence economy, urbanized highly industrial society).

The perceived difference ascribed by others may result in stigmatization. Stigma occurs when a quality identifiable in an individual or setting is undervalued, and negative attributions are applied to a person, object, or event by others (Goffman, 1963). It is a cultural product that does not exist independently of the social actors who construe persons, objects, or events in negative ways. Stigma is produced by collective judgments, such as those associated with medical diagnostic categories (Fabrega, 1990, 1991; Kleinman, Keusch, & Wilentz, 2006). Disability is one such judgment that is stigmatizing, and, consequently, individuals with disabilities may experience significant attitudinal barriers to community participation.

As sociocultural structures become more inclusive, however, the designation of atypical conditions as disabilities becomes less prevalent, and individuals who were typically excluded claim their participation space and are perceived as more similar to others (and less negatively evaluated). For example, in highly industrialized cultures or communities, advanced technology increases the activity and participation capacity among those previously excluded due to an ostensible disability. There has been a rapid deployment of computerized tools in industrialized countries that allow, for example, persons with hearing and speech impairments to communicate with levels of sophistication previously unimagined in the workplace. "Kneeling buses" are another example of a sociostructural structure that has improved the capacity of people with restricted mobility to move around in the community for work and leisure purposes.

These developments highlight the importance of understanding disability from an interactive person–environment perspective within the context of cultural facilitators or enablers. Technological innovations have the potential over time to reduce overall disability, even in the presence of significant bodily or mental impairment.

Promoting social practices that are more accommodating of diversity in human attributes would obviate the use of disability as a service delivery category. Human rights perspectives to social services (United Nations, 2007) present a challenge to cultures that categorize, stigmatize, and marginalize others believed to be different due to imputed disability.

Disability and Culture

Culture is, by definition, "something that is shared amongst people belonging to the same socially defined and recognized group" (Levine, Park, & Kim, 2007, p. 207). In short, culture is something people have in common with certain others. A local culture is comprised of situated or customized ways of doing things, including evaluating behavior and deciding on the worth of practices. Culture is evident in customs of appropriate dress and manners, forms of speech, ways of addressing people, and habits. As such, there are cultural ways of defining functioning, disability, and health, and culturally driven approaches to addressing the health and rehabilitation needs of persons with disabilities. For example, in contrast to the medical approach to explaining disability, many cultures perceive the origin of disability from a metaphysical-spiritual realm. Examples of cultures that value metaphysical explanations for health and well-being include traditionalist African Americans (Mpofu & Harley, 2002), Mexican Americans (Adkins & Young, 1976), Native Americans (Locust, 1988), Hispanic/Latino Americans (Mpofu, Beck, & Weinrach, 2004), and some Southeast Asian groups

(Chan, 1986). Further, for some cultures, disability is a condition that should not be altered as it is considered to be predetermined by fate and not amenable to adaptive device (Sotnik & Jezewski, 2005). In some African and Indian cultures, certain types of disability may be perceived worthy of reverence and those with such disabilities are highly respected.

Immigrant persons from culturally and linguistically diverse backgrounds (CALD) may experience disability and rehabilitation or health care practices differently than those of the majority culture, which could limit their participation in health care (Hwang & Mpofu, 2010; Zea, Belgrave, Townsend, Jarama, & Banks, 1996). For example, in the United States, persons of color experience lower access to health care relative to their peers with disabilities who hold the majority culture status (Atkins & Wright, 1980; Dodd, Nelson, Ostwald, & Fischer, 1991; Donnell, 2008; Dziekan & Okocha, 1993; Faubion, Calico, & Roessler, 1998; Smart & Smart, 1994; Wilson, 2000; Wilson, Harley, & Alston, 2001). Filipino Australians with children with intellectual disabilities perceived child care services as relatively inaccessible to them or to lack cultural responsiveness. These differences in perceived and actual opportunity to participate in life situations reflects the need to better understand the impact of cultural environments on rehabilitation practices. Cultural environments for health care are grounded in worldviews or philosophies.

Cultural Foundations of Rehabilitation

Culturally loaded rehabilitation philosophies drive service provision in the global context (Sotnik & Jezewski, 2005). According to Sotnik and Jezewski, "disability service systems can be considered as entities that, similar to a country or ethnic enclave, embody a philosophy, values, policies, and practices" (p. 28). In the United States, for example, rehabilitation practice is grounded in an individualistic value orientation that rewards self-determination, professional achievement, and self-sufficiency (Sotnik & Jezewski, 2005). It has a sociocultural history based on an economic model designed to enable veterans with war-related disabilities to become employed. These influences can be most pointedly identified in the U.S. public Vocational Rehabilitation (VR) program's establishment of job placement as the sole criteria for successful outcome. Those who achieve this outcome likely consist of individuals who believe in the same values as those underlying the VR system. Such standards may conflict with those of a family from another culture that believes to subsist for a living would result in loss of face or shame for the collective (Chen & Huo, 2009).

The U.S. rehabilitation system assumes a scientific approach to problem-solving and disability explanation (Mpofu & Harley, 2002; Sotnik & Jezewski, 2005) that is integrally tied to the field's long history of relying on a medical orientation, aligned with the modernist social ideology that embraces categories, diagnoses, and outcomes. This ideology is most clearly evident in contemporary health care systems that use classifications to produce medical and psychiatric diagnoses that are rarely examined for cultural sensitivity (Mezzich et al., 1999; Mzimukulu & Simbayi, 2006; Parker, Cheah, & Roy, 2001). According to Mezzich et al. (1999, p. 458), "culture provides the matrix of the interpersonal situation of the diagnostic interview… [it] informs the overall conceptualization of diagnostic systems, which are children of their time and circumstances."

Often, rehabilitation clients transact with alternative cultural worlds to access services to meet their needs. For instance, rehabilitation clients may be relatively successful in seeking services from both spiritual or faith-based therapies, herbal therapies, and movement therapies, in addition to modern medically oriented treatments (Mzimukulu & Simbayi, 2006; WHO, 2001b). Rosaldo (1989) referred to the experience of accessing health services involving the negotiation of contrasting worldviews as "border crossings." In the rehabilitation services context, the notion of border crossing is particularly apt in highlighting the significance of how cultural orientations may influence the extent to which clients from CALD backgrounds engage providers. Clients may weigh the evidence from alternative therapies differently than would the providers of particular therapies. Disability and rehabilitation care constructs may not translate equivalently between and even within client groups and provider settings (Mpofu & Ortiz, 2009; Osterlind, Mpofu, & Oakland, 2010). The criteria for acceptability and perceived relevance of these cross-over, alternative rehabilitative and health services, will influence adherence, follow-through and outcomes (Mpofu, 2006). Rehabilitation service providers need to be conscious of exchanges in which border crossings are occurring, given the distinct possibility that health and rehabilitation practices may be less effective due to the contradictions or misunderstandings of cultural meanings that remain unrecognized and therefore unaddressed.

In the absence of supporting research evidence, the best guide available for negotiating border crossings is the notion of *cultural safety*. Cultural safety was proposed in the 1980s in Aotearoa, New Zealand (New Zealand Psychologists Registration Board, 2006; Wepa, 2010). Cultural safety in rehabilitation care occurs when collaborative rehabilitation practices with clients are prioritized by health care providers to allow mutual learning by both the client and provider. The process involves learning about the best ways to meet a client's rehabilitation needs, and recognizing clients as experts regarding their rehabilitation service needs and alternative ways to meet those needs (see also Mpofu, Crystal, & Feist-Price, 2000). To illustrate, there are many cultures in which having a male health professional work with a female client is considered not culturally safe practice. Thus, rehabilitation service agencies working with clients from culturally conservative communities may seek to enhance cultural safety by routinely allocating female counselors to female clients and male counselors to male clients. The development of rehabilitation care protocols to ensure cultural safety is a step in the right direction.

Rehabilitation services that take into account clients' cultural safety minimize the potential for client disempowerment through cultural appropriation (Mpofu et al., 1998). *Cultural appropriation* occurs when rehabilitation service providers, in acquiring information about CALD clients ostensibly to "empower" or enable participation, may instead produce paradoxical effects in disempowering the clients by commodifying their clients' experiences (Greaves, 1994, 1995; Mpofu et al., 1998). Commodification is a process in which the lived experiences of different and marginalized others are made the objects of undue curiosity or scrutiny by socially privileged others for the material and intellectual gratification of the latter. Negative consequences from commodification include cultural insensitivity (Alston & Bell, 1996; Szymanski & Trueba, 1994; Tichenor, Thomas, & Kravetz, 1975) and treating persons with disabilities as products in a rehabilitation industry (Albrecht, 1992; Mpofu et al., 1998). The adoption of a human rights perspective to disability as a basis for rehabilitation services would minimize the commodification of people with disabilities (see also United Nations, 2008).

Best Practices in Rehabilitation Interventions with People with Disabilities

The category of disability does not necessarily enable full participation by those who transact differently with the environment because of a perceived impairment. Sociocultural environments designed for universal access would obviate the need to label others because of environmental barriers to their participation. "It is the collective responsibility of society at large to make the environmental modifications necessary for full participation of people with disabilities in all areas of social life" (WHO, 2001, p. 15). Many of the issues faced by those affected by disability are human rights violations and go beyond medically managed service delivery. Indeed, attempts to manage disability from a primarily impairment-oriented approach is likely to be inadequate. Consideration of cultural context is important for the provision of services to facilitate the participation of people with disabilities in preferred life situations (Chan, Tarvydas, Blalock, Strauser, & Atkins, 2009).

Of particular importance is the field's lack of evidenced-based practice for persons from CALD backgrounds. In the United States or other Western settings, practitioners have historically provided services to clients based on monocultural frameworks using methods more suited for the white, middle-class majority (Sue & Sue, 2003). Indeed, best practice is culturally competent practice, which requires practitioners and scholars to integrate (or use in conjunction with) counseling techniques/theoretical frameworks that are based on the majority with multicultural counseling theory (Mpofu et al., 2004). Mpofu et al. (2004) suggested that "it is more realistic to perceive mainstream and minority counseling approaches on a continuum, with some aspects of mainstream counseling applicable to working with minority clients and vice versa" (p. 398). Addressing both mainstream and minority context issues for and with the client would maximize the chances for effective participation by those with disability.

Practitioners must incorporate cultural sensitivity and safety practices into rehabilitation service provision (Cottone & Tarvydas, 2007; Remley & Herlihy, 2005). For instance, practitioners should consider the interlinking of disability status, personal factors, and environmental influences in the design, implementation, and evaluation of rehabilitation services (Mpofu & Conyers, 2004). Persons with disabilities often have multiple cultural affiliations (i.e., race, ethnicity, gender, socioeconomic status, sexual orientation) that, together with impairment, may influence how they participate in preferred life situations. Overlapping identities from disability, personal, and environmental contexts contribute to choices and opportunities for participation.

Representation theory offers a model with which to conceptualize working with clients with disabilities who are from CALD backgrounds (Mpofu & Conyers, 2004). Representation theory has been associated with minority group membership and refers to "communities of interest who share a similar set of economic and social handicaps that have arisen from a history of unfair discrimination by the majority" (p. 143). This model suggests that negotiating the characteristics of a minority status in one area may have a successful impact or outcome on another minority status held by the same individual. For example, a female feminist activist with a disability who is successful in advocating for women's rights may also be successful in self-advocacy for disability rights. Rehabilitation practitioners can help to facilitate this process by working with the client to build his or her self-efficacy. This model also emphasizes that practitioners, especially of different racial, ethnic, or cultural background, should minimize the effects of *tokenism* (the overrepresentation of minority group members that may lead to increased scrutiny) by involving persons of a similar worldview, family, and friends in the rehabilitation process, to minimize feelings of isolation and ensure that the client's needs will be addressed (Mpofu & Conyers, 2002).

Rehabilitation practitioners should facilitate a structured, open forum for the client and practitioner to discuss sociocultural differences (Mpofu et al., 2000; Mpofu et al., 2004; Wepa, 2010). This structured forum facilitates mutual decision-making, negotiation, rapport and mutual trust, which in turn, may prevent the early dropout rate of clients from culturally diverse backgrounds. For example, when a client's spiritual and/or religious beliefs are central to his or her way of life (Sue & Sue, 2003), the rehabilitation practitioner should work with the individual to develop and facilitate interventions sensitive to the individual's beliefs. This rationale implies the use of approaches to transform fixed ideas into tentative formulations to allow the client to actively engage in the process as a collaborative partner. Counselors adopting such positions can often be heard using words and phrases like "I wonder if," "maybe," "perhaps this might be worth considering," and "help me to understand what you are going through," in contrast to "I know," "I'm sure," or "I know exactly how you feel." Communicating that one does not fully understand, and being prepared to acknowledge one's lack of knowledge of cultural norms with regards to how illness or disability is understood

within that culture, is fundamental to building trust and mutual respect within a multicultural setting (Donnell, Robertson, & Tansey, 2010).

A collaborative, tentative approach is particularly effective when opposing points of view arise because it allows the client the opportunity to verbalize thoughts and feelings in order to reconcile the dilemma and move forward in achieving desired rehabilitation goals. Finally, to facilitate a culturally sensitive dialogue and communication process, rehabilitation practitioners should use disability terminology that is understandable to the client and his or her family (Mpofu et al., 2004). In addition, family members should not translate or interpret; trained personnel should be employed for these roles to reduce the possibility of misinterpretation between the client and counselor (Mpofu et al., 2004).

Directions for Future Research

Rehabilitation researchers share a common goal of optimizing the lives of persons living with disabilities (Bartlett et al., 2006). However, rehabilitation research has been driven predominantly by "disability" as the primary multicultural factor, thus rendering a limited body of research that considers the intersection of disability and other equally salient cultural characteristics. Multicultural rehabilitation research generally falls into one of the following categories: studies that (a) examine the characteristics of distinct cultural groups in order to identify within-group determinants rehabilitation outcomes; (b) look at the relationships of demographic/ethnographic variables to rehabilitation outcomes in samples of people with heterogeneous or specific disabilities; and (c) investigate the relationship of multicultural counseling competency (MCC) to rehabilitation-related outcomes.

Within-Group Determinants of Rehabilitation Outcomes

With regards to the first category, a few studies have provided empirical support for cultural characteristics of particular groups in relationship to rehabilitation outcomes. For example, studies find that social support and the role of family are especially important psychosocial resources that should be considered in the rehabilitation process of African Americans with disabilities (Belgrave & Gilbert, 1989; Belgrave & Moorman-Lewis, 1986; Miller, 1986). Specifically, Alston and Turner (1994) identified family (i.e., nuclear, extended, and external family) as a key determinant of healthy psychosocial adjustment for African Americans with disabilities. They found a moderate to high relationship between adjustment to disability and family characteristics (i.e., cohesion, achievement orientation, and moral-religious emphasis). In addition, Alston and Turner (1994) found that their *four family strengths* model which includes kinship bonds, role flexibility, strong religious orientation, and strong work and education ethics, explained 73% of the variance in adjustment among African Americans with disabilities.

In a study using Wright's (1983) model of adjustment to disability, Belgrave (1991) found that social support was one of three variables (social support, self-esteem, perception of disability severity) that predicted adjustment to disability among African Americans with disabilities, accounting for 71% of the variance in adjustment. Belgrave and colleagues also compared the relationship among social support, coping, and depression in Latinos and African Americans with disabilities (Zea, Belgrave, Townsend, Jarama, & Banks, 1996) and found that social support and perception of disability were significantly related to depression for both groups. For Latinos, coping, social support, and perception of disability severity accounted for 62% of the variance in depression scores, and for African Americans, coping, social support, and type of disability explained 44% of the variance in depression scores.

Wallander's risk–resilience model (Wallander, Varni, Babani, Banis, DeHaan, & Wilcox, 1989) was applied by Jarama and Belgrave (2002) to better understand the rehabilitation process of African Americans with a disability. Originally developed to explain child, adolescent, and family adjustment to disability, Wallander's risk–resilience model postulates that resiliency factors mediate the relationship between risk factors and adjustment. Jarama and Belgrave (2002) found that 41% of the variance in depression scores and 36% of the variance in anxiety scores was accounted for by constructs proposed by the model. Specifically, functional limitations, stress, coping, and social support predicted rehabilitation adjustment for African Americans with disabilities.

In sum, research that focuses specifically on individuals with disabilities who belong to more than one cultural minority group is truly needed because the risk for experiencing multiple negative experiences or "double" discrimination and stigmatization is significant (Brodwin, 1995) and arguably moderates rehabilitation success and health care outcomes. This stigmatization is evident by the numerous studies revealing poor rehabilitation outcomes among clients from culturally diverse backgrounds (e.g., Atkins & Wright, 1980; Dodd et al., 1991; Dziekan & Okocha, 1993; Faubion et al., 1998; Smart & Smart, 1994; Wilson, 2000; Wilson et al., 2001). It is also well known that ethnic minorities have poorer health outcomes than majority groups in Western culture, and, even though there is an attenuated need, they are also underusers of relevant health and welfare services (see Murphy, 1977, for a teasing out of the relevant issues).

Cultural diversity and Rehabilitation Outcomes

Limited research examines cultural identity and rehabilitation outcomes (Mpofu & Harley, 2006). A related study conducted by Alston (2003) investigated the differences in the level of racial identity and cultural mistrust for African Americans with and without successful VR outcomes using public rehabilitation services. A significant difference between groups was found on the internalization status only, with the group of African Americans closed successfully having higher scores. In contrast, there were no significant differences in scores between the groups for pre-encounter, encounter, and immersion statuses. These findings suggest that client characteristics, such as healthy racial identity, may facilitate rehabilitation success (Mpofu & Harley, 2006). Given the myriad of psychosocial and environmental challenges associated with disability adjustment (e.g., feelings of loss, architectural barriers, societal ignorance/fear), it is likely that a healthy level of racial identity development, including self-acceptance and admiration, could positively influence rehabilitation outcomes. Indeed, a client with racial membership confusion and insecurities may experience negative emotions (Cross, 1971, 1978) that would likely spill over into difficulties in adjusting to another identity.

Studies investigating the role of demographic and ethnographic factors in rehabilitation provide a superficial understanding of multicultural characteristics in rehabilitation and are therefore not recommended as a tool for better understanding the complex role of cultural factors in rehabilitation. These studies typically control for demographic/ethnographic variables as a method of improving the explanatory power of the primary variables under study; they do not explain the processes that result in observed differences in rehabilitation outcomes, although understanding these processes would be key to the design of effective rehabilitation interventions for specific client groups. The most useful findings from these studies are those that shed light on demographic groups that are at high risk of rehabilitation failure. For example, Li and Moore (1998) studied correlates of acceptance and found that age, marital status and income correlated with adjustment scores, suggesting that those who are older, not married and have lower income are at risk for lower levels of adjustment. Studies examining gender differences in adjustment to disability typically focus on a specific disability group such as adults with chronic pain, spinal cord injury, or multiple sclerosis. For example, Hampton and Crystal (1999) found significant gender differences in adjustment scores among adult VR clients with various disabilities, with women reporting lower adjustment scores than men (Livneh, 1986; Lunsky, 2003). Post hoc explanations for observed differences tend to raise more questions than answers.

Training in Multicultural Counseling Skills

The importance of training rehabilitation professionals in multicultural competent counseling (MCC) is repeatedly emphasized in the literature (Atkins, 1996; Chan, Leahy, Saunders, Tarvydas, Ferrin, & Lee, 2003; Niemeier, Burnett, & Whitaker, 2003; Olkin, 2002; Reid, 2002). Studies show that MCC training affects rehabilitation counselor performance, self-reported cultural competency, and the relationship of cultural competency to client outcomes. For example, Wheaton and Granello (1998) investigated the role of multicultural training on counselor competency and found that training increased the amount of multicultural counseling skills. Similarly, Bellini (2002) found a positive relationship between graduate-level multicultural courses and workshops on counselor's self-reported cultural competencies. Counselors from CALD backgrounds see themselves as having high levels of cultural competency (Holcomb-McCoy & Myers, 1998; Lee & Richardson, 1991; Wheaton & Granello, 1998). This self-perception may be explained by the fact that counselors from CALD backgrounds function with cultural awareness in daily experiences or with "greater valuation" of cultural diversity (Bellini, 2002, p. 74). Nonetheless, Matrone and Leahy (2005) found that client characteristics explained client rehabilitation outcomes more than did counselor MCC competencies.

The value of MCC training appears to be overstated, and the evidence that participation in such training programs produces MCC in participants is lacking (Kleinman, 2006). However, understanding the client's alliance with the rehabilitation service provider is key to successful rehabilitation outcomes (Matrone & Leahy, 2005; Wampold, 2010, 2001). The importance of practitioners reviewing and reflecting on their communication practices in attempting to serve clients whose cultural and linguistic backgrounds are different from their own cannot be overstated. Multicultural training is a first step toward effective, reflective practice with CALD clients, but the quality of the relationship between provider and client is key.

Conclusion

Rehabilitation practices are influenced by cultural historical factors germane to geopolitical regions. The uneven development of health care services across the globe also contributes to the cultural-historical differences in the nature, type, and quality of rehabilitation services offered across nations and regions. Rehabilitation interventions need to address relevant cultural aspects that underlie perceived relevance and appropriateness of the services.

Disability is a product of culture. It is not a necessary or inevitable category for describing the diversity of human characteristics. Disability is an interpretation imputed on others with atypical development by social agencies. As people with disabilities are enabled in their participation of life situations, the category of disability as a human service criteria may become redundant. The universal design of environments for participation in the context of a human rights perspective is significant in bringing about a sociocultural context in which differences in human attributes are accepted and supported.

Cultural safety in the delivery of rehabilitation services is an ethical imperative. Lessons for multicultural rehabilitation practice continue to evolve over time. The fact that disability is less about the person with an impairment than about sociocultural barriers to participation (through the ascription of disability) suggests that rehabilitation service options to circumvent barriers are possible. Biopsychosocial models of disability, functioning, and health as proposed by the WHO (i.e., ICF) provide a useful framework for understanding disability in diverse human cultures, and for the design and implementation of culturally appropriate interventions. Involving people with disabilities in rehabilitation research, education, and training would add to enhanced cultural safety of rehabilitation interventions by building into services insider perspectives regarding the disability experience and qualities to support participation needs among those with disabilities.

References

Adkins, P. G., & Young, R. G. (1976). Cultural perceptions in the treatment of handicapped school children of Mexican-American parentage. *Journal of Research and Development in Education, 9*(4), 83–90.

Albrecht, G. T. (1992). The social meaning of impairment and interpretation of disability. In G. L. Albrecht (Ed.), *The disability business in America* (pp. 67–90). Newbury Park, CA: Sage.

Alston, R. J. (2003). Racial identity and cultural mistrust among African American recipients of rehabilitation services: An exploratory study. *International Journal of Rehabilitation Research, 26*, 289–295.

Alston, R. J., & Bell, T. J. (1996). Cultural mistrust and the rehabilitation enigma for African Americans. *Journal of Rehabilitation, 62*, 16–20.

Alston, R. J., & Turner, W. L. (1994). A family strengths model of adjustment to disability for African American clients. *Journal of Counseling and Development, 72*, 378–383.

Atkins, B. J. (1996). Envisioning the future: Diversity in rehabilitation. *Rehabilitation Education, 10*, 211–223.

Atkins, B. J., & Wright, G. N. (1980). Vocational rehabilitation of Blacks. *Journal of Rehabilitation, 46*, 42–26.

Bartlett, D., Macnab, J., Macarthur, C., Mandich, A., Magill-Evans, J., Young, N., et al. (2006). Advancing rehabilitation research: An interactionist perspective to guide question and design. *Disability and Rehabilitation, 28*, 1169–1176.

Belgrave, F. Z. (1991). Psychosocial predictors of adjustment to disability in African Americans. *Journal of Rehabilitation, 57*, 37–40.

Belgrave, F. Z., & Gilbert, S. K. (1989). Health care adherence of persons with sickle cell disease: The role of social support. *The Annals of the New York Academy of Sciences, 565*, 369–370.

Belgrave, F. Z., & Moorman-Lewis, D. (1986). The role of social support in disease severity in chronically ill Black patients. In S. Walker, F. Z. Belgrave, A. M. Banner, & R. W. Nicholls (Eds.), *Equal to the challenge—Perspectives, problems, and strategies in the rehabilitation of the nonwhite disabled*. Washington, DC: Bureau of Educational Research, Howard University.

Bellini, J. (2002). Correlates of multicultural counseling competencies of vocational rehabilitation counselors. *Rehabilitation Counseling Bulletin, 45*, 66–75.

Blanchard, J., & Lurie, N. (2004). R-E-S-P-E-C-T: Patient reports of disrespect in the health care setting and its impact on care. *Journal of Family Practice, 53*, 721–730.

Brodwin, M. G. (1995). Barriers to multicultural understanding: Improving university rehabilitation counselor education programs. *Rehabilitation and Diversity: New Challenges, New Opportunities*, 39–45.

Chan, F., Leahy, M.J., Saunders, J.L., Tarvydas, V.M., Ferrin, J.M., & Lee, G. (2003). Training needs of certified rehabilitation counselors for contemporary practice. *Rehabilitation Counseling Bulletin, 46*, 82–91.

Chan, F., Tarvydas, V., Blalock, K., Strauser, D., & Atkins, B. J. (2009). Unifying and elevating rehabilitation counseling through model-driven, diversity-sensitive evidence-based practice. *Rehabilitation Counseling Bulletin, 52*, 114–119.

Chen, H. Z., & Huo, H. H. (2009). Promoting the development of independent living of individuals with disabilities: Current issues and considerations for the future. *Journal of Mental Retardation ROC, 25*, 23–28.

Chimedza, R. M., & Peters, S. (1999). Disabled people's quest for social justice in Zimbabwe. In F. Armstrong, & L. Barton (Eds.), *Disability, human rights and education* (pp. 7–23). Buckingham, UK: Open University Press.

Cottone, R. R., & Tarvydas, V. M. (2007). *Counseling ethics and decision making*. Upper Saddle River, NJ: Pearson.

Cross, W. E. (1971). The Negro-to-Black conversion experience. Toward a psychology of Black liberation. *Black World, 20*, 13–27.

Cross, W. E. (1978). The Thomas and Cross models of psychological nigrescence: A literature review. *Journal of Black Psychology, 4*, 13–31.

Dell Orto, A. E. (2003). Coping with the enormity of illness and disability. In R. P. Marinelli, & A. E. Dell Orto (Eds.), *The psychological and social impact of disability* (3rd ed., pp. 333–335). New York: Springer Publishing Co.

Dodd, J. M., Nelson, J. R., Ostwald, S. W., & Fisher, J. (1991). Rehabilitation counselor education programs' response to cultural pluralism. *Journal of Applied Rehabilitation Counseling, 22*, 46–48.

Donnell, C. M. (2008). Examining multicultural counseling competencies of rehabilitation counseling graduate students. *Rehabilitation Education, 22*, 47–58.

Donnell, C. M., Robertson, S. L., & Tansey, T. N. (2010). Measures of culture and diversity in rehabilitation and health assessment. In E. Mpofu, & T. Oakland (Eds.), Measures of culture and diversity in rehabilitation and health assessment. (pp. 67–92). New York: Springer.

Dziekan, K. I., & Okocha, A. G. (1993). Accessibility of rehabilitation services: Comparison by racial-ethnic status. *Rehabilitation Counseling Bulletin, 36*, 84–95.

Faubion, C. W., Calico, J., & Roessler, R. T. (1998). Meeting the needs of underserved populations: Vocational rehabilitation and the Cherokee Nation 130 Project. *Rehabilitation Counseling Bulletin, 41*, 173–189.

Fabrega, H. (1990). Psychiatric stigma in the classical and medieval period: A review of the literature. *Comprehensive Psychiatry, 31*, 289–306.

Fabrega, H. (1991). The culture and history of psychiatric stigma in early modern and modern western societies: A review of recent literature. *Comprehensive Psychiatry, 32*, 97–119.

Goffman, E. (1963). Stigma: Notes on the management of spoiled identity. Englewood Cliffs, NJ: Prentice hall.

Greaves, T. C. (1994). *Intellectual property rights of indigenous people: A source book*. Oklahoma City: Society for Applied Anthropology.

Greaves, T. C. (1995). Cultural rights and ethnography. *Bulletin of the General Anthropology Division, 1*, 1–6.

Hampton, N. Z., & Crystal, R. (1999). Gender differences in acceptance of disabilities among vocational rehabilitation consumers. *Journal of Applied Rehabilitation Counseling, 30*, 16–21.

Haviland, M. G., Morales, L. S., Dial, T. H., & Pincus, H. A. (2005). Race/ethnicity socioeconomic status, and satisfaction with health care. *American Journal of Medical Quality, 20*, 195–203.

Holcomb-McCoy, C. C., & Myers, J. E. (1998). Multicultural competence and counselor training: A national survey. *Journal of Counseling and Development, 77*, 294–302.

Hwang, K., & Mpofu, E. (2010). Health care quality assessments. In E. Mpofu, & T. Oakland (Eds.), *Rehabilitation and health assessment: Applying ICF guidelines* (pp. 141–161). New York: Springer.

ILO, UNESCO & WHO. (2004). *CBR A strategy for rehabilitation, equalization of opportunities, poverty reduction and social inclusion of people with disabilities.* Joint Position Paper. Geneva: World Health Organization.

Jarama, S. L., & Belgrave, F. Z. (2002). A model of mental health adjustment among African Americans with disabilities. *Journal of Social and Clinical Psychology, 21,* 323–342.

Kleinman, A., Keusch, G. T., & Wilentz, J. (2006). Stigma and global health: Developing a research agenda. *The Lancet, 367,* 525–527

Llewellyn, G., Madden, R., Bretnall, J., Lukersmith, S., Mpofu, E., Bundy, A., et al. (2010). *Developing a disability and development research agenda for Asia and the Pacific.* The University of Sydney and RMIT University.

Lee, C. C., & Richardson, B. L. (1991). Promise and pitfalls of multicultural counseling. In C. C. Lee, & B. L. Richardson (Eds.), Multicultural issues in counseling: New Approaches to diversity (pp. 3–9). Alexandria, VA: American Counseling Association.

Levine, T., Park, H. S., & Kim, R. K. (2007). Some conceptual and theoretical challenges for cross-cultural communication research in the 21st century. *Journal of Intercultural Communication Research, 36*(3), 205–221.

Li, L., & Moore, D. M. (1998). Acceptance of disability and its correlates. *The Journal of Social Psychology, 138,* 13–25.

Livneh, H. (1986). A unified approach to existing models of adaptation to disability: Part I-A model adaptation. *Journal of Applied Rehabilitation Counseling, 17,* 5–16.

Locust, C. (1988). Wounding the spirit: Discrimination and traditional American belief systems. *Harvard Review, 58*(3), 315–330.

Lunsky, Y. (2003). Depressive symptoms in intellectual disability: Does gender play a role? *Journal of Intellectual disability Research, 47,* 417–427.

Madden, R., Glozier, N., Mpofu, E., & Llewellyn, G. (2010). *Eligibility, ICF and UN Convention: Australian perspectives.* The University of Sydney.

Matrone, K. F., & Leahy, M. J. (2005). The relationship between vocational rehabilitation client outcomes and rehabilitation counselor multicultural counseling competencies. *Rehabilitation Counseling Bulletin, 48,* 233–244.

Merrill, R. M., & Allen, E. W. (2003). Racial and ethnic disparities in satisfaction with doctors and health providers in the United States. *Ethnicity and Disease, 13,* 429–498.

Mezzich, J. E., Kirmayer, L. J., Kleinman, A., Fabrega, H., Parron, D. L., Good, B., et al. (1999). The place of culture in DSMIV. *Journal of Nervous and Mental Disease, 187*(8), 457–464.

Miller, S. (1986). Patients' perceptions of their adjustment to disability and social support in a community-based teaching hospital. In S. Walker, F. Z. Belgrave, A. M. Banner, & R. W. Nicholls (Eds.), *Equal to the challenge—Perspectives, problems, and strategies in the rehabilitation of the nonwhite disabled* (pp. 22–38). Washington, DC: Bureau of Educational Research, Howard University.

Murphy, H. B. M. (1977). Migration, culture and mental illness. *Psychological Medicine, 7,* 667–687.

Mpofu, E. (2006). Majority world health care traditions intersect indigenous and complimentary and alternative medicine. *International Journal of Disability, Development and Education, 53,* 375–380.

Mpofu, E., Beck, R., & Weinrach, S. G. (2004). Multicultural rehabilitation counseling: Challenges and strategies. In F. Chan, N. Berven, & K. Thomas (Eds.), *Counseling theories and techniques for rehabilitation health professionals* (pp. 386–402). New York: Springer.

Mpofu, E., Bishop, M., Hirschi, A. & Hawkins, T. (2010). Assessment of values. In E. Mpofu, & T. Oakland (Eds.), *Rehabilitation and health assessment: Applying ICF guidelines* (pp. 381–407). New York: Springer.

Mpofu, E., & Conyers, L. M. (2002). Application of tokenism theory to enhancing quality in rehabilitation services. *Journal of Applied Rehabilitation Counseling, 33*(2), 31–38.

Mpofu, E., & Conyers, L. M. (2004). A representational theory perspective of minority status and people with disabilities: Implications for rehabilitation education and practice. *Rehabilitation Counseling Bulletin, 47*(3), 142–151.

Mpofu, E., Crystal, R., & Feist-Price, S. (2000). Tokenism among rehabilitation clients: Implications for rehabilitation education. *Rehabilitation Education, 14,* 243–256

Mpofu, E., & Harley, D. A. (2002). Disability and rehabilitation in Zimbabwe: Lessons and implications for rehabilitation practice in the U.S. *Journal of Rehabilitation, 68*(4), 26–33.

Mpofu, E., & Harley, D. R. (2006). Racial and disability identity: Implications for the career counseling of African Americans with disabilities. *Rehabilitation Counseling Bulletin, 50,* 14–23.

Mpofu, E., Jelsma, J., Maart, S., Levers, L. L., Montsi, M. M. R, Tlabiwe, P., & Mupawose, A. (2007). Rehabilitation in seven sub-Saharan African countries: Personnel, education and training. *Rehabilitation Education, 21,* 223–230.

Mpofu, E., & Ortiz, J. (2009). Equitable assessment practices in diverse contexts. In E. Grigorenko (Ed.), *Multicultural psychoeducational assessment* (pp. 41–76). New York: Springer.

Mpofu, E., Thomas, K., & Thompson, D. (1998). Cultural appropriation and rehabilitation counseling: Implications for rehabilitation education. *Rehabilitation Education, 12,* 205–216.

Mzimukulu, K. G., & Simbayi, L. C. (2006). Perspectives and practices of Xhosa-speaking African traditional healers when managing psychosis. *International Journal of Disability, Development and Education, 53,* 401–417.

New Zealand Psychologists Registration Board. (2006). *Standards and procedures for the accreditation of qualifications leading to registration as a psychologist in New Zealand.* Wellington: Author.

Niemeier, J. P., Burnett, D. M., & Whitaker, D. A. (2003). Cultural competence in the multidisciplinary rehabilitation setting: Are we falling short of meeting needs? *Archives of Physical Medicine and Rehabilitation, 94,* 1240–1245.

Olkin, R. (2002). Could you hold the door for me? Including disability in diversity. *Cultural Diversity and Ethnic Minority Psychology, 8,* 130–137.

Osterlind, S. J., Mpofu, E., & Oakland, T. (2010). Item response theory and computer adaptive testing. In E. Mpofu, & T. Oakland (Eds.), *Rehabilitation and health assessment: Applying ICF guidelines* (pp. 95–119). New York: Springer.

Reid, P. T. (2002). Multicultural psychology: Bringing together gender and ethnicity. *Cultural Diversity and Ethnic Minority Psychology, 8,* 103–114.

Parker, G., Cheah, Y. C., & Roy, K. (2001). Do the Chinese somatize depression? A cross-cultural study. *Social Psychiatry and Psychiatric Epidemiology, 36,* 287–293.

Rosaldo, R. (1989). *Culture and truth: The remaking of social analysis.* Boston: Beacon Press.

Remley, T. P., & Herlihy, B. (2005). *Ethical, legal, and professional issues in counselling.* Upper Saddle River, NJ: Pearson.

Smart, J. F., & Smart, D. W. (1994). Rehabilitation of Hispanics: Implications for training and educating service providers. *Rehabilitation Education, 8,* 360–368.

Sotnik, P., & Jezewski, M. A. (2005). Disability service providers as culture brokers. In J. H. Stone (Ed.), *Culture and disability* (pp. 31–64). Thousand Oaks, CA: Sage.

Sue, D. W., & Sue, D. (2003). *Counseling the culturally diverse: Theory and practice.* New York: Wiley.

Szymanski, E. M., & Trueba, H. T. (1994). Castification of people with disabilities: Potential disempowering aspects of classification in disability services. *Journal of Rehabilitation, 60,* 12–20.

Tichenor, D. F., Thomas, K. R., & Kravets, S. P. (1975). Client-counselor congruence in perceiving handicapping problems. *Rehabilitation Counseling Bulletin, 19,* 299–304.

United Nations. (2007). *UN Convention on the Rights of Persons with Disabilities.* Retrieved October 2011, from http://www.un.org/depts/dhl/resguide/resins.htm

United Nations. (2008). *Mainstreaming disability in the development agenda* (E/CN.5/2008/6). Retrieved October 2011, from www.un.org/disabilities/documents/reports/e-cn5-2008-6.doc

Wallander, J. L., Varni, J. W., Babani, L., Banis, H. T., DeHaan, C., & Wilcox, K. T. (1989). Disability parameters, chronic strain, and adaptation of physically handicapped children and their mothers. *Journal of Pediatric Psychology, 14,* 23–42.

Wampold, B., E. (2001). *The great psychotherapy debate: Models, methods and findings.* Mahwah, NJ & London: Lawrence Erlbaum.

Wampold, B. (2010). *The basics of psychotherapy: An introduction to theory and practice.* Washington, DC: American Psychological Association.

Wepa, D. (2010). *Cultural safety in Aotearoa New Zealand.* Retrieved September 21, 2010 from http://www.mdaa.org.au/archive/06/wepa.ppt277,22,Slide 22

Wheaton, J. E., & Granello, D. H. (1998). The multicultural counseling competencies of state vocational rehabilitation counselors. *Rehabilitation Education, 12,* 51–64.

Wilson, K. B. (2000). Predicting vocational rehabilitation eligibility based on race, education, work status, and source of support and application. *Rehabilitation Counseling Bulletin, 43,* 97–105.

Wilson, K. B., Harley, D. A., & Alston, R. J. (2001). Race as a correlate of vocational rehabilitation acceptance. Revisited. *Journal of Rehabilitation, 67,* 35–41.

World Health Organization (WHO). (1999). *ICIDH-2: International classification of impairments, disabilities and handicaps: A manual of classification relating to the consequences of disease.* Geneva: Author.

World Health Organization (WHO). (2001a). *International Classification of Functioning, Disability and Health.* Geneva: Author.

World Health Organization (WHO). (2001b). *Legal status of traditional medicines and complementary/alternative medicine: A worldwide review.* Retrieved July 1, 2006, from http://whqlibdoc.who.int/hq/2001/WHO_EDM_TRM_2001.2.pdf

WHO, ILO, UNESCO. (2004). *CBR: A strategy for rehabilitation, equalization of opportunities, poverty reduction and social inclusion of people with disabilities.* Joint position paper. International Labour Organization, United Nations Educational, Scientific and Cultural Organization and the World Health Organization. Geneva: Author.

Wright, B. A. (1983). *Physical disability: A psychosocial approach* (2nd ed.). New York: Harper & Row.

Zea, M.C., Belgrave, F.Z., Townsend, T.G., Jarama, S.L., & Banks, S.R. (1996). The influence of social support and active coping on depression among African Americans and Latinos with disabilities. *Rehabilitation Psychology, 41,* 225–42.

Rehabilitation Psychology and Global Health

Malcolm MacLachlan

Abstract

This chapter considers the role of rehabilitation psychology in the context of global health. It begins by reviewing the relationship between rehabilitation psychology and disability, public health, and global health. We then consider the situation of people with disabilities in low-income countries. Having described the scale of the difficulties facing rehabilitation within the broader context of global health, we then explore the international aid and development "architecture"—the organizations and policies—that seek to assist people with disabilities in low-income countries. Given the scale of the demand and the resources available to address them, much of the rehabilitation psychology–related work undertaken has been at the level of policy, systems strengthening, and organizational development, rather than at the level of individual interventions. We review work on improving access to health care, on how the human resources for the health crisis affects rehabilitation in low-income countries, and how advocacy and networking are being used to provide a stronger and more effective evidence base for addressing the challenges facing people with disabilities in low-income countries in general, and Africa in particular. Finally, we consider how rehabilitation psychology can address content, process, and context challenges of working in low- income countries and suggest that closer collaboration with the emerging field of humanitarian work psychology may be fruitful.

Key Words: Rehabilitation, disability, psychology, global health, public health, health services, international aid, poverty reduction, human rights, policy, access, advocacy, inclusion, empowerment, development, humanitarian.

Disability and Global Health

The American Psychological Association (2010) defines rehabilitation psychology as "that area of psychological practice concerned with assisting individuals with disabilities (congenital or acquired) in achieving optimal psychological, physical, and social functioning. Rehabilitation psychologists consider the entire network of biological, psychological, social, environmental and political factors that affect the functioning of persons with disabilities. Rehabilitation psychologists are active in the areas of clinical practice, research, advocacy, administration, and education." This very broad scope of rehabilitation psychology has been developed, and applied, mostly in high-income countries. The interdisciplinary nature of rehabilitation psychology has emerged as being critically important: according to the Council of Specialities within Professional Psychology (2010), rehabilitation psychology "consistently involves interdisciplinary teamwork as a condition of practice and services within a network of biological, psychological, social, environmental and political considerations in order to achieve optimal rehabilitation goals."

Although there are considerable cultural and contextual differences in the ways in which chronic disease and disability present, are experienced and responded to (MacLachlan, 2004, 2006), many of the clinical interventions developed by rehabilitation psychologists and others may well have widespread application. Evidence-based practice, applied reflexively and sensitively to situations quite different from that in which previous research has been conducted, holds great promise for people marginalized by socioeconomic, geographical, political, or other circumstances. In this chapter, we will, however, focus more on the contribution that rehabilitation psychology can make to organizational processes, health systems, policy development, and advocacy that seek to promote greater functioning, inclusion, and participation of people with disabilities in society, and especially in low-income countries where people with disabilities are among the poorest of the poor (MacLachlan & Swartz, 2009). The right to appropriate health care in contexts of extreme poverty, marginalization, and disadvantage is a primary concern of the global health movement.

Public Health, International Health, and Global Health

Public health has traditionally focused on the prevention of mortality, morbidity, and disability, but has been silent on how to help those who are not prevented from living with disability. This is ironic because public health interventions and medical technologies have created what Oeffinger et al. (1998) have described as "an epidemic of survival" in which people escape death through living with disability. Although this effect may be considerably smaller in low-income countries, the moral responsibility of health services in addressing the consequences of their actions similarly applies.

Lollar and Crews suggest that public health has been slow to respond to the health needs of people with disabilities for several reasons. First, the conventional public health emphasis on reducing mortality, morbidity, and disability has "led to a mindset that equates disability with a failure of the public health system—specifically, to prevent conditions associate with disability" (Lollar & Crews, 2003, p. 198). The consequence of this has been that public health has found it difficult to frame a public health role toward people with disabilities. In addition, lack of a standard classification and coding scheme that allows public health practitioners and researchers to gather data and assess the multidimensional nature of disability—similar to International Classification of Diseases (ICD) classification for mortality and morbidity—has been problematic. Lollar and Crews are critical of the lack of public health research on health issues related to disability, such as the natural course of "secondary conditions" or studies of the efficacy of interventions to prevent them.

Although the conceptual confusion between disability and mortality is perhaps waning, this insight is not, in itself, new. Over a decade ago, Chamie (1995) stated that disability is not synonymous with illness, and that morbidity is only one factor in a plethora of causes of disability. Furthermore, although morbidity or injury may be risk factors for disability, the possibility of ameliorating their consequences, using interventions that prevent them developing into disability, is increasingly being recognized (MacLachlan, De Silva, Patel, & Devane, 2009). Increasingly, it is acknowledged that disability and health are not mutually exclusive, but often coexist with the same person and/or community and must, therefore, be equitably addressed within the same health service (MacLachlan, 2004). As this becomes clearer, so too does the role for public health in contributing to enhancing the quality of life for people with disabilities, just as for anyone else.

The idea that public health interventions could contribute to the prevention of secondary health conditions and so lead to greater efficiencies in the health system is also gathering greater traction. As Lollar and Crews conclude: "Public health is now moving into a new era of emphasis—one in which people with disabilities are included as an integral part of the public, a population group that needs attention in order to eliminate disparities" (2003, p. 204). By providing an evidence base to inform policy decisions that seek to promote universal and equitable access to health care, rehabilitation psychology can make an important contribution to these exciting and overdue developments.

Debate about the demarcations and uniqueness of public health, international health, and global health continues, but their nuances are beyond the scope of this chapter. However, some distinguishing features seem clear and relevant to rehabilitation and disability in low-income countries. The impetus for the development of public health in Europe was the need to address infectious epidemics, poor sanitation, and unsafe living conditions, particularly associated with greater industrialization. Public health's focus was on community health and the national structures needed to sustain it. International health, although adopting much of the same ethos and techniques as European public health, was particularly concerned with death and disease "over there"—tropical diseases in foreign countries—and thrived during the late 19th century as a concomitant of European colonization (MacLachlan, 2003).

Global health's geographical reach is much more ambitious, seeing all diseases, disorders, and disabilities as having commonalities across the globe and, yet, having distinct specifics in terms of local settings and conditions. Global health also aspires to cooperation at the international level, rather than just between governments. Global health has placed special significance on the idea of the right to health for all and, therefore, on the importance of equal and equitable access to health for all (although people may not have a right to "health" per se; the argument is that they have a right of access to health services that are appropriate to their needs; see later MacLachlan & Mannan, 2011). Finally, the range of disciplines that can make a legitimate claim to relevance is arguably greater for global health than for public or international health, with the former admitting a much greater range of social sciences, "voices" in order to recognize the broader social determinants of health (Koplan et al., 2009). In summary then, global health addresses the effects of globalization on health; this ranges from increased viral mobility with more people traveling greater distances, to the increased mobility of health workers being drawn toward rich countries with relatively less health burden and away from poorer countries with a relatively greater health burden, to the effects of social inequality and absolute poverty on health and health care. Although global health has relevance to all countries, it has a particular focus on low- and middle-income countries and on marginalized and vulnerable groups.

Disability Models and Rehabilitation

The medical model of disability has been interpreted as problematizing the individual and seeing them as being "deficient" in certain respects (Shakespeare, 2007). However, this "individualized" view is not restricted to medicine, and many psychological interventions inevitably, also, target individuals in terms of their reactions to or attempts at coping with the experience of disability. It is, therefore, important to note that people with disabilities are individuals and have individual challenges in achieving an acceptable quality of life, some of which may be related to specific sensory, physical, intellectual, or psychological aspects of their disability.

The "charity" view of people with disabilities is that they are in need of help and deserving of our sympathy and compassion. It is important to recognize that the lives of some individuals with disabilities have benefited from interventions and supports motivated by people—sometimes explicitly, sometimes implicitly—adopting these views. It is, also, a view historically associated with some nongovernmental and, particularly, faith-based organizations working in low-income countries, many of which have also done, and continue to do, a great deal of good, often in the absence of any alternative services.

The "social model" of disability has sought to emancipate people with disabilities by focusing attention on the extent to which society constructs barriers—physical, social, political, and psychological—to the participation of people with disabilities in society: society disables people by being more cognizant of, structured for, and adapted to the needs of some rather than others. This view is seen in the World Bank's (2008) definition of disability as a result of the interaction between people with different levels of functioning and an environment that does not take these differences into account.

The human rights approach, as embodied in the United Nations Convention on the Rights of Persons with Disabilities (see later), asserts the right of people with disabilities to have the same demands for recognition, dignity, inclusion, and participation in society as anyone else. In effect, it requires society to be organized for people with disabilities to the same extent that it is organized for people without disabilities. The "capabilities approach" (Sen, 1992) fits well with this view. Sen uses the term "functionings" to describe the range of things a person values being or doing; for example, being well nourished or driving a car. He uses the term "capabilities" to describe the range of functionings that a person can feasibly achieve in his or her current situation. Sen (1992) argues that international development should be about increasing people's "freedom," by broadening the range of capabilities—or possibilities—they have. The capabilities approach fits well with the human rights aspirations of marginalized groups, including people with disabilities (Borg, 2011).

The field of global health endorses the social model of disability, the need for the attainment of human rights, and the empowerment of people to expand their capabilities (MacLachlan & Swartz, 2009). These aspirations are not necessarily to be contrasted with more individual approaches, as doing so may, in fact, diminish the very challenging reality of an individual's particular life circumstances, including the nature of his or her physical embodiment (MacLachlan, 2004). The social and medical models, therefore, need to be better integrated

(Shakespeare, 2007), a challenge beyond the scope of this chapter but certainly one that global health can contribute to and that should be addressed.

Here we present three brief examples that illustrate how, in reality, these various models and approaches interplay in the lives of people with disabilities living in low-income country settings. These examples, based on real events, illustrate the link between availability of human resources and community-based rehabilitation (CBR).

- A mother who has a 7-year-old child with severe cerebral palsy often needs to take her child to the local clinic because of recurring upper respiratory tract infections. The child is too big to carry, and it costs up to 12% of the annual household income to pay for transport and fees for every visit to the clinic. The mother thus only takes the child when the illness gets really severe. This results in the child suffering from pneumonia and loss of energy, and not progressing in her development.

- An elderly woman, who is supported with a meagre income from her children, has severe rheumatoid arthritis and struggles to get to the clinic for her regular check-ups and her repeat medication. The cost of getting to the clinic is high for the woman, both financially and in terms of effort. Therefore, she only goes to the clinic every now and then, rather than regularly. She experiences significant pain and loss of mobility when she is not on her medication.

- A blind teenage girl attends the local voluntary counseling and testing clinic for advice on how to protect her from HIV infection. The clinic staff tells her she is not at risk—the assumption being that blind people do not have sexual lives. They tell her to forget about HIV and send her away without any information or counseling. When questioned further, the clinic staff say that the pamphlets they have are all printed and are, therefore, of no use to the girl.

What each of the people have in common are the experiences of physical and functional *impairments* involving an organ or body part; *activity limitation* involving the whole body or person; and *participation restrictions* involving the person in his or her environment. These three concepts are at the core of the International Classification of Functioning, Disability, and Health (ICF), which represented a paradigm shift by conceptualizing disability along a *continuum*. The ICF acknowledges that every human being experiences some degree of disability during his or her lifespan and, thus, recognizes that disability is a universal experience and not just one that happens to a minority of the population (see World Health Assembly, 2001).

Health is increasingly seen as a matter of optimal human functioning, rather than simply the absence of disease, disorder, or even disability—thus recognizing that many people with disabilities can lead very healthy lives. Within the context of health and rehabilitation services, it is also increasingly important to recognize that rather than seeing disability as a "health problem," people with disabilities have a right to health and to rehabilitative services that can contribute to achieving the "highest attainable standard of health" (as indicated in the United Nations Convention [UNCRPD], see below). Focus is, thus, shifting in health provision toward *inclusive health* (MacLachlan, Kasnabis, & Mannan, 2012) and away from *special treatment* to *equal treatment* (Reinhardt et al., 2009).

In line with these recent shifts—still often occurring more in theory than in practice—in orientation toward people with disability accessing health and rehabilitation services, it has been argued that professional associations (e.g., the International Society of Physical & Rehabilitation Medicine [ISPRM]), which have a traditional mandate to promote the professional and scientific aspects of their discipline, should also adopt a much more explicit humanitarian or civil society mission, especially in low-income countries (Rheinhardt et al., 2009). This should apply equally to societies of rehabilitation psychology which, arguably, have a much broader skill set to contribute to global health challenges than do many others.

The degree to which geographically and socially disparate peoples—including people with disabilities—can now share similar "spaces" though internet, global telecommunications, mass media, and information technologies brings greater opportunities and greater obligations. Professional bodies may choose to reach out to those most marginalized, deprived, and left wanting by a system of globalization that embraces and even promotes uneven distributions of resources and power, in order to promote political dominance (MacLachlan, Carr, & McAuliffe, 2010; Marmot, 2005; Reinhardt et al., 2009). Such views suggest that poverty is not simply a by-product of inaction, but that it is often a predictable consequence of actions that do not prioritize the lives of the most disempowed and disadvantaged. In low-income countries, people with disabilities often constitute the poorest of the poor.

Disability and Poverty

The case studies presented above also illustrate how poverty is an overarching theme for people with disabilities in low-income countries. The United Nations have recognized that the estimated 1 billion people with disabilities constitutes the world's largest minority (WHO & World Bank, 2011), of which 80% live in low-income countries. Of the 200 million children reported to be living with disabilities, few of those living in developing countries have access to health and rehabilitation or support services, with one in five people living below the poverty line having a disability and 80% of persons with disabilities living in low-income countries on less than 1 Euro per day.

The United Nations Special Rapporteur for Disability has stated that there are 62 countries with no effective health and rehabilitation services (United Nations Special Rapporteur on Disability, 2007) and the World Health Organization (WHO) has found that only 5–15% of persons with disabilities can access assistive devices in low-income countries (World Health Organization [WHO], 2009), with only 3% of all persons with disabilities getting the rehabilitation services they actually need (UNICEF, 1999). Of concern, the WHO also notes that the number of persons with disabilities is rising due to conflict, malnutrition, accidents, violence, communicable and noncommunicable diseases (including HIV/AIDS), ageing, and natural disasters. Interestingly, however, although persons with disabilities are found to be at higher risk of exposure to HIV, little attention has been paid to the relationship between HIV and disability (UNAIDS, 2009).

Research on living conditions of persons with disabilities in Namibia, Zimbabwe, Malawi, and Zambia has documented that people with disabilities and their families have poorer living conditions than persons without disabilities, and problems include those of economic and material poverty, low levels of participation in education and employment, and poorer social and health conditions (Eide, Nhiwatiwa, Muderedzi, & Loeb, 2003; Eide, van Rooy, & Loeb, 2003; Loeb & Eide, 2004). This much more complex, multidimensional understanding of the well-being of people with disabilities living in poverty chimes with the view that poverty alleviation must address more than income and consumption and reach further to encompass health, education, social, and political participation, as well as security, environmental quality, and basic human and social rights (Wolfensohn & Bourguignon, 2004). Other studies indicate that sociocultural factors are crucial and that women with disabilities and children are particularly vulnerable to exclusion, discrimination, and stigma (Groce, 2003). It is also clear that, especially in resource-poor settings, the extended family plays a considerable role in coping with the challenges that confront persons with disabilities (Grut & Ingstad, 2006).

The International Aid Architecture for Disability and Rehabilitation

Within the context of global health, rehabilitative interventions are often facilitated through civil society organizations (sometimes also referred to as nongovernmental organizations or NGOs), including disabled peoples organizations (DPOs) and bilateral (between two parties) and multilateral (between multiple parties) organizations. The way in which these organizations are structured may be referred to as "the architecture of international aid"; although the term "architecture" possibly implies a greater degree of design than is characteristic of the plethora of organizations—sometimes working in harmony and sometimes not—in the aid world (MacLachlan, Carr, & McAuliffe, 2010).

Multilateral organizations working in disability and rehabilitation—such as the WHO, International Labour Organization (ILO), the World Bank, and the United Nations Educational, Scientific and Cultural Organization (UNESCO)—attempt to establish policy instruments that create an international environment that is likely to facilitate improvements in the quality of life for people with disabilities on a worldwide basis. These policies relate to a very broad range of activities, including clinical services, employment opportunities, economic empowerment and entrepreneurship, education, transport, and so on. Such policies are intended to guide not only nation states but also individual organizations working within them. Some of the most significant policy instruments recently developed in the sphere of disability and rehabilitation—within the context of global health—are briefly described here.

A United Nations Decade for Persons with Disabilities

The United Nations declared 1982–1992 as the Decade for People with Disabilities, in the hope that it would focus attention on the need to address the causes of disability and the social exclusion that is often a consequence of disability, and encourage the meaningful integration of disability issues into national development processes. Although that initiative did produce some important successes—for instance, the formulation of the Standard Rules on the Equalization of Opportunities for Persons with Disabilities and the creation of an increased number of DPOs—it fell far short of its ambitious objectives. There were various reasons for this, including a lack of adequate funding, poor monitoring of funding, and a lack of real commitment from many governments. This lack of governmental commitment may have been related to rather decontextualized aspirations during the United Nations Decade. So, for instance, the government of Mozambique has argued in its own disability policy initiative that "a global approach to the problems of disability was used, and the solutions that were offered were general and global or based on the assumption of the availability of economic and technical resources, which later was found not to be the case" (Republic of Mozambique, 2006; p. 7).

At a regional level, the Organization of African Unity (OAU) adopted the African Decade of Persons with Disabilities (1999–2009) at its Algiers session in 1999. In 2002, in Durban, the African Union adopted the Continental Plan of Action for the African Decade of Persons with Disabilities. The Secretariat is mandated to facilitate the implementation of the Continental Plan of Action. It seeks to build capacity, both in its own services and among its member organizations; to formulate and implement national policies, legislation, and programs that will promote the full and equal participation of persons with disabilities; and to lobby and advocate for inclusive planning and implementation of disability programs at regional and continental levels. In recognition of the valuable work of the African Decade, as well as the considerable challenges still facing people with disabilities, the African Union has recently extended the Secretariat's mandate for another 10 years—a second decade, up to 2019. The energy, vision, advocacy, and political wisdom of the Secretariat of the African Decade of Persons with Disabilities will play a key role in realizing some of the disability-related policy instruments on the African continent.

The United Nations Convention on the Rights of Persons with Disabilities

This ground-breaking convention seeks to address discrimination, change perceptions, and combat stereotypes and prejudices. It focuses particular attention on the rights of disabled women and children, as they have been particularly marginalized. With regard to health (Article 25), the convention states that "persons with disabilities have the right to the enjoyment of the highest attainable standard of health without discrimination on the basis of disability," and this means that persons with disabilities should have "the same range, quality or standard of free or affordable health care and programs as provided to other persons, including in the area of sexual and reproductive health and population-based public health programs" (see also UNCRPD Article 26 Habilitation & Rehabilitation). The most problematic phrase of Article 25, from a global health perspective is, of course, "highest attainable standards." Do resource constraints necessarily put limits on rights, or, more particularly, on those rights to be realized? Or are there some rights that simply must be realized, with resource constraints being less of a determining factor than resource allocation: for instance, expenditure on the military versus on the poor or on health?

In the context of international aid, it is worth noting that Article 32 of the Convention states that "Countries are to provide development assistance in efforts by developing countries to put into practice the Convention." A review of the inclusion of disability and rehabilitation in aid and development policies is beyond our scope here. However, it may be instructive to consider how Article 32 resonates with an example of international aid for the European Union, the world's largest multilateral donor. The European Commission's Guidance Note on Disability and Development for European Union Delegations and Services (European Commission, 2004) calls for the inclusion of disability in health projects and in health research. It states that "there is a need to mainstream disability issues across all relevant programs and projects and to have specific projects for disabled people. This means that disability concerns should be recognized in the main EU funding programs" (European Commission, 2004, p. 12). The European Commission recognizes a clear link between the issue of disability and the basic principles of the European Community's Development Policy: promotion of human rights, poverty eradication, and action to combat inequality; stating "it is essential that the EU in all its development cooperation initiatives recognizes the needs and rights of people with disabilities. Disability should be adequately reflected within country strategy processes and EU documentation" (European Commission, 2004, p. 12).

The Commission's Guidance Note stresses that the European Union is committed to poverty reduction, as expressed in the Millennium Development

Goals (MDGs), and acknowledges that "This goal cannot be met without considering the needs of disabled people, yet disabled people are still not sufficiently included in international development work funded by the EU" (p. 3). Most emphatically, the Commission argues "If the interests of disabled people are not recognized then the key goal of poverty reduction in developing countries will not be achieved" (p. 3) and further that "If sustainable poverty reduction is to be achieved, *disability needs to be addressed by* sensitizing people active in *development work funded by the EU* to these issues" (p. 3 emphasis added). Not only in the case of the European Commission, but also with other development agencies, disability is finding a place on the development agenda.

The Millennium Development Goals

The MDGs are an internationally agreed set of targets that governments and aid agencies have agreed are a priority to achieve by 2015. Although in most cases this will not be possible, they are influential in terms of guiding the overall direction of aid expenditure and development projects. The eight goals, with an accompanying 18 targets and 48 indicators are, unfortunately, silent on people with disability or rehabilitation services. Although it is regrettable that disability is not mentioned in any of the MDGs, it is now becoming increasingly recognized that achieving the MDGs will not be possible unless an explicit disability dimension is incorporated into them. For instance, the White Paper on Irish Aid (Government of Ireland, 2006, p. 116) states "It is clear now that, if the Millennium Development Goals are to be achieved, the needs of disabled people must be considered alongside other development challenges by national governments, donors, international organizations and NGOs." This is also evident in the decision of AusAid, the official Australian government aid program, to make disability one of the three areas that its program has an explicit focus on in its international development efforts.

The lack of explicit reference to disability in the MDGs could make disability invisible from a policy perspective and, in doing so, undermine the prospects of achieving them. However, the Secretariat of the African Decade of Persons with Disabilities (2002) has argued persuasively that achieving each of the MDGs requires incorporation of disability-related aspects of the MDGs. For instance, the eradication of extreme poverty and hunger (MDG1) will be possible only through recognizing that people with disabilities and their families represent a very substantial proportion of the poorest of the poor. A reduction in child mortality (MDG4) must combat the under-5 mortality of disabled children, which can be as high as 80% in some regions of Africa. Similarly, the improvement in maternal health (MDG5) will be achieved only by addressing the disabling impairments associated with pregnancy and childbirth, affecting up to 20 million women a year. And to combat HIV/AIDS, malaria, and other diseases (MDG6), we will need to account for the fact that disabled people are particularly vulnerable to these diseases (which are also a major cause of disabling impairments) (Secretariat of the African Decade, 2002).

The Bamako Call

IJsselmuiden and Matlin (2006) acknowledge that the scope of conventional health research is broad, including biomedical and public health research, research on health policy and systems, environmental health, science and technology, and operational research, as well as social and behavioral sciences. However, they argue that the range of research needed to protect and promote health and reduce disease is, in fact, much broader than this: "the fields of interest span the relationships between health and, among many others, social, economic, political, legal, agricultural and environmental factors" (p. 4). For example, major health gains have been made possible through civil engineering improvements in water quality, sanitation, and housing conditions, in addition to medicines and health care. The Bamako Call to Action on Research for Health (Toumani Touré, 2008) arose from a meeting of Ministers of Health, Education, Science, and Technology, Foreign Affairs and International Cooperation, in Bamako, Mali, 2008. It sought to incorporate a much greater range of research disciplines in the pursuit of health and to promote cross-fertilization between them.

The Bamako Call states that: "The nature of research and innovation for health improvement, especially in the context of the United Nations Millennium Development Goals, is not sufficiently inter-disciplinary and inter-sectoral; there is a need to mobilize all relevant sectors (public, private, civil society) to work together in effective and equitable partnerships to find needed solutions" (Recognition Statement 5). This revision, addressing how research for health is conducted, is certainly ambitious. In practice, it means working across disciplines, ministries, and sectors. It also means working at various levels within these disciplines—for instance, working at the policy, organizational, and service delivery levels. Rehabilitation psychology is one of the few disciplines that can provide the range of skills necessary to do this. However, a major difficulty with the Bamako Call's lofty ideals is concretizing them into practical action. One of the few and most recent opportunities to do this has been presented in the form of new guidelines for working with people with disabilities through CBR, particularly in low-income countries.

The Community-Based Rehabilitation Guidelines

Inspired by the "Health for All" ethos of the Alma-Ata declaration (WHO, 1978), the WHO promoted CBR as a strategy within general community development for rehabilitation, equalization of opportunities, and social inclusion of all children and adults with disabilities (ILO, UNESCO, WHO, 2004). Community-based rehabilitation is aligned with international conventions, guidelines, and strategies, in particular the UNCRPD. The CBR Guidelines provide new ideas on how CBR can be used as a tool in operationalizing the UNCRPD and promoting more inclusive MDGs,

highlighting the crucial importance of the inclusion and participation of persons with disabilities and their contributions in the development of their societies.

The guidelines have five major components: health, education, livelihood, social inclusion, and empowerment (see Figure 31.1). Beside these five components, the Guidelines also focus on management of some special scenarios: HIV/AIDS, leprosy, and mental health, as well as CBR in crisis situations. As can be seen in Figure 31.1, the guidelines place rehabilitation in a much stronger educational, empowerment, and psychosocial context than has previously been the case. They thus beckon many of the skills associated with rehabilitation psychology, to which we shall return. Finally, and related to the idea of the socioeconomic empowerment of people with disabilities, we consider one more critical policy instrument within the context of national development and low-income countries.

Poverty Reduction Strategy Papers

The MDGs set goals for general "development" in poor countries. The World Bank and International Monetary Fund have established various aid instruments to support the establishment of these goals.

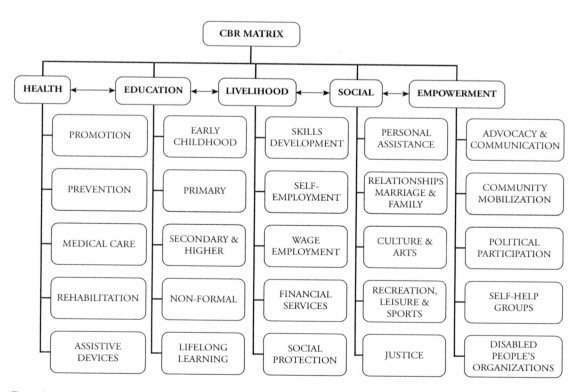

Figure 31.1 Matrix summarizing the guidelines for community-based rehabilitation. (WHO, 2010).

Poverty reduction strategy papers (PRSP) are one such instrument, and these enable countries to obtain debt relief and to access World Bank/IMF credits. Poverty reduction strategy papers have become the main multilateral mechanisms for providing development aid to the world's poorest countries. In effect, they are national plans to reduce poverty. The idea is that a variety of stakeholders participate in the drawing up of the paper, with the paper reflecting stakeholder consensus and outlining priority actions to be taken. The PRSP process is meant to be country-driven and country-owned, results-orientated, comprehensive, partnership-orientated, based on a medium and long-term perspective, and have the participation of a broad range of stakeholders. The PRSP is not an isolated tool, but rather linked to other national and international strategies and policies (for instance, sector-wide approaches [SAPs] and sector investment programmes [SIPs]) and is now in use in over 70 countries (Handicap International, 2006). Unfortunately, disability issues have, on the whole, been poorly served by PRSPs (Secretariat of the African Decade of Persons with Disability, 2007).

Poverty reduction strategy papers should outline the process that led to the formation of the PRSP, outline the poverty profile of the country, set targets and priorities within the proposed policy measures, and provide a plan for monitoring and evaluation (World Bank, 2007). Where disability has been included in the PRSP processes, this inclusion has tended to revolve around the concept of charity; however, where DPOs have been involved, the inclusion of disability has referred instead to education, training, employment, and to broader participation and access to services (Handicap International, 2006). A critical issue, then, is to work out just how to get disability on the development agenda. Poverty reduction strategy papers act as an agreed agenda for what should be funded over a 3- to 5-year period and thus constitute a strong mechanism for "selecting in" or "selecting out" (excluding) many worthy and competing interests. If practitioners want to get support and funding for new disability or rehabilitation services, then getting the need for such developments on the country's PRSP is of critical importance. Without doing so, funders may be reluctant to support such service developments, or, if they do happen, they may operate outside the health and rehabilitation system in general, thus failing to capitalize on the potential for over-all system strengthening and potentially actually diminishing the capacity of the broader health system (MacLachlan, Carr, & McAuliffe, 2010).

The above calls, conventions, guidelines, guidance notes, goals, and papers represent a highly selected sampling of international aid and development instruments; they are reviewed here because they are seen as having particular relevance to disability and rehabilitation. The launch of the 2011 World Report on Disability gives further impetus to strengthen the focus on disability and rehabilitation within global health, and, hopefully, also on global health within rehabilitation psychology. It provides an up-to-date and global purview of development and challenges in the field. In the next section, we consider some broad challenges for people with disabilities in low-income countries and the possible contributions that rehabilitation psychology can make.

Challenges in Global Health and Rehabilitation
Conceptualizing Access

Although access is often difficult for people with disabilities even in wealthy countries, in poorer countries, the challenges tend to be ever greater, physically, financially, and attitudinally. MacLachlan and Mannan (2012a) have argued that the General Comment of the United Nations Committee on Economic, Social, and Cultural Rights (2002) can be applied to health care access to better understand facilitators and barriers. The indicators of good services, as outlined in the General Comment, encompass four intersecting elements. *Accessibility* refers to the need for health facilities, goods, and services to be accessible to everyone without discrimination and within the jurisdiction of the State. This first element of accessibility can be further broken down into the related dimensions of nondiscrimination, physical accessibility, economic accessibility (affordability), and information accessibility. The second element stressed in the General Comment, *availability*, concerns the quantity of services available; well-functioning public health and health care facilities and associated goods (such as medicines) and services (such as prenatal examinations), as well as programs (such as nutritional support), have to be available to the general public in sufficient quantity to meet their needs. The third element, *acceptability*, stresses that all health facilities, goods, and services must be respectful of medical ethics, be culturally appropriate, and sensitive to gender and life cycle requirements, as well as designed to respect confidentiality and improve the health status of those concerned. The fourth and final element of the General Comment refers to *quality*, by which is meant that health facilities, goods, and services must be scientifically and clinically appropriate to provide services of good quality. This final element is, perhaps, the least well developed but one of the most important and strongly related to the drive for more evidence-based practice. The scientist-practitioner ethos of rehabilitation psychology is especially well suited to addressing this need, and the strong research focus of rehabilitation psychology may be of particular benefit to efforts directed at research capacity building and overall health and rehabilitation systems strengthening.

MacLachlan, Mannan, and McAuliffe (2011) also argue, from a health systems perspective, that the extent to which the health service needs of persons with disability are met is an ideal probe to research, monitor, and evaluate health, development, and equity in low-income country health systems in general. The experiences that persons with disabilities have of their respective health systems exposes system limitations more lucidly than perhaps those of any other service users. The experience of people with disability can thus be used to probe broader systemic issues concerning health care delivery and integrates with complementary services provided by other ministries—for instance, those concerning social welfare, transport, or economic development.

ACCESS AND HIERARCHY

One approach to increasing access on the ground is using what is referred to as the *BIAS FREE framework*. Eichler and Burke's (2006) BIAS FREE seeks to increase access by promoting human rights and social inclusion. They recognize that many biases and prejudices derive from social hierarchies. The BIAS FREE framework is designed to identify biases that derive from "any and all social hierarchies." BIAS FREE stands for Building an Integrative Analytical System for Recognizing and Eliminating Inequities. It addresses the intersection of biases that derive from hierarchies based on disability, ethnicity, gender, age, class, caste, socioeconomic status, religion, sexual orientation, geographical location, and immigrant/refugee status, among others. The framework helps people explore how hierarchies play out in their overall well-being and functioning. The framework is also a useful instrument for addressing accessibility in existing facilities and health systems and has been used by its authors for this purpose in low-income settings with some success (see Eichler & Burke, 2006).

ACCESS AND POLICY

Although access needs to be addressed in terms of service delivery on the ground in health care facilities it also has to become a salient issue in society more broadly. In the latter case, this means having health care policies that promote accessibility as a primary goal: if social inclusion and human rights do not underpin policy formation, it is unlikely they will be seen in service delivery. EquiFrame is a policy analysis instrument designed to evaluate the extent to which social inclusion is promoted and human rights are upheld within health policy documents and to offer guidelines for further development and revision, where appropriate (Amin et al., 2011; MacLachlan et al., 2012; Mannan, Amin, MacLachlan, & the EquitAble Consortium, 2011). It details 21 core concepts of human rights in analyzing health policies. Concepts include quality, efficiency, and access, as well as individualized and appropriate services, service coordination and collaboration, service integration, and cultural responsiveness. EquiFrame also considers the coverage of 12 vulnerable groups (including ethnic minorities, displaced populations, those living away from services, those suffering from chronic illness, and people with disabilities). EquiFrame facilitates policy analysis and benchmarking against other policies, nationally and internationally. Figure 31.2 shows the extent to which over 50 policies across four countries addressed different vulnerable groups. It can be

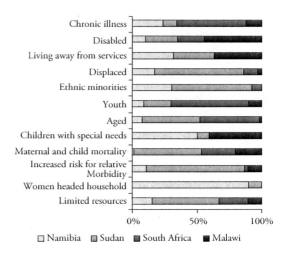

Figure 31.2 The relative frequency of mention of different vulnerable groups in health policies across four countries (expressed as a percentage). From Mannan, H., Amin, M., MacLachlan, M., & the EquitAble Consortium. (2011). *The EquiFrame manual: A tool for evaluating and promoting the inclusion of vulnerable groups and core concepts of human rights in health policy documents.* Dublin: Global Health Press.

seen that the relative prominence given to people with disability and other vulnerable groups varies considerably. Although the reasons for some variations are clear (for instance, displaced people), for others, the variation may reflect factors relevant to marginalization within the countries. Such an analysis reminds us that people with disabilities may also constitute other vulnerable groups (ethnic minorities, those living away from services), and they must compete with such groups both for health policy attention, greater resources, and access to services. Ultimately, EquiFrame allows us to evaluate—to measure—the extent of inclusion and prominence of rights accorded to people with disabilities. This is important, as, according to the old adage, "what gets measured, gets done."

EquiFrame is one aspect of the larger EquitAble project (see www.EquitableProject.org) that also includes intensive ethnographic case studies of service users and nonusers, as well as an extensive survey of 8,000 households across very different African cultures and contexts. It will provide critical evidence in identifying the barriers to accessing health care services for people with disabilities where there are a large number of internally displaced people (e.g., Sudan); where there are those suffering with chronic poverty and a high burden of other diseases (e.g., Malawi); where there are a highly dispersed populations (e.g., Namibia); and where, despite relative wealth, huge inequalities exist post-apartheid (e.g., South Africa). It is hoped that the results will help to develop a model of health care access that is applicable across a range of situations.

A FRAMEWORK FOR ACCESS

A very provisional framework for exploring access to health and rehabilitation services—especially in low-income settings—is the *reason-inclination-means-receptiveness-effectiveness-follow-up* (RIMREF) framework (MacLachlan & Mannan, 2011). It outlines some key features of access that are logically apparent. In describing these, we are referring only to "conventional" ("Western style") health care, but these would also apply, at least in some respects, to "alternative" or "traditional" health care (MacLachlan, 2006). First, we suggest that there needs to be a perceived *reason* to access health care; that is, a problem for which access to health care can provide some help. Then, there has to be an *inclination* to access health care; some people, perhaps for religious or other reasons, may not wish to use health care facilities, despite their availability. Assuming that there is a reason and

an inclination, then, next there must be *means* for getting the service. This could include transport or the cost of seeing a clinician, for instance. With sufficient means to be at the health facility, the staff should then be *receptive* to the person attending, not disadvantaging them because of non–health related characteristics or attributes such as poverty, ethnicity, disability, or gender. The treatment offered must then be acceptable, which is defined as "the social and cultural distance between health care systems and their users" (Gilson & Schneider, 2009, p. 28), and this, along with the treatment's intrinsic efficacy, will determine its overall *effectiveness*. There should also be *follow-up* of the person in his or her community. Such follow-up provides more accurate evaluation of the longer term effectiveness of interventions and may prevent the reoccurrence of problems or the development of secondary or iatrogenic complications, and it may help to develop the outreach function of accessible health care. This sort of framework offers the possibility of helping to contextualize more conventional health-seeking behavior models, such as the *theory of reasoned action* (Fishbein & Ajzen, 1975).

The Human Resources for Health Crisis

Health service providers (psychologists, doctors, nurses, occupational therapists, physiotherapists) are the personification of a health system's core values—they are the human link that connects knowledge to health action (World Health Report, 2006). Developing capable, motivated, and well-supported health workers is essential for achieving national and global health goals. However, there is a crisis in human resources for health, with 75 countries having fewer than 2.5 health workers per 1,000 population, which is the minimum number estimated as necessary to deliver basic health services (Joint Learning Initiative, 2005). The WHO's Maximizing Positive Synergies Collaborative Group (2009) noted a global deficit of trained health workers of over 4 million, while suggesting that "new strategies are needed to improve staff retention that integrate in-service training of existing staff members with long-term investment in development. The production of new health workers through pre-service education needs greater attention and resources" (p. 2157). The Global Health Workforce Alliance (2007) suggested that Africa needs 1.5 million new workers to be trained to address current shortfalls in its health systems (p. 2157), whereas others predict a shortage of conventionally trained nurses and physicians of 800,000 in sub-Saharan

Africa alone, by the MDGs target date of 2015 (Scheffler, Mahoney, Fulton, Dal Poz, & Preker, 2009).

High-income countries with high salaries and attractive living conditions are attracting qualified doctors and nurses (the vast majority of the "health professionals" with internationally recognized qualifications in low-income countries) from low-income countries to fill gaps in their own human health resources pool. The emigration of skilled labor in search of better returns on knowledge, skills, qualifications, and competencies is depleting human capital in many low-income countries (Lowell & Findlay, 2001). While low-income countries have limited resources for training health care professionals, the migration of those who are trained to conventional international standards has made dependence on such cadres increasingly precarious (McAuliffe & MacLachlan, 2005). Beyond the nation-level shortages, imbalances in geographic distributions, especially between rural and urban areas, exacerbate the human health resources crisis (Dussault & Franceschini, 2006). The migration of health professionals from one geographical region to another, from the public to the private sector, from areas of generalization to areas of specialization, from clinical to nonclinical fields, and from one country to another affects the capacity of the health system to maintain adequate coverage, access, and utilization of services (Awases, Gbary, Nyoni, & Chatora, 2004; Padarath et al., 2003).

Health worker migration may be conceptualized as being influenced by a combination of factors that either "push" professionals away from source countries or "pull" them to a recipient country. Push and pull factors refer to influences that are felt by professionals within the source country that either create an impetus to leave or an attraction to seek work in a recipient country. Efforts to address the workforce crisis include increased remuneration through salary top-ups, locum, rural allowances, and other forms of financial incentives. However, there is growing evidence that other factors in the work environment may also be acting as strong push factors. Workload and staff shortages are contributing to burnout, high absenteeism, stress, depression, low morale, and demotivation, and are responsible for driving workers out of the public sector (Sanders & Lloyd, 2005). Poor working conditions are reported to seriously undermine health system performance by thwarting staff morale and motivation, and directly contributing to problems in recruitment and retention (Troy, Wyness, & McAuliffe, 2007). The more

human face of staff and funding shortages is illustrated here, in the form of three brief case studies that show how severely a lack of skilled staff may disadvantage people with disabilities in low-income countries.

Case Study 1: Mabvuto

Mabvuto worked for a mining company and was involved in an accident in which his spine was crushed, resulting in paralysis below the waist. The company's insurance policy covered 3 months' rehabilitation, and Mabvuto benefited from good inpatient rehabilitation services and was provided with a wheelchair on discharge. Three months after returning home to a remote area with poor roads, one of the supporting spars on his wheelchair broke. A neighbor kindly brought the wheelchair to the nearest welder, who fixed it, but left the sitting position at a slightly different angle. Mabvuto subsequently developed pressure sores and back pain and started to feel down. Eleven months after discharge, and after suffering from an untreated chronic urinary tract infection, Mabvuto died in considerable pain.

Although Mabvuto got good inpatient rehabilitation, there was nobody to follow him up in the community. Simple knowledge about the importance of sitting positions and the use of appropriate technology and the timely treatment of pressure sores and urinary tract infection would have saved his life, enhanced his quality of life, and contributed to addressing his right to health.

Case Study 2: Washeila

Washeila's mother and father were laborers in a vineyard and were paid, in part, with alcohol. Washeila's birth was not planned, and her mother consumed significant amounts of alcohol during her pregnancy. As a result, Washeila was born with an intellectual disability and was not felt likely to benefit from schooling. Washeila's difficulties communicating became increasingly frustrating and were often associated with anger, aggression, and self-harming, distressing her parents and siblings. Ultimately, Washeila was admitted to a children's home on a long-term basis.

Information about risk factors during pregnancy might have prevented Washeila's disability. Advocacy for her right to education may have helped her learn how to communicate more effectively, and facilitation of the development of coping skills for the family could have prevented her subsequent institutionalization. All of these services could have been provided through one worker, but none of these needs was addressed by anybody.

Case Study 3: Precious

Precious was born with a club foot, which was taken to signify bad fortune, attributable, some people said, to her mother's alleged infidelity. Precious' father left to live with another woman, and Precious' mother became reclusive and somewhat resentful toward her. Precious was kept indoors, and her mother, being nonetheless attentive to her needs, had to earn what she could by exchanging sex for food and firewood. A community nurse heard about Precious and was able to arrange for corrective surgery. When Precious went away for surgery, neighbors were told that she had died. After intensive inpatient therapy Precious was ready to come back home but her mother felt it was best, both for Precious and for herself, that she not come back. Social workers could not find Precious' mother and believe that she moved away.

Community education about the cause and meaning of disability could have challenged the stigma often associated with cultural explanations of it. Early screening of children could have prevented Precious' mother struggling so desperately to cope and prevented the disintegration of the family. Had a CBR worker been present in the area, he or she would have addressed these problems and liaised with the community nurse.

So, while rehabilitation services may be lacking, so too are "habilitation" services that facilitate people to live with dignity and respect in a community. However, often it is not the know-how that is lacking, but the human resources to provide relatively minimal interventions that can empower individuals, families, and communities to improve their lives. Rehabilitation and habilitation should go hand-in-hand, having restorative and adaptive functions, as well as community development and social inclusion functions, as described in the guidelines for CBR launched in Abuja, in 2010.

Persons with disabilities in low-income countries may need to travel great distances from their homes to consult specialized staff. Although many countries do provide rehabilitation programs, a gulf often exists between the provision of these services and the percentage of the population receiving them (WHO, 2001). Assistive devices are often not available, and there are inadequate systems for delivery, adaptation, and maintenance (Eide & Øderud, 2009; Borg, Lindström, & Larsson 2009). Many personnel working in the disability field have received little or no relevant formal training. Additionally, resources are wasted by not involving persons with

disabilities, their families, and their organizations in the planning of programs and education (WHO, 2001). A recent expert opinion exercise on identifying research priorities in the field of disability (Tomlinson et al., 2009) has ranked creation of sustainable rehabilitation systems in low- and middle-income countries highly, along with research on strategies to improve primary health care systems to increase early detection and referral.

Domestic resources in many countries may not be sufficient to support scaling up the health workforce to the levels required to address population needs (Joint Learning Initiative, 2005). It has therefore been suggested that countries need to move away from the expensive production of clinically oriented health professionals to focus instead on the more pragmatic production of health workers appropriate to their burden of disease, availability of resources, and minimum standards of care (Huddart & Picazo, 2003).

Indeed, this strategy has already been adopted by several countries that are increasingly relying on so-called "mid-level cadres," such as medical assistants, clinical officers, and enrolled nurses (who have shorter lengths of training than doctors or registered nurses) to provide health care (Buchan & Dal Poz, 2003). In addition, a recent review of mid-level health workers (WHO, 2008) suggests that more than 100 different categories of mid-level workers have been used to provide health care, particularly to underserved communities, and that the use of mid-level workers has been widening in both high- and low-income countries. Although the review notes that utilization, skills, length of training, and management practices vary quite substantially across cadres and countries, it highlights the success of Asian countries in developing a large number of local mid-level worker categories, from birth attendants to health assistants, who are not modeled on traditional health professions but rather respond to specific country needs. In many of the poorest countries, there will be no psychologist with expertise in rehabilitation and the prospect of developing such a profession would be quite unrealistic, at least in the short to medium term. However, innovative human resource strategies do offer rehabilitation psychologists a real opportunity to contribute to service development.

Recent studies provide strong evidence for the clinical efficacy (Chilopora et al., 2007; McCord, Mbaruku, Pereira, Nzabuhakwa, & Bergstrom, 2009) and economic value (Kruk, Pereira, Vaz, Bergström, & Galea, 2007) of mid-level cadres, with most of this research being undertaken in the area of emergency obstetrics care. Given such positive indicators, it is important to recruit, retain, and support these cadres to build the capacity of health systems—including perhaps rehabilitation—in low-income countries.

Figure 31.3 illustrates the WHO's working concept of *task shifting*, in which specific tasks can be reallocated from personnel with longer training to personnel with shorter and more restricted training focused on specific tasks. However, the optimal means of identifying the most appropriate types of task to be shifted from one cadre to another have yet to be fully developed because, to date, such task shifting has been more based on service needs rather than job analysis, skill set specification, or educational and capability levels. This sort of analysis—part and parcel of organizational psychology and perhaps some of rehabilitation psychology practice—is essential in order to identify appropriate types of task shifting, where appropriate decision-making and patient/client safety is combined with technical efficacy (MacLachlan, Mannan, & McAuliffe, 2010).

Dubois and Singh's (2009) call for us to think less about "staff types" and more about "staff member's skills," arguing that "in order to use human resources most effectively, health care organizations must consider a more systematic approach—one that accounts for factors beyond narrowly defined human resources management practices

and includes organizational and institutional conditions" (p. 1). Dubois and Singh also discuss the importance of "skill management," which they see as an organization's ability to optimize the use of its workforce, seeking to "optimise patients' outcomes while ensuring the most effective, flexible and cost-effective use of human resources" (p. 13). This may involve both *role enhancement* (assuming a higher range of responsibilities) and *role enlargement* (assuming more responsibilities, usually at the same level), each of which can act as motivational factors, if appropriately managed.

Clearly, an array of rehabilitation psychology skills might be appropriately shifted to low-cadre practitioners. But it may also be the case that rehabilitation psychology has an important role to play in identifying the most appropriate skills that can be shifted from other professions in the rehabilitation field. Of course, such an approach is fraught with political and professional sensitivities and rivalries—one reason why it should be approached in as scientific and evidence-based a manner as possible, employing the skills of job analysis, job specification, and so on.

We have already described the new guidelines for CBR, which acknowledge the interdependence of health and education, income, and social context (such as transport, stigma, and welfare provision), as well as the importance of personal agency for people with disabilities and disabled people's organizations. However, implementation of these new guidelines must not only address the shortage of staff, but also the vastly expanded range of skills that will be required for those trying to put the guidelines into practice. Here, too, the need for an evidence-based approach is paramount and is an area where rehabilitation psychology has much to offer (see Figure 31.4) both in terms of increasing the opportunity for better service delivery by alternative rehabilitation workers and by redesigning how these services are delivered, and by whom (MacLachlan, Mannan, & McAuliffe, 2010).

Advocacy and Networking

The A-PODD Project (African Policy on Disability & Development—www.a-podd.org) is exploring the extent to which DPOs have been involved in the process of developing PRPSs in Uganda, Sierra Leone, Ethiopia, and Malawi. Data gathering has included the use of a range of techniques from key informant interviews and focus groups, to the organizational psychology techniques of critical incidents analysis, the nominal group

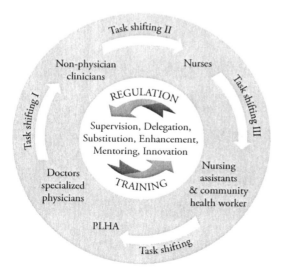

Figure 31.3 Illustration of the World Health Organization (WHO) concept of task shifting. From World Health Organization. (2007). *Task shifting to tackle health worker shortages.* Geneva: WHO.

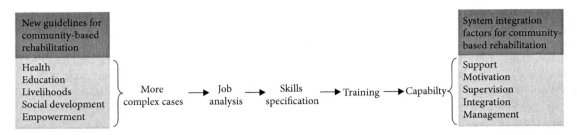

Figure 31.4 Integrative staff skill mix requirements for community-based rehabilitation and important associated factors for system integration. Reproduced with permission from MacLachlan, M., Mannan, H., & McAuliffe, E. (2011). Staff skills not staff types for community based rehabilitation. *Lancet*, 37(9782), 1988–1989.

technique, and force field analysis, as well as substantial documentary analysis. Figure 31.5 helps to illustrate how these psychological research techniques can contribute to developing an evidence base that can be useful in advocacy-related work to influence development policy. We have been trying to identify when, where, and how disability issues get to influence policy making and how to overcome some of the barriers that prevent them having more influence (see, for instance, Wazakili et al., 2011). We are particularly interested in the extent to which research evidence is used to make decisions about practice and policy. Early indications are that relevant research evidence—even when it does exist—is rarely used by advocacy groups and is rarely influential for decision makers. However, a lack of research evidence may be used as a rationale for postponing or avoiding a decision. Of course, this is also the case in health systems that are much better resourced (Lavis et al., 2005).

One attempt to address the lack of a link between evidence and action for people with

disability in Africa has been the establishment of AfriNEAD (African Network for Evidence to Action on Disability), founded in 2007, through its first international symposium in Cape Town. This network deliberately targets an array of stakeholders that rarely come together: people with disabilities themselves, policy makers, activists, practitioners, researchers, and academics. One of the major challenges is the vastly different capacity to engage in research production and utilization, both across these different groups and across different countries in Africa itself. Nonetheless, the meetings do give a platform for the presentation and discussion of an evolving evidence base (Mji, Gcaza, Swartz, MacLachlan, & Hutton, 2011; Mji, MacLachlan, Melling-Williams, & Gcaza, 2009).

AfriNEAD has tried to capitalize on the cultural principle of *ubuntu* (or its linguistic variations as used in many African countries), which refers to a social system of inter-relatedness, in which a person's sense of humanity is determined not so much by his or her personal qualities, but to a much greater

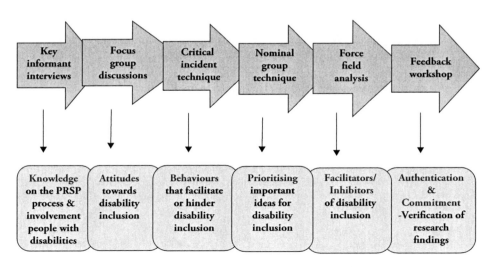

Figure 31.5 Research sequence used in the African Policy on Disability and Development (A-PODD) project.

extent in terms of how he or she relates to all in the community (Mji et al., 2011). The idea that "a person is a person through other persons" encapsulates the essence of the *ubuntu* philosophy, contrasting sharply with more individualized Western views of the self (MacLachlan, 2006). In such a social system, therefore, the idea that people with disabilities should strive for "independence" may be questionable. *Ubuntu* is a more interconnected way of being, locating people not as independent entities striving for self-actualization, but as interdependent beings who are part of a collectively derived identity, recognized through their contribution to others and to the common good of "all" (Mbigi & Maree, 1995). Of course, such a concept may be over reified and overly romanticized, and it may apply more to members of one's own in-group than to society in general. However, at culturally salient symbolic levels, although it would be naïve to assume that cultural values apply equally to all or that they do not change over time (MacLachlan, 2006), *ubuntu* offers a powerful and culturally resonant symbol for groups and networks trying to address the challenges facing people with disabilities across many African countries (Mji et al., 2011).

Process, Context, and Content in Rehabilitation and Global Health

Researching and practising rehabilitation psychology in low-income countries presents some challenges not usually encountered in richer countries. As well as knowing *what* (in terms of specific interventions) should be done to help a person or a situation, just *how* it can get done, or to what extent local contexts and cultures may modify its effect may need to be considered (MacLachlan, 2009a). For instance, in the field of prosthetic devices and their use in low-income countries (see Borg, 2011), we would need to combine different types of knowledge to produce an effective intervention. The *content knowledge* on prosthetic prescription and how to use prosthetics to provide possible personal gains for individuals would need to be applied through *process knowledge*. For example, how such services are set up—whether they are targeted through specific NGOs or if there is a well-developed interface between community and rehabilitative health care services—may have implications for the provision, servicing, and replacement of such devices and, therefore, the mobility of their users. Equally, *context knowledge* of, say, resources and attitudes toward people with disabilities may play a significant role in the extent to which people with disabilities are

included or excluded from mainstream society and from other support services that must work together for their well-being.

Process knowledge, in terms of international aid, may also extend to examining the way in which aid is structured both locally and regionally and, indeed, how international NGOs and DPOs operate more generally and internationally. The organization of international aid is fraught with very complex human dynamics that, at least in some instances, seem to work against their stated aims (see, for example, MacLachlan, Carr, & McAuliffe, 2010; Carr, McWha, MacLachlan, & Furnham, 2010). Although a review of these factors is beyond the scope of this chapter (see Carr, MacLachlan, & Furnham, 2012), the importance of establishing whether the sort of aid delivered, and the way in which it is delivered, is enabling and empowering for people with or without disabilities is certainly of relevance to rehabilitation psychology in such contexts.

Context knowledge is concerned with trying to understand how people and place affect action, in particular, this concerns how being a member of a vulnerable group, such as people with disabilities or a member of an ethnic minority, affects interventions that seem to work with other groups. It is also concerned with the influence of place. For instance, living in an urban slum, in an agriculturally degraded area, in a politically fragile state, or in an area that has just come through a natural disaster, are all likely to have significant effects on interventions that may work well in other situations.

Humanitarian work psychology is a new area of psychology that seeks to apply psychology to these and related challenges. It seeks to apply work, industrial, and organizational psychology evidence and ideas to situations of humanitarian concern and to develop a broader psychological understanding of humanitarian work content, process, and context (see Berry et al., 2011; Carr et al., 2008; Carr et al., 2012). Organizational psychology has often been associated with corporate wealth creation rather than poverty reduction in resource-poor contexts, yet many of the skills are applicable to both, and some of them overlap with skills relevant to rehabilitation psychology, particularly the "psychological, social, environmental and political factors that affect the functioning of persons with disabilities" (American Psychological Association, 2010). Each also recognizes that individuals are part of wider systems and require their needs to be met systemically, as we have noted already. Humanitarian work psychology may be of particular relevance to people with disabilities through helping them to achieve the aspirations inculcated in the ILO's agenda for "Decent Work" for all, but it may also help to inform organizational aspects of the delivery of rehabilitation services or advocacy efforts. A stronger interplay between these two areas of psychology may well be beneficial to people with disabilities in low-income countries.

Conclusion

Rehabilitation psychology has much to offer global health, particularly in addressing the needs of people with disabilities in low-income countries. The UNCRPD 2007 is now enshrined in international law, establishing obligations and aspirations for the achievement of human rights. The guidelines for CBR, launched in 2010, offer a means of realizing the United Nations Convention and of contributing to achieving the MDGs. In combination with these initiatives, the World Report on Disability, 2011, gives much greater—and a much needed—impetus to action in this area, particularly in low- and middle-income countries. Rehabilitation psychology can contribute to these challenges, and now is an opportune time for the development of new initiatives, particularly collaborative initiatives with partners in poorer countries (MacLachlan & Mannan, 2012a).

Within the policy realm, it is important to ensure that the challenges confronting people with disabilities and people with chronic illnesses are addressed in health policies and other policies related to livelihood, education, employment, and empowerment. It is also very important that such policies outline just how progress will be measured and how monitoring and evaluation will be undertaken at the level of individuals and communities, as well as at the level of service provision. Currently, many policies are weak with regard to social inclusion, often neglecting vulnerable or marginalized groups, and policies also often express little intention to monitor or evaluate outcomes (MacLachlan, 2012).

At the level of practice, many more interventions incorporating evidence-based rehabilitation psychology are needed. Given the greatly constrained financial and human resource situation in many poor countries, such interventions will need to be delivered by an alternative cadre of rehabilitation workers and perhaps supported remotely by rehabilitation psychologists. Closely linked to practice is the need to strengthen research capacity to trial and evaluate interventions, across practice, policy, and advocacy.

Great challenges also exist in terms of advocacy, and especially in addressing the stigma associated with disability in many low-income countries. Without meaningful participation, clinically sound interventions are unlikely to realize their potential in terms of improving the quality of people's lives and securing their human rights. Perhaps more than elsewhere, in poor countries there is a great need for those working within different models of disability to work more closely together (for instance, clinical interventions and advocacy initiatives).

As well as addressing these "content" issues (policy, practice, advocacy), rehabilitation psychology—and psychology in general—has much to contribute to understanding context issues. For example, how does culture or extreme poverty, for example, influence the effects of interventions that work well elsewhere? We need to understand more about how context moderates or mediates interventions. Process issues, such as what sort of delivery or support mechanisms work best, either in terms of specific disability and rehabilitation projects or more broadly in terms of international aid, are also critical areas where rehabilitation psychology has much to offer.

Although rehabilitation psychology has much to offer global health, it will quickly become apparent to anyone working in low-income countries that it also has much to learn from low-income countries. Often, these challenges are also much closer to home than we acknowledge. The global health ethos sees health as being determined by the same sort of factors globally—poverty, access, disempowerment—while recognizing that the degree and form of manifestation vary locally. By better understanding the situations of others, we also better understand our own.

Acknowledgments

I would like to thank my colleagues and collaborators for allowing me to report on some of our joint work from the EquitAble (www.equitableproject.org) and A-PODD (www.A-PODD.org) consortia and, most especially, Hasheem Mannan and Gubela Mji. I am also grateful to members of the Humanitarian Work Psychology network (http://www.humworkpsych.org) and the African Network for Evidence to Action on Disability (www.Afrinead.org) for many helpful discussions related to issues discussed in this chapter. I would like also to thank Tsitsi Chataika for drawing Figure 31.5, Margie

Schneider for her contribution to the first set of case studies, and Marcella Maughan for proofing this chapter. Much of the research reported in this chapter has been funded by Irish Aid (including the Health Research Board) and the European Union's Framework Seven Programme, for which I am very grateful.

References

American Psychological Association. (2010). *Division of rehabilitation psychology's definition of rehabilitation psychology.* Retrieved May 12, 2010 from www.apadivisions.org/division-22/index.aspx

Amin, M., MacLachlan, M., Mannan, H., El Tayeb, S., El Khatim, A., Swartz, L., et al. (2011). Core concepts of human rights and the inclusion of vulnerable groups in the HIV/AIDS, tuberculosis and malaria policies of Malawi, Sudan, South Africa and Namibia: An agenda for the global fund. *Health and Human Rights, 13*(2), 1–20.

Awases, M., Gbary, A., Nyoni, J., & Chatora, R. (2004). *Migration of health professionals in six countries: A synthesis report.* Brazzaville, ROC: World Health Organization.

Berry, M. O., Reichman, W., Klobasb, J., MacLachlan, M., Hui, H. C., & Carr, S. C. (2011). Humanitarian work psychology: The contributions of organizational psychology to poverty reduction. *Journal of Economic Psychology, 32*, 240–247.

Borg, J. (2011). *Assistive technology, human rights and poverty in developing countries: Perspectives based on a study in Bangladesh.* PhD thesis, Department of Social Medicine and Global Health, Lund University, Sweden.

Borg, J., Lindstrøm, A., & Larsson, S. (2009). Assistive technology in developing countries: National and international responsibilities to implement the Convention on the Rights of Persons with Disabilities. *Lancet, 374*, 1863–1865.

Buchan, J. M. D., & Dal Poz, M. R. (2003). Role definition, skill mix, multi skilling and 'new workers'. In P. Ferrinho, M. Dal Poz (Eds.), *Towards a global workforce strategy* (pp. 275–300). Antwerp: ITG Press.

Carr, S. C., & MacLachlan, M. (2005). *Knowledge flows and capacity development.* Special Issue of Higher Education Policy. Paris: UNESCO/IAU/Palgrave.

Carr, S. C., MacLachlan, M., & Furnham, A. (Eds.). (2012). *Humanitarian work psychology.* London: Palgrave.

Carr, S. C., MacLachlan, M., Reichman, W., Klobas, J., Berry, M. O., & Furnham, A. (2008). Organizational psychology and poverty reduction: Where supply meets demand. *Journal of Organizational Behavior, 29*, 843–851.

Carr, S. C., McWha, I., MacLachlan, M., & Furnham, A. (2010). International-local remuneration differences across six countries: Do they undermine poverty reduction work? *International Journal of Psychology, 45*, 321–340.

Chamie, M. (1995). What does morbidity have to do with disability? *Disability and Rehabilitation, 17*(7), 323–337.

Chilopora, G., Pereira, C., Kamwendo, F., Chimbiri, A., Malunga, E., & Bergström, S. (2007). Postoperative outcome of caesarean sections and other major emergency obstetric surgery by clinical officers and medical officers in Malawi. *Human Resource Health, 5*, 17.

Council of Specialities within Professional Psychology. (2010). *Definition of rehabilitation psychology.* Retrieved May 12, 2010 from http://cospp.org/resources

Dubois, C. A., & Singh, D. (2009). From staff mix to skill mix and beyond: Towards a systematic approach to health workforce management. *Human Resources for Health, 7*(87).

Dussault, G., & Franceschini, M. C. (2006), Not enough there, too many here: Understanding geographical imbalances in the distribution of the health workforce. *Human Resources for Health, 4*, 12.

Eichler, M., Burke, M. A. (2006). The BIAS FREE Framework: A new analytical tool for global health research. *Canadian Journal of Public Health, 97*(1), 63–68.

Eide, A. H., Nhiwatiwa, S., Muderedzi, J., & Loeb, M. E. (2003). *Living conditions among people with activity limitations in Zimbabwe. A representative regional survey.* SINTEF report no. STF78A034512. Oslo: SINTEF Unimed.

Eide, A. H., & Øderud, T. (2009). Disability and assistive technology in low-income countries. In M. Maclachlan, & L. Swartz (Eds.), *Disability and international development: Towards inclusive global health* (pp. 149–160). New York: Springer.

Eide, A. H., van Rooy, G., & Loeb, M. (2003) *Living conditions among people with disabilities in Namibia. A national, representative study.* SINTEF Report no. STF 78 A034503. Oslo: SINTEF Unimed.

European Commission. (2004). *Guidance note on disability and development for European Union delegations and services.* Brussels: European Directorate-General for Development.

Fishbein, M., & Ajzen, I. (1975). *Belief, attitude, intention, and behavior: An introduction to theory and research.* Reading, MA: Addison-Wesley.

Gilson, L., & Schneider, H. (2009). Understanding health service access: Concepts and experience. *Global Forum Update on Research for Health, 4*, 28–32.

Global Health Workforce Alliance. (2007). *Global atlas of the health workforce.* Geneva: WHO.

Government of Ireland. (2006). *White paper on Irish Aid.* Dublin: Government of Ireland.

Groce, N. (2003). HIV/AIDS and persons with disability: Overlooked and at grave risk. *The Lancet, 361*, 1401–1402.

Grut, L., & Ingstad, B. (2006). *This is my life- living with a disability in Yemen: A qualitative study.* Oslo: Sintef Health Research.

Handicap International. (2006). *Making PRSPs inclusive.* Munich: Handicap International.

Huddart, J., & Picazo, O. (2003). *The health sector human resources crisis in Africa.* An issues paper. Washington, DC: US Agency for International Development, Bureau for Africa, Office of Sustainable Development.

IJsselmuiden, C., & Matlin, S. (2006). *Why health research?* Geneva: Research for Health Policy Briefings, Council on Heath Research for Development & Global Forum for Health Research.

ILO, UNESCO, WHO. (2004). *CBR: A strategy for rehabilitation, equalization of opportunities, poverty reduction and social inclusion of people with disabilities.* Joint position paper. Retrieved May 19, 2010 from www.who.int/disabilities/publications/cbr/en/index.html

Joint Learning Initiative. (2005). *Human resources for health: Overcoming the crisis.* Cambridge, MA: Harvard University Press.

Koplan, J. P., Bond, T. C., Merson, M. H., Reddy, K. S., Rodriguez, M. H., Sewankwambo, N. K., et al. (2009). Towards a common definition of global health. *Lancet, 373*, 1993–1995.

Kruk, M. E., Pereira, C., Vaz, F., Bergström, S., & Galea, S. (2007). Economic evaluation of surgically trained assistant medical officers in performing major obstetric surgery in Mozambique. *British Journal of Obstetrics and Gynaecology, 114*, 1253–1260.

Lavis, J., Davies, H., Oxman, A., Denis, J. L., Golden-Biddle, K., & Ferlie, E. (2005). Towards systematic reviews that inform health care management and policy making. *Journal of Health Service Research Policy, 10* (Suppl 1), 35–48.

Loeb, M., & Eide, A. H. (Eds.). (2004). *Living conditions among people with activity limitations in Malawi.* SINTEF Report no. STF78 A044511. Oslo: SINTEF Health Research.

Lollar, D. J., & Crews, J. E. (2003). Redefining the role of public health in disability. *Annual Review of Public Health, 24,* 195–208.

Lowell, B. L., & Findlay, A. (2001). *Migration of highly skilled persons from developing countries: Impact and policy responses.* International Migration Papers 44. Geneva: International Labour Office, International Migration Branch.

MacLachlan, M. (2003). Health, empowerment and culture. In M. Murray (Ed.), *Critical health psychology* (pp. 110–117). London: Sage.

MacLachlan, M. (2004). *Embodiment: Clinical, critical and cultural perspectives on health and illness.* Milton Keynes, UK: Open University Press.

MacLachlan, M. (2006). *Culture and health: A critical perspective towards global health* (2nd ed.). Chichester, UK: Wiley.

MacLachlan, M. (2009a). Rethinking global health research: Towards integrative expertise. *Globalization and Health, 5,* 6.

MacLachlan, M. (2012). Community based rehabilitation and inclusive health: a way forward. *Statement to the United Nations Commission for Social Development.* United Nations, New York, February 2.

MacLachlan, M., Amin, M., Mannan, H., El Tayeb, S., El Khatim, A., Swartz, L., et al. (2012). *Inclusion and human rights in African health policies: Using EquiFrame for comparative and benchmarking analysis of 50 policies from Malawi, Sudan, South Africa and Namibia.* Manuscript submitted for publication.

MacLachlan, M., Carr, S. C., McWha, I. (2008). *Interdisciplinary research for development: A workbook on content and process challenges.* New Delhi: Global Development Network.

MacLachlan, M., De Silva, M., Patal, V., & Devine, D. (2009). Preventative psychosocial interventions: Who, what and when? *Open Rehabilitation, 2,* 86–88.

MacLachlan, M., Kasnabis, C., & Mannan, H. (2012). Inclusive health. *Tropical Medicine and International Health, 17,* 139–141.

MacLachlan, M., & Mannan, H. (2012a). Health care access. In M. Juergensmeyer, et al. (Eds.), *Encyclopaedia of global studies.* London: Sage Publishers.

MacLachlan, M., & Mannan, H. (2012b). The World Report on Disability and its implications for Rehabilitation Psychology. Manuscript submitted for publication.

MacLachlan, M., Mannan, H., Amin, M., Dube, A. K., Eide, A., Munthali, A., et al. (2007). *EquitAble: Enabling universal and equitable access to healthcare for vulnerable people in resource poor settings in Africa.* Submission to the European Union Framework Seven Programme.

MacLachlan, M., Mannan, H., & McAuliffe, E. (2011). Staff skills not staff types for community based rehabilitation. *Lancet, 377,* 1988–1989.

MacLachlan, M., Mannan, H., & McAuliffe, E. (2011). Access to healthcare of persons with disabilities as an indicator of equity in health systems. *Open Medicine, 5*(1), 414.

MacLachlan, M., Carr, S. C., & McAuliffe, E. (2010). *The aid triangle: The human dynamics of dominance, justice and identity.* London: Zed.

MacLachlan, M., & Swartz, L. (2009). *Disability and international development: Towards inclusive global health.* New York: Springer.

Mannan, H., Amin, M., MacLachlan M., & the EquitAble Consortium. (2011). *The EquiFrame Manual: A tool for evaluating and promoting the inclusion of vulnerable groups and core concepts of human rights in health policy documents.* Dublin: Global Health Press.

Marmot, M. (2005). Social determinants of health inequalities. *Lancet, 365,* 1099–1104.

Mbigi, L., & Maree, J. (1995). *Ubuntu. The spirit of African transformation management.* Randburg, South Africa: Knowledge Resources.

McAuilffe, E., & MacLachlan, M. (2005). Turning the ebbing tide: Knowledge flows and health in low-income countries. *Higher Education Policy, 18,* 231–242.

McCord, C., Mbaruku, G., Pereira, C., Nzabuhakwa, C., & Bergstrom, S. (2009). The quality of emergency obstetrical surgery by assistant medical officers in Tanzanian district hospitals. *Health Affairs, 28*(5), w876–w885.

Mji, G., Gcaza, S., Swartz, L., MacLachlan, M., & Hutton, B. (2011). An African way of networking around disability. *Disability and Society, 26,* 365–368.

Mji, G., MacLachlan, M., Melling-Williams, N., & Gcaza, S. (2009). Realising the rights of disabled people in Africa: An introduction to the special issue. *Disability and Rehabilitation, 31*(1), 1–6.

Oeffinger, K. C., Eshelman, D. A., Tomlinson, G. E., & Buchanan, G. R. (1998). Programs for adult survivors of childhood cancer. *Journal of Clinical Oncology, 16,* 2864–2867.

Padarath, A., Chamberlain, C., McCoy, D., Ntuli, A., Rowson, M., & Loewenson, R. (2003). *Health personnel in Southern Africa: Confronting maldistribution and brain drain.* Equinet Discussion Paper Series, 3. Durban, SA: Health Systems Trust.

Reinhardt, J. D., von Groote, P. M., DeLisa, J. A., Melvin, J. L., Bickenbach, J. E., & Stucki, G. (2009). International nongovernmental organizations in the emerging world society: The example of ISPRM. *Journal of Rehabilitation Medicine, 41,* 810–822.

Republic of Mozambique. (2006). *Poverty reduction strategy paper.* Maputo: Author.

Sanders, D., & Lloyd, B. (2005). Human resources: International contexts. In P. Ijumba, & P. Barron (Eds.), *South African health review 2005* (pp. 76–87). Durban, SA: Health Systems Trust.

Secretariat of the African Decade of Persons with Disabilities (SADPD). (2002). *Continental plan of action for the African decade of persons with disabilities.* Cape Town: SADPD.

Secretariat of the African Decade of Persons with Disabilities (SADPD). (2007). *Lessons learned from lobbying in Uganda.* Retrieved May 10, 2010 from www. africandecade.org/ articles/lessons-learned-from-lobbying-in-uganda/

Sen, A. (1992). *Inequality re-examined.* Oxford: Oxford University Press.

Scheffler, R. M., Mahoney, C. B., Fulton, B. D., Dal Poz, M. R., & Preker, A. S. (2009). Estimates of health care professional shortages in Sub-Saharan Africa by 2015. *Health Affairs, 28*(5), w849–w862. doi: 10.1377/hlthaff.28.5.w849

Shakespeare, T. (2007). *Disability rights and wrongs.* London: Routledge.

Tomlinson, M., Swartz, L., Officer, A., Chan, K. Y., Rudan, I., & Saxena, S. (2009). Research priorities for health of people with disabilities: An expert opinion exercise. *The Lancet, 374*(9704), 1857–1862.

Toumani Touré, A. (2008). *The Bamako call to action: Research for health.* Retrieved February 20, 2009 from www.who.int/entity/rpc/news/Bamako%20call%20to%20action%20-%20thelancet%20281108.pdf

Troy, P., Wyness, L., & McAuliffe, E. (2007). Nurses' experiences of recruitment and migration from developing countries: A phenomenological approach. *Human Resources for Health, 5*, 15.

UNAIDS. (2009). *Policy brief on disability and HIV.* New York: United Nations.

UNICEF. (1999). *An overview of young people living with disabilities: Their needs and their rights, UNICEF Inter-Divisional Working Group on Young People Programme Division.* New York: UNICEF.

United Nations. (2006). United Nations convention on the rights of persons with disabilities. Retrieved May 10, 2010 from www.un.org/disabilities/default.asp?navid=12&pid=150

United Nations. (2007). *Convention on the rights of persons with disabilities.* Retrieved May 28, 2008 from www.un.org/disabilities/convention/conventionfull.shtml United Nations Committee on Economic Social and Cultural Rights. (2002). *International covenant on economic, social and cultural rights.* Retrieved May 10, 2010 from www.un.org/millennium/law/iv-3.htm

United Nations Special Rapporteur on Disability. (2007). *Statement of the special rapporteur on disability to the 45th session of the Commission for Social Development.* New York: UN.

Wazakili, M., Chataika, T., Mji, G., Dube, A. K., & MacLachlan, M. (2011). Influencing poverty reduction policy in Africa. In A. Eide, & B. Ingsted (Eds.), *Poverty and disability* (pp. 14–29). London: Polity Press.

Wolfensohn, J., & Bourguignon, F. (2004). *Development and poverty reduction: Looking back, looking ahead.* Washington, DC: World Bank.

World Bank. (2007). *World Bank PRSP sourcebook.* Retrieved May 10, 2010 from http://go.worldbank.org/3I8LYLXO80)

World Bank. (2008). *What is disability?* Retrieved May 10, 2010 from http://go.worldbank.org/OCFI93GX30

World Health Assembly. (2001). *International classification of functioning, disability, and health.* Retrieved May 28, 2008 from http://www.who.int/classifications/icf/site/whares/wha-en.pdf

World Health Organization. (1978). *Declaration of Alma-Ata: International conference on primary health care.* Alma-Ata, USSR, September 6–12, 1978. Retrieved May 10, 2010 from www.who.int/hpr/NPH/docs/declaration_almaata.pdf

World Health Organization. (2001). *Rethinking care from the perspective of disabled people.* Geneva: WHO.

World Health Organization (2006). The World Health Report 2006. Geneva: WHO.

World Health Organization. (2007). *Task shifting to tackle health worker shortages.* Geneva: WHO.

World Health Organization. (2008). Mid-level Health Workers. The state of the evidence on programmes, activities, costs and impact on health outcomes A literature review. Geneva: WHO.

World Health Organization. (2010). Community-Based Rehabilitation: CBR Guidelines. Geneva: WHO.

World Health Organization & World Bank. (2011). World Report on Disability. Geneva: WHO.

World Health Organization Maximizing Positive Synergies Collaborative Group. (2009). An assessment of interactions between global health initiatives and country health systems. *Lancet, 373*, 2137–2169.

Rehabilitation Psychology: The Continuing Challenge

Paul Kennedy

Abstract

This book has explored a range of applied psychological models, the factors associated with adjustment, and the predictors of health outcomes. There is a need to move away from linear models and include broader themes, such as, genetic, social, and environmental factors. Although research is increasing in volume, we also need to be aware of engaging in initiatives that foster translational research. This afterword reports on a number of suggestions to enhance outcomes and value for rehabilitation providers. It highlights the remaining opportunities to develop the discipline and practice of rehabilitation psychology to address the challenges of the 21st century.

Key Words: Biopsychosocial, translational research, global perspective, outcomes, lived experience.

We are now into the fourth decade of applied research in rehabilitation psychology. Researchers and practitioners have used a range of models, methods, and health conditions to demonstrate the clinical importance of the biopsychosocial perspective. This model provides the conceptual basis for the integration of biological, psychological, and social variables. So, the earlier optimism of Frank, Gluck, and Buckelew (1990) in heralding rehabilitation psychology as psychology's greatest opportunity has been vindicated. In this book, we have explored a range of applied psychological models, the factors associated with adjustment, and the predictors of health outcomes. However, there is a continuing need to develop our models further and build up partnerships across health and behavioural disciplines to build on our understanding of the etiology, maintenance, and amelioration of chronic health conditions.

There is also a requirement to consider the global impact and cross-cultural factors associated with health concerns. We need to move away from linear modeling to include the vast repertoire of genetic, biopsychosocial, and environmental factors associated with disease, disability, and adjustment. In chapter 4 of this volume, Livneh and Martz (Livneh & Martin, 2012) conclude that we need to explore the reciprocal nature of coping and adaptation, develop a more integrated approach to the measurement of these concepts, and investigate more causal predictors of adaptive outcomes. This book also reveals how rehabilitation psychology has contributed to the management and understanding of a broad range of health conditions across the lifespan. The success of the biopsychosocial mission resulted in a greater understanding by health commissioners and health care providers of the important role of biopsychosocial factors and of the potential contribution of rehabilitation psychologists. Although the research output has increased considerably, we need to remind ourselves of the significance of engaging in initiatives to foster translational research by building on partnerships with practitioners and exploring the application of interventions across a variety of treatment paradigms and settings. Economic concerns have always been with us but not more so than in this second decade of the 21st century. A continued challenge for rehabilitation psychologists is to produce definitive evidence on the cost-effectiveness of rehabilitation psychology interventions.

A further issue for rehabilitation psychologists, as highlighted in chapter 11 of this volume by Gerstenecker and Mast (2012), concerns the challenge of managing chronic conditions across the lifespan. Demographic indicators demonstrate that new treatment and research paradigms are required to ensure that we can maximally benefit from our findings and put them into practice. The mechanisms that enhance adjustment and functional improvement deserve further study. The association between socioeconomic status and physical health is robust, and the psychosocial resources that play a critical mediating role in health have their origins in childhood (Mathews, Gallow, & Taylor, 2010). However, much has yet to be learned regarding the psychosocial pathways that connect socioeconomic status and health. It is also necessary to have a broader global perspective of socioeconomic status that incorporates the world's varied economies, communities, and cultures.

In relation to considering outcomes, Benté (2005) suggests the following steps for rehabilitation providers to provide ever-increasing value to the patients and communities being served. These include ceasing to defend outcomes in the presence of poorly designed processes; looking to research to determine which processes are supported by evidence; standardizing practitioner processes to support evidence-based performance; rigorously and honestly measuring the key processes and making the results known to all practitioners, regardless of how painful these findings may be and regardless of how good their outcomes may appear; focusing on and using process measures to drive meaningful re-engineering of the rehabilitation process; and, finally, encouraging and fostering organizational and individual transparency by sharing process measurement results with providers, commissioners, accreditation organizations, and service users.

Finally, this book provides clear indicators of the remaining opportunities to develop the discipline and practice of rehabilitation psychology. Cox, Hess, Hibbard, Layman, and Stewart (2010) conclude that rehabilitation psychology is ready to address the continuing challenges of ageing, war, illness, and catastrophes in this century. There is no shortage of psychological need, our evidence base has matured and developed, and practice and professional training is more effective and refined. For the future, it is vital that we build on our partnerships with health care practitioners, service users, and researchers across the health domains, health sciences, and chronic health conditions. This book demonstrates how energetic rehabilitation psychologists can influence research, practice, and the experience of health care for people with chronic conditions; however, there remains the challenge to ensure that resources, research funds, and service developments continue to expand. We need to provide leadership in the applied domain to make certain that research is translated into practice to improve the lived experience of ill health and disability.

References

Benté, J. R. (2005). Performance measurement, healthcare policy and implications for rehabilitation services. *Rehabilitation Psychology, 50*(1), 87–93.

Cox, D. R., Hess, D. W., Hibbard, M. R., Layman, D. E., & Stewart, R. K. (2010). Specialty practice in rehabilitation psychology. *Professional Psychology: Research and Practice, 41*(1), 82–88.

Frank, R. G., Gluck, J. P., & Buckelew, S. P. (1990). Rehabilitation: Psychology's greatest opportunity? *American Psychologist, 45*(6), 757–761.

Gerstenecker, A. T., & Mast, B. T. (2012). Aging, rehabilitation, and psychology. In P. Kennedy (Ed.), *The Oxford Handbook of Rehabilitation Psychology* (Chapter 12, pp. 211–234). New York: Oxford University Press.

Livneh, H., & Martz, E. (2012). Adjustment to chronic illness and disability: theoretical perspectives, empirical findings, and unresolved issues. In P. Kennedy (Ed.), *The Oxford Handbook of Rehabilitation Psychology* (Chapter 4, pp. 47–87). New York: Oxford University Press.

Mathews, K. A., Gallow, L. C., & Taylor, S. E. (2010). Are psychosocial factors mediators of social economic status and health connections? *Annals of the New York Academy of Sciences, 1186*, 146–173.

INDEX

Note: Page numbers followed by "*f*" and "*t*" refer to figures and tables, respectively.

interventions (*cont.*)
  complex health, 99
  comprehensive-holistic, 267
  computer-based, 283
  depression, 197–99
  emotional disorders, 267
  executive function, 265–66
  holistic, 266–67
  language, 264–65
  learning theory and, 34
  lifestyle, 530–31
  memory, 265
  for MS, 225–26
  MS caregiver, 226–27
  organizational, 241
  in PR, 326
  praxis, 264
  problem-solving, 38–39
  in PRPs, 326–28
  psychoeducational, 166
  for SCI, 292–94
  self-awareness, 266
  for stroke, 240–45
  targeting, 342–43
  TBI, 263–67
  visuospatial, 264
  weight-loss, 532
interviews, 163–64, 381
An Introduction to the Vocational
    Rehabilitation Process (McGowan
    & Porter), 12
IOM. *See* Institute of Medicine
IPEs. *See* individual plans for employment
IPT. *See* interpersonal therapy
Iraq War, 280–81
Ireland, 22
IRT. *See* item response therapy
ischemic heart disease, 4
Israel, 23–24
issue-specific family counseling model
    (ICFM), 177–78
item response therapy (IRT), 104

J
James, William, 288
Japan, 24
job placement assistance, 459–61,
    460*t*, 462
job training programs, 458–59
Journal of Rehabilitation Psychology, 23

K
Kaiser Permanente, 514–15
Katz, Shlomo, 24
Kazan Psychoanalytic Association, 274–75
kidneys, 369–70, 372
Kojima-Cassels, Yoko, 24
Kravetz, Shlomo, 24
Kuhn, Herb, 280
Kurtzke Expanded Disability Status Scale,
    212–13
Labby, David, 111
Ladieu, Gloria, 18

language
  CP and, 181
  deficits, 282
  interventions, 264–65
laughing, pathological, 215–16
laws, 426–27. *See also* legislation
  social inclusion, 465–66
LDL. *See* low-density lipoprotein
learned nonuse, 34, 422
learning
  CP and, 180–82
  disabilities, 477
  errorless, 244
  Pavlovian, 300
  theory, 33–35, 266
LEARN Institute for Lifestyle
    Management, 532
left ventricular assist device (LVAD),
    371, 434
legislation trends, 515–16
length of stay, 278
leprosy, 25, 561
lesions, 211
Leviton, Gloria, 18
Lewin, Kurt, 12, 18, 49
Lewinian field theory, 36
Lezak, Muriel, 5–6
life-expectancy, 4
Life Satisfaction Inventory (LSI), 56
Life Satisfaction Survey (LSS), 56
Life Situation Questionnaire, 56
Lifespan Respite Care Act, 161–62
Life Stress Monitoring Program, 342
lifestyle behaviors, 526
  assessments and, 529–30
  clinical implications of, 537
  disease prevention through, 527
  research, 536–37
  sedentary, 527
limb activation, 283
literacy services, 460*t*
livers, 369*f*, 370
Lives of a Cell (Thomas), 275
Living Well with a Disability, 497
locus of control (LOC), 66–67, 76, 240
Lofquist, Lloyd, 12
long-term potentiation (LTP), 300
Lorig, Kate, 496
low-density lipoprotein (LDL), 388
LSI. *See* Life Satisfaction Inventory
LSS. *See* Life Satisfaction Survey
LTP. *See* long-term potentiation
lung transplant, 371
Luria, Alexander, 37–38, 274–75
LVAD. *See* left ventricular assist device

M
magical thinking, 381
magnetic resonance imaging (MRI), 211
maintenance services, 461*t*
major affective disorder (MDD), 435
maladaptive cognitions, 302
malaria, 561

Malec, James, 98
malpractice litigation, 434
managed care, 19–20
The Man with a Shattered World (Luria,
    Solotaroff, & Sacks), 275
marriage, 291
Mason, Pip, 504
master's degree programs, 425
mastery, sense of, 476, 478–79
Mayo Clinic, 514–15
Mayo Older Adult Normative Study
    (MOANS), 196
Mayo Older African American Normative
    Studies (MOAANS), 196
MBBT. *See* mindfulness-based breathing
    therapy
MBMD. *See* Millon Behavioral Medicine
    Diagnostic
MBSR. *See* mindfulness-based stress
    reduction
MCC. *See* multicultural counseling
    competency
McGovern, Robert, 6
McGowan, John, 12
McMaster University, 388
MDD. *See* major affective disorder
MDGs. *See* Millennium Development
    Goals
MDT. *See* multidisciplinary team
meaning-making, 222, 357
measurements
  anxiety, 72
  behavioral, 117–18
  challenges, 102–5
  of DC, 69
  depression, 72
  dietary intake, 530
  of employment outcomes, 464–65
  of environment, 118
  levels, 253
  outcome, 97
  of physical activity, 530
  of resilience, 484
  scalable focus, 113
  selection, 103
  sensitivity, 102–3
Measure of End-stage Liver Disease
    (MELD) score, 372
Meat, Eggs, Dairy, Frying foods, In baked
    goods, Convenience foods, Table
    fats, and Snacks (MEDFICTS), 530
Meat, Egg yolks, Dairy, Invisible fat,
    Cooking/table fats, Snacks
    (MEDICS), 530
MEDFICTS. *See* Meat, Eggs, Dairy,
    Frying foods, In baked goods,
    Convenience foods, Table fats, and
    Snacks
Medicaid, 511, 516–18
Medicaid Global Payment System
    Demonstration Project, 517
medical care model, 520
medical compliance, 374